Medical Language For Modern Health Care

Fourth Edition

David M. Allan, MA, MD

Rachel C. Basco, MS, RRT
Bossier Parish Community College

Mc
Graw
Hill
Education

MEDICAL LANGUAGE FOR MODERN HEALTH CARE, FOURTH EDITION

Published by McGraw-Hill Education, 2 Penn Plaza, New York, NY 10121. Copyright ©2019
by McGraw-Hill Education. All rights reserved. Printed in the United States of America.
Previous editions ©2014, 2011, and 2008. No part of this publication may be reproduced
or distributed in any form or by any means, or stored in a database or retrieval system,
without the prior written consent of McGraw-Hill Education, including, but not limited to,
in any network or other electronic storage or transmission, or broadcast for distance learning.

Some ancillaries, including electronic and print components, may not be available to customers outside
the United States.

This book is printed on acid-free paper.

1 2 3 4 5 6 7 8 9 LMN 21 20 19 18

ISBN 978-1-260-08493-1
MHID 1-260-08493-0

www.mhhe.com

David Allan

David Allan received his medical training at Cambridge University and Guy's Hospital in England. He was Chief Resident in Pediatrics at Bellevue Hospital in New York City before moving to San Diego, California.

Dr. Allan has worked as a family physician in England, a pediatrician in San Diego, and Associate Dean at the University of California, San Diego School of Medicine. He has designed, written, and produced more than 100 award-winning multimedia programs with virtual reality as their conceptual base. Dr. Allan resides happily in San Diego and enjoys the warmth of the people, the weather, and the beaches.

Rachel Curran Basco

Rachel Basco earned her BS in Cardiopulmonary Science and MS in Health Sciences from Louisiana State University Health Science Center, School of Allied Health Professions (SAHP). She worked as a registered respiratory therapist for ten years and then began her career in college instruction in respiratory therapy at LSU-SAHP in Shreveport, LA. She then found her interest to be in nonclinical education and began instructing biology courses at Bossier Parish Community College (BPCC) in Bossier City, LA.

Ms. Basco's interest in online learning developed, leading to the completion of a graduate certificate in Instructional Design from the University of Wisconsin–Stout. She is employed full-time as a project director but also as an online adjunct instructor in medical terminology at BPCC. She is in the dissertation phase for her EdD at Louisiana Tech University in Ruston, LA, with a focus on higher education policy analysis.

Ms. Basco resides in Shreveport with her husband and children. While very busy with her family, work, and studies, Rachel always finds time to visit her relatives in her home state of Wisconsin.

BRIEF CONTENTS

We wish to acknowledge with great appreciation the most valuable contributions that Karen Lockyer, BA, RHIT, CPC, made to the first three editions of this book. Karen's expertise and knowledge were intrinsic to the foundation of the book's approach. The text wouldn't be what it has become without her involvement. Her high standards, devotion, and skills are missed in this edition.

We also would like to thank the extraordinary efforts of a talented group of individuals at McGraw-Hill Education who made this textbook and its ancillaries come together: our managing director, Thomas Timp; William Mulford, our senior brand manager; Yvonne Lloyd and Christine Scheid, our senior product developers; Valerie Kramer, our marketing manager; Tara McDermott, our senior designer; Katherine Ward, our digital product analyst; Jessica Portz and Kelly Hart, our core project managers; Brent dela Cruz, our senior content project manager; Susan Culbertson, our senior buyer; and Melissa Homer, our content licensing specialist.

We are indebted to the following individual, who helped develop, critique, and shape the ancillary package: Mirella Pardee, the University of Toledo.

We would like to recognize the valuable contributions of those who helped guide our developmental decisions with their insightful reviews and suggestions:

Previous Edition Reviewers

Dr. Irfan Akhtar
Career Institute of Health and Technology

Jessica Lynn Alexander, BS, MN
Mississippi University for Women

Suzanne Allen, RMA, RPT
Sanford-Brown Institute

Theresa Louise Allyn, BS, MEd
Edmonds Community College

Emil Asdurian, MA
Bramson ORT College

Dr. Joseph H. Balatbat
Sanford-Brown Institute

Rachel Curran Basco, MHS, RRT-NPS
Bossier Parish Community College

Nina Beaman, MS, RNC-AWHC, CMA (AAMA)
Bryant & Stratton College

Ruth Berger, RS, RHIA
Chippewa Valley Technical College

Carole Berube, MA, MSN, BSN, RN
Bristol Community College

Jean L. Bucher, BA, MSEd
Clark College

Ruth A. Bush, PhD, MPH
San Diego Mesa College

Robin L. Cavallo, RN, BSN
Montgomery County Community College

Jean M. Chenu, MS
Genesee Community College

Carolyn Sue Coleman, LPN, AS
National College

Lucinda A. Conley, RHIT
Ozarka College

Mary Alice Conrad, ADN
Delaware Technical and Community College

Lynn M. Egler, RMA, AHI, CPhT
Dorsey Schools

Robert Edward Fanger, BS, MEd
Del Mar College

William C. Fiala, BS, MA
University of Akron, Allied Health Department

Nancy Gacke, BA
Southeast Technical Institute

Leslie Harbers, BSN, RMA
National College

Betty Hassler, RN, RMA
National College

Katherine Hawkins, BS, MS
Ivy Tech Community College

Mary W. Hood, MS, ARRT(R)(CT)
William Rainey Harper College

Harold N. Horn
Lincoln Land Community College

Bud W. Hunton, MA
Sinclair Community College

Judy Hurtt, MEd
East Central Community College

Carol Lee Jarrell, MLT, AHI
Brown Mackie College

Sherry Jones, COTA/L
Sinclair Community College

Timothy J. Jones, MA
Oklahoma City Community College

Judith Karls, RN, BSN, MSEd
Madison Area Technical College

Cathy Kelley-Arney, CMA, MLTC, BSHS
National College and National College of Business and Technology

Heather Kies, MHA, CMA (AAMA)
Goodwin College

Crystal Kitchens, CMT, MA
Richland Community College

Barbara Klomp, BA, RT(R)
Macomb Community College

Naomi Kupfer, CMA
Heritage College

LM Liggan, MEd, C-AHI, RMA
Director of Health Care Education, National College

Susan Long, BS
Ogeechee Technical College

Ann M. Lunde, BS, CMT
Waubonsee Community College

James M. Lynch, MD
Florida Southern College

Loreen W. MacNichol, CMRS, RMC
Andover College

Allan L. Markezich, PhD
Black Hawk College

Heather Marti
Carrington College

Amie L. Mayhall, MBA, CCA
Olney Central College

David McBride, BA, MA, RT(R)(CT)(MR)
Westmoreland County Community College

Mindy S. McDonald, CMA (AAMA)
University of Northwestern Ohio

Elizabeth L. Miller, CPC, CMA
Probill PMCC

Steve G. Moon, MS, FAMI, CMI
The Ohio State University

Deborah M. Mullen, CCS-P, CPC, CPC-I
Probill PMCC

Charlotte Susie Myers, MA
Kansas City Community College

Eva Oltman, Med, CPC-I, CPC, CMA, EMT
Jefferson Community and Technical College

Gail P. Orr, BA
National College

Mirella G. Pardee, MSN, MA, RN
University of Toledo

Judith L. Paulsen, BA
Vatterott College

Pamela K. Roemershauser, CPC
MedVance Institute

Patricia L. Sell, AAS, BS, MSEd
National College

Shirley J. Shaw, MA
Northland Pioneer College

Gene Simon, RHIA, RMD
Florida Career College

Donna J. Slovensky, PhD, RHIA, FAHIMA
University of Alabama at Birmingham

Christine Sproles, RN, BSN, MS
Pensacola Christian College

Susan Stockmaster, MHS, CMA (AAMA)
Trident Technical College

Diane Swift, RHIT
State Fair Community College

Margaret A. Tiemann, RN, BS
St. Charles Community College

Rita F. Waller, MSN, RRT
Augusta Technical College

Kathryn Whitley, RN, MSN, NP-C
Patrick Henry Community College

Cassandra E. Williams, MS, RHIA
Ogeechee Technical College

Kari Williams, BS, DC
Front Range Community College

Marsha L. Wilson, MA, BS, MEd
Clarian Health Sciences Education Center

James R. Woods, MS, RRT, RPFT
Florida Community College

Carole A. Zeglin, MSEd, BS, MT, RMA
Westmoreland County Community College

Medical Reviewers

Marie Atkinson, MD
Wayne State University School of Medicine Department of Neurology

Courtney L. Barr, MPH, MD
University of Missouri School of Medicine Department of OB/GYN

Toby C. Campbell, MD, MSCI
University of Wisconsin–Madison, Carbone Cancer Center Department of Hematology/Oncology

Lawrence S. Chan, MD
University of Illinois College of Medicine Department of Dermatology

Dawn Belt Davis, MD, PhD
University of Wisconsin–Madison Department of Endocrinology

Julie A. Kovach, MD, FACC, FASE
Wayne State University School of Medicine Division of Cardiology, Department of Medicine

Noelle K. LoConte, MD
University of Wisconsin–Madison Department of Medicine, Section of Hematology/Oncology

Barry Newman, MD
PC Tech

Abdul Ghani Sankri-Tarbichi, MD
Wayne State University School of Medicine

Scott E. Van Valin, MD
Medical College of Wisconsin Department of Orthopaedic Surgery

Damandeep S. Walia, MD
The University of Kansas Medical Center Division of Allergy, Clinical Immunology & Rheumatology

Jennifer M. Weiss, MD
University of Wisconsin School of Medicine and Public Health

Fred Arthur Zar, MD
University of Illinois at Chicago Department of Medicine

Giancarlo F. Zuliani, MD
Wayne State University School of Medicine Department of Otolaryngology–Head and Neck Surgery

TEACHING AND LEARNING SUPPLEMENTS

The **Instructor's Manual** (available online through Connect) is an invaluable resource for new and experienced medical terminology instructors. All of the components of the *Medical Language for Modern Health Care* textbook program are designed to be coherent and connected in order to create a consistent environment in which students can learn medical terminology. The Instructor's Manual shows how each component of the textbook program works to support and reinforce the content and strengths of the other components, from art and exercises to content and test bank questions.

The Instructor's Manual contains the following sections:

- **Your Medical Terminology Course—An Introduction to Teaching Medical Terminology**

  The Instructor's Manual contains:

  - A helpful introduction to teaching medical terminology.
  - Information about student learning styles and corresponding instructor strategies.
  - Innovative learning activities.
  - Assessment techniques and strategies.
  - Classroom management tips.
  - Techniques for teaching limited-English-proficiency students.

- **Lesson Planning Guide**

  In addition, the Instructor's Manual contains a Lesson Planning Guide for each of the lessons in the book. Each lesson plan contains a step-by-step teaching plan and master copies of handouts. These lessons may be used alone or combined to accommodate different class schedules. The lessons can easily be revised to reflect your preferred topic or sequence, or to add or delete topics entirely. Each of the lesson plans is designed to be used with a corresponding PowerPoint® presentation that is available on the Online Learning Center, discussed as follows.

  The **Online Learning Center, Instructor Resources** also contains:

- **McGraw-Hill's Test Generator.** This flexible electronic testing program allows instructors to create tests from book-specific items. It accommodates a wide range of question types, and instructors may add their own questions. Multiple versions of a test can be created, and any test can be exported for use with course management systems such as WebCT, Blackboard, or PageOut. The program is available for Windows and Macintosh environments.

- **PowerPoint® Lecture Outlines.** PowerPoint lectures with speaking notes are available for the chapters in the textbook. The PowerPoint presentations, which combine art and lecture notes, are designed to help instructors discuss with students the important points of the lessons. The slides are customizable, allowing instructors to modify lectures to ensure that the needs of their unique students and curricula are met.

- **Image Bank.** The image bank features selected textbook images.

- **BodyAnimat3D.** Integrated 3D animations help students visualize the most difficult concepts, with pre- and post-assessment questions for every animation.

HOW TO TEACH MEDICAL TERMINOLOGY

The **Online Course for Instructors to Support** *Medical Language for Modern Health Care* is found in the Instructor Resources section of the Online Learning Center.

The **How to Teach Medical Terminology** course guidelines provide instructors with the introductory knowledge and resources they need to begin using the *Medical Language for Modern Health Care* textbook and related materials effectively. This course is designed to cover the "basics" of how to teach medical terminology effectively.

The How to Teach Medical Terminology online course allows instructors to choose for themselves which module they wish to take, or they may opt to take a self-assessment survey that will recommend one of the three modules.

- **Module 1** is designed for the inexperienced instructor.
- **Module 2** is designed for the instructor who has previous classroom experience but has never taught medical terminology.
- **Module 3** is designed for the experienced medical terminology instructor who has not previously used a contextualized approach to teaching the subject.

McGraw-Hill Connect® is a highly reliable, easy-to-use homework and learning management solution that utilizes learning science and award-winning adaptive tools to improve student results.

Homework and Adaptive Learning

- Connect's assignments help students contextualize what they've learned through application, so they can better understand the material and think critically.

- Connect will create a personalized study path customized to individual student needs through SmartBook®.

- SmartBook helps students study more efficiently by delivering an interactive reading experience through adaptive highlighting and review.

Over **7 billion questions** have been answered, making McGraw-Hill Education products more intelligent, reliable, and precise.

Connect's Impact on Retention Rates, Pass Rates, and Average Exam Scores

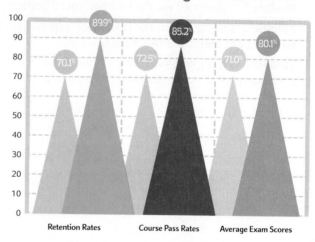

without Connect   with Connect

Using **Connect** improves retention rates by **19.8** percentage points, passing rates by **12.7** percentage points, and exam scores by **9.1** percentage points.

73% of instructors who use **Connect** require it; instructor satisfaction **increases** by 28% when **Connect** is required.

Quality Content and Learning Resources

- Connect content is authored by the world's best subject matter experts, and is available to your class through a simple and intuitive interface.

- The Connect eBook makes it easy for students to access their reading material on smartphones and tablets. They can study on the go and don't need internet access to use the eBook as a reference, with full functionality.

- Multimedia content such as videos, simulations, and games drive student engagement and critical thinking skills.

Robust Analytics and Reporting

- Connect Insight® generates easy-to-read reports on individual students, the class as a whole, and on specific assignments.

- The Connect Insight dashboard delivers data on performance, study behavior, and effort. Instructors can quickly identify students who struggle and focus on material that the class has yet to master.

- Connect automatically grades assignments and quizzes, providing easy-to-read reports on individual and class performance.

©Hero Images/Getty Images

Impact on Final Course Grade Distribution

without Connect		with Connect
22.9%	A	31.0%
27.4%	B	34.3%
22.9%	C	18.7%
11.5%	D	6.1%
15.4%	F	9.9%

More students earn **As** and **Bs** when they use **Connect**.

Trusted Service and Support

- Connect integrates with your LMS to provide single sign-on and automatic syncing of grades. Integration with Blackboard®, D2L®, and Canvas also provides automatic syncing of the course calendar and assignment-level linking.

- Connect offers comprehensive service, support, and training throughout every phase of your implementation.

- If you're looking for some guidance on how to use Connect, or want to learn tips and tricks from super users, you can find tutorials as you work. Our Digital Faculty Consultants and Student Ambassadors offer insight into how to achieve the results you want with Connect.

©2014 Nucleus Medical Media

What's New in the Fourth Edition

- The content is focused on the terminology of anatomy and physiology, diseases, disorders, symptoms, diagnostic and therapeutic procedures, and pharmacology. The content is now more concise and up-to-date with new terms.

- Each content area and exercise set is tagged with its corresponding chapter learning outcome (LO).

- Over 50% of the book's artwork and photos have been replaced with more current and relevant images.

- The terms defined in this book have been reviewed for relevance against the provisional new ICD-10.

- In each of the chapters on body systems new sections detailing diagnostic procedures, therapeutic procedures and pharmacology have been added.

The abbreviation LO stands for a chapter learning outcome or goal that can be achieved by a learner during the chapter. Each LO is linked to appropriate major headings on each page of text.

Chapter Learning Outcomes

Your journey through this book, and your externship at Fulwood Medical Center, begins with getting to know the surroundings in which you will experience medical language.
In order to get the most out of your experience, you need to be able to:

LO W.1 Establish a commitment to learn medical terminology.

LO W.2 Understand how the contextual approach of this book promotes active learning.

LO W.3 Differentiate the roles of the health care team in different medical specialties.

LO W.4 Recognize the knowledge and skills you will need to be an active learner.

LO W.5 Describe the importance of effective organizational strategies and study habits.

LO W.6 Utilize the pedagogic devices used in each chapter and lesson to understand the concepts being taught.

 Case Report (CR) W.1

You are

. . . a student preparing for a career as a health professional. As part of your training program, you must complete a supervised **externship.** You have just arrived at Fulwood Medical Center for your first day as an **extern.** You are glad to have this opportunity: Fulwood is a busy medical center with highly skilled, compassionate staff members. Between attending classes at night, working during the day, and raising two children, you have a full schedule. However, the knowledge and skills you are learning in your studies and at Fulwood will prepare you for a successful future.

Lesson W.1
WELCOME

Active Conceptual Learning

Lesson Objectives

The information in this
lesson will enable you to:

W.1.1 Understand the reasons
for learning medical
terminology in order
to communicate and
document information
effectively as a health
professional.

W.1.2 Describe the
conceptual approach
used in the book and
how it motivates your
learning.

W.1.3 Understand the
concept and structure
of a health care team.

W.1.4 Determine how to
be an active learner
and how to actively
experience medical
language.

LO W.1 Why You Should Learn Medical Terminology

Medical terminology is not just another subject for which you memorize the facts and then forget them when you move on to your next course. Medical language will be used throughout your studies, as well as every day on your job. Your understanding of medical terminology will make you a successful student and health professional.

Even beyond your career goals, everyone becomes a patient at one time or another. You also may accompany an elderly parent, a friend, or a child to a doctor or emergency room. Knowing medical terminology makes it easier for you to communicate with physicians and use the Internet to research health information—and ultimately to become a proactive medical consumer.

Figure W.1 shows an electronic report of a patient's condition, which is something you must be able to understand as a health professional. Terms like **dyspnea**, **pleuritic, effusion**, and **neutrophils** are used every day in medical language.

Health care professionals use specific terms to describe and talk about objects and situations they encounter each day. Like every language, medical terminology changes constantly as new knowledge is discovered. For example, in the world of genetics, the terminology used today was unheard of a decade ago. Medical terms quickly become outdated as new information makes its debut. **Consumption** is now known as **tuberculosis**, **grippe** as **influenza**, and **whooping cough** as **pertussis**.

Modern medical terminology is a language constructed over centuries, using words and elements from Greek and Latin origins as its building blocks. Some 15,000 or more words are formed from 1,200 Greek and Latin roots. It serves as an international language, enabling medical scientists from different countries and in different medical fields to communicate with a common understanding.

In your world as a health care professional, medical terminology enables you to communicate with your team leader, with other health care professionals on your team, and with other professionals in different disciplines outside your team. Understanding medical terminology also enables you to translate the medical terms into language your patients can understand, thus improving the quality of their care and demonstrating your professionalism.

In short, if you can't speak the language, you can't join the club.

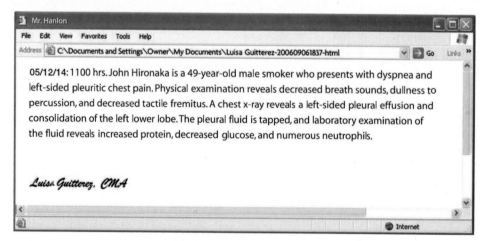

▲ **Figure W.1** Electronic Report of a Patient's Condition.

LO W.2 The Contextual Approach to Learning

When medical terms are separated from their intended context, it is easy to lose sight of how important it is to use them accurately and precisely. Learning medical terminology in the context of the medical setting reinforces the importance of correct usage and precision in communication.

In every chapter and lesson in this book, the learner steps into the role of a health professional working in a situation that is relevant to the medical specialty associated with the body system being studied in that chapter. You will learn the medical terminology used in that medical specialty and body system through the context of anatomy and physiology, pathology, and therapeutic and diagnostic procedures and tests.

Patient case reports and documentation are used to illustrate the real-life application of medical terminology in modern health care, to care for and communicate with patients, and to interact with other members of the health care team.

Fulwood Medical Center is the realistic health care setting in which these interactions take place. It consists of a medical office building and an attached 250-bed hospital. The office building houses physicians practicing primary care, the major medical and surgical specialties, and some complementary medicine therapies—in all, nearly 100 physicians in 25 specialty areas. The hospital and the medical offices share pharmacy, laboratory, radiology, physical therapy, health education, and cafeteria facilities, but they have separate main entrances. A directory on the wall near the hospital lobby lists all the departments and doctors and their locations *(Figure W.2)*.

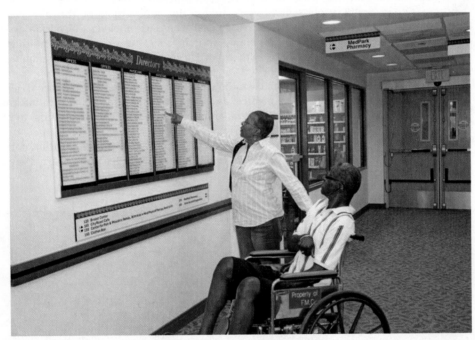

▲ **Figure W.2** An office directory can help orient visitors within the medical office complex. ©McGraw-Hill Education/Rick Brady, photographer

▲ **Figure W.3** A busy medical practice at Fulwood Medical Center. ©McGraw-Hill Education/Rick Brady, photographer

▲ **Figure W.4** A primary care physician oversees the health concerns of patients and refers patients to specialists when necessary. ©McGraw-Hill Education/Rick Brady, photographer

LO W.3 The Health Care Team

A variety of health professionals make up the teams caring for patients in each medical specialty. As a **health professional,** you are part of a team of medical and other professionals who provide health care services designed to improve patients' health and well-being in each medical specialty and setting *(Figure W.3).*

The team leader is a medical doctor, or physician, who can be an **MD** (doctor of medicine) or a **DO** (doctor of osteopathy). Most **managed care systems** require the patient to have a **primary care physician (PCP)** *(Figure W.4).* This PCP, who may be a **family practitioner, internist,** or **pediatrician** (a doctor for children), is responsible for the overall care of the patient. In managed care delivery systems, such as Health Maintenance Organizations (HMOs) and Preferred Provider Organizations (PPOs), the PCP acts as the gatekeeper for the patient to enter the system, supervising all care the patient receives.

If needed medical care is beyond the expertise of the PCP, the patient is referred to a medical specialist *(Figure W.4),* whose expertise is based on a specific body system or even a part of a body system. For example, a **cardiologist** has expertise in diseases of the heart and vascular system, a **dermatologist** specializes in diseases of the skin, and an **orthopedist** specializes in problems with the musculoskeletal system. A **gastroenterologist** is an expert in diseases of the whole digestive system, whereas a **colorectal surgeon** specializes only in diseases of the lower gastrointestinal tract.

Other health professionals work under the supervision of the physician and provide direct care to the patient *(Figure W.5).* These can include a **physician assistant, nurse practitioner, medical assistant,** and, in specialty areas, different therapists, technologists, and technicians with expertise in the use of specific therapeutic and diagnostic tools.

Still other health professionals on the team provide indirect patient care *(Figure W.6).* These include **administrative medical assistants, transcriptionists, health information technicians, medical insurance billers,** and **coders,** all of whom are essential to providing high-quality patient care.

As you study the language of each medical specialty at Fulwood Medical Center, you also will meet the members of each specialty's health care team and learn more about their roles in caring for the patient.

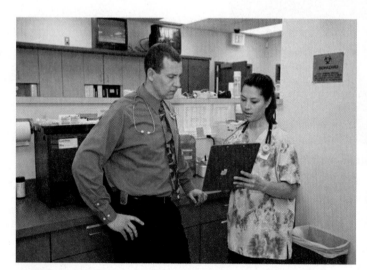

▲ **Figure W.5** Physicians, nurses, and medical assistants provide direct care to patients. ©McGraw-Hill Education/Rick Brady, photographer

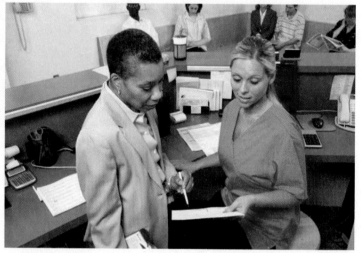

▲ **Figure W.6** Administrative medical assistants are among the health professionals who provide indirect care to patients. ©McGraw-Hill Education/Rick Brady, photographer

LO W.4 Being an Active Learner

Medical terms provide health care professionals a way to communicate with each other and document the care they provide. To provide effective patient care, all health care professionals must be fluent in medical language. One misused or misspelled medical term on a patient record can cause errors that can result in injury or death to patients, incorrect coding or billing of medical claims, and possible fraud charges. The patient care record is a legal document as well as a clinical document.

When the medical terms are separated from their intended context, as they are in other medical terminology textbooks, it is easy to lose sight of how important it is to use these medical terms accurately and precisely. Learning medical terminology in the context of the medical setting reinforces the importance of correct usage and precision in communication.

During your time at Fulwood Medical Center, you will *experience* medical language. Just as in a real medical center, you will encounter and apply medical terminology in a variety of ways. Actively experiencing medical language will help ensure that you are truly learning, and not simply memorizing, the medical terms in each chapter. Memorizing a term allows you to use it in the same situation (for example, repeating a definition) but doesn't help you apply it in new situations. Whether you are reading chart notes in a patient's medical record or a description of the treatment prescribed by a physician, you will see medical terms being used for the purpose they were intended.

This book goes beyond simply presenting and defining new medical terms. Fulwood Medical Center, with its wide range of patient cases and health professionals and its realistic medical environment, allows you to encounter and discover terms the way they are used in real life—in different medical settings. Experiencing medical language in this context bridges the gap between what you learn in the classroom and what really happens in the clinical setting.

As you progress through this book,

- You will encounter, and be asked to interact with, patients and health care professionals.

- You will analyze medical records and documentation.

- You will be introduced to diagnostic and therapeutic methods and the pathophysiology of disease.

- You will be able to see how all of these activities depend on effective communication, accurate comprehension, and precise use of medical language.

▲ **Figure W.7** A CMA **communicates with a patient.** ©Rocketclips, Inc./ Shutterstock.com RF

▲ **Figure W.8** One of your responsibilities may be to read the results of diagnostic tests, such as this blood sugar reading.
©McGraw-Hill Education/Rick Brady, photographer

LO W.4 Being an Active Learner

Below are just a few of the ways you will use medical language on your first day at Fulwood.

Listening and Speaking

You will

- Listen to patients as they describe their medical history and explain their symptoms *(Figure W.7)*. A conversation between Luisa Guitterez, a Certified Medical Assistant (CMA), and Mrs. Martha Jones, a patient, follows:

    Luisa Guitterez, CMA: "Mrs. Jones, I'm Luisa, an assistant to Dr. Lee. The receptionist noticed that you were looking pale and sweaty and notified Dr. Lee."

    Mrs. Jones: "In the rush to get here this morning, Luisa, I didn't have time to eat breakfast. I'm not feeling so well right now. . . . I'm diabetic, you know."

    Luisa Guitterez, CMA: "Dr. Lee has asked me to test your blood sugar level. As a diabetic, you've done this many times yourself, I'm sure."

- Listen to and carry out physicians' instructions and information concerning patient care.
- Speak to physicians and other health care professionals, report information, and ask questions.
- Talk with patients in the course of patient encounters and phone calls, including giving instructions and answering questions about the physician's prescribed treatment plans.
- Document your interaction with the patient.

Reading

You will

- Read physicians' comments and treatment plans in patient medical records and case reports.
- Read the results of physical examinations, procedures, and laboratory and diagnostic tests *(Figure W.8)*.

Writing

You will

- Document actions taken by yourself and other members of the health care team.
- Proofread medical documentation to ensure its accuracy.

Thinking Critically

You will

- Evaluate medical documentation for accuracy.
- Translate technical medical communication into words patients can understand.
- Analyze and understand unfamiliar medical terms using the strategies presented in this book.

Learning from Patient Cases

You will encounter realistic patient cases throughout this book. These cases ask you to step into the role of a health care professional *(You are . . .)* and focus on a real patient with real health care needs *(Your patient is . . .).*

Taking full advantage of the patient cases in this book allows you to

- Experience various health care careers.
- Examine the roles you may fill to provide care for patients.
- See the types of documentation needed in these situations.
- Become acquainted with medical terminology in real-life settings.
- Recognize that every interaction with a patient is a learning experience.

Applying What You Learn

Throughout each chapter, you will be asked to apply and practice what you are learning. These application opportunities are designed to help you practice using medical terms in a variety of ways and for a variety of purposes. Specifically, the exercises will require you to perform tasks you would perform on the job, such as *listening and speaking, reading, writing,* and *thinking critically.* They are designed to help you move beyond simple memorization and become fluent in the language of modern health care.

Exercises

A. Each encounter with medical language improves your ability to (a) understand the medical terms you hear, (b) speak accurately and precisely using medical terms, (c) write accurately and precisely using the appropriate medical terms, (d) read and understand medical terms, and (e) think critically about the medical terms you experience. *These five skills are very important for all health care professionals. It is important to be able to identify experiences that build your knowledge and skill with medical language. Write the letter of the skill or skills being used in each blank below. More than one skill may be needed for each activity.* **LO W.4**

Skills: **a.** Understand spoken medical terms.

          b. Speak accurately and precisely using medical terms.

          c. Write accurately and precisely using medical terms

          d. Read and understand medical terms.

          e. Think critically about medical language.

_____   **1.** Answering a patient's questions about the physician's diagnosis and instructions.

_____   **2.** Taking a phone message when a specialist calls from another facility and has information concerning one of the patients of a physician in your facility.

_____   **3.** Proofreading an insurance claim form.

_____   **4.** Teaching a patient with special nutritional needs how to modify her diet.

_____   **5.** Using the Internet and textbooks to learn more about a disease or condition.

▲ **Figure W.12** Being a good listener is important to success. ©Hemera Technologies/Getty Images RF

LO W.4 Being an Active Learner (continued)

As you will find out in your externship at Fulwood Medical Center, true learning is active. You can't sit back and let someone else pour knowledge into your head. You need to play the various health care professional roles you'll assume at Fulwood and work to get as much from them as you can. Simply attending your medical terminology class is another valuable thing you can do to help yourself. However, it doesn't end there. Here are more ways you can be an active learner and get the most out of your studies.

Getting the Most Out of Lectures

1. **Prepare.** You'll be amazed at how much easier it is to understand the material when you have previewed the chapter before going to class. If you find it difficult to carve out the time, simply arrive at class 5 to 15 minutes earlier than usual and skim the chapter before the lecture begins. This will at least give you an overview of what may be discussed.

2. **Be a good listener.** Most people think they are good listeners, but few really are *(Figure W.12)*. Are you?

   - You can't listen if you are talking or text messaging or looking at your cell phone.
   - You can't listen if you are daydreaming or dozing.
   - Listening and comprehending are two different things. If you don't understand something the instructor is saying, ask a question or jot a note and visit the instructor after class. Don't feel intimidated: You probably aren't the only person who "doesn't get it."

3. **Take good notes.** Here are some tips for successful note-taking:
   - Use a standard-size notebook or, better yet, a three-ring binder with loose-leaf paper. The binder will allow you to organize and integrate your notes and handouts.
   - Use a standard black or blue ink pen to take your initial notes. You can annotate later using a pencil, which can be erased if necessary.
   - Start a new page with each lecture or note-taking session.
   - Label each page of your notes with the date and a heading.
   - Focus on the main points, and try to use an outline format to take notes. This will help you capture key ideas and organize subpoints.
   - Review and edit your notes shortly after class—at least within 24 hours—to make sure they make sense. You also may want to compare your notes with those of a study partner later to make sure neither of you has missed anything.

Getting the Most Out of Reading

1. **Concentrate on what you are reading.** Survey the titles, outcomes, objectives, and headings in each chapter, and look at the visuals to identify what the chapter is all about.
2. **Use the SQ3R** (see the Study Hint) to help you read actively.
3. **Take notes on key ideas** in the reading.
4. **Write down any questions** you have.
5. **Discuss what you have read** with your study partner.

 Study Hints

The SQ3R Model for Reading is a successful equation for studying:
Survey what you are going to read.
Question what you are going to learn after the preview.
Read—Read the assignment.
Recite—Stop every once in a while, look up from the book, and put what you've just read into your own words.
Review—After you've finished, review the main points.

Performing Well on Tests

1. **Always read the directions.** If you are unsure, ask. Find out if there is a penalty for guessing. If there is not, try to answer every question on the test even if you have to guess at some.

2. **Before you begin, scan the entire test** so that you know how long it is and what types of activities and questions it contains.

3. **Answer the easy questions or sections first** so that you get as much of the exam finished as possible if difficult questions slow you down.

   - When answering multiple-choice questions, eliminate each incorrect option until you are left with the answer that seems most correct to you.

   - When answering matching questions, match all items you know first; then do your best with the ones that remain.

   - When answering essay questions, reword the question as a statement to be sure you have answered it. Give enough examples and explanation to support your points.

4. **Once you have finished the test, use any extra time to check that you have answered all questions.** If you still have time after checking for completion, reread the questions and recheck your answers.

Studying with a Partner or Group

1. **Get a study partner.** *Schedule fixed* study dates. Talk through the concepts, compare notes, and quiz each other. Studying with a partner can be fun. Think of it this way: You are multitasking, layering study time and social time. Just be sure the social time doesn't squeeze out the study time.

2. **Don't take advantage of your study partner.** If you can't make a study date or attend a class, let your partner know. You won't have a study partner—or a friend—much longer if it isn't a mutually beneficial arrangement.

3. **Establish a study group.** Choose a few students in the class, including your study partner, with whom to study on a regular basis. Having a group in addition to a study partner ensures that you will still be able to study with others if your partner has to miss a session.

Exercises

A. Budgeting your time is key to being able to take care of your priorities. *Follow these steps with the list of tasks you need to get done.* **LO W.5**

1. Rank each of the tasks in the table in order of its priority (e.g., 1 is the highest priority, 2 is next highest, and so on).

2. On a separate sheet of paper, plan a weekly schedule that will help you accomplish these tasks. Include all seven days of the week, and block off the days in hourly increments.

3. Keep in mind that while some activities have set times, others can be flexible. Also consider that activities like studying and household tasks will need to be done for a period of time *every day*, not just once a week.

   (Note: There is no one "correct" answer to this exercise; however, it is beneficial to see how other students in the class chose to budget their time. Be creative but realistic. Don't forget to budget for travel time between tasks if needed.)

Weekly Tasks

Studying for Medical Terminology _____	Errands (groceries, etc.) _____	Leisure time _____
Sleep _____	Family time _____	Household chores _____
Medical Terminology class (Tuesday and Thursday 6:30–9:30 p.m.) _____	Work (8:00–3:30 daily) _____	Meals, including preparation & cleanup _____
Church and/or hobbies _____	Exercise _____	Grooming _____

Now that you understand what it takes to be successful, you are ready to move through this textbook and engage in an externship at Fulwood Medical Center.

Lesson W.2

Learning Medical Language

Keynote

As novelist Lillian Smith once said, **"When you stop learning, stop listening, stop looking and asking questions, always new questions, then it is time to die."**

"I don't think much of a man who is not wiser today than he was yesterday."
—Abraham Lincoln

LO W.5 Learning Medical Language

Your current training in medical terminology is necessary for you to be able to continue your education in health care, but school is just one of the many places where you acquire knowledge. Each time you solve a problem in life, such as working through an argument with a friend or helping your child perform better in school, the knowledge you gain is *your own* answer to *your own* problem. This type of knowledge—discovered through experience—is genuine, real, and trustworthy for you. It is not determined by some distant authority, like what you learn in school. Your medical terminology instructor isn't likely to ask a test question on how to unclog your sink. Instead, this type of learning is driven by your needs and goals. The knowledge you gain from solving your own problems, whether by yourself or with the help of other people or resources, motivates you to learn even more and helps you grow as a person and as a professional.

When you are working as a health care professional, your ongoing education is an integral and inseparable part of your work activities. You'll need additional classroom training to keep your skills and professional knowledge up to date. You'll also continue to learn on your own through experience. As a health care professional, every time you interact with a patient, read a report, or talk with your team leader or peers, you are given another opportunity to learn *(Figure W.9)*.

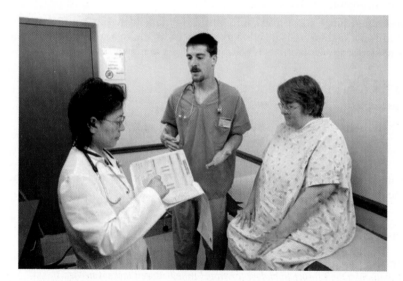

▲ **Figure W.9** Learning doesn't stop when you leave the classroom; every time you interact with other health care professionals and patients, you have the opportunity to learn something. ©McGraw-Hill Education/Rick Brady, photographer

Case Report (CR) W.1 *(Continued)*

Your first day at Fulwood Medical Center went very well. The supervisor, Rosana Rice, gave you a tour of the facilities and introduced you to several health care professionals with whom you will be working. Ms. Rice discussed your duties and her expectations of you, and she asked you to review your plan for keeping up with your studies. Now it's late evening, and you have yet to feed your kids and get them into bed—not to mention pick up around the house, pay bills, and, oh yes, review a whole chapter in your medical terminology textbook to prepare for a test in class tomorrow night. How are you going to get everything done?

LO W.5 Study Strategies and Habits

If you know you have a test every Thursday night, ask your spouse, mother, sister, or friend or someone in your support group to take care of the children on Wednesday night so you can get to a quiet place and dedicate the evening to studying. A support group of family and friends is essential to your success, so look for ways to surround yourself with people you can trust and rely on.

In addition to support, you will need to evaluate and

- Recognize the stresses you are experiencing.
- Determine what you can change because the situation, people, and events are making excessive demands on you.
- Prioritize your schedule in your head or on paper and complete each task in the proper order of importance.
- Find ways to give yourself a break from stressful situations.

The next section contains strategies that will help you get focused. It will help you learn how to manage your time and your studies to succeed—but this lesson can't do it alone. You are what you put into your studies. You have a lot of time and money invested in your education. Don't waste it by putting in half the effort. Succeeding in this class, and in life, requires the following:

- Commit your time and perseverance to learning.
- Know how to motivate yourself.
- Get organized.
- Schedule and manage your time.
- Be an active learner.

The rest of this chapter will help you learn how to be effective in these areas. As you encounter new learning situations during your externship at Fulwood, you will be prepared to handle them.

Exercises

A. Reflect on the idea of lifelong learning and how you can make it work for you to enrich your life's experience. *Think about one instance in your life when something you learned (by yourself, from another person, from research, etc.) became the foundation upon which you built further learning and information. Some examples are how to paint a room, clean a fish, use a computer, and cook a meal. Briefly describe that here.* **LO W.5**

1. What I learned, and how I learned it:

_____

_____

2. Now describe why you need to be committed to learning from everyday experiences on the job, and explain how that can help you in your career.

_____

_____

_____

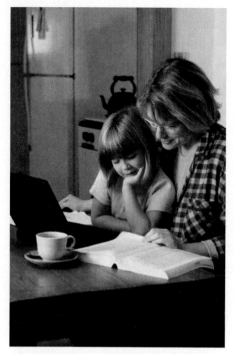

▲ **Figure W.10** Identify your own personal preferences for learning, and seek out the resources that will best help you with your studies. Recognize your weaknesses, and try to compensate for or work to improve them. ©Scott T. Baxter/Getty Images RF

LO W.5 Study Strategies and Habits (continued)

Committing Yourself to Learning: Your Time and Perseverance

Understanding—and mastering—what you learn in the classroom will take time and patience. Nothing worthwhile comes easily. Be committed to your studies, and you will reap the benefits in the long run. Consider this: Your training in health care is the foundation of your future career. If the foundation is poorly built, it will lead to difficulties later.

Knowing and Motivating Yourself

What type of learner are you? When are you most productive? Know yourself and your limits, and work within them *(Figure W.10)*. Think about how to motivate yourself to prioritize your studies and achieve your goals. You are the one who benefits most from your success. If you lack self-motivation and drive, you are the first person who suffers.

Know your learning style. Just as there are many types of learners, there is no right or wrong way of learning. In which of the following categories do you see yourself?

Visual learner. You respond best to seeing processes and information. Take advantage of the strengths of your learning style by doing the following:

- Focus on text illustrations and charts, as well as course handouts.

- Check to see if there are animations on the course or text website to help you.

- Consider drawing diagrams in your notes to illustrate concepts.

- Use the contextual and labeling exercises at McGraw-Hill Connect.

Auditory learner. You work best by listening to processes and information. Take advantage of the strengths of your learning style by doing the following:

- Listen carefully to—and possibly tape record (with instructor permission)—the lecture.

- Talk information through with a study partner.

- Listen to audio pronunciations of terms at McGraw-Hill Connect.

Tactile/kinesthetic learner. Hands-on learning works best for you. Take advantage of the strengths of your learning style by doing the following:

- Apply what you have learned in a role-play or realistic scenario.

- Think of ways to apply your critical thinking skills in application-based ways.

- The Online Learning Center and McGraw-Hill Connect also will help you.

In addition to these suggestions, here are a few helpful hints for students of all learning styles:

- Ask questions to make sure you understand what you hear, read, and do.

- Rephrase what you have heard in lectures and read in the text as you talk with your peers.

- Study with a partner to help you stay committed and double-check your understanding of concepts.

Getting Organized

It seems the more organized you are, the easier things come. Take time now to analyze your life and your study habits to help you get organized now, and you'll find you have a little more time—and a lot less stress as the class progresses.

Find a calendar system that works for you. The best kind is one that you can take with you everywhere. To be truly organized, you should integrate all aspects of your life into this one calendar—school, work, family, and leisure *(Figure W.11)*. Some people also find it helpful to have an additional monthly calendar posted in a convenient place (for example, on the refrigerator) for "at a glance" dates and to have a visual of what is to come. If you do this, be sure you are consistently synchronizing both calendars so that you do not miss anything. (More tips for organizing your calendar can be found in the following Scheduling and Managing Your Time section.) Some sample entries follow:

▲ **Figure W.11** Use a daily planner to help you organize school, work, family, and leisure time. ©Vstock LLC/Tetra Images/Corbis RF

Thursday

- Work from 8:00 a.m. to 3:30 p.m.
- Doctor's appointment from 4:00 to 4:45
- Dinner from 5:15 to 6:15
- Class from 6:30 to 9:30
- Study from 10:00 to 10:30

Keep everything for your course or courses in one place—and at your fingertips. A three-ring binder works well because it allows you to add or organize handouts and notes from class in any order you prefer. Incorporating your own custom tabs helps you flip instantly to the material you need.

Find your space. Find a place that helps you be organized and focused. If it is a desk or table at home, keep it clean. Clutter adds confusion and stress, and it wastes time. If there are small children in your home, be sure your study materials are kept out of their reach. If your study space is at the library or a relative's house, keep a backpack or bag fully stocked with your text, binder or notes, pens, highlighters, sticky notes, phone numbers of study partners, and anything else you might need.

Scheduling and Managing Your Time

There is never enough time in the week to get everything done, and managing your time is one of the most difficult tasks to successfully master. Valuable time slips through your fingers so easily. Here are just a few ways time slips away unnoticed:

- **Procrastination**—putting off tasks simply because you don't feel in the mood to do them right away.
- **Distraction**—getting sidetracked by the endless variety of other things that seem easier (or more fun) to do.
- **Underestimating the value of small bits of time**—thinking it isn't worth doing any work because you have something else to do, or someplace else to be, in 20 minutes or so.

Just as you make choices about where to spend your money and how to get the best value for your dollar, you do the same with your time. In order to get the most out of your externship at Fulwood Medical Center and out of your life in general, you have to spend your time wisely. You may be able to save money for future use, but you *can't* store away time to use later. However, you *can* plan how you will spend your time in a way that maximizes the quality and the quantity of things you can get done in a day, week, month, or year. If you're like most people, you may not have a good idea of how your time is actually being used.

Keynote

We all lead busy lives, but we all make choices as to how we spend our time. Choose wisely, and make the most of every minute you have.

Exercises

A. Take time to assess your learning style, and use that to aid your study and classroom habits. *Identify the type of learner you are, and briefly describe which of the strengths in that style work best for you.* **LO W.5**

1. I am a _____ learner.

2. This works best for me:

_____

_____

_____

LO W.5 Study Strategies and Habits (continued)

Ten Steps to a Study Schedule That Works

Making a study schedule you will actually follow means knowing yourself and your limits. Implement the following tips to develop a schedule that works for you.

1. **Study when you are most productive.** When are you most productive? Are you a night owl or an early bird? Plan to study when you are most alert and can have uninterrupted segments of time. This could include a quick 5-minute review before class or a 1-hour problem-solving study session with a friend.

2. **Create a set study time for yourself daily.** Having a set schedule means making a commitment to studying. Write your study time on your calendar, and do not schedule other activities during this time.

3. **Schedule study time using shorter, focused blocks with small breaks.** Studying a little each day rather than cramming the night before a test is a much more effective use of your time. Doing this helps you learn the material and store it in your long-term memory, not just memorize it and forget it after the test. Also, you will be less fatigued and less likely to procrastinate.

4. **Plan time for family, leisure, friends, exercise, and sleep.** Studying should be your main focus, but you need to balance your time—and your life.

5. **Log your projects and homework deadlines.** Record all due dates, tests, and projects in your personal calendar so that you know what is coming. If you have a large writing project, break the assignment down into smaller targets. Set a goal for the first draft, second draft, and final copy, and record each of these deadlines in your calendar.

6. **Try to complete tasks ahead of schedule.** This will give you a chance to carefully review your work before you hand it in. You'll feel less stressed in the end.

7. **Prioritize.** In your calendar or planner, highlight or number key projects. Do them first; then cross them off when they are completed. Give yourself a pat on the back for getting them done.

8. **Review and reprioritize daily.** Check your scheduled activities each day, and adjust them if priorities have changed.

9. **Resist distractions.** Don't let unscheduled activities take you away from designated study time. The Internet is a notorious time-waster. It is easy to lose hours surfing the web or instant messaging. It's just as easy to let a 5-minute phone call with a friend turn into a 3-hour conversation. Stick to your schedule.

10. **Multitask when possible.** You may find a lot of extra time you didn't think you had. Review material or deconstruct medical terms in your head while walking to class, while doing laundry, or during "mental down time." (*Note:* Mental down time does *not* mean in the middle of a lecture.)

How to Set Yourself Up for Success

1. Don't skip class and always be on time.

2. Allow enough time to study. Schedule studying on your calendar so you won't run out of time right before a test or assignment.

3. Get a good night's sleep.

4. Ask questions and participate in class. If you have a question, someone else probably does too.

5. Take advantage of instructor office hours. If you are an online student, be sure to contact your instructor when you need additional assistance.

6. Exam preparation should be an ongoing activity. Make sure you complete your homework, and take advantage of online activities that will enhance the learning process.

7. The learning outcomes at the beginning of every chapter summarize what you must understand by the end of that chapter. Use the book and digital resources to ensure you understand the chapter material.

8. Take notes in class. Your instructor will often provide tips for remembering difficult concepts or alert you to what will be on your exams.

Good luck on your journey to mastering the language of medicine!

Study Hints

Use previous quizzes and tests as study materials. Be certain you find out the correct answer for each question you answered incorrectly. Learn from your mistakes. These questions may appear on the final exam in one form or another.

As a way to review before a test, write 10 sample questions that might appear on the test. Ask your study partner or study group to write their 10 questions. Compare questions, and try to answer every question correctly. Subject matter that you have all included in a sample question is probably important enough to be on the test.

Keynotes

Additional points to remember about your study schedule:

- Be realistic when planning—know your limits and priorities.
- Be prepared for the unexpected (child's illness, your illness, overtime at work, inclement weather), which will leave any well-planned schedule in shambles.
- Reprioritize daily on the basis of schedule disruptions and other conflicts.
- Keep the overall picture in mind, and set long- and short-term goals (what you need to get done this week, this month, before the end of the semester, and so on).
- Form a support group.

Exercises

A. Be honest with yourself and self-assess. *Are you guilty of any of the self-defeating tendencies described earlier? If so, determine to change at least one bad habit before this course begins.* **LO W.5**

1. The habit I would most like to change is

_____

2. I recognize that if I change this habit, the *benefit* to me will be

_____

Remember: Your instructor puts time and effort into preparing this class and marking tests. You need to devote your time and energy to the class as well.

LO W.6 Innovative Learning Aids in This Book

Each chapter is structured around a consistent and unique framework of learning devices including vivid illustrations, photographs, specific content tables, Word Analysis and Definition (WAD) tables, Case Reports, and contextual placements. No matter what the subject matter of a chapter, the structure enables you to develop a consistent learning strategy, making *Medical Language for Modern Health Care 4e* a superior learning tool.

You Are . . . Your Patient Is

Each chapter opens by placing you in the role of a health professional related to the specialty and associated body systems and areas covered by the chapter. You also are introduced to a patient and given information about the patient's case.

Chapter Learning Outcomes

At the same time, **Chapter Learning Outcomes** let you know what you will learn in each chapter. This technique immediately engages you, motivating you to read on to learn how a particular patient's case (and the health care provider's role in the patient's care) relates to the medical terminology being introduced in the chapter.

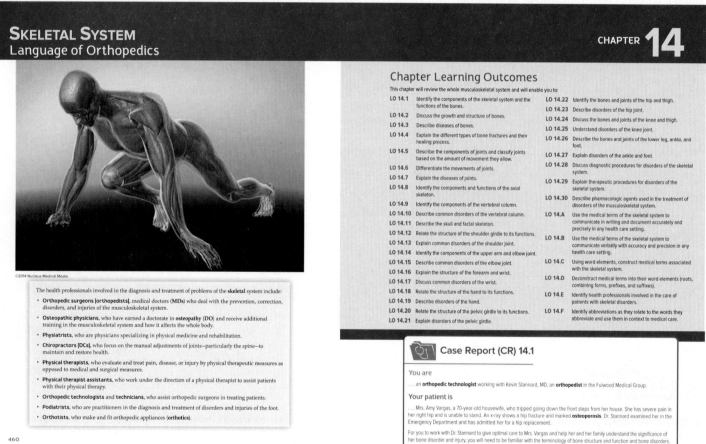

SKELETAL SYSTEM
Language of Orthopedics

CHAPTER 14

©2014 Nucleus Medical Media

The health professionals involved in the diagnosis and treatment of problems of the **skeletal** system include:

- **Orthopedic surgeons (orthopedists)**, medical doctors **(MDs)** who deal with the prevention, correction, disorders, and injuries of the musculoskeletal system.
- **Osteopathic physicians**, who have earned a doctorate in **osteopathy (DO)** and receive additional training in the musculoskeletal system and how it affects the whole body.
- **Physiatrists**, who are physicians specializing in physical medicine and rehabilitation.
- **Chiropractors (DCs)**, who focus on the manual adjustments of joints—particularly the spine—to maintain and restore health.
- **Physical therapists**, who evaluate and treat pain, disease, or injury by physical therapeutic measures as opposed to medical and surgical measures.
- **Physical therapist assistants**, who work under the direction of a physical therapist to assist patients with their physical therapy.
- **Orthopedic technologists** and **technicians**, who assist orthopedic surgeons in treating patients.
- **Podiatrists**, who are practitioners in the diagnosis and treatment of disorders and injuries of the foot.
- **Orthotists**, who make and fit orthopedic appliances (**orthotics**).

Chapter Learning Outcomes

This chapter will review the whole musculoskeletal system and will enable you to:

LO 14.1 Identify the components of the skeletal system and the functions of the bones.	**LO 14.22** Identify the bones and joints of the hip and thigh.
LO 14.2 Discuss the growth and structure of bones.	**LO 14.23** Describe disorders of the hip joint.
LO 14.3 Describe diseases of bones.	**LO 14.24** Discuss the bones and joints of the knee and thigh.
LO 14.4 Explain the different types of bone fractures and their healing process.	**LO 14.25** Understand disorders of the knee joint.
LO 14.5 Describe the components of joints and classify joints based on the amount of movement they allow.	**LO 14.26** Describe the bones and joints of the lower leg, ankle, and foot.
LO 14.6 Differentiate the movements of joints.	**LO 14.27** Explain disorders of the ankle and foot.
LO 14.7 Explain the diseases of joints.	**LO 14.28** Discuss diagnostic procedures for disorders of the skeletal system.
LO 14.8 Identify the components and functions of the axial skeleton.	**LO 14.29** Explain therapeutic procedures for disorders of the skeletal system.
LO 14.9 Identify the components of the vertebral column.	**LO 14.30** Describe pharmacologic agents used in the treatment of disorders of the musculoskeletal system.
LO 14.10 Describe common disorders of the vertebral column.	**LO 14.A** Use the medical terms of the skeletal system to communicate in writing and document accurately and precisely in any health care setting.
LO 14.11 Describe the skull and facial skeleton.	
LO 14.12 Relate the structure of the shoulder girdle to its functions.	**LO 14.B** Use the medical terms of the skeletal system to communicate verbally with accuracy and precision in any health care setting.
LO 14.13 Explain common disorders of the shoulder joint.	
LO 14.14 Identify the components of the upper arm and elbow joint.	**LO 14.C** Using word elements, construct medical terms associated with the skeletal system.
LO 14.15 Describe common disorders of the elbow joint.	
LO 14.16 Explain the structure of the forearm and wrist.	**LO 14.D** Deconstruct medical terms into their word elements (roots, combining forms, prefixes, and suffixes).
LO 14.17 Discuss common disorders of the wrist.	
LO 14.18 Relate the structure of the hand to its functions.	**LO 14.E** Identify health professionals involved in the care of patients with skeletal disorders.
LO 14.19 Describe disorders of the hand.	
LO 14.20 Relate the structure of the pelvic girdle to its functions.	**LO 14.F** Identify abbreviations as they relate to the words they abbreviate and use them in context to medical care.
LO 14.21 Explain disorders of the pelvic girdle.	

Case Report (CR) 14.1

You are

. . . an **orthopedic technologist** working with Kevin Stannard, MD, an **orthopedist** in the Fulwood Medical Group.

Your patient is

. . . Mrs. Amy Vargas, a 70-year-old housewife, who tripped going down the front steps from her house. She has severe pain in her right hip and is unable to stand. An x-ray shows a hip fracture and marked **osteoporosis**. Dr. Stannard examined her in the Emergency Department and has admitted her for a hip replacement.

For you to work with Dr. Stannard to give optimal care to Mrs. Vargas and help her and her family understand the significance of her bone disorder and injury, you will need to be familiar with the terminology of bone structure and function and bone disorders.

460

Lesson-Based Organization

The chapter content is broken down into chunks, or lessons, in order to help you digest new information and relate it to previously learned information. Rather than containing many various topics within a chapter, these lessons group the chapter material into logical, streamlined learning units designed to help you achieve the chapter outcomes. Lessons within a chapter build on one another to form a cohesive, coherent experience for the learner.

Each lesson is based on specific lesson **objectives** designed to support your achievement of the overall **chapter learning outcomes.** Each lesson in a chapter contains an introduction, lesson objectives, lesson topics, Word Analysis and Definition boxes, and lesson exercises. Within each lesson, all topics and information are presented in **self-contained two-page spreads.** This means you do not have to flip back and forth to see figures on one page that are described on another. Each section of information and every exercise are tagged with the appropriate chapter learning outcome (LO).

Word Analysis and Definition Boxes

The medical terms covered in each lesson are introduced in context, either within a patient case or in the lesson topics. To facilitate easy reference and review, the terms also are listed in boxes as a group. The **Word Analysis and Definition (WAD) boxes** list the term and its pronunciation, elements, and definition in a concise, color-coded, at-a-glance format.

Exercises

A. Describe how the lesson-based organization of the material will help you learn more efficiently. LO W.6

1. _____

B. Detail how to use the chapter Learning Outcomes to develop a study outline for the chapter material. LO W.6

1. _____

Exercises

A. Identify the structures that make up the knee joint. *Given the description, identify the structure that makes up the knee joint. Fill in the blanks.* **LO 14.24**

1. This cartilage is tough and functions to cushion and add stability to the joint. _____

2. This bone protects the anterior portion of the knee joint. It is embedded in a tendon. _____

3. The femur articulates with this leg bone. _____

4. This lower leg bone is on the lateral side of the leg. _____

5. Ligaments that form a "cross" are termed _____ ligaments.

6. Ligaments that stabilize the knee joints on the lateral and medial sides are termed _____ ligaments.

B. Use medical terminology in written documentation. *June has come to the emergency department complaining of sudden knee pain. After reading the description, insert the medical term that correctly replaces the description.* **LO 14.25, 14.A**

June has just recently taken up the sport of running. She ran too many miles her first week, causing a sharp pain to develop in front of her kneecap **1.**(_____). The physician believes that the pain is due to a softening of the cartilage **2.**(_____) of the kneecap. June thought it best to not run long distances, and instead practice sprinting with sudden stopping and starting. This resulted in an over flexion of her knee **3.**(_____), which caused a sudden tearing of her ACL.

LESSON 14.4 Appendicular Skeleton **491**

LO W.6 Innovative Learning Aids (continued)

Section and Chapter-End Exercises

Each spread ends with exercises designed to allow you to check your basic understanding of the terms you just learned. These checkpoints can be used by instructors as assignments or in-class activities or by students for self-evaluation.

At the end of each chapter, you will find chapter review of exercises that ask you to apply what you learned in all the lessons of a chapter. These exercises reinforce learning of each chapter's terms and help you go beyond mere memorization to think critically about the medical language you use. In addition to reviewing and recalling the definitions of terms learned in the chapter, you will be asked to use medical terms in new and different ways.

Study Hint Boxes

Study Hint boxes are found throughout the exercise sections. They reinforce, and remind you to use, basic study skills.

Chapter 1 Review

The Anatomy of Medical Terms

E. Use your newly acquired knowledge of medical language to correctly answer the following questions. Let the roots and combining forms be your guide. Choose the correct answer to complete each statement. (LO 1.1, 1.2)

1. This term means one who studies the skin.
   a. dermatologist
   b. urologist
   c. neurologist

2. This term relates to the intestines and the stomach.
   a. gastroenterology
   b. cardiology
   c. dermatology

3. This term relates to the process of breathing.
   a. apex
   b. toxic
   c. respiratory

4. This term relates to the stomach.
   a. gastritis
   b. gynecology
   c. dermatitis

5. This term relates to a joint.
   a. urethritis
   b. arthritis
   c. neuralgia

F. Use the correct medical term to complete the sentence. Use the words to complete each sentence below. Fill in the blanks. (LO 1.1, 1.4)

bladder   breech   cardiologist   ileum   ilium   kidney   lymph   malleolus   trapezium   ureter   urethra

1. A _____ is a specialist in the care of the heart.

2. The _____ is a tube from the kidney to the bladder.

3. Urology is the study of diseases of the _____ and _____.

4. A segment of the small intestine is the _____.

5. _____ means the buttocks, not the head, present first at delivery.

6. _____ is the tube from the bladder to the outside.

7. _____ is a fluid collected from body tissues.

8. A bone in the wrist is the _____.

9. The bony protuberance at the ankle is the _____.

10. The _____ is a bone in the pelvis.

16   CHAPTER 1 REVIEW The Anatomy of Medical Terms

G. Case report questions. Read Case Report 1.4. You should feel more comfortable with the medical terminology now and will be able to answer the questions that follow. (LO 1.4)

Case Report (CR) 1.4

You are

. . . a medical assistant employed by Russell Gordon, MD, a primary care physician at Fulwood Medical Center.

Your patient is

. . . Mrs. Connie Bishop, a 55-year-old woman who presents with a swelling in her lower abdomen and shortness of breath. She has no gynecologic or gastroenterologic symptoms. Her previous medical history shows recurrent dermatitis of her hands since a teenager and an arthroscopy for a knee injury at age 40. Physical examination reveals a circular mass 6 inches in diameter in the left lower quadrant of her abdomen. There is no abnormality in her respiratory or cardiovascular system.

Your role is to maintain her medical record and document her care, assist Dr. Gordon during his examinations, explain the examination and treatment procedures to Mrs. Bishop, and facilitate her referral for specialist care.

> **Study Hint**
> Many elements have more than one meaning. You must know the different meanings because that will make a difference in the use of the medical term.

1. What type of skin problem has Mrs. Bishop had since she was a teenager? _____

2. Which term in the case study means *pertaining to the stomach and small intestines*? _____

3. Her knee injury required what type of procedure? _____

4. Does she have any issues with her lungs or heart? (yes or no) _____

5. Do her symptoms indicate a possible problem with her ileum? (yes or no) _____

H. Because much of clinical documentation centers on surgeries, knowledge of surgical suffixes is most important—especially for coders. (LO 1.2)

Matching
Match the definition in the first column the correct term it is describing in the second column.

Term	Meaning
_____ 1. scopy	A. surgical repair
_____ 2. desis	B. visual examination
_____ 3. plasty	C. surgical fixation

Combine these suffixes with the combining form arthr/o and fill in the blanks with the correct medical term.

4. The surgeon wants a closer look inside Mr. Parker's knee so he is scheduled for an _____ tomorrow morning.

5. Mary Collins has torn her knee ligaments playing high school basketball. Her treatment plan includes scheduling an _____ to reattach them. (fixation)

6. June Larkin had a bad skiing accident while on vacation. Her tendons and ligaments in her knee will require extensive surgery to get her walking again without crutches. She needs an _____. (repair)

Congratulations! You are on your way to learning medical terminology.

CHAPTER 1 REVIEW The Anatomy of Medical Terms   17

Vivid Illustrations and Photos

Colorful, precise anatomical illustrations and photos lend a realistic view of body structures and correlate to the clinical context of the lessons.

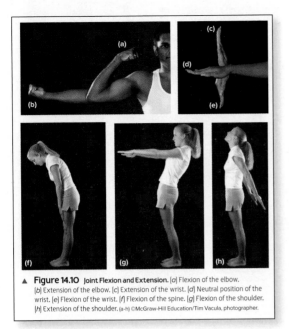

▲ **Figure 14.10** Joint Flexion and Extension. (*a*) Flexion of the elbow. (*b*) Extension of the elbow. (*c*) Extension of the wrist. (*d*) Neutral position of the wrist. (*e*) Flexion of the wrist. (*f*) Flexion of the spine. (*g*) Flexion of the shoulder. (*h*) Extension of the shoulder. (a-h) ©McGraw-Hill Education/Tim Vacula, photographer.

▲ **Figure 14.25** Hip Joint. (*a*) Right frontal view of a section of hip joint. (*b*) Ligaments of hip joint.

▲ **Figure 14.29** Total-Hip Replacement. Colored x-ray of prosthetic hip. ©AJPhoto/ Photo Researchers, Inc.

Exercises

A. Pick one of the photos above and explain how it helps you understand the material better. LO W.6

1. _____

_____

_____

B. Practice precision in medical terminology. *Choose any five terms in the illustration of the hip joint above. See the term, hear it, and write it down. Make sure you spell it correctly.* **LO W.6**

1. _____

2. _____

3. _____

4. _____

5. _____

LO W.6 Innovative Learning Aids (continued)

Tables
Meaningful tables aid in summarizing concepts and lesson topics.

▲ **Figure 14.7** Healing of Bone Fracture.

LO 14.4 Bone Fractures
A fracture is a break of a bone and can have a traumatic or pathological reason for occurring. The types of bone fractures are shown in *Figure 14.6* and described in *Table 14.1*.

Healing of Fractures
Uncomplicated fractures take 8 to 12 weeks to heal.

Step 1: When a bone is fractured, blood vessels bleed into the fracture site, forming a **hematoma** (*Figure 14.7a*).

Step 2: A few days after the fracture (Fx), osteoblasts move into the hematoma and start to produce new bone. This is called a **callus** (*Figure 14.7b*).

▲ **Figure 14.6** Bone Fractures.

Step 3: Osteoblasts produce immature, lacy, **cancellous** (spongy) bone that replaces the callus (*Figure 14.7c*).

Step 4: Osteoblasts continue to produce bone cells. They produce compact bone and fuse the bone segments together (*Figure 14.7d*).

Abbreviation	
Fx	fracture

Table 14.1 Classification of Bone Fractures

Name	Description	Reference
Closed	A bone is broken, but the skin is not broken.	Figure 14.6b, c, d, f, and g
Open	A fragment of the fractured bone breaks the skin, or a wound extends to the site of the fracture.	Figure 14.6e
Displaced	The fractured bone parts are out of alignment.	Figure 14.6e
Complete	A bone is broken into at least two fragments.	Figure 14.6a
Incomplete	The fracture does not extend completely across the bone; it can be **hairline** (as in a stress fracture in the foot when there is no separation of the two fragments).	Figure 14.6a
Comminuted	The bone breaks into several pieces, usually two major pieces and several smaller fragments.	Figure 14.6b
Transverse	The fracture is at a right angle to the long axis of the bone.	Figure 14.6b
Impacted	One bone fragment is driven into the other, with resulting shortening of a limb.	Figure 14.6c
Spiral	The fracture spirals around the long axis of the bone.	Figure 14.6d
Oblique	A diagonal fracture runs across the long axis of the bone.	Figure 14.6d
Linear	The fracture runs parallel to the long axis of the bone.	Figure 14.6f
Greenstick (closed)	This is a partial fracture: one side breaks, the other bends.	Figure 14.6g
Pathologic	The fracture occurs in an area of bone weakened by disease (such as cancer). Also called stress fracture.	—
Compression	The fracture occurs in a vertebra from trauma or pathology, leading to the vertebra being crushed.	—

Keynotes and Abbreviations
Keynote and Abbreviation boxes offer you additional information correlating with the lesson.

▲ **Figure 14.2** Femur: Long Bone of the Thigh.
(a) ©McGraw-Hill Education/Christine Eckel, photographer.

LO 14.2 Bone Growth and Structure

Bone Growth
Factors that affect bone growth include

1. **Genes.** Genes determine the size and shape of bones and the ultimate adult height.
2. **Nutrition.** Calcium and phosphorus are needed to develop good bone density.
3. **Exercise.** Exercise increases bone density and total bone mass.
4. **Mineral deposition.** Calcium and phosphate are taken from plasma and deposited in bone.
5. **Mineral resorption.** Calcium and phosphate are released from bone back into the plasma when they are needed elsewhere. For example, calcium is needed for muscle contraction, communication between neurons, and blood clotting. Phosphate is a component of deoxyribonucleic acid (DNA) and ribonucleic acid (RNA).
6. **Vitamins.** Vitamin A activates **osteoblasts**; vitamin C is essential for collagen synthesis; vitamin D stimulates absorption of calcium and phosphate, its transport, and its deposition into bones.
7. **Hormones.** For example, growth hormone stimulates the epiphyseal plate to calcify, and estrogen and testosterone accelerate bone growth after puberty and maintain bone density (*see Chapter 17*).

Structure of Bones
Long bones are the most common type of bone in the body (*Figure 14.2a*).

The shaft of a long bone is called the **diaphysis**. Each end of the bone is called the **epiphysis** and is expanded to provide extra surface area for the attachment of ligaments and tendons.

Sandwiched between the diaphysis and epiphysis is a thin area called the **metaphysis**. Thin layers of cartilage cells in the **epiphyseal plate** enable the diaphysis (bone shaft) to grow in length. When growth stops, compact bone grows into the epiphyseal plate and forms the **epiphyseal line** (*Figure 14.2b*).

A tough connective tissue sheath called **periosteum** covers the outer surface of all bones and is attached to the compact or **cortical** bone by tough collagen fibers. The periosteum protects the bone and anchors blood vessels and nerves to the surface of the bone.

The hollow cylinder inside the diaphysis is called the **medullary cavity**. It contains bone **marrow** and is lined by a thin membrane called the **endosteum**. The marrow is a fatty tissue that contains blood cells in different stages of development (*see Chapter 11*).

The endosteum and periosteum contain **osteoblasts**, cells that produce the matrix of new bone tissue. This process is called **osteogenesis**. Bone **matrix** consists of cells, collagen fibers, a gel that supports and suspends the fibers, and calcium phosphate crystals that give bone its hardness.

When osteoblasts are incorporated into the new bone, they become **osteocytes**. These cells, which maintain the matrix, reside in small spaces in the matrix called **lacunae**.

Osteoclasts are produced by the bone marrow. They dissolve calcium, phosphorus, and the organic components of the bone matrix. There is a continual balancing act going on as osteoclasts remove matrix and osteoblasts produce matrix. If osteoclasts outperform the osteoblasts, then **osteoporosis** occurs, as with Mrs. Vargas.

All bones are well supplied with blood (*Figure 14.3*). The blood vessels travel through the bone in a system of small **central (haversian) canals**. Because of its good blood supply, bone heals well.

▲ **Figure 14.3** Blood Supply to Bone.

Keynote
Minerals are deposited in bone when the supply is ample and released when they are needed elsewhere.

Case Report (CR) 14.2 (continued)
By age 65, more than 80% of people have some degree of joint degeneration. Mr. Johnson had always been very physically active, putting a lot of pressure on his weight-bearing joints. At different times in his life, he had been overweight, adding to the pressure.

X-rays of his lower back showed **osteoarthritis** of his lower lumbar intervertebral joints and marked osteoarthritis of his left hip joint (*Figure 14.12a and b*). He received a left total-hip replacement (**THR**) and physiotherapy (**PT**) for his lower back.

LO 14.7 Diseases of Joints
Osteoarthritis (OA) is caused by the breakdown and eventual destruction of cartilage in a joint. It develops as a result of wear and tear and is most common in the weight-bearing joints: the knee, hip, and lower back (*Figure 14.12a*). Because it is a wear-and-tear disease, it is sometimes called **degenerative joint disease (DJD)**. The degenerative process begins in the articular cartilage, which cracks and frays, eventually exposing the underlying bone.

Rheumatoid arthritis (RA) is a chronic, inflammatory disease that can affect many joints, causing deformity and disability. In *Figure 14.12b*, the hand deformities of RA—swelling of the **metacarpophalangeal (MCP)** and **proximal interphalangeal (PIP)** joints with **ulnar deviation** of the fingers—are shown. The disease process initially causes inflammation of the synovial membrane and then spreads to all other parts of the joint. Rheumatoid arthritis is three times as common in women and often begins in the thirties and forties.

Bursitis is inflammation of a **bursa** that can result from overuse of a joint, repeated trauma, or diseases such as RA.

Abbreviations	
DJD	degenerative joint disease
MCP	metacarpophalangeal
OA	osteoarthritis
PIP	proximal interphalangeal
PT	physiotherapy (physical therapy)
RA	rheumatoid arthritis
THR	total-hip replacement

▲ **Figure 14.12** Arthritis. (a) Magnetic resonance imaging (MRI) scan of lumbar vertebrae showing degenerative changes due to osteoarthritis. (b) Rheumatoid arthritis of the hands (a) ©Du Cane Medical Imaging Ltd./Photo Researchers, Inc. (b) ©VisualDx

©2014 Nucleus Medical Media

Chapter Learning Outcomes

The technical language of medicine has been developed logically from Latin and Greek roots because it is in Latin and Greek cultures that the concept of treating patients began. This medical language provides all the health professionals involved in the care of a patient with the ability to communicate with each other by using medical terms with precise meanings. To be a qualified health professional it is necessary to be able to speak the language of medicine.

Medical terms are built from individual parts, or elements, that form the anatomy of the word. The information in this chapter will enable you to:

LO 1.1 Recognize the logic of the language of medicine in individual medical terms.

LO 1.2 Identify the roots and combining forms of medical terms.

LO 1.3 Demonstrate the importance of suffixes and prefixes in forming medical terms.

LO 1.4 Identify medical terms taken directly from Greek, Latin, or Old English words.

LO 1.5 Differentiate between medical terms that are spelled and/or pronounced similarly.

 ## Case Report (CR) 1.1

You are

. . . a **respiratory therapist** working with Tavis Senko, MD, a **pulmonologist** at Fulwood Medical Center.

You are communicating with

. . . Mrs. Sandra Schwartz, a 43-year-old woman referred to Dr. Senko by her primary care physician, Dr. Andrew McDonald, an **internist**. Mrs. Schwartz has a persistent abnormality on her chest x-ray. You have been asked to determine her **pulmonary** function prior to a scheduled **bronchoscopy**.

This summary of a Case Report

. . . illustrates for you the use of some simple medical terms. Modern health care and medicine have their own language. The medical terms all have precise meanings, which enable you, as a health professional, to communicate clearly and accurately with other health professionals involved in the care of a patient. This communication is critical for patient safety and the delivery of high-quality patient care.

From her medical records, you can see that 2 months ago Mrs. Schwartz developed a right upper lobe (RUL) **pneumonia**. After treatment with an **antibiotic**, a follow-up chest x-ray (CXR) showed some residual collapse in the right upper lobe and a small right **pneumothorax**. Mrs. Schwartz has smoked a pack a day since she was a teenager. Dr. Senko is concerned that she has lung cancer and has scheduled her for a **bronchoscopy**.

The Construction of Medical Words

Lesson Objectives

Your confidence in using and understanding the medical terms in this book will increase as you become familiar with the logic of how these terms are constructed. The information in this lesson will enable you to:

1.1.1 Build and construct medical terms using their elements.

1.1.2 Select and identify the meaning of essential medical term roots.

1.1.3 Define the elements combining vowel and combining form.

1.1.4 Identify the combining vowel and combining form of essential medical terms.

1.1.5 Define the elements suffix and prefix.

1.1.6 Select and identify the meaning of the suffixes and prefixes of essential medical terms.

ROOTS:

- A root is the constant foundation and core of a medical term.
- Roots are usually of Greek or Latin origin.
- All medical terms have *one* or *more* roots.
- A root can appear anywhere in the term.
- More than one root can have the same meaning.
- A root plus a combining vowel creates a combining form.

LO 1.1 The Logic of Medical Terminology

Understanding and being comfortable with the technical language of medicine are keys to a successful career as a health professional. Your ability to use and understand the technical language to communicate verbally and in writing are essential for patient safety, high-quality patient care, precise interaction with other health professionals, and your own self-esteem as a health professional.

Your confidence in using medical terms will increase as you understand the logic of how each term is built from its individual parts, or elements. In addition, understanding the logic of this process will help you analyze or deconstruct an unknown medical term and break it down into its elements so that its meaning can be understood.

The **elements** of a medical term are its roots, suffixes, and prefixes, and the vast majority of these elements are derived from Latin and Greek origins. Throughout this book, when words are broken down, the elements will be color coded.

LO 1.2 Roots

Every medical term has a root—the element that provides the core meaning of the word. For example, in Case Report 1.1:

- The word *pneumonia* has the root *pneumon-*, taken from the Greek word meaning *lung* or *air*. The Greek root *pneum-* also means lung or air. *Pneumonia* is an infection of the lung tissue.
- Dr. Tavis Senko is a *pulmonologist*. The root *pulmon-* is taken from the Latin word meaning *lung*. A *pulmonologist* is a specialist who treats lung diseases.

LO 1.2 Combining Forms

Roots are often joined to other elements in a medical term by adding a combining vowel, such as the letter "o," to the end of the root, like *pneum-*, to form pneum/o-.

Throughout this book, whenever a term is presented, a slash (/) will be used to separate the combining vowel from the root. Other examples of this approach are as follows:

- Adding the combining vowel "o" to the Latin root *pulmon-* makes the combining form *pulmon/o-*.

Any vowel, "a," "e," "i," "o," or "u," can be used as a combining vowel.

- The root *respir-* means *to breathe*. Adding the combining vowel "a" makes the combining form *respir/a-*.

- The root *bronch-* is derived from the Greek word for *windpipe* and is one of the two subdivisions of the trachea that carry air to and from the lungs. Adding the combining vowel "o" to the root *bronch-* makes the combining form *bronch/o-*.

Many medical terms contain more than one root; when two roots occur together, they are always joined by a combining vowel, as in the following example:

- The word **hemopneumothorax** has the root *hem-*, from the Greek word meaning *blood*; the root *pneum-*, from the Greek word meaning *air* or *lung*; and the suffix *-thorax*, from the Greek word meaning *chest*. The combining vowel "o" is added to these two roots to make the combining forms *hem/o* and *pneum/o-*. A combining vowel is used to join a root (*pneum-*) to a suffix that begins with a consonant (*-thorax*). A **hemopneumothorax** is the presence of air and blood in the space that surrounds the lungs in the chest. As blood and air fill the pleural cavity, the lungs cannot expand and respiration is not possible, thus forcing the affected lung to collapse.

COMBINING FORMS:
- Combine a root and a combining vowel.
- Can be attached to another root or combining form.
- Can precede another word element called a suffix.
- Can follow a prefix.

Keynote

- Throughout this book, look for the following patterns:
  - Roots, combining forms, and combining vowels will be colored pink.
  - Prefixes will be colored green.
  - Suffixes will be colored blue.
- Different roots can have the same meaning. *Pulmon-* and *pneumon-* both mean *lung, air.*

Exercises

A. Review what you have just learned about roots and combining forms. *Select the correct answer to the statement.* **LO 1.1**

~~root~~   ~~combining form~~   ~~combining vowel~~   ~~suffix~~   ~~prefix~~

1. Roots and combining forms can go before a __SUFFIX__.

2. This element does not have a meaning; it serves to make the word easier to pronounce: __COMbining VOWEl__

3. A __prefix__ can go before a root.

4. The __COMbining form__ is the root plus a combining vowel.

B. Identify the word parts of a medical term. *Use the provided medical term to correctly answer the questions.* **LO 1.2**

1. In the word **pneumonia,** the root is:
   - **a.** *pneum-*   **b.** *pneumon-*   **c.** *-ia*   **d.** *-nia*

2. In the medical term **pulmonologist,** the root is:
   - **a.** *pulm-*   **b.** *pulmon-*   **c.** *-logist*   **d.** *-gist*

3. The combining vowel in the medical term **respiratory** is:
   - **a.** *-a-*   **b.** *-o-*   **c.** *-i-*   **d.** *-e-*

▲ **Figure 1.1** Dermatitis due to a latex glove.
©Dr. P. Marazzi/Photo Researchers, Inc.

 Case Report (CR) 1.2

You are

. . . a **genetic** nurse working with **geneticist** Ingrid Hughes, MD, PhD, in the Genetics Department at Fulwood Medical Center.

Your patient is

. . . Mrs. Geraldine Long, a 37-year-old administrative assistant who has been referred by primary care physician Susan Lee, MD. Mrs. Long has twin girls who are 12 years old. She is an award-winning ballroom dancer who does not smoke, drinks alcohol occasionally, and rehearses her dance routines four or five days each week. Her mother, aged 62, is being treated for ovarian cancer. Her mother's sister is being treated for breast cancer and has been found to carry a **gene mutation** associated with breast cancer. Mrs. Long's **mammogram** is normal. She has requested **genetic screening**.

LO 1.3 Suffixes

In the above Case Report 1.2 , the root genet-, meaning origin or gene, is teamed with the suffix -ic, which means *pertaining to,* to form the word genetic, *pertaining to a gene.* Again, the root genet- is teamed with the suffix -ics, which means *knowledge of,* to form the word **genetics**, *the knowledge of or the science of the inheritance of characteristics.* Also, the root genet- can be teamed with two suffixes, -ic, pertaining to, and -ist, *a specialist,* to form the word geneticist, *pertaining to a specialist in genetics.* There can be more than one suffix in a single word.

Using the combining form of cardi/o, in the medical specialty of cardiology, a cardiologist will often diagnose a cardiopathy. The suffix -logy, which means *study of;* the suffix -logist, which means *one who studies* or *a specialist;* and the suffix -pathy, which means *disease,* all give different meanings in the sentence "in the specialty of cardiology, a cardiologist will often diagnose a cardiopathy."

Another example of the use of suffixes is in the medical specialty of dermatology, when a dermatologist will often diagnose a case of dermatitis *(Table 1.1, Figure 1.1).*

Table 1.1 Use of Suffixes

Complete Word	Root or Combining Form	Suffix	Meaning of Suffix	Meaning of Word
dermatitis	dermat-	-itis	*inflammation*	*inflammation of the skin*
dermatologist	dermat/o-	-logist	*one who studies*	*one who studies the skin, specialist in dermatology*
dermatology	dermat/o-	-logy	*study of*	*study of the skin*

In *dermatitis,* the suffix -itis starts with a vowel, so there is no need for a combining vowel, and the suffix is attached directly to the root.

In a different example of the use of suffixes, an orthopedic surgeon operating on a joint can perform an arthroscopy, an arthrodesis, or an arthroplasty, all different operations with different outcomes, as shown in *Table 1.2.*

Table 1.2 Different Meanings of Suffixes

Complete Word	Combining Form	Suffix	Meaning of Suffix	Meaning of Word
arthroscopy	arthr/o-	-scopy	*visual examination*	*visual examination of a joint*
arthrodesis	arthr/o-	-desis	*fixation*	*fixation of a joint*
arthroplasty	arthr/o-	-plasty	*surgical repair*	*repair of a joint*

You always need a combining vowel before a suffix that begins with a consonant (e.g., dermatology, arthroplasty).

Classification of Suffixes

One strategy to help you understand medical terms is to divide suffixes into different types, such as diagnostic, surgical, pathologic, and descriptive or adjectival.

Diagnostic Suffixes

This group of suffixes, when added to a root or combining form, produces a medical term that is a diagnosis or a procedure or test to identify the nature of an illness.

The roots/combining forms hem/o and hemat/o both mean *blood*. Adding diagnostic suffixes can produce a variety of diagnostic medical terms throughout the body systems *(Table 1.3)*.

▲ **Figure 1.2** Hematoma (black eye) following a fall. ©Dr. P. Marazzi/Photo Researchers, Inc.

Table 1.3 Diagnostic Suffixes

Diagnostic Suffix	Meaning of Suffix	Word Example	Meaning of Word Example
-chezia	pass a stool	hemat/ochezia	passage of a bloody stool
-crit	to separate	hemat/ocrit	percentage of red blood cells in the blood
-gram	record	cardi/ogram	record derived from the heart
-graph	instrument for recording	cardi/ograph	instrument for recording the heart
-lysis	destruction	hem/olysis	destruction of red blood cells
-oma	tumor, mass	hematoma (Figure 1.2)	collection of blood in a tissue
-philia	attraction	hem/ophilia	an inherited blood disease
-ptysis	spit	hem/optysis	to cough up bloody sputum
-rrhage	to flow profusely	hem/orrhage	to bleed profusely
-rrhoid	to flow	hem/orrhoid	painful anal swelling of venous blood
-uria	urine	hematuria	blood in the urine

As you go through each body system in the book, there will be additional diagnostic suffixes you will learn in relation to the actual diagnoses made at that point in the book.

Surgical Suffixes

When added to a root or combining form, surgical suffixes produce medical terms that describe the invasive surgical procedure performed on the body *(Table 1.4)*.

Table 1.4 Surgical Suffixes

Surgical Suffix	Meaning of Suffix	Word Example	Meaning of Surgical Procedure
-centesis	surgical puncture	arthr/ocentesis	surgical puncture of a joint space with a needle
-desis	fixation	arthr/odesis	surgical fixation of the bones of a joint
-ectomy	surgical removal	appendectomy	surgical removal of the appendix
-plasty	surgical repair	rhin/oplasty	surgical repair of the nose
-rrhaphy	surgical suture	herni/orrhaphy	surgical suture of a hernia
-stomy	surgical formation of an opening	trache/ostomy	surgical formation of an artificial opening into the trachea into which a tube is inserted
-tomy	surgical incision	trache/otomy	surgical incision into the trachea
-tripsy	crushing	lith/otripsy	crushing of a stone (calculus), e.g., in the ureters

Pathologic Suffixes

When added to a **root** or **combining form**, this type of **suffix** produces a medical term that describes a symptom or sign of a disease process *(Table 1.5)*.

Table 1.5 Pathologic Suffixes

Pathologic Suffix	Meaning of Suffix	Word Example	Meaning of Pathologic Term
-algia	pain	arthralgia	pain in a joint(s)
-ectasis	dilation	bronchiectasis	chronic dilation of bronchi
-edema	accumulation of fluid in tissues	lymphedema	swelling in tissues as a result of obstruction of lymphatic vessels
-emesis	vomiting	hematemesis	vomiting of blood
-genesis	form, produce	oste/ogenesis	formation of new bone
-itis	inflammation	cystitis	inflammation of the urinary bladder
-oma	tumor, mass	hematoma	mass of blood leaked outside blood vessels into tissues
-osis	abnormal condition	cyanosis	dark blue coloration of blood due to lack of oxygen
-pathy	disease	neur/opathy	any disease of the nervous system
-penia	deficiency, lack of	erythr/openia	decrease in red blood cells
-phobia	fear of	agoraphobia	an unfounded fear of public places that arouses a state of panic
-stenosis	narrowing	arteri/ostenosis	abnormal narrowing of an artery

Adjectival Suffixes

As you learn new medical terms in each body system chapter in this book, you will see that there are 28 **suffixes** that mean *pertaining to.* These **suffixes** are used as adjectives to describe the **root**. Examples of adjectival **suffixes** are:

- **-ac cardiac** pertaining to the heart
- **-ary pulmonary** pertaining to the lungs
- **-ior posterior** pertaining to the back of the body

Those 28 **suffixes** are listed in the Keynote on this page.

Noun Suffixes

Several **suffixes** do not fall under any of the earlier classifications but maintain the **root** or **combining form** as a noun *(Table 1.6)*.

Table 1.6 Noun Suffixes

Noun Suffix	Meaning of Suffix	Word Example	Meaning of Word Example
-iatry	treatment, medical specialty	psychiatry	diagnosis and treatment of mental disorders
-ician	expert, specialist	pediatrician	medical specialist in children's development and disorders
-icle	small, minute	ossicle (Figure 1.3)	small bone, relating to the three small bones in the middle ear
-ist	expert, specialist	dentist	specialist in disorders of the orofacial complex
-istry	medical specialty	dentistry	specialty in disorders of the orofacial complex
-ole	small, minute	arteriole	small artery
-ule	small, minute	venule	small vein

Note that in *Table 1.6*, three **suffixes** mean "small," two **suffixes** mean "specialist," and two **suffixes** mean "medical specialty."

Ossicles

▲ **Figure 1.3** Ossicles of the middle ear. ©VEM/Photo Researchers, Inc.

Keynote

Adjectival **suffixes** meaning *pertaining to:*

-ac, -al, -ale, -alis, -ar, -aris, -ary, -atic, -ative, -eal, -ent, -etic, -ial, -ic, -ica, -ical, -ine, -ior, -iosum, -ious, -istic, -ius, -nic, -ous, -tic, -tiz, -tous, -us.

LO 1.3 Prefixes

Prefixes are added directly to the root or combining form and do not require combining vowels.

For example, you can add the different prefixes peri- and endo- to the same root, cardi-, to produce the different words pericardium and endocardium, which have very different meanings, as shown in *Table 1.7*.

Table 1.7 Use of Prefixes

Complete Word	Prefix	Meaning of Prefix	Meaning of Word
pericardium	peri-	around	structure around the heart
endocardium	endo-	inside	structure inside the heart

Note that -um is a suffix meaning *structure*.

Similarly, epigastric, hypogastric, and endogastric all have the same root, gastr-, but because of the different prefixes, epi-, hypo-, and endo-, have very different meanings, as shown in *Table 1.8*.

Table 1.8 Different Meanings of Prefixes

Complete Word	Prefix	Meaning of Prefix	Meaning of Word
epigastric	epi-	above	pertaining to above the stomach
hypogastric	hypo-	below	pertaining to below the stomach
endogastric	endo-	inside	pertaining to inside the stomach

Note that -ic is a suffix meaning *pertaining to*.

Exercises

A. Building onto the elements of roots, combining vowels, and combining forms are the prefixes and suffixes of medical terminology. *Prefixes and suffixes are additional word elements that give further meaning to a root or combining form. Develop your knowledge of more word elements with the following exercise. Choose T if the statement is true. Choose F if the statement is false.* **LO 1.1, 1.2, 1.3**

1. In a medical term, the suffix will always appear at the end. (T) F

2. Every medical term has to have a prefix. T (F)

3. In the terms arthroscopy and arthrodesis, the combining form is the same, but the suffix is different. T (F)

4. If a suffix begins with a consonant, you will need a combining vowel before it. (T) F

B. Identify the meaning of the word by the suffix. *The medical terms below are commonly used by people who are not necessarily in the medical field. Using what you may already know, identify the meaning of the suffix of medical terms. Match the definition on the left with the correct term it is describing on the right.* **LO 1.3**

1. _____ a specialist   a. agoraphobia

2. _____ afraid of   b. pneumonectomy

3. _____ study of   c. dentist

4. _____ removal of   d. dermatitis

5. _____ inflammation of   e. biology

Your learning goal is to understand the logic of medical language.

LO 1.3 Prefixes (continued)

Classification of Prefixes

Many **prefixes** can be classified into **prefixes** of position, **prefixes** of number or measurement, and **prefixes** of direction (*Tables 1.9, 1.10, 1.11*).

Table 1.9 Prefixes of Position

Position Prefix	Meaning of Prefix	Word Example	Meaning of Medical Term
ante-	before, forward	antevert	to tilt forward, as a uterus can
anti-	against	antibiotic	an agent that can destroy bacteria and other microorganisms
circum-	around	circumcision	to cut around the penis to remove the foreskin
endo-	inside, inner	endocrine	a gland that secretes directly into the blood
epi-	above, over, upon	epidermis	the top layer of the skin
exo-	outside, outward	exocrine	a gland that excretes outwardly through ducts
hyper-	above, excessive	hypertrophy	increase in size
hypo-	below	hypodermis	tissue layer below the top layer of the skin
inter-	between	intercostal	the space between two ribs
intra-	inside, within	intradermal (Figure 1.4)	within the skin
para-	adjacent, alongside	paranoid	having delusions of persecution
peri-	around	perinatal	around the time of birth
post-	after	postnatal	after the time of birth
pre-	before	prenatal	before the time of birth
retro-	backward	retrovert	to tilt backward, as a uterus can
supra-	above, excessive	suprapubic	above the pubic bone
trans-	across, through	transdermal	going across or through the skin
ultra-	higher, beyond	ultrasound (Figure 1.5)	very high-frequency sound waves

Table 1.10 Prefixes of Number and Measurement

Measurement Prefix	Meaning of Prefix	Word Example	Meaning of Medical Term
bi-	two, twice, double	bilateral	pertaining to or related to two sides of the body
brady-	slow	bradycardia	slow heart rate
di-	two	diplegia	paralysis of corresponding parts on both sides of the body
eu-	normal	eupnea	normal breathing
hemi-	half	hemiparesis	weakness of one side (half) of the body
macro-	large	macrocyte	large red blood cell
micro-	small	microcyte	small red blood cell
mono-	single, one	monocyte	white blood cell with a single nucleus
multi-	many	multipara	woman who has given birth at least twice
pan-	all	pancytopenia	deficiency of all types of blood cells
poly-	excessive	polyuria	excessive production of urine
primi-	first	primipara	woman who has given birth for the first time
quadri-	four	quadriplegia	paralysis of all four limbs
tachy-	rapid	tachycardia	rapid heart rate
tri-	three	tricuspid	having three points—a tricuspid heart valve has three flaps
uni-	single, one	unipolar	pertaining to one pole; neuron having a single process

▲ **Figure 1.4** **Intradermal injection.** ©Andrew Aitchison/Contributor/Getty Images

▲ **Figure 1.5** **Obstetric ultrasonography of a 22-year-old woman.** The 12-week-old fetus is *in brown*. The placenta is *in green*. ©Warrick G./Photo Researchers, Inc.

Table 1.11 Prefixes of Direction and Location

Directional Prefix	Meaning of Prefix	Medical Term Example	Meaning of Medical Term
ab-	away from	abduction	action of moving away from the midline
ad-	toward	adduction	action of moving toward the midline
ante-	coming before, in front of	antevert	to tilt forward
post-	coming after, behind	postnatal	occurring after birth
sub-	under, beneath	subdural	in the space under the dura mater
syn-	coming together	synapse	junction between two nerve cells

Exercises

A. Review the prefixes and terms in Table 1.9. *Select the correct answer to complete each statement.* **LO 1.3**

1. The location of the tumor was *above the pubic bone.* The tumor is located _____.
   - **a.** hypogastric
   - **b.** transdermal
   - **c.** suprapubic
   - **d.** ultrasonic

2. The *transdermal* route of drug administration goes:
   - **a.** through the skin.
   - **b.** in an IV.
   - **c.** through the mouth.
   - **d.** in the rectum.

3. *Postpartum* occurs
   - **a.** before delivery.
   - **b.** during delivery.
   - **c.** after delivery.

4. *Retroverted* means
   - **a.** tilted sideways.
   - **b.** tilted forward.
   - **c.** tilted backward.

B. Answer the following questions regarding the proper use of prefixes. *Choose T if the statement is True. Choose F if the statement is False.* **LO 1.3**

1. They usually appear in the beginning of a term.	T	F
2. They can attach to a root or combining form.	T	F
3. Every term must have a prefix.	T	F
4. Some terms can have more than one prefix.	T	F
5. A prefix can designate number or location.	T	F

Lesson 1.2

Unique Medical Words

 Case Report (CR) 1.3

You are

. . . a **medical** assistant working for Russell Gordon, MD, a primary **care** physician at Fulwood Medical Center.

Your patient is

. . . Mr. William Doyle, a 72-year-old retired long-distance truck driver and a lifetime pack-a-day smoker. He is complaining of shortness of **breath**, increased **cough**, and production of sticky yellow **mucus**. In his medical **record**, you see that he has had stones in both ureters and is frequently a **patient** in the urology department, and that he has had both **knees** replaced. You begin to examine him.

LO 1.4 Greek, Latin, and Old English Words

Case Report 1.3 features several medical terms taken directly from Latin or Greek words or from Old English terms that do not break down (deconstruct) into word elements. Several of them are also used in general language outside of medicine. These medical terms in Case Report 1.3 are:

- **medical**, from a Latin term meaning *to heal;* it means *pertaining to the practice of medicine.*
- **care**, an Old English word meaning *to worry;* when you care for your patients, you look after them and are concerned about them.
- **breath**, an Old English word meaning *a single cycle of inhaling and exhaling.*
- **cough**, an Old English word meaning *to expel breath from the lungs.*
- **mucus**, a Latin word for *a clear, sticky secretion.*
- **record**, a Latin word meaning *to remember;* a medical *record* is a written account of a patient's medical history.
- **patient**, an Old English term meaning *to suffer* or *undergo;* the term refers to a person who is under medical or surgical treatment.
- **knee**, an Old English word meaning *an angular shape;* today it refers to the **joint** (a Latin word for junction) between the upper and lower leg.

Other examples not used in Case Report 1.3 include:

- **apex**, a Latin word meaning *tip* or *summit* (as in Mount Everest); the apex of the heart is the downward-pointing tip of the cone-shaped heart.
- **patent**, a Latin word meaning *open* or *exposed;* a *patent* blood vessel is open to the circulation of freely flowing blood. (Note the difference in the word **patient**).
- **quadrant**, a Latin word meaning *a quarter;* the abdomen is divided into four *quadrants* by horizontal and vertical planes that intersect at the umbilicus.
- **umbilicus**, which is a Latin word for the *navel or belly button.*
- **toxin**, a Greek word meaning *poison;* a *toxin* is a poisonous substance formed by a cell, such as a bacterium.
- **lymph**, a Latin word meaning *clear spring water; lymph* is a clear, shimmering fluid collected from the body tissues.
- **breech**, an Old English word meaning *buttocks;* in obstetrics, a fetus is in a *breech* presentation when the buttocks, rather than the head, are the presenting part at delivery.
- **specialist**, a Latin word meaning *of a given species;* a *specialist* devotes professional attention to a particular subject area.

LO 1.5 Terms That Are Alike

Precision in both written and verbal communication is essential for a health professional, with great attention given to detail. There are many words in the medical language that are very similar to each other in both their spelling and pronunciation. Examples are

- **ilium**, pronounced **ill-ee-um**, a bone in the pelvis
- **ileum**, pronounced the same way, **ill-ee-um**, a segment of the small intestine
- **ureter**, the tube from the kidney to the bladder
- **urethra**, the tube from the bladder to the outside
- **trapezius**, a muscle in the back
- **trapezium**, a bone in the wrist
- **malleus**, a small bone in the middle ear
- **malleolus**, a bony protuberance at the ankle
- **neurology**, the study of diseases of the nervous system
- **urology**, the study of diseases of the kidney and bladder

Exercises

A. The following medical terms are all of Greek or Latin origin. *Match the definition on the left with the correct term it is describing on the right.* **LO 1.4**

_____ **1.** tip or summit   **a.** patent

_____ **2.** buttocks   **b.** mucus

_____ **3.** poison   **c.** apex

_____ **4.** clear, sticky secretion   **d.** breech

_____ **5.** open   **e.** toxin

B. Choose the correct spelling of medical terms taken directly from Greek, Latin, or Old English words. **LO 1.4**

1. A tube from the bladder to the outside.

    a. ureethra   **b.** urethra   **c.** ureter   **d.** ureetere

2. The study of the diseases of the nervous system.

    a. urology   **b.** ureology   **c.** neurlogy   **d.** neurology

3. A muscle in the back.

    a. ilium   **b.** ileum   **c.** trapezius   **d.** trapezium

4. A small bone in the middle ear.

    a. ileum   **b.** ilium   **c.** malleolus   **d.** malleus

The Anatomy of Medical Terms

Challenge Your Knowledge

A. Identify the statements below as either true or false. Choose T if the statement is true. Choose F if the statement is false. **(LO 1.1)**

1. A term never has more than one root.   T   F

2. Some terms will have no combining vowel.   T   F

3. A combining vowel changes the meaning of the word.   T   F

4. A vowel must always be present in a combining form.   T   F

B. The root/combining form is the core meaning of the word. Choose the correct definition for the root/combining form for each term. **(LO 1.2)**

1. The term *hypogastric* relates to under or below the

   a. chest.

   b. skin.

   c. stomach.

   d. lungs.

2. The term *neuralgia* means pain in a

   a. nerve.

   b. joint.

   c. heart.

   d. cell.

3. The term *subdermal* means pertaining to below the

   a. chest.

   b. skin.

   c. stomach.

   d. lungs.

4. The term *cardiac* means pertaining to the

   a. lungs.

   b. joints.

   c. kidneys.

   d. heart.

5. The term *arthritis* means inflammation of the

   a. lungs.

   b. joints.

   c. kidneys.

   d. heart.

6. The term *erythrocyte* means cell that is

   a. large.

   b. round.

   c. red.

   d. swollen.

7. The term *bronchitis* means inflammation of a

   a. kidney.

   b. eye.

   c. bronchus.

   d. joint.

8. The term *hematology* means the study of

   a. blood.

   b. skin.

   c. the heart.

   d. the mind.

C. Match the Greek/Latin elements in the first column with their meanings in the second column. (LO 1.2, 1.4)

_____ 1. pneum

_____ 2. hemat

_____ 3. lymph

_____ 4. thorax

_____ 5. arthr

_____ 6. respir

_____ 7. mucus

_____ 8. patent

_____ 9. toxin

_____ 10. apex

_____ 11. dermat

_____ 12. breech

a. to breathe

b. open

c. clear, sticky secretion

d. tip or summit

e. buttocks

f. chest

g. skin

h. joint

i. blood

j. air, lung

k. clear spring water

l. poison

D. Spelling is most important in medical terminology. For example, **ilium** and **ileum** may be similar in appearance and sound, but the difference of one letter makes each a different body part. Select the correct spelling for the following terms. **(LO 1.4, 1.5)**

1. The _____ of the small intestine was infected.

   a. ileum   **b.** ilium   **c.** illium

2. The _____ system keeps you breathing.

   a. respieratory   **b.** respiratory   **c.** resspiratory

3. Inflammation of the heart is _____.

   a. carditus   **b.** carditis   **c.** cardiitis

4. A muscle in the back is the _____.

   a. trapeze   **b.** trapezium   **c.** trapezius

5. A bony protuberance in your ankle is the _____.

   a. maleus   **b.** malius   **c.** malleolus

The Anatomy of Medical Terms

E. Use your newly acquired knowledge of medical language to correctly answer the following questions. Let the roots and combining forms be your guide. Choose the correct answer to complete each statement. **(LO 1.1, 1.2)**

1. This term means one who studies the skin.

   a. dermatologist

   b. urologist

   c. neurologist

2. This term relates to the intestines and the stomach.

   a. gastroenterology

   b. cardiology

   c. dermatology

3. This term relates to the process of breathing.

   a. apex

   b. toxic

   c. respiratory

4. This term relates to the stomach.

   a. gastritis

   b. gynecology

   c. dermatitis

5. This term relates to a joint.

   a. urethritis

   b. arthritis

   c. neuralgia

F. Use the correct medical term to complete the sentence. Use the words to complete each sentence below. Fill in the blanks. **(LO 1.1, 1.4)**

| bladder | breech | cardiologist | ileum | ilium | kidney | lymph | malleolus | trapezium | ureter | urethra |

1. A _____ is a specialist in the care of the heart.

2. The _____ is a tube from the kidney to the bladder.

3. Urology is the study of diseases of the _____ and _____.

4. A segment of the small intestine is the _____.

5. _____ means the buttocks, not the head, present first at delivery.

6. _____ is the tube from the bladder to the outside.

7. _____ is a fluid collected from body tissues.

8. A bone in the wrist is the _____.

9. The bony protuberance at the ankle is the _____.

10. The _____ is a bone in the pelvis.

G. Case report questions. Read Case Report 1.4. You should feel more comfortable with the medical terminology now and will be able to answer the questions that follow. **(LO 1.4)**

Case Report (CR) 1.4

You are

. . . a medical assistant employed by Russell Gordon, MD, a primary care physician at Fulwood Medical Center.

Study Hint
Many elements have more than one meaning. You must know the different meanings because that will make a difference in the use of the medical term.

Your patient is

. . . Mrs. Connie Bishop, a 55-year-old woman who presents with a swelling in her lower abdomen and shortness of breath. She has no gynecologic or gastroenterologic symptoms. Her previous medical history shows recurrent dermatitis of her hands since a teenager and an arthroscopy for a knee injury at age 40. Physical examination reveals a circular mass 6 inches in diameter in the left lower quadrant of her abdomen. There is no abnormality in her respiratory or cardiovascular system.

Your role is to maintain her medical record and document her care, assist Dr. Gordon during his examinations, explain the examination and treatment procedures to Mrs. Bishop, and facilitate her referral for specialist care.

1. What type of skin problem has Mrs. Bishop had since she was a teenager? _____

2. Which term in the case study means *pertaining to the stomach and small intestines*? _____

3. Her knee injury required what type of procedure? _____

4. Does she have any issues with her lungs or heart? (yes or no) _____

5. Do her symptoms indicate a possible problem with her ileum? (yes or no) _____

H. Because much of clinical documentation centers on surgeries, knowledge of surgical suffixes is most important—especially for coders. (LO 1.2)

Matching
Match the definition in the first column with the correct term it is describing in the second column.

Term	Meaning
_____ 1. scopy	A. surgical repair
_____ 2. desis	B. visual examination
_____ 3. plasty	C. surgical fixation

Combine these suffixes with the combining form arthr/o and fill in the blanks with the correct medical term.

4. The surgeon wants a closer look inside Mr. Parker's knee so he is scheduled for an _____ tomorrow morning.

5. Mary Collins has torn her knee ligaments playing high school basketball. Her treatment plan includes scheduling an _____ to reattach them. (fixation)

6. June Larkin had a bad skiing accident while on vacation. Her tendons and ligaments in her knee will require extensive surgery to get her walking again without crutches. She needs an _____. (repair)

Congratulations! You are on your way to learning medical terminology.

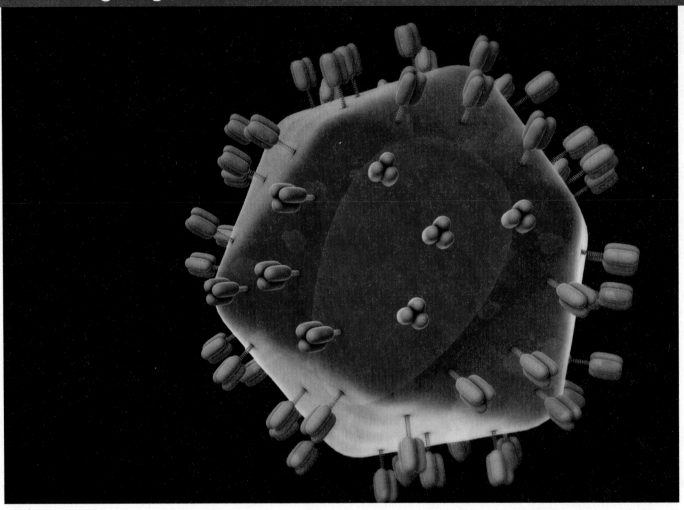

©2014 Nucleus Medical Media

Chapter Learning Outcomes

LO 2.1 Deconstruct a medical term into its basic elements.

LO 2.2 Use word elements to identify or construct a medical term.

LO 2.3 Connect the singular and plural components of medical terms.

LO 2.4 Employ the phonetic system used to pronounce medical terms.

LO 2.5 Use Word Analysis and Definition boxes to describe the phonetic pronunciation, word elements, and definition of terms used in the book.

LO 2.6 Communicate with precision in both written and verbal communication in all health care fields.

 ## Case Report (CR) 2.1

You are

. . . an emergency medical technician **(EMT)** employed in the Emergency Department at Fulwood Medical Center.

Your patient is

. . . Barbara Rotelli, a 17-year-old woman, who presents with **pyrexia** and shaking chills. On her medical record, you read that her physical examination reveals splinter **hemorrhages** under her fingernails and a heart **murmur**. There is blood in her urine. She had **dental** surgery four days ago. A provisional **diagnosis** is made of acute **endocarditis**. You are to prepare her for admission to intensive care.

Lesson 2.1

Word Analysis and Definition

Lesson Objectives

When you see a medical term you do not understand, the first step you can take to analyze, decipher, or deconstruct the term is to break it down into its component elements, or parts. In this lesson, you will learn to:

2.1.1 Deconstruct a medical term into its word elements.

2.1.2 Use the word elements to identify the medical term.

Abbreviation

EMT	emergency medical technician

LO 2.1, 2.2, 2.5 Word Analysis and Definition

For words you need to define, first identify the suffix.

For example, in the term **endocarditis**, the suffix at the end of the word is -itis, which means *inflammation*.

That leaves **endocard-**. You have learned that -card- is a root meaning *heart*. So now you have *inflammation of the heart*.

Card — itis = **inflammation of the heart**

That leaves endo-, a prefix meaning *inside*. So now you can assemble the pieces together to form the word meaning *inflammation of the inside of the heart*:

You also have learned that the suffix -um means *a structure*. So changing the suffix to **endocardium** would be the structure that lines the inside of the heart.

Therefore, you can understand that **endocarditis** is used to mean that the endocardium lining the heart has become inflamed or infected. Both -card- and -cardi- are roots meaning *heart*.

Another example is the word **hemorrhage**, used in CR 2.1 in the opening spread of this chapter. The suffix -rrhage following the combining vowel "o" is borrowed from the Greek word meaning *to flow profusely*. The combining form hem/o- is from the Greek word for *blood*. The elements of the medical term **hemorrhage** are assembled together and used to mean *profuse bleeding*.

In this book, when the medical terms are broken down into their elements, a hyphen is used to isolate each major element and to identify its position in the whole word.

When a combining form is used, the combining vowel is separated from the root by a slash (/).

One of the key design concepts of this book is that all the textual and visual information you need for any given topic will be on the two-page spread open in front of you. As part of this, in the top right-hand quarter of the two-page spread will be a box designed to give you the elements, definition, and pronunciation (covered in Lesson 2.2) of every new medical term that appears in the two pages you are reviewing. For example, the box will look like the box at the top of the next page, which refers to the medical terms used on these two pages and to the boldfaced terms in the Case Report at the beginning of the chapter. This box is a Word Analysis and Definition box, called a WAD for short.

S = Suffix   P = Prefix   R = Root   R/CF = Combining Form

WORD	PRONUNCIATION	ELEMENTS		DEFINITION
dental	**DEN**-tal	S/ R/	-al *pertaining to* **dent-** *tooth*	Pertaining to the teeth
diagnosis (noun) diagnoses (pl) diagnostic (adj) (**Note:** The "is" in gnosis is deleted to allow the word to flow.)	die-ag-**NO**-sis die-ag-**NO**-seez die-ag-**NOS**-tik	P/ R/ S/	**dia-** *complete* **-gnosis** *knowledge of an abnormal condition* -tic *pertaining to*	The determination of the nature of a disease, injury or congenital defect Pertaining to or a diagnosis
diagnose (verb)	die-ag-**NOSE**	R/	**-gnose** *recognize an abnormal condition*	To make a diagnosis
endocarditis	**EN**-doh-kar-**DIE**-tis	S/ P/ R/	-itis *inflammation* **endo-** *within, inner* **-card-** *heart*	Inflammation of the lining of the heart
endocardium	**EN**-doh-**KAR**-dee-um	S/ P/ R/	-um *structure* **endo-** *within, inner* **-cardi-** *heart*	The inside lining of the heart
hemorrhage	**HEM**-oh-raj	S/ R/CF	-rrhage *to flow profusely* **hem/o-** *blood*	To bleed profusely
murmur	**MUR**-mur		Latin *murmur*	Abnormal sound heard on auscultation of the heart or blood vessels
pyrexia	pie-**REK**-see-ah	S/ R/	-ia *condition* **pyrex-** *fever, heat*	An abnormally high body temperature or fever

Many of the exercises at the end of each spread are based on information found in the Word Analysis and Definition box (WAD) or in the reading.

Exercises

A. To analyze a medical term, simply break the elements down (deconstruct them) into their basic forms. *To construct a new term, take the appropriate elements, put them in the correct position in the term, and build your term.* **Note:** *Remember that not every term will have all elements present at the same time.* **LO 2.1, LO 2.2**

1. **To deconstruct:** Take the medical term **endocarditis** and break it down into elements.

   The prefix _____ means _____.

   The root _____ means _____.

   The suffix _____ means _____.

2. **To construct:** Take the following elements and construct a new term with them.

   The element *"um"* means _____. What type of word element is this? _____

   The element *"endo"* means _____. What type of word element is this? _____

   The element *"cardi"* means _____. What type of word element is this? _____

Lesson 2.2

Plurals and Pronunciation

Lesson Objectives

In your career as a health professional, the correct, precise pronunciation of medical terms is an essential part of your daily life and of your self-esteem. It is also critical for patient safety and high-quality patient care. The information in this lesson will enable you to:

2.2.1 Connect the singular and plural components of medical terms.

2.2.2 Employ the system for describing pronunciation used in the textbook.

2.2.3 Verbalize the pronunciation of common medical terms.

LO 2.3 Plurals

When you change a medical term from singular to plural, it is not as simple as adding an s, as you often can in the English language. Unfortunately, in medical terms, the end of the word changes in ways that were logical in Latin and Greek but have to be learned by memory in English. This is shown in *Table 2.1*.

Table 2.1 Singular and Plural Forms

Singular Ending	Plural Ending	Examples	Singular Ending	Plural Ending	Examples
-a		axilla	-on		ganglion
	-ae	axillae		-a	ganglia
-ax		thorax	-um		septum
	-aces	thoraces		-a	septa
-en		lumen	-us**		viscus
	-ina	lumina		-era	viscera
-ex		cortex	-us**		villus
	-ices	cortices		-i	villi
-is*		diagnosis	-us**		corpus
	-es	diagnoses		-ora	corpora
-is*		epididymis	-x		phalanx
	-ides	epididymides		-ges	phalanges
-ix		appendix	-y		ovary
	-ices	appendices		-ies	ovaries
-ma		carcinoma	-yx		calyx
	-mata	carcinomata		-ices	calices

* **Note:** *both singular terms can end in -is. You have to know on a case-by-case basis which singular terms change to -es and which ones change to -ides.*
***The same applies to the singular terms ending in -us—some will form plurals with -era, -i, or -ora.*

LO 2.4 Pronunciation

In your role as a health professional, pronouncing medical terms correctly and precisely is not only about understanding conversations with your peers or a physician. It is also a matter of ensuring patient safety and providing high-quality patient care.

Correct pronunciation is essential so that other health professionals with whom you are working can understand what you are saying. Throughout this textbook, the pronunciation of each medical term will be written out phonetically using modern English forms. The part(s) of the word to which you give the strongest, or primary, emphasis is (are) written in bold, uppercase letters.

For example, the term **gastroenterology** will be phonetically written **GAS**-troh-en-ter-**OL**-oh-gee, whereas the term **gastritis**, which means *inflammation of the stomach*, will be phonetically written as gas-**TRY**-tis. **Hemorrhage** will be written as **HEM**-oh-raj, whereas the term **hemostasis**, which means *the stopping of bleeding*, will be written he-moh-**STAY**-sis.

The only way you can learn how to pronounce medical terms is to say them repeatedly and have your pronunciation checked against a standard, which is found in McGraw-Hill Connect.

Exercises

A. Forming plurals of medical terms will be less difficult if you follow the rules and apply them correctly. *The rules are given to you in the following chart—practice changing the medical terms from singular to plural. Fill in the chart.* **LO 2.3**

Singular	Plural	Singular Term	Plural Term
-a	-ae	axilla	1.
-um	-a	septum	2.
-ax	-aces	thorax	3.
-en	-ina	lumen	4.
-ex	-ices	cortex	5.
-is	-es	diagnosis	6.
-on	-a	ganglion	7.
-us	-i	villus	8.
-ix	-ices	appendix	9.
-x	-ges	phalanx	10.

Lesson 2.3
WORD ANALYSIS AND COMMUNICATION

Precision in Communication

This year in the United States, more than 400,000 people will die because of drug reactions and medical errors. Many of these deaths are due to inaccurate or imprecise written or verbal communications between the different members of the health care team. You can avoid making errors in your own communications, and this lesson will help you do that by enabling you to:

2.3.1 Communicate with precision both verbally and in writing.

2.3.2 Use word analysis to ensure the precise use of words.

Keynote

- Communicate verbally and in writing with attention to detail, accuracy, and precision.

- When you understand the individual word elements that make up a medical term, you are better able to understand clearly the medical terms you are using.

Abbreviation

stat   immediately, at once

 Case Report (CR) 2.2

You are
. . . a radiology technician working in the Radiology Department of Fulwood Medical Center.

Your patient is
. . . Mrs. Matilda Morones, a 38-year-old woman who presents with sudden onset of severe, **colicky** right-flank pain and pain in her **urethra** as she passes urine.

The physical examination revealed that Mrs. Morones is in severe distress, with marked tenderness in the right **costovertebral** angle and in the right lower quadrant of her **abdomen**. **Microscopy** of her urine showed numerous red blood cells. The **stat abdominal** x-ray you have taken reveals a **radiopaque** stone in the right **ureter**. She has now become faint and is in **hypotension**.

How are you going to communicate Mrs. Morones' condition as you ask for help and then document her condition and your response?

LO 2.6 Precision in Communication

In Case Report 2.2, if **hypotension** (low blood pressure) is confused with **hypertension** (high blood pressure), incorrect treatments could be prescribed. Confusing Mrs. Morones' **ureter** (the tube from the kidney to the bladder) with her **urethra** (the tube from the bladder to the outside) could lead to disastrous consequences.

Being a health professional requires the utmost attention to detail and precision, both in written documentation and in verbal communication. A patient's life could be in your hands. In addition, the medical record in which you document a patient's care and your actions is a legal document. It can be used in court as evidence in professional medical liability cases. Any incorrect spelling can reflect badly on the whole health care team.

LO 2.5 Use of Word Analysis

In Case Report 2.2, **ureter** (you-RET-er) and **urethra** (you-REE-thra) are both simple words with no prefix, combining vowel, or suffix. They are derived from the Greek word for *urine*. They are similar words but have very different anatomic locations (*Chapter 6*).

To deconstruct the word **hypotension** (HIGH-poh-TEN-shun), start with the suffix -ion, which means *a condition*. Next, the prefix hypo- means *below* or *less than normal*. The root -tens- is from the Latin word for *pressure*. Place the pieces together to form a word meaning *condition of below-normal pressure*, or low blood pressure.

To deconstruct the term **costovertebral** (koss-toh-ver-TEE-bral), start with the suffix -al, which means *pertaining to*. Separated by the combining vowel "o" are two roots, cost- and -vertebr-. The combining form cost/o- is from the Latin word for *a rib*. -Vertebr- is from the Latin word for *backbone or spine*. So you have *pertaining to the rib and the spine*.

The **costovertebral angle** is the angle pertaining to or between the 12th rib and the spine. This angle is a surface anatomy marking for the kidney.

WORD	PRONUNCIATION		ELEMENTS	DEFINITION
abdomen	**AB**-doh-men		Latin *abdomen*	The part of the trunk that lies between the thorax and the pelvis
abdominal	ab-**DOM**-in-al	S/ R/	-al *pertaining to* **abdomin-** *abdomen*	Pertaining to the abdomen
colic	**KOL**-ik	S/ R/	-ic *pertaining to* **col-** *colon*	Pertaining to the colon or spasmodic pain in the abdomen.
colicky	**KOL**-icky	S/	-icky *arising from*	Pain in the colon
costovertebral	kos-toe-**VER**-teh-bral	S/ R/CF R/	-al *pertaining to* **cost/o-** *rib* **-vertebr-** *spine*	Pertaining to the rib and spine
hypertension	**HIGH**-per-**TEN**-shun	S/ P/ R/	-ion *action, condition* **hyper-** *excessive* **-tens-** *pressure*	Persistent high arterial blood pressure
hypotension	**HIGH**-poh-**TEN**-shun	P/	**hypo-** *low, below*	Persistent low arterial blood pressure
radiopaque	ray-dee-oh-**PAKE**	S/ R/CF	-paque *shady* **radi/o-** *radiation*	Impenetrable by x-rays or other forms of radiation
ureter (**Note:** Two "e"s = two tubes.)	you-**RET**-er		Greek *urinary canal*	Tube that connects the kidney to the urinary bladder
urethra	you-**REE**-thra		Greek *urethra*	Canal leading from the urinary bladder to the outside

Exercises

A. Precision in communication. *Verbal and written communication must always be precise and accurate for patient safety and legal requirements. Develop your eyes' and ears' ability to distinguish correct pronunciations, word choice, and spelling to ensure documentation and communication accuracy. Fill in the following blanks:* **LO 2.6**

1. If the doctor tells you a patient's blood pressure readings are elevated, does the patient have **hypertension** or **hypotension**?

    _____

2. Would you describe pain in the colon as **colic** or **colicky**?

    _____

3. Does urine travel from a kidney to the bladder through a **ureter** or **urethra**?

    _____

4. Does a patient with a kidney infection need to see a **urologist** or a **neurologist**?

    _____

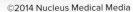

Chapter 2 Review

©2014 Nucleus Medical Media

Word Analysis and Communication

Challenge Your Knowledge

A. **The answer to this question can be retrieved from the WAD in Lesson 2.2.** Select the correct answer to the statement. **(LO 2.3, 2.6)**

    1. *Costovertebral* pertains to the

        a. rib and colon.

        b. heart and rib cage.

        c. rib and spine.

        d. lung and rib.

        e. rib and kidney.

B. **Recall your pronunciation.** Select the correct answer that completes each statement. **(LO 2.4, 2.5)**

    1. What is the correct pronunciation of *pyrexia*?

        a. pie-RECK-si-a

        b. PIE-RECK-ci-a

        c. PY-rek-sia

        d. pie-REK-see-ah

        e. py-rek-SEE-ah

    2. What is the correct pronunciation of *costovertebral*?

        a. KOSTO-ver-TREE-bral

        b. cost-o-VER-tre-bal

        c. kos-toe-VER-teh-bral

        d. COSTO-ver-tree-bral

        e. kosto-ver-tree-BAL

    3. What is the correct pronunciation of *radiopaque*?

        a. ray-dee-oh-PAKE

        b. ra-di-o-PAKE

        c. RADIOH-plaque

        d. radio-PAKE

        e. ray-DI-o-pake

C. **To help you master plurals, practice changing singular endings to plural and plural endings to singular in the following exercise.** If you are given a singular word, change it to plural. If you are given a plural word, change it to singular. <u>The first one is done for you.</u> **(LO 2.3)**

Word	Singular	Plural
1. carcinomata	carcinoma	_____
2. ovaries	_____	_____
3. ganglia	_____	_____
4. lumen	_____	_____
5. villi	_____	_____
6. cortices	_____	_____
7. calyx	_____	_____
8. epididymis	_____	_____
9. axilla	_____	_____
10. viscus	_____	_____
11. appendices	_____	_____
12. corpora	_____	_____
13. diagnoses	_____	_____
14. thoraces	_____	_____

D. **Precision in documentation means using the correct form of the term, as well as the correct term.** Medical terms can take the forms of noun (thing), verb (action), or adjective (description). Fill in the blank with the correct term. **(LO 2.6)**

diagnosis   diagnose   diagnostic   diagnoses

1. After performing several _____ tests, the physician has confirmed his _____.

2. In addition to her diabetes, the patient has several other _____.

3. The physician was unable to _____ the patient's condition because the patient refused the prescribed tests.

Word Analysis and Communication

E. **Use the appropriate medical language to answer the questions.** Select the correct answer that completes each statement or answers each question. **(LO 2.1, 2.2)**

1. Which one of the following terms is an x-ray technician likely to use?

   a. hypertension

   b. radiopaque

   c. hypotension

   d. pyrexia

   e. hemorrhage

2. Which one of the following terms would describe the condition of a person with an increased body temperature?

   a. pyrexia

   b. fainting

   c. hemorrhage

   d. murmur

   e. endocardium

3. Inflammation of the lining of the heart is

   a. cardiology.

   b. cardiac.

   c. endocarditis.

   d. cardiologist.

   e. endocardium.

4. Which term might be used to describe an area of the ribcage?

   a. hypertensive

   b. urethra

   c. hypotensive

   d. costovertebral

   e. ureter

5. Which one of the following terms would a heart specialist use to describe a heart condition?

   a. radiopaque

   b. urethra

   c. murmur

   d. abdominal

   e. dermatitis

F. Use the word elements to identify the correct medical term. Select the correct answer to answer each question. **(LO 2.2)**

1. Which medical term has an element meaning *to flow profusely*?

   a. dentistry

   b. endocardium

   c. hemorrhage

   d. pyrexia

   e. diagnosis

2. Which medical term has an element meaning *a structure*?

   a. endocarditis

   b. cardiologist

   c. endocardium

   d. dental

   e. cardiology

3. Which medical term has an element meaning *condition*?

   a. pyrexia

   b. murmur

   c. diagnoses

   d. hemostasis

   e. gastroenterology

4. Which medical term has an element meaning *inflammation*?

   a. gastroenterologist

   b. gastritis

   c. gastrologist

   d. gastric

   e. gastrology

5. Which medical term has an element meaning *knowledge of an abnormal condition*?

   a. murmur

   b. diagnosis

   c. convulsion

   d. seizure

   e. pyrexia

©2014 Nucleus Medical Media

Word Analysis and Communication

G. Speak and spell with precision in medical communication. All terms in the WAD boxes are spelled phonetically to make them easier for you to learn to pronounce. Be sure you can speak them correctly as well as spell them correctly! Practice, practice, practice. Choose the best answer, and then fill in the blanks. **(LO 2.5, 2.6)**

1. The correct pronunciation for an inflammation of the heart is

   a. EN-do-kar-di-tis   **b.** en-**DO**-kard-itis   **c. EN**-doh-kar-**DIE**-tis

   The correct spelling of this term is _____.

2. An abnormally high body temperature is

   a. pie-**REK**-see-ah   **b. PIE**-rek-seeah   **c.** pie-**REK**-see-**AH**

   The correct spelling of this term is _____.

3. Profuse bleeding is termed a

   a. HEM-oh-raj   **b.** hem-**OH**-raj   **c. HEM**-oh-**RAJ**

   The correct spelling of this term is _____.

H. Case report questions. This Case Report is taken from the beginning of Chapter 2. You should feel more comfortable with the medical terminology now. Read the report again, and you will be able to answer the questions that follow. **(LO 2.1, 2.2)**

Case Report (CR) 2.1

You are

. . . an **EMT** employed in the Emergency Department at Fulwood Medical Center.

Your patient is

. . . Barbara Rotelli, a 17-year-old woman, who presents with **pyrexia** and shaking chills. On her medical record, you read that her physical examination reveals splinter **hemorrhages** under her fingernails and a heart **murmur**. There is blood in her urine. She had **dental** surgery four days ago. A provisional **diagnosis** is made of acute **endocarditis**. You are to prepare her for admission to intensive care.

1. *Pyrexia* has an element that means *fever* or *heat*. What is that element? _____

2. What is a *heart murmur*? _____

3. *Endocarditis* has a prefix that means _____

I. Spelling comprehension. Select the correct spelling of the term. (**LO 2.6**)

1. **a.** pyrexcia   **b.** pyrexia   **c.** pirixia   **d.** pyrixea   **e.** pirexia

2. **a.** murmur   **b.** mermer   **c.** murmer   **d.** mirmur   **e.** mumur

3. **a.** endocardites   **b.** endocarditis   **c.** endocaritis   **d.** endoarites   **e.** endacardites

4. **a.** hemorrhege   **b.** hemorrage   **c.** hemmorrhage   **d.** hemmorage   **e.** hemorrhage

5. **a.** dintal   **b.** dental   **c.** dentel   **d.** dendal   **e.** denttal

6. **a.** diagnosis   **b.** deagnossis   **c.** diagnnosis   **d.** diaggnosis   **e.** diagnosiss

7. **a.** hypotenssion   **b.** hopotension   **c.** hypotension   **d.** hypotennsion   **e.** hipotension

8. **a.** costovertebrral   **b.** costovertebral   **c.** costoverrtibral   **d.** castovertebal   **e.** costovertebal

9. **a.** hemostassis   **b.** hemostasis   **c.** hematsasis   **d.** hemmostassis   **e.** hemastasis

10. **a.** urethrra   **b.** ureathra   **c.** urettra   **d.** ureathrra   **e.** urethra

J. Provide the correct spelling of the term based on the meaning provided below. Fill in the blank with the correct term. (**LO 2.2**)

Meaning	Term
1. abnormally high fever	_____
2. pertaining to the ribs and spine	_____
3. stopping bleeding	_____
4. abnormal heart sound	_____
5. low blood pressure	_____
6. canal that leads to the outside	_____
7. determination of the cause of a disease	_____
8. pertaining to the teeth	_____
9. to bleed profusely	_____
10. inflammation of the inside of the heart	_____

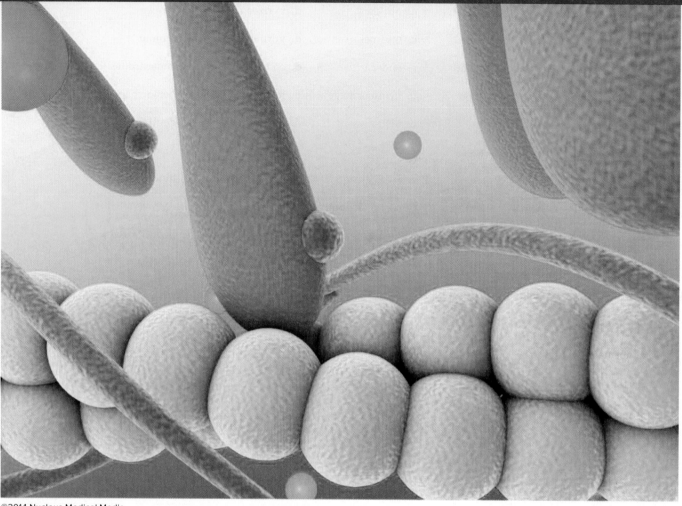

©2014 Nucleus Medical Media

Chapter Learning Outcomes

Each of us begins as a **zygote** and becomes a whole person. Effective medical diagnosis and treatment recognizes that each **organ**, **tissue**, and **cell** in our body functions in harmony with and affects every other organ, tissue, and cell. Our whole body also includes our thoughts, emotions, and perceptions that affect our health, disease, and recovery. This concept of treating the body as a whole is called **holistic** and requires you to be able to:

LO 3.1   Identify the elements that compose the body.

LO 3.2   Discuss the structure and functions of cells.

LO 3.3   Describe the four primary tissue groups found in the body.

LO 3.4   Differentiate the different organ systems and their major organs.

LO 3.5   Explain the structure and functions of deoxyribonucleic acid (DNA).

LO 3.6   Discuss the roles of genes in heredity.

LO 3.7   Define medical genetics and its applications in modern medicine.

LO 3.8   Relate the advantages of personalized and predictive medicine to modern health care.

LO 3.9   Differentiate the different anatomic positions, planes, and directions of the body.

LO 3.10 Map the body cavities.

LO 3.11 Describe the abdominal quadrants and the nine regions of the abdomen.

LO 3.A   Use medical terms pertaining to the body as a whole to communicate and document in writing accurately and precisely in any health care setting.

LO 3.B   Use medical terms pertaining to the body as a whole to communicate verbally with accuracy and precision in any health care setting.

LO 3.C   Using word elements, construct medical terms associated with the body systems.

LO 3.D   Deconstruct medical terms related to the body system as a whole into their word elements (roots, combining forms, prefixes, and suffixes).

LO 3.E   Identify abbreviations as they relate to the words they abbreviate and use them in the correct context of medical care.

 ## Case Report (CR) 3.1

You are

. . . a certified medical assistant (CMA) employed as an in vitro fertilization coordinator in the Assisted Reproduction Clinic at Fulwood Medical Center.

Your patient is

. . . Mrs. Mary Arnold, a 35-year-old woman who has been unable to conceive. **In vitro fertilization (IVF)** was recommended. After **hormone** therapy, several healthy and mature eggs were recovered from her **ovary**. The eggs were combined with her husband's **sperm** in a laboratory dish where **fertilization** occurred to form a single cell, called a **zygote**. The cells were allowed to divide for 5 days to become **blastocysts**, and then four blastocysts were implanted in her **uterus**.

Your role is to guide, counsel, and support Mrs. Arnold and her husband through the implementation and follow-up for the IVF process.

Lesson 3.1

Organization of the Body

Lesson Objectives

Lesson Objectives

All the elements of your body interact with one another to enable your body to be in constant change as it reacts to the environment, to the nourishment you give it, and to the thoughts and emotions that you express to it.

To understand the structure and function of your body, you need to be able to use correct medical terminology to:

3.1.1 Define the medical terms associated with the structures and functions of organ systems and organs.

3.1.2 List the four primary groups of tissue and describe their functions.

3.1.3 Identify the structure and functions of the components of a cell.

LO 3.1 Composition of the Body

- The whole body or organism is composed of **organ** systems.
  - Organ systems are composed of **organs.**
    - Organs are composed of **tissues**.
      - Tissues are composed of **cells**.
        - Cells are composed in part of **organelles**.
          - Organelles are composed of **molecules**.
            - Molecules are composed of **atoms**.
              - The **nucleus** of a cell directs all the activities of a cell.

Organism   Body system   Organ   Tissue   Cell   Organelle   Molecule   Atom

Abbreviation	
IVF	in vitro fertilization

LO 3.2 The Cell

This single fertilized cell, the **zygote**, is the result of the **fertilization** of an egg **(oocyte)** by a sperm and is the origin of every cell in your body *(Figure 3.1)*. The oocyte divides and multiplies into millions of cells that are the basic unit of every tissue and organ. The structure and all of the functions of your tissues and organs are due to their cells. The **cell** is the basic unit of life. **Cytology** is the study of this cell structure and function. Your understanding of the cell will form the basis for your knowledge of the anatomy and physiology of every tissue and organ.

▲ **Figure 3.1** Fertilization of egg by single sperm.
©Francis Leroy, Biocosmos/ Photo Researchers, Inc.

 Case Report 3.1 *(Continued)*

Mrs. Arnold achieved pregnancy and delivered a healthy girl at term.

WORD	PRONUNCIATION		ELEMENTS	DEFINITION
atom	**AT**-om		Greek *indivisible*	A small unit of matter
blastocyst	**BLAS**-toe-sist	R/CF S/	blast/o *immature cell* -cyst *cyst, sac, bladder*	First 2 weeks of the developing embryo
cell cellular (adj) cytology	SELL **SELL**-you-lar **SIGH**-tol-oh-gee	 S/ R/ S/ R/CF	Latin *a storeroom* -ar *pertaining to* cellul- *small cell* -logy *study of* cyt/o- *cell*	The smallest unit capable of independent existence Pertaining to a cell Study of the cell
fertilization fertilize (verb)	**FER**-til-eye-**ZAY**-shun **FER**-til-ize	S/ R/	-ation *process* fertiliz- *to bear*	Union of a male sperm and a female egg
molecule molecular (adj) (**Note:** The two suffixes are joined by two vowels, therefore the e in *ule* is not used.)	**MOLL**-eh-kyul mo-**LEK**-you-lar	S/ R/ S/	-ule *small* molec- *mass* -ar *pertaining to*	Very small particle consisting of two or more atoms held tightly together
oocyte	**OH**-oh-site	R/ R/CF	-cyte *cell* o/o- *egg*	Female egg cell
organ organelle	**OR**-gan **OR**-gah-nell	 S/ R/	Latin *instrument, tool* -elle *small* organ- *organ*	Structure with specific functions in a body system Part of a cell having a specialized function(s)
tissue	**TISH**-you		Latin *to weave*	Collection of similar cells
vitro in vitro fertilization (IVF)	**VEE**-troh IN **VEE**-troh **FER**-til-eye-**ZAY**-shun		Latin *glass*	Process of combining a sperm and egg in a laboratory dish and placing resulting embryos inside a uterus
zygote	**ZYE**-goat		Greek *yoked*	Cell resulting from the union of the sperm and egg

Exercises

A. As you begin your study of *medical language*, it is important to realize the logic of how terms are formed. *Elements are building blocks. There is always a root, but you may not see the root in the same position in every term. Not every term requires a prefix and/or a suffix. Build your terms after first reviewing the above WAD box. Fill in the blanks.* **LO 3.1, 3.2, 3C**

> 💡 **Study Hint**
> Notice the position of the root in questions 1, 2, and 3. A root can appear at the end of a term or at the beginning of a term, as well as in the middle of a term (its usual place).

1. The female egg cell is known as an _____ / _____ / _____

2. This term does not start with a prefix; it starts with a combining form and ends with a suffix. Study of the cell: _____ / _____ / _____

3. This term also begins with a combining form, which is a root plus a combining vowel. The term ends with a suffix. Pertaining to the cell: _____ / _____

Structure and Functions of Cells

As the zygote divides, every cell derived from it becomes a small, complex factory that carries out these **basic functions of life:**

• Estimates of the total number of cells in the human body vary from 50 trillion to 70 trillion cells.

• The number of cells in your own body is constantly changing, as cells die and new cells take their place.

• In addition to your own cells, there are 10 times as many microorganisms (bacterial and fungal cells) residing on the skin, in saliva, in the conjunctiva, in the vagina, and in the gastrointestinal tract.

• These microorganisms (normal flora) participate in maintaining normal health, and under normal circumstances do not cause disease.

- *Manufacture* of proteins and lipids
- *Production* and use of energy
- *Communication* with other cells
- *Replication* of **deoxyribonucleic acid (DNA)**
- *Reproduction*

All your cells contain a fluid called **cytosol (intracellular** fluid) surrounded by a **cell membrane** (*Figure 3.2*). A single cell may have 10 billion protein molecules inside it.

The cell membrane is made of proteins and lipids and allows water, oxygen, glucose, **electrolytes, steroids,** and alcohol to pass through it. On the outside of the cell membrane are receptors that bind to chemical messengers, such as **hormones** sent by other cells. These are the chemical signals by which your cells communicate with each other. The **cytoplasm** is a clear, gelatinous substance containing cytosol and crowded with different organelles. **Organelles** are small structures that carry out special **metabolic** tasks, the chemical processes that occur in the cell. Examples of organelles are

- **Nucleus**
- Endoplasmic reticulum
- Golgi complex or apparatus
- **Mitochondria**

- **Nucleolus**
- Ribosomes
- Lysosomes

These are defined and their functions detailed in the succeeding pages.

Organelles

The **nucleus** is the largest organelle and located between the cell membrane and the cytoplasm. (*Figure 3.2*). It directs all the activities of the cell. Most of your cells have one nucleus; red blood cells have none, and some liver cells and muscle cells contain many nuclei. The nucleus is surrounded by its own membrane, which has small openings called *pores*. Every minute, hundreds of molecules pass through the pores. These molecules include the raw materials for the DNA and ribonucleic (RNA) synthesis that is ongoing inside the nucleus. Forty-six molecules of DNA and their associated **proteins** are packed into each nucleus as thin strands called **chromatin**. When cells divide, the chromatin condenses to form 46 more densely coiled bodies called **chromosomes**. This **synthesis** is described in more detail in the next lesson.

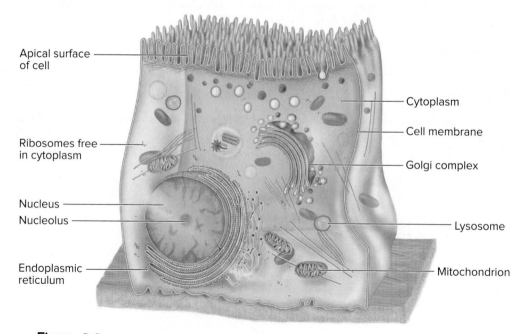

Apical surface of cell

Cytoplasm

Cell membrane

Ribosomes free in cytoplasm

Golgi complex

Nucleus

Nucleolus

Lysosome

Endoplasmic reticulum

Mitochondrion

▲ **Figure 3.2** Structure of a representative cell.

WORD	PRONUNCIATION	ELEMENTS		DEFINITION
chromatin	**KROH**-ma-tin	S/ R/	-in *substance, chemical compound* chromat- *color*	Substance composed of DNA that forms chromosomes during cell division
chromosome	**KROH**-moh-sohm	S/ R/CF	-some *body* chrom/o- *color*	Body in the nucleus that contains DNA and genes
cytoplasm	**SIGH**-toh-plazm	S/ R/	-plasm *something formed* cyt/o- *cell*	Clear, gelatinous substance that forms the substance of a cell except for the nucleus
cytosol	**SIGH**-toh-sawl	S/	-sol *solution*	Liquid portion of the cell
deoxyribonucleic acid (DNA)	dee-**OCK**-see-**RYE**-boh-noo-**KLEE**-ik **ASS**-id		**deoxyribose** *sugar* **nucleic acid** *protein*	Source of hereditary characteristics found in chromosomes
electrolyte	ee-**LEK**-troh-lite	S/ R/CF	-lyte *soluble* electr/o- *electric*	Substance that, when dissolved in a suitable medium, forms electrically charged particles
hormone hormonal (adj)	**HOR**-mohn hor-**MOHN**-al		Greek *set in motion*	Chemical formed in one tissue or organ and carried by the blood to stimulate or inhibit a function of another tissue or organ
intracellular	in-trah-**SELL**-you-lar	S/ P/ R/	-ar *pertaining to* intra- *within* -cellul- *small cell*	Within the cell
membrane membranous (adj)	**MEM**-brain **MEM**-brah-nus		Latin *parchment*	Thin layer of tissue covering a structure or cavity
metabolism metabolic (adj)	meh-**TAB**-oh-lizm met-ah-**BOL**-ik	S/ R/ S/	-ism *condition* metabol- *change* -ic *pertaining to*	The constantly changing physical and chemical processes occurring in the cell Pertaining to metabolism
nucleolus	nyu-**KLEE**-oh-lus	S/ R/CF	-lus *small* nucle/o- *nucleus*	Small mass within the nucleus
nucleus nuclear (adj) nuclei (pl)	**NYU**-klee-us **NYU**-klee-ar **NYU**-klee-eye	S/ R/	-us *pertaining to* nucle- *nucleus*	Functional center of a cell or structure
steroid steroidal (adj)	**STER**-oyd **STER**-oy-dal	S/ R/	-oid *resemble* ster- *solid*	Large family of chemical substances found in many drugs, hormones, and body components
synthesis	**SIN**-the-sis	P/ R/	syn *together* thesis *to arrange*	The process of building a compound from different elements

Exercises

A. Continue building your knowledge of elements. *Add the elements that will complete this medical term. Fill in the blanks.* **LO 3.2, 3.C**

1. Within the cell   _____/cellul/ _____

2. Substance of a cell except for the nucleus   _____/ _____/plasm

3. Chemical substance found in drugs   _____/oid

B. Seek and find in the above WAD the medical term that is defined as follows. *Fill in the blank with the correct term.* **LO 3.1, 3.2, 3.A**

1. small organ _____

2. thin layer of tissue covering a structure or cavity _____

3. electrically charged particles _____

4. functional center of a cell or structure _____

Nucleus —————————————

Nucleolus ————————————

Chromatin ————————————

Rough endoplasmic ————————
reticulum (ER)

Ribosomes on ————————
rough ER

▲ **Figure 3.3** The nucleus.

Structure and Functions of Cells (continued)

Ribosomes are organelles involved in the manufacture of **protein** from simple materials. This process is called **anabolism**.

Each nucleus (*Figure 3.3*) contains a **nucleolus**, a small dense body composed of RNA and protein. It manufactures ribosomes that migrate through the nuclear membrane pores into the cytoplasm.

The **endoplasmic reticulum** is an organelle that manufactures steroids, cholesterol and other lipids, and proteins. It also detoxifies alcohol and other drugs.

Lysosomes are organelles that are the garbage disposal units of the cell. They digest and dispose of worn-out organelles as part of the process of cell death. They also digest foreign particles and bacteria.

Mitochondria (**mitochondrion**, singular) are the powerhouses of the cells. They extract energy by breaking down compounds such as glucose and fat. This process is called **catabolism**. The energy is used to do the work of the cell: for example, to make a muscle contract.

WORD	PRONUNCIATION		ELEMENTS	DEFINITION
anabolism	an-**AB**-oh-lizm	S/ R/	-ism *condition* anabol- *build up*	The buildup of complex substances in the cell from simpler ones as a part of metabolism
carbohydrate	kar-boh-**HIGH**-drate	S/ R/CF R/	-ate *composed of, pertaining to* carb/o- *carbon* -hydr- *water*	Group of organic food compounds that includes sugars, starch, glycogen, and cellulose
catabolism	kah-**TAB**-oh-lizm	S/ R/	-ism *condition* catabol- *break down*	Breakdown of complex substances into simpler ones as a part of metabolism
centriole	**SEN**-tree-ole		Greek *center*	A paired organelle lying in cytoplasm near the nucleus
lysosome	**LIE**-soh-sohm	S/ R/CF	-some *body* lys/o- *decompose*	Enzyme that digests foreign material and worn-out cell components
mitochondrion mitochondria (pl)	my-toe-**KON**-dree-on my-toe-**KON**-dree-ah	S/ R/CF R	-ion *action, condition* mit/o- *thread* -chondr- *cartilage, rib, granule*	Organelle that generates, stores, and releases energy for cell activities
protein	**PRO**-teen	S/ R/CF	-in *substance, chemical compound* prot/e- *first*	Class of food substances based on amino acids
ribosome	**RYE**-bo-sohm	S/ R/CF	-some *body* rib/o- *like a rib*	Structure in the cell that assembles amino acids into protein

Exercises

A. Continue analyzing the logic of medical language. *Fill in the blanks.* **LO 3.2, 3.D**

1. Which term in the above WAD refers to an enzyme? _____

2. Find a term in the above WAD that contains an element that means *water.* _____

3. Which term in the above WAD refers to breaking substances down? _____

B. Identify the meaning of the word elements. *Knowing the meaning of the word elements will help you to quickly define medical terms. Select the correct answer to each question.* **LO 3.C**

1. The word element that means *body* is:

    a. *prot/e*

    b. *lys/o*

    c. *-some*

    d. *anabol-*

2. The word element that means *water* is:

    a. *hydr-*

    b. *-ism*

    c. *rib/o*

    d. *-ate*

3. The word element that means *decompose:*

    a. *prot/e*

    b. *lys/o*

    c. *-some*

    d. *carb/o*

Case Report (CR) 3.2

You are

. . . a physical therapy assistant employed in the Rehabilitation Unit in Fulwood Medical Center.

Your patient is

. . . Mr. Richard Josen, a 22-year-old man who injured tissues in his left knee playing football *(Figure 3.4)*.

Using arthroscopy, the orthopedic surgeon removed Mr. Josen's torn **anterior cruciate ligament** (ACL) and replaced it with a graft from his patellar ligament. The torn medial collateral ligament was sutured together. The tear in his medial meniscus was repaired. His rehabilitation, in which you play a key role, focuses on strengthening the **muscles** around his knee joint and helping him regain joint mobility.

Anterior cruciate ligament (torn)
Medial collateral ligament (torn)
Medial meniscus (torn)
Patellar ligament (cut)

Femur
Quadriceps muscle
Patella
Synovial fluid
Cartilage
Synovial membrane
Tibia
Patellar ligament

(a) Injury to Mr. Josen's left knee

(b) Normal knee

▲ **Figure 3.4 Knee anatomy.**

LO 3.3 Tissues

The knee contains examples of all the different major groups of tissue and will be used in this lesson to illustrate the relation of structure to function in the different tissues. To understand the condition of the 22-year-old in Case Report 3.2, you need a knowledge of tissue structure and function. Ultimately, this is important for your understanding of the anatomy and physiology of organs, organ systems, and the whole body.

Tissues hold your body together. The many tissues of your body have different structures for specialized functions. The different tissues are made of similar cells with unique materials around them that are manufactured by the cells. **Histology** is the study of the structure and function of tissues. The four primary tissue groups are outlined in *Table 3.1*.

Table 3.1 The Four Primary Tissue Groups

Type	Function	Location
Connective	Bind, support, protect, fill spaces, store fat	Widely distributed throughout the body; for example, in blood, bone, cartilage, and fat
Epithelial	Protect, **secrete**, absorb, **excrete**	Cover body surface, cover and line internal organs, compose glands
Muscle	Movement	Attached to bones, in the walls of hollow internal organs, and in the heart
Nervous	Transmit impulses for coordination, sensory reception, motor actions	Brain, spinal cord, nerves

WORD	PRONUNCIATION	ELEMENTS		DEFINITION
epithelium	ep-ih-**THEE**-lee-um	S/ P/ R/CF	-um *structure* epi- *upon* -thel/i- *nipple*	Tissue that covers surfaces or lines cavities
epithelial (adj)	ep-ih-**THEE**-lee-al	S/	-al *pertaining to*	Pertaining to epithelium
excrete	eks-**KREET**		Latin *separate*	To pass waste products of metabolism out of the body
excretion (noun)	eks-**KREE**-shun			Removal of waste products of metabolism out of the body
histology	his-**TOL**-oh-jee	S/ R/CF	-logy *study of* hist/o- *tissue*	Structure and function of cells, tissues, and organs
histologist	his-**TOL**-oh-jist	S/	-logist *one who studies*	Specialist in the structure and function of cells, tissues, and organs
ligament	**LIG**-ah-ment		Latin *band*	Band of fibrous tissue connecting two structures
muscle	**MUSS**-el		Latin *muscle*	A tissue consisting of contractile cells
secrete secretion (noun)	se-**KREET** se-**KREE**-shun		Latin *release*	To produce a chemical substance in a cell and release it from the cell

Exercises

A. Define words with a Latin meaning. *Not all terms can be deconstructed into word elements. Match each term on the left with its correct meaning on the right.* **LO 3.2, 3.A**

_____ **1.** secrete

_____ **2.** ligament

_____ **3.** muscle

_____ **4.** excrete

A. tissue made of contractile cells

B. to produce and release a chemical substance from a cell

C. to pass waste products out of the body

D. band of fibrous tissue

B. Define word elements. *Given the word element, identify its meaning.* **LO 3.D**

1. The meaning of the word element -*logy:*
   a. pertaining to
   b. composed of
   c. one who studies
   d. study of

2. The meaning of the word element -*al:*
   a. pertaining to
   b. composed of
   c. structure
   d. study of

3. The meaning of the word element -*logist:*
   a. one who studies
   b. tissue
   c. upon
   d. structure

LO 3.3 Connective Tissues in the Knee Joint

- **Bone** is the hardest connective tissue due to the presence of calcium mineral salts, mostly calcium phosphate. Cells that make up bone tissue are
  - **Osteoblasts** deposit bone **matrix** *(Figure 3.5)* in concentric patterns around a central canal containing a blood vessel. As a result, every osteoblast is close to a supply of **nutrients** from the blood.
  - **Osteocytes** are former osteoblasts that maintain the bone matrix.
  - **Osteoclasts** dissolve the bone matrix to release calcium and phosphate into the blood when these chemicals are needed elsewhere.
- **Cartilage** has a flexible, rubbery matrix that allows it, as a meniscus, to function as a shock absorber and as a gliding surface where two bones meet to form a joint. Cartilage also forms the shape of your ear, the tip of your nose, and your larynx. Cartilage has very few blood vessels and heals poorly or not at all. Cells of cartilage include
  - Chrondroblasts, which deposit the cartilage matrix.
  - Chrondrocytes, which are former chondroblasts that maintain the cartilage matrix.
  - Fibers, which give the cartilage strength and flexibility.
- **Ligaments** are strips or bands of fibrous connective tissue *(Figure 3.6)*. Cells called **fibroblasts** form a gelatinous (jellylike) matrix and closely packed, parallel **collagen** fibers. These fibers provide the strength the ligament needs. Their blood supply is poor, so they do not heal well without surgery.
- **Tendons** are thick, strong ligaments that attach muscles to bone.
- The **joint capsule** of the knee joint is attached to the tibia and femur, encloses the joint cavity, and is made of thin, collagenous fibrous connective tissue. It is strengthened by fibers that extend over it from the ligaments and muscles surrounding the knee joint. These features are common to most joints.
- The inner surface of many joint capsules is lined with **synovial membrane,** which secretes **synovial fluid.** This fluid is a slippery lubricant retained in the joint cavity by the capsule. It has a texture similar to raw egg white. It makes joint movement almost friction-free and distributes nutrients to the cartilage on the joint surfaces of bone.
- **Muscle** tissue stabilizes the knee joint. Extensions of the tendons of the *quadriceps femoris,* the large muscle in front of the thigh, and of the *semimembranosus muscle* on the rear of the thigh, are major stabilizers. The muscles themselves respectively extend and flex the joint. The structure and functions of these and other skeletal muscles are described in *Chapter 14.*
- **Nervous** tissue extensively supplies all the knee structures, which is why a knee injury is excruciatingly painful. The structure and functions of nervous tissue are described in *Chapter 9.*

LM 400×

▲ **Figure 3.5** Bone tissue.
©McGraw-Hill Education/Al Telser, photographer.

Posterior view

▲ **Figure 3.6** Ligaments of the knee joint.

LO 3.3, 3.A
Word Analysis and Definition

S = Suffix   P = Prefix   R = Root   R/CF = Combining Form

WORD	PRONUNCIATION	ELEMENTS		DEFINITION
capsule capsular (adj)	**KAP**-syul **KAP**-syu-lar	S/ R/ S/	-ule *little* caps- *box* -ar *pertaining to*	Fibrous tissue layer surrounding a joint or some other structure Pertaining to a capsule
cartilage	**KAR**-tih-lage		Latin *gristle*	Nonvascular firm, connective tissue found mostly in joints
chondroblast	**KON**-droh-blast	S/ R/CF	-blast *germ cell* chondr/o- *cartilage*	Cartilage-forming cell.
chondrocyte	**KON**-droh-site	S/	-cyte *cell*	Cartilage cell.
collagen	**KOL**-ah-jen	S/ R/CF	-gen *produce, form* coll/a- *glue*	Major protein of connective tissue, cartilage, and bone
fibroblast	**FIE**-bro-blast	S/ R/CF	-blast *germ cell* fibr/o- *fiber*	Cell that forms collagen fibers
matrix	**MAY**-triks		Latin "mater" *mother*	Substance that surrounds cells, is manufactured by the cells, and holds them together
nutrient	**NYU**-tree-ent	S/ R/	-ent *end result* nutri- *nourish*	A substance in food required for normal physiologic function
osteoblast	**OS**-tee-oh-blast	S/ R/CF	-blast *germ cell* oste/o- *bone*	Bone-forming cell
osteoclast osteocyte	**OS**-tee-oh-klast **OS**-tee-oh-site	S/ S/	-clast *break* -cyte *cell*	Bone-removing cell Bone-maintaining cell
synovial (adj)	si-**NOH**-vee-al	S/ R/CF	-al *pertaining to* synov/i- *synovial membrane*	Pertaining to synovial fluid and synovial membrane
tendon	**TEN**-dun		Latin *sinew*	Fibrous band that connects muscle to bone

Exercises

A. Understanding elements is the key to a large medical vocabulary. *Work with the following exercise to increase your knowledge of medical language. Fill in the blanks.* **LO 3.3**

osteoblast   osteoclast   osteocyte

1. These terms all refer to (select one)   a. cartilage   b. bone   c. collagen   The element they have in common is: _____.

2. The element that changes in every term is the (select one):   P   R   CF   S

3. The suffix in the WAD that means *germ cell* is: _____.

4. The suffix in the WAD that means *break* is: _____.

5. The suffix in the WAD that means *cell* is: _____.

B. Match the appropriate medical term in the first column to the descriptions given in the second column. LO 3.3

_____	**1.** synovial	**a.**	bone forming cell
_____	**2.** meniscus	**b.**	connects muscle to bone
_____	**3.** tendon	**c.**	slippery lubricant
_____	**4.** osteoblast	**d.**	shock absorber

LESSON 3.1 Organization of the Body   43

Case Report (CR) 3.3

Fulwood Medical Center

An 84-year-old man with advanced Parkinson disease was having difficulty breathing because his stooped posture was compressing his lungs and his muscle spasticity made respiration more difficult. A bout of influenza increased his breathing difficulty, and a tracheostomy tube was inserted to help him breathe. He then became unable to swallow, and a feeding tube was inserted. Because of hypertrophy of his prostate, he developed a **urinary** tract infection. This led to septicemia. The bloodborne infection attacked his kidneys, heart, and lungs, leading to failure of these organs and their organ systems and, ultimately, death.

▲ **Figure 3.7** Organs of the urinary system.
©McGraw-Hill Education

LO 3.4 Organs and Organ Systems

Organs

An **organ** is a structure composed of several tissues that work together to carry out specific functions. For example, the skin is an organ that has different tissues in it such as epithelial cells, hair, nails, and glands.

Each organ has well-defined anatomic boundaries separating it from adjacent structures and performs a particular function. The different organs in an organ system are usually interconnected. For example, in the urinary organ system, the organs are the kidneys, ureters, bladder, and urethra, and they are all connected (*Figure 3.7*) as they work to eliminate fluid waste from the body. See *Table 3.2* to review the organs of each body system.

Organ Systems

An **organ system** is a group of organs with a specific collective function, such as digestion, circulation, or respiration. For example, the nose, pharynx, larynx, trachea, and bronchi work together to achieve the total function of respiration.

The body has 11 organ systems, shown in *Table 3.2*. The muscle and skeleton can be considered one organ system, the musculoskeletal system.

All your organ systems work together to ensure that your body's internal environment remains relatively constant. This process is called **homeostasis**. For example, your digestive, respiratory, and circulatory organ systems work together so that (a) every cell in your body receives adequate nutrients and oxygen and (b) waste products from the breakdown of these nutrients during cell metabolism are removed. Your cells can then function normally. Disease affecting an organ or organ system disrupts this game plan of homeostasis.

As described in Case Report 3.3, when organs and organ systems do not function in an integrated way, a person can die.

Table 3.2 Organ Systems

Organ System	Major Organs	Major Functions
Integumentary	Skin, hair, nails, sweat glands, sebaceous glands	Protect tissues, regulate body temperature, support sensory receptors
Skeletal	Bones, ligaments, cartilages, tendons	Provide framework, protect soft tissues, provide attachments for muscles, produce blood cells, store inorganic salts
Muscular	Muscles	Cause movements, maintain posture, produce body heat
Nervous	Brain, spinal cord, nerves, sense organs	Detect changes, receive and interpret sensory information, stimulate muscles and glands
Endocrine	Glands that secrete hormones: pituitary, thyroid, parathyroid, adrenal, pancreas, ovaries, testes, pineal, thymus	Control metabolic activities of organs and structures
Cardiovascular	Heart, blood vessels	Move blood and transport substances throughout body
Lymphatic	Lymph vessels and nodes, thymus, spleen	Return tissue fluid to the blood, carry certain absorbed food molecules, defend body against infection
Digestive	Mouth, tongue, teeth, salivary glands, pharynx, esophagus, stomach, liver, gallbladder, pancreas, small and large intestines	Receive, break down, and absorb food; eliminate unabsorbed material
Respiratory	Nasal cavity, pharynx, larynx, trachea, bronchi, lungs	Control Intake and output of air, exchange gases between air and blood
Urinary	Kidneys, ureters, urinary bladder, urethra	Remove wastes from blood, maintain water and electrolyte balance, store and transport urine
Reproductive	*Male:* scrotum, testes, epididymides, vas deferens, seminal vesicles, prostate, bulbourethral glands, urethra, penis	Produce and maintain sperm cells, transfer sperm cells into female reproductive tract, secrete male hormones
	Female: ovaries, uterine (fallopian) tubes, uterus, vagina, vulva	Produce and maintain egg cells, receive sperm cells, support development of an embryo, function in birth process, secrete female hormones

WORD	PRONUNCIATION	ELEMENTS		DEFINITION
cardiovascular	KAR-dee-oh-VAS-kyu-lar	S/ R/CF R/	-ar *pertaining to* cardi/o- *heart* -vascul- *blood vessel*	Pertaining to the heart and blood vessels
digestive	die-JEST-iv	S/ R/	-ive *nature of* digest- *to break down*	Pertaining to the breakdown of food into elements suitable for cell metabolism
endocrine	EN-doh-krin	P/ R/CF	endo- *within* -crin/e *secrete*	Pertaining to a gland that produces an internal or hormonal secretion
homeostasis (**Note:** *Hemo*stasis is very different.)	ho-mee-oh-STAY-sis	S/ R/CF	-stasis *stand still, control* home/o- *the same*	Stability or equilibrium of a system or the body's internal environment
integumentary	in-TEG-you-MEN-tah-ree	S/ R/	-ary *pertaining to* integument- *covering of the body*	Pertaining to the covering of the body (the skin)
lymphatic	lim-FAT-ik	S/ R/	-atic *pertaining to* lymph- *lymph*	Pertaining to lymph or the lymphatic system
muscular	MUSS-kyu-lar	S/ R/	-ar *pertaining to* muscul- *muscle*	Pertaining to muscle or muscles
nervous	NER-vus		Latin *nerve*	Pertaining to a nerve
organ	OR-gan		Greek *instrument*	Structure with specific functions in a body system
reproductive	ree-pro-DUC-tiv	S/ P/ R/	-ive *nature of, pertaining to* re- *again* -product- *lead forth*	Relating to the process by which organisms produce offspring
respiratory	RES-pir-ah-TOR-ee	S/ P/ R/CF	-tory *relating to* re- *again* -spir/a *to breathe*	Relating to the process of exchanging oxygen and carbon dioxide
skeletal	SKEL-eh-tal	S/ R/	-al *pertaining to* -skelet- *skeleton*	Pertaining to the bony skeleton
urinary	YUR-in-ary	S/ R/	-ary *pertaining to* urin- *urine*	Pertaining to urine

Exercises

A. Use your knowledge of the building blocks of terms, and deconstruct the following terms into their basic elements. *This will give you a better picture of how the words were formed. Fill in the blanks. The first one is done for you.* **LO 3.D**

1. homeostasis   home/o/stasis

2. urinary   _____ / _____

3. cardiovascular   _____ / _____ / _____ / _____

4. respiratory   _____ / _____ / _____ / _____

Basic Genetics

LO 3.5, 3.6 DNA and Genes

Inside the cell nucleus are packed 46 molecules of **deoxyribonucleic acid (DNA)** as thin strands called **chromatin**. When cells divide, the chromatin condenses with **histone** proteins to form 23 pairs (46 total) of densely coiled bodies called **chromosomes**. Twenty-two of these pairs look the same in both males and females. In the 23rd pair, females have two copies of the X chromosome; males have one X and one Y. The picture of the human chromosomes lined up in pairs is called a **karyotype** *(Figure 3.8)*.

The information in DNA is stored as a code of four chemical bases: adenine (A), guanine (G), cytosine (C), and thymine (T). The total human DNA contains about 3 billion bases, and more than 99% of those bases are the same in all people. The sequence of these bases determines the building and maintaining of the organism's cells, similar to the way in which letters of the alphabet appear in order to form words and sentences.

(a) **(b)**

▲ **Figure 3.8** Human karyotype. (a) ©Kateryna Kon/Shutterstock.com RF

(b) ©Kateryna Kon/Shutterstock.com RF

The **chromosomal** DNA bases pair with each other—A with T and C with G—and are attached to a sugar molecule and a phosphate molecule. A base, sugar, and phosphate form a **nucleotide**. Nucleotides are arranged in two long strands to form a spiral called a double **helix**.

The nuclear DNA in the chromosomes is the **hereditary** material, each unit of which is called a **gene**. The genes act as instructions to make molecules of different proteins. Each person has two copies of each gene, one inherited from each parent. Most genes are the same in all people; only less than one percent is slightly different between people. These small differences contribute to each person's unique physical features. Humans are thought to have between 20,000 and 25,000 genes. This total is called the **genome**.

Mitosis

The critical property of DNA is that it can **replicate**, make copies of itself, so that when cells divide, each new cell has an exact copy of the DNA present in the old cell. This cell division is called **mitosis**, in which a cell duplicates all of its contents, including its chromosomes, to form two identical daughter cells. When mitosis is not performed correctly, abnormal cells, such as cancer cells, can result.

Mutations and Epigenetic Changes

A permanent alteration of the nucleotide sequence of the genome of an organism is called a **mutation**. Mutations may or may not produce visible changes in the observable characteristics (**phenotype**) of an organism. Mutations play a part in both normal and abnormal biological processes including evolution, cancer, and the development of the immune system.

Chemical compounds that become added to single genes can regulate their activity to produce modifications known as **epigenetic** changes. These changes can remain as cells divide and can be inherited through generations. Environmental influences from pollution, drugs, pharmaceuticals, aging, and diets can also produce epigenetic modifications, such as cancers, mental disorders, and degenerative and metabolic disorders.

WORD	PRONUNCIATION		ELEMENTS	DEFINITION
chromatin	**KROH**-ma-tin	S/ R/CF	-tin *pertaining to* chrom/a- *color*	DNA that forms chromosomes during cell division
chromosome	**KROH**-moh-sohm	R/CF R/	chrom/o- *color* -some *body*	The body in the cell nucleus that carries the genes
chromosomal (adj)	**KROH**-moh-**SO**-mal	S/	-al *pertaining to*	Pertaining to a chromosome
deoxyribonucleic acid (DNA)	dee-**OCK**-see-**RYE**-boh-noo-**KLEE**-ik **ASS**-id	S/ P/ P/ R/ R/ R/	-ic *pertaining to* de- *without* -oxy- *oxygen* -ribo- *ribose* -nucle- *nucleus* acid *acid, low pH*	The chemical repository of hereditary characteristics
epigenetics	**EP**-ih-jeh-**NET**-iks	S/ P/ R/	-etics *pertaining to* epi- *above, over* -gen- *to create*	The study of disorders produced by the effects of chemical compounds (e.g., pollutants) or environmental influences (such as diet) on genes
gene	JEEN		Greek *birth*	The functional unit of heredity on a chromosome
genetic (adj)	jeh-**NET**-ik	R/ R/	-etic *pertaining to* gen- *to create*	Pertaining to genetics
genome	**JEE**-nome		-ome *body*	A complete set of chromosomes
helix	**HEE**-liks		Greek *a coil*	A spiral of nucleotides in the structure of DNA
heredity	heh-**RED**-ih-tee	S/	Latin *an heir*	The transmission of characteristics from parent to offspring
hereditary	heh-**RED**-ih-ter-ee	R/	-ary *pertaining to* heredit- *inherited through genes*	Transmissible from parent to offspring
histone	**HIS**-tone	S/ R/	-one *chemical* hist- *tissue*	A simple protein found in the cell nucleus
karyotype	**KAIR**-ee-oh-type	S/ R/CF	-type *model* kary/o- *nucleus*	The chromosome characteristics of an individual cell
mitosis	my-**TOE**-sis		Greek *thread*	Cell division to create two identical cells, each with 46 chromosomes
mutation	myu-**TAY**-shun		Latin *to change*	A permanent alteration in the nucleotide sequence of the genome
nucleotide	**NYU**-klee-oh-tide	R/CF R/	nucle/o- *nucleus* -tide *time*	Combination of a DNA base, a sugar molecule, and a phosphate molecule
phenotype	**FEE**-noh-type	S/ R/CF	-type *model* phen/o- *appearance*	Manifestation of a genome
replicate	**REP**-lih-kate		Latin *a reply*	To produce an exact copy

Exercises

A. Use your knowledge of medical terminology related to genetics. *Insert the correct term in the appropriate statement.* **LO 3.5**

gene   genome   mitosis   chromosome   chromatin

1. When the cell is maintaining normal function, DNA and proteins are contained within thin strands of _____ _____.

2. When the cell is dividing, DNA wraps around the proteins and is contained within densely coiled bodies called _____ _____.

3. The unit of nuclear DNA in the chromosomes is called a _____.

4. A _____ is a complete set of chromosomes.

5. The process of _____ occurs when a cell creates an exact copy of itself and divides into two identical cells.

Lesson 3.3

THE BODY AS A WHOLE

Genetic Medicine

Case Report (CR) 3.4

You are

. . . a physician's assistant (PA) in the Genetic Counseling Clinic at Fulwood Medical Center.

Your patient is

. . . Mrs. Patricia Bennet, a 52-year-old office manager with two daughters, aged 30 and 25. Mrs. Bennett's sister, aged 55, recently had a mastectomy for breast cancer and is now receiving chemotherapy. Their mother died of ovarian cancer in her late fifties. Mrs. Bennet wants to know her risk for breast or ovarian cancer, what she can do to prevent it, and what her daughters' risks are.

Abbreviations

ADHD attention deficit hyperactivity disorder

BRCA breast cancer

LO 3.7, 3.8 Genetic Medicine

Medical genetics is the application of genetics to medical care. Genetic medicine is the newer term for medical genetics and incorporates areas such as gene therapy, personalized (precise) medicine, and predictive medicine.

Every person has a unique variation of the human genome and an individual's health stems from this genetic variation interacting with behaviors (drinking, smoking, etc.) and influences from the environment (chemical pollution in some form). Knowing the genetic makeup will enable more accurate diagnoses to be made, the source of the disease to be understood, and earlier, more accurate treatments or the prevention of progression of the disease provided. This concept is called *personalized medicine.*

One way that the biological variant is seen is responsiveness to drugs. Attention deficit hyperactivity disorder (ADHD) medications only work for one out of ten preschoolers, cancer drugs are effective for only one out of four patients, and depression drugs work for six out of ten patients. The drug Tamoxifen used to be prescribed to women with a form of breast cancer (BRCA), but 65% developed resistance to it. These women were found to have a mutation in their CYP2D6 gene that made Tamoxifen an ineffective treatment.

Personalized medicine can assist with preventive care. Women, such as Patricia Bennet in Case Report 3.4, are already being genotyped for mutations in the BRCA1 and BRCA2 genes if they have a family history of breast or ovarian cancer. In Mrs. Bennet's case, she is positive for both mutations and is now considering surgical measures that can then be taken to prevent the disease from developing. Her daughters have appointments to receive genetic testing in their own health plans.

Cytogenetics is the study of chromosome abnormalities to determine a cause for developmental delay, mental retardation, birth defects, and **dysmorphic** features, and chromosomal abnormalities are often detected in cancer cells.

Gene therapy is an experimental technique to replace a mutated gene that causes disease with a healthy copy, inactivate a mutated gene that is functioning improperly, or introduce a new gene into the body to prevent or help cure a disease. The **therapeutic** genes are introduced into body cells, and some 600 clinical trials utilizing this form of therapy are underway in the United States.

Predictive medicine looks at the probability of a disease and allows preventive measures to be taken. Examples are newborn screening to identify genetic disorders that can be treated early in life, and **prenatal** testing to look for diseases and conditions in an **embryo** or **fetus** whose parents have an increased risk of having a baby with a genetic or chromosomal disorder.

WORD	PRONUNCIATION		ELEMENTS	DEFINITION
cytogenetics	SIGH-toh-jeh-NET-iks	S/ R/CF R/	-etics *pertaining to* cyto- *cell* -gen- *create*	Study of chromosomal abnormalities in a cell
dysmorphology	dis-mor-FOLL-oh-jee	S/ P/ R/CF	-logy *study of* dys- *difficult, bad* -morph/o- *form*	The study of developmental structural defects
dysmorphic	dis-MOR-fik	S/	-ic *pertaining to*	Possessing a developmental structural defect
embryo	EM-bree-oh		Greek *a young one*	Developing organism from conception until the end of the eighth week
fetus	FEE-tus		Latin *offspring*	Human organism from the end of the eighth week to birth
predictive	pree-DIK-tiv	S/ P/ R/	-ive *quality of* pre- *before* -dict- *consent*	The likelihood of a disease or disorder being present or occurring in the future
prenatal	pree-NAY-tal	S/ P/ R/	-al *pertaining to* pre- *before* -nat- *born*	Before birth
therapy therapeutic	THAIR-ah-pee THAIR-ah-PYU-tik		Greek *medical treatment* Greek *curing of a disorder or disease*	Systematic treatment of a disease, dysfunction, or disorder Curing or capable of curing a disorder or disease

Exercises

A. Discuss the applications of medical genetics. *Choose the correct answer to complete the following statements.* **LO 3.7**

1. The replacement of a mutated gene with a healthy copy is termed:
   a. predictive medicine
   b. cytogenetics
   c. gene therapy
   d. personalized medicine

2. The study of chromosome abnormalities in a cell is:
   a. cytogenetics
   b. dysmorphology
   c. prenatal therapy
   d. precise medicine

3. _____ medicine uses genetics to determine accurate treatments for an existing condition.
   a. Personalized
   b. Preventative
   c. Cytogenetic
   d. Predictive

B. Not all terms can be deconstructed. *It is sometimes necessary to memorize the medical terms of Greek and Latin origin. Given the definition, provide the term that is being described. Fill in the blanks.* **LO 3.7, 3.A**

1. Systematic treatment of a disease, dysfunction, or disorder. _____

2. Human organism from conception to the end of the eighth week. _____

3. Human organism from the end of the eighth week to birth. _____

4. Curing or capable of curing a disorder or disease. _____

Anatomic Position, Planes, and Directions

Terms have been developed over the past several thousand years to enable you to describe clearly where different anatomic structures and lesions are in relation to each other. To communicate effectively with other health professionals, it is critical that you are able to use the terminology to describe these positions and relative positions. To do this, you need to be able to use correct medical terminology to:

3.4.1 Define the fundamental anatomic position on which all descriptions of anatomic locations are based.

3.4.2 Describe the different anatomic planes and directions.

3.4.3 Locate the body cavities.

3.4.4 Identify the four abdominal quadrants and nine abdominal regions.

LO 3.9 Anatomic Position

When all **anatomic** descriptions are used, it is assumed that the body is in the anatomic position. The body is standing erect with feet flat on the floor, face and eyes facing forward, and arms at the sides with the palms facing forward *(Figure 3.9)*.

When your palms face forward, the forearm is **supine**. When you lie down flat on your back, you are supine. When your palms face backward, the forearm is **prone**. When you lie down flat on your abdomen, you are prone.

LO 3.9 Directional Terms

Directional terms describe the position of one structure or part of the body relative to another; for example, **cephalic** vs. **caudal**, **ventral** vs. **dorsal**, and **proximal** vs. **distal**. These directional terms are shown in *Figures 3.9* and *3.10*.

LO 3.9 Anatomic Planes

Different views of the body are based on imaginary "slices" producing flat surfaces that pass through the body *(Figure 3.11)*. The three major anatomic planes are

- **Transverse** or **horizontal**—a plane passing across the body parallel to the floor and perpendicular to the body's long axis. It divides the body into an upper (**superior**) portion and a lower (**inferior**) portion.
- **Sagittal**—a vertical plane that divides the body into right and left portions.
- **Frontal** or **coronal**—a vertical plane that divides the body into front (**anterior**) and back (**posterior**) portions.

> ### 💡 Study Hint
>
> Help your memory with little tricks of association for medical terms. *Example:* The medical term *supine* has the word *up* in it. The meaning of supine is *lying with the face and the anterior part of the body UP*. Associate UP with s**UP**ine, and you will have no trouble remembering its definition.
>
> Then associate the opposite term, and you will know the meaning of *prone* as well.

▲ **Figure 3.9** Anatomic position with directional terms. ©McGraw-Hill Education/ Joe DeGrandis, photogrpaher.

▲ **Figure 3.10** Directional terms. ©Aaron Roeth Photography

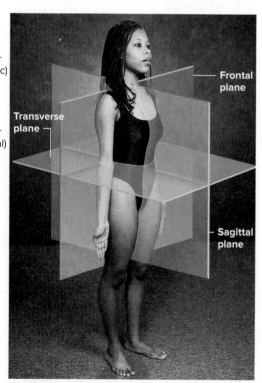

▲ **Figure 3.11** Anatomic planes. ©McGraw-Hill Education/Joe DeGrandis, photogrpaher.

WORD	PRONUNCIATION	ELEMENTS		DEFINITION
anatomy	ah-**NAT**-oh-mee	S/ P/ R/	-y *process* ana- *apart from* -tom- *section*	Study of the structures of the human body
anatomic (adj)	an-ah-**TOM**-ik	S/	-ic *pertaining to*	Pertaining to anatomy
anterior (opposite of posterior)	an-**TER**-ee-or	S/ R/	-ior *pertaining to* anter- *coming before*	Front surface of body; situated in front
caudal (opposite of cephalic)	**KAW**-dal	S/ R/	-al *pertaining to* caud- *tail*	Pertaining to or nearer to the tail
cephalic (opposite of caudal)	se-**FAL**-ik	S/ R/	-ic *pertaining to* cephal- *head*	Pertaining to or nearer to the head
coronal (equivalent to frontal)	**KOR**-oh-nal	S/ R/	-al *pertaining to* coron- *crown*	Pertaining to the vertical plane dividing the body into anterior and posterior portions
distal (opposite of proximal)	**DISS**-tal	S/ R/	-al *pertaining to* dist- *away from the center*	Situated away from the center of the body
dorsal (equivalent to posterior)	**DOR**-sal	S/ R/	-al *pertaining to* dors- *back*	Pertaining to the back or situated behind
frontal (equivalent to coronal)	**FRON**-tal	S/ R/	-al *pertaining to* front- *front*	In front; relating to the anterior part of the body
inferior (opposite of superior)	in-**FEE**-ree-or	S/ R/	-ior *pertaining to* infer- *below*	Situated below
posterior (opposite of anterior)	pos-**TER**-ee-or	S/ R/	-ior *pertaining to* poster- *coming behind*	Pertaining to the back surface of the body; situated behind
prone (opposite of supine)	PRONE		Latin *bending forward*	Lying face-down, flat on your abdomen
proximal (opposite of distal)	**PROK**-sih-mal	S/ R/	-al *pertaining to* proxim- *nearest*	Situated nearest the center of the body
sagittal	**SAJ**-ih-tal	S/ R/	-al *pertaining to* sagitt- *arrow*	Pertaining to the vertical plane through the body, dividing it into right and left portions
superior (opposite of inferior)	soo-**PEE**-ree-or	S/ R/	-ior *pertaining to* super- *above*	Situated above
supine (opposite of prone)	soo-**PINE**		Latin *bend backward*	Lying face-up, flat on your spine
transverse	trans-**VERS**		Latin *crosswise*	Pertaining to the horizontal plane dividing the body into upper and lower portions
ventral (equivalent to anterior)	**VEN**-tral	S/ R/	-al *pertaining to* ventr- *belly*	Pertaining to the abdomen or situated nearer the surface of the abdomen

Exercises

A. Identify directional terms. *Identify the term that has the opposite meaning. Fill in the blank.* **LO 3.9, 3.C**

1. ventral _____

2. caudal _____

3. distal _____

4. posterior _____

5. superior _____

> ### Study Hint
> Terms will be easier to remember if you study them in *pairs of opposites*.

B. Identify the planes of the body. *Identify the plane that is being described. Fill in the blank.* **LO 3.9**

1. This plane divides the body into right and left sides: _____

2. This plane is also known as the frontal plane: _____

3. This plane is also known as the horizontal plane: _____

► Figure 3.12 Body
cavities. (a) lateral view;
(b) frontal view.

Cranial cavity

Spinal cavity

Thoracic cavity

Diaphragm

Abdominal cavity

Abdominopelvic cavity

Pelvic cavity

Mediastinum
Pleural cavity
Pericardial cavity
Diaphragm
Abdominal cavity
Pelvic cavity
Thoracic cavity
Abdominopelvic cavity

(a) Lateral view   **(b) Frontal view**

LO 3.10 Body Cavities

The body contains many **cavities**. Some, like the nasal cavity, open to the outside. Five cavities do not open to the outside and are shown in *Figure 3.12*.

- **Cranial** cavity—contains the brain within the skull.
- **Thoracic** cavity—contains the heart, lungs, thymus gland, trachea, and esophagus, as well as numerous blood vessels and nerves.
- **Abdominal** cavity—is separated from the thoracic cavity by the **diaphragm** and contains the stomach, intestines, liver, spleen, pancreas, and kidneys.
- **Pelvic** cavity—is surrounded by the pelvic bones and contains the urinary bladder, part of the large intestine, the rectum, the anus, and the internal reproductive organs.
- **Spinal** cavity—contains the spinal cord.

The abdominal cavity and pelvic cavity are collectively referred to as the **abdominopelvic** cavity.

Abbreviations	
LLQ	left lower quadrant
LUQ	left upper quadrant
RLQ	right lower quadrant
RUQ	right upper quadrant

LO 3.11 Abdominal Quadrants and Regions

One way of referring to the locations of abdominal structures and to the site of abdominal pain and other abnormalities is to divide the abdominal region into **quadrants**, as shown in *Figure 3.13a*. The locations are **right upper quadrant (RUQ), left upper quadrant (LUQ), right lower quadrant (RLQ),** and **left lower quadrant (LLQ).** Each quadrant has a three-letter abbreviation as shown—for example, RUQ.

The **abdomen** can also be divided into nine **regions** *(Figure 3.13b)*. The central region is called the **umbilical** region, as it is located around the **umbilicus**. The areas above and below that region are named relative to the stomach—**epigastric**, above the stomach, and **hypogastric**, below the stomach.

The six remaining regions are on the right and left sides of these three central regions. The upper regions on either side of the epigastric region, which sit below the ribs, are named the right and left **hypochondriac** regions. The regions on either side of the umbilical region are named the right and left **lumbar** regions (according to the area of the spine nearby). The regions on either side of the hypogastric region are named the right and left **inguinal** (groin) regions.

▼ Figure 3.13 Regional
anatomy. (a) ©McGraw-
Hill Education/JW Ramsey,
photographer. (b) ©McGraw-
Hill Education/JW Ramsey,
photographer.

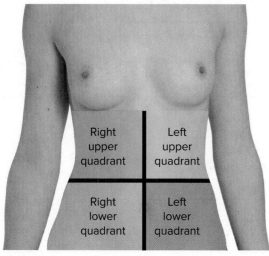

Right upper quadrant

Left upper quadrant

Right lower quadrant

Left lower quadrant

(a) Abdominal quadrants

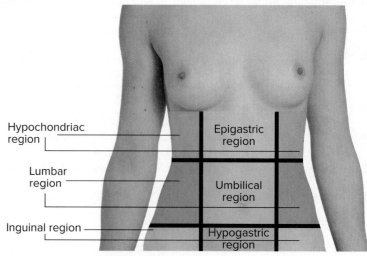

Hypochondriac region

Lumbar region

Inguinal region

Epigastric region

Umbilical region

Hypogastric region

(b) Abdominal regions

WORD	PRONUNCIATION		ELEMENTS	DEFINITION
abdomen	**AB**-doh-men		Latin *abdomen*	Part of the trunk between the thorax and the pelvis
abdominal (adj)	ab-**DOM**-in-al	S/	-al *pertaining to*	Pertaining to the abdomen
		R/	abdomin- *abdomen*	
abdominopelvic	ab-**DOM**-ih-noh-**PEL**-vik	S/	-ic *pertaining to*	Pertaining to the abdomen and pelvis
		R/CF	abdomin/o- *abdomen*	
		R/	-pelv- *pelvis*	
cavity	**KAV**-ih-tee		Latin *hollow place*	Hollow space or body compartment
cavities (pl)	**KAV**-ih-tees			
cranial	**KRAY**-nee-al	S/	-al *pertaining to*	Pertaining to the skull
		R/CF	cran/i- *skull*	
diaphragm	**DIE**-ah-fram		Greek *diaphragm, fence*	The musculomembranous partition separating the abdominal and thoracic cavities
epigastric	ep-ih-**GAS**-trik	S/	-ic *pertaining to*	Pertaining to the abdominal region above the stomach
		P/	epi- *above*	
		R/	gastr- *stomach*	The upper central region of the abdomen located
epigastrium (noun)	ep-ih-**GAS**-tree-um	S/	-ium *structure*	between the costal margins and the subcostal plane
hypochondriac	high-poh-**KON**-dree-ack	S/	-ac *pertaining to*	Pertaining to below the cartilage below the ribs
		P/	hypo- *below*	
		R/	-chondr- *cartilage*	
hypogastric	high-poh-**GAS**-trik	S/	-ic *pertaining to*	Pertaining to the abdominal region below the stomach
		P/	hypo- *below*	
		R/	-gastr- *stomach*	
inguinal	**IN**-gwin-a	S/	-al *pertaining to*	Pertaining to the groin
		R/	inguin- *groin*	
lumbar	**LUM**-bar	S/	-ar *pertaining to*	Pertaining to the region in the back and sides between the ribs and pelvis
		R/	lumb- *lower back, loin*	
pelvic	**PEL**-vic	S/	-ic *pertaining to*	Pertaining to the pubic bone
		R/	pelv- *pelvis*	
quadrant	**KWAD**-rant		Latin *one quarter*	One-quarter of a circle
umbilical	um-**BIL**-ih-kal	S/	-al *pertaining to*	Pertaining to or around the umbilicus or the center of the abdomen
umbilicus (noun)	um-**BIL**-ih-kus	R/	umbilic- *belly button (navel)*	Pit in the abdomen where the umbilical cord entered the fetus

Exercises

A. Take a closer look at the breakdown of medical terms. *The medical term is given to you. Break it down into elements with a slash (/). See how the combination of elements will give you the meaning of the entire term.* <u>The first one is done for you.</u> *Fill in the blanks.* **LO 3.11, 3.D**

1. *epigastrium*

$$\frac{epi}{above} \Big/ \frac{gastr}{stomach} \Big/ \frac{ium}{structure}$$

2. *hypogastric*

_____ / _____ / _____

3. *abdominopelvic*

_____ / _____ / _____

> 💡 **Study Hint**
> Remember to start with the suffix and work back to the front of the term.

B. Create medical terms related to the body cavities. *Fill in the blank with the missing word elements.* **LO 3.10, 3.11, 3.C**

1. The quadrants mark the areas of the _____ /al cavity.

2. The center of the abdominal regions is the _____ /al region.

The Body as a Whole
Challenge Your Knowledge

A. **Demonstrate your knowledge of directional terms and abbreviations by identifying the correct choice.** Select the correct answer that completes each statement. (**LO 3.9, 3.11, 3.E**)

1. The epigastric region is _____ the stomach.

   a. above

   b. below

2. Therefore, the epigastric region is _____ to the stomach.

   a. superior

   b. inferior

3. The umbilical region is so named because it is in the _____ of the abdomen.

   a. center

   b. back

4. The umbilical region is _____ to the epigastric region.

   a. inferior

   b. superior

5. In the abbreviation LLQ, the first "L" means _____.

   a. lower

   b. left

6. The spine is _____ to the heart.

   a. anterior

   b. posterior

7. The nose is _____ to the chin.

   a. superior

   b. inferior

8. The umbilicus is _____ to the spine.

   a. dorsal

   b. ventral

9. The toes are _____ to the knee.

   a. distal

   b. proximal

B. **Latin and Greek terms.** There is no easy way to remember these—you just have to know them so that you can relate to their meanings. Match the terms in 1–10 to the meanings in a-j. (**LO 3.2, 3.3, 3.6, 3.A**)

_____ 1. secrete

_____ 2. helix

_____ 3. hormone

_____ 4. ligament

_____ 5. cell

_____ 6. matrix

_____ 7. mutation

_____ 8. membrane

_____ 9. cartilage

_____ 10. tendon

a. a storeroom

b. to change

c. gristle

d. release

e. band

f. coil

g. mother

h. to set in motion

i. sinew

j. parchment

C. Knowledge of anatomic locations on the body will make your communications with other health professionals precise. Challenge yourself with the following questions. Choose T if the statement is true. Choose F if the statement is false. (LO 3.9, 3.10, 3.11)

1. Standing erect with feet flat on the floor, face and eyes facing forward, and arms at the side with palms facing forward is the anatomical position.   T   F

2. A transverse plane is a horizontal plane.   T   F

3. Frontal and sagittal planes are both vertical planes.   T   F

4. Inferior is situated above another part of the body.   T   F

5. *Dorsal* means the same as *anterior.*   T   F

6. The abdominal cavity contains the urinary bladder.   T   F

7. The thoracic cavity is superior to the pelvic cavity, and the pelvic cavity is inferior to the abdominal cavity.   T   F

8. The diaphragm divides the pelvic cavity and the abdominal cavity.   T   F

9. In RUQ, "Q" means *quadrant.*   T   F

10. The RUQ and the LUQ are divided by a sagittal plane.   T   F

D. What am I? Fill in the blanks with the correct answers. (LO 3.1, 3.2, 3.4)

1. Anabolism + catabolism = _____.

2. The largest organelle that directs all the activities of the cell is the _____.

3. This forms the tip of your nose, the shape of your ear, and the larynx: _____.

4. The relatively constant internal environment in the body is _____.

5. Standing erect, with feet flat on the floor, face and eyes facing forward, and arms at the side, palms facing

   forward is _____.

©2014 Nucleus Medical Media

The Body as a Whole

E. Use the language of anatomy to answer the questions. Select the correct answer to each question. **(LO 3.9)**

1. Which of the following medical terms is NOT an anatomic plane?

   a. transverse   **d.** supine

   b. frontal   **e.** coronal

   c. sagittal

2. Which of the following medical terms is NOT a correct pair of opposites?

   a. anterior   posterior

   b. inferior   superior

   c. dorsal   proximal

   d. prone   supine

   e. caudal   cephalic

3. Which of the following medical terms has an element meaning *nearest*?

   a. ventral   **d.** sagittal

   b. proximal   **e.** superior

   c. supine

4. Which of the following terms means the same thing as *coronal*?

   a. frontal   **d.** dorsal

   b. superior   **e.** cephalic

   c. ventral

5. If dorsal is *equivalent to* posterior, it means they are

   a. nouns.   **d.** the same.

   b. verbs.   **e.** the opposite.

   c. adjectives.

F. Anatomic positions and planes. You must know anatomic positions to prepare a patient for any type of procedure or surgery. Anatomic planes can help define radiologic studies. Using this knowledge, fill in each blank with the correct term that completes each statement. **(LO 3.9)**

1. The surgeon needs his patient in the _____ position to remove a lesion on his back.

2. To prepare for a knee arthroscopy, the patient will be in the _____ position.

3. When the palms of the hands are faced up, the forearms are in the _____ position.

4. A plane that divides the body into an upper, or superior, portion and a lower, or inferior, portion is called a _____ plane.

5. A frontal plane can also be called a _____ plane.

G. Use the language of anatomy to answer the following questions about the cell. Select the correct answer that completes each statement or answers each question. (LO 3.2)

1. Which one of the following medical terms is *not* an organelle?

   a. lysosomes   d. sulcus

   b. nucleolus   e. mitochondria

   c. endoplasmic reticulum

2. The fluid contained inside the cell is

   a. cytoplasm.   d. synovial fluid.

   b. endoplasm.   e. plasma.

   c. ectoplasm.

3. What surrounds and protects the cell?

   a. Golgi complex   d. ribosomes

   b. endoplasmic reticulum   e. cell membrane

   c. lysosomes

4. What are the chemical messenger cells called?

   a. lymphocytes   d. hormones

   b. erythrocytes   e. minerals

   c. electrolytes

5. What type of tasks do organelles carry out?

   a. excretory   d. communicative

   b. sensory   e. reproductive

   c. metabolic

H. Build medical terms using your knowledge of elements and their proper position in a medical term. Fill in the blanks. (LO 3.1, 3.2, 3.11, 3.C)

1. Small mass   molec/_____

2. Pertaining to below the stomach   _____ / _____ /ic

3. Manifestation of a genome   _____ /o/type

4. Pertaining to urine   urin/_____

5. A change in condition (when the elements are taken literally)   _____ /ism

6. Small organ   organ/_____

7. Small nucleus   nucle/o/_____

8. Enzyme that digests foreign material   lys/o/_____

I. Body cavities. The organ is given to you in the following chart. Fill in the chart. Organize the terms in the correct body cavity, and then place the organ in the correct body system. Note: There are two answers to every question. (LO 3.4, 3.10, 3.A)

Organ	Body Cavity	Body System
brain	1.	2.
gallbladder	3.	4.
heart	5.	6.
kidneys	7.	8.
lungs	9.	10.
pituitary	11.	12.
prostate	13.	14.
spleen	15.	16.
uterus	17.	18.

The Body as a Whole

J. **Multiple choice is the format used for most national certification examinations.** Choose the correct answer to the statement or question. **(LO 3.2, 3.3, 3.4, 3.7, 3.8)**

1. The single, fertilized cell is called the

   a. mitochondria.

   b. ribosome.

   c. organelle.

   d. zygote.

   e. blastocyst.

2. The word *membrane* means

   a. small organ.

   b. fluid inside a cell.

   c. thin layer of tissue.

   d. chemical substance.

   e. molecule with electrical charge.

3. Possessing a developmental structural defect is

   a. mutation.

   b. anatomic.

   c. dysmorphic.

   d. metabolic.

   e. phenotype.

4. Which of the following functions as a shock absorber?

   a. cartilage

   b. muscle

   c. tendon

   d. ligament

   e. blood vessel

5. The prefix *endo-* means

   a. outside.

   b. within.

   c. around.

   d. behind.

   e. across.

6. The study of the function of tissues is called

   a. cytology.

   b. cardiology.

   c. dermatology.

   d. histology.

   e. gastroenterology.

7. The type of cell that forms cartilage is a

   a. chondroblast.

   b. chondrocyte.

   c. osteocyte.

   d. osteoclast.

   d. osteoblast.

8. How many quadrants are in the abdominal region?

   a. one

   b. two

   c. three

   d. four

   e. five

9. *Hypogastric* refers to a

   a. body region.

   b. body opening.

   c. body quadrant.

   d. body cavity.

   e. body plane.

10. What forms the gliding surface where two bones meet to form a joint?

   a. cartilage

   b. blood vessels

   c. collagen

   d. ligaments

   e. lymph

K. Spelling comprehension. Select the correct spelling of the term. **(LO 3.A)**

1. **a.** organale   **b.** orgenele   **c.** organelle   **d.** orgenelle   **e.** organel

2. **a.** sinovial   **b.** sinnovial   **c.** synoveal   **d.** synevial   **e.** synovial

3. **a.** rybosome   **b.** ribosonme   **c.** rhibosome   **d.** ribosome   **e.** rhybosone

4. **a.** diaphram   **b.** diaphrame   **c.** diaphragm   **d.** deaphragm   **e.** diafragm

5. **a.** feneotyp   **b.** feenotipe   **c.** pheneotype   **d.** pheenotype   **e.** phenotype

6. **a.** nucklii   **b.** nucleei   **c.** nuclei   **d.** neuclei   **e.** nucklie

7. **a.** zygoat   **b.** zigote   **c.** zygote   **d.** zigotte   **e.** zygoate

8. **a.** endockrine   **b.** endocrine   **c.** endoccrine   **d.** endockryne   **e.** endocrin

9. **a.** osteocyte   **b.** osteoscyte   **c.** osteyosite   **d.** osteeoscite   **e.** osteasyte

10. **a.** histology   **b.** historyology   **c.** hystology   **d.** hestology   **e.** historology

L. Discuss the body cavities. Place each organ in the correct body cavity. Fill in the blanks. **(LO 3.4, 3.10)**

1. stomach   cavity: _____

2. spinal cord   cavity: _____

3. bladder   cavity: _____

4. pancreas   cavity: _____

5. thymus gland   cavity: _____

The Body as a Whole

M. **Comprehend, spell, and write medical terms pertaining to the body as a whole so that you communicate and document accurately and precisely in any health care setting.** You are given the meaning of the term. Spell it correctly and write it on the line. (**LO 3.2, 3.7, 3.9, 3.11, 3.A**)

1. muscle separating the thoracic and abdominal cavities _____

2. abdominal region above the stomach _____

3. in the body system building path, what organelles are composed of _____

4. a group of organic food compounds that includes sugar and starch _____

5. pertaining to, or nearer, the head _____

6. the chromosome characteristics of an individual cell _____

7. the manifestation of a genome _____

8. study of disorders produced by the effects of pollutants or diet on genes _____

N. **Describe the medical terms for the different anatomic positions, planes, and directions of the body.** Identify which of the following terms apply to anatomic position, planes, or directions of the body. Select the correct choice. (**LO 3.9**)

1. caudal

   a. anatomic position

   b. planes

   c. directions

2. transverse

   a. anatomic position

   b. planes

   c. directions

3. superior

   a. anatomic position

   b. planes

   c. directions

4. prone

   a. anatomic position

   b. planes

   c. directions

5. distal

   a. anatomic position

   b. planes

   c. directions

O. Apply correct medical terms to the anatomy and physiology of the body as a whole. Choose T if the answer is True. Choose F if the answer is False. (**LO 3.4**)

1. Muscles are in the immune system.		T	F
2. The reproductive system vocabulary is divided into male and female terms.		T	F
3. Teeth are considered part of the digestive system.		T	F
4. One of the functions of the urinary system is to remove wastes from the blood.		T	F
5. Muscles are in the immune system.		T	F

©2014 Nucleus Medical Media

Health professionals involved in the care of patients with dermatological diseases include

- **Dermatologists**, who are medical specialists in diseases of the skin.

- **Dermatopathologists**, who are medical specialists in dermatology and surgical pathology and who focus on the study of cutaneous diseases at a microscopic level.

- **Cosmetic surgeons**, who are board certified by the American Board of Cosmetic Surgery to enhance appearance through elective surgical and medical procedures.

- **Plastic surgeons**, who are board certified by the American Board of Plastic Surgery to reconstruct facial and body defects due to birth disorders, trauma, burns, and disease.

- **Nurse practitioners** and **physician assistants**, who with extensive training and experience in dermatology work under the supervision of dermatologists.

- **Estheticians**, also called *skin care therapists*, who perform various cosmetic procedures for the treatment of the skin. They do not diagnose, prescribe medications, or suggest treatments.

Chapter Learning Outcomes

In addition to anticipating Dr. Echols' needs for equipment to **biopsy**, diagnose, and treat the lesions of Mr. Rod Andrews in Case Report 4.1, you also have to be able to communicate clearly with her in medical terms and to understand her language as she communicates with you and the patient about the **etiology** (cause) and structure of the lesions. You will then need to document the medical history and treatment and communicate clearly with the patient about his treatment and **prognosis**.

To perform these tasks you must be able to:

LO 4.1   Explain the functions of the skin.

LO 4.2   Define the regions of the skin surface area and their percentage of the total surface area.

LO 4.3   Describe the structure of the skin: epidermis, dermis, hypodermis.

LO 4.4   Discuss common disorders of the skin.

LO 4.5   Describe the anatomy and physiology of the accessory skin organs.

LO 4.6   Identify disorders of the accessory skin organs.

LO 4.7   Discuss wounds and burns of the skin.

LO 4.8   Describe the process of healing and repair of the skin.

LO 4.9   Discuss the diagnostic procedures used in dermatology.

LO 4.10 Describe the therapeutic procedures used in dermatology.

LO 4.11 Define the types of pharmacologic agents used in dermatology.

LO 4.A   Use the medical terms of dermatology to communicate and document in writing accurately and precisely in any health care setting.

LO 4.B   Use the medical terms of dermatology to communicate verbally with accuracy and precision in any health care setting.

LO 4.C   Using word elements, construct medical terms associated with dermatology.

LO 4.D   Deconstruct medical terms associated with dermatology into their word elements (roots, combining forms, prefixes, and suffixes.)

LO 4.E   Identify health professionals involved in the care of patients with conditions related to dermatology.

LO 4.F   Identify and use correctly abbreviations of terms used in dermatology.

 ## Case Report (CR) 4.1

You are

. . . a clinical medical assistant working in the office of **dermatologist** Dr. Lenore Echols, a member of the Fulwood Medical Group.

Your patient is

. . . Mr. Rod Andrews, a 60-year-old man, who shows you three skin lesions— two on his left forearm and one on the back of his left hand. On questioning him, you learn that he has been living for the past 10 years in Arizona and has returned to the area to be near his daughter and young grandchildren. You find no other skin lesions on his body.

Lesson 4.1

Functions and Structure of the Skin

Lesson Objectives

The three lesions on Mr. Andrews' arm and hand developed in the superficial layer of the skin called the epidermis. This lesson looks at the structure and functions of the skin and at diseases of the epidermis so that you will be able to:

4.1.1 Discuss the functions and structure of the skin.

4.1.2 List the layers of the skin.

4.1.3 Name the tissues in the different layers of the skin.

4.1.4 Identify the functions of the different layers of the skin.

4.1.5 Describe disorders affecting the superficial layers of the skin, including cancers.

4.1.6 Apply correct medical terminology to the anatomy, physiology, and disorders of the superficial layers of the skin.

Keynotes

- The skin is the largest and most vulnerable organ in the body.
- There are four combining forms for skin:
  - *cutane/o*
  - *derm/a*
  - *dermat/o*
  - *derm/o*

Case Report (CR) 4.1 *(Continued)*

When Dr. Echols examined Mr. Andrews, she determined clinically that two of his lesions were basal cell **carcinomas** and she treated them with **cryosurgery**. She believed that the third lesion was a **squamous cell** carcinoma, and she performed a **biopsy removal** of that **lesion**. You sent it to the laboratory with a request for **pathological** diagnosis and determination of whether the lesion had been completely removed. This is done by ensuring that a normal skin margin completely surrounds the lesion when it is examined under the microscope.

LO 4.1, 4.2 Functions of the Skin

The **integumentary system** consists of the skin and its associated organs. The skin is also known as the **cutaneous** membrane. The cutaneous membrane is made up the **epidermis**, **dermis**, and **hypodermis** *(Figure 4.1)*. The study and treatment of the integumentary system is called **dermatology**. This organ system receives more medical and personal attention than any other organ system. Your understanding of its structure and functions will be used every day in your professional and personal life.

The skin is the largest organ in your body and accounts for 7% to 8% of body weight. The skin is the most vulnerable of all your organs because it is continually exposed to chemicals, trauma, infection, radiation, temperature change, humidity variation, and all the pollution of modern life. The skin is an important part of a person's self-image and an important part of total patient care.

The skin is a barrier that is not easily broken. Few infectious organisms can penetrate the skin on their own. Those that do use accidental breaks in the skin or rely on animals such as mosquitoes, fleas, or ticks to puncture the skin to allow access for the infectious organisms. The skin is also a barrier to solar radiation, including ultraviolet (UV) rays.

A summary of the functions of the skin:

- **Protection.** The skin is a physical barrier against injury, chemicals, ultraviolet rays, microbes, and toxins.
- **Water resistance.** You don't swell up every time you take a bath because your skin is water resistant. It also prevents water from leaking out from the body tissues.
- **Temperature regulation.** A network of capillaries in the skin opens up or dilates (vasodilation) when your body is too hot so that the blood flow increases and the heat from the blood dissipates through your skin. When your body is cold, the capillary network narrows (vasoconstriction), blood flow decreases, and heat is retained in your body.
- **Vitamin D synthesis.** As little as 15 to 30 minutes of sunlight daily allows your skin cells to initiate the metabolism of vitamin D, which is essential for bone growth and maintenance.
- **Sensation.** Nerve endings that detect touch, pressure, heat, cold, pain, vibration, and tissue injury are particularly numerous on your face, fingers, palms, soles, nipples, and genitals.
- **Excretion and secretion.** Water and small amounts of waste products from cell metabolism are lost through the skin by excretion (the process of removal of waste products from the body) and by secretion (the process of producing and releasing a substance by a tissue or organ of the body) from your sweat glands.
- **Social functions.** The skin reflects your emotions, blushing when you are self-conscious, going pale when you are frightened, wrinkling when you dislike something.

Epidermis

Dermis

Hypodermis (subcutaneous fat)

Cutaneous blood vessels

▲ **Figure 4.1** Structure of the cutaneous membrane.

64   CHAPTER 4 Integumentary System The Language of Dermatology

WORD	PRONUNCIATION		ELEMENTS	DEFINITION
biopsy	**BI**-op-see	S/ R/CF	-opsy *to view* bio- *life*	Removing tissue from a living person for laboratory examination
biopsy removal	**BI**-op-see re-**MUV**-al			Used for small tumors when complete removal provides tissue for a biopsy and cures the lesion
carcinoma	kar-sih-**NOH**-mah	S/ R/	-oma *tumor, mass* carcin- *cancer*	A malignant and invasive epithelial tumor
cryosurgery	cry-oh-**SUR**-jer-ee	S/ R/CF R/	-ery *process of* cry/o- *icy cold* -surg- *operate*	Use of liquid nitrogen or argon gas in a probe to freeze and kill abnormal tissue
cutaneous	kyu-**TAY**-nee-us	S/ R/CF	-us *pertaining to* cutane/o- *skin*	Pertaining to the skin
dermis dermal (adj)	**DER**-miss **DER**-mal		Greek *skin*	Connective tissue layer of the skin beneath the epidermis
dermatology	der-mah-**TOL**-oh-jee	S/ R/CF	-logy *study of* dermat/o- *skin*	Medical specialty concerned with disorders of the skin
dermatologist	der-mah-**TOL**-oh-jist	S/	-logist *one who studies*	Medical specialist in diseases of the skin
epidermis	ep-ih-**DER**-miss	P/ R/	epi- *upon* -dermis *skin*	Top layer of the skin
esthetics esthetician	es-**THET**-iks es-the-**TI**-shun	S/ R/	Greek *sensation* -ician *specialist* esthet- *beauty*	Concerned with beauty A therapist who enhances the beauty of the skin
integument	in-**TEG**-you-ment		Latin *a covering*	Organ system that covers the body, the skin being the main organ within the system
integumentary (adj)	in-**TEG**-you-**MEN**-tah-ree	S/ R/	-ary *pertaining to* integument- *covering of the body*	Pertaining to the covering of the body
lesion	**LEE**-zhun		Latin *injury*	Pathological change or injury in a tissue
microscope	**MY**-kroh-skope	P/ R/	micro- *small* -scope *instrument for viewing*	Instrument for viewing something small that cannot be seen in detail by the naked eye
microscopic (adj)	**MY**-kroh-**SKOP**-ik	S/	-ic *pertaining to*	Visible only with the aid of a microscope
pathology	pa-**THOL**-oh-jee	S/ R/CF R/	-logy *study of* path/o- *disease* -log- *to study*	Medical specialty dealing with the structural and functional changes of a disease process or the cause, development, and structural changes in disease
pathologic (adj)	path-oh-**LOJ**-ik	S/	-ic *pertaining to*	Pertaing to the changes in the body induced by disease
squamous cell	**SKWAY**-mus **SELL**		Latin *scaly*	Flat, scalelike epithelial cell

Exercises

A. Review the above WAD before starting this exercise. *Build your knowledge of the elements in the language of dermatology. Choose the best answer.* **LO 4.D**

1. The suffix *-oma* can mean tumor or

   a. gland   **b.** mass   **c.** cancer

2. Choose the term that has a word element meaning *study of:*

   a. dermatology   **b.** dermatologist   **c.** dermatitist

3. *Cryo-* is a combining form that signifies

   a. location   **b.** color   **c.** temperature

4. The term **cutaneous** means *pertaining to*

   a. skin   **b.** mass   **c.** tumor

Dr. Echols learned that Mr. Andrews had driven extensively in Arizona while wearing a short-sleeved shirt. His left forearm and hand were exposed to sunlight through the untinted car window to his left. This was an important factor in causing his skin cancers, all of which responded to the appropriate treatment.

Keynote

The skin provides protection, contains sensory organs, and helps control body temperature.

Keynotes

• The stratum granulosum waterproofs the skin.
• The stratum spinosum holds the epidermis together.

LO 4.3 Structure of the Skin

Epidermis

The three lesions that Mr. Andrews had were present in the **epidermis**, the most superficial layer of his skin. This layer

• Protects underlying structures.
• Withstands the toxic pollution of modern life.
• Sheds its superficial cells and renews them continually throughout life.
• Provides a waterproof barrier.

The epidermis is an **epithelial** tissue, which consists of four to five layers of cells, most of which are **keratinocytes**. Keratinocytes are formed in the bottommost layer of the epidermis, **stratum basale**, and then pushed up (migrate) to the topmost layer of the epidermis, the **stratum corneum** *(Figure 4.2)*. The palms of the hands and the soles of the feet have five layers; all other areas of the body have four. From superficial to deep, these layers are:

• **Stratum corneum:** a layer of compact, dead cells packed with **keratin**. These dead cells have no nuclei and are continually shed. Keratin is a tough, scaly protein that is also the basis for hair and nails.
• **Stratum lucidum:** only found in the palm of the hands and the soles of the feet, it is a thin translucent layer of cells. These cells, **keratinocytes**, are filled with a protein that becomes keratin.
• **Stratum granulosum:** these keratinocytes produce a fatty mixture that covers the surface of the cells and waterproofs them. This waterproof barrier not only stops water from getting in and out but also cuts off the supply of nutrients to the keratinocytes above it and they die.
• **Stratum spinosum:** the keratinocytes contain nuclei and are firmly attached to each other by numerous spines (hence "spinosum"). This enables the epidermis to be firm and strong.
• **Stratum basale:** a single layer of cells that form the keratinocytes. This layer also contains **melanocytes**, which produce the dark pigment **melanin**, and the tactile (touch) cells attached to sensory nerve fibers. The process by which keratinocytes migrate from this layer to the skin's surface, where they are shed as dead cells, takes about a month.

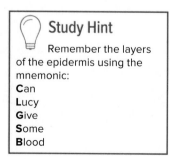

Study Hint

Remember the layers of the epidermis using the mnemonic:
Can
Lucy
Give
Some
Blood

▲ **Figure 4.2** Epidermis.

WORD	PRONUNCIATION		ELEMENTS	DEFINITION
epithelial (adj)	ep-ih-**THEE**-lee-al	S/ P/ R/CF	-al *pertaining to* epi- *upon* -thel/i- *nipple*	Relating to or consisting of epithelium
epithelium	ep-ih-**THEE**-lee-um	S/	-um *tissue*	Tissue that covers surfaces or lines cavities
keratin keratinocyte	**KER**-ah-tin ke-**RAT**-in-oh-site	 S/ R/CF	**Greek** *keratin* -cyte *cell* keratin/o- *keratin*	Protein found in the dead outer layer of skin and in nails and hair Cell producing a tough, horny protein (keratin) in the process of differentiating into the dead cells of the stratum corneum
melanin melanocyte	**MEL**-ah-nin **MEL**-an-oh-cyte	 S/ R/CF	Greek *black* -cyte *cell* melan/o- *black*	Black pigment found in skin, hair, retina Cell that synthesizes (produces) melanin
stratum strata (pl) stratum basale	**STRAH**-tum **STRAH**-tah **STRAH**-tum ba-**SAL**-eh	S/ R/ R/	-um *structure* strat- *layer* basal/e *deepest part*	A layer of tissue Deepest layer of the epidermis, from which the other cells originate and migrate
stratum corneum	**STRAH**-tum **COR**-nee-um	R/	corne- *having a horn*	Outermost layer of the epidermis that has cells containing keratin; the layer is tough and thick, like a horn
stratum granulosum	**STRAH**-tum gran-you-**LOH**-sum	S/ R/	-sum *pick up* granul/o- *small grain*	Layer of the epidermis where the cells contain granules of lipids
stratum lucidum	**STRAH**-tum **LOO**-si-dum	R/	lucid- *clear*	Layer of the epidermis only found on the palms of the hands and the soles of the feet
stratum spinosum	**STRAH**-tum spy-**NOH**-sum	S/	Latin *spiny*	Layer of the epidermis where the cells appear to have spines
tactile	**TAK**-tile		Latin *to touch*	Relating to touch

Exercises

A. Apply the correct rule for plurals and form the plural of the term. LO 4.A

1. There are many (strata/stratum) of the epidermis.

2. The most superficial layer of the epidermis, (strata/stratum) corneum, contains only dead keratinocytes.

B. Number the layers of the epidermis in the correct order, from superficial to deep. The most superficial layer is "1"; the deepest layer is "5." LO 4.3

_____ stratum lucidum

_____ stratum basale

_____ stratum granulosum

_____ stratum corneum

_____ stratum spinosum

C. Deconstruct medical terms to determine their meaning. *Identify the meaning of the word elements in each term.* **LO 4.D**

1. The root in the term **melanocyte** means:

   a. layer   **b.** color   **c.** spiny   **d.** cell   **e.** touch

2. The root in the term **lucidum** means:

   a. layer   **b.** pertaining to   **c.** structure   **d.** protein   **e.** clear

3. The suffix -*cyte* means:

   a. structure   **b.** pertaining to   **c.** small   **d.** state of   **e.** cell

LO 4.3 Structure of the Skin (continued)

Dermis

Figure 4.3 shows that the **dermis** is a much thicker tissue layer than the epidermis. The dermis is a type of connective tissue consisting mainly of **collagen**, a type of protein fiber produced by **fibroblasts**. Collagen provides strength and flexibility to the cutaneous membrane. The dermis is well supplied with blood vessels and nerves and contains the accessory skin organs: sweat glands, sebaceous glands, hair follicles, and nail roots. The accessory skin organs will be discussed later in this chapter. The boundary between the dermis and the epidermis is distinct: irregular and wavy.

Abbreviation	
SC	subcutaneous

Hypodermis

The **hypodermis**, the layer beneath the dermis, is the site of **subcutaneous** fat (**adipose** tissue). It is also called the **subcutaneous tissue layer** and is often referred to as **SC** in clinical documentation.

Epidermis

Dermis

Hypodermis

Sensory nerves

Motor nerve

▲ **Figure 4.3** Dermis and its organs.

WORD	PRONUNCIATION	ELEMENTS		DEFINITION
adipose	**ADD**-i-pose	S/ R/	-ose *condition* adip- *fat*	Containing fat
collagen	**KOL**-ah-jen	S/ R/	-gen *producing* coll/a- *glue*	Major protein of connective tissue, cartilage, and bone
fibroblast	**FIE**-bro-blast	S/ R/CF	-blast *germ cell* fibr/o- *fiber*	Cell that forms collagen fibers
hypodermis	high-poh-**DER**-miss	P/ R/	hypo- *below* -dermis *skin*	Tissue layer below the dermis
hypodermic (adj)	high-poh-**DER**-mik	S/ R/	-ic *pertaining to* -derm- *skin*	Beneath the skin
subcutaneous hypodermic (syn)	sub-kew-**TAY**-nee-us	S/ P/ R/CF	-ous *pertaining to* sub- *below* -cutan/e- *skin*	Below the skin

Exercises

A. The following definitions represent medical terms found in the above WAD. *Find the missing elements and build the terms. Fill in the blanks.* **LO 4.3, 4.C**

1. pertaining to below the skin: _____/derm/_____

2. containing fat: adip/_____

3. pertaining to below the skin: _____/cutane/_____

B. Answer the following questions regarding terms relating to the structure of the skin. LO 4.3

1. The type of cells that produce fibers is called a:

   a. melanocyte

   b. keratinocyte

   c. fibroblast

   d. adipose

   e. stratum

> **Study Hint**
> Whenever there are two or more terms with the same meaning, you must know all of them.

2. The type of connective tissue found in the hypodermis:

   a. epithelium

   b. collagen

   c. adipose

   d. keratin

Lesson 4.2

INTEGUMENTARY SYSTEM

Disorders of the Skin

Lesson Objectives

This lesson will enable you to use correct medical terminology to:

4.2.1 Describe common disorders of the skin.

4.2.2 Identify the different types of infections of the skin.

LO 4.4 Disorders of the Skin

Carcinomas

The **squamous cell carcinoma** *(Figure 4.4)* that Mr. Andrews (Case Report 4.1) had on his hand arose from keratinocytes in the stratum spinosum in the skin on the back of the hand, face, and ears, areas exposed to sunlight. It responds well to surgical removal but can **metastasize** (spread) to lymph glands if neglected.

Mr. Andrews's **basal cell carcinoma** *(Figure 4.5)* began in the cells of the stratum basale and invaded the dermis and epidermis. It is the most common skin cancer and is also the least dangerous because it does not metastasize.

Sunlight can also be an irritant to the skin, not only by burning it but by leading to cancer when there is excessive exposure, as it did for Mr. Andrews. Any congenital lesion of the skin, including various types of birthmarks and all **moles**, is referred to as a **nevus**.

Malignant melanoma *(Figure 4.6)* is the least common skin cancer but is the most deadly. It arises from the melanocytes in the stratum basale. It metastasizes quickly and is fatal if neglected.

▲ **Figure 4.4** Squamous cell carcinoma. ©BioPhoto Associates/Photo Researchers, Inc.

▲ **Figure 4.5** Basal cell carcinoma. ©BioPhoto Associates/ Photo Researchers, Inc.

▲ **Figure 4.6** Malignant melanoma. ©James Stevenson/Photo Researchers, Inc.

WORD	PRONUNCIATION	ELEMENTS		DEFINITION
basal	BAY-sal	S/ R/	-al *pertaining to* bas- *lower part*	Pertaining to the lower part of a structure
carcinoma	kar-sih-NOH-mah	S/ R/	-oma *tumor, mass* carcin- *cancer*	A malignant epithelial tumor
decubitus ulcer	de-KYU-bit-us UL-ser	P/ R/ R/	de- *from* -cubitus *lying down* ulcer *sore*	Sore caused by lying down for long periods of time
malignant	mah-LIG-nant	S/ R/	-ant *pertaining to* malign- *harmful*	Having the properties of being locally invasive and able to spread to distant parts of the body
melanoma	MEL-ah-NO-mah	S/ R/	-oma *tumor, mass* melan- *black*	Malignant tumor formed from cells that produce the pigment melanin
metastasis	meh-TAS-tah-sis	P/ R/	meta- *beyond* -stasis *stay in one place*	Spread of a disease from one part of the body to another
metastasize	meh-TAS-tah-size	S/ R/	-ize *affect in a specific way* -stat- *stand still*	To spread to distant parts
mole	MOLE		Latin *spot*	Benign localized area of melanin-producing cells
nevus nevi (pl)	NEE-vus NEE-vie		Latin *mole, birthmark*	Congenital or acquired lesion of the skin
squamous	SKWAY-mus		Latin *scaly*	Flat, scalelike epithelial cell

Exercises

A. Demonstrate that you are able to spell medical terms related to disorders of the skin. *Fill in the blank.* **LO 4.4, 4.A**

1. The medical term that means the same as *mole* is _____.

2. A cancerous tumor originating in the deepest layer of the epidermis is termed a _____ cell carcinoma.

3. The plural form of the term *nevus* is _____.

4. A _____ is a malignant tumor of cells that produce melanin.

Case Report (CR) 4.2

Fulwood Medical Center

Mrs. Rose McGinnis, a 72-year-old widow, was in a nursing home for the past 6 months. She was unable to get out of bed since surgery to repair a broken hip. She was depressed and difficult to feed and nurse. Two months ago, she developed **decubitus ulcers** over her buttocks and left heel. The ulcer over her buttocks became infected with a methicillin-resistant *Staphylococcus aureus* (MRSA). Staphylococcal septicemia ensued, and she died.

Pressure Sores

▲ **Figure 4.7** Decubitus ulcer on heel.
©Medical-on-line/Alamy

When a patient lies in one position for a long period, the pressure between the bed and bony body projections, like the lower spine or heel, cuts off the blood supply to the skin and **decubitus (pressure) ulcers** can appear *(Figure 4.7)*. The protective function of the skin is broken, and germs can enter the body. Pressure sores begin as a reddened area of the skin. With continued pressure on the skin overlying the bony structure, the epidermis may form blisters and erode (wear away). If the pressure continues, the dermis wears away, and then the hypodermis. If it continues, the muscles and bones can be affected. Other major factors in the breakdown of Rose's skin were that it was thin and dry because of aging. Also, her poor nutritional status had depleted the fatty protective layer in the hypodermis under the skin.

Allergic Reactions

Case Report (CR) 4.3

Fulwood Medical Center

Ms. Cheryl Fox is a 37-year-old nursing assistant working in a surgical unit in Fulwood Medical Center. Recently her fingers became red and itchy, with occasional **vesicles**. She also noticed irritation and swelling of her earlobes and a generalized **pruritus**. Over the weekend, both the itching and the rash on her hands worsened. A patch test by her dermatologist showed her to be **allergic** to nickel in rings that she wore on both hands and in her earrings. She wore these only on weekends and not during her workdays.

▲ **Figure 4.8** Dermatitis of ear due to nickel sensitivity. ©Dr. P. Marazzi/SPL/Photo Researchers, Inc.

Ms. Fox had a **dermatitis** *(Figure 4.8)* resulting from direct exposure to an irritating agent. In her case, it was not just a reaction to an irritant. Her form of **atopic (allergic) dermatitis** develops when the body becomes sensitive to an **allergen**. **Allergenic** agents include latex, nickel in jewelry, or poison ivy. This whole-body involvement was shown by her systemic symptoms of pruritus distant from the local irritant site. She has stopped wearing the rings and earrings at any time.

Eczema is a general term used for inflamed, itchy skin conditions. When the itchy skin is scratched, it becomes **excoriated** and produces the dry, red, scaly patches characteristic of eczema. Continued scratching can cause the rash to "weep" **serous** fluid that can lead to crusting of the area. There are numerous types of eczema, the most common type being **atopic** dermatitis, which is caused by an allergic reaction, such as that from which Ms. Fox suffers when she developed an **allergy** to nickel. Her vesicles were filled with a serous fluid.

Ichthyosis is a condition of dry, scaly skin. The skin is flaky and resembles the skin of a fish. This condition is usually inherited, but it also can be acquired.

S = Suffix   P = Prefix   R = Root   R/CF = Combining Form

WORD	PRONUNCIATION	ELEMENTS		DEFINITION
allergen allergenic (adj) allergy allergic (adj)	**AL**-er-jen al-er-**JEN**-ik **AL**-er-jee ah-**LER**-jik	S/ R/ S/	**-gen** *producing* **allerg-** *allergy* Greek *other work* **-ic** *pertaining to*	Substance producing a hypersensitivity (allergic) reaction Hypersensitivity to an allergen Pertaining to any response stimulated by an allergen
atopy atopic	**AY**-toh-pee ay-**TOP**-ik		Greek *strangeness*	State of hypersensitivity to an allergen; allergic
dermatitis	der-mah-**TYE**-tis	S/ R/	**-itis** *inflammation* **dermat-** *skin*	Inflammation of the skin
eczema eczematous (adj)	**EK**-zeh-mah ek-**ZEM**-ah-tus	 S/ R/	Greek *to boil or ferment* **-tous** *pertaining to* **eczema-** *eczema*	Inflammatory skin disease often with a serous discharge Pertaining to or resembling eczema
excoriate excoriation (noun)	eks-**KOR**-ee-ate eks-**KOR**-ee-**AY**-shun	S/ P/ R/ S/	**-ate** *composed of, pertaining to* **ex-** *away from, out of* **-cori-** *skin* **-ation** *process*	To scratch Scratch mark
ichthyosis	ik-thee-**OH**-sis	S/ R/	**-osis** *condition* **ichthy-** *fish*	Scaling and dryness of the skin
latex	**LAY**-tecks		Latin *liquid*	Manufactured from the milky liquid in rubber plants; used for gloves in patient care
pruritus pruritic (adj)	proo-**RYE**-tus proo-**RIT**-ik		Latin *to itch*	Itching Itchy
serous	**SEER**-us		Latin *serum*	Thicker and less transparent than water
vesicle	**VES**-ih-kull		Latin *small sac*	Small sac containing liquid; for example, a blister

Exercises

A. Medical terms can have small differences that make them entirely new words. *Fill in the blanks with the correct terms.* **LO 4.4, 4.A**

allergens   allergenic   allergy   allergic

1. After many _____ tests, it was determined that she was _____ to mold.

2. There were too many _____ substances in the carpet, therefore it was removed from the room.

3. Dust mites, peanuts, and pollen can be _____ to some people.

B. One of the following terms is a noun (person, place, or thing), and the other term is a verb (action).
Identify the noun and verb. **LO 4.4, 4.A**

1. Excori**ate**   Noun or verb: _____

2. Excori**ation**   Noun or verb: _____

▲ **Figure 4.9** Shingles. ©VisualDx

▲ **Figure 4.10** Tinea pedis between toes. ©SPL/Photo Researchers, Inc.

▲ **Figure 4.11** Oral thrush. ©Dr. P. Marazzi/ SPL/Photo Researchers, Inc.

▲ **Figure 4.12** House dust mite. ©Meckes/Ottawa/Photo Researchers, Inc.

LO 4.4 Disorders of the Skin (continued)

Skin Infections

The skin is also susceptible to many different types of infections. The following are examples.

Viral Infections

Warts (verrucas) are caused by the human papillomavirus invading the epidermis and causing the outer epidermal cells to produce a roughened projection from the skin surface. Human papillomavirus is discussed extensively in *Chapter 8.*

Varicella-zoster virus causes **chickenpox** in unvaccinated people, forming macules, papules, and vesicles. The virus can then remain dormant in the peripheral nerves for decades before erupting as the painful vesicles of **herpes zoster (shingles)** *(Figure 4.9).*

Fungal Infections

Tinea is a general term for a group of related skin infections caused by different species of fungi. The fungi live on, and are strictly confined to, the nonliving stratum corneum and its derivatives, hair and nails, where keratin provides their food. The different types of tinea take their name from the location of the infection.

Tinea pedis, athlete's foot, causes itching, redness, and peeling of the foot, particularly between the toes *(Figure 4.10).* **Tinea capitis** describes infection of the scalp (ringworm); **tinea corporis** is the name for infections of the body. **Tinea cruris** ("jock itch") is the name for infections of the groin. The fungus spreads from animals, from the soil, and by direct contact with infected individuals. **Tinea versicolor** is characterized by brown and white patches on the trunk.

The yeastlike fungus **Candida** can produce recurrent infections of the skin, nails, and mucous membranes. The first sign can be a recurrent diaper rash or **thrush** in infants. Older children can show recurrent or persistent lesions on the scalp. In adults, chronic **candidiasis** can affect the mouth (**thrush**) *(Figure 4.11)* and vagina, as well as the skin. It can also be associated with diseases of the immune system *(see Chapter 12).*

Parasitic Infestations

A **parasite** is an organism that lives in contact with and feeds off another organism (host). This process is called an **infestation**. It is different from an **infection**.

Lice are small, wingless, blood-sucking parasites that produce the disease **pediculosis** by attaching their eggs (nits) to hair and clothing *(Table 4.1).*

Scabies ("itch mites") produce an intense, itching rash, often in the genital area, waist, breast, and armpits. The mites live and lay eggs under the skin.

The skin normally sheds its cells. These tiny specks form some of the dust on our furniture, floors, and carpets. The house dust mite *(Figure 4.12)* thrives on the keratin of these cells and lives well on carpets, upholstery, pillows, and mattresses. Many people are allergic to the inhaled feces of these parasites.

Bacterial Infections

Staphylococcus aureus (commonly called *staph*) is the most common bacterium to invade the skin and is the cause of pimples, boils, **carbuncles**, and **impetigo**. It can infect hair follicles and the surrounding tissues to produce **furuncles** and carbuncles. Staph can cause a **cellulitis** of the epidermis and dermis.

Necrotizing fasciitis is caused when some strains of staph and strep produce enzymes that are very toxic and digest the connective tissues and spread into muscle layers.

Table 4.1 Pediculosis

Louse (lice, pl)	Attachment of Eggs	Disease
Pediculus capitis	Hair of scalp	Pediculosis capitis
Phthirus pubis (crab-shaped)	Pubic hair	Pediculosis cruris (crabs)
Pediculus humanus	Clothing, body hair	Pediculosis corporis

WORD	PRONUNCIATION		ELEMENTS	DEFINITION
Candida candidiasis thrush	**KAN**-did-ah can-dih-**DIE**-ah-sis THRUSH	S/ R/	Latin *dazzling white* -iasis *condition, state of* candid- *Candida*	A yeastlike fungus Infection with the yeastlike fungus *Candida* Infection with *Candida albicans*
carbuncle	**KAR**-bunk-ul		Latin *carbuncle*	Infection composed of many furuncles in a small area, often on the back of the neck
cellulitis	sell-you-**LIE**-tis	S/ R/	-itis *inflammation* cellul- *small cell*	Infection of subcutaneous connective tissue
furuncle	**FU**-rung-kel		Latin *a boil*	An infected hair follicle that spreads into the tissues around the follicle
herpes zoster shingles (syn)	**HER**-pees **ZOS**-ter		**herpes** *to creep or spread* **zoster** *belt, girdle*	Painful eruption of vesicles that follows a dermatome or nerve root on one side of the body
impetigo	im-peh-**TIE**-go		Latin *scabby eruption*	Infection of the skin that produces thick, yellow crusts
infection	in-**FEK**-shun	S/ R/	-ion *process* infect- *tainted, internal invasion*	Invasion of the body by disease-producing microorganisms
infestation	in-fes-**TAY**-shun	S/ R/	-ation *process* infest- *invade*	Act of being invaded on the skin by a troublesome other species, such as a parasite
louse lice (pl)	LOWSE LICE		Old English *louse*	Parasitic insect
necrotizing fasciitis	neh-kroh-**TIZE**-ing fash-eh-**EYE**-tis	S/ R/CF S/ S/ R/CF	-ing *quality of* necr/o- *death* -tiz- *pertaining to* -itis *inflammation* fasc/i – *fascia*	Inflammation of fascia, producing death of the tissue
parasite	**PAR**-ah-site		Greek *guest*	An organism that attaches itself to, lives on or in, and derives its nutrition from another species
pediculosis	peh-dick-you-**LOH**-sis	S/ R/	-osis *condition* pedicul- *louse*	An infestation with lice
scabies	**SKAY**-bees		Latin *to scratch*	Skin disease produced by mites
tinea	**TIN**-ee-ah		Latin *worm*	General term for a group of related skin infections caused by different species of fungi
tinea capitis	**TIN**-ee-ah **CAP**-it-us	S/ R/	-is *pertaining to* capit- *head*	Fungal infection of the scalp
tinea corporis	**TIN**-ee-ah **KOR**-por-is	S/ R/	-is *pertaining to* corpor- *body*	Fungal infection of the body
tinea cruris	**TIN**-ee-ah **KROO**-ris	S/ R/	-is *pertaining to* crur- *leg*	Fungal infection of the groin
tinea versicolor	**TIN**-ee-ah **VERSE**-ih-col-or	R/CF R/	vers/i- *to turn* -color *color*	Fungal infection of the trunk in which the skin loses pigmentation
verruca	ver-**ROO**-cah		Latin *wart*	Wart caused by a virus

Exercises

A. Demonstrate that you are able to spell medical terms related to disorders of the skin. *Fill in the blanks.* **LO 4.4**

1. A condition caused by lice infestation: _____

2. Inflammation of a small cell: _____

B. The terms for skin conditions are similar. *It is important to know the specific differences in skin conditions. Fill in the blanks.* **LO 4.4**

1. One infected hair follicle that spreads to surrounding tissues: _____

2. A small area of many infected hair follicles: _____

3. Skin infection characterized by thick, yellow crusts: _____

4. Skin infection caused by mites: _____

5. Skin infection caused by fungus (nonspecific): _____

6. Infection caused by the fungus *Candida* (two terms mean the same thing): _____ and _____

▲ **Figure 4.13** Systemic lupus erythematosus. ©Dr. P. Marazzi/SPL/Photo Researchers, Inc.

▲ **Figure 4.14** Scleroderma. ©SPL/Science Source

▲ **Figure 4.15** Psoriasis. ©Dave Bolton/ Getty Images RF

LO 4.4 Diseases of the Skin

Collagen Diseases

Collagen, a fibrous protein, accounts for 30% of total body protein. Therefore, collagen diseases can have a dramatic effect all over the body. Collagen diseases, **autoimmune** or otherwise, attack collagen or other components of connective tissue.

Systemic lupus erythematosus (SLE), an autoimmune disease, occurs most commonly in women and produces characteristic skin lesions. A butterfly-shaped red rash on both cheeks joined across the bridge of the nose is commonly seen (*Figure 4.13*). It is associated with fever, fatigue, joint pains, and multiple internal organ involvement.

Rosacea produces a facial rash similar to that of SLE, and the underlying capillaries become enlarged and show through the skin. It is thought to be worsened by alcohol and spicy food. Its etiology is unknown. It has no **systemic** complications.

Scleroderma is a chronic, persistent autoimmune disease, occurring more often in women and characterized by hardening and shrinking of the skin that makes it feel leathery (*Figure 4.14*). Joints show swelling, pain, and stiffness. Internal organs such as the heart, lungs, kidneys, and digestive tract can be involved in a similar process. The etiology is unknown, and there is no effective treatment.

Other Skin Diseases

Psoriasis (*Figure 4.15*) is marked by itchy, flaky, red patches of skin of various sizes covered with white or silvery scales. It appears most commonly on the scalp, elbows, and knees. Its cause is unknown.

Vitiligo produces pale, irregular patches of skin. It is thought to have an autoimmune etiology.

Skin Manifestations of Internal Disease

Signs of the presence of cancer inside the body are often shown by skin lesions, even before the cancer has produced **symptoms** or been diagnosed.

Dermatomyositis (*Figure 4.16*) is often associated with ovarian cancer, which can appear within 4 to 5 years after the skin disease is diagnosed. It is an inflammatory condition causing symptoms of muscle weakness and a characteristic skin rash found around the eyes.

▲ **Figure 4.16** Periorbital rash of dermatomyositis. ©Medical-on-line/Alamy

Study Hint

There are many different suffixes that mean *pertaining to*. Some have been introduced in the next WAD.

WORD	PRONUNCIATION	ELEMENTS		DEFINITION
autoimmune	aw-toh-im-YUNE	P/ R/CF	**auto-** *self, same* **-immune** *immune response*	Immune reaction directed against a person's own tissue.
dermatomyositis	**DER**-mah-toh-**MY**-oh-site-is	S/ R/CF R/	**-itis** *inflammation* **dermat/o-** *skin* **-myos-** *muscle*	Inflammation of the skin and muscles
psoriasis	so-**RYE**-ah-sis		Greek *the itch*	Rash characterized by reddish, silver-scaled patches
rosacea	roh-**ZAY**-she-ah		Latin *rosy*	Persistent erythematous rash of the central face
scleroderma	sklair-oh-**DERM**-ah	S/ R/CF	**-derma** *skin* **scler/o-** *hard*	Thickening and hardening of the skin due to new collagen formation
sign (objective) symptom (subjective) symptomatic (adj)	SINE **SIMP**-tum simp-toh-**MAT**-ik	S/ R/	Latin *mark* Greek *sign* **-ic** *pertaining to* **symptomat-** *symptoms*	Physical evidence of a disease process Departure from normal health experienced by the patient Pertaining to the symptoms of a disease
systemic lupus erythematosus	sis-**TEM**-ik **LOO**-pus er-ih-**THEE**-mah-toh-sus	S/ R/ S/ R/	**-ic** *pertaining to* **system-** *body system* **lupus** *wolf* **-osus** *condition* **erythemat-** *redness*	Inflammatory connective tissue disease affecting the whole body
vitiligo	vit-ill-**EYE**-go		Latin *skin blemish*	Nonpigmented white patches on otherwise normal skin

Exercises

A. Building medical terms and taking them apart force you to focus on the elements they contain. *Understanding elements is the key to increasing your medical vocabulary. Deconstruct the following terms to increase your knowledge of their elements.* **LO 4.4, 4.D**

1. In the term **erythematosus,** the root means:

    a. condition of   **b.** blemish   **c.** red   **d.** inflammation

2. In the term **symptomatic,** the suffix means:

    a. pertaining to   **b.** inflammation   **c.** painful   **d.** condition of

3. In the term **dermatomyositis,** the word element that means *skin* is a:

    a. root/combining form   **b.** prefix   **c.** suffix

4. In the term **autoimmune,** the word element that means *self* is a:

    a. root/combining form   **b.** prefix   **c.** suffix

Accessory Skin Organs

Lesson Objectives

Hair follicles and their associated sebaceous glands, sweat glands, and nails are organs located in your skin. They each have specific anatomical and physiologic characteristics. You must understand their roles in the different functions of the skin and in diseases that affect the skin. This lesson will enable you to use correct medical terminology to:

4.3.1 Name the associated skin organs.

4.3.2 Identify the anatomy and physiology of the associated skin organs.

4.3.3 Match the structures of the different organs to their functions.

4.3.4 Describe disorders affecting the associated skin organs.

4.3.5 Explain the etiology of disorders affecting the associated skin organs.

 Case Report (CR) 4.4

You are

. . . a medical assistant working with Lenore Echols, MD, a dermatologist in Fulwood Medical Center.

Your patient is

. . . Wayne Winter, an 18-year-old man, who has been accepted to college in the fall.

He has had acne since the age of 15 and has tried numerous over-the-counter products. Retinoic acid has also been unsuccessful. He has numerous **comedones**, **papules**, **pustules**, and scars on his face and forehead with severe **cystic** lesions and scars on his back. His social life is nonexistent, and he is teased by his peers. He wishes to change all this before he gets to college.

Your role is to document his care and explain to him how to use the medications Dr. Echols prescribes, what their effects will be, and his prognosis.

LO 4.5, 4.6 Hair Follicles and Sebaceous Glands

Each hair follicle has a **sebaceous gland** opening into it *(Figure 4.17)*. The gland secretes into the follicle a mixture of oily, acidic **sebum** and broken-down cells from the base of the gland.

Around puberty, **androgens** are thought to trigger excessive production of sebum from the glands, which then brings excessive numbers of broken-down cells toward the skin surface. This blocks the follicle, forming a **comedo** (whitehead or blackhead). Comedones can stay closed, leading to **papules**, or can **rupture**, allowing bacteria to get in and produce **pustules**. These are the classic signs of **acne**, which is said to affect, in different degrees, about 85% of people between 12 and 25 years *(Figure 4.18)*. For many acne patients, treatment is difficult during puberty and the face can be scarred.

A different skin problem involving the sebaceous glands is **seborrheic dermatitis.** The glands are thought to be inflamed and to produce a different sebum. The skin around the face and scalp is reddened and covered with yellow, greasy scales. In infants, this condition is called cradle cap. Seborrheic dermatitis of the scalp produces dandruff. **Dandruff** is clumps of these keratinocytes stuck together with **sebum,** oil from **sebaceous** glands.

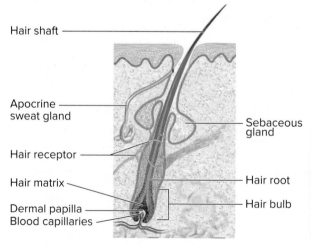

Hair shaft

Apocrine sweat gland

Hair receptor

Hair matrix

Dermal papilla
Blood capillaries

Sebaceous gland

Hair root

Hair bulb

▲ **Figure 4.17** Hair follicle and sebaceous gland.

▲ **Figure 4.18** Acne. ©Teim/Shutterstock. com RF

WORD	PRONUNCIATION		ELEMENTS	DEFINITION
acne	**AK**-nee		Greek *point*	Inflammatory disease of sebaceous glands and hair follicles
androgen	**AN**-droh-jen	S/ R/CF	**-gen** *to produce* **andr/o-** *male*	Hormone that promotes masculine characteristics
comedo comedones (pl)	**KOM**-ee-doh		Latin *eat up*	A whitehead or blackhead caused by too much sebum and too many keratin cells blocking the hair follicle
cyst cystic (adj)	SIST **SIS**-tik	S/ R/	Greek *sac, bladder* **-ic** *pertaining to* **cyst-** *cyst, bladder*	An abnormal, fluid-containing sac Relating to a cyst
dandruff	**DAN**-druff		Old English *scurf*	Seborrheic scales from the scalp
papule	**PAP**-yul		Latin *pimple*	Small, circumscribed elevation on the skin
pustule	**PUS**-tyul		Latin *pustule*	Small protuberance on the skin that contains pus
rupture	**RUP**-tyur		Latin *break*	Break or tear of any organ or body part
sebaceous glands sebum	se-**BAY**-shus GLANDZ **SEE**-bum	S/ R	**-ous** *pertaining to* **sebace-** *sebum* Latin *wax*	Glands in the dermis that open into hair follicles and secrete an oily fluid called sebum. Waxy secretion of the sebaceous glands
seborrhea	seb-oh-**REE**-ah	S/ R/CF	**-rrhea** *flow* **seb/o-** *sebum*	Excessive amount of sebum
seborrheic (adj)	seb-oh-**REE**-ik	S/	**-ic** *pertaining to*	Pertaining to seborrhea

Exercises

A. Recognize the causes and disorders related to the hair follicles and sebaceous glands. *Match the term to their correct.* **LO 4.6, 4.A**

_____ **1.** sebum

_____ **2.** cyst

_____ **3.** pustule

_____ **4.** acne

_____ **5.** comedo

_____ **6.** dandruff

_____ **7.** rupture

_____ **8.** androgen

_____ **9.** papule

_____ **10.** seborrhea

a. point

b. containing pus

c. whitehead, blackhead

d. wax

e. sac, bladder

f. hormone that promotes masculine characteristics

g. excessive amount of sebum

h. break or tear of any organ or part

i. seborrheic scales from the scalp

j. small, circumscribed elevation of the skin

B. Indicate if the statement is true or false. LO 4.6, 4.A

1. A *pustule* is filled with pus.   True   False

2. *Acne* is a degenerative disease of the skin.   True   False

3. A *cystic lesion* is filled with hard, packed cells.   True   False

4. A *comedo* can be either a whitehead or a blackhead.   True   False

LO 4.5, 4.6 Accessory Skin Organs (continued)

Hair

Keynotes

- Genes, hormones, and pigment determine hair characteristics.
- Body hair has no specific function.

Each hair, no matter where it is on your body or scalp, originates from epidermal cells at the base (matrix) of a hair follicle. As these cells divide and grow, they push older cells upward away from the source of nutrition in the hair papilla *(Figure 4.19)*. The cells become keratinized and die. They rest for a while; and when a new hair is formed, the old, dead hair is pushed out and drops off.

In cross-section, each hair has three layers *(Figure 4.20)*. Its core, the **medulla**, is composed of loosely arranged cells containing a flexible keratin. The **cortex** is composed of densely packed cells with a harder keratin that gives hair its stiffness. These cells also contain pigment. The outer **cuticle** is a single layer of scaly, dead keratin cells.

Straight hair is round in cross-section *(Figure 4.20a and b)*. Curly hair is oval *(Figure 4.20c and d)*. Two pigments derived from **melanin** (**eumelanin** and **pheomelanin**) give hair its natural color. Black and dark brown hair have a lot of a dark form of the pigment eumelanin in the cells of the cortex *(Figure 4.20b)*. Blonde hair has little of this dark pigment but a lighter form of pheomelanin *(Figure 4.20a)*. Red hair has a lot of the lighter pigment *(Figure 4.20c)*. White or gray hair has little pigment *(Figure 4.20d)*.

A problem with the scalp hair follicle occurs in men when a combination of genetic influence and excess testosterone produces "top of the head" baldness. In most people, aging causes **alopecia**, thinning of the hair and baldness as the follicles shrink and produce thin, wispy hairs.

Scalp hair is thick enough to retain heat. Body hair has no specific function in our present evolution because, in most people, it is too thin to retain heat. Beard, pubic, and **axillary** (armpit) hair reflect sexual maturity. Stronger hairs guard the nostrils and ears to prevent foreign particles from entering. Similarly, eyelashes protect the eyes, and eyebrows help keep perspiration from running into the eyes.

Melanin is in the black skin melanocytes of dark-skinned people and is the pigment generated by sunbathing and tanning. The absence of melanin produces **albinism**.

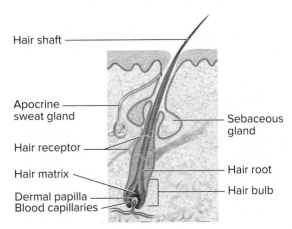

Hair shaft

Apocrine sweat gland

Hair receptor

Hair matrix

Dermal papilla
Blood capillaries

Sebaceous gland

Hair root

Hair bulb

▲ **Figure 4.19** Hair follicle.

(a) (b) (c) (d)

Cuticle — Cortex
— Medulla
— Eumelanin
— Pheomelanin

Air

Eumelanin

Pheomelanin

(a) (b) (c) (d)

▲ **Figure 4.20** Basis of hair color and texture. a.©McGraw-Hill Education/Joe DeGrandis, photographer. b.©McGraw-Hill Education/Joe DeGrandis, photographer. c.©McGraw-Hill Education/Joe DeGrandis, photographer. d.©McGraw-Hill Education/Joe DeGrandis, photographer.

WORD	PRONUNCIATION		ELEMENTS	DEFINITION
albinism	AL-bih-nizm	S/	-ism *condition*	Genetic disorder with lack of melanin
albino	al-BY-no	R/CF	albin/o- *white*	Person with albinism
alopecia	al-oh-PEE-shah		Greek *mange*	Partial or complete loss of hair, naturally or from medication
axilla	AK-sill-ah		Greek *region under a bird's wing*	Medical name for the armpit
axillae (pl)	AK-sill-ee			
axillary (adj)	AK-sill-air-ee			Pertaining to the axilla
cortex	KOR-teks		Latin *outer covering*	Outer portion of an organ, such as bone
cortical (adj)	KOR-tih-kal			Gray covering of cerebral hemispheres
cortices (pl)	KOR-tih-sees			
cuticle	KEW-tih-cul		Diminutive of cutis *skin*	Nonliving epidermis at the base of the fingernails and toenails, and the outer layer of hair
medulla	meh-DULL-ah		French *middle*	Central portion of a structure surrounded by cortex
medullary (adj)	meh-DULL-eh-ree			
melanin	MEL-ah-nin		Greek *black*	Black pigment found in skin, hair, and retina
eumelanin	YOU-mel-ah-nin	P/	eu- *good, normal*	The dark form of the pigment melanin
		R/	-melanin *black*	
pheomelanin	FEE-oh-mel-ah-nin	P/	pheo- *gray*	The lighter form of melanin

Exercises

A. A good review of the above WAD will aid you in answering the following questions about the language of dermatology. *Fill in the blanks regarding statements about the hair.* **LO 4.5, 4.6**

1. The root melanin denotes the color _____.

2. The medical term for *armpit* is _____.

3. The plural form of *cortex* is _____.

4. The central portion of a structure is the _____, which means _____.

5. The outer portion of an organ is the _____.

6. The medical term for baldness is _____.

7. *Alopecia* can result from natural causes or from _____.

B. The following nouns all have an adjectival form. *Fill in the blanks.* **LO 4.A**

1. Noun: axilla   Adjective: _____

2. Noun: cortex   Adjective: _____

3. Noun: medulla   Adjective: _____

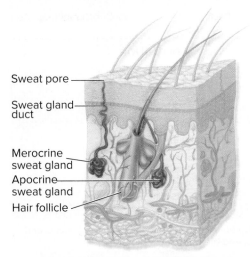

▲ Figure 4.21 Sweat glands.

Sweat pore
Sweat gland duct
Merocrine sweat gland
Apocrine sweat gland
Hair follicle

Free edge
Nail body
Nail fold
Nail groove
Lunula
Eponychium (cuticle)

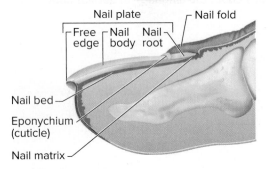

Nail plate
Free edge
Nail body
Nail root
Nail fold
Nail bed
Eponychium (cuticle)
Nail matrix

▲ FIGURE 4.22 Anatomy of a fingernail.

Sweat Glands

You have 3 million to 4 million **eccrine** (**merocrine**) sweat glands *(Figure 4.21)* scattered all over your skin, with higher concentrations on your palms, soles, and forehead.

Their main function is to produce the watery perspiration (sweat) that cools your body. Your sweat is 99% water; the rest is made up of electrolytes such as sodium chloride, which gives the sweat its salty taste. Some waste products of cell metabolism are also secreted.

In the dermis, the sweat gland is a coiled tube lined with epithelial cells that secrete the sweat. Around the tube, muscle cells contract to squeeze the sweat up the tube directly to the surface of the skin. Perspiration is a normal process to cool the body and remove waste products. An excessive amount of sweating, as seen with very stressful situations or medical conditions, such as a myocardial infarction (heart attack), is termed **diaphoresis**.

In your armpits (axillae), around your nipples, in your groin, and around your anus, **apocrine** sweat glands produce a thick, cloudy secretion that interacts with normal skin bacteria to produce a distinct, noticeable smell. The ducts of these glands lead directly into hair follicles *(see Figure 4.21)*. They respond to sexual stimulation and stress and secrete chemicals called **pheromones**, which have an effect on the sexual behavior of other people.

Ceruminous glands are found in the external ear canal, where their secretions combine with sebum and dead epidermal cells to form earwax (**cerumen**). This wax waterproofs the external ear canal and kills bacteria.

Sweat gland functions are severely affected in a group of diseases termed *ectodermal dysplasia*, manifested in the reduction or absence of sweat. They can be involved in the infections that engulf the nearby hair follicles and sebaceous glands.

Mammary glands, a type of modified sweat gland, serve a distinct purpose in reproduction and are therefore discussed in *Chapter 8* under the female reproductive system.

Nails

Nails are formed from the stratum corneum of the epidermis. They consist of closely packed, thin, dead cells that are filled with parallel fibers of hard keratin.

Fingernails grow about 1 mm per week. New cells are added by cell division in the nail **matrix**, which is protected by the nail fold of skin and the cuticle at the base of the nail *(Figure 4.22)*. The nail rests on the nail bed, which consists of the living layers of the epidermis and the strata basale, spinosum, and granulosum.

Diseases of Nails

Fifty percent of all nail disorders are caused by fungal infections and are labeled **onychomycosis** *(Figure 4.23)*. They begin in nails constantly exposed to moisture and warmth; for example, in warm shoes when associated with poor foot hygiene, in the hands of a restaurant dishwasher, under artificial fingernails, and in pedicure bowls if they are not sanitized. The fungus grows under the nail and leads to brittle cracked nails that separate from the underlying nail bed.

Paronychia *(Figure 4.24)* is a bacterial infection, usually staphylococcal, of the base of the nail. The nail fold and cuticle become swollen, red, and painful, and pus forms under the nail and can escape at the side of the nail.

The nail of the big toe can grow into the skin at the side of the nail, particularly if pressured by tight, narrow shoes. Infection can then get underneath this ingrown toenail.

The nails can reflect systemic illness. In anemia, the nail bed is pale, and the nails can become spoon-shaped. In conditions producing chronic **hypoxia**, the fingers, toes, and nails become clubbed. **Malnutrition** or severe illness can produce horizontal white lines in the nails.

▲ FIGURE 4.23 Onychomycosis (fungal infection). ©Dr. Harout Taniellian/ Photo Researchers, Inc.

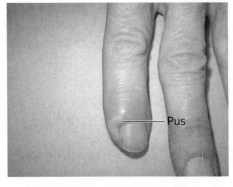

Pus

▲ FIGURE 4.24 Paronychia, with pus at the corner of the nail bed. ©VisualDx

WORD	PRONUNCIATION	ELEMENTS		DEFINITION
apocrine	AP-oh-krin	P/ R/	apo- *different from* -crine *secrete*	Apocrine sweat glands open into the hair follicle
cerumen ceruminous (adj)	seh-ROO-men seh-ROO-mih-nus		Latin *wax*	Waxy secretion of the ceruminous glands of the external ear
diaphoretic	DIE-ah-foh-RET-ic	S/ R/	-etic *pertaining to* diaphor- *sweat*	Pertaining to sweat or perspiration
diaphoresis	DIE-ah-foh-REE-sis	S/	-esis *abnormal condition*	Abnormal amount of sweat or perspiration
eccrine	EK-rin		Greek *to secrete*	Coiled sweat gland that occurs in skin all over the body
hypoxia	high-POCK-see-ah	S/ P/ R/	-ia *condition* hyp- *below* -ox- *oxygen*	Decrease below normal levels of oxygen in tissues, gases, or blood
hypoxic (adj)	high-POCK-sik	S/	-ic *pertaining to*	Deficient in oxygen
malnutrition	mal-nyu-TRISH-un	S/ P/ R/	-ion *process* mal- *bad, inadequate* -nutrit- *nourishment*	Inadequate nutrition from poor diet or inadequate absorption of nutrients
matrix matrices (pl)	MAY-triks		Latin *womb*	Substance that surrounds cells, is manufactured by the cells, and holds them together
merocrine	MARE-oh-krin	P/ R/	mero- *partial* -crine *secrete*	Another name for eccrine
onychomycosis	oh-ni-koh-my-KOH-sis	S/ R/CF R/	-osis *condition* onych/o- *nail* -myc- *fungus*	Condition of a fungus infection in a nail
paronychia	par-oh-NICK-ee-ah	S/ P/ R/	-ia *condition* para- *alongside* -onych- *nail* (**Note:** *The vowel "a" at the end of para- is dropped to make the composite word flow more easily.*)	Infection alongside the nail
pheromone (*Note: The hor in hor- mone is dropped to ease pronunciation*)	FER-oh-moan	P/ R/	pher- *carrying* -hormone *excite, stimulate*	Substance that carries and generates a physical attraction for other people

Exercises

A. Work on understanding the meanings of the elements. *From the given definition, construct medical terms relating the WAD above. Fill in the blanks.* **LO 4.6, 4.C**

1. Fungal infection of the nail: onych/o/_____ /osis

2. Coiled sweat gland that occurs all over the body: mer/o/_____

3. Substance that carries and generates attraction for other people: _____ /omone

4. Infection alongside the nail: par/_____ /ia

B. Answer the following questions about the medical terms in the above WAD relating to diseases of the nail.
Fill in the blanks. **LO 4.6, 4.A**

paronychia   onychomycosis   hypoxia   malnutrition

1. Clubbing of the nails can occur with chronic _____.

2. An infection alongside the nail is termed _____.

3. A fungal infection of the nails is termed _____.

4. A person suffering from _____ may have visible white lines in the nail bed.

Lesson 4.4

INTEGUMENTARY SYSTEM

Burns and Injuries to the Skin

Lesson Objectives

You have learned that a major role of the skin is protection of your internal organs. In the previous lessons, you have seen the effects of infectious agents on the skin. In this lesson, you will learn the effects of direct injury to the skin, and you will be able to use correct medical terminology to:

4.4.1 Distinguish the four types of burns.

4.4.2 Describe the inflammatory process of the skin when it is injured.

4.4.3 Explain the process of healing and repair of the skin.

4.4.4 Describe wounds, burns, and the process of healing and repair.

4.4.5 Describe the Rule of Nines for estimating the surface area of the six different regions of the skin.

Case Report (CR) 4.5

You are

. . . a burn technologist employed in the Burn Unit at Fulwood Medical Center.

Your patient is

. . . Mr. Steven Hapgood, a 52-year-old man, admitted to the Fulwood Burn Unit with severe burns over his face, chest, and abdomen.

After an evening of drinking, Mr. Hapgood was smoking in bed and fell asleep. His next-door neighbors in the apartment building smelled smoke and called 911. In the Burn Unit, his initial treatment included large volumes of intravenous (IV) fluids to prevent **shock**.

Your role will be to participate in Mr. Hapgood's care as a member of the Burn Unit team and to document the care and his response to it. Mr. Hapgood's burns were mostly third degree. The protective ability of the skin to prevent water loss had been removed, as had the skin barrier against infection. The burned, dead tissue forms an **eschar** that can have toxic effects on the digestive, respiratory, and cardiovascular systems. The eschar was surgically removed by **debridement**.

LO 4.7 Burns

Burns are the leading cause of *accidental* death. The immediate threats to life are from fluid loss, infection, and the systemic effects of burned dead tissue.

Burns are classified according to the depth of tissue involved *(Figure 4.25)*:

- **First-degree (superficial) burns** involve only the epidermis and produce inflammation with redness, pain, and slight **edema**. Healing occurs in 3 to 5 days without scarring.

- **Second-degree (partial-thickness) burns** involve the epidermis and dermis but leave some of the dermis intact. They produce redness, blisters, and more severe pain. Healing occurs in 2 to 3 weeks with minimal scarring.

- **Third-degree (full-thickness) burns** involve the epidermis, dermis, and subcutaneous tissues, which are often completely destroyed. Healing takes a long time and involves using skin grafts.

- **Fourth-degree burns** destroy all layers of the skin and involve tendons, muscles, and sometimes bones.

(a) First degree (superficial)

(b) Second degree (partial thickness)

(c) Third degree (full thickness)

▲ **FIGURE 4.25** Degrees of burns. (a).©Sheila Terry/Photo Researchers, Inc. (b).©Dr. P. Marazzi/SPL/Photo Researchers, Inc. (c).©John Radcliffe Hospital/Photo Researchers, Inc.

WORD	PRONUNCIATION	ELEMENTS		DEFINITION
debridement	day-**BREED**-mon	S/ P/ R/	**-ment** *resulting state* **de-** *take away* **-bride-** *rubbish*	The removal of injured or necrotic tissue
edema edematous (adj)	ee-**DEE**-mah ee-**DEM**-ah-tus	S/ R/	Greek *swelling* **-tous** *pertaining to* **edema-** *swelling*	Excessive collection of fluid in cells and tissues Marked by edema
eschar	**ESS**-kar		Greek *scab of a burn*	The burned, dead tissue lying on top of third-degree burns
shock	SHOCK		German *to clash*	Sudden physical or mental collapse or circulatory collapse

Exercises

A. Define the terms associated with burn injuries. *Match the terms in the first column with their correct definition in the second column.* **LO 4.7**

_____ 1. regenerate

_____ 2. eschar

_____ 3. debridement

_____ 4. shock

_____ 5. edema

a. sudden physical collapse

b. burned, dead tissue

c. excessive collection of fluid in cells and tissues

d. to reconstitute a lost part

e. removal of injured or necrotic tissue

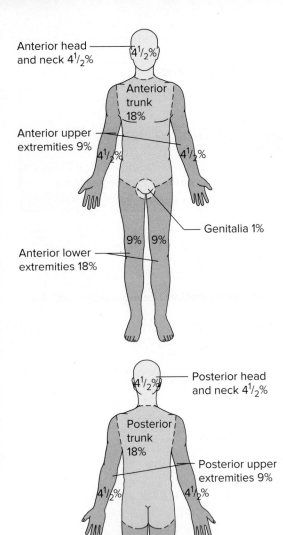

Anterior head
and neck 4¹/₂%

(4¹/₂%)

Anterior
trunk
18%

Anterior upper
extremities 9%

4¹/₂%   4¹/₂%

Genitalia 1%

Anterior lower
extremities 18%

9% 9%

Posterior head
and neck 4¹/₂%

4¹/₂%

Posterior
trunk
18%

Posterior upper
extremities 9%

4¹/₂%   4¹/₂%

Posterior lower
extremities 18%

9% 9%

▲ **Figure 4.26** Rule of Nines.

LO 4.7 Burns (continued)

Burn injury to the lungs through damage from heat or smoke inhalation is responsible for 60% or more of fatalities from burns.

In partial-thickness burns, **regeneration** of the skin can occur from remaining cells in the stratum basale, from residual hair follicles and sweat glands, and from the edges of the burned area. In full-thickness burns, there is no dermal tissue left for regeneration, and skin grafts are needed. The ideal graft is an **autograft** taken from another location on the patient. It is not rejected by the immune system. Mr. Hapgood had autografts taken from his unburned legs and back.

If the patient's burns are too extensive, **allografts** from another person are needed. These are provided by skin banks and are taken from deceased people (cadavers). A **homograft** is another name for an allograft. A **xenograft**, or **heterograft**, is a graft from another species, for example, pigs.

Artificial skin is being developed commercially and can stimulate the growth of connective tissues from the patient's underlying tissue.

LO 4.2 Regions of Skin Surface Area

The skin's surface area can be divided into six regions, each one of which is a fraction or multiple of 9% of the total surface area. This is called the Rule of Nines *(Figure 4.26)*.

The treatment and prognosis for a burn patient depend, in part, on the extent of the body surface that is affected. This is estimated by applying the Rule of Nines to determine the percentage of the skin's surface affected by burns:

- Head and neck are assigned 9% (4½% anterior and 4½% posterior).

- Each arm is 9% (4½% anterior and 4½% posterior).

- Each leg is 18% (9% anterior and 9% posterior).

- The anterior trunk is 18%.

- The posterior trunk is 18%.

- The genitalia are 1%.

WORD	PRONUNCIATION		ELEMENTS	DEFINITION
allograft	AL-oh-graft	P/	allo- *other*	Skin graft from another person or cadaver
		R/	-graft *transplant*	
homograft (syn)	HOH-moh-graft	P/	homo- *same, alike*	
autograft	AWE-toh-graft	P/	auto- *self*	A graft using tissue taken from the individual who is receiving the graft
		R/	-graft *transplant*	
regenerate	ree-JEN-eh-rate	S/	-ate *composed of*	To reconstitute a lost part
		P/	re- *again*	
		R/	-gener- *produce*	
regeneration (noun)	ree-JEN-eh-RAY-shun	S/	-ation *process*	Reconstitution of a lost part
xenograft	ZEN-oh-graft	P/	xeno- *foreign*	A graft from another species
		R/	-graft *transplant*	
heterograft (syn)	HET-er-oh-graft	P/	hetero- *different*	

Exercises

A. Compare and contrast the meanings of word elements that describe the types of skin grafts.
Fill in the blank with the correct term. **LO 4.7, 4.A**

1. A graft from another species is a **xenograft** and a _____.

2. A graft from another person is an **allograft** and a _____.

3. A graft taken from one part a person's body and placed elsewhere on the same body: _____

B. Remembering the meaning of the word element can help you easily identify the type of skin grafts.
Match the prefix to its meaning. **LO 4.7, 4.A**

_____ **1.** *hetero-*   **a.** other

_____ **2.** *allo-*   **b.** same, alike

_____ **3.** *xeno-*   **c.** self

_____ **4.** *homo-*   **d.** different

_____ **5.** *auto-*   **e.** foreign

C. Refer to Case Report 4.5 and to the information presented on the previous page to answer the following questions. **LO 4.7, 4.A**

1. The material removed via debridement is termed: _____

2. How deep were the majority of Mr. Hapgood's burns?

   a. partial-thickness

   b. superficial

   c. full-thickness

3. The first treatment Mr. Hapgood received in the Burn Unit was fluid replacement to prevent:

   a. infection

   b. toxicity

   c. shock

   d. hypoxia

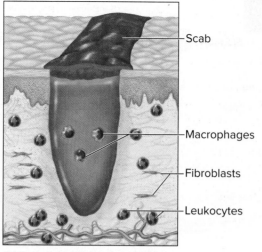

Scab

Macrophages

Fibroblasts

Leukocytes

(a) Bleeding into the wound

(b) Scab formation and macrophage activity

▲ **FIGURE 4.27** Wound healing.

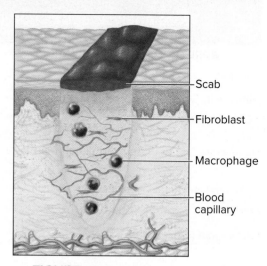

Scab

Fibroblast

Macrophage

Blood capillary

▲ **FIGURE 4.28** Formation of granulation tissue.

Epidermal growth

Scar tissue (fibrosis)

▲ **FIGURE 4.29** Scar formation.

▲ **FIGURE 4.30** A keloid of the earlobe. **This scar resulted from piercing the ear for earrings.** ©BSIP/Contributor/Getty Images

LO 4.8 Wounds and Tissue Repair

If you cut yourself with paper and produce a shallow **laceration** primarily in the epidermis, the epithelial cells along its edges will divide rapidly and fill in the gap. An adhesive bandage helps the process by pulling the edges together.

If you cut yourself more deeply, extending the **wound** into the dermis or hypodermis, or if a surgeon makes an **incision**, then blood vessels in the dermis break and blood escapes into the wound *(Figure 4.27a)*.

This escaped blood forms a **clot** in the wound. The clot consists of protein (**fibrin**) together with **platelets** (also called **thrombocytes**), blood cells, and dried tissue fluids trapped in the fibers. **Macrophages** come into the wound with the escaped blood. They digest and clean up the tissue debris. The surface of the clot dries and hardens in the air to form a **scab**. The scab seals and protects the wound from becoming infected *(Figure 4.27b)*.

The clot begins to be invaded by new capillaries from the surrounding dermis. Three or four days after the injury, fibroblasts migrate into the wound and form new collagen fibers that pull the wound together. This soft tissue in the wound is called **granulation tissue** and in unsutured wounds takes a couple of weeks to completely form *(Figure 4.28)*.

As healing continues, surface epithelial cells from the edges of the wound migrate into the area underneath the scab. As this new epithelium thickens, the scab loosens and falls off. Inside the wound, new collagen fibers formed by the fibroblasts form a **scar** to replace the granulation tissue *(Figure 4.29)*. In unsutured wounds, this takes up to a month to complete.

Suturing brings together the edges of the wound to enhance tissue healing. It also reduces the risk of infection and the amount of scarring. A liquid skin adhesive can sometimes be used in place of **sutures**. Some sutures eventually dissolve, avoiding the need for suture removal. The scar formation and remodeling process may go on for more than a year.

In some people, there is excessive fibrosis and scar tissue formation, producing raised, irregular, lumpy, shiny scars called **keloids** *(Figure 4.30)*. They can extend beyond the edges of the original wound and often return if they are surgically removed. They are most common on the upper body and earlobes.

Surgery on the skin is now being performed using light beams called **lasers**. These beams of light can be focused precisely to vaporize specific lesions on the superficial layers of the skin. The beams remove lesions and create a fresh surface over which new skin can grow. Healing takes 10 to 15 days and goes through the process described above, with clotting and scabbing.

A superficial scraping of the skin, a mucous membrane, or the cornea *(see Chapter 16)* is called an **abrasion**.

WORD	PRONUNCIATION		ELEMENTS	DEFINITION
abrasion	ah-**BRAY**-shun		Latin *to scrape*	Area of skin or mucous membrane that has been scraped off
clot	KLOT		German *to block*	The mass of fibrin and cells that is produced in a wound
fibrin fibrous (adj)	**FIE**-brin **FIE**-brus	S/ R/	Latin *fiber* -ous *pertaining to* fibr- *fiber*	Stringy protein fiber that is a component of a blood clot Tissue containing fibroblasts and fibers
granulation	gran-you-**LAY**-shun	S/ R/	-ation *process* granul- *small grain*	New fibrous tissue formed during wound healing
incision	in-**SIZH**-un	S/ R/	-ion *action, condition* incis- *cut into*	A cut or surgical wound
keloid	**KEY**-loyd		Greek *stain*	Raised, irregular, lumpy, shiny scar due to excess collagen fiber production during healing of a wound
laceration	lass-eh-**RAY**-shun	S/ R/	-ation *process* lacer- *to tear*	A tear of the skin
laser	**LAY**-zer		acronym for **L**ight **A**mplification by **S**timulated **E**mission of **R**adiation	Intense, narrow beam of monochromatic light
macrophage	**MAK**-roh-fayj	P/ R/	macro- *large* -phage *to eat*	Large white blood cell that removes bacteria, foreign particles, and dead cells
platelet (also called thrombocyte)	**PLAYT**-let		Greek *small plate*	Cell fragment involved in clotting process
scab	SKAB		Old English *crust*	Crust that forms over a wound or sore during healing
scar	SKAR		Greek *scab*	Fibrotic seam that forms when a wound heals
suture	**SOO**-chur		Latin *seam*	Stitch to hold the edges of a wound together
wound	WOOND		Old English *wound*	Any injury that interrupts the continuity of skin or a mucous membrane

Exercises

A. Review the above WAD before starting this exercise—the elements and definitions will help you work out the answers.
Put on your thinking cap. Fill in the blanks. **LO 4.8, 4.A**

1. Reorder these terms into the order of their occurrence. Place a 1 for the process that occurs first, ending with 4 for the process that occurs last.

   _____scab   _____scar   _____clot   _____wound

2. An excess amount of scar tissue is termed a _____.

3. What is the soft tissue in the wound-healing process called? _____

4. The type of cell that produces collagen is a _____.

5. A scraping of the skin is termed an _____.

6. A tear in the skin is termed a _____.

7. What is another name for a stitch used to close a wound? _____

Congratulations! You have mastered these terms.

Lesson 4.5

Procedures and Pharmacology

LO 4.9 Diagnostic Procedures

The most important procedures in making a diagnosis of a skin lesion are a careful history of the etiology and progression of the lesion and a careful visual examination to define the clinical appearance of the lesion.

Diascopy, in which a finger or a microscope slide is pressed against a lesion to see if it blanches, helps define a vascular (inflammatory) lesion, which blanches, from a hemorrhagic lesion (petechia or purpura) which does not blanch.

Microscopic examination of skin scrapings helps diagnose fungal infections and scabies. Tzank testing by scraping the base of vesicles and staining them with a Giemsa stain shows multinucleated giant cells of herpes simplex or zoster under microscopy.

Cultures using swabs taken from lesions and implanted in the appropriate growth medium are utilized to diagnose some viruses (e.g., herpes simplex) and certain bacteria.

Biopsy (Bx) of a skin lesion using a punch biopsy, excision of a whole lesion, or shaving of the lesion for microscopic examination is valuable in diagnosing malignancies, fungal diseases, and immune diseases.

Wood's light (black light) is used to define the borders of pigmented lesions before excision, show the presence of *Pseudomonas* infection (**fluoresces** green), and distinguish the **hypopigmentation** of vitiligo, which fluoresces a deep ivory white.

LO 4.10 Therapeutic Procedures

Photodynamic therapy (PDT) in a series of sessions exposes the skin in acne to a high-intensity blue light and creates a toxic environment in which bacteria in the sebaceous glands cannot live. In addition to treating acne, PDT can be used to treat precancerous lesions called **actinic keratoses**, which have the potential to develop into squamous cell carcinomas.

Laser therapy is used for the management of birthmarks, vascular lesions, warts, and skin disorders like vitiligo.

Chemical peels are performed on the face, neck, or hands. An acid solution such as glycolic acid, salicylic acid, or carbolic acid (phenol) is applied to small areas of skin to reduce fine facial lines and wrinkles, treat sun damage, and reduce age spots and dark patches (**melasma**).

Cryotherapy is used frequently to treat acne, scars, sebaceous plaques, and some skin cancers. Liquid nitrogen is sprayed onto the affected area of skin to cause peeling or scabbing.

Used purely for **cosmetic** procedures, Botox is a prescription medicine that blocks signals from nerves to muscles. When injected into superficial muscles, the injected muscle can no longer contract, causing facial wrinkles and lines to temporarily relax and soften.

Dermal fillers such as Restylane and Juvederm help to diminish facial lines and wrinkles by restoring subcutaneous volume and fullness to the face as subcutaneous fat is lost in the natural aging process.

WORD	PRONUNCIATION	ELEMENTS		DEFINITION
actinic	ak-**TIN**-ik	S/ R/	-ic *pertaining to* actin- *ray*	Pertaining to the sun
cosmetic	koz-**MET**-ik		Greek *an adornment*	A concern for appearance
cryotherapy	**CRY**-oh-**THAIR**-ah pee	P/ R/	cryo- *cold* -therapy *medical treatment*	The use of cold in the treatment of disease
culture	**KUL**-chur		Latin *tillage*	The growth of microorganisms on or in media
diascopy	di-**AS**-koh-pee	P/ R/	dia- *through* scopy *to examine, to view*	Examination of superficial skin lesions with pressure
fluoresce	flor-**ESS**		Greek *bright color*	Emit a bright-colored light when irradiated with ultraviolet or violet-blue rays
keratosis keratoses (pl)	ker-ah-**TOH**-sis ker-ah-**TOH**-seez	S/ R/	-osis *condition* kerat- *horny*	Epidermal lesion of circumscribed overgrowth of the horny layer
melasma	meh-**LAZ**-mah		Greek *black spot*	Patchy pigmentation of the skin
pigment hypopigmentation	**PIG**-ment **HIGH**-poh-pig-men-**TAY**-shun	 S/ P/ R/	Latin *paint* -ation *process* hypo- *below normal* -pigment- *color*	A coloring matter or stain Below normal melanin relative to the surrounding skin

Exercises

A. Identify the proper diagnostic procedure or treatment for each condition. *Use the words from the provided word bank to complete the sentences. Fill in the blank.* **LO 4.9, 4.10, 4.A**

diascopy   Juvederm   cryotherapy   Botox   fluoresce

1. Injecting _____ into the skin will fill areas to reduce the appearance of aging.

2. Acne can be treated with _____ to freeze the cells of the affected area.

3. Pigmented or hypopigmented areas can be better seen when they _____ with Wood's light.

4. Pressing on an area of skin to see if it blanches is termed _____.

5. The injection of _____ can reduce the appearance of wrinkles by paralyzing the affected muscles.

B. Defining the meaning of word elements can help you to quickly decipher the meaning of medical terms. *Choose the correct answer to each question.* **LO 4.D**

1. The word element that means *cold:*

   a. *dia-*   **b.** *-therapy*   **c.** *cry/o-*   **d.** *hypo-*

2. The word element *dia-* means:

   a. to view   **b.** through   **c.** light   **d.** two

3. The word element *-scopy* means:

   a. to view   **b.** scrape   **c.** suture   **d.** inject

4. The suffix that means *condition of* is:

   a. *-osis*   **b.** *-ic*   **c.** *-itis*   **d.** *-al*

LO 4.11 Dermatologic Pharmacology

A wide range of **topical pharmacologic** agents of different types can be used in the treatment of skin lesions either to relieve symptoms or to cure the disease.

- **Anesthetics**: topical agents that relieve pain or itching on the skin's surface. Benzocaine is used for this purpose as a numbing **cream.** It is used prior to injections, for oral ulcers, for hemorrhoids, and for infant teething.

- **Antibacterials:** topical agents that eliminate bacteria that cause skin lesions. Neomycin **ointment** is commonly used.

- **Antifungals:** topical agents that eliminate or inhibit the growth of fungi. Nystatin (*Mycostatin,Nilstat*) is used as a cream or ointment. Terbinafine (*Lamisil*) is used as a cream or ointment. Clotrimazole (*Canesten, Clomazol*) and ketaconazole (*Ketopine, Daktagold*) are *imadazoles* available in creams, sprays, **lotions,** and **shampoos.** Amphotericin B (*Fungizone*) is used locally to treat oral candidiasis (thrush), and in IV therapy for systemic fungal infections.

- **Antipruritics**: topical lotions, ointments, creams, or sprays that relieve itching. **Corticosteroids** such as hydrocortisone are most frequently used.

- **Keratolytics:** topical agents that peel away the skin's stratum corneum from the other epidermal layers. Salicylic acid is used for this purpose in the treatment of acne, psoriasis, ichthyoses, and dandruff. It is available in the form of wipes, creams, **lotions, gels,** ointments, and **shampoos** in strengths varying from 3% to 20%.

- **Parasiticides:** topical agents that kill parasites living on the skin. Hexachlorocyclohexane (*Lindane 1%*) is used in lotion or shampoo form to kill lice if other methods have failed.

- **Retinoids**: derivatives of retinoic acid (vitamin A) used under the strict supervision of a physician in the treatment of acne, sun spots, and psoriasis. Tretinoin (*Retin-A*) is used topically for acne; isoretinoin (*Accutane*) is taken orally for severe acne; etretinate (*Tegison*) is taken orally to treat severe psoriasis; and adapalene (*Differin*) is used topically for psoriasis.

Classes of Topical Medications

Solutions are usually a powder dissolved in water or alcohol.

Lotions are usually a powder mixed with oil and water to be thicker than a solution.

Gels are a semisolid **emulsion** in an alcohol base

Creams are an emulsion of oil and water that is thicker than a lotion and holds its shape when removed from its container. They penetrate the outer stratum corneum layer of skin.

Ointments are a homogenous semisolid preparation, 80% a thick oil and 20% water, that lies on the skin. They can also be used on the mucous membranes of the eye, vulva, anus, and nose, and are emulsifiable with the mucous membrane secretions.

Transdermal patches are a very precise time-released method to deliver a drug. Release of the drug can be controlled by **diffusion** through the adhesive that covers the whole patch or through a membrane with adhesive only on the patch rim.

WORD	PRONUNCIATION	ELEMENTS		DEFINITION
anesthetic	an-es-**THET**-ik	S/ P/ R/	-ic *pertaining to* an- *without* -esthet- *sensation,* *perception*	Substance that takes away feeling and pain.
antibacterial	**AN**-tee-bak-**TEER**-ee-al	S/ P/ R/CF	-al *pertaining to* anti- *against* -bacter/i-	Destroying or preventing the growth of bacteria
antifungal antipruritic	**AN**-tee-**FUN**-gul **AN**-tee-pru-**RIT**-ik	R/ S/ P/ R/	fung- *fungus* -ic *pertaining to* anti- *against* -prurit- *itch*	Destroying or preventing the growth of a fungus Medication against itching
cream	KREEM		Latin *thick juice*	A semisolid emulsion
diffusion	dih-**FYU**-zhun	S/ R/	-ion *process* diffus- *movement*	The process by which small particles move between tissues
emulsion	ee-**MUL**-shun	S/ R/	-ion *process* emuls- *suspension in a* *liquid*	Very small particles suspended in a solution
keratolytic	**KER**-ah-toh-**LIT**-ik	S/ R/CF R/	-ic *pertaining to* kerat/o- *horn* -lyt- *loosening*	Causing separation or loosening of the horny layer (stratum corneum) of the skin
parasiticide	par-ah-**SIT**-ih-side	S/ R/CF	-cide *to kill* parasit/i *parasite*	Agent that destroys parasites
retinoid	**RET**-ih-noyd		Derived from retinoic acid	A cream that is a derivative of vitamin A used to treat acne and wrinkles
topical	**TOP**-ih-kal	S/ R/	-al *pertaining to* topic- *local*	Medication applied to the skin to obtain a local effect

Exercises

A. Practice your *language of pharmacology* by correctly filling in the blanks of patient documentation. LO 4.11, 4.A

Mrs. Robison brought in her 8-year-old daughter to the doctor because the child had a red ring–like rash on her scalp. Dr. Palmer examined the child and diagnosed her with tinea capitis. She prescribed clotrimazole cream to be applied to the site twice daily for 6 weeks.

1. Dr. Palmer prescribed an _____ cream to cure the patient's tinea capitis.

2. She prefers to provide _____ application of the medication because it stays local to the site of the infection.

B. Define the classes of topical medications. *Topical medications come in a variety of forms to best deliver medication to the skin. Match the description of the form of the medication to its term.* **LO 4.11**

Term	Meaning
_____ 1. gel	a. adhesive membrane attached to the surface of the skin
_____ 2. lotion	b. semisolid emulsion in an alcohol base
_____ 3. ointment	c. powder dissolved in alcohol or water
_____ 4. transdermal patch	d. powder mixed with oil and water; thicker than a solution
_____ 5. solution	e. semisolid preparation of oil and waer

Integumentary System

Challenge Your Knowledge

A. Match the type of skin graft with its correct definition. The definitions can be used more than once. (**LO 4.7**)

_____ 1. homograft

_____ 2. autograft

_____ 3. allograft

_____ 4. xenograft

_____ 5. heterograft

a. skin graft taken from the individual who is receiving the graft

b. skin graft from another person or cadaver

c. a graft from another species

B. Plurals. Follow the rules and form the plurals for the following terms. (**LO 4.A, 4.B**)

1. papilla   Plural: _____

2. matrix   Plural: _____

3. cortex   Plural: _____

4. axilla   Plural: _____

C. Abbreviations appear in written documentation and must be used correctly. From the sentences, give the abbreviation of the description in italics. (**LO 4.F**)

1. Please inject the medication *into the hypodermis.*

_____

2. The antibiotic will be injected *into the muscle* of the buttock.

_____

D. Skin diseases can affect any and all parts of the body. Some skin diseases are an early manifestation of a more serious internal problem. Match the symptom or association in the left column with the correct medical term in the right column. You have more answer choices than you need. (**LO 4.4, 4.6**)

_____ 1. cause unknown; silvery scales

_____ 2. butterfly rash

_____ 3. associated with ovarian cancer

_____ 4. enlarged capillaries show through skin

_____ 5. pale patches of skin

_____ 6. shrinking of skin; hardening

a. pemphigus vulgaris

b. vitiligo

c. rosacea

d. psoriasis

e. seborrheic lesions

f. scleroderma

g. systemic lupus erythematosus

h. herpes zoster

i. dermatomyositis

E. Case report questions. Reread Case Report 4.5. You should feel more comfortable with the medical terminology now and will be able to answer the questions that follow. (**LO 4.2, 4.7, 4.A**)

Case Report (CR) 4.5

You are

. . . a burn technologist employed in the Burn Unit at Fulwood Medical Center.

Your patient is

. . . Mr. Steven Hapgood, a 52-year-old man, admitted to the Fulwood Burn Unit with severe burns over his face, chest, and abdomen.

After an evening of drinking, Mr. Hapgood was smoking in bed and fell asleep. His next-door neighbors in the apartment building smelled smoke and called 911. In the Burn Unit, his initial treatment included large volumes of intravenous fluids to prevent shock.

Your role will be to participate in Mr. Hapgood's care as a member of the Burn Unit team and to document the care and his response to it. Mr. Hapgood's burns were mostly third-degree. The protective ability of the skin to prevent water loss had been removed, as had the skin barrier against infection. The burned, dead tissue forms an eschar that can have toxic effects on the digestive, respiratory, and cardiovascular systems. The eschar was surgically removed by debridement.

---

1. Based on the Rule of Nines, approximately what percent of Mr. Hapgood's body was burned?

   a. 16%   **b.** 18%   **c.** 20%   **d.** 22%

2. The first treatment that Mr. Hapgood received was:

   a. CPR   **b.** removal of the eschar   **c.** IV fluids   **d.** skin grafts   **e.** wound therapy

3. _____ is the medical term for burned, dead tissue lying on top of third-degree burns.

   a. Eschar   **b.** Wheal   **c.** Vesicle   **d.** Eczema   **e.** Vitiligo

4. His burns involved only the:

   a. epidermis   **c.** epidermis, dermis, and hypodermis

   b. epidermis and dermis   **d.** epidermis, dermis, hypodermis, and muscles

5. Mr. Hapgood's loss of skin makes him at increased risk of:

   a. ulcers   **b.** infection   **c.** furuncles   **d.** wheals

F. Use your knowledge of the language of dermatology to make the connection with the following medical terms. Match the medical terms in the left column with the descriptions in the right column. (**LO 4.4, 4.6, 4.A**)

   _____ **1.** pruritus   **a.** can infiltrate or metastasize

   _____ **2.** edema   **b.** body as a whole

   _____ **3.** malignancy   **c.** swelling

   _____ **4.** systematic   **d.** to scratch

   _____ **5.** excoriate   **e.** itching

Integumentary System

G. **Identify the correct dermatologic condition or procedure.** Choose the correct answer. (LO 4.1–4.11, 4.F)

1. Use of liquid nitrogen to freeze or kill abnormal tissue is called:

   a. biopsy

   b. patch test

   c. cryosurgery

   d. hypodermic injection

   e. infestation

2. A laceration that is *superficial* is not very:

   a. swollen

   b. edematous

   c. deep

   d. purulent

   e. infected

3. Keratinized stratified squamous epithelium is:

   a. stratum corneum

   b. dandruff

   c. hair follicle

   d. sweat

   e. dermatitis

4. An ointment, cream, or spray prescribed to relieve itching is called:

   a. antifungal

   b. keratolytic

   c. antipruritic

   d. retinoid

   e. antibacterial

5. Subcutaneous fat is another name for:

   a. epidermis

   b. hypodermis

   c. dermis

   d. adipose tissue

   e. follicles

6. A congenital lesion of the skin, including birthmarks and moles, is called a:

   a. macule

   b. papule

   c. vesicle

   d. nevus

   e. melanoma

7. Another name for a pressure ulcer is:

   a. eczema

   b. excoriation

   c. decubitus

   d. edematous

   e. serous

8. Strep enzymes digest connective tissue and spread into muscle layers in:

   a. lesions

   b. atopic dermatitis

   c. cellulitis

   d. ulcers

   e. necrotizing fasciitis

9. The medical term for shingles is:

   a. eczema

   b. herpes zoster

   c. impetigo

   d. candidiasis

   e. pediculosis

10. A facial butterfly rash is associated with which autoimmune disease?

   a. SC

   b. HIV

   c. SLE

   d. TB

   e. MRSA

H. **Medical terms that are nouns can also have an adjectival form that must be used in some cases.** Test your knowledge of the correct form of the term to use in the following sentences. **(LO 4.A)**

1. This puncture wound has completely penetrated the _____.

   a. dermis   **b.** dermal

2. This burn wound has completely penetrated the _____ layer of skin.

   a. dermis   **b.** dermal

3. Please take this specimen to the _____ department.

   a. pathological   **b.** pathology

4. The _____ diagnosis has not yet been determined.

   a. pathological   **b.** pathology

5. The _____ properties of the aloe lotion reduced the pain in the sunburn.

   a. anesthesia   **b.** anesthetic

I. **Build your medical language of dermatology.** Complete the medical terms by filling in the blanks. The first one has been done for you. **(4.4, 4.11, 4.A, 4.C)**

1. Study of disorders of the skin   dermato/*logy*

2. To scratch the skin   ex/_____/ate

3. Sore caused by lying in bed   _____/cubitus

4. Infestation with lice   _____/osis

5. Takes away feeling and pain   an/_____/ia

6. Medication against itching   anti/_____/ic

Integumentary System

J. Apply your knowledge of the language of dermatology to the following Case Report. Use Case Report 4.3 to correctly answer each question or complete each statement below. **(LO 4.4, 4.5, 4.A)**

 ### Case Report (CCR) 4.3

Ms. Cheryl Fox is a 37-year-old nursing assistant working in a surgical unit in Fulwood Medical Center. Recently her fingers have become red and itchy, with occasional vesicles. She has also noticed irritation and swelling of her earlobes and a generalized pruritus. Over the weekend, both the itching and the rash on her hands worsened. A patch test by her dermatologist showed her to be allergic to nickel in rings that she wears on both hands and in her earrings. She wore these on weekends and not during her workdays.

---

1. What diagnostic test did Ms. Fox have to determine the cause of her condition?

    a. itching   **b.** patch test   **c.** nickel   **d.** blood serum

2. Identify her symptoms. Choose all that apply.

    a. vesicle   **b.** pruritus   **c.** allergies   **d.** swelling

3. What part of her body was edematous?

    a. fingers   **b.** earlobes   **c.** abdomen   **d.** toes

4. Write the term in the above Case Report that means *itching:* _____

5. What is the *allergen* that Ms. Fox is allergic to? _____

6. A likely diagnosis for Ms. Fox would be:

    a. melanoma   **b.** dermatitis   **c.** vitiligo   **d.** candidiasis

K. Terminology challenge. Use the following medical terms to complete the sentences. **(LO 4.A)**

metastasis   **metastasize**   **metastatic**

1. The surgeon predicted that the lesion would _____ to the liver.

2. The _____ lesion received radiation therapy, while the primary lesion was surgically removed.

3. The pathology report confirmed that there was no _____ of the lesion.

L. Identify the type of secretions from each gland of the integumentary system. Match the secretion with the gland type. **(LO 4.5)**

    _____ **1.** cerumen   **a.** sweat at groin and armpits

    _____ **2.** milk   **b.** ear wax

    _____ **3.** apocrine   **c.** typical sweat

    _____ **4.** eccrine   **d.** mammary

M. **Write the term for the condition that is being described.** Interpret each statement that may be given to you from a patient to the correct medical term. Fill in the blank. (**LO 4.4, 4.6, 4.8**)

1. "My child fell off his skateboard and scraped off a lot of skin from her leg." She has a large _____.

2. "I was cutting up vegetables and accidentally gave myself a deep cut to my hand." He has a _____.

3. "After my cut on my arm, I developed a large, thickened, shiny scar." He has developed a _____.

4. "My daughter has several patches of skin that do not have any pigment." She may have a condition called _____.

N. **Identify the correct topical skin treatment for each condition.** Choose the best answer for each question. (**LO 4.11**)

1. A treatment to kill lice:

   a. antipruritic   **b.** keralytic   **c.** retinoid   **d.** parasiticide

2. A cream that would relieve itching due to allergies:

   a. retinoid   **b.** corticosteroid   **c.** antifungal   **d.** antibacterial

3. A topical treatment for tinea pedis is a(n) _____ cream:

   a. parasiticide   **b.** antibacterial   **c.** antifungal   **d.** anesthetic

4. A topical treatment for acne is a(n) _____ cream:

   a. retinoid   **b.** corticosteroid   **c.** antifungal   **d.** antibacterial

O. **Identify the health professionals involved in the care of dermatological patients.** From the given description, choose the medical professional that would be involved in the care of the patient. Fill in the blank. (**LO 4.E**)

dermatologist   **nurse practitioner**   **dermatopathologist**   **plastic surgeon**   **esthetician**

1. Uses a microscope to examine a skin sample: _____

2. Medical specialist in the care and diagnosis of skin disorders: _____

3. Utilizes corrective surgery to correct deformities due to injury or birth defects: _____

4. Professional who uses cosmetic procedures to beautify the skin: _____

5. Works under the direction of a physician to treat skin disorders: _____

DIGESTIVE SYSTEM
The Language of Gastroenterology

©2014 Nucleus Medical Media

In your future career as a health professional, you may work directly or indirectly with one or more of the health professionals involved in **gastroenterology**:

- **Gastroenterologists** are medical specialists in the field of gastroenterology.

- **Proctologists** are surgical specialists in diseases of the anus and rectum.

- **Dentists** are licensed practitioners in the anatomy, physiology, and pathology of the oral-facial complex.

- **Periodontists** are specialists in diseases of the tissues surrounding the teeth.

- **Nutritionists** are professionals who prevent and treat illness by promoting healthy eating habits.

- **Dieticians** manage food services systems and promote sound eating habits.

Chapter Learning Outcomes

As a medical **transcriptionist**, you and all the other health professionals directly and indirectly involved with Mrs. Jones's care need to be able to:

LO 5.1 Describe the alimentary canal and its accessory organs.

LO 5.2 Discuss the functions of the digestive system.

LO 5.3 Describe overall disorders of the alimentary system to include gastrointestinal bleeding.

LO 5.4 Relate the anatomy of the mouth to the function of mastication.

LO 5.5 Describe disorders of the mouth.

LO 5.6 Relate the anatomy of the pharynx and esophagus to the function of swallowing.

LO 5.7 Describe disorders of the esophagus.

LO 5.8 Relate the anatomy of the stomach and small intestine to the process of digestion.

LO 5.9 Discuss disorders of the stomach and small intestine.

LO 5.10 Relate the anatomy of the liver, gallbladder, and pancreas to their functions in digestion.

LO 5.11 Discuss disorders of the liver, gallbladder, and pancreas that affect digestion.

LO 5.12 Explain the digestion and absorption of proteins, carbohydrates, and fats.

LO 5.13 Discuss malabsorption syndromes and their diagnoses.

LO 5.14 Relate the anatomy of the large intestine to its functions.

LO 5.15 Discuss disorders of the large intestine.

LO 5.16 Describe diagnostic procedures used in gastroenterology.

LO 5.17 Discuss therapeutic procedures used in gastroenterology.

LO 5.18 Define the types of pharmacologic agents used in gastroenterology.

LO 5.A Use the medical terms of gastroenterology to communicate and document in writing accurately and precisely in any health care setting.

LO 5.B Use the medical terms of gastroenterology to communicate verbally with accuracy and precision in any health care setting.

LO 5.C Construct medical terms associated with gastroenterology using word elements (roots, combining forms, prefixes, and suffixes).

LO 5.D Deconstruct medical terms associated with gastroenterology into their word element (roots, combining forms, prefixes, and suffixes).

LO 5.E Use approved abbreviations of medical terms associated with gastroenterology in the correct context of medical care.

LO 5.F Identify health professionals involved in treating gastroenterological patients.

Fulwood Medical Center
3333 Medical Parkway, Fulwood, MI 01234
555-247-6100

Department of: **Bariatric** Surgery

To: Charles Leavenworth, MD
Medical Director
Lombard Insurance Company

From: Stewart Walsh, MD, FACS
Chief of Surgery
Center for Bariatric Surgery
Fulwood Medical Center

10/06/17

Dear Doctor Leavenworth,

Request for authorization of surgery

Re: Mrs. Martha Jones
Subscriber ID 056437

Mrs. Jones is a 52-year-old former waitress, recently divorced. She is 5 feet 4 inches tall and weighs 275 pounds. She has type 2 diabetes with frequent episodes of hypoglycemia and also ketoacidosis, requiring three different hospitalizations. She now has diabetic retinopathy and peripheral vasculitis. Complicating this is hypertension (185/110), coronary artery disease, and pulmonary edema. Exercise is out of the question because she has marked osteoarthritis of her knees and hips. Mrs. Jones is now housebound, dependent on transportation to our medical center. In spite of monthly meetings with our nutritionist, she has gained 25 pounds in the past 6 months.

At a case conference earlier today, we all recognized that unless we were able to reduce and control her weight, we had no hope of controlling any of her other multiple problems.

Therefore, I am proposing to perform a **Roux-en-Y gastric** bypass using a laparoscopic approach. We will need to admit her 2 days prior to surgery to control her blood sugar and cardiovascular problems and anticipate that she will remain in the hospital for 2 days after surgery, barring any complications. My surgical technologist and I have spent time with Mrs. Jones explaining the procedure and its risks, and she is aware and accepting of these. She is also very aware of the necessary follow-up to the procedure and the counseling required for a new lifestyle.

We believe not only that this is an essential procedure medically but that it will reduce in the long term the financial burden of her multiple therapies and improve the quality of the patient's life. Enclosed is supportive documentation of her current history and medical problems.

Your company has designated our hospital as a Center of Excellence for weight-loss surgery, and I look forward to your prompt agreement with this approach for this patient.

Sincerely,

Stewart Walsh, MD, FACS
Chief of Surgery
Fulwood Medical Center

Case Report (CR) 5.1

You are

. . . a medical **transcriptionist** at Fulwood Medical Center.

One of your physicians

. . . Dr. Stewart Walsh, has dictated the letter at left to request authorization for a procedure.

Lesson 5.1

DIGESTIVE SYSTEM

The Digestive System

Lesson Objectives

There are basic elements of anatomy, physiology, and medical terminology that apply throughout the different parts of the digestive system. These elements are discussed in this lesson. That information will enable you to:

5.1.1 Select the correct medical terminology to describe the structure and functions of the digestive system.

5.1.2 List the organs and accessory organs of the digestive system.

5.1.3 Discuss the basic processes of digestion.

Abbreviation

GI	gastrointestinal

LO 5.1 Digestive Tract and Accessory Organs

Every cell in your body requires a constant supply of nourishment. The cells cannot travel, so the nourishment has to be brought to them in a form that can be absorbed across their cell membrane. The foods that you ingest cannot be used in their existing form by the cells. The digestive system, through its alimentary canal, breaks down the nutrients in the food into elements that can be transported to the cells via the blood and **lymphatics**. This physical breakdown of food into smaller sizes and the chemical change of food into the basic elements of lipids, amino acids, and sugars is termed **digestion**. These elements can then be transported across the cell membrane into the cell.

The **digestive system** consists of the digestive tract (**alimentary canal**), which is a hollow tube that extends from the **mouth** to the **anus,** and **accessory organs** connected to the digestive tract to assist in digestion. The accessory organs project into or secrete liquids into the the digestive tract.

The term **gastrointestinal (GI)** technically refers to the stomach and **intestines** but is often used to mean the whole digestive system. **Gastroenterology** is the study of the digestive system. A **gastroenterologist** is a physician who specializes in the digestive system.

The alimentary canal *(Figure 5.1)* includes the

- **Mouth**
- Small **intestine**
- Stomach
- **Esophagus**
- Pharynx
- Large **intestine**

The **accessory organs** of digestion include the

- Teeth
- Gallbladder
- Liver
- Salivary glands
- Tongue
- Pancreas

Case Report (CR) 5.1 *(continued)*

In Mrs. Martha Jones's case, the **Roux-en-Y** procedure reduced the size of her available stomach from 2 quarts to 2 ounces. This resulted in her being able to eat less and to absorb less. She had no complications from the **laparoscopic** procedure. In the succeeding 2 months, she lost 15 pounds in weight.

▲ **Figure 5.1** **Digestive Tract.**

WORD	PRONUNCIATION	ELEMENTS		DEFINITION
alimentary	al-ih-**MEN**-tar-ee	S/ R/	-ary *pertaining to* aliment- *nourishment*	Pertaining to the digestive tract
bariatric	bar-ee-**AT**-rik	S/ R/	-atric *treatment* bari- *weight*	Treatment of obesity
digestion	die-**JEST**-shun	S/ R/	-ion *action* digest- *to break down*	Breakdown of food into elements suitable for cell metabolism
digestive (adj)	die-**JEST**-iv	S/	-ive *nature of*	Pertaining to digestion
esophagus	ee-**SOF**-ah-gus		Greek *gullet*	Tube linking the pharynx and the stomach
gastric	**GAS**-trik	S/ R/	-ic *pertaining to* gastr- *stomach*	Pertaining to the stomach
gastroenterology	**GAS**-troh-en-ter-**OL**-oh-gee	S/ R/CF R/CF	-logy *study of* gastr/o- *stomach* -enter/o- *intestine*	Medical specialty of the stomach and intestines
gastroenterologist gastrointestinal (GI)	**GAS**-troh-en-ter-**OL**-oh-jist **GAS**-troh-in-**TESS**-tin-al	S/ S/ R/CF R/	-logist *one who studies* -al *pertaining to* gastr/o- *stomach* -intestin- *gut, intestine*	Medical specialist in gastroenterology Pertaining to the stomach and intestines
intestine intestinal (adj)	in-**TES**-tin in-**TES**-tin-al	S/ R/	-al *pertaining to* intestin- *intestine, gut*	The digestive tube from stomach to anus
laparoscopy	lap-ah-**ROS**-koh-pee	S/ R/CF	-scopy *to view* lapar/o- *abdomen in general*	Examination of the contents of the abdomen using an endoscope
laparoscope	**LAP**-ah-roh-skope	S/	-scope *instrument for viewing*	Instrument (endoscope) used for viewing the abdominal contents
laparoscopic (adj)	**LAP**-ah-rah-**SKOP**-ik	S/	-ic *pertaining to*	Pertaining to laparoscopy
lymph	LIMF		Latin *spring water*	A clear fluid collected from tissues and transported by vessels to venous circulation
lymphatic (adj)	lim-**FAT**-ik	S/ R/	-atic *pertaining to* lymph- *lymph*	Pertaining to lymph
mouth	MOWTH		Old English *mouth*	External opening of a cavity or canal
Roux-en-Y	**ROO**-on-Y		César Roux, a Swiss surgeon, 1857–1934	Surgical procedure to reduce the size of the stomach
symptom	**SIMP**-tum		Greek *sign*	Departure from the normal experienced by a patient.
symptomatic	simp-toh-**MAT**-ik	S/ R/	-ic *pertaining to* symptomat- *symptom*	Pertaining to the symptoms of a disease
transcript	**TRAN**-skript	P/ R/	trans- *across, through* -script *writing, thing copied*	An exact copy or reproduction
transcription	tran-**SCRIP**-shun	S/	-ion *action, condition*	The action of making a copy of dictated material
transcriptionist	tran-**SCRIP**-shun-ist	S/	-ist *a specialist in*	One who makes a copy of dictated material

Exercises

A. Analyzing the elements can tell you a lot about a medical term. *Review the above WAD box before you start the exercise. Fill in the blanks.* **LO 5.1, 5.A, 5.D, 5.F**

1. Analyzing the two combining forms shows that the term **gastroenterology** relates to the _____ and the _____.

2. In the term **gastric,** the root _____ has the same meaning as the combining form _____ in the term **gastroenterology.**

3. _____ symptoms pertain to the stomach only. Because Mrs. Jones had stomach and intestinal problems, her symptoms can be described as _____. For this condition, she will need a specialist in the study of the stomach and intestines, a field known as _____. This type of physician is referred to as a _____.

LO 5.2 Functions of the Digestive System

1. **Ingestion**—the selective intake of food into the mouth.

2. **Propulsion**—the movement of food from the mouth to the anus *(Figure 5.2)*. Normally, this takes 24 to 36 hours. **Deglutition**, or swallowing, moves the **bolus** of food from the mouth into the esophagus. **Peristalsis**, or waves of contraction and relaxation, moves material through most of the alimentary canal. **Segmental contractions** in the small intestine move food back and forth to mix it with digestive secretions.

3. **Digestion**—the breakdown of foods into forms that can be transported to and absorbed into cells. This process has two components:

   a. **Mechanical digestion** breaks larger pieces of food into smaller ones without altering their chemical composition. This process exposes a larger surface area of the food to the action of digestive enzymes with which to interact.

   b. **Chemical digestion** breaks down large molecules of food into smaller and simpler chemicals. This process is carried out by digestive enzymes produced by the salivary glands, stomach, small intestine, and pancreas.

   The digestive enzymes have three main groups:

   - **Amylases** that digest carbohydrates into sugars
   - **Lipases** that digest fats into fatty acids
   - **Proteases** that digest proteins into amino acids

4. **Secretion**—the addition throughout the digestive tract of secretions that lubricate, liquefy, and digest the food. Mucus lubricates the food and the lining of the tract. Water liquefies the food to make it easier to digest and absorb. Enzymes digest the food.

5. **Absorption**—the movement of nutrient molecules out of the digestive tract and through the epithelial cells lining the tract into the blood or lymph for transportation to body cells.

6. **Elimination**—the process by which the unabsorbed residue of food is removed from the body.

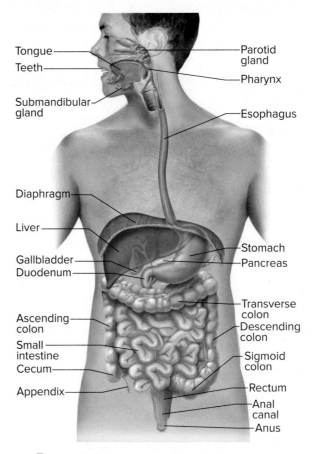

▲ **Figure 5.2** The Digestive System.

WORD	PRONUNCIATION		ELEMENTS	DEFINITION
absorption absorb (verb)	ab-**SORP**-shun ab-**SORB**		Latin *to swallow*	Uptake of nutrients and water by cells in the GI tract
amylase	**AM**-il-aze	S/ R/	-**ase** *enzyme* **amyl-** *starch*	Enzyme that breaks down starch
bolus	**BOH**-lus		Greek *lump*	Single mass of a substance
contraction	kon-**TRAKT**-shun	S/ R/	-**ion** *action* **contract-** *to shorten*	A shortening of a muscle, which increases tension
contract	kon-**TRAKT**		Latin *draw together*	To shorten
deglutition	dee-glue-**TISH**-un	S/ R/	-**ion** *action* **deglutit-** *to swallow*	The act of swallowing
elimination	e-lim-ih-**NAY**-shun	S/ R/	-**ation** *process* **elimin-** *throw away*	Removal of waste material from the digestive tract
ingestion	in-**JEST**-shun	S/ R/	-**ion** *action* **ingest-** *carry in*	Intake of food or drink into the digestive tract
lipase	**LIE**-paze	S/ R/	-**ase** *enzyme* **lip-** *fat*	Enzyme that breaks down fat
peristalsis	per-ih-**STAL**-sis	P/ R/	**peri-** *around* -**stalsis** *constrict*	Waves of alternate contraction and relaxation of alimentary canal wall to move food through the digestive tract
protease	**PROH**-tee-aze	S/ R/CF	-**ase** *enzyme* **prot/e-** *protein*	Enzyme that breaks down protein
secrete secretion (noun)	seh-**KREET** seh-**KREE**-shun		Latin *to separate*	To release or give off, as substances produced by cells Production by a cell or gland
segment segmental (adj)	**SEG**-ment seg-**MENT**-al	S/ R/	Latin *to cut* -**al** *pertaining to* **segment-** *section*	A section of an organ or structure Pertaining to a segment

Exercises

A. The body process or action has been described for you. *Match the definition in the left column to the correct medical term in the right column.* **LO 5.2, 5.A**

_____ 1. Swallowing

_____ 2. Helps lubricate, liquefy, and digest food

_____ 3. Increased muscular tension

_____ 4. Removal of waste material

a. contraction

b. elimination

c. deglutition

d. secretion

B. Build the medical terms by filling in their missing elements. LO 5.2, 5.C

1. Enzyme that breaks down protein: _____/ase

2. Removal of waste material from the digestive tract: _____/ation

3. Enzyme that breaks down fat: lip/_____

4. Enzyme that breaks down starch: _____/ase

5. Pertaining to a section of an organ or structure: _____/al

6. Waves that move food in intestines: peri/_____.

LO 5.3 Overall Digestive System Disorders

A large number of disorders produce symptoms from the gastrointestinal tract but have no specific lesions discoverable in any part of the tract. These disorders include:

- **Food intolerance** has gastrointestinal symptoms such as bloating, cramps, gas, heartburn, diarrhea, and general nonspecific symptoms such as irritability and headache. It is usually diagnosed by keeping a food diary to identify which foods are triggering the symptoms so that they can be avoided.

- **Food allergies** are estimated by the Centers for Disease Control and Prevention (CDC) to affect 4 to 6% of children and 4% of adults. An **allergic** reaction to food occurs when the immune system (see Chapter 12) overreacts to a food, identifying it as a danger, and triggering a protective response. A food that triggers only mild symptoms on one occasion can cause severe symptoms on another occasion. Gastrointestinal symptoms involve vomiting, stomach cramps, and difficulty swallowing. Eight types of food account for 90% of all allergic food reactions: eggs, milk, peanuts, tree nuts, fish, shellfish, wheat, and soy. Skin-prick tests and blood tests can indicate whether food-specific **immunoglobulin** E (IgE) **antibodies** are present in the body. Management of the allergy is to avoid consuming the food.

- **Irritable bowel syndrome** (IBS) is a symptom-based diagnosis with chronic abdominal pain, abdominal discomfort, bloating, and either diarrhea or **constipation**. There is no known organic cause and routine testing shows no abnormality. Dietary adjustments involving fiber intake and psychological interventions can help.

- **Inflammatory bowel disease** (IBD) involves chronic inflammation of all or part of the digestive tract, but primarily includes ulcerative colitis and Crohn's disease (see Lesson 5.5 of this chapter).

- **Aging** has less effect on the digestive system than on other organ systems. In the small intestine, **lactase** levels (see Lesson 5.3 of this chapter) decrease, leading to intolerance of dairy products (**lactose** intolerance). In the large intestine, there is a slight slowing of the movement of contents, leading to constipation.

Gastrointestinal Bleeding

Bleeding can occur anywhere in the gastrointestinal (GI) tract from a variety of causes, as described in the preceding sections. The bleeding can be internal and painless. It can present in different ways to provide a clue to the site of bleeding:

- **Hematemesis**—the vomiting of bright red blood, which indicates an upper GI source of ongoing bleeding (esophagus, stomach, duodenum).

- **Vomiting of "coffee grounds" (coffee ground emesis)**—occurs when bleeding from an upper GI source has slowed or stopped; red hemoglobin has been converted to brown hematin by gastric acids.

- **Hematochezia**—the passage of bright red bloody stools, which usually indicates lower GI bowel bleeding from the sigmoid colon, rectum, or anus.

- **Melena**—the passage of black tarry stools, which usually indicates upper GI bleeding. The blood is digested and hemoglobin is oxidized as it passes through the intestine to produce the black color. Melena can continue for several days after a severe hemorrhage.

- **Occult blood**—no bleeding seen in the stool, but a chemical fecal occult blood test (**Hemoccult test**) is positive. The chronic source of the bleeding can be anywhere in the GI tract.

    Consuming black licorice, Pepto-Bismol, or blueberries can produce black stools.

Abbreviations

CDC	Centers for Disease Control and Prevention
GI	gastrointestinal
IBD	inflammatory bowel disease
IBS	irritable bowel syndrome
IgE	immunoglobulin E

LO 5.3, 5.A
Word Analysis and Definition

S = Suffix   P = Prefix   R = Root   R/CF = Combining Form

WORD	PRONUNCIATION	ELEMENTS		DEFINITION
aging	**A**-jing		Latin *old*	The process of growing old
allergy	**AL**-er-jee	P/	**all** *other*	An acquired sensitivity to certain proteins
		R/	**-ergy** *process of working*	
		R/	**-erg** *work*	
allergen	**AL**-er-jen	R/	**-gen** *to produce*	The substance that incites an allergic reaction
allergic (adj)	Ah-**LER**-jick	S/	**-ic** *pertaining to*	Relating to any response to an allergen
antibody	**AN**-tih-body	P/	**anti-** *against*	Protein produced in response to an antigen
antibodies (pl)	**AN**-tih-bod-ees	R/	**-body** *substance*	
antigen	**AN**-tih-jen	P/	**anti-** *against*	Substance capable of triggering an immune response
		R/	**-gen** *to produce*	
constipation	kon-stih-**PAY**-shun	S/	**-ation** *process*	Hard, infrequent bowel movements
		R/	**constip-** *press together*	
emesis	**EM**-eh-sis		Greek *vomiting*	Condition of vomiting
hematemesis	he-mah-**TEM**-eh-sis	R/	**hemat-** *blood*	Vomiting of red blood
		S/	**emesis** *vomiting*	
hematochezia	he-mat-oh-**KEY**-zee-ah	S/	**-chezia** *pass a stool*	The passage of red, bloody stools
		R/CF	**hemat/o-** *blood*	
immunoglobulin	**IM**-you-noh-**GLOB**-you-lin	S/	**-in** *chemical compound*	Specific protein evoked by an antigen; all
		R/CF	**immun/o-** *immune response*	antibodies are immunoglobulins
		R/	**-globul-** *protein*	
intolerance	in-**TOL**-er-ance		Latin *unable to cope with*	Inability of the small intestine to metabolize a particular dietary constituent
intolerant (adv)	in-**TOL**-er-ant			Possessing intolerance
lactose	**LAK**-toes	S/	**-ose** *condition*	The disaccharide in cow's milk
		R/	**lact-** *milk*	
lactase	**LAK**-tase	S/	**-ase** *enzyme*	Enzyme that breaks down lactose to glucose and galactose
melena	mel-**EN**-ah		Greek *black*	The passage of black, tarry stools
occult	oh-**KULT**		Latin *to hide*	Not visible on the surface
Hemoccult test	**HEEM**-oh-kult TEST			Trade name for a fecal occult blood test
vomit (verb)	**VAH**-mit		Latin *to spew forth, discharge*	Expel contents from the stomach, though the esophagus, and out the mouth
vomit (noun)				Matter vomited from the stomach

Exercises

A. Abbreviations used in general disorders of the gastrointestinal system. *Healthcare providers often use abbreviations when communicating verbally and in writing. Fill in the blank with the correct abbreviation from the provided word bank.* **LO 5.3, 5.A, 5.E**

IBD   IBS   GI

1. The patient has been diagnosed with ulcerative colitis, and therefore has a form of _____.

2. A problem of the digestive tract would be considered to be a _____ disorder.

3. A patient complaining of unpredictable bouts of diarrhea that had no known cause was diagnosed with _____.

B. Describe disorders of the gastrointestinal system. *Determine if the statements are accurate. Choose T if the statement is true, choose F if the statement is false.* **LO 5.3**

1. A food allergy involves the immune system.   T   F

2. A lack of a digestive enzyme causes a food allergy.   T   F

3. Melena is a sign of active bleeding.   T   F

4. Aging has the least effect on the digestive system compared to the other body systems.   T   F

5. Hematochezia is a sign of active bleeding.   T   F

Lesson 5.2
DIGESTIVE SYSTEM

Mouth, Pharynx, and Esophagus

Lesson Objectives

When you pop a piece of chicken and some vegetables into your mouth, you start a cascade of digestive tract events that occur during the following 24 to 36 hours. In this chapter, you will follow a meal of chicken and vegetables as it goes through the digestive tract. In this lesson, you will review the first stages in the cascade while the food is in the mouth and then is swallowed. The information in this lesson will enable you to:

5.2.1 Select the correct medical terminology to describe the anatomy, physiology, and disorders of the mouth, pharynx, and esophagus.

5.2.2 Identify the structure and functions of the teeth, tongue, and salivary glands.

5.2.3 Describe the composition and functions of saliva.

5.2.4 Describe the process and outcomes of mastication and deglutition.

5.2.5 Discuss some common disorders of the mouth, pharynx, and esophagus.

Case Report (CR) 5.2

You are
. . . a Certified Medical Assistant working with Susan Lee, MD, a primary care physician at Fulwood Medical Center.

Your patient is
. . . Mrs. Helen Schreiber, a 45-year-old high school principal. Your task is to document her care.

Documentation

Mrs. Helen Schreiber, a 45-year-old high school principal, presents with a 6-month history of dry mouth, bleeding gums, and difficulty in chewing and swallowing food.

Questioning by Dr. Susan Lee, her primary care physician, reveals that she also has dry eyes, is having pain in some joints of both hands, and has felt fatigued. Her previous medical history is uneventful. Physical examination shows a dry mouth, mild **gingivitis,** and an **ulcer** on the back of the lower lip. Her salivary glands are not swollen. Her eyes show no **ulceration** or conjunctivitis. The metacarpophalangeal joints of both index fingers are swollen, stiff, and tender. All other systems show no abnormality.

Initial laboratory reports show anemia, decreased **WBC** count, and an elevated **ESR.** Dr. Lee made a provisional diagnosis of **Sjögren syndrome.** The results of blood studies for **SSA** and **SSB** antibodies (Sjögren syndrome antibodies A and B) and for rheumatoid factor titers are pending, as are x-rays of her hands.

Mrs. Schreiber was given advice about symptomatic treatment for her dry mouth and will be seen again in 1 week.

Luisa Guitterez, **CMA** 06/12/12, 1530 hrs.

LO 5.4 The Mouth and Mastication

The mouth, or **oral** cavity *(Figure 5.3)*, is the entrance to your digestive tract and is the first site of mechanical digestion (through **mastication**, chewing) and of chemical digestion (through an enzyme in saliva).

The cheeks contain the buccinator muscles. These muscles hold the chicken and vegetables in place while you chew and your teeth crush and tear them.

The roof of the mouth is called the **palate**. The anterior two-thirds is the bony hard palate. The posterior one-third is the muscular soft palate. The hard palate is covered with folds of epithelium called **rugae**, which assist the tongue to manipulate food for mechanical and chemical digestion prior to swallowing. The soft palate has a projection called the **uvula** that closes off the nasopharynx during swallowing.

The **tongue** *(Figure 5.4)* moves food around your mouth and helps the cheeks, lips, and gums hold the food in place while you chew it. Small, rough, raised areas on the tongue, called **papillae**, contain some 4,000 **taste buds** that react to the chemical nature of the food to give you the different sensations of **taste**. A taste bud cell lives for 7 to 10 days and is then replaced.

Abbreviations

CMA	Certified Medical Assistant
ESR	erythrocyte sedimentation rate
SSA	Sjögren syndrome antibody A
SSB	Sjögren syndrome antibody B
WBC	white blood cell

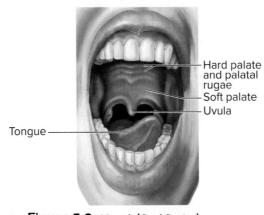

▲ **Figure 5.3** Mouth (Oral Cavity).

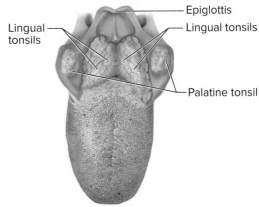

▲ **Figure 5.4** Tongue.

WORD	PRONUNCIATION	ELEMENTS		DEFINITION
masticate mastication (noun)	**MAS**-tih-kate mas-tih-**KAY**-shun	S/ R/	-ate *composed of, pertaining to* **mastic-** *chew*	To chew
oral	**OR**-al	S/ R/	-al *pertaining to* or- *mouth*	Pertaining to the mouth
palate	**PAL**-uht		Latin *palate*	Roof of the mouth
papilla papillae (pl)	pah-**PILL**-ah pah-**PILL**-ee		Latin *small pimple*	Any small projection
ruga rugae (pl)	**ROO**-gah **ROO**-gee		Latin *wrinkle*	A fold, ridge, or crease
taste	TAYST		Latin *to taste*	Sensation from chemicals on the taste buds
tongue	TUNG		Latin *tongue*	Mobile muscle mass in mouth; bears the taste buds
uvula	**YOU**-vyu-lah		Latin *grape*	Fleshy projection of the soft palate

Exercises

A. Many medical terms have Latin origins and cannot be deconstructed. *Use the terms from the above WAD to complete the sentences. Fill in the blank.* **LO 5.4, 5.A**

1. The roof of the mouth is termed the _____.

2. During swallowing, the _____ covers the entrance to the nose from the back of the throat.

3. Taste buds are located on the sides of the tongue's _____.

4. The _____ that covers the hard palate aid in mechanical digestion of food.

B. After reading Case Report (CR) 5.2, answer the following questions. LO 5.5

1. Which of the following is a sign that the physician noted?

   a. difficulty chewing

   b. gingivitis

   c. dry mouth

   d. headache

2. The patient was diagnosed with:

   a. Sjögren syndrome

   b. rheumatoid arthritis

   c. ulcerative colitis

   d. irritable bowel syndrome

3. Blood tests that were used to diagnose her disorder included:

   a. electrolytes

   b. platelet count

   c. pregnancy test

   d. Sjögren syndrome antibodies A and B

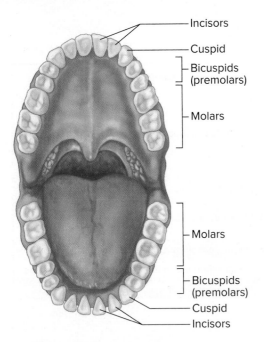

▲ **Figure 5.5** Adult Teeth.

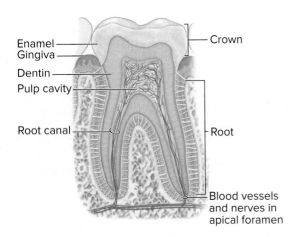

▲ **Figure 5.6** Anatomy of a Molar.

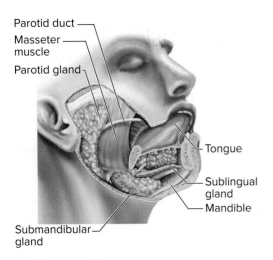

▲ **Figure 5.7** Salivary Glands.

LO 5.4 The Mouth and Mastication (continued)

Adult Teeth

The normal adult has 32 teeth, 16 rooted in the upper jaw (maxilla) and 16 in the lower jaw (mandible). The teeth are the hardest structures in your body, and different teeth *(Figure 5.5)* are designed to handle food in different ways. The eight **incisors** are shaped like a chisel to slice and cut into food. The four **cuspids** have a pointed tip for puncturing and tearing. The eight **bicuspids** and twelve **molars** have flattened surfaces for grinding and crushing food. Your wisdom teeth are molars.

Each tooth has two main parts:

- The **crown**, which projects above the gum and is covered in **enamel**, the hardest substance in the body.
- The **root**, which anchors the tooth to the jaw.

The bulk of the tooth is composed of **dentin**, a substance like bone but harder *(Figure 5.6)*. The dentin surrounds a central **pulp cavity** that contains blood vessels, nerves, and connective tissue. The blood vessels and nerves reach this cavity from the jaw through tubular **root canals**. The **gingiva** is a soft pink tissue that surrounds and attaches to teeth and the jaw bones. The area around the tooth is referred to as the **periodontal region.**

Salivary Glands

Salivary glands secrete saliva. The two **parotid** glands, the two **submandibular** glands, the two **sublingual glands** *(Figure 5.7)*, and numerous minor salivary glands scattered in the mucosa of the tongue and cheeks secrete more than a quart of saliva each day.

Saliva is 95% water, and its functions are to

- Begin starch digestion with the **enzyme amylase.**
- Begin fat digestion with the enzyme **lipase.**
- Prevent the growth of bacteria in the mouth with the enzyme **lysozyme** and the protective **immunoglobulin A (IgA)** *(see Chapter 12).*
- Produce **mucus** to lubricate food to make it easier to swallow.

Imagine that you are eating a piece of chicken with some vegetables. By the end of the mastication process, the chicken has been torn and ground into small pieces by your teeth, and its fat has begun to be digested by the lipase in your saliva. The vegetables have been ground into small pieces as well, and the starch in them has begun to be digested by the amylase in your saliva. The food has been lubricated, mixed together, and formed into a bolus ready to be swallowed.

> **Case Report (CR) 5.2** *(continued)*
>
> Mrs. Helen Schreiber has Sjögren syndrome, an autoimmune disease *(see Chapter 12)* that affects her salivary glands, stopping production of saliva. This leads to a dry mouth, difficulty in swallowing, and increased bacterial activity in the mouth, causing gingivitis. It is associated with dry eyes and with rheumatoid arthritis, which is beginning in her hands. There is no known cure, and treatment is **symptomatic**.

S = Suffix   P = Prefix   R = Root   R/CF = Combining Form

WORD	PRONUNCIATION	ELEMENTS		DEFINITION
bicuspid (also called premolar)	by-KUSS-pid	S/ P/ R/	-id *having a particular quality* bi- *two* -cusp- *point*	Having two points; a bicuspid (premolar) tooth has two points
crown	KROWN		Latin *crown*	Part of the tooth above the gum
cuspid	KUSS-pid	S/ R/	-id *having a particular quality* cusp- *point*	Tooth with one point
dentin (also spelled dentine)	DEN-tin	S/ R/	-in *substance, chemical compound* dent- *tooth*	Dense, ivory-like substance located under the enamel in a tooth
enamel	ee-NAM-el		French *enamel*	Hard substance covering a tooth
enzyme	EN-zime	P/ R/	en- *in* -zyme *fermenting, enzyme*	Protein that induces changes in other substances
gingiva gingival (adj)	JIN-jih-vah JIN-jih-vul	S/ R/	Latin *gum* -al *pertaining to* gingiv- *gums*	Tissue surrounding teeth and covering the jaw Pertaining to the gums
incisor	in-SIGH-zor		Latin *to cut into*	Chisel-shaped tooth
lysozyme	LIE-soh-zime	S/ R/CF	-zyme *enzyme* lys/o- *dissolve*	Enzyme that dissolves the cell walls of bacteria
molar	MOH-lar		Latin *millstone*	One of six teeth in each jaw that grind food
parotid	pah-ROT-id	S/ P/ R/	-id *having a particular quality* par- *beside* -ot- *ear*	Parotid gland is the salivary gland beside the ear
periodontal	PER-ee-oh-DON-tal	S/ P/ R/	-al *pertaining to* peri- *around* -odont- *tooth*	Around a tooth
pulp	PULP		Latin *flesh*	Dental pulp is the connective tissue in the cavity in the center of the tooth
root	ROOT		Old English *beginning*	Fundamental or beginning part of a structure
saliva salivary (adj)	sa-LIE-vah SAL-ih-var-ee	S/ R/	Latin *spit* -ary *pertaining to* saliv- *saliva*	Secretion in the mouth from salivary glands Pertaining to saliva
sublingual	sub-LING-wal	S/ P/ R/	-al *pertaining to* sub- *underneath* -lingu- *tongue*	Pertaining to underneath the tongue
submandibular	sub-man-DIB-you-lar	S/ P/ R/	-ar *pertaining to* sub- *underneath* -mandibul- *the jaw*	Pertaining to underneath the mandible
symptom symptomatic asymptomatic	SIMP-tum simp-toe-MAT-ik	S/ R/ P/	Greek *sign* -ic *pertaining to* symptomat- *symptom* a- *without*	Departure from the normal experienced by the patient Pertaining to the symptoms of a disease Absence of symptoms

Exercises

A. Study the terms and elements in the above WAD. *Notice that some terms are formed with only a prefix and a root, while others are formed with a root and a suffix. Write the correct element on each blank that needs an element.* **LO 5.4, 5.A, 5.D**

1   submandibular _____/_____ /_____
                        P   R   S

2.   sublingual _____/_____ /_____
                     P   R   S

▲ **Figure 5.8** **Dental Caries.** Child with dental caries. ©Ted Croll/Science Source

▲ **Figure 5.9** **Cold Sores.** Ulcer inside lower lip. ©defun/Getty Images RF

▲ **Figure 5.10** **Oral Thrush.** ©Medical-on-line/Alamy

Abbreviations	
HIV	human immunodeficiency virus
HSV-1	herpes simplex virus, type 1

LO 5.5 Disorders of the Mouth

An accumulation of dental **plaque** (a collection of oral microorganisms and their products) or **dental calculus (tartar),** calcified deposits at the gingival margin of the teeth, is a precursor to dental disease.

Dental caries, tooth decay and cavity formation, is an erosion of the tooth surface caused by bacteria *(Figure 5.8)*. If untreated, it can lead to an **abscess** at the root of the tooth. **Gingivitis** is an infection of the gums. **Periodontal disease** occurs when the gums and the jawbone are involved in a disease process. In **periodontitis**, infection causes the gums to pull away from the teeth, forming pockets that become infected. The infection can spread to the underlying bone. Infection of the gums with a purulent discharge is called **pyorrhea**.

The term **stomatitis** is used for any infection of the mouth. The most common infections are

- **Mouth ulcers**, also called **canker** sores, which are erosions of the mucous membrane lining the mouth. The most common type are **aphthous ulcers**, which occur in clusters of small ulcers and last for 3 or 4 days. They are usually related to stress or illness. Ulcers can also be caused by trauma.

- **Cold sores,** also known as fever blisters *(Figure 5.9)*, which are recurrent ulcers of the lips, lining of the mouth, and gums due to infection with the virus **herpes simplex type 1 (HSV-1).**

- **Thrush** *(Figure 5.10)*, an infection occurring anywhere in the mouth and caused by the fungus *Candida albicans*. This fungus typically is found in the mouth, but it can multiply out of control as a result of prolonged antibiotic or steroid treatment, cancer chemotherapy, or diabetes. A newborn baby can acquire oral thrush from the mother's vaginal yeast infection during the birth process.

- **Leukoplakia**, a white plaque seen anywhere in the mouth. It is more common in the elderly, it is often associated with smoking or chewing tobacco, and approximately 3% turn into oral cancer. Patients whose immune systems are compromised (for example, with **human immunodeficiency virus [HIV]**) are susceptible to leukoplakia.

- **Oral cancer** *(Figure 5.11)*, which is mostly squamous cell **carcinoma**, occurring often on the lip. Eighty percent of oral cancers are associated with smoking or chewing tobacco. Metastasis occurs to lymph nodes, bone, lung, and liver. The 5-year survival rate is only 51%.

- **Halitosis**, the medical term for bad breath, which can be found in association with any of the above mouth disorders.

- **Glossodynia**, a painful burning sensation of the tongue. It occurs in postmenopausal women. Its etiology is unknown, and there is no successful treatment.

- **Cleft palate,** a congenital fissure in the median line of the palate. It is often associated with a cleft lip.

- **Sjögren syndrome**, an autoimmune disease that attacks the glands that produce saliva and tears. Symptoms include dry mouth and eyes. It is associated with other autoimmune diseases, such as rheumatoid arthritis.

— Cancer

▲ **Figure 5.11** **Oral Cancer.** Cancer of the tongue. ©Clinica Claros/Science Source

WORD	PRONUNCIATION	ELEMENTS		DEFINITION
abscess	**AB**-sess		Latin *a going away*	A collection of pus.
aphthous ulcer	**AF**-thus **UL**-ser		Greek *ulcer*	Painful small oral ulcer (canker sore)
canker; canker sore (also called **mouth ulcer**)	**KANG**-ker SOAR		Latin *crab*	Nonmedical term for aphthous ulcer
carcinoma	kar-sih-**NOH**-mah	S/ R/	**-oma** *tumor, mass* **carcin-** *cancer*	A cancerous (malignant) and invasive epithelial tumor.
caries	**KARE**-eez		Latin *dry rot*	Bacterial destruction of teeth
gingivitis	jin-jih-**VIE**-tis	S/ R/	**-itis** *inflammation* **gingiv-** *gums*	Inflammation of the gums
gingivectomy	jin-jih-**VEC**-toe-mee	S/	**-ectomy** *surgical excision*	Surgical removal of diseased gum tissue
glossodynia	gloss-oh-**DIN**-ee-ah	S/ R/CF	**-dynia** *pain* **gloss/o-** *tongue*	Painful, burning tongue
halitosis	hal-ih-**TOE**-sis	S/ R/	**-osis** *condition* **halit-** *breath*	Bad odor of the breath
leukoplakia	loo-koh-**PLAY**-kee-ah	S/ R/CF R/	**-ia** *condition* **leuk/o-** *white* **-plak-** *plate, plaque*	White patch on oral mucous membrane, often precancerous
periodontics	**PER**-ee-oh-**DON**-tiks	S/ P/ R/	**-ics** *knowledge of* **peri-** *around* **-odont-** *tooth*	Branch of dentistry specializing in disorders of tissues around the teeth
periodontist periodontitis	**PER**-ee-oh-**DON**-tist **PER**-ee-oh-don-**TIE**-tis	S/ S/	**-ist** *specialist* **-itis** *inflammation*	Specialist in periodontics Inflammation of tissues around a tooth
plaque	PLAK		French *plate*	Patch of abnormal tissue
pyorrhea	pie-oh-**REE**-ah	S/ R/CF	**-rrhea** *flow* **py/o-** *pus*	Purulent discharge
Sjögren syndrome	**SHOW**-gren **SIN**-drome		Henrik Sjögren, 1889–1986, Swedish ophthalmologist	Autoimmune disease that attacks the glands that produce saliva and tears
stomatitis	**STOW**-ma-**TIE**-tis	S/ R/	**-itis** *inflammation* **stomat-** *mouth*	A general term given to any infection of the mouth.
syndrome	**SIN**-drome	P/ R/	**syn-** *together* **-drome** *course*	A collection of signs and symptoms that typify a disease.
tartar (also called **dental calculus**)	**TAR**-tar		Latin *crust on wine casks*	Calcified deposit at the gingival margin of the teeth
thrush	THRUSH		Root unknown	Infection with *Candida albicans*
ulcer ulceration	**ULL**-cer ull-cer-**A**-shun	S/ R/	**-ation** *a process* **ulcer-** *a sore*	Erosion of an area of skin or mucosa Formation of an ulcer

Exercises

A. Enter the correct suffix to complete the medical terms. *Fill in the blanks.* LO 5.5, 5.A, 5.C, 5.F

1. Inflammation of the gums — gingiv/_____
2. Specialized branch of dentistry — periodont/_____
3. Painful, burning tongue — glosso/_____
4. Inflammation around a tooth — periodont/_____
5. Bad breath — halit/_____
6. Purulent discharge — pyo/_____
7. Precancerous white patches — leukoplak/_____

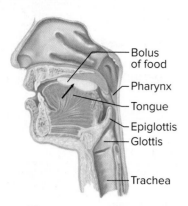

- Bolus of food
- Pharynx
- Tongue
- Epiglottis
- Glottis
- Trachea

▲ **Figure 5.12** **Deglutition** (Swallowing): Phase One.

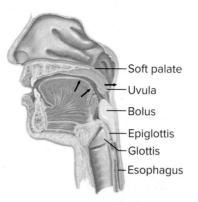

- Soft palate
- Uvula
- Bolus
- Epiglottis
- Glottis
- Esophagus

▲ **Figure 5.13** **Deglutition** (Swallowing): Phase Two.

- Epiglottis
- Bolus now in esophagus

▲ **Figure 5.14** **Deglutition** (Swallowing): Phase Three.

- Bolus
- Stomach
- Cardiac (esophageal) sphincter

▲ **Figure 5.15** **Deglutition** (Swallowing): Phase Four.

Abbreviation

GERD gastroesophageal reflux disease

LO 5.6 Deglutition (Swallowing)—Pharynx and Esophagus

The pieces of chicken and vegetables that you ingested have now been sliced and ground into small particles by the teeth, partially digested and lubricated by saliva, and rolled into a bolus between the tongue and the hard palate, the bony roof of the mouth *(Figure 5.12)*. The bolus is now ready to be swallowed **(deglutition).**

- **Phase One.** As you swallow, the bolus of food is pushed backward by your tongue into the **oropharynx**. Once the bolus is in your oropharynx, the tongue contracts against the hard palate and pushes up the soft palate and uvula to close off the **nasopharynx** at the back of the nose. This prevents food from going up into your nasopharynx and nose *(see Figure 5.12).*

- **Phase Two.** Surrounding the oropharynx are circular muscles called **constrictors.** These muscles contract, forcing the bolus down through the laryngopharynx toward the **esophagus** and pushing the **epiglottis** closed so that food cannot enter the airways to the lungs, the larynx, and trachea *(Figure 5.13).*

- **Phase Three.** When the bolus reaches the lower end of the **pharynx**, the upper **esophageal sphincter** relaxes and the bolus enters the esophagus, where contractions of the muscles in the wall move the bolus toward the stomach *(Figure 5.14).*

- **Phase Four.** The esophageal sphincter at the lower end of the esophagus **(cardiac sphincter)** relaxes to allow the bolus to enter the stomach *(Figure 5.15).*

The **esophagus** *(Figure 5.16)* is a tube 9 to 10 inches long; it pierces the diaphragm at the esophageal **hiatus** to go from the thoracic cavity to the abdominal cavity.

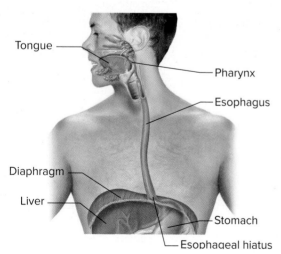

- Tongue
- Pharynx
- Esophagus
- Diaphragm
- Liver
- Stomach
- Esophageal hiatus

▲ **Figure 5.16** **Esophagus.**

LO 5.7 Disorders of the Esophagus

Esophagitis is inflammation of the lining of the esophagus that produces a **postprandial** burning chest pain **(heartburn),** pain on swallowing, and occasional vomiting of blood **(hematemesis).** The most common cause is **reflux** of the stomach's acid contents into the esophagus, **gastroesophageal reflux disease (GERD). Regurgitation** of stomach contents into the mouth **(water brash)** can occur with resulting hypersalivation.

- **Hiatal hernia** occurs when a portion of the stomach protrudes **(herniates)** through the diaphragm alongside the esophagus at the esophageal **hiatus.** Reflux of acid stomach contents into the esophagus causes an **esophagitis.** Surgical repair sometimes is necessary and is called a **herniorrhaphy.**

- **Esophageal varices** are **varicose** veins of the esophagus. They are **asymptomatic** until they rupture, causing massive bleeding and hematemesis. They are a complication of cirrhosis of the liver *(see Lesson 5.4).*

- **Cancer of the esophagus** arises from the lining of the tube. Symptoms are difficulty in swallowing **(dysphagia),** a burning sensation in the chest, and weight loss. Risk factors include cigarettes, alcohol, betel nut chewing, and esophageal reflux.

WORD	PRONUNCIATION	ELEMENTS		DEFINITION
constrictor	kon-**STRIK**-tore	S/ R/	**-or** *a doer, one who does, that which does something* **constrict-** *narrow, to narrow*	Muscle that contracts or compresses an organ
deglutition	dee-glue-**TISH**-un		Latin *to swallow*	The act of swallowing
dysphagia	dis-**FAY**-jee-ah	P/ R/	**dys-** *difficult* **-phagia** *swallowing*	Difficulty in swallowing
emesis hematemesis	**EM**-eh-sis he-mah-**TEM**-eh-sis	S/ R/	**-emesis** *to vomit* **hemat-** *blood*	Vomiting Vomiting of red blood
epiglottis	ep-ih-**GLOT**-is	P/ R/	**epi-** *above* **-glottis** *windpipe*	Leaf-shaped plate of cartilage that shuts off larynx during swallowing
esophagus esophageal (adj) esophagitis	ee-**SOF**-ah-gus ee-**SOF**-ah-**JEE**-al ee-**SOF**-ah-**JIE**-tis	 S/ R/ S/	Greek *gullet* **-eal** *pertaining to* **esophag-** *esophagus* **-itis** *inflammation*	Tube linking the pharynx and stomach Pertaining to the esophagus Inflammation of the lining of the esophagus
gastroesophageal	**GAS**-troh-ee-sof-ah-**JEE**-al	S/ R/CF R/CF	**-al** *pertaining to* **gastr/o** *stomach* **-esophag/e** *esophagus*	Pertaining to the stomach and esophagus
hernia herniorrhaphy herniate (verb)	**HER**-nee-ah **HER**-nee-**OR**-ah-fee **HER**-nee-ate	 S/ R/CF S/	Latin *rupture* **-rrhaphy** *suture* **herni/o-** *hernia* **-ate** *pertaining to*	Protrusion of a structure through the tissue that normally contains it Repair of a hernia To protrude
hiatus hiatal (adj)	high-**AY**-tus high-**AY**-tal	 S/ R/	Latin *an aperture* **-al** *pertaining to* **hiat-** *aperture*	An opening through a structure Pertaining to an opening through a structure
nasopharynx	**NAY**-zoh-**FAIR**-inks	R/CF R/	**nas/o-** *nose* **-pharynx** *throat*	Region of the pharynx at the back of the nose and above the soft palate
oropharynx	**OR**-oh-**FAIR**-inks	R/CF R/	**or/o-** *mouth* **-pharynx** *throat*	Region at the back of the mouth between the soft palate and the tip of the epiglottis
pharynx	**FAIR**-inks		Greek *throat*	Air tube from the back of the nose to the larynx
postprandial	post-**PRAN**-dee-al	S/ P/ R/	**-ial** *pertaining to* **post-** *after* **-prand-** *meal*	Following a meal
reflux	**REE**-fluks	P/ R/	**re-** *back* **-flux** *flow*	Backward flow
regurgitation	ree-gur-jih-**TAY**-shun	S/ P/ R/	**-ation** *process* **re-** *back* **-gurgit-** *flood*	Expelling contents of the stomach into the mouth, short of vomiting
sphincter	**SFINK**-ter		Greek *band, lace, or anything that binds tight*	Bank of muscle that encircles an opening; when it contracts, the opening squeezes closed.
varix varices (pl) varicose (adj)	**VAIR**-iks **VAIR**-ih-seez **VAIR**-ih-kos		Latin *dilated vein*	Dilated, tortuous vein Characterized by or affected with varices

Exercises

A. Some of the terms in this chapter are particularly hard to spell and pronounce. *Select the correct spelling for the medical term(s) that complete each sentence.* **LO 5.6, 5.7, 5.A**

1. (Hyatus/Hiatus) is the Latin word for *opening* and is the opening through the diaphragm for the (esophagis/esophagus).

2. The (eppiglotis/epiglottis) is a leaf-shaped plate of cartilage that acts to cover the opening of the (larynix/larynx) during deglutition.

3. Medication may be ordered (postprandially/postperandially), meaning *taken after meals.*

4. (Hemotemasis/Hematemesis) is the (vomiting/vomitting) of blood.

5. (Esophagitis/Esophogitis) can be caused by reflux disease.

6. (Varricces/Varices) is the plural of (varix/varex) and means *dilated, tortuous vein.* The adjective is (varicose/varricose).

Lesson 5.3

DIGESTIVE SYSTEM

Digestion—Stomach and Small Intestine

Lesson Objectives

The bolus of food that you swallowed has passed down the esophagus. It now enters the stomach, and the process of digestion begins in earnest. The stomach continues the mechanical breakdown of the food particles and begins the chemical digestion of protein and fats. It is in the small intestine that the greatest amount of digestion and absorption occurs. The information in this lesson will enable you to:

5.3.1 Describe the process of digestion in the small intestine.

5.3.2 Describe the layers of the wall of the small intestine.

5.3.3 Describe the secretions of the stomach and their functions.

5.3.4 Discuss the secretions of the small intestine and their functions.

5.3.5 Explain how food is propelled through the stomach and small intestine.

5.3.6 Describe how the breakdown products of digestion are absorbed from the small intestine.

Abbreviations

EMR	emergency medical responder
ER	emergency room
HCl	hydrochloric acid

Case Report (CR) 5.3

You are

. . . an **EMR** working in the Emergency Department at Fulwood Medical Center.

Your patient is

. . . Mrs. Jan Stark, a 36-year-old pottery maker. Your task is to document her visit.

Documentation

Mrs. Jan Stark, a 36-year-old pottery maker, was admitted to the Emergency Department at 2015 hrs.

She stated that she had passed between 20 and 30 watery, gray stools in the previous 24 hours. She had not passed urine for more than 12 hours. She was markedly **dehydrated** and responded well to infusion of lactated Ringer solution and then D5NS (5% dextrose in normal 0.9% saline).

Questioning revealed that, for the past 10 years, she has had spasmodic episodes of diarrhea and flatulence associated with severe headaches and fatigue. During those episodes, her stools were greasy and pale. In the past 3 or 4 months, she has had some difficulties with fine movements as she works on her pottery wheel and has had tingling in her fingers and toes.

Dr. Homer Hilinski, emergency physician, believes her **dehydration** is a result of a **malabsorption syndrome.** An appointment has been made for her to see Dr. Cameron Grabowski, gastroenterologist, tomorrow. She was discharged to her husband's care at midnight. She has been advised to stay on fluids only and to return to the Emergency Room (**ER**) if the diarrhea returns.

Sunil Patel, EMT-1. 10/21/12, 0100 hrs.

LO 5.8 Digestion in the Stomach

The stomach's peristaltic contractions mix different boluses of food together and also push the more liquid contents toward the **pylorus** *(Figure 5.17)*. These contractions and the digestive process work on the boluses of food to produce a mixture of semidigested food called **chyme.**

The cells of the lining of the stomach secrete the following:

- **Mucin**—continues to lubricate food and protects the stomach lining. Mucin combines with the other secretions to become **mucus.**
- **Hydrochloric acid (HCl)**—breaks up the

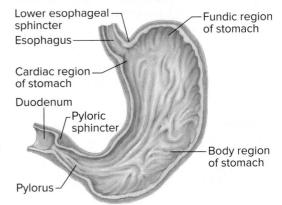

▲ **Figure 5.17** Stomach.

connective tissue of the chicken and the cell walls of the vegetables that you ingested a few seconds ago. It also destroys any pathogens that enter your stomach along with the food you eat.

- **Pepsinogen**—is converted by hydrochloric acid to **pepsin,** an active enzyme that starts to digest the protein in the chicken and vegetables.
- **Intrinsic factor**—is essential for the absorption of vitamin B_{12} in the small intestine. Neither chicken nor vegetables contain this factor.
- **Chemical messengers**—stimulate other cells in the gastric mucosa. One of these messengers, **gastrin,** stimulates both the production of HCl and pepsinogen by the stomach cells and the peristaltic contractions of the stomach.

Liquids exit the stomach within 1½ to 2 hours after ingestion. A typical meal like your chicken and vegetables takes 3 to 4 hours to exit. The resulting chyme is held in the pylorus. Peristaltic waves squirt 2 to 3 mL of the chyme at a time through the **pyloric sphincter** into the **duodenum.**

Anywhere from 40 minutes to 2 hours after consuming that chicken and vegetable dinner mentioned earlier, your food is partially digested by the salivary and stomach enzymes described previously.

WORD	PRONUNCIATION	ELEMENTS		DEFINITION
chyme	KIME		Greek *juice*	Semifluid, partially digested food passed from the stomach into the duodenum
dehydration	dee-high-**DRAY**-shun	S/ P/ R/	-ation *a process* de- *without* -hydr- *water*	Process of losing body water
duodenum	du-oh-**DEE**-num	S/ R/	-um *structure* duoden- *Latin for twelve*	The first part of the small intestine; approximately 12 finger-breadths (9 to 10 inches) in length
duodenal (adj)	du-oh-**DEE**-nal	S/	-al *pertaining to*	Pertaining to the duodenum
gastrin	**GAS**-trin	S/ R/	-in *substance* gastr- *stomach*	Hormone secreted in the stomach that stimulates secretion of HCl and increases gastric motility
hydrochloric acid (HCl)	high-droh-**KLOR**-ic **ASS**-id	S/ R/CF R/	-ic *pertaining to* hydr/o- *water* -chlor- *green*	The acid of gastric juice
intrinsic factor	in-**TRIN**-sik **FAK**-tor	S/ R/ R/	-ic *pertaining to* intrins- *on the inside* factor *maker*	Substance secreted by the stomach that is necessary for the absorption of vitamin B_{12}
malabsorption	mal-ab-**SORP**-shun	S/ P/ R/	-ion *action, condition* mal- *bad* -absorpt- *to swallow*	Inadequate gastrointestinal absorption of nutrients
mucus	**MYU**-kus		Latin *slime*	Sticky secretion of cells in mucous membranes
mucous (adj)	**MYU**-kus	S/ R/	-ous *pertaining to* muc- *mucus*	Relating to mucus or the mucosa
mucin	**MYU**-sin	S/	-in *chemical compound*	Protein element of mucus
pepsin	**PEP**-sin		Greek *to digest*	Enzyme produced by the stomach that breaks down protein
pepsinogen	pep-**SIN**-oh-jen	S/ R/CF	-gen *produce* pepsin/o- *pepsin*	Enzyme converted by HCl in stomach to pepsin
pylorus	pie-**LOR**-us	S/ R/	-us *pertaining to* pylor- *gate*	Exit area of the stomach proximal to the duodenum
pyloric (adj)	pie-**LOR**-ik	S/	-ic *pertaining to*	Pertaining to the pylorus

Exercises

A. After reading Case Report 5.3 on the opposite page, answer the following questions. *Select the correct answer that completes each statement or answers the question.* **LO 5.8, 5.A**

1. Mrs. Stark's dehydration was due to:

   a. excessive urination   **b.** not drinking enough fluids   **c.** her intestines not absorbing water

   d. inflammation of her stomach

2. How was Mrs. Stark's infusion administered?

   a. through her veins   **b.** via a tube to her stomach   **c.** she drank the fluid   **d.** through her rectum

3. Dr. Grabowski is a specialist in the treatment of disorders of the:

   a. mouth   **b.** stomach and intestines   **c.** stomach only   **d.** liver

B. Define the actions of the secretions of the stomach. *Match the secretion in the first column with its function listed in the second column.* **LO 5.8**

_____ **1.** intrinsic factor

_____ **2.** pepsin

_____ **3.** mucus

_____ **4.** hydrochloric acid

a. protects the lining of the stomach

b. destroys pathogens

c. allows for absorption of vitamin B_{12}

d. enzyme that breaks down protein

Gastroesophageal reflux disease (GERD) is the regurgitation of stomach contents back into the esophagus, often when a person is lying down at night. The patient experiences burning sensations in the chest and mouth from the acidity of the regurgitation. The acidity can also irritate and ulcerate the lining of the esophagus, causing it to bleed. Scar tissue can form and cause an esophageal **stricture,** with difficulty in swallowing (dysphagia).

Vomiting can result from distention or irritation of any part of the digestive tract. A message is sent via the **vagus** nerve to the vomiting center in the brain, which, in turn, stimulates the muscles of the diaphragm and abdominal wall to forcefully contract and expel the stomach contents upward into the esophagus and out the mouth.

Gastritis is an inflammation of the lining of the stomach, producing symptoms of epigastric pain, a feeling of fullness, nausea, and occasional bleeding. Gastritis can be caused by common medications such as aspirin and nonsteroidal anti-inflammatory drugs (**NSAIDs**), by radiotherapy and chemotherapy, and by alcohol and smoking. Treatment is directed at removing the factors causing the gastritis by acid neutralization and suppression of gastric acid

Peptic ulcers occur in the stomach and duodenum when the balance between the acid gastric juices and the protection of the mucosal lining breaks down, causing an **erosion** of the lining by the acid *(Figure 5.18)*. Most peptic ulcers are caused by the bacterium *Helicobacter pylori (H. pylori),* which produces enzymes that weaken the protective mucus. These ulcers respond to an antibiotic. Use of NSAIDs increases the incidence of peptic ulcers, particularly in the elderly. **Dyspepsia**, epigastric pain with bloating and nausea, is the most common symptom.

Gastric ulcers are peptic ulcers occurring in the stomach. Symptoms are epigastric burning pain after food, nausea, vomiting, and belching. Bleeding can occur from **erosion** of a blood vessel. If untreated, the ulcer can erode through the entire wall, causing a **perforation**.

Gastric cancer can be asymptomatic for a long period and then cause **indigestion, anorexia**, abdominal pain, and weight loss. It affects men twice as often as women. It metastasizes to lymph nodes, liver, peritoneum, chest, and brain.

▲ **Figure 5.18 Bleeding Peptic Ulcer.**
The yellow floor of the ulcer shows black
blood clots. Fresh blood is around the ulcer
margin. ©CNRI/SPL/Photo Researchers Inc.

WORD	PRONUNCIATION	ELEMENTS		DEFINITION
anorexia	an-oh-**RECK**-see-ah	S/ P/ R/	-ia *condition* an- *without* -orex- *appetite*	Severe lack of appetite; or an aversion to food
dyspepsia	dis-**PEP**-see-ah	S/ P/ R/	-ia *condition* dys- *difficult, bad* -peps- *digestion*	"Upset stomach," epigastric pain, nausea, and gas
erosion	ee-**ROH**-shun		Latin *to gnaw away*	A shallow ulcer in the lining of a structure
gastritis	gas-**TRY**-tis	S/ R/	-itis *inflammation* gastr- *stomach*	Inflammation of the lining of the stomach
peptic	**PEP**-tik	S/ R/	-ic *pertaining to* pept- *digest*	Relating to the stomach and duodenum
perforation	per-foh-**RAY**-shun	S/ R/	-ion *action* perforat- *bore through*	Erosion that progresses to become a hole through the wall of a structure
vagus	**VAY**-gus		Latin *wandering*	Tenth (X) cranial nerve; supplies many different organs throughout the body

Exercises

A. Deconstruct the following medical terms into basic elements. *The definitions of the elements will help you understand the meaning of the term. Select the correct answer that completes each statement.* **LO 5.9, 5.A, 5.D**

1. The meaning of the prefix in the medical term **dyspepsia** is:

   a. digestion

   b. condition

   c. difficult

   d. stomach

2. The meaning of the root in the medical term **peptic** is:

   a. pump

   b. digestion

   c. ulcer

   d. digest

3. The meaning of the suffix in the medical term **perforation** is:

   a. action

   b. condition

   c. pertaining to

   d. inflammation

4. The meaning of the root in the medical term **anorexia** is:

   a. digestion

   b. stomach

   c. without

   d. appetite

B. Given the description of a disorder of the stomach, give the condition. *Fill in the blank.* **LO 5.9, 5.A, 5.E**

1. This condition can be caused by *Helicobacter pylori*: _____ ulcer

2. Inflammation of the lining of the stomach: _____

3. Regurgitation of the stomach contents back into the esophagus (write the abbreviation): _____

Lumen

Serosa

Plica

Mucosa

Submucosa

Muscularis

Villus

Blood vessels

▲ **Figure 5.19** **Tissue Layers of Digestive Tract.** An example of the most typical histologic structure of the tract.

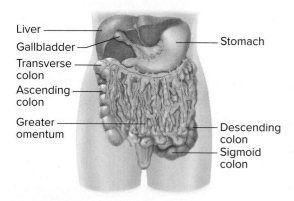

Liver

Gallbladder

Transverse colon

Ascending colon

Greater omentum

Stomach

Descending colon

Sigmoid colon

▲ **Figure 5.20** Greater Omentum.

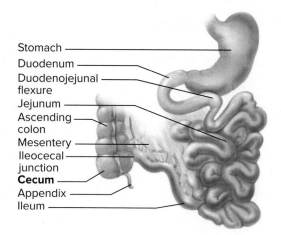

Stomach

Duodenum

Duodenojejunal flexure

Jejunum

Ascending colon

Mesentery

Ileocecal junction

Cecum

Appendix

Ileum

▲ **Figure 5.21** Small Intestine.

LO 5.8 Small Intestine

The small intestine, called "small" because of its diameter, finishes the process of chemical digestion and is responsible for the absorption of most of the nutrients.

Four major layers are present in the wall of the small intestine and in all areas of the digestive tract *(Figure 5.19)*:

1. **Mucosa**, or mucous membrane—the layer containing the epithelial cells that line the tract, intestinal glands that secrete the digestive enzymes, and supportive connective tissue. Fingerlike shapes of mucosa called **villi** project into the lumen of the intestine.

2. **Submucosa**—a thick connective tissue layer containing blood vessels, lymphatic vessels, and nerves.

3. **Muscularis**—an inner, circular layer of smooth muscle and an outer longitudinal layer of smooth muscle. When the inner circular layer contracts, it decreases the diameter of the tract. When the outer longitudinal layer contracts, it shortens the tract. These two movements create peristalsis and segmental contractions.

4. **Serosa**—an outermost layer of thin connective tissue and a single layer of epithelial cells.

Most of the digestive organs lie within the abdominal cavity *(see Chapter 3)*, which is lined by a moist serous membrane called the **peritoneum**. **Parietal** peritoneum lines the wall of the abdominal cavity. **Visceral** peritoneum (a serosa) covers the external surface of the digestive organs.

The intestines are suspended from the back wall of the abdominal cavity by a translucent membrane called the **mesentery**, a continuation of the peritoneum. A fatty portion of the mesentery, called the **greater omentum** *(Figure 5.20)*, hangs like an apron in front of all the intestines.

The small intestine *(Figure 5.21)* occupies much of the abdominal cavity, extends from the pylorus of the stomach to the beginning of the large intestine, and has three segments:

1. The **duodenum** is the first 9 to 10 inches of the small intestine. It receives chyme from the stomach, together with pancreatic juices and bile. Here, stomach acid is neutralized, fats are broken up by the bile acids, and pancreatic enzymes take over chemical digestion.

2. The **jejunum** makes up about 40% of the small intestine's length. It is the primary region for chemical digestion and nutrient absorption.

3. The **ileum** makes up about 55% of the small intestine's length. It ends at the **ileocecal** valve, a sphincter that controls entry into the large intestine.

From the duodenum to the middle of the ileum, the lining of the small intestine is folded into circular folds called **plicae**. Along their surface, the plicae have tiny fingerlike villi. The plicae and villi increase the surface area over which secretions can act on the food and through which nutrients can be absorbed. The folds also act as "speed bumps" to slow down the movement of chyme through the small intestine. The cells at the tip of the villi are shed and renewed every 3 or 4 days.

Digestion in the Small Intestine

After leaving the stomach as chyme, the food spends 3 to 5 hours in the small intestine, from which most of the nutrients are absorbed.

Secretion from the small intestine cells is mostly water, mucus, and enzymes. Peristaltic movements of the small intestine have three functions:

1. To mix chyme with intestinal and pancreatic juices and with bile.

2. To churn chyme to make contact with the mucosa for digestion and absorption.

3. To move the residue toward the large intestine.

Anywhere from four to six hours after consuming that chicken and vegetable dinner mentioned earlier, your food has passed through the small intestine and is ready to be moved into the large intestine. Most of the protein, carbohydrate, and fat of your meal has been broken down by enzymes into basic nutrients and absorbed into your bloodstream.

WORD	PRONUNCIATION		ELEMENTS	DEFINITION
duodenum	du-oh-DEE-num	S/ R/	-um *structure* duoden- Latin for *twelve*	The first part of the small intestine; approximately 12 finger-breadths (9 to 10 inches) in length.
ileum ileocecal	ILL-ee-um ILL-ee-oh-SEE-cal	 S/ R/CF R/	Latin *to roll up* -al *pertaining to* ile/o- *ileum* -cec- *cecum*	Third portion of the small intestine Pertaining to the junction of the ileum and cecum (the first part of the large intestine)
jejunum jejunal (adj)	je-JEW-num je-JEW-nal	 R/ S/	Latin *empty* jejun *empty* -al *pertaining to*	Segment of small intestine between the duodenum and the ileum where most of the nutrients are absorbed Pertaining to the jejunum
mesentery mesenteric (adj)	MESS-en-ter-ree MESS-en-ter-ik	P/ R/ S/	mes- *middle* -entery *intestine* -ic *pertaining to*	A double layer of peritoneum enclosing the abdominal viscera Pertaining to the mesentery
mucosa (another name for mucous membrane) mucosal (adj) submucosa	myu-KOH-sah myu-KOH-sal sub-mew-KOH-sa	 S/ P/ R/	Latin *mucus* -al *pertaining to* sub- *under* -mucosa *lining of a cavity*	Lining of a tubular structure Pertaining to the mucosa Tissue layer underneath the mucosa
muscularis	muss-kyu-LAR-is	S/ R/	-aris *pertaining to* muscul- *muscle*	The muscular layer of a hollow organ or tube
omentum omental (adj)	oh-MEN-tum oh-MEN-tal	 S/	Latin *membrane that drapes over the intestines* -al *pertaining to*	Membrane that drapes over the intestines Pertaining to the omentum
parietal	pah-RYE-eh-tal	S/ R/	-al *pertaining to* pariet- *wall*	Pertaining to the wall of an organ or a body cavity
peritoneum peritoneal (adj)	per-ih-toh-NEE-um per-ih-toh-NEE-al	 S/	Latin *to stretch over* -al *pertaining to*	Membrane that lines the abdominal cavity Pertaining to the peritoneum
plica plicae (pl)	PLEE-cah PLEE-key		Latin *fold*	Fold in a mucous membrane
serosa serosal (adj)	seh-ROH-sa seh-ROH-sal	 S/ R/	Latin *serous, watery* -al *pertaining to* seros- *watery consistency*	Outermost covering of the alimentary tract Pertaining to serosa
villus villi (pl)	VILL-us VILL-eye		Latin *shaggy hair*	Thin, hairlike projection, particularly of a mucous membrane lining a cavity
viscus (Note: Viscous is pronounced the same but means something *sticky*.) viscera (pl) visceral (adj)	VISS-kus VISS-er-ah VISS-er-al	 R/ S/	Latin *internal organ* viscer- *soft parts* -al *pertaining to*	Hollow, walled, internal organ Internal organs, particularly in the abdomen Pertaining to the internal organs

Exercises

A. Greek and Latin terms do not deconstruct into basic elements, so you must know them for what they are. *Build your knowledge of these terms by matching the phrase in the left column to the correct medical term in the right column.* **LO 5.8, 5.A**

_____ 1. To roll up   a. viscus

_____ 2. Membrane that drapes over the intestines   b. peritoneum

_____ 3. Watery   c. mucosa

_____ 4. Shaggy hair   d. plica

_____ 5. Internal organ   e. omentum

_____ 6. Fold   f. ileum

_____ 7. Empty   g. serosa

_____ 8. To stretch over   h. villus

_____ 9. Lining of a tubular structure   i. jejunum

LO 5.9 Disorders of the Small Intestine

The absorption of nutrients occurs primarily through the small intestine. **Impairment of absorption,** including Crohn's disease and lactose intolerance, is covered in *Lesson 5.5* of this chapter.

Infections of the small intestine are common and are caused by a variety of agents:

- **Gastroenteritis**, or inflammation of the stomach and small intestine, can result in acute vomiting and diarrhea. It can be caused by a variety of viruses and bacteria (including, occasionally, the parasite *Giardia lamblia*) and is initiated by contact with contaminated food (food poisoning) and water.

- Bleeding from the small intestine is usually caused by a **duodenal ulcer.**

- **Celiac disease** is an allergy to gluten, which is a protein contained in wheat, rye, barley, and other grains. Celiac disease *(Figure 5.22)* damages the lining of the small intestine and can cause abdominal swelling, gas, pain, weight loss, fatigue, and weakness. Treatment is a strict gluten-free diet.

- An **intussusception** occurs when a part of the small intestine slides into a neighboring portion of the small intestine—much like the way that parts of a collapsible telescope slide into each other. Eighty percent of intussusceptions can be cured with an enema; the remaining 20% require surgical intervention.

- **Ileus** is a disruption of the normal peristaltic ability of the small intestine. It can be caused by a bowel obstruction or by intestinal paralysis. Risk factors for **paralytic ileus** include GI surgery, diabetic ketoacidosis *(see Chapter 17)*, peritonitis, and medications, such as opiates.

- **Cancer** of the small intestine occurs infrequently compared with tumors in other parts of the GI tract. An **adenocarcinoma** is the most common malignant tumor of the small bowel.

▲ **Figure 5.22** **Photomicrograph of Celiac Disease Showing Atrophy of Duodenal Villi.** ©Biophoto Associates/Photo Researchers, Inc.

WORD	PRONUNCIATION	ELEMENTS		DEFINITION
celiac	**SEE**-lee-ack	S/ R/	-ac *pertaining to* celi- *abdomen*	Relating to the abdominal cavity
celiac disease	**SEE**-lee-ack diz-**EEZ**	P/ R/	dis- *apart* -ease *normal function*	Disease caused by a sensitivity to gluten
constipation	kon-stih-**PAY**-shun	S/ R/	-ation *process* constip- *press together*	Hard, infrequent bowel movements
diarrhea	die-ah-**REE**-ah	P/ S/	dia- *complete* -rrhea *flow*	Abnormally frequent and loose stools
gastroenteritis	**GAS**-troh-en-ter-**I**-tis	S/ R/CF R/	-itis *inflammation* gastr/o- *stomach* -enter- *intestine*	Inflammation of the stomach and intestines
Giardia	jee-**AR**-dee-ah	S/	Alfred Giard, 1846–1908, French biologist	Parasite that can affect the small intestine
ileus	**ILL**-ee-us		Greek *intestinal colic*	Dynamic or mechanical obstruction of the small intestine
intussusception	**IN**-tuss-sus-**SEP**-shun	S/ P/ R/	-ion *action* intus- *within* -suscept- *to take up*	The slippage of one part of the bowel inside another, causing obstruction

Exercises

A. Match the disorder of the small intestine in column one with the statement describing it in column two. LO 5.9, 5.A

_____ 1. ileus

_____ 2. constipation

_____ 3. celiac disease

_____ 4. *Giardia lamblia*

_____ 5. intussusception

a. Parasite that causes gastroenteritis

b. Part of the small intestine slides into a neighboring part

c. Disruption of the normal peristalsis of the small intestine

d. Hard, infrequent bowel movements

e. Allergy to gluten

B. Use your knowledge of the small intestine and answer the questions. *Choose T if the statement is true. Chosse F if the statement is false.* **LO 5.9, 5.A**

1. People with constipation complain of frequent trips to the bathroom to pass soft stools.   T   F

2. Gastroenteritis can result in acute vomiting and diarrhea.   T   F

3. Bleeding from the small intestine is usually from an infection.   T   F

4. Cancer of the small intestine is a common occurrence.   T   F

5. Risk factors for paralytic ileus include GI surgery, diabetic ketoacidosis, and medicines such as opiates.   T   F

Lesson 5.4

DIGESTIVE SYSTEM

Digestion–Liver, Gallbladder, and Pancreas

The liver and pancreas secrete enzymes that are responsible for most of the digestion that occurs in the small intestine. You must understand the function of these enzymes as they relate to digestion, and you will need to be able to:

5.4.1 Use correct medical terminology to describe the anatomy, physiology, and common disorders of the liver, gallbladder, bile ducts, and pancreas.

5.4.2 Identify the functions of the liver, gallbladder, bile ducts, and pancreas.

5.4.3 Describe the functions of the digestive secretions of the liver and pancreas.

5.4.4 Explain common disorders of the liver, gallbladder, bile ducts, and pancreas.

Sternum   5th rib

Liver

▲ **Figure 5.23** Location of Liver.

Keynote

Only the production of bile relates the liver to digestion.

Case Report (CR) 5.4

You are

... a Certified Medical Assistant working with Susan Lee, MD, a primary care physician at Fulwood Medical Center.

Your patient is

... Mrs. Sandra Jacobs, a 46-year-old mother of four. Your task is to document her care.

Documentation

Mrs. Sandra Jacobs, a 46-year-old mother of four, presents in Dr. Susan Lee's primary care clinic with episodes of crampy pain in her right upper quadrant associated with nausea and vomiting. The pain often occurs after eating fast food. She has not noticed fever or jaundice. Physical examination reveals an obese white woman with a positive **Murphy sign**. Her blood pressure (BP) is 170/90, and she has slight pedal edema. A **provisional diagnosis** of **gallstones** has been made. She has been referred for an ultrasound examination, and an appointment has been made to see Dr. Stewart Walsh in the Surgery Department.

I explained to her the etiology of her gallstones and the need for surgical removal of the gallbladder, and I discussed with her a low-fat, 1500-calorie diet sheet.

Luisa Guitterez, CMA. 06/12/12, 1430 hrs.

LO 5.10 Liver

The **liver**, the body's largest *internal* organ, is a complex structure located under the right ribs and below the diaphragm *(Figure 5.23)*.

The liver has multiple functions, including to:

- **Manufacture** and **excrete bile**. Although it contains no digestive enzymes, bile plays key roles in digestion. It neutralizes the acidic chyme so that pancreatic enzymes can function. Bile salts **emulsify** fat. **Bile acids** are synthesized from **cholesterol**, and bile also contains cholesterol and fat-soluble vitamins.

- **Remove** the pigment **bilirubin** from the bloodstream and excrete it in bile. Bilirubin is produced as a breakdown product of hemoglobin during phagocytosis by macrophages in the spleen and liver. It is dark yellow and is responsible for the brown color of feces and for the yellow color of skin in **jaundice**.

- **Remove** excess glucose (sugar) from the blood and store it as **glycogen** and release glucose when needed by the body.

- **Convert** proteins and fats into glucose, a process called **gluconeogenesis**.

- **Store** fat and the fat-soluble vitamins A, D, E, and K.

- **Manufacture** blood proteins, including those necessary for clotting *(see Chapter 11)*.

- **Remove** toxins from the blood.

A major reason that the liver can perform all these functions is that venous blood is returned from all the small intestines to join into the **portal vein** that takes the blood directly to the liver.

The liver cells **secrete** bile into narrow channels that converge on the underside of the liver to form the common **hepatic duct.**

Several hours after consuming that chicken and vegetable dinner mentioned earlier, the bile manufactured by the liver neutralizes the acidic chyme and emulsifies the fat.

WORD	PRONUNCIATION		ELEMENTS	DEFINITION
bile bile acids biliary (adj)	BILE BILE **ASS**-ids **BILL**-ee-air-ee	 S/ R/CF	Latin *bile* -ary *pertaining to* bil/i- *bile*	Fluid secreted by the liver into the duodenum Steroids synthesized from cholesterol Pertaining to bile or the biliary tract
bilirubin	bill-ee-**RU**-bin	S/ R/CF	-rubin *rust colored* bil/i- *bile*	Bile pigment formed in the liver from hemoglobin
cholesterol	koh-**LESS**-ter-ol	S/ R/CF	-sterol *steroid* chol/e- *bile*	Steroid formed in liver cells; the most abundant steroid in tissues, which circulates in the plasma attached to proteins of different densities
emulsify emulsion (noun)	eh-**MUL**-sih-fie eh-**MUL**-shun	S/ R/ S/	-ify *to become* emuls- *suspend in a liquid* -sion *state, condition*	Break up into very small droplets to suspend in a solution (emulsion) System containing two liquids, one of which is in the form of small globules that are dispersed throughout the other
gallstone	**GAWL**-stone	R/ R/	gall- *bile* -stone *pebble*	Hard mass of cholesterol, calcium, and bilirubin that can be formed in the gallbladder and bile duct
gluconeogenesis	**GLU**-koh-nee-oh-**JEN**-eh-sis	S/ R/CF P/	-genesis *creation* gluc/o- *sugar* -neo- *new*	Formation of glucose from noncarbohydrate sources
glycogen	**GLIE**-koh-jen	S/ R/CF	-gen *produce, create* glyc/o- *sugar*	The body's principal carbohydrate reserve, stored in the liver and skeletal muscle
hepatic hepatitis	hep-**AT**-ik hep-ah-**TIE**-tis	S/ R/ S/	-ic *pertaining to* hepat- *liver* -itis *inflammation*	Pertaining to the liver Inflammation of the liver
jaundice	**JAWN**-dis		French *yellow*	Yellow staining of tissues with bile pigments, including bilirubin
liver	**LIV**-er		Old English *liver*	Body's largest internal organ, located in right upper quadrant of abdomen
Murphy sign	**MUR**-fee SINE		John B. Murphy, 1857–1916, Chicago surgeon	Tenderness in the right subcostal area on inspiration, associated with acute cholecystitis
pancreas	**PAN**-kree-as		Greek *sweetbread*	Lobulated gland, the head of which is tucked into the curve of the duodenum
portal vein	**POR**-tal VANE		Latin *gate*	The vein that carries blood from the intestines to the liver
provisional diagnosis (also called **preliminary** diagnosis)	proh-**VISH**-un-al die-ag-**NOH**-sis	S R/ P/ R/	-al *pertaining to* provision- *provide* dia- *complete* -gnosis *knowledge*	A temporary diagnosis pending further examination or testing The determination of the cause of a disease

Exercises

A. Use this exercise as a quick review of the elements related to the liver. *Select the correct answer that completes each statement.* **LO 5.10, 5.D**

1. In the term **hepatic**, the root means

   a. pancreas   **b.** stomach   **c.** liver

2. The term **gallstone** is composed of

   a. root + combining form   **b.** root + root   **c.** root + suffix

3. The term **biliary** is composed of a

   a. prefix + root   **b.** root + suffix   **c.** combining form + suffix

4. In the term **gluconeogenesis**, *neo* means

   a. never   **b.** new   **c.** negative

Abbreviations

ALP	alkaline phosphatase
ALT	alanine aminotrans-ferase (also known as SGPT)
AST	aspartate aminotrans-ferase (also known as SGOT)
GGT	gamma-glutamyl transpeptidase
HAV	hepatitis A virus
HBV	hepatitis B virus
HCV	hepatitis C virus
HDV	hepatitis D virus
LFT	liver function test
SGOT	serum glutamic oxaloacetic acid transaminase (also known as AST)
SGPT	serum glutamic-pyruvic transaminase (also known as ALT)

LO 5.11 Disorders of the Liver

Hepatitis is an inflammation of the liver causing jaundice. Viral hepatitis is the most common cause of hepatitis and is related to three major types of virus:

1. **Hepatitis A virus (HAV)** is highly contagious and causes a mild to severe infection. It is transmitted by the **fecal-oral route** through contaminated food. It frequently occurs in schools, camps, and institutions.

2. **Hepatitis B virus (HBV)** is transmitted through contact with blood, semen, vaginal secretions, saliva, or a needle prick and through sharing contaminated needles. Some people become chronic carriers of the virus in their blood.

3. **Hepatitis C virus (HCV)** is transmitted by blood-to-blood contact; it is often asymptomatic. It can be cured in 51% of patients with antiviral treatment but can progress to chronic hepatitis and cirrhosis.

4. **Hepatitis D virus (HDV)** can occur only in the presence of HBV. In 2017 outbreaks of HDV infection have been seen in homeless populations.

5. **Hepatitis E** is similar to hepatitis A and occurs mostly in underdeveloped countries.

Other causes of hepatitis include abuse of alcohol; autoimmune hepatitis; metabolic disorders such as Wilson's disease and diabetes mellitus; other viruses, such as mononucleosis and cytomegalovirus; and drugs such as acetaminophen.

Symptoms include nausea, vomiting and loss of appetite, joint pain, and sore muscles. Signs include jaundice, fever, and tenderness in the right upper quadrant of the abdomen.

Chronic hepatitis occurs when the acute hepatitis is not healed after 6 months. It progresses slowly, can last for years, and is difficult to treat.

Cirrhosis of the liver is a chronic, irreversible disease, replacing normal liver cells with hard, fibrous scar tissue *(Figure 5.24)*. It is the seventh leading cause of death in the United States. The most common cause of **cirrhosis** is alcoholism. In cirrhosis, the damage sustained to the liver is irreversible, and there is no known cure. Treatment is symptomatic. When cirrhosis blocks the flow of blood in the portal vein, the back-pressure produces **ascites,** an accumulation of fluid in the abdominal cavity.

Cancer of the liver as a primary cancer typically arises in patients with chronic liver disease, usually from HBV infection. A more common form of liver cancer is secondary deposits of metastases from a primary cancer in the colon, lung, breast, or prostate.

Hemochromatosis is caused by the absorption of too much iron, which is stored throughout the body, mostly in the liver, and can lead to liver failure.

▲ **Figure 5.24** Cirrhosis of Liver.
©Biophoto Associates/Science Source

Hyperbilirubinemia, too much bilirubin in the blood, is caused when red cells break down, producing the yellow pigment **bilirubin.** Newborn babies cannot get rid of the bilirubin easily and it can build up in the blood and other tissues, producing a yellow discoloration of the skin and eyes called **jaundice.** About 60% of term newborns and 80% of premature babies develop hyperbilirubinemia. There are several causes of this condition:

- **Physiologic jaundice,** a "normal" response in the first few days of life.

- **Breast milk jaundice,** which occurs in about 2% of breastfed babies, peaking around 2 weeks of age and persisting up to 3 to 12 weeks. No treatment is necessary.

- **Breast feeding failure jaundice,** when there is difficulty establishing breast feeding, resulting in dehydration, decreased urine production, and build up of bilirubin in the blood and tissues. It goes away once breast feeding is established.

- **Hemolytic disease of the newborn (Rh disease)** *(see Chapter 11)* produces jaundice as too many red blood cells (**RBCs**) break down and release bilirubin to cause jaundice.

- **Inadequate liver function** due to infection or other rare problems, which can also produce jaundice.

Wilson disease is the retention of too much copper in the liver and also can lead to liver failure.

Word Analysis and Definition

S = Suffix   P = Prefix   R = Root   R/CF = Combining Form

WORD	PRONUNCIATION		ELEMENTS	DEFINITION
alanine aminotransferase (ALT)	**AL**-ah-neen ah-**MEE**-noh-**TRANS**-fer-aze	S/ R/CF R/	**alanine** *an amino acid* **-ase** *enzyme* **amin/o-** *nitrogen compound* **-transfer-** *carry* **aspartate** *an amino acid*	Enzymes that are found in liver cells and leak out into the bloodstream when the cells are damaged, enabling liver damage to be diagnosed
aspartate aminotransferase (AST)	as-**PAR**-tate			A salt of aspartic acid
ascites	ah-**SIGH**-teez	S/ R/	**-ites** *associated with* **asc-** *belly*	Accumulation of fluid in the abdominal cavity
cholestatic	koh-les-**TAT**-ik	S/ R/CF R/	**-ic** *pertaining to* **chol/e-** *bile* **-stat-** *standing still*	Stopping the flow of bile
cirrhosis	sir-**ROH**-sis	S/ R/	**-osis** *condition* **cirrh-** *yellow*	Extensive fibrotic liver disease
hemochromatosis	**HEE**-moh-kroh-mah-**TOH**-sis	S/ R/CF R/	**-osis** *condition* **hem/o-** *blood* **-chromat-** *color*	Dangerously high levels of iron in the body with deposition of iron pigments in tissues
hepatitis	hep-ah-**TIE**-tis	S/ R/	**-itis** *inflammation* **hepat** *liver*	Inflammation of the liver
phosphatase	**FOS**-fah-tase	S/ R/	**-ase** *enzyme* **phosphat-** *phosphorus*	Enzyme that liberates phosphorus
Wilson disease			Samuel Alexander Kinnier Wilson, 1878–1937, British neurologist	Genetic disorder in which copper accumulates in the body, which can lead to liver failure

Exercises

A. Work on recognizing the elements contained in the above WAD. *Know the medical terms in which they will appear.*
Fill in the chart. **LO 5.3, 5.11, 5.C**

Element	Meaning of Element	Type of Element (Prefix, Root, Combining Form, Suffix)	Medical Term Containing This Element
osis	1.	2.	3.
hemo	4.	5.	6.
asc	7.	8.	9.
cirrh	10.	11.	12.
chole	13.	14.	15.
ase	16.	17.	18.

Inferior vena cava   Bare area

Gallbladder

(a)

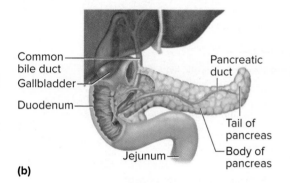

Common bile duct
Gallbladder
Duodenum

Pancreatic duct

Tail of pancreas

Jejunum

Body of pancreas

(b)

▲ **Figure 5.25** **Gallbladder and Biliary Tract.** (a) Underside of liver. (b) Anatomy of gallbladder, pancreas, and biliary tract.

Keynotes

- Between meals, the gallbladder absorbs water and electrolytes from the bile and concentrates it 10 to 20 times.
- Jaundice is caused by bilirubin in the tissues.

Abbreviations

RBC   red blood cell

LO 5.10 Gallbladder and Biliary Tract

On the underside of the liver is the **gallbladder** *(Figure 5.25a)*, which stores and concentrates the bile that the liver produces. The **cystic duct** from the gallbladder joins with the **hepatic duct** to form the **common bile duct.** The system of ducts to get the bile from the liver to the duodenum is called the **biliary tract** *(Figure 5.25b)*.

When acid and fat arrive in the duodenum, cells in the lining of the duodenum secrete a hormone, **cholecystokinin**, which causes the gallbladder to contract and force bile into the bile duct and, from there, into the duodenum. Cholecystokinin also stimulates the production of pancreatic enzymes.

LO 5.11 Disorders of the Gallbladder

Gallstones (cholelithiasis) can form in the gallbladder from excess cholesterol, bile salts, and bile pigment *(Figure 5.26)*. The stones can vary in size and number. Risk factors are **obesity**, high-cholesterol diets, multiple pregnancies, and rapid weight loss. Mrs. Jacobs presented in the Emergency Department with the classic gallstone symptoms of severe waves of right upper quadrant pain (**biliary colic**), nausea, and vomiting. **Cholelithotomy** is the operative removal of one or more gallstones. If small stones become impacted in the common bile duct, this is called **choledocholithiasis**. This can cause biliary colic and jaundice (see the following).

Cholecystitis is an acute or chronic inflammation of the gallbladder usually associated with cholelithiasis and obstruction of the cystic duct with a stone. Acute colicky pain in the right upper quadrant with nausea and vomiting are followed by jaundice, dark urine (because bilirubin backs up into the blood and is excreted by the kidneys), and pale-colored stools (because bilirubin cannot get into the duodenum).

Jaundice (icterus) is a symptom of many different diseases in the biliary tract and liver. It is a yellow discoloration of the skin and sclera of the eyes *(see Chapter 16)* caused by deposits of bilirubin just below the outer layers of the skin. Bilirubin is a breakdown product of hemoglobin that occurs as old **red blood cells (RBCs)** are destroyed. Bilirubin is removed from the bloodstream by the liver and excreted in bile.

Jaundice occurs when there is an increased concentration of bilirubin circulating in the bloodstream. There are three categories of disease that cause jaundice:

1. **Obstructive jaundice** is a result of the blockage of bile between the liver and the duodenum, usually due to gallstones in the common bile duct or to a carcinoma of the head of the pancreas impinging on the common duct.

2. **Hemolytic jaundice** results from an accelerated destruction of RBCs such that the liver cannot remove the excess bilirubin fast enough. This is most often seen in newborn infants with hemolytic jaundice due to blood group incompatibility between mother and infant.

3. **Hepatocellular jaundice** occurs when an infection or poison injures the liver cells, preventing the removal of bilirubin from the blood. This occurs in viral hepatitis.

▲ **Figure 5.26** **Gallstones.** ©SIU Biomedical/Photo Researchers, Inc.

WORD	PRONUNCIATION	ELEMENTS		DEFINITION
biliary colic	**BILL**-ee-air-ee **KOL**-ik	S/ R/CF S/ R/	-ary *pertaining to* bil/i- *bile* -ic *pertaining to* col- *colon*	Severe waves of pain in the right upper quadrant due to a gallstone blocking the bile duct
cholecystitis	**KOH**-leh-sis-**TIE**-tis	S/ R/CF R/	-itis *inflammation* chol/e *bile* -cyst- *bladder*	Inflammation of the gallbladder
cholecystokinin	**KOH**-leh-sis-toh-**KIE**-nin	S/ R/CF R/CF	-kinin *move in* chol/e- *bile* -cyst/o- *bladder*	Hormone secreted by the lining of the intestine that stimulates secretion of pancreatic enzymes and contraction of the gallbladder
choledocholithiasis	koh-leh-**DOH**-koh-lih-**THIGH**-ah-sis	S/ R/CF	-iasis *condition* choledoch/o- *common bile duct*	Presence of a gallstone(s) in the common bile duct
cholelithiasis	**KOH**-leh-lih-**THIGH**-ah-sis	R/ S/ R/CF	-lith- *stone* -iasis *condition* chol/e- *bile*	Condition of having bile stones (gallstones)
gallbladder	**GAWL**-blad-er	R/	gall- *bile* Old English *bladder*	Receptacle on inferior surface of the liver for storing bile
hemolysis	hee-**MOL**-ih-sis	S/ R/CF	-lysis *destroy* hem/o- *blood*	Destruction of RBCs so that hemoglobin is liberated
hemolytic (adj)	hee-moh-**LIT**-ik	S/ R/	-tic *pertaining to* -ly- *break down*	Pertaining to the process of destruction of RBCs
hepatocellular	**HEP**-ah-toh-**SELL**-you-lar	S/ R/CF R/	-ar *pertaining to* hepat/o- *liver* -cellul- *small cell*	Pertaining to liver cells
icterus jaundice	**ICK**-ter-us **JAWN**-dis		Greek *jaundice* French *yellowness*	Yellow staining of tissues with bile pigments, including bilirubin.
obesity	oh-**BEE**-sih-tee		Latin *fat*	Excessive amount of fat in the body

Exercise

A. In this exercise, the root or combining form remains the same, but the addition of other elements will construct entirely different medical terms. *Use this group of elements, in addition to* **chol/e**, *to form the medical terms that are defined. Some elements you will use more than once; some elements you will not use at all. Fill in the blanks.* **LO 5.11, 5.C**

1. The element *chol/e* means _____.

2. The element *choledoch/o* means _____.

Add these elements to **chol/e** *or* **choledoch/o** *to form the medical terms defined as follows:*

lith	**lysis**	**iasis**	**graphy**	**osis**	**cyst**
kinin	**nephr/o**	**cyst/o**	**hemat/o**	**itis**	

3. Condition of gallstones in the common bile duct _____

4. Condition of having bile stones (gallstones) _____

5. Inflammation of the gallbladder _____

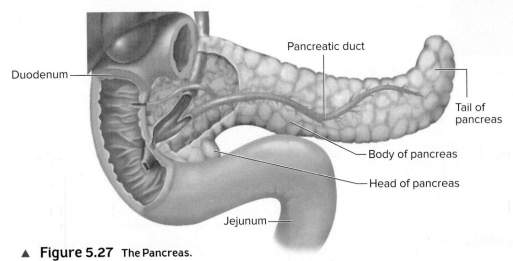

Duodenum

Pancreatic duct

Tail of pancreas

Body of pancreas

Head of pancreas

Jejunum

▲ **Figure 5.27** The Pancreas.

Pancreatic islet

Alpha cells (secrete glucagon)

Beta cells (secrete insulin)

Vein

} Lobule

To bloodstream (Endocrine)

Interlobular duct

To pancreatic duct (Exocrine)

Acinar cells (secrete enzymes)

▲ **Figure 5.28** Exocrine and Endocrine Aspects of Pancreas.

LO 5.10 Pancreas

The **pancreas** (*Figure 5.27*) is a spongy gland, the head of which is encircled by the duodenum. Most of the pancreas secretes digestive juices; this is a part of the pancreas called an **exocrine gland** (*Figure 5.28*), and the **pancreatic** digestive juices formed in the **acinar cells of the exocrine part of the pancreas** are excreted through the pancreatic duct. The pancreatic duct joins the common bile duct shortly before it opens into the duodenum (*Figure 5.27*). Pancreatic and bile juices then enter the duodenum.

In the same parts of the pancreas as those in which pancreatic enzymes are produced, pancreatic **islet cells** secrete the hormones insulin and glucagon (*see Chapter 17*), which go directly into the bloodstream. This part of the pancreas is an **endocrine gland** (*Figure 5.28*). Thus, the pancreas is both an exocrine and endocrine gland.

The exocrine pancreatic juices contain:

1. **Electrolytes**, including the alkaline sodium bicarbonate, that make the pancreatic juice alkaline and help neutralize the acid chyme as it comes from the stomach.

2. **Enzymes:**
   - **Amylase** breaks down the **polysaccharide** starch into **disaccharides** and **monosaccharides**.
   - **Lipase** breaks down **triglyceride** fat molecules into **fatty acids** and **monoglycerides**.
   - **Trypsin**, **chymotrypsin**, and **carboxypeptidase** split proteins into their amino acids.

Pancreatic exocrine secretions are regulated by both the nervous and endocrine systems. While food is being digested in the stomach, nervous impulses stimulate the pancreas to produce its juices. When chyme enters the duodenum, the hormone **secretin**, produced in the duodenal mucosa, stimulates the pancreas to produce large volumes of watery fluid. Another hormone, cholecystokinin, is produced in the intestinal mucosa to stimulate production of pancreatic enzymes. Both hormones travel from the intestine via the bloodstream to the pancreas.

LO 5.11 Disorders of the Pancreas

Pancreatitis is inflammation of the pancreas. The acute disease ranges from a mild, self-limiting episode to an acute life-threatening emergency with severe abdominal pain, nausea, vomiting, and a rapid fall in blood pressure. In the **chronic** form, there is a progressive destruction of pancreatic tissue leading to **malabsorption** and **diabetes**. Factors in the development of pancreatitis are biliary tract disease, gallstones, and alcoholism. The pancreatic enzyme trypsin builds up and digests parts of the pancreas, causing the intense pain.

Pancreatic cancer is the fourth-leading cause of cancer-related death. It occurs twice as often in males as in females. Incidence peaks in the 40- to 60-year-old range. The cancer can be asymptomatic in its early stages and is difficult to detect. The treatment is surgical resection of the pancreas.

Diabetes, in which endocrine insulin production is shut down or severely reduced or its effects are resisted by body cells, is discussed in *Chapter 17*.

Cystic fibrosis (CF) is an inherited disease that becomes apparent in infancy or childhood. It affects exocrine glands in multiple body systems, including the respiratory and digestive systems.

Keynote

The prognosis of pancreatic cancer is poor, with only a 15% to 20% 5-year survival rate.

Abbreviation

CF   cystic fibrosis

S = Suffix   P = Prefix   R = Root   R/CF = Combining Form

WORD	PRONUNCIATION	ELEMENTS		DEFINITION
acinar cells	ASS-in-ar SELLS	S/ R/	-ar *pertaining to* acin- *grape*	Enzyme-secreting cells of the pancreas
carboxypeptidase	kar-box-ee-**PEP**-tid-ase	S/ R/ R/	-ase *enzyme* carboxy- *group of organic* *compounds* -peptid- *digestion*	Enzyme that breaks down protein
cystic fibrosis (CF)	**SIS**-tik fie-**BROH**-sis	S/ R/ S/ R/CF	-ic *pertaining to* cyst- *bladder* -sis *condition* fibr/o *fiber*	Genetic condition in which thick mucus obstructs the pancreas so that digestive enzymes do not reach the small intestine.
endocrine gland	**EN**-doh-krin GLAND	P/ R/	endo- *within* -crine *secrete*	A gland that produces an internal or hormonal secretion and secretes it into the bloodstream
exocrine gland	**EK**-soh-krin GLAND	P/ R/	exo- *outward* -crine *secrete*	A gland that secretes outwardly through excretory ducts
fatty acid	**FAT**-ee **ASS**-id		Old English *fat* Latin *sour*	An acid obtained from the hydrolysis of fats
islet cells	**EYE**-let SELLS		islet *small island*	Hormone-secreting cells of the pancreas
monoglyceride	mon-oh-**GLISS**-eh-ride	S/ P/ R/	-ide *having a particular* *quality* mono- *one* -glycer- *glycerol*	A fatty substance with a single fatty acid
triglyceride	trie-**GLISS**-eh-ride	P/	tri- *three*	Substance with three fatty acids
monosaccharide	**MON**-oh-**SACK**-ah-ride	S/	-ide *having a particular* *quality*	Simplest form of sugar; for example, glucose
disaccharide	die-**SACK**-ah-ride	P/ R/ P/	mono- *one* -sacchar- *sugar* di- *two*	A combination of two monosaccharides; for example, table sugar
polysaccharide	pol-ee-**SACK**-ah-ride	P/	poly- *many*	A combination of many saccharides; for example, starch
pancreas	**PAN**-kree-as		Greek *sweetbread*	Lobulated gland, the head of which is tucked into the curve of the duodenum
pancreatic (adj)	pan-kree-**AT**-ik	S/ R/	-ic *pertaining to* pancreat- *pancreas*	Pertaining to the pancreas
pancreatitis	**PAN**-kree-ah-**TIE**-tis	S/	-itis *inflammation*	Inflammation of the pancreas
secretin	se-**KREE**-tin	S/ R/	-in *substance, chemical* *compound* secret- *separate*	Hormone produced by duodenum to stimulate pancreatic juice
trypsin	**TRIP**-sin	S/ R/	-in *substance, chemical* *compound* tryps- *friction*	Enzyme that breaks down protein
chymotrypsin	kie-moh-**TRIP**-sin	R/CF	chym/o- *chyme*	Trypsin found in chyme

Exercises

A. Describe the anatomy and function of the pancreas. *Choose the correct answer to the following questions.* **LO 5.10**

1. The exocrine function of the pancreas is the secretion of:

   a. bile   **b.** insulin   **c.** glucagon   **d.** pancreatic juice

2. On the pH scale, pancreatic juice is:

   a. alkaline   **b.** acidic

3. The pancreas is:

   a. in the left lower quadrant   **b.** superior to the diaphragm   **c.** surrounded by the curve of the duodenum   **d.** lateral to the stomach

B. Define the disorders of the pancreas. *Match the disorder of the pancreas with its correct description.* **LO 5.11**

_____ 1. cystic fibrosis   **a.** lack of insulin production

_____ 2. pancreatitis   **b.** genetic condition affecting the pancreas

_____ 3. diabetes   **c.** can be caused by biliary disease, gallstones, or alcholism

Lesson 5.5

DIGESTIVE SYSTEM

Absorption and Malabsorption

Lesson Objectives

In the previous lessons in this chapter, you have learned the digestive secretions of the different segments of the digestive tract, liver, and pancreas. This information can now be brought together to review the overall process of digestion so that you will be able to:

5.5.1 Describe chemical digestion, absorption, and malabsorption.

5.5.2 Describe disorders of chemical digestion and absorption.

Keynotes

- Proteins are broken down into amino acids.
- Minerals are electrolytes.

LO 5.12 Chemical Digestion, Absorption, and Transport

When the remains of the chicken and vegetable arrive in your duodenum, they have been reduced to very small particles by **mastication** and gastric **peristalsis**, and they have been mixed with other food to form boluses. Thus far, 10% of their carbohydrates has been partially digested by salivary **amylase**, operating mostly in the mouth; 10% to 15% of their protein has been partially digested by **proteases** in the stomach; and 10% of their fats has been digested by the salivary **lipase** operating in the stomach.

Carbohydrates are ingested in three forms:

1. **Polysaccharides**, such as starches.

2. **Disaccharides**, such as sucrose (table sugar) and lactose (milk sugar).

3. **Monosaccharides**, such as glucose (the basic sugar), fructose (found in fruits), and galactose (found in milk).

In the small intestine, polysaccharides are broken down by pancreatic amylase into disaccharides *(Figure 5.29)*. Disaccharides are broken down to monosaccharides by maltase and dextrinase, enzymes secreted by the cells lining the villi of the small intestine.

The monosaccharides are taken up by the lining cells and transferred to the capillaries of the villi. They are then carried by the portal vein to the liver, where the nonglucose sugars are converted to glucose.

Proteins arrive in the duodenum and small intestine only 10% to 20% digested by gastric pepsin. Enzymes attached to the villi of the small intestine, together with the pancreatic enzyme trypsin, break down the remaining proteins to **amino acids**.

The amino acids are taken in by the epithelial cells of the small intestine, released into the capillaries of the villi, and carried away in the hepatic portal circulation. They are transported into cells all over the body, to be used as building blocks for new tissue formation.

Lipids (including fats) enter the duodenum and small intestine as large globules that have to be emulsified by bile salts into smaller droplets so that pancreatic lipase can digest the fats into very small droplets of free fatty acids and monoglycerides. There is enough pancreatic lipase in the duodenum to digest average amounts of fat within 1 or 2 minutes.

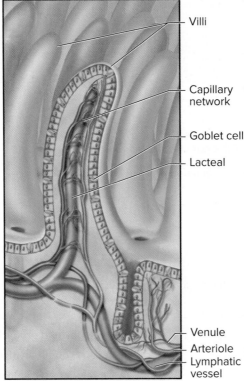

The very small droplets are absorbed by the intestinal cells and then taken into the lymphatic system by the **lacteals** inside the villi. The white, fatty lymphatic **chyle** eventually reaches the thoracic duct and is transferred into the left subclavian vein of the bloodstream. The chyle is carried by the blood and stored in adipose tissue.

The fat-soluble vitamins (A, D, E, and K) are absorbed with the lipids.

Water that is ingested is 92% absorbed by the small intestine and taken into the bloodstream through the capillaries in the villi *(Figure 5.30)*. Water-soluble vitamins (C and the B-complex) are absorbed with water with the exception of vitamin B_{12}. This is a large molecule that has to bind with intrinsic factor from the stomach so that cells in the distant ileum can receive it and pass it through to the bloodstream.

Minerals are absorbed along the whole length of the small intestine. Iron and calcium are absorbed according to the body's needs. The other minerals are absorbed regardless of need, and the kidneys excrete the surplus.

Figure 5.30 labels: Villi; Capillary network; Goblet cell; Lacteal; Venule; Arteriole; Lymphatic vessel

▲ **Figure 5.30** Intestinal Villi.

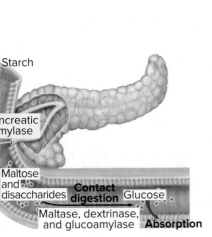

Labels: Starch; Pancreatic amylase; Maltose and disaccharides; Contact digestion; Glucose; Maltase, dextrinase, and glucoamylase; **Absorption**

▲ **Figure 5.29** Starch Digestion in the Small Intestine.

WORD	PRONUNCIATION	ELEMENTS		DEFINITION
amino acid	ah-**MEE**-noh **ASS**-id	R/CF	**amin/o** *nitrogen compound* **acid** Latin *sour*	The basic building block of protein
carbohydrate	kar-boh-**HIGH**-drate	S/ R/CF R/	**-ate** *composed of* **carb/o-** *carbon* **-hydr-** *water*	Group of organic food compounds that includes sugars, starch, glycogen, and cellulose
chyle (contrast **chyme**, p. 122)	KILE		Greek *juice*	A milky fluid that results from the digestion and absorption of fats in the small intestine
lacteal	**LAK**-tee-al	S/ R/CF	**-al** *pertaining to* **lact/e-** *milk*	A lymphatic vessel carrying chyle away from the intestine
lipid	**LIP**-id		Greek *fat*	General term for all types of fatty compounds; for example, cholesterol, triglycerides, and fatty acids
mineral	**MIN**-er-al	S/ R/	**-al** *pertaining to* **miner-** *mines*	Inorganic compound usually found in earth's crust
protein	**PRO**-teen		Greek *first, primary*	Class of food substances based on amino acids

Exercises

A. Apply your medical vocabulary to answer the following questions about digestion. *Select the correct answer that completes each statement.* **LO 5.12**

1. The suffix that is used to form the names of enzymes is

   a. *-ic*   **b.** *-al*   **c.** *-ase*   **d.** *-ous*   **e.** *-ion*

2. Which of the following terms means *a milky fluid resulting from the digestion and absorption of fats in the small intestine*?

   a. lipid   **b.** chyme   **c.** protease   **d.** chyle   **e.** lacteal

3. The group of organic food compounds that includes sugars, starch, glycogen, and cellulose is

   a. proteins   **b.** fats   **c.** lipids   **d.** carbohydrates   **e.** calories

4. The root *hydr-* means

   A. blood   **b.** juice   **c.** water   **d.** milk   **e.** bile

B. Apply your medical vocabulary to answer the following questions about digestion. *Select the correct answer that completes each statement.* **LO 5.12**

1. The general term for all fatty compounds is

   a. bile   **b.** protein   **c.** carbohydrate   **d.** lipid   **e.** protease

2. What is another name for a mineral?

   a. enzyme   **b.** electrolyte   **c.** lipid   **d.** hormone   **e.** fatty acid

3. The majority of water is absorbed in the:

   a. pancreas   **b.** stomach   **c.** small intestine   **d.** large intestine

- In malnutrition, the body breaks down its own tissues to meet its nutritional and metabolic needs.

- Milk sugar is lactose. The enzyme lactase breaks down lactose to glucose.

- Diarrhea is caused by irritation of the intestinal lining so that feces pass through the intestine too quickly for adequate amounts of water to be reabsorbed.

 ## Case Report (CR) 5.3 (continued)

Mrs. Jan Stark, who presented in the Emergency Department with dehydration, was found to have **celiac disease**, a sensitivity to the protein **gluten** that is found in wheat, rye, and barley. This disease involves the destruction of epithelial cells of the digestive tract lining, so intestinal enzymes are not being produced and absorption is not taking place.

Her difficulties with fine motor movement were the result of a **neuropathy** caused by vitamin B_{12} deficiency because of the lack of intrinsic factor to enable B_{12} to be absorbed. The diagnosis was made by an intestinal biopsy through oral endoscopy. A diet free of such gluten-containing foods as breads, cereals, cookies, and beer relieved her symptoms.

LO 5.13 Disorders of Absorption

Malabsorption syndromes refer to a group of diseases in which intestinal absorption of nutrients is impaired.

Malnutrition can arise from malabsorption or from insufficient food intake as a result of famine, poverty, loss of appetite due to cancer, or terminal illness. Many of the poor and elderly in this country suffer from malnutrition.

Lactose intolerance occurs when the small intestine is not producing sufficient **lactase** to break down the milk sugar lactose. The result is **diarrhea** and cramps. Lactase can be taken in pill form before eating dairy products, and/or lactose can be avoided by using soy products rather than milk products.

Crohn's disease (or **regional enteritis**) is an inflammation of the small intestine (frequently in the ileum) and occasionally also in the large intestine. The symptoms are abdominal pain, diarrhea, fatigue, and weight loss. Malabsorption is common, and children with Crohn's disease may have delayed development and stunted growth.

Constipation occurs when fecal movement through the large intestine is slow, causing too much water to be reabsorbed by the large intestine. The feces become hardened. Factors causing constipation are lack of dietary fiber, lack of exercise, and emotional upset.

Gastroenteritis (stomach "flu") is an infection of the stomach and intestine that can be caused by a large variety of bacteria and viruses. It causes vomiting, diarrhea, and fever. An outbreak of gastroenteritis can sometimes be traced to contaminated food or water. The Norwalk virus and rotaviruses are major causes of diarrhea in infants and children.

Dysentery is a severe form of bacterial gastroenteritis with blood and mucus in frequent, watery stools. It can lead to dehydration.

WORD	PRONUNCIATION		ELEMENTS	DEFINITION
celiac celiac disease	**SEE**-lee-ack **SEE**-lee-ack diz-**EEZ**	S/ R/ P/ R/	-ac *pertaining to* celi- *abdomen* dis- *apart* -ease *normal function*	Relating to the abdominal cavity Disease caused by sensitivity to gluten
constipation	kon-stih-**PAY**-shun	S/ R/	-ation *process* constip- *press together*	Hard, infrequent bowel movements
Crohn's disease (also called **regional enteritis**)	KRONES diz-**EEZ** **REE**-jun-al en-ter-**EYE**-tis		Burrill Crohn, 1884–1993, New York gastroenterologist	Inflammatory bowel disease with narrowing and thickening of the terminal small bowel
diarrhea	die-ah-**REE**-ah	P/ S/	dia- *complete, through* -rrhea *flow, discharge*	Abnormally frequent and loose stools
dysentery	**DIS**-en-tare-ee	P/ R/	dys- *bad, difficult* -entery *intestine*	Disease with diarrhea, bowel spasms, fever, and dehydration
gastroenteritis	**GAS**-troh-en-ter-**EYE**-tis	S/ R/CF R/	-itis *inflammation* gastr/o- *stomach* -enter- *intestine*	Inflammation of the stomach and intestines
gluten	**GLU**-ten		Latin *glue*	Insoluble protein found in wheat, barley, and oats
intolerance	in-**TOL**-er-ance		Latin *unable to cope with*	Inability of the small intestine to digest and dispose of a particular dietary constituent
lactose **lactase**	**LAK**-toes **LAK**-tase	S/ R/	-ase *enzyme* lact- *milk*	The disaccharide found in cow's milk Enzyme that breaks down lactose to glucose and galactose

Exercises

A. Study the terms and elements in the above WAD. *Notice that some terms are formed with only a prefix and a root, while others are formed with a root and a suffix.* **The only element that needs to be present in every term is a root or combining form.** *The definitions for the terms are given, as well as the element placement in the term. Write the correct element on each blank.* **LO 5.13, 5.D**

1. Abnormally frequent and loose stools _____ / _____

2. Infrequent bowel movements _____ / _____

3. Enzyme that breaks down lactose _____ / _____

4. Relating to the abdominal cavity _____ / _____

5. Disease with fever, diarrhea, and bowel spasms _____ / _____

Lesson 5.6

DIGESTIVE SYSTEM

Elimination and the Large Intestine

Lesson Objectives

After the nutrients have been digested and absorbed in the small intestine, the residual materials have to be prepared in the large intestine for elimination from the body. The information in this lesson will enable you to:

5.6.1   Describe the anatomy and physiology of the large intestine.

5.6.2   Relate the structure of the large intestine to its functions.

5.6.3   Discuss common disorders of the large intestine.

Keynote

A sphincter is a ring of smooth muscle that forms a one-way valve.

LO 5.14 Structure and Functions of the Large Intestine

Structure of the Large Intestine

The **large intestine** is so named because its diameter is much greater than that of the small intestine. It forms a **perimeter** in the abdominal cavity around the central mass of the small intestine *(Figure 5.31)*.

At the junction between the small and large intestines, a ring of smooth muscle called the **ileocecal sphincter** forms a one-way valve. This allows **chyme** to pass into the large intestine and prevents the contents of the large intestine from backing up into the ileum.

At the beginning of the large intestine, the **cecum** is a pouch in the lower right quadrant of the abdomen *(Figure 5.31)*. A narrow tube with a closed end, the **vermiform appendix**, projects downward from the cecum. The function of the appendix is not known.

The **ascending colon** begins at the cecum and extends upward until, just underneath the liver, it makes a sharp left turn at the hepatic **flexure** and becomes the transverse colon. At the left side of the abdomen, near the spleen at the splenic flexure, the transverse colon turns downward to form the descending colon. At the pelvic brim, the **descending** colon makes an S-shaped curve, the **sigmoid** colon, which descends in the pelvis to become the **rectum** and then the **anal canal.**

The rectum has three transverse folds, rectal valves that enable it to retain feces while passing gas (**flatus**). Intestinal gas is 90% nitrogen and oxygen, ingested while breathing and eating, together with methane, hydrogen, sulfites, and carbon dioxide contributed from bacterial fermentation of undigested food. This yields pungent ammonia and foul-smelling hydrogen sulfide to give gas and feces their characteristic odor.

The anal canal is the last 1 to 2 inches of the large intestine, opening to the outside as the **anus.** The mucous membrane is folded into six to eight longitudinal **anal columns. Feces** pressing against the columns causes them to produce more mucus to lubricate the canal during **defecation.** Two **sphincter** muscles guard the anus *(Figure 5.32)*: an internal sphincter, composed of smooth muscle from the intestinal wall, and an external sphincter, composed of skeletal muscle that you can control voluntarily.

Functions of the Large Intestine

- **Absorption** of water and electrolytes. The large intestine receives more than 1 L (1.05 quarts) of chyme each day from the small intestine and reabsorbs water and electrolytes to reduce the volume to 100 to 150 mL of feces to be eliminated by **defecation**.
- **Secretion** of mucus that protects the intestinal wall and holds particles of **fecal** matter together.
- **Digestion** by the bacteria that inhabit the large intestine of any food remnants that have escaped the digestive enzymes of the small intestine.
- **Peristalsis,** which, in the large intestine, happens only a few times a day to produce mass movements toward the rectum. Often when you ingest food into your stomach, your **gastrocolic reflex** will generate a mass movement of feces.
- **Elimination** of materials that were not digested or absorbed.

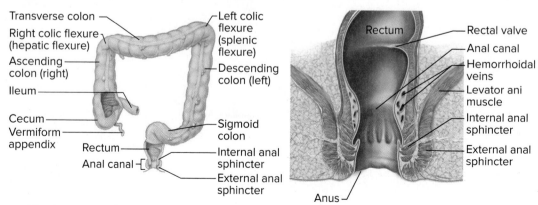

▲ **Figure 5.31** **Large Intestine.** Anatomy of the large intestine.

▲ **Figure 5.32** **Anal Canal**

WORD	PRONUNCIATION	ELEMENTS		DEFINITION
anus	AY-nuss		Latin *ring*	Terminal opening of the digestive tract through which feces are discharged
anal (adj)	AY-nal	S/ R/CF	al *pertaining to* an/o *anus*	Pertaining to the anus
appendix vermiform	ah-PEN-dicks VER-mih-form		Latin *appendage* Latin *wormlike*	Small blind projection from the pouch of the cecum Worm shaped; used as a descriptor for the appendix
cecum	SEE-kum		Latin *blind*	Blind pouch that is the first part of the large intestine
colon colic	KOH-lon KOL-ik	S/ R/	Greek *colon* -ic *pertaining to* col- *colon*	The large intestine, extending from the cecum to the rectum Spasmodic, crampy pains in the abdomen
feces fecal (adj)	FEE-sees FEE-kal	S/ R/	Latin *dregs* -al *pertaining to* fec- *feces*	Undigested, waste material discharged from the bowel Pertaining to feces
defecation	def-eh-KAY-shun	S/ P/	-ation *process* de- *from, out of*	Evacuation of feces from the rectum and anus
defecate (verb)	DEF-eh-kate	S/	-ate *process*	Process of defecation
flatus flatulence flatulent (adj)	FLAY-tus FLAT-you-lents FLAT-you-lent	S/ R/	Latin *blowing* -ence *forming* flatul- *excessive gas*	Gas or air expelled through the anus Excessive amount of gas in the stomach and intestines
flexure	FLECK-shur		Latin *bend*	A bend in a structure
gastrocolic reflex	gas-troh-KOL-ik REE-fleks	S/ R/CF R/ R/	-ic *pertaining to* gastr/o- *stomach* -col- *colon* reflex *bend back*	Mass movement of feces in the colon and the desire to defecate caused by taking food into stomach
ileocecal sphincter	ILL-ee-oh-SEE-cal SFINK-ter	S/ R/CF R/	-al *pertaining to* ile/o- *ileum* -cec- *cecum* sphincter Greek *band*	Band of muscle that encircles the junction of the ileum and cecum
perimeter	peh-RIM-eh-ter	P/ R/	peri- *around* -meter *measure*	An edge or border
rectum rectal (adj)	RECK-tum RECK-tal	S/ R/	Latin *straight* -al *pertaining to* rect- *rectum*	Terminal part of the colon from the sigmoid to the anal canal Pertaining to the rectum
sigmoid	SIG-moyd	S/ R/	-oid *resembling* sigm- Greek *letter "S"*	Sigmoid colon is shaped like an "S"

Exercises

A. Memorizing the meaning of word elements will help you to understand the meaning of many medical terms. *Match the word element in the first column with its correct meaning in in the second column.* **LO 5.14**

_____ **1.** *sigm-*

_____ **2.** *peri-*

_____ **3.** *col-*

_____ **4.** *-ence*

_____ **5.** *meter-*

a. forming

b. colon

c. measure

d. Greek letter "S"

e. around

> 💡 **Study Hint**
>
> il**e**um = int**e**stine
> Il**i**um hip
> Both terms are pronounced the same, but they are spelled differently. Be precise!

B. Some words cannot be deconstructed. *Correctly complete each sentence with the term from the WAD above. Use the italicized word as a clue to the correct term. Fill in the blank.* **LO 5.14**

1. The *blind* pouch of the large intestine is the _____.

2. The structure of the large intestine that is shaped like a *ring* is the _____.

3. The appendix has a *wormlike* appearance, and therefore is often termed as the _____ appendix.

4. The large intestine has several *bends* that are each termed as a _____.

LO 5.15 Disorders of the Large Intestine and Anal Canal

Disorders of the Large Intestine

Appendicitis is the most common cause of acute abdominal pain in the right lower quadrant. On palpation, tenderness over the **McBurney point**, one-third the distance from the anterior superior iliac crest to the umbilicus *(see Chapter 3)*, suggests appendicitis. If neglected, the inflamed appendix can rupture, leading to **peritonitis**. This is strongly suggested by the presence of *rebound tenderness*, in which a stab of severe pain is produced when the abdominal wall, which has been pressed in slowly, is released rapidly. A surgical appendectomy, usually performed through laparoscopy, is the treatment for appendicitis.

Diverticulosis is the presence of small pouches (**diverticula**) bulging outward through weak spots in the lining of the large intestine *(Figure 5.33)*. They are asymptomatic until the pouches become infected and inflamed, a condition called **diverticulitis**. This condition causes abdominal pain, vomiting, constipation, and fever. Complications, such as perforation and abscess formation, can occur. The most likely cause of diverticular disease (diverticulosis and diverticulitis) is a low-fiber diet.

Ulcerative colitis is an extensive inflammation and ulceration of the lining of the large intestine. It produces bouts of bloody diarrhea, crampy pain, and often weight loss and electrolyte imbalance.

Irritable bowel syndrome (IBS) is an increasingly common large-**bowel** disorder, presenting with crampy pains, gas, and changes in bowel habits to either constipation or diarrhea. There are no anatomic changes seen in the bowel, and the cause is unknown.

Polyps are masses of tissue arising from the wall of the large intestine and other tubelike structures that protrude into the bowel **lumen**. They vary in size and shape. Most are benign. Endoscopic biopsy can determine if they are **precancerous** or cancerous.

Colon and **rectal cancers** *(Figure 5.34)* are the second leading cause of cancer deaths after lung cancer. The majority occur in the rectum and sigmoid colon. These cancers spread by:

1. Direct extension through the bowel wall.
2. **Metastasis** to regional lymph nodes.
3. Moving down the lumen of the bowel.
4. Bloodborne **metastases** to liver, lung, bone, and brain.

Obstruction of the large bowel can be caused by cancers, large polyps, or diverticulitis.

Intussusception is a form of obstruction whereby a tumor in the lumen of the bowel, together with its segment of bowel, is telescoped into the immediately distal segment of bowel.

Proctitis is inflammation of the lining of the rectum, often associated with ulcerative colitis, Crohn's disease, or radiation therapy. Symptoms are **anorectal** pain, rectal bleeding, and excess mucus in the **stool.**

Disorders of the Anal Canal

Hemorrhoids are dilated veins in the submucosa of the anal canal, often associated with pregnancy, chronic constipation, diarrhea, or aging. They protrude into the anal canal (internal hemorrhoid) or bulge out along the edge of the anus (external hemorrhoid) producing pain and bright red blood from the anus. A thrombosed hemorrhoid, in which blood has clotted, is very painful.

Anal fissures are tears in the lining of the anal canal, such as may occur with difficult **bowel** movements (BMs).

Anal fistulas occur following abscesses in the anal glands. The anal canal has six or seven glands in the posterior canal that secrete mucus to lubricate the canal. If the glands become infected, abscesses form that, when they heal, can form a passage (fistula) between the anal canal and the skin outside the anus.

Diverticula

▲ **Figure 5.33** Barium Enema Showing **Diverticulosis** ©Susan Leavine/Photo Researchers Inc.

▲ **Figure 5.34** Barium Enema Showing Cancer of the Colon (orange area)
©SPL/Photo Researchers, Inc.

Abbreviations

BM	bowel movement
IBS	irritable bowel syndrome

WORD	PRONUNCIATION	ELEMENTS		DEFINITION
appendicitis	ah-pen-dih-**SIGH**-tis	S/ S/ R/	-ic- *pertaining to* -itis *inflammation* append- *appendix*	Inflammation of the appendix
bowel	**BOUGH**-el		Latin *sausage*	Another name for intestine
colitis	koh-**LIE**-tis	S/ R/	-itis *inflammation* col- *colon*	Inflammation of the colon
diverticulum diverticula (pl) diverticulosis	die-ver-**TICK**-you-lum die-ver-**TICK**-you-lah **DIE**-ver-tick-you-**LOH**-sis	S/ R/ S/	-um *tissue* diverticul- *byroad* -osis *condition*	A pouchlike opening or sac from a tubular structure (e.g., gut) Presence of a number of small pouches in the wall of the large intestine
diverticulitis	**DIE**-ver-tick-you-**LIE**-tis	S/	-itis *inflammation*	Inflammation of the diverticula
fissure	**FISH**-ur		Latin *slit*	Deep furrow or cleft
fistula	**FIS**-tyu-lah		Latin *pipe, tube*	Abnormal passage
hemorrhoid hemorrhoids (pl) hemorrhoidectomy	**HEM**-oh-royd **HEM**-oh-roy-**DEK**-toh-me	S/ R/CF S/	-rrhoid *flow* hem/o- *blood* -ectomy *excision*	Dilated rectal vein producing painful anal swelling Surgical removal of hemorrhoids
intussusception	**IN**-tuss-sus-**SEP**-shun	S/ P/ R/	-ion *action* intus- *within* -suscept- *to take up*	The slipping of one part of bowel inside another to cause obstruction
lumen	**LOO**-men		Latin *light, window*	The interior space of a tubelike structure
McBurney point	mack-**BUR**-nee POYNT		Charles McBurney, 1845–1913, New York surgeon	One-third the distance from the anterior superior iliac spine to the umbilicus
metastasis metastases (pl)	meh-**TAS**-tah-sis meh-**TAS**-tah-seez	P/ R/	meta- *beyond* -stasis *placement*	Spread of a disease from one part of the body to another
peritoneum	per-ih-toh-**NEE**-um	S/ R/CF	-um *tissue* periton/e- *stretch over*	Membrane that lines the abdominal cavity
peritoneal (adj) peritonitis	**PER**-ih-toe-**NEE**-al **PER**-ih-toh-**NIE**-tis	S/ S/	-al *pertaining to* -itis *inflammation*	Pertaining to the peritoneum Inflammation of the peritoneum
polyp	**POL**-ip		Latin *foot, stalk*	Mass of tissue that projects into the lumen of a hollow organ
polyposis polypectomy	pol-ih-**POH**-sis pol-ip-**ECK**-toh-mee	S/ R/ S/	-osis *condition* polyp- *polyp* -ectomy *excision*	Presence of several polyps Excision or removal of a polyp
precancerous	pree-**KAN**-sir-us	S/ P/ R/	-ous *pertaining to* pre- *before* -cancer- *cancer*	Lesion from which a cancer can develop
proctitis	prok-**TIE**-tis	S/ R/	-itis *inflammation* proct- *anus and rectum*	Inflammation of the lining of the rectum
ulcerative	**UL**-sir-ah-tiv	S/ R/	-ative *quality of* ulcer- *a sore*	Marked by an ulcer or ulcers

Exercise

A. This exercise focuses on the suffixes in the above WAD. *The suffix is your first clue to the meaning of a medical term. Match the word element in the first column with its correct meaning in the second column. Some answers you will use twice because more than one suffix can have the same meaning. One answer will not be used at all.* **LO 5.15**

_____ **1.** –um

_____ **2.** –ous

_____ **3.** –osis

_____ **4.** –ion

_____ **5.** –itis

_____ **6.** –rrhoid

_____ **7.** –ative

_____ **8.** –al

_____ **9.** –ectomy

a. flow

b. action

c. inflammation

d. tissue

e. pertaining to

f. condition

g. excision

h. quality of

i. study of

Procedures and Pharmacology of the Digestive System

LO 5.16 Diagnostic Procedures

Nasogastric aspiration and lavage are used to detect upper GI bleeding. The presence of bright red blood in the lavage material indicates active upper GI bleeding; "coffee grounds" indicate the bleeding has slowed or stopped.

Enteroscopy uses an oral, flexible **endoscope** containing light-transmitting fibers or a video transmitter to visualize and biopsy tumors and ulcers and to control bleeding from the esophagus, stomach, and duodenum. Visualization of the stomach is called **gastroscopy**; visualization of the esophagus, stomach, and duodenum is called **panendoscopy**.

Capsule endoscopy enables examination of the entire small intestine by ingesting a pill-sized video capsule with its own camera and light source that sends images to a data recorder worn on the patient's belt.

Double balloon endoscopy uses two balloons at the tip of the endoscope that are inflated sequentially to move the endoscope further into the small intestine than with a usual endoscope.

Upper GI tract barium x-rays (barium swallow) use barium sulfate, a contrast material, to study the distal esophagus, the stomach, and duodenum. They are less accurate than enteroscopy at identifying bleeding lesions.

Angiography uses injected dye to highlight blood vessels and is used to detect the site of bleeding in the GI tract.

In a **digital rectal examination** the physician palpates the rectum and prostate gland with a gloved, lubricated index finger to determine the presence of lesions.

Proctoscopy is procedure performed with a proctoscope that allows for the visual examination of the anus, rectum and sigmoid colon to look for diseases, causes of rectal bleeding or check on abnormal results seen during a barium enema.

Fecal occult blood test (Hemoccult) is used to detect the presence in the stool of blood not visible to the naked eye. It is a good first screening test for cancer of the large intestine.

Anoscopy is an examination of the anus and lower rectum using a rigid instrument. Flexible **sigmoidoscopy** examines the rectum and sigmoid colon and **flexible colonoscopy** examines the whole length of the colon.

In a **barium swallow,** the patient ingests barium sulfate, a contrast material, to show details of the pharynx and esophagus on x-ray.

In a **barium meal,** barium sulfate is used to study the distal esophagus, stomach, and duodenum on x-ray (*Figure 5.35*).

Barium enema uses the contrast material barium sulfate, which is injected into the large intestine as an enema and x-ray films are taken (*Figure 5.36*).

Pyloric sphincter — Pylorus of stomach

Jejunum — Duodenum

▲ **Figure 5.35** **Barium meal showing pylorus and duodenum.** ©Collection CNRI/Phototake/Alamy

Descending colon

Cecum

Appendix

Sigmoid colon

▲ **Figure 5.36** **Barium enema of the large intestine** ©CNRI/Photo Researchers, Inc.

LO 5.11 Liver Function Tests

Liver function tests (LFTs) are a group of tests to show how well your liver is functioning. They are divided into four categories:

1. Measuring liver proteins in blood serum
   - Measuring proteins, albumin, and globulin *(see Chapter 7)*, which are low when there is liver damage.

2. Measuring liver enzymes in blood serum
   - Measuring enzymes made in the liver, known as **transaminases,** including **alanine aminotransferase (ALT;** also known as **serum glutamic-pyruvic transaminase,** or **SGPT)** and **aspartate aminotransferase (AST;** also known as **serum glutamic oxaloacetic acid transaminase,** or **SGOT).** Elevated levels of these enzymes in the blood indicate liver damage.

3. Measuring cholestatic liver enzymes in the blood serum
   - Measuring **alkaline phosphatase (ALP),** which metabolizes phosphorus and makes energy available for the body. Elevated blood levels are found in liver and biliary tract disorders.
   - Measuring **gamma-glutamyl transpeptidase (GGT),** which is elevated in liver disease.

4. Measuring bilirubin in the bloodstream
   - **Bilirubin** is formed in the liver from hemoglobin and secreted into the biliary system. If the liver is damaged, bilirubin can leak out into the bloodstream, producing elevated levels and jaundice.

WORD	PRONUNCIATION	ELEMENTS		DEFINITION
angiography	an-jee-**OG**-rah-fee	S/	-graphy *process of recording*	Process of recording the image of blood vessels after injection of contrast material
		R/CF	angio- *blood vessel*	
anoscopy	**A**-nos-koh-pee	S/	-scopy *to examine*	Endoscopic examination of the anus
		R/CF	an/o- *anus*	
aspiration	**AS**-pih-**RAY**-shun	S/	-ion *process*	Removal by suction of fluid or gas from a body cavity
		R/CF	aspirat- *to breathe on*	
cholangiography	**KOH**-lan-jee-**OG**-rah-fee	S/	-graphy *process of recording*	X-ray of the bile ducts after injection or ingestion of a contrast medium
		R/	chol- *bile*	
		R/CF	-angi/o- *blood vessel, lymph vessel*	
colonoscopy	koh-lon-**OSS**-koh-pee	S/	-scopy *to examine*	Endoscopic examination of the colon
		R/CF	colon/o *colon*	
digital	**DIJ**-ih-tal	S/	-al *pertaining to*	Pertaining to a finger or toe
		R/	digit- *finger or toe*	
endoscope	**EN**-doh-skope	P/	endo- *within, inside*	Instrument to examine the inside of a tubular or hollow organ
		R/	-scope *instrument for viewing*	
endoscopic (adj)	**EN**-doh-**SKOP**-ik	S/	-ic *pertaining to*	Pertaining to the use of an endoscope
endoscopy	en-**DOSS**-koh-pee	S/	-scopy *to examine*	The use of an endoscope
enema	**EN**-eh-mah		Greek *injection*	An injection of fluid into the rectum
enteroscopy	en-ter-**OSS**-koh-pee	S/	-scopy *to examine, to view*	The examination of the lining of the digestive tract
		R/CF	enter/o- *intestine*	
gastroscope	**GAS**-troh-skope	S/	-scope *instrument for viewing*	Instrument to view the inside of the stomach
		R/CF	gastr/o *stomach*	
gastroscopy	gas-**TROS**-koh-pee	S/	-scopy *to examine*	Endoscopic examination of the stomach
ileoscopy	ill-ee-**OS**-koh-pee	S/	-scopy *to examine*	Endoscopic examination of the ileum
		R/CF	ile/o- *ileum*	
lavage	lah-**VAHZH**		Latin *to wash*	Washing out of a hollow cavity, tube, or organ
panendoscopy	pan-en-**DOS**-koh-pee	S/	-scopy *to examine*	Endoscopic examination of the esophagus, stomach and duodenum
		P/	pan *all*	
		P/	-endo- *inside*	
proctoscopy	prok-**TOSS**-koh-pee	S/	-scopy *to examine*	Examination of the inside of the anus and the rectum by proctoscope or rectoscope
		R/CF	proct/o- *anus and rectum*	
resection	ree-**SEK**-shun	S/	-ion *action, condition*	Removal of a specific part of an organ or structure
resect (verb)		P/	re- *back*	
		R/	-sect- *cut off*	
sigmoidoscopy	sig-moi-**DOS**-koh-pee	S/	-scopy *to examine*	Endoscopic examination of the sigmoid colon
		R/CF	sigmoid/o- *sigmoid colon*	

Exercises

A. Utilize the correct terms for patient documentation. *When communicating verbally and in writing, it is crucial to use correct medical terminology. Using the terms provided below, fill in the blanks with the correct term. Not all terms will be used.* **LO 5.16, 5.A, 5.F**

endoscopy   proctoscopy   colonoscopy   enema   gastroenterologist   sigmoidoscopy   barium   angiography

A patient was complaining of blood in his stool. The physician requested that you schedule a **(1)**_____ **(2)**_____ with the radiology department. One week later, the test results came back and were inconclusive.
The physician decided that further tests were needed, and therefore wished to view the inside of the intestines. Because the physician believed the source of the bleeding was in the large intestine, she ordered a **(3)**_____. The medical assistant called the hospital's **(4)**_____ department.

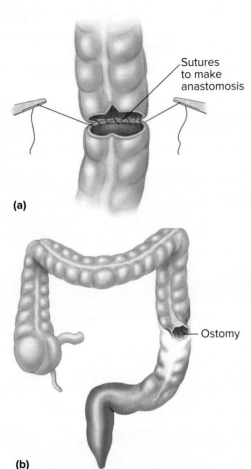

Sutures to make anastomosis

(a)

Ostomy

(b)

▲ **Figure 5.37** Intestinal Resections.

Abbreviations	
ERCP	endoscopic retrograde cholangiopancreatography
EUS	endoscopic ultrasound

LO 5.17 Therapeutic Procedures

Many of the diagnostic procedures in the previous section can also be used as therapeutic procedures. For example, endoscopy can be used to remove polyps, biopsy suspicious lesions, stop bleeding, and be used as screening procedures for cancer.

Alternatively, food can be inserted directly into the stomach via a **nasogastric** or stomach tube, when medically indicated.

Laparoscopy uses a thin, lighted tube inserted through an **incision** in the abdominal wall to examine abdominal and pelvic organs. Biopsy samples can be taken through the **laparoscope,** and in many cases surgery can be performed instead of using a much larger incision. Laparoscopy is done to check for and remove abnormal tumors; **ligate** Fallopian tubes; fix **hiatal** and **inguinal hernias**; and remove such organs as the uterus, spleen, gallbladder, ovaries, or appendix. **Resection** of the colon can also be performed **laparoscopically.**

Intestinal resections are used to surgically remove diseased portions of the intestine. The remaining portions of the intestine can be joined back together through an **anastomosis** *(Figure 5.37a)*. If there is insufficient bowel remaining for an anastomosis, an **ostomy** *(Figure 5.37b)* can be performed, where the end of the bowel opens onto the skin at a **stoma**. **Ileostomy** and **colostomy** are two such procedures.

Endoscopic retrograde cholangiopancreatography (ERCP) is used to diagnose and treat problems in the biliary ductal system. Through an endoscope, the physician can see the inside of the duodenum and inject radiographic contrast dye into the biliary tract ducts. Gallstones and cancer can be treated with this technique.

Pancreas endoscopic ultrasound (EUS) is a type of endoscopic examination that enables detailed imaging and analysis of the pancreas. A thin tube tipped with an ultrasound probe is inserted through the mouth down into the stomach and the first part of the small intestine. The probe emits sound waves that bounce off surrounding structures, and these sound waves are recaptured by the probe and converted to black and white images that can be interpreted by the physician. EUS is of great value in assessing pancreatic tumors and cysts and acute and chronic pancreatitis.

Gastric cancer is usually treated with **resection** and chemotherapy.

WORD	PRONUNCIATION		ELEMENTS	DEFINITION
appendectomy	ah-pen-**DEK**-toh-mee	S/ R/	-ectomy *surgical excision* append- *appendix*	Surgical removal of the appendix
anastomosis **anastomoses** (pl)	ah-**NAS**-to-**MOH**-sis ah-**NAS**-to-**MOH**-seez	S/ R/	-osis *condition* anastom- *join together*	A surgically made union between two tubular structures
cholecystectomy	**KOH**-leh-sis-**TEK**-toh-mee	S/ R/CF R/	-ectomy *surgical excision* chol/e- *bile* -cyst- *bladder*	Surgical removal of the gallbladder
cholelithotomy	**KOH**-leh-lih-**THOT**-oh-mee	S/ R/	-otomy *surgical incision* -lith- *stone*	Surgical incision to remove a gallstone(s)
hernia	**HER**-nee-ah		Latin *rupture*	Protrusion of a structure through the tissue that normally contains it
hiatal	high-**AY**-tal	S/ R/	-al *pertaining to* hiat- *aperture*	Pertaining to an opening through a structure
inguinal	**IN**-gwin-al	S/ R/	-al *pertaining to* inguin- *groin*	Pertaining to the groin
ostomy (Note: an "s" is removed for the purpose of spelling)	**OS**-toh-mee	S/ R/	-stomy *new opening* os- *mouth*	Surgery to create an artificial opening into a tubular structure
colostomy	ko-**LOS**-toh-mee	R/	col- *colon*	Artificial opening from the colon to the outside of the body
ileostomy	ill-ee-**OS**-toh-mee	R/	ile- *ileum*	Artificial opening from the ileum to the outside of the body
pancreatography	**PAN**-kree-ah-**TOG**-raff-ee	S/ R/CF	-graphy *process of recording* pancreat/o *pancreas*	Process of recording the structure of the pancreas
retrograde	**RET**-roh-grade	P/ R/	retro- *backward* -grade *going*	Reversal of a normal flow
stoma	**STOH**-mah		Greek *mouth*	Artificial opening
ultrasound	**UL**-trah-sownd	P/ R/	ultra- *higher* -sound *noise*	Very-high-frequency sound waves

Exercises

A. Use word elements to build medical terms. Many therapeutic procedures differ by one word element. *Given the definition of the procedure, provide the correct word element to create the medical term. Fill in the blank.* **LO 5.17, 5.C**

1. Surgical incision to remove a gallstone: cholelitho/_____

2. Surgical removal of the appendix: _____ /ectomy

3. Surgery to create an opening from a tubular structure to the outside: _____ /tomy

4. Surgical removal of the gallbladder: chole/_____ /ectomy

5. Artificial opening from the ileum to the outside of the body: ile/_____ /tomy

B. Deconstruct medical terms to determine their meanings. *By knowing the meaning of word elements, you can decipher the meaning of the medical term. Choose the correct answer for each question.* **LO 5.17, 5.D, 5.E**

1. In the procedure ERCP, the "E" stands for

   a. enteric   **b.** echo   **c.** endoscopic   **d.** electrical

2. In the procedure of inserting a nasogastric tube, the practitioner inserts the tube through the

   a. nose   **b.** mouth   **c.** stomach   **d.** rectum

3. In the procedure ERCP, the "C" tells you that the organ being treated is the

   a. stomach   **b.** pancreas   **c.** biliary ducts   **d.** duodenum

4. In an anastomosis, the root means

   a. removal   **b.** creation of an opening   **c.** join together   **d.** incision

LO 5.18 Gastrointestinal Drugs

Drugs to Treat Excess Gastric Acid

Antacids, which are taken orally, neutralize gastric acid and relieve heartburn and acid indigestion. Examples of antacids include:

- aluminum hydroxide and magnesium hydroxide (*Maalox, Mylanta*)
- magnesium hydroxide (*Milk of Magnesia*)
- calcium carbonate (*Tums, Rolaids*)

Histamine-2 receptor antagonists (H$_2$-blockers) block signals that tell the stomach cells to produce acid. They are used to treat gastroesophageal reflux (GERD) and esophagitis (*see Lesson 5.2*). Examples include:

- cimetidine (*Tagamet*)
- famotidine (*Pepcid*)
- ranitidine (*Zantac*)
- nizatidine (*Axid*)

Less potent OTC variants of these drugs are also available.

Proton pump inhibitors (PPIs) suppress gastric acid secretion in the lining of the stomach by blocking the secretion of gastric acid from the cells into the lumen of the stomach. Examples include:

- omeprazole (*Prilosec*)
- lansoprazole (*Prevacid*)
- esomeprazole (*Nexium*)

A new form of PPI called imidazopyridine (*Tenatoprazole*) appears to be extremely effective in reducing gastric acid.

Misoprostol (*Cytotec*) inhibits the secretion of gastric acid and is approved for the prevention of **nonsteroidal anti-inflammatory drug (NSAID)**–induced gastric acid.

Sucralfate (*Carafate*) reacts with gastric acid (hydrogen chloride [**HCl**]) to form a paste that binds to stomach mucosal cells and inhibits the **diffusion** of acid into the stomach lumen. It also forms a protective barrier on the surface of an ulcer. Its main use is in the **prophylaxis** of stress ulcers.

Anti–H. pylori therapy for the treatment of peptic ulcer and chronic gastritis is given with a combination of two antibiotics (for example, amoxicillin [generic] and clarithromycin [generic]) and a proton pump inhibitor.

Drugs to Treat Nausea and Vomiting

Antiemetics, drugs that are effective against vomiting and nausea, are used to treat motion sickness and the side effects of opioid analgesics, general anesthetics, and chemotherapy. The types of antiemetics include:

- **Serotonin antagonists,** which block serotonin receptors in the CNS and GI tract. They are used to treat postoperative and chemotherapy nausea and vomiting. Examples include dolasetron (*Anzemet*), granisetron (*Kytril*), and ondansetron (*Zofran*).
- **Dopamine antagonists,** which act in the brain. They are inexpensive but have an extensive side-effect profile and have been replaced by serotonin antagonists. Examples include chlorpromazine (*Thorazine*) and prochlorperazine (*Compazine*).
- **Antihistamines,** which are used to treat motion sickness, morning sickness in pregnancy, and opioid nausea. Examples include diphenhydramine (*Benadryl*) and promethazine (*Phenergan*).
- **Cannabinoids,** which are used in patients with **cachexia** or who are unresponsive to other antiemetics. Examples include cannabis (medical marijuana) and dronabinol (*Marinol*).

Drugs to Treat Constipation

Laxative drugs are used to treat chronic constipation:

- If increased water and fiber are unsuccessful, OTC forms of magnesium hydroxide are the first-line agents to be used.
- Lubiprostone (*Resolor*) has received FDA approval; it acts on the epithelial cells of the GI tract to produce a chloride-rich fluid that softens the **stool** and increases bowel **motility**.

Drugs to Treat Diarrhea

Antidiarrheal drugs are widely available OTC. Examples include loperamide (*Imodium A-D, Maalox*), which reduces bowel motility; bismuth subsalicylate (*Pepto-Bismol*), which decreases the secretion of fluid into the intestine; and attapulgite (*Kaopectate*), which pulls diarrhea-causing substances away from the GI tract; as well as enzymes and nutrients. A combination of diphenyloxylate and atropine (*Lomotil*), a Schedule V drug, reduces bowel motility.

Abbreviations	
H$_2$-blocker	histamine-2 receptor antagonist
PPI	proton pump inhibitor

WORD	PRONUNCIATION	ELEMENTS		DEFINITION
antidiarrheal	**AN**-tee-die-ah-**REE**-al	S/ P/ P/ S/	**-al** *pertaining to* **anti-** *against* **-dia-** *complete, through* **-rrhea** *flow, discharge*	Drug that prevents abnormally frequent and loose stools
antiemetic	**AN**-tee-eh-**MEH**-tik	P/ R/	**anti-** *against* **-emetic** *causing vomiting*	Agent that prevents vomiting
antihistamine	an-tee-**HISS**-tah-meen	P/ R/ R/CF	**anti-** *against* **-hist-** *tissue* **-amine** *nitrogen compound*	Drug that can be used to treat allergic symptoms or prevent vomiting
cachexia	kah-**KEK**-see-ah	P/ R/	**cach-** *bad* **-exia** *condition of body*	A general weight loss and wasting of the body
cannabinoid	can-**AH**-bi-noyd	S/ R/	**-oid** *resembling* **cannabin-** *hemp*	A group of chemical compounds, some of which increase appetite and others treat nausea and vomiting
laxative	**LAK**-sah-tiv	S/ R/CF	**-tive** *pertaining to* **lax/a-** *looseness*	An oral agent that promotes the expulsion of feces
motility	moh-**TILL**-ih-tee	S/ R/	**-ility** *condition, state of* **mot-** *to move*	The ability for spontaneous movement
proton pump inhibitor (PPI)	**PROH**-ton PUMP in-**HIB**-ih-tor	R/ R/ S/ R/	**proton** *first* **pump** *pump* **-or** *a doer* **inhibit-** *repress*	Agent that blocks production of gastric acid
stool	STOOL		Old English *a seat*	The matter discharged in one movement of the bowels

Exercise

A. Read the statements carefully and match them with the right drugs. *Match the definition in the first column with the correct medication it is describing in the second column.* **LO 5.18**

_____ 1. used to suppress gastric acid secretions   **a.** Maalox

_____ 2. used to treat opioid nausea   **b.** Imodium

_____ 3. neutralizes gastric acid and relieves heartburn   **c.** Tagamet

_____ 4. used for treatment of postoperative nausea   **d.** Nexium

_____ 5. antidiarrheal drug   **e.** Benadryl

_____ 6. blocks production of stomach acid   **f.** Zofran

Chapter 5 Review

© 2014 Nucleus Medical Media

Digestive System
Challenge Your Knowledge

A. **A dental assistant, or anyone working in an Oral Surgery Department, needs to have a thorough knowledge of the mouth and the mastication process.** Your knowledge of medical terms will help you communicate with the dentist or oral surgeon and the patients. Match the definition in the first column with the correct structure it is describing in the second column. **(LO 5.1, 5.4, 5.5)**

_____ 1. Grind and crush food   **a.** mouth

_____ 2. Projects above the gum/covered with enamel   **b.** pulp cavity

_____ 3. Wrinkle   **c.** root canal

_____ 4. Destroys tooth enamel and dentin   **d.** caries

_____ 5. Contains blood vessels, nerves, tissue   **e.** root

_____ 6. Harder than bone   **f.** gingivitis

_____ 7. Oral cavity   **g.** papillae

_____ 8. Dental decay   **h.** crown

_____ 9. Anchors tooth to jaw   **i.** tartar

_____ 10. Inflammation of the gum   **j.** rugae

_____ 11. Nerves reach the tooth through this   **k.** bicuspids and molars

_____ 12. Contain the taste buds   **l.** dentin

B. **A medical term that is a noun can also have an adjective form.** Each statement has the noun form in parentheses; you must fill in the correct form of the adjective on the blank. Fill in the blanks. **(LO 5.A)**

1. The patient's (digestion) _____ symptoms were resolved with the new medication.

2. Due to an obstruction, the (pylorus) _____ sphincter was necrotic.

3. The (feces) _____ sample showed the presence of blood.

4. The patient is suffering from (pancreas) _____ cancer.

5. The (saliva) _____ gland was removed and sent to pathology.

6. Due to infection, the patient's (intestine) _____ surgery has been postponed until next week.

7. (Hemolysis) _____ jaundice results from RBC destruction and excess bilirubin.

8. The patient's (esophagus) _____ varices were bleeding.

9. The (laparoscope) _____ surgery poses less risk to the patient.

10. The (segment) _____ resection of the intestine is scheduled for later today.

C. Abbreviations. Choose the abbreviation that is best described in the statement, and fill it in on the blank provided. There are more answers than questions. Fill in the blanks. **(LO 5.1, 5.2, 5.7, 5.11, 5.16, 5.E)**

GI   SSA   GERD   BMI   HAV   SGOT   CF   BM

1. Final act of elimination   Abbreviation: _____

2. Backing up into the esophagus   Abbreviation: _____

3. Digestive system component   Abbreviation: _____

4. Liver disease indicator   Abbreviation:_____

5. Inherited disease that affects exocrine glands   Abbreviation: _____

D. Be aware of singular and plural terms. Insert the correct medical terms in the blanks; watch for spelling. You will not use all the terms. **(LO 5.3)**

diverticulitis   **diverticulum**   **diverticulosis**   **diverticula**

1. What starts out as a single _____ can be followed by many other _____.

The condition of having a number of these small pouches in the wall of the intestine is known as _____.

Should these pouches become inflamed, _____ will result.

metastasses   **metastases**   **metastize**   **metastasis**

2. What was originally thought to be a single _____ to the patient's lung was proved to be multiple

_____ to lung, kidney, and bone.

polypectomy   **polyposis**   **polyp (singular)**

3. The first polyp was found on sigmoidoscopy. A follow-up colonoscopy 6 months later found several more (plural)

_____ in the large intestine. Diagnosis is _____. Proposed

treatment is _____.

peritoneum   **peritonitis**   **peritoneal**

4. The _____ laceration sliced completely through the _____. Because of an

infection in the wound, the patient developed _____.

Digestive System

E. **Word elements are the keys to unlocking medical terms.** Assess your knowledge of elements with this exercise. **(LO 5.D)**

1. Where is the inflammation in **hepatitis**?

   a. belly

   b. liver

   c. pancreas

   d. mouth

   e. intestine

2. In the term **submucosa,** the prefix means

   a. over

   b. under

   c. around

   d. inside

   e. across

3. The color denoted in the term **leukoplakia** is

   a. green

   b. black

   c. white

   d. yellow

   e. red

4. The element **os** means

   a. stomach

   b. mouth

   c. eye

   d. liver

   e. ear

5. If the root **cyst** means *bladder,* what is a **cystectomy**?

   a. bladder irrigation

   b. bladder removal

   c. bladder examination

   d. bladder laceration

   e. bladder hemorrhage

6. If a medication is given **postprandially,** you will take it after

   a. exercise

   b. drinking water

   c. a meal

   d. a vitamin

   e. waking up

7. **Gingivitis** has a root that means

   a. opening

   b. teeth

   c. gum

   d. decay

   e. enzyme

8. A **cholecystectomy** is

   a. a procedure

   b. a diagnosis

   c. an inflammation

   d. a discharge

   e. an instrument

9. What is the adjective used to describe a dilated, tortuous vein?

   a. adipose

   b. varicose

   c. edematous

   d. pyloric

   e. segmental

10. On the basis of the suffix, you know that the **peritoneum** will be

    a. an opening

    b. an incision

    c. a structure

    d. a tumor

    e. a matrix

F. Deconstruct. Deconstruct the following medical terms related to the digestive system. Write each element in the appropriate area of the chart. If a term does not have a particular element, write n/a. Fill in the blanks. The first one has been done for you. **(LO 5.4, 5.9, 5.15, 5.D)**

Medical Term	Prefix	Meaning of Prefix	Root	Meaning of Root	Suffix	Meaning of Suffix	Meaning of Term
stomatitis	1. n/a	2. n/a	3. stom	4. mouth	5. itis	6. inflammation	7. Inflammation of the mucous membrane of the mouth
sublingual	8.	9.	10.	11.	12.	13.	14.
dyspepsia	15.	16.	17.	18.	19.	20.	21.
intussusception	22.	23.	24.	25.	26.	27.	28.
flatulence	29.	30.	31.	32.	33.	34.	35.

G. Check the accuracy of your chart documentation. The following patients have presented to the gastroenterology clinic today. Can you correctly complete their documentation? Fill in the blanks. **(LO 5.3, 5.16)**

1. Caroline Mason presents today with severe _____ (vomiting of blood), which has been getting progressively worse. _____ (looking within by a scope) reveals _____ -atous (swollen) _____ (pertaining to the esophagus) _____ (dilated veins).

2. Andrew Baker reported to the Fulwood Emergency Room yesterday with symptoms of _____ (following a meal) burning chest pain and _____ (vomiting of blood). Dr. Lee admitted him to the GI service for further diagnostic tests and possible surgery.

H. Medical abbreviations must be interpreted correctly to ensure precision in communication and patient safety. Match the correct abbreviation in the first column to the defined meanings in the second column. **(LO 5.1, 5.4, 5.18, 5.E)**

_____ **1.** CF

_____ **2.** IBS

_____ **3.** GI

_____ **4.** PPI

_____ **5.** NSAIDs

a. use increases incidence of peptic ulcers

b. blocks production of gastric acid

c. an intestinal diagnosis

d. an inherited disease

e. refers to two specific organs

Digestive System

I. **Can you interpret the following colonoscopy report for this patient?** If you need to, consult a dictionary or your glossary for additional help. Fill in the blanks. (**LO 5.14, 5.16, 5.D**)

Preoperative Diagnosis: History of (H/O) multiple colonic polyps.

Postoperative Diagnosis: Normal colon.

In the left lateral position, the colonoscope was advanced into the rectum without difficulty. Examination of the rectum was normal. The sigmoid and descending colon revealed extensive diverticular disease but no evidence of colonic polyp disease. The transverse colon was examined to the hepatic flexure. There were no abnormalities of the transverse colon. The ascending colon was examined to the ileocecal valve. There were no abnormalities of the ascending colon. The patient tolerated the procedure well and was discharged from the endoscopy suite in good condition. In view of his age and a clean colonoscopy, I have recommended no further surveillance.

1. Analyze the prefixes. What is the difference between the pre- and postoperative diagnoses?

   pre- = _____ post- = _____

2. Describe the left lateral position:

   a. side

   b. belly

   c. back

3. What instrument was used for this procedure? _____

4. Deconstruct **diverticulosis.** Suffix:_____; Root/Combining Form: _____

5. Define **polyp.**

   a. mass of tissue projecting into hollow organ

   b. erosion of tissue causing bleeding

   c. bulging of veins

   d. death of tissue wall

J. **Precision in documentation.** Get the stone in the right place: **cholelithiasis** or **choledocholithiasis**? Make the correct choice of medical terminology for the digestive system. Fill in the blanks. (**LO 5.11**)

1. The patient's films revealed a stone in the common bile duct.

   Diagnosis:

   _____

2. The presence of a stone in the patient's gallbladder was confirmed by the radiologist.

   Diagnosis:

   _____

K. Supply the missing element that will complete the medical term. Fill in the blanks. The first one is done for you. **(LO 5.6, 5.15, 5.16 5.C)**

1. Inflammation of the appendix

    appendic / <u> itis   </u>

2. Part of the colon shaped like an "S"

    sigm / _____

3. Pertaining to the anus

    an / _____

4. Excessive amount of gas

    flatul / _____

5. Inflammation of the anus and rectum

    _____ / itis

6. Presence of polyps

    polyp / _____

7. Examination of the contents of the abdomen using an endoscope

    /o / scopy / _____

8. Evacuation of feces from the rectum and anus

    de / fec / _____

9. An edge or a border

    peri / _____

10. Inflammation of the colon

    / itis / _____

L. Many medical terms that are nouns also have an adjectival form. Correctly apply these six medical terms to the following sentences. Fill in the blanks. **(LO 5.3, 5.A)**

mucous   mucin   mucus   mucosal   mucosa   submucosa

1. The lining of a tubular structure is referred to as the _____.

2. A sticky film containing mucin is _____.

3. The term for *pertaining to* the mucosa is _____.

4. The tissue layer beneath the mucosa is the _____.

5. _____ is a secretion from the mucosal glands.

6. _____ means *relating to mucus or the mucosa.*

Digestive System

M. **After reading Case Report 5.4, answer the following questions.** Select the correct answer to complete each statement or answer each question. **(LO 5.3, 5.13, 5.15, 5.E)**

 ## Case Report (CR) 5.4

You are

. . . a Certified Medical Assistant working with Susan Lee, MD, a primary care physician at Fulwood Medical Center.

Your patient is

. . . Mrs. Sandra Jacobs, a 46-year-old mother of four. Your task is to document her care.

Documentation

Mrs. Sandra Jacobs, a 46-year-old mother of four, presents in Dr. Susan Lee's primary care clinic with episodes of crampy pain in her right upper quadrant associated with nausea and vomiting. The pain often occurs after eating fast food. She has not noticed fever or jaundice. Physical examination reveals an obese white woman with a positive **Murphy sign.** Her BP is 170/90. A provisional diagnosis of **gallstones** has been made. She has been referred for an ultrasound examination, and an appointment has been made to see Dr. Stewart Walsh in the Surgery Department.

I explained to her the etiology of her gallstones and the need for surgical removal of the stones, and I discussed with her a low-fat, 1500-calorie diet sheet.

Luisa Guitterez, CMA. 10/12/12, 1430 hrs.

---

1. In which quadrant is Mrs. Jacobs having pain?

   a. LUQ

   b. LLQ

   c. RUQ

   d. RLQ

2. The fact that she does not have jaundice rules out a disorder of the:

   a. stomach

   b. liver

   c. gallbladder

   d. pancreas

3. What is a *positive Murphy sign*?

   a. pain in the right upper quadrant

   b. accumulation of fluid in the peritoneum

   c. blood in the stool

   d. vomit that appears as coffee grounds

4. What additional diagnostic procedure is she scheduled for?

   a. sigmoidoscopy

   b. cholecystectomy

   c. barium enema

   d. ultrasound

N. **Medications used to treat disorders of the gastrointestinal tract.** Select the correct answer that will complete each statement. **(LO 5.18)**

1. Antihistamines treat

   a. diarrhea

   b. constipation

   c. nausea and vomiting

   d. excess gastric acid

2. Imodium A-D® treats

   a. diarrhea

   b. constipation

   c. nausea and vomiting

   d. excess gastric acid

3. Histamine-2 blockers treat

   a. diarrhea

   b. constipation

   c. nausea and vomiting

   d. excess gastric acid

4. Proton pump inhibitors treat

   a. diarrhea

   b. constipation

   c. nausea and vomiting

   d. excess gastric acid

5. Laxative drugs treat

   a. diarrhea

   b. constipation

   c. nausea and vomiting

   d. excess gastric acid

©2014 Nucleus Medical Media

Health professionals involved in the diagnosis and treatment of patients with problems with the urinary system include

- **Urologists**, who are specialists in the diagnosis and treatment of patients with diseases of the urinary system.

- **Nephrologists**, who are specialists in the diagnosis and treatment of diseases of the kidney.

- **Urologic nurses and nurse practitioners**, who are registered nurses with advanced academic and clinical experience in urology.

Chapter Learning Outcomes

In order to define and understand the areas of concern about Mr. Hughes' postoperative state in Case Report 6.1 and to understand the conditions of all your **urinary** system patients, you need to be able to:

LO 6.1 Describe the structure and functions of the urinary system.

LO 6.2 Relate the structure of the kidney to its functions.

LO 6.3 Explain disorders of the kidneys.

LO 6.4 Discuss the structure and function of the ureters.

LO 6.5 Explain the disorders of the ureters.

LO 6.6 Relate the structure of the urinary bladder and urethra to their functions.

LO 6.7 Describe disorders of the urinary bladder and urethra.

LO 6.8 Explain the diagnostic procedures used for urinary system disorders.

LO 6.9 Discuss the therapeutic procedures used for urinary system disorders.

LO 6.10 Describe the pharmacologic agents used in the treatment of urinary system disorders.

LO 6.A Use the medical terms of urology to communicate in writing and to document the terms of urology accurately and precisely in any health care setting.

LO 6.B Use the medical terms of urology to communicate verbally with accuracy and precision in any health care setting.

LO 6.C Using word elements, construct medical terms associated with urology.

LO 6.D Deconstruct medical terms associated with urology into their word elements.

LO 6.E Identify health professionals involved in the care of urologic patients.

LO 6.F Use approved abbreviations for urologic terms correctly.

Case Report (CR) 6.1

You are

. . . a surgical physician assistant working with **urologist** Phillip Johnson, MD, at Fulwood Medical Center.

Your patient is

. . . Mr. Nelson Hughes, a 58-year-old school principal. You are making your afternoon hospital visits to Dr. Johnson's patients. Earlier today you assisted at Mr. Hughes's surgery. A **laparoscopic radical nephrectomy** for a **tumor-nodes-metastases (TNM) stage II renal cell carcinoma** (cancer) with no evidence of local invasion or lymph node involvement (**metastasis**) was performed.

Your job is to assess Mr. Hughes's postoperative state and determine whether postoperative complications exist.

Lesson 6.1
URINARY SYSTEM

Urinary System and Kidneys

Lesson Objectives

Although the respiratory system (*see Chapter 13*) excretes carbon dioxide and water; the integumentary system (*see Chapter 4*) excretes water, inorganic salts, and lactic acid in sweat; and the digestive tract (*see Chapter 5*) excretes water, salts, lipids, bile pigments, and other wastes, the urinary system carries the major burden of excretion. Within the urinary system, the kidneys are the agents that eliminate the waste products. If the kidneys fail to function, the other three systems of excretion are not able to replace them. Therefore, the kidney is a vital organ, and it brings with it a whole new set of terminology.

In this lesson, the information will enable you to:

6.1.1 Detail the urinary system.

6.1.2 Identify the location and anatomic features of the kidney.

6.1.3 Describe the functions of the kidney.

6.1.4 Map the flow of fluid through the renal filtration process.

6.1.5 Explain how common disorders of the kidneys affect health.

Abbreviations

IVP	intravenous pyelogram
TNM	tumor, nodes, and metastases (tumor staging method)

Keynotes

- **Urology** is the medical specialty of the diagnosis and treatment of diseases of the urinary system.
- The **kidney** is the major organ that eliminates the waste products of cellular metabolism.

LO 6.1 Urinary System

The urinary system (*Figure 6.1*) consists of six organs:

- Two kidneys **KID**-nees **(2)**
- A single **urinary bladder (1)**
- Two **ureters (2)**
- A single **urethra (1)**

The process of removing metabolic waste is called **excretion**. It is an essential process in maintaining homeostasis (*see Chapter 3*). The metabolic wastes include carbon dioxide from cellular respiration, excess water and electrolytes, **nitrogenous** compounds from the breakdown of proteins, and **urea**. If these wastes are not eliminated, they poison the whole body.

In the body's cells, protein is broken down (*see Chapter 3*) into **amino acids**. When an amino acid is broken down, **ammonia** is produced. Ammonia is extremely toxic to cells. The liver quickly converts it to the less toxic urea, which is **excreted** by the kidneys in the form of **urine**.

Labels: Inferior vena cava, Adrenal gland, Kidney, Aorta, Ureter, **Urinary bladder**, Urethra

(a) (b)

▲ **Figure 6.1** **The Urinary System.** (a) Major organs. (b) Structures of the urinary system are visible in this colored **intravenous pyelogram** (IVP). (b) ©CNRI/SPL/Photo Researchers, Inc.

WORD	PRONUNCIATION		ELEMENTS	DEFINITION
amino acid	ah-**MEE**-noh **ASS**-id	R/CF	**amin/o** nitrogen containing **acid** Latin sour	The basic building block for protein
ammonia	ah-**MOHN**-ih-ah	S/ R/	**-ia** condition **ammon-** ammonia	Toxic breakdown product of amino acids
bladder	**BLAD**-er		Old English bladder	Hollow sac that holds fluid; for example, urine or bile
excretion excrete (verb)	eks-**KREE**-shun eks-**KREET**		Latin remove	Removal of waste products of metabolism out of the body To pass out of the body the waste products of metabolism
kidney	**KID**-nee		Greek kidney	Organ of excretion
nephrology	neh-**FROL**-oh-jee	S/ R/	**-logy** study of **nephr/o** kidney	Medical specialty of diseases of the kidney
nephrologist	neh-**FROL**-oh-jist	S/	**-logist** one who studies, specialist	Medical specialist in diseases of the kidney
nitrogenous	ni-**TROJ**-en-us	S/ R/CF R/	**-ous** pertaining to **nitr/o-** nitrogen **-gen-** create	Containing or generating nitrogen
renal	**REE**-nal	S/ R/	**-al** pertaining to **ren-** kidney	Pertaining to the kidney
urea	you-**REE**-ah		Greek urine	End product of nitrogen metabolism expelled in urine
ureter (**Note:** Two "e's" = two tubes.)	you-**REET**-er		Greek urinary canal	Tube that connects the kidney to the urinary bladder (Note: The roots for **urethra** and **ureter** are different.)
ureteral (adj)	you-**REE**-ter-al	S/ R/	**-al** pertaining to **ureter-** ureter	Pertaining to the ureter
urethra (**Note:** One "e" = one tube.)	you-**REE**-thra		Greek urethra	Canal leading from the bladder to outside (Note: The roots for **urethra** and **ureter** are different.)
urethral (adj)	you-**REE**-thral	S/ R/	**-al** pertaining to **urethr-** urethra	Pertaining to the urethra
urine urinary (adj)	**YUR**-in **YUR**-in-air-ee	S/ R/	Latin urine **-ary** pertaining to **urin-** urine	Fluid and dissolved substances excreted by kidney Pertaining to urine
urinate (verb)	**YUR**-in-ate	S/	**-ate** composed of, pertaining to	To pass urine
urination	yur-ih-**NAY**-shun	S/	**-ation** process	The act of passing urine
urology	you-**ROL**-oh-jee	S/ R/CF	**-logy** study of **ur/o-** urinary system	Medical specialty of disorders of the urinary system
urologist urologic (adj)	you-**ROL**-oh-jist yur-roh-**LOJ**-ik	S/ S/	**-logist** one who studies **-ic** pertaining to	Medical specialist in disorders of the urinary system Pertaining to urology

Exercises

A. The same but different. *More than one word element can have the same meaning. In this body system, **nephr/o** and **ren-** both mean kidney. The elements are not interchangeable—one particular element will be used for a specific term. You need to know them individually. Fill in the blanks. Read carefully!* **LO 6.1, 6.D, 6.E**

1. Medical specialist in kidney treatment   _____ / _____ / _____

2. Medical specialty in kidney diseases   _____ / _____ / _____

3. Pertaining to the kidney   _____ / _____

> **Study Hint**
> You are keeping a list in the back of your text for all the suffixes meaning *pertaining to*. You should also keep a separate list of various elements like *ren* and *nephr/o* that have the same meaning but generate their own medical terms.

B. Employ the *language of urology* to correctly match the medical term to the brief description. **LO 6.1, 6.A**

_____ 1. hollow sac that holds fluids   **a.** kidney

_____ 2. organ of excretion   **b.** ureter

_____ 3. connects kidney to bladder   **c.** urethra

_____ 4. canal leading from bladder to outside the body   **d.** bladder

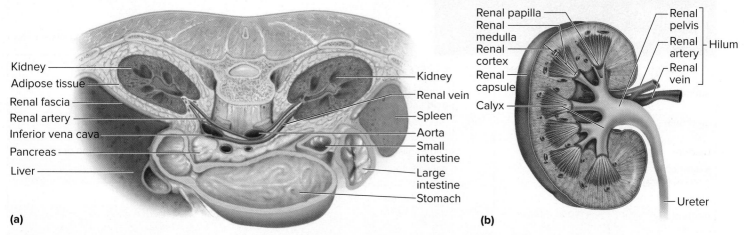

▲ **Figure 6.2** **Kidney.** (a) Transverse section of abdomen showing position of kidneys. (b) Longitudinal section of a kidney.

LO 6.2 Anatomy and Physiology of the Kidneys

Each kidney is a bean-shaped organ about the size of a clenched fist. It is located on either side of the vertebral column behind the peritoneum and lies against the deep muscles of the back. The left kidney is behind the spleen, and the right kidney is behind and below the liver *(Figure 6.2a)*.

Waste-laden blood enters the kidney at its **hilum** *(Figure 6.2b)* through the renal artery. Excess water, urea, and other waste products are **filtered** from the blood by the kidney, collected in the ureter, and carried off to the bladder through the renal pelvis at the hilum. The filtered blood exits through the renal vein at the hilum.

Each kidney has three regions *(see Figure 6.2b)*:

- An outer renal **cortex**—containing about 1 million **nephrons**, the basic filtration unit of the kidney.
- An inner renal **medulla**—containing the collecting ducts, which merge together to form about 30 papillary ducts, that enter into a **calyx**.
- A central renal **pelvis**—a funnel-shaped structure into which the calyces open, and which forms the ureter.

In the cortex, the renal artery divides into smaller and smaller arterioles, each of which enters a nephron and divides into a network of approximately 50 capillaries, known as a **glomerulus**. Each glomerulus is encased in the **glomerular capsule.** Because the blood is under pressure and the capillaries and glomerular capsule are **permeable**, much of the fluid from the blood filters through the capillary wall and glomerular capsule into the renal tubule, which includes the **nephron loop,** sometimes called the **loop of Henle** *(Figure 6.3)*.

This **filtrate** entering the renal tubule contains water, urea, glucose, electrolytes, amino acids, and vitamins. Red blood cells, platelets, and plasma proteins are too large to pass through the capillary membrane, and they remain in the blood.

Approximately 180 liters (45 gallons) of filtrate are formed each day. As the filtrate passes down the renal tubule, over 90% of the water is returned to the blood by **reabsorption**. Glucose and minerals are also returned to the blood. Some residual wastes in the blood are secreted from the blood into the tubule. These interchanges between the filtrate in the tubule and the blood are made possible by a mesh of capillaries that surrounds the renal tubule *(Figure 6.3)*. The material that remains in the tubule is urine. It consists of excess water, electrolytes, and urea.

The renal tubules merge to form collecting ducts *(Figure 6.3)* that merge into the calyces and then form the **renal pelvis** and become the **ureter.**

Purified blood is returned from the **peritubular** mesh of capillaries to the circulatory system through the renal vein.

Keynote

The functions of the kidneys are to:

- **Filter** blood to eliminate wastes.
- **Regulate** blood volume and pressure by eliminating or conserving water as necessary.
- **Maintain homeostasis** by controlling the quantities of water and electrolytes that are eliminated.
- **Secrete** the enzyme **renin**, which raises arterial blood pressure.
- **Secrete** the hormone **erythropoietin**, which acts on the bone to release red blood cells.
- **Synthesize vitamin D** to contribute to maintaining normal blood calcium levels.

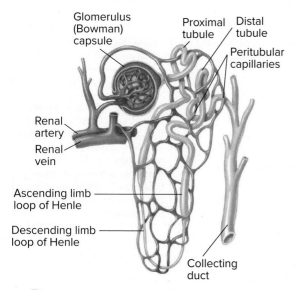

▲ **Figure 6.3** **Glomerulus and Renal Tubule.**

WORD	PRONUNCIATION		ELEMENTS	DEFINITION
calyx calyces (pl)	**KAY**-licks **KAY**-lih-sees		Greek *cup of a flower*	Funnel-shaped structure
cortex cortices (pl) cortical (adj)	**KOR**-teks **KOR**-tih-sees **KOR**-tih-kal	 S/ R/	Latin *tree bark* -ical *pertaining to* cort- *cortex*	Outer portion of an organ Pertaining to the cortex
erythropoietin	eh-**RITH**-roh-**POY**-ee-tin	S/ R/	-poietin *the maker* erythr/o- *red*	Protein secreted by the kidney that stimulates red blood cell production
filter	**FIL**-ter		Latin *to filter through the material felt*	A porous substance through which a liquid or gas is passed to separate out contained particles; or to use a filter
filtrate	**FIL**-trate	S/ R/	-ate *composed of, pertaining to* filtr- *strain through*	That which has passed through a filter
filtration	fil-**TRAY**-shun	S/	-ation *process*	Process of passing liquid through a filter
glomerulus glomeruli (pl) glomerular (adj)	glo-**MER**-you-lus glo-**MER**-you-lee glo-**MER**-you-lar	 R/ S/	Latin *small ball of yarn* gomerul- *glomerulus* -ar *pertaining to*	Plexus of capillaries; part of a nephron Pertaining to or affecting a glomerulus or glomeruli
hilum hila (pl)	**HIGH**-lum **HIGH**-lah		Latin *small bit*	The part where the nerves and blood vessels enter and leave an organ
medulla	meh-**DULL**-ah		French *middle*	Central portion of a structure surrounded by cortex
nephron nephron loop (loop of Henle)	**NEF**-ron **NEF**-ron LOOP LOOP of **HEN**-lee		Greek *kidney* Friedrich Henle, 1809–1885, German anatomist, pathologist, and histologist	Filtration unit of the kidney; glomerulus + renal tubule Part of the renal tubule where reabsorption occurs
pelvis	**PEL**-vis		Latin *basin*	A cup-shaped cavity, as in the pelvis of the kidney
peritubular	**PER**-ih-**TOO**-byu-lar	S/ P/ R/	-ar *pertaining to* peri- *around* -tubul- *small tube*	Surrounding the small renal tubules
permeable	**PER**-mee-ah-bull	S/ R/CF	-able *capable of* perm/e- *pass through*	Allowing passage of substances through a membrane
semipermeable impermeable	sem-ee-**PER**-me-ah-bull im-**PER**-me-ah-bull	P/ P/	semi- *half* im- *not, in*	Freely permeable to water but not to solutes When nothing is allowed passage
reabsorption (**Note:** This term has two prefixes.)	ree-ab-**SORP**-shun	S/ P/ P/ R/	-ion *process* re- *back* -ab- *away from* -sorpt- *swallow*	The taking back into the blood of substances that had previously been filtered out from it
renin	**REE**-nin	S/ R/	-in *substance* ren- *kidney*	Enzyme secreted by the kidney that causes vasoconstriction

Exercises

A. Deconstruct the following medical terms into their basic elements. *Fill in the blanks.* **LO 6.2, 6.D**

1. Passage of a substance through a filter   _____ / _____

2. Enzyme that causes vasoconstriction   _____ / _____

3. Surrounding the small renal tubules   _____ / _____ / _____

4. Blood that reclaims previously filtered substances   _____ / _____ / _____

B. Three of these terms refer to the regions of the kidney. *Choose the correct three terms and match them to the region.* **LO 6.1, 6.2**

peritubular   cortex   glomerular capsule   pelvis   nephron loop   medulla

1. outer region   _____

2. inner region   _____

3. central region   _____

Abbreviations

AIDS	acquired immunodeficiency syndrome
HIV	human immunodeficiency virus
UTI	urinary tract infection

Keynotes

- Of all renal cancers, 25% to 30% relate directly to smoking.
- As little as 1 mL of blood will turn the urine red.
- Hematuria can be caused by a lesion anywhere in the urinary system.
- The acute form of glomerulonephritis has a 100% recovery rate.
- Acute interstitial nephritis causes 15% of cases of acute renal failure.

Case Report (CR) 6.1 *(Continued)*

Mr. Nelson Hughes had been well until a few months before his surgery, when he noticed a vague, aching pain in his left loin. One week before surgery, he suddenly passed bright red urine. **Urinalysis** showed red blood cells (RBCs) (**hematuria**). Physical examination revealed an enlarged left kidney. IVP and other imaging tests showed a tumor 3 inches in diameter in the center of the left kidney. Bone scan was normal, indicating no **metastases** to bone.

LO 6.3 Disorders of the Kidneys

Renal cell carcinoma is the most common form of kidney cancer and occurs twice as often in men as in women. The cancer develops in the lining cells of the renal tubules, which is why Mr. Hughes had hematuria.

Nephroblastoma, or **Wilms tumor**, is a malignant kidney tumor of childhood, usually appearing between ages 3 and 8 years.

Benign kidney tumors, such as **renal adenoma,** are usually asymptomatic, are discovered incidentally, and are not life-threatening.

Acute glomerulonephritis is an inflammation of the glomerulus. It damages the glomerular capillaries, allows protein and red blood cells to leak into the urine, and interferes with the clearance of waste products. In its acute form, it can develop rapidly after an episode of strep throat infection, most often in children. The *Streptococcus* bacteria do not invade the kidney but stimulate the immune system to overproduce antibodies that damage the glomeruli.

Chronic glomerulonephritis can occur with no history of kidney disease and present as kidney failure. It also occurs in **diabetic nephropathy** and can be associated with autoimmune diseases such as lupus erythematosus; HIV can cause glomerular disease even before developing into AIDS.

Nephrotic syndrome involves large amounts of protein leaking out into the urine so that the level of protein in the blood falls. The types of nephrotic syndrome are described in *Table 6.1*. The most obvious symptom is fluid retention with edema of the ankles and legs.

Interstitial nephritis is an inflammation of the spaces between the renal tubules. Most often it is acute and temporary. It can be an allergic reaction to or a side effect of drugs such as penicillin or ampicillin, NSAIDs, and diuretics. Treatment is directed to the underlying disease. Temporary **dialysis** may be necessary.

Pyelitis is inflammation of the renal pelvis due to bacterial infection. If pyelitis is not effectively treated, it often progresses to **pyelonephritis**, an infection of the renal pelvis and kidney tissue. Most often it occurs as part of a total **urinary tract infection (UTI),** commencing in the urinary bladder. It has a high mortality rate in the elderly and in people with a compromised immune system *(see Chapter 4)*. It requires aggressive antibiotic therapy.

Table 6.1 Types of Nephrotic Syndrome

Disease (as Seen on Biopsy)	Description
Minimal change disease	Most common in children; responds to steroids
Focal segmental glomerulosclerosis (FSGS)	Cause unknown; little response to treatment
Membranous nephropathy	Cause unknown; may respond to immunosuppressive treatment
Diabetes	Occurs if blood sugar has been poorly controlled

WORD	PRONUNCIATION	ELEMENTS		DEFINITION
adenoma	AD-eh-NOH-mah	S/	-oma *tumor*	Benign tumor that originates from glandular tissue.
		R/	aden- *gland*	
carcinoma	kar-sih-NOH-mah	S/	-oma *tumor*	A cancerous (malignant) and invasive epithelial tumor.
		R/	carcin- *cancer*	
glomerulonephritis	glo-MER-you-loh-nef-RIE-tis	S/	-itis *inflammation*	Infection of the glomeruli of the kidney
		R/CF	glomerul/o- *glomerulus*	
		R/	-nephr- *kidney*	
interstitial	in-ter-STISH-al	S/	-ial *pertaining to*	Pertaining to the spaces between cells in a tissue or organ
		P/	inter- *between*	
		R/	-stit- *space*	
nephritis	neh-FRIE-tis	S/	-itis *inflammation*	Inflammation of the kidney
		R/	nephr- *kidney*	
nephroblastoma	NEF-roh-blas-TOH-mah	S/	-oma *tumor, mass*	Cancerous kidney tumor of childhood
		R/CF	nephr/o- *kidney*	
		R/	-blast- *embryonic, immature cell*	
Wilms tumor (syn)	WILMZ TOO-mor		Max Wilms, 1867–1918, German surgeon	
nephropathy	neh-FROP-ah-thee	S/	-pathy *disease*	Any disease of the kidney
		R/CF	nephr/o- *kidney*	
nephrotic syndrome	neh-FROT-ik SIN-drome	S/	-tic *pertaining to*	Glomerular disease with marked loss of protein
		R/CF	nephr/o- *kidney*	
nephrosis (syn)	neh-FRO-sis	S/	-osis *condition*	
pyelitis	pie-eh-LIE-tis	S/	-itis *inflammation*	Inflammation of renal pelvis
		R/	pyel- *renal pelvis*	
pyelonephritis	PIE-eh-loh-neh-FRIE-tis	R/CF	pyel/o- *renal pelvis*	Inflammation of the kidney and renal pelvis
		R/	-nephr- *kidney*	

Exercises

A. After reading Case Report 6.1, answer the following questions. LO 6.3

1. "Bright red urine" would indicate the presence of _____ in the urine.

2. Mr. Hughes complained of pain in the loin. Which of the following statements best describes the location of the loin?

   a. upper back   **b.** lower back   **c.** pelvic region   **d.** upper chest   **e.** lower chest

3. Is a patient's pain considered to be a sign or a symptom?

   a. sign   **b.** symptom

4. Has the cancer spread to other parts of the body?

   a. Yes   **b.** No

B. Differentiate the types of kidney disorders. *Match the kidney disorder in the first column with its correct description in the second column.* **LO 6.3**

Term	Meaning
_____ **1.** renal adenoma	**a.** condition only diagnosed in children
_____ **2.** nephroblastoma	**b.** malignant condition of the kidney; develops in the cells of the renal tubules
_____ **3.** nephrotic syndrome	**c.** can develop as a result of strep throat infection
_____ **4.** renal cell carcinoma	**d.** benign and usually asymptomatic
_____ **5.** acute glomerulonephritis	**e.** condition that causes leakage of proteins into the urine; edema of the ankles and legs is a common sign

Hypertension, with its high blood pressure, can damage the renal arterioles and glomeruli, causing them to thicken and narrow. This reduces their capability to remove wastes and excess water, which can cause the blood pressure (**BP**) to rise even more.

Polycystic kidney disease (PKD) is an inherited disease. Large, fluid-filled cysts grow within the kidneys and press against the kidney tissue. Finally, the kidneys cannot function effectively.

Acute renal failure (ARF) makes the kidneys suddenly stop filtering waste products from the blood. The causes of acute renal failure include:

- **Severe burns, trauma,** or **complicated surgery**—with a drastic drop in blood pressure and the release of myoglobin from injured muscles (*see Chapter 14*). Myoglobin lodges in the renal tubules and blocks the flow of urine.
- **Drugs**—including pain medications such as aspirin and ibuprofen, antibiotics such as streptomycin and gentamicin, and contrast dyes used in angiography.
- **Toxins**—such as heavy metals (mercury is one) and excessive alcohol.
- **Systemic infections**—septicemia.
- **Blood disorders**—such as idiopathic thrombocytopenic purpura or disseminated intravascular coagulation (*see Chapter 11*).

Chronic renal failure (CRF), or **chronic kidney disease (CKD),** is a gradual loss of renal function. Symptoms and signs may not appear until kidney function is less than 25% of normal.

The causes of chronic renal failure include **diabetes**—type 1 and type 2 (*see Chapter 17*); **hypertension; kidney diseases;** and **lead poisoning.**

End-stage renal disease (ESRD) means the kidneys are functioning at less than 10% of their normal capacity. At this point, life cannot be sustained, and either dialysis or kidney **transplant** is needed.

The signs and symptoms of kidney failure can include **oliguria** (reduction of urine output), **anuria** (cessation of urine output), confusion, seizures, and coma due to the buildup of toxins.

Hematuria (blood in the urine) can be caused by lesions anywhere in the urinary system; this includes trauma (including long-distance running), infections, medications (such as quinine and phenytoin), and congenital diseases (such as sickle cell anemia). In **microscopic hematuria,** the urine is not red, and red blood cells can be seen only under a microscope or identified by a urine dipstick. Normal urine contains no blood. Excessive consumption of beets, rhubarb, and red food coloring can cause urine to be colored red. This is not hematuria. Also, in the collection of urine from a woman during menstruation, the urine can be contaminated with blood, giving the impression of hematuria.

Azotemia is the buildup of urea (nitrogenous waste products) in the blood. **Uremia** is the complex of symptoms resulting from excess nitrogenous waste products in the blood, as seen in renal failure.

WORD	PRONUNCIATION	ELEMENTS		DEFINITION
anuria	an-**YOU**-ree-ah	S/ P/ R/	-ia *condition* an- *lack of, without* -ur- *urine*	Absence of urine production
azotemia	az-oh-**TEE**-mee-ah	S/ R/	-emia *blood condition* azot- *nitrogen*	Excess nitrogenous waste products (urea) in the blood
hematuria	hee-mah-**TYU**-ree-ah	S/ R/ R/	-ia *condition* hemat- *blood* -ur- *urine*	Blood in the urine
hypertension	**HIGH**-per-**TEN**-shun	S/ P/ R/	-ion *action, condition* hyper- *excessive* -tens- *pressure*	Persistent high arterial blood pressure.
oliguria	ol-ih-**GYUR**-ee-ah	S/ P/ R/	-ia *condition* olig- *scanty* -ur- *urine*	Scanty production of urine
polycystic	pol-ee-**SIS**-tik	S/ P/ R/	-ic *pertaining to* poly- *many* -cyst- *bladder, cyst*	Composed of many cysts
proteinuria	pro-tee-**NYU**-ree-ah	S/ R/ R/	-ia *condition* protein- *protein* -ur- *urine*	Presence of protein in urine.
uremia	you-**REE**-mee-ah	S/ R/	-emia *blood condition* ur- *urine*	A condition caused by excess urea and other nitrogenous wastes in the blood.

Exercises

A. Abbreviations are commonly used in written and verbal communication. *Demonstrate your understanding of kidney disorders by selecting the correct kidney disorder abbreviation that completes each sentence.* **LO 6.3, 6.F**

CRF   ARF   PKD   ESRD

1. An athlete has sprained her knee. She self-treats it with very large doses of ibuprofen, which can lead to _____.

2. Diabetes that is not well managed can lead to _____.

3. An inherited disease in which fluid-filled sacs are present within the kidney is known as _____.

B. Identify the meanings of the word elements in each term. *Recalling the meanings of word elements aids in determining the definition of medical terms.* **LO 6.3, 6.D**

1. The meaning of the prefix in the term *hypertension* is:

   a. pressure   **b.** condition   **c.** excessive   **d.** low

2. The meaning of the prefix in the term *oliguria* is:

   a. urine   **b.** scanty   **c.** condition   **d.** blood

3. The meaning of the suffix in the term *hematuria* is:

   a. urine   **b.** condition   **c.** blood   **d.** inflammation

4. The root *azot-* means:

   a. nitrogen   **b.** protein   **c.** sugar   **d.** without

5. The prefix *poly-* means:

   a. sac   **b.** fluid   **c.** scanty   **d.** many

Lesson 6.2

Ureters and Associated Disorders

Lesson Objectives

6.2.1 Identify the structure of the ureters.

6.2.2 Relate the functions of the ureters to their structure.

6.2.3 Describe disorders of the ureters.

Abbreviations

EMT-P	emergency medical technician–paramedic
ESWL	extracorporeal shock wave lithotripsy
IV	intravenous
IVP	intravenous pyelogram
KUB	x-ray of abdomen to show **k**idneys, **u**reters, and **b**ladder
VS	vital signs

Keynotes

- The muscle wall of the bladder acts as a sphincter around the ureters to prevent **reflux** of urine.

- The presence of urine in the renal pelvis initiates **peristalsis** of the ureters.

Renal calculi

Kidney

Ureter

Urinary bladder

Renal calculus

Urethra

▲ **Figure 6.4** Renal Calculi. Calculi can become lodged at different sites in the ureters.

Case Report (CR) 6.2

You are

. . . an Emergency Medical Technician–Paramedic (**EMT-P**), working in the Emergency Department of Fulwood Medical Center.

Your patient is

. . . Mr. Justin Leandro, a 37-year-old construction worker who is complaining of a sudden onset of excruciating pain in his right abdomen and back an hour previously while at work. The pain is **spasmodic** and radiates down into his groin. He has vomited once and keeps having the urge to urinate but cannot. He has no previous medical history of significance.

Vital signs (VS) T 99.4°F, P 92, R 20, BP 130/86. Abdomen slightly distended, with tenderness in the right upper and lower quadrants and flank. A dipstick test showed blood in his urine.

Provisional diagnosis: stone in right ureter. An **IV** line was inserted, and 2 mg morphine sulfate given by IV push at 1540. He is going to x-ray stat for **KUB** and **IVP.**

LO 6.4 Function and Structure of the Ureters

Each **ureter** is a muscular tube, about 10 inches long (25.5 cm) and ¼ inch (0.6 cm) wide, that carries urine from the renal pelvis to the urinary bladder. It lies on the posterior abdominal wall, which is why Mr. Leandro had pain in his back. It passes behind the bladder and enters it on its posterior inferior surface, which is why the pain radiated into his groin.

Each ureter passes obliquely through the muscle wall of the bladder. As pressure builds in a filling bladder, the muscle wall compresses the ureter and prevents urine from being forced back up the ureter to the kidneys (**reflux**).

In addition to gravity pulling the urine from the renal pelvis to the bladder, **peristaltic** waves in the muscular wall of the ureter, beginning at the renal pelvis, squeeze urine down the ureter and squirt the urine into the bladder. The peristaltic waves are **intermittent**, which is why Mr. Leandro's pain was spasmodic.

Case Report (CR) 6.2 *(continued)*

X-ray of Mr. Leandro's kidneys, ureters, and bladder (**KUB**) showed a suspicious lesion halfway down his right ureter, and the **pyelogram (IVP)** confirmed that this was a renal stone blocking the ureter.

The stone (**calculus**) was large enough to be lodged in the ureter, blocking the flow of urine, and, because of the back-flow pressure, causing the renal pelvis to dilate (**hydronephrosis** of the kidney).

LO 6.3, 6.5 Nephrolithiasis

Stones (**calculi**) begin in the pelvis of the kidney as a tiny grain of undissolved material, usually a mineral called calcium oxalate (*Figure 6.4*). When the urine flows out of the kidney, the grain of material is left behind. Over time, more material is deposited and a stone is formed. The presence of stones is called **nephrolithiasis**.

Most stones enter the ureter while they are still small enough to pass down the ureter into the bladder and out of the body in urine.

WORD	PRONUNCIATION	ELEMENTS		DEFINITION
calculus calculi (pl)	KAL-kyu-lus KAL-kyu-lie		Latin *pebble*	Small stone
hydronephrosis	HIGH-droh-neh-FROH-sis	S/ P/ R/CF	-osis *condition* hydro- *water* -nephr/o- *kidney*	Dilation of pelvis and calyces of a kidney
hydronephrotic (adj)	HIGH-droh-neh-FROT-ik	S/	-tic *pertaining to*	Pertaining to or suffering from the dilation of the pelvis and calyces of the kidney
intermittent	IN-ter-MIT-ent	S/ P/ R/	-ent *end result* inter- *between* -mitt- *send*	Alternately ceasing and beginning again
nephrolithiasis	NEF-roh-lih-THIGH-ah-sis	S/ R/CF R/	-iasis *condition* nephr/o- *kidney* -lith- *stone*	Presence of a kidney stone
peristalsis	per-ih-STAL-sis	P/ R/	peri- *around* -stalsis *constrict*	Waves of alternate contraction and relaxation along a tube to move its contents onward
peristaltic (adj)	per-ih-STAL-tik	S/	-tic *pertaining to*	Pertaining to peristalsis
reflux	REE-fluks	P/ R/	re- *back* -flux *flow*	Backward flow
spasmodic (**Note:** One "m" is taken out.)	spaz-MOD-ik	S/ R/ R/	-ic *pertaining to* spasm- *spasm* -mod- *nature, form*	Having intermittent spasms or contractions

Exercises

A. After reading both parts of Case Report 6.2, answer the following questions. LO 6.3, 6.5

1. If Mr. Leandro's pain had a "sudden onset," is it acute or chronic? _____

2. The medical term for *blood in the urine* is: _____

3. What does **spasmodic** mean?

    a. dull

    b. sharp

    c. constant

    d. intermittent

4. The medical term that defines his provisional diagnosis is: _____

> **Study Hint**
> Review the WAD again. Find the suffixes *-ic* and *-tic*, which both mean *pertaining to*. Add these to your list.

Urinary Bladder and Urethra

Lesson Objectives

The urinary bladder is a temporary storage place for urine before it is voided through the urethra. A moderately full bladder contains about 500 mL (1 pint) of urine. The maximum capacity of the bladder is around 750 to 800 mL (1.5 pints). Urination, or emptying of the bladder, is also called *micturition* or *voiding*. The information in this lesson will enable you to use correct medical terminology to:

6.3.1 Describe the structure and functions of the urinary bladder.

6.3.2 Contrast the differences in structure of the male and female urethras.

6.3.3 Explain the greater incidence of urinary tract infections in the female.

6.3.4 Discuss common disorders of the bladder and urethra.

Abbreviation

HPI	history of present illness

Case Report (CR) 6.3

You are

. . . a medical assistant working in the office of Dr. Susan Lee, a primary care physician at Fulwood Medical Center.

Your patient is

. . . Mrs. Caroline Dobson, a 32-year-old housewife. You have asked her to describe the reason for her visit to the office today.

Patient Interview

Mrs. Dobson:

"Since yesterday afternoon I've had a lot of pain low down in my belly and in my lower back. I keep having to go to the bathroom every hour or so to pee. It's often difficult to start, and it burns as it comes out. I've had this problem twice before when I was pregnant with my two kids, so I've started drinking cranberry juice. I've been shivering since I woke up this morning, and the last urine I passed was pink. Was that due to the cranberry juice?"

LO 6.6 Urinary Bladder and Urethra

The **urinary bladder** is a hollow, muscular organ on the floor of the pelvic cavity, posterior to the pubic symphysis *(Figure 6.5)*. When the bladder is distended, it rises upward and can be palpated above the symphysis pubis.

Urethra

The final passageway for the urine to escape to the outside is the **urethra**, a thin-walled tube that takes urine from the floor of the bladder to the outside. At the base of the bladder, the muscular wall is thickened to form the **internal urethral sphincter**. As the urethra passes through the skeletal muscles of the pelvic floor, the **external urethral sphincter** provides voluntary control of **micturition**.

In the female *(see Figure 6.6)*, the urethra is only about 1.5 inches long, and it opens to the outside anterior to the vagina (see *Figure 6.7*). In the male *(Figure 6.5)*, the urethra is 7 to 8 inches in length and passes through the penis. In both the male and the female, the opening of the urethra to the outside is called the **external urinary meatus**.

Micturition

When the bladder contains about 200 mL of urine, stretch receptors in its wall trigger the **micturition reflex**. However, voluntary control of the external sphincter can keep that sphincter contracted and can hold urine in the bladder until you decide to urinate. The passage of urine can be described as **urination**, **micturition**, or **voiding**.

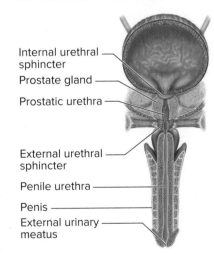

Internal urethral sphincter
Prostate gland
Prostatic urethra
External urethral sphincter
Penile urethra
Penis
External urinary meatus

▲ **Figure 6.5** Male Urinary Bladder and Urethra.

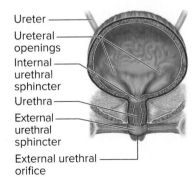

Ureter
Ureteral openings
Internal urethral sphincter
Urethra
External urethral sphincter
External urethral orifice

▲ **Figure 6.6** Female Urinary Bladder and Urethra.

WORD	PRONUNCIATION		ELEMENTS	DEFINITION
meatus	mee-**AY**-tus		Latin *a passage*	The external opening of a passage
micturition	mik-choo-**RISH**-un	S/	-ition *process*	Act of passing urine
		R/	**mictur**- *pass urine*	
micturate	**MIK**-choo-rate	S/	-ate *composed of, pertaining to*	Pass urine
reflex	**REE**-fleks		Latin *to bend back*	An involuntary response to a stimulus
sphincter	**SFINK**-ter		Greek *band*	Band of muscle that encircles an opening; when the muscle contracts, the opening squeezes closed
urination	yur-ih-**NAY**-shun	S/	-ation *process*	The passing of urine
void	VOYD		Latin *to empty*	To evacuate urine or feces

Exercises

A. Describe the structures of the bladder and urethra. *Indicate if the following statements are accurate. If the statement is true, choose T. If the statement is false, choose F.* **LO 6.6**

1. The length of the urethra is the same for males and females.   T   F

2. Micturition, voiding, and urination are synonyms.   T   F

3. Humans have control over the micturition reflex.   T   F

4. In both males and females, urine exits the urinary meatus.   T   F

5. There are two urethral sphincters.   T   F

6. The presence of 100ml of urine in the bladder triggers the urge to void.   T   F

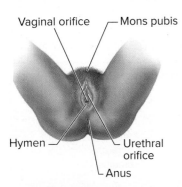

Vaginal orifice — Mons pubis

Hymen —

Urethral orifice

Anus

▲ **Figure 6.7** **Female External Genitalia.**

Keynotes

- Ten million doctor visits each year in the United States are for UTIs.
- Aging itself is not a cause of urinary incontinence.
- Incontinence is not a way of life. It can be helped.
- Cigarette smoking contributes to more than 50% of bladder cancers.
- Bladder cancer is more common in men than women. It is the fourth most common cancer in men and the eighth in women *(see Chapter 20).*

Abbreviations

UTI urinary tract infection

Keynote

The prostate gland and its disorders are detailed in Chapter 7

LO 6.7 Disorders of the Urinary Bladder and Urethra

Urinary Tract Infection

A **urinary tract infection (UTI)** occurs when bacteria invade and multiply in the urinary tract. The portal of entry for the bacteria is through the urethra. Because the female urethra is shorter than the male urethra and opens to the surface near the anus *(Figure 6.7)*, bacteria from the **gastrointestinal** tract can more easily invade the female urethra. This is why women are more prone than men to UTIs. Once UTIs have occurred, they often recur.

Infection of the urethra is called **urethritis**; infection of the urinary bladder is **cystitis**. If cystitis is untreated, infection can spread up the ureters to the renal pelvis, causing **pyelitis**, and carry on to reach the renal cortex and nephrons, causing pyelonephritis.

The diagnosis can be made through urinalysis. Culture of the organism and testing of its sensitivity to different antibiotics enables appropriate antibiotic therapy to be prescribed. Cranberry juice makes the urine more acidic? so that bacteria have difficulty multiplying, and chemicals in the juice make the bladder more slippery so that bacteria can't stick to it.

Case Report (CR) 6.3 *(continued)*

Mrs. Dobson described many of the symptoms of cystitis. She had **suprapubic** and low-back pain. She had increased **frequency** of micturition with **dysuria** and had difficulty in and burning on micturition. Her pink urine is probably hematuria.

Urinary Incontinence

Loss of control of your bladder is called **urinary incontinence.** The result is wet clothes. About 12 million adults in America have urinary incontinence. It is most common in women over the age of 50 years.

There are four types of urinary incontinence:

- **Stress incontinence.** Urine leaks because of sudden pressure on the lower stomach muscles when you cough, laugh, sneeze, lift something heavy, or exercise. It is most common in women, with previous pregnancy and childbirth being risk factors.
- **Urge incontinence.** The need to urinate comes on too fast for you to get to the toilet. It is often **idiopathic** but can be associated with UTI, diabetes, stroke, Alzheimer and Parkinson disease, or bladder cancer.
- **Overflow incontinence.** Small amounts of urine leak from a bladder that is always full because you cannot empty it. This occurs when an enlarged prostate gland or tumor blocks the outflow of urine from the bladder. It also occurs in spinal cord injuries and as a side effect of some medications.
- **Functional incontinence.** You cannot get to the toilet in time because of arthritis or any other disease that makes moving quickly difficult.

Urinary retention is the abnormal, involuntary holding of urine in the bladder. **Acute retention** can be caused by an obstruction in the urinary system; for example, an enlarged prostate in the male *(see Chapter 7)* or neurologic problems such as multiple sclerosis. It can be a side effect of anticholinergic drugs that include tricyclic antidepressants *(see Chapter 18).* **Chronic retention** can be caused by untreated obstructions in the urinary tract such as an enlarged prostate.

Transitional cell carcinoma is the most common type of bladder cancer, arising in the transitional cells of the lining of the bladder. A primary symptom of bladder cancer is **hematuria.**

Methods of Urine Collection

- **Random collection** is taken with no precautions regarding contamination. It is often used for collecting samples for drug testing.
- **Early morning collection** is used to determine the ability of the kidneys to concentrate urine following overnight dehydration.
- **Clean-catch, midstream specimen** is collected after the external urethral meatus is cleaned. The first part of the urine is passed, and a sterile collecting vessel is introduced into the urinary stream to collect the last part.
- **Twenty-four-hour collection** is used to determine the amount of protein being excreted and to estimate the kidneys' filtration ability.
- **Suprapubic transabdominal needle aspiration** of the bladder is used in newborns and small infants to obtain a pure sample of urine.
- **Catheterization of the bladder** can be used as a last resort to obtain a urine specimen. A soft plastic or rubber tube (catheter) is inserted through the urethra into the bladder to drain and collect urine.

WORD	PRONUNCIATION	ELEMENTS		DEFINITION
cystitis	sis-**TIE**-tis	S/ R/	**-itis** *inflammation* **cyst-** *bladder*	Inflammation of the urinary bladder
dysuria	dis-**YOU**-ree-ah	S/ P/ R/	**-ia** *condition* **dys-** *bad, difficult* **-ur-** *urinary system*	Difficulty or pain with urination
frequency	**FREE**-kwen-see	S/ R/	**-ency** *state of, quality of* **frequ-** *repeated, often*	The number of times something happens in a given time (e.g., passing urine)
idiopathic	**ID**-ih-oh-**PATH**-ik	S/ R/CF R/	**-ic** *pertaining to* **idi/o-** *personal, distinct* **-path-** *disease*	Pertaining to a disease of unknown etiology
incontinence	in-**KON**-tin-ens	S/ P/ R/	**-ence** *state of, quality of* **in-** *in, not* **-contin-** *hold together*	Inability to prevent discharge of urine or feces
incontinent	in-**KON**-tin-ent	S/	**-ent** *pertaining to, end result*	Denoting incontinence
retention	ree-**TEN**-shun		Latin *hold back*	A holding in of what should normally be discharged (e.g., urine)
suprapubic	**SOO**-prah-**PYU**-bik	S/ P/ R/	**-ic** *pertaining to* **supra-** *above* **-pub-** *pubis*	Above the symphysis pubis

Exercises

A. Define the different types of disorders related to the urinary bladder and urethra. *Choose the correct answer that completes each statement.* **LO 6.7**

1. The portal of entry for bacteria to infect the urinary bladder is the:

   a. urethra   **b.** ureter   **c.** blood   **d.** kidney

2. The medical term that defines *infection of the bladder* is:

   a. pyelitis   **b.** cystitis   **c.** incontinence   **d.** retention

3. Diagnosis of a bladder infection is confirmed via:

   a. blood test   **b.** x-ray of the bladder   **c.** ultrasound   **d.** urinalysis

4. The medical term *incontinence* is defined as a(n)

   a. inability to empty the bladder   **b.** loss of the micturition reflex

   c. loss of bladder control   **d.** infection of the bladder and urethra

5. A primary symptom of bladder cancer is

   a. urea in the blood   **b.** inability to empty the bladder

   c. blood in the urine   **d.** pain with urination

B. Describe the different types of urinary incontinence. *Match the type of incontinence in column one with its correct definition in the second column.* **LO 6.7**

Term	Meaning
_____ 1. overflow incontinence	**a.** urine leaks because the need to urinate comes on too fast to make it to the toilet in time to void
_____ 2. stress incontinence	**b.** urine leaks because the bladder is always full
_____ 3. functional incontinence	**c.** urine leaks because another condition prevents the person from reaching the toilet in time to void
_____ 4. urge incontinence	**d.** urine leaks due to sudden pressure, like a cough

Lesson 6.4

Diagnostic Procedures and Pharmacology

Abbreviations

CT	computed tomography
KUB	x-ray of kidneys, ureters, and bladder
MRI	magnetic resonance imaging
SG	specific gravity
TNM	tumor, nodes, metastases
UA	urinalysis
VCUG	voiding cystourethrogram

LO 6.8 Diagnostic Procedures

Urinalysis

A **dipstick** (a plastic strip bearing paper squares of reagent) is the most cost-effective method of screening urine *(Figure 6.8)*. After the stick is dipped in the urine specimen, the color change in each segment of the dipstick is compared to a color chart on the container. Dipsticks can screen for pH, specific gravity, protein, blood, glucose, ketones, bilirubin, **nitrite**, and leukocyte esterase (see the following).

Routine urinalysis (UA) in the laboratory can include the following tests:

- **Visual observation** examines **color** and **clarity.** Normal urine is pale yellow or amber in color and clear. Cloudiness indicates excess cells or cellular material. Red and cloudy indicates red blood cells.
- **Odor** of normal urine has a slight "nutty" scent. Infected urine has a foul odor. **Ketosis** gives urine a fruity odor.
- **pH** measures how acidic or alkaline urine is *(see Chapter 3).*
- **Specific gravity (SG)** measures how dilute or concentrated the urine is.
- **Protein** is not detected normally in urine. Its presence **(proteinuria)** indicates infection or urinary tract disease.
- **Glucose** in the urine **(glycosuria)** is a spillover into the urine when the nephrons are damaged or diseased or blood sugar is high in uncontrolled diabetes.
- **Ketones** are present in the urine in **diabetic ketoacidosis** *(see Chapter 17)* or in starvation.
- **Leukocyte esterase** indicates the presence of white blood cells (WBCs) in the urine, which in turn can indicate a UTI.
- **Urine culture** from a clean-catch specimen is the definitive test for a UTI.

Microscopic urinalysis is performed on the solids deposited by centrifuging a specimen of urine. It can reveal **red blood cells (RBCs), WBCs,** renal tubular epithelial cells stuck together to form **casts,** WBCs stuck together to form casts, and bacteria.

Other Diagnostic Procedures

- **KUB.** An x-ray of the abdomen that shows the kidneys, ureters, and bladder.
- **IVP.** A contrast material containing iodine is injected intravenously, and its progress through the urinary tract is then recorded on a series of rapid x-ray images.
- **Retrograde pyelogram.** Contrast material is injected through a urinary catheter into the ureters to locate stones and other obstructions.
  - **Voiding cystourethrogram (VCUG).** Contrast material is inserted into the bladder through a catheter and x-rays are taken as the patient urinates.
  - **Computed tomography (CT) scan.** X-ray images show cross-sectional views of the kidneys and bladder.
  - **Magnetic resonance imaging (MRI).** Magnetic fields are used to generate cross-sectional images of the urinary tract.
  - **Ultrasound imaging.** High-frequency sound waves and computer generated noninvasive images of the kidneys.
  - **Renal angiogram.** X-rays with contrast material are used to assess blood flow to the kidneys.
  - **Cystoscopy.** A pencil-thin, flexible, tubelike optical instrument (**cystoscope**) is inserted through the urethra into the bladder to examine directly the lining of the bladder to determine the causes of hematuria, urinary frequency, urgency, incontinence or urinary retention, and to take a biopsy if needed. Cystoscopy with biopsy is the definitive test for bladder cancer.

▲ **Figure 6.8** Urinalysis Dipstick Being Compared Against Color Chart on Container. ©Saturn Stills/SPL/Photo Researchers, Inc.

WORD	PRONUNCIATION		ELEMENTS	DEFINITION
cast	KAST		Latin *pure*	A cylindrical mold formed by materials in kidney tubules
cystoscope	**SIS**-toh-skope	S/	**-scope** *instrument for viewing*	An endoscope to view the inside of the bladder
		R/CF	**cyst/o** *bladder*	
cystoscopy	sis-**TOS**-koh-pee	S/	**-scopy** *to examine*	The process of using a cystoscope
cystourethrogram	sis-toh-you-**REETH**-roh-gram	S/	**-gram** *a record*	X-ray image during voiding to show structure and function of bladder and urethra
		R/CF	**cyst/o-** *bladder*	
		R/CF	**-urethr/o-** *urethra*	
glycosuria (*Note:* The "s" is added to make the word flow.)	**GLIE**-koh-**SYU**-ree-ah	S/	**-ia** *condition*	Presence of glucose in urine
		R/CF	**glyc/o-** *glucose*	
		R/	**-ur-** *urinary system*	
ketone	**KEY**-tone		Greek *acetone*	Chemical formed in uncontrolled diabetes or in starvation
ketosis	key-**TOH**-sis	S/	**-sis** *condition*	Excess production of ketones
		R/CF	**ket/o-** *ketones*	
ketoacidosis	**KEY**-toh-as-ih-**DOH**-sis	R/CF	**-acid/o-** *acid, low pH*	Excessive production of ketones, making the blood acidic
nitrite	**NIE**-trite		Greek *niter, saltpeter*	Chemical formed in urine by *Escherichia coli (E. coli)* and other microorganisms
proteinuria	pro-tee-**NYU**-ree-ah	R/	**protein-** *protein*	Presence of protein in urine
		R/	**-uria** *urine*	
pyelogram	**PIE**-el-oh-gram	S/	**-gram** *recording*	X-ray image of renal pelvis and ureters
		R/CF	**pyel/o-** *renal pelvis*	
retrograde	**RET**-roh-grade	P/	**retro-** *backward*	Reversal of a normal flow; for example, back from the bladder into the ureters
		R/	**-grade** *going*	
stage	STAJ		Latin *status, to stand*	A description of the distribution and extent of dissemination of a cancer disease process
urinalysis	you-rih-**NAL**-ih-sis	S/	**-lysis** *to separate*	Examination of urine to separate it into its elements and define their kind and/or quantity
		R/CF	**urin/a-** *urine*	

Exercises

A. Apply your knowledge of medical language to this exercise. *All the questions can be answered using terms from this spread.*
Select the best answer. **LO 6.8**

1. An x-ray image taken during voiding:

   a. retrograde   **b.** pyelogram   **c.** KUB   **d.** cystourethrogram

2. Presence of sugar in urine:

   a. hematuria   **b.** polyuria   **c.** glycosuria   **d.** proteinuria

3. Reversal of normal flow:

   a. reflex   **b.** retrograde   **c.** regenerate   **d.** retention

4. Excessive ketones in the blood, making it acidic:

   a. ketosis   **b.** ketoacidosis   **c.** ketone

5. Separating urine into its elements:

   a. urinalysis   **b.** cystourethrogram   **c.** retrograde   **d.** pyelogram

LO 6.9 Therapeutic Procedures

Renal Stones

For renal stones that do not pass down the ureter into the bladder and out of the body in urine, there are several treatment options:

- **Watchful waiting.** With pain medication to relieve symptoms, the hope is that the stone can be passed.
- **Extracorporeal shock wave lithotripsy (ESWL).** With ESWL, a machine called a **lithotripter** from outside the body generates sound waves that crumble the stone into small pieces that can pass down the ureter into the bladder and be voided.
- **Ureteroscopy.** A small, flexible **ureteroscope** is passed through the urethra and bladder into the ureter. Devices can be passed through the endoscope to remove or fragment the stone.
- **Percutaneous nephrolithotomy.** A **nephroscope** is inserted through the skin and into the kidney to locate and remove the stone.
- **Open surgery.** A surgical incision is made to expose the ureter and remove the stone; this is rarely done.

Kidney Failure

Dialysis is an artificial method of removing waste materials and excess fluid from the blood in end-stage renal disease. It is not a cure, but can prolong life. There are several types of kidney dialysis: In treatment of acute renal failure (ARF), the goal is to treat the underlying disease. Dialysis may be necessary while the kidneys are healing.

- **Hemodialysis** (*Figure 6.9*) filters the blood through an artificial kidney machine (**dialyzer**). Most patients require 12 hours of dialysis weekly, usually in three sessions.
- **Peritoneal dialysis** uses a solution that is infused into and drained out of the patient's abdominal cavity through a small flexible catheter implanted into the patient's abdominal cavity. The dialysis solution extracts wastes and excess fluid from the blood through the network of capillaries in the peritoneal lining of the abdominal cavity.
- **Continuous ambulatory peritoneal dialysis (CAPD)** (*Figure 6.10*) is performed by the patient at home usually four times each day, seven days a week.
- **Continuous cycling peritoneal dialysis (CCPD)** uses a machine to automatically infuse dialysis solution into and out of the abdominal cavity during sleep.

A **kidney transplant** provides a better quality of life than dialysis, provided a suitable donor can be found (see Chapter 12). A **sibling** or blood relative can often qualify as a donor. If not, tissue banks across the country can search for a kidney from an accident victim or a donor who has died.

Urinary Bladder

Cystoscopy can be used therapeutically to remove stones and to perform a transurethral resection of the prostate (**TURP**) to remove tissue from the inner portion of the prostate gland in men with benign prostatic hyperplasia (**BPH**).

For acute or chronic lower urinary tract obstruction in which the urethra is blocked, a flexible urethral catheter (**Foley catheter**) is passed into the bladder. The catheter can be left indwelling, or the patient can perform clean intermittent catheterization. If a Foley catheter cannot be passed, a suprapubic tube can be placed through the lower anterior abdominal wall into the bladder.

Treatment for urinary incontinence depends on the cause. If a medical or surgical problem is present, then the incontinence can go away when the problem is treated. **Bladder training** and **biofeedback** lengthen the time between the urges to go to the toilet. **Kegel exercises** strengthen the muscles of the pelvic floor. Medications, for example oxybutynin, are used for urge incontinence. Surgery can pull up the bladder and secure it if pelvic floor muscles are weak (**cystopexy**). Absorbent underclothing is available.

▲ **Figure 6.9** Hemodialysis.

▲ **Figure 6.10** Continuous Ambulatory Peritoneal Dialysis. ©Medical-on-Line/Alamy

LO 6.9, 6.A
Word Analysis and Definition

S = Suffix   P = Prefix   R = Root   R/CF = Combining Form

WORD	PRONUNCIATION	ELEMENTS		DEFINITION
ambulatory	**AM**-byu-lah-tor-ee	S/ R/	-ory *relating to* ambulat- *walk*	Relating to walking
catheter	**KATH**-eh-ter		Greek *to send down*	Hollow tube that allows passage of fluid into or out of a body cavity, organ, or vessel.
cystopexy	**SIS**-toh-pek-see	S/ R/CF	-pexy *surgical fixation* cyst/o- *bladder*	Surgical procedure to support the urinary bladder
dialysis dialyzer hemodialysis	die-**AL**-ih-sis die-**A**-lie-zer **HEE**-moh-die-**AL**-ih-sis	P/ R/ S/ R/CF	dia- *complete* -lysis *to separate* -lyzer *separator* hem/o *blood*	An artificial method of filtration to remove excess waste materials and water from the body. Machine that performs dialysis. An artificial machine-based method to remove wastes from the blood
extracorporeal	**EKS**-trah-kor-**POH**-ree-al	S/ P/ R/	-eal *pertaining to* extra- *outside* -corpor- *body*	Outside the body
Kegel exercises	**KEE**-gal **EKS**-er-size-ez		Arnold Kegel, 1894–1981, American gynecologist	Contraction and relaxation of the pelvic floor muscles to improve urethral and rectal sphincter function
lithotripsy lithotripter	**LITH**-oh-trip-see **LITH**-oh–trip-ter	S/ R/CF S/	-tripsy *to crush* lith/o- *stone* -tripter *crusher*	Crushing stones by sound waves Instrument that generates the sound waves
nephrolithotomy	**NEF**-roh-lih-**THOT**-oh-mee	S/ R/CF R/CF	-tomy *surgical incision* nephr/o- *kidney* lith/o- *stone*	Incision to remove a renal stone
nephroscope nephroscopy	**NEF**-roh-skope neh-**FROS**-koh-pee	S/ R/CF S/	-scope *instrument for viewing* nephr/o- *kidney* -scopy *to examine*	Endoscope to view the inside of the kidney Visual examination of the kidney
percutaneous	**PER**-kyu-**TAY**-nee-us	S/ P/ R/CF	-us *pertaining to* per- *through* cutane/o- *skin*	Pertaining to through the skin
transplant	**TRANZ**-plant	P/ R/	trans- *across* -plant *insert, plant*	The act of transferring tissue from one person to another
ureteroscope ureteroscopy	you-**REE**-ter-oh-skope you-**REE**-ter-**OS**-koh-pee	S/ R/CF S/	-scope *instrument for viewing* ureter/o *ureter* -scopy *to examine*	Endoscope to view the inside of the ureter Endoscopic examination of the inside of the ureter

Exercises

A. Abbreviations are used in written and verbal communication. *Complete each sentence with the correct abbreviations. Use the provided abbreviations to fill in the blanks.* **LO 6.9, 6.A, 6.F**

BPH	CAPD	CCPD	ESWL	TURP

1. The nephrologist recommended that the patient have _____ to assist in the passing of his kidney stones.

2. Because of his _____, Mr. Plaza suffered from overflow incontinence.

3. Mrs. Doskos prefers to receive her dialysis while she sleeps, and therefore the nephrologist recommended _____ to dialyze her blood.

4. _____ is used to remove sections of an enlarged prostate.

5. _____ allows the patient to walk around while receiving dialysis.

B. Construct terms using word elements. *Given the definition, complete each medical term with the correct missing element. Fill in the blank. The first one has been done for you.* **LO 6.9, 6.A, 6.C**

1. Relating to walking   <u>ambulat</u>/ory

2. Surgical procedure to support the urinary bladder.   cysto/ _____

3. Visual examination of the kidney.   _____ /scopy

4. Pertaining to through the skin.   _____ /cutaneo/us

5. Incision to remove a stone.   nephro/litho/ _____

6. Artificial method to remove wastes from the blood.   _____ /dia/lysis

LO 6.10 Pharmacology of the Urinary System

There are several distinct classes of drugs with different effects on the urinary system.

Diuretics

Diuretic drugs increase urine output by the kidney—they promote this **diuresis** by altering how the kidney handles sodium. If the kidney excretes more sodium, then water excretion will also increase. **Loop diuretics** such as furosemide (*Lasix*) are more powerful than **thiazide** diuretics such as hydrochlorthiazide, which is available as a **generic** drug. The most frequent problem with both forms of diuretics is **hypokalemia**, and potassium supplements are usually prescribed with them. Acetazolamide (*Diamox*) is a weak diuretic that also lowers the intraocular pressure in glaucoma (*see Chapter 16*).

Renal Drugs

Pyelonephritis, which is inflammation of the pelvis of the kidney usually spreading from a **urinary tract infection (UTI)**, is treated aggressively with antibiotics, such as an aminoglycoside (*Gentamycin*) together with ampicillin or ceftriaxone (*Rocephin*).

Nephrotic syndrome is treated initially with corticosteroids (*Prednisolone*) and cytostatic drugs, such as cyclophosphamide (*Cytoxan*) and cyclosporine (*Cyclosporin A*), are used for relapses.

Renal cell carcinoma is treated surgically with radical nephrectomy. As renal cell carcinoma is resistant to both radiation and chemotherapy, metastases are treated with targeted therapies using drugs such as temsirolimus (*Torisel*) and bevacizumab (*Avastin*). Despite these drugs, the overall survival rate has not improved much.

Renal transplant patients receive a regimen of drugs to prevent rejection. The most common regimen is a cocktail of tacrolimus (*Prograf*), mycophenolate (*Cellcept*), and prednisone (generic).

Nonrenal Urinary Tract Drugs

Antibiotics are the usual treatment for UTIs no matter in which part of the urinary system the infection is located (*see Lesson 6.3*). The specific antibiotic to be used is determined by the **sensitivity** of the organism obtained by **culture** of the urine specimen. UTIs, including **cystitis**, are treated with antibiotics, such as trimethoprim (*Trimpex, Primsol*), nitrofurantoin (*Furadantin, Macrobid*), or one of the many cephalosporins. Infections that spread from the urinary tract to the epididymis (epididymitis) and the testes (orchitis) are treated with cefalexin or ciprofloxacin.

In patients with chronic renal disease and diminished renal function, dosing of renally excreted drugs should be adjusted by reducing the dose, increasing the dosing interval, or both. Drugs that have to be adjusted include antihypertensive agents, hypoglycemic agents, antimicrobials, analgesics, NSAIDs, and many herbal products.

A **urinary analgesic** phenazopyridine (*Pyridium*), a dye, is used to provide symptomatic relief in acute cystitis and is often prescribed after the use of an indwelling Foley catheter, cystoscopy, or urinary bladder surgery. It produces a vivid dark orange to red color in the urine.

Alpha-blocking agents (**alpha-blockers**) relax smooth muscle in the body. They can be used to relax the smooth muscle in the ureters and make them wider to help a kidney stone pass more easily.

There are no reliable medications that can prevent renal stones from forming, though alkalinization of the urine with acetazolamide (*Diamox*) can help.

WORD	PRONUNCIATION	ELEMENTS		DEFINITION
alpha-blocking agent alpha-blockers	**AL**-fah **BLOK**-ing **A**-jent		**alpha-** Greek *first letter* **block** French *inhibit*	Drugs that relax smooth muscle
analgesia	an-al-**JEE**-zee-ah	S/ P/ R/	**-ia** *condition* **an-** *without* **-alges-** *sensation of pain*	State in which pain is reduced
analgesic	an-al-**JEE**-zic	S/	**-ic** *pertaining to*	Substance that produces analgesia
culture	**KUL**-chur		Latin *to till*	The reproduction of microorganisms (e.g., bacteria) on or in various media
diuresis (Note: the a is dropped)	die-you-**REE**-sis	S/ P/ R/	**-esis** *abnormal condition* **dia-** *complete* **-ur-** *urinary system*	Excretion of large volumes of urine
diuretic (adj)	die-you-**REH**-tik	S/	**-etic** *pertaining to*	Agent that increases urine output
generic	je-**NEHR**-ik	S/ R/	**-ic** *pertaining to* **gener-** *birth*	A nonproprietary name for a drug
hypokalemia	**HIGH**-poh-kah-**LEE**-mee-ah	S/ P/ R/	**-emia** *blood condition* **hypo-** *below, low* **-kal-** *potassium*	Low concentration of potassium in the blood
sensitivity	sen-si-**TIV**-ih-tee	S/ R/	**-ity** *condition, state* **sensitiv-** *feeling*	Denoting the susceptibility of a microorganism to inhibition or destruction by a given antibiotic

Exercises

A. Demonstrate the proper use of medical terms. *Suffixes change the meanings of words and how they are to be used in verbal and written communication. Complete each sentence with the proper term provided in parentheses. Fill in the blank.* **LO 6.10, 6.A**

1. The _____ (**diuretic/diuresis**) medication was given to increase Mrs. Bienvenue's urinary output.

2. The patient needed _____ (**analgesia/analgesic**) to relieve the moderate pain caused by the cystitis.

3. Morphine relieves pain and therefore is an _____ (**analgesia/analgesic**).

4. The nephrologist recommend that _____ (**diuretic/diuresis**) be utilized to quickly relieve the excess fluid in the patient's interstitial tissues.

B. Identify the purpose and effects of medications used to treat urinary system conditions. *Select the term that correctly answers each question.* **LO 6.10, 6.F**

1. In order to choose the correct antibiotic, the physician must order a urine:

   a. blocker   **b.** culture   **c.** analgesic   **d.** chemotherapeutic

2. A side effect of some diuretics is:

   a. hypokalemia   **b.** carcinoma   **c.** bacterial infection   **d.** analgesia

3. The usual treatment for an UTI is:

   a. radiation   **b.** diuresis   **c.** surgery   **d.** antibiotics

4. A dye that produces an analgesic effect in the urinary system is:

   a. ibuprofen   **b.** aspirin   **c.** phenazopyridine   **d.** cyclophosphamide

LO 6.10 Urologic Drugs (continued)

Drugs for Sexually Transmitted Diseases

Sexually transmitted diseases (STDs) are caused by a variety of organisms in both men and women and primarily affect the **genitalia**. They require different drug treatments, depending on the organism.

- **Chlamydia** is treated with a single dose of azithromycin (*Zithromax* and others) or a week of doxycycline (*Vibramycin* and others) in both sexes.

- **Trichomoniasis** is treated with metronidazole (*Flagyl*) or tinidazole (*Tindamax*).

- **Gonorrhea** has become resistant to most classes of antibiotics except cephalosporins, such as ceftriaxone (*Rocephin*) and cefixime (*Suprax*).

- **Bacterial vaginosis** is treated with metronidazole (*Flagyl*) or clindamycin (*Cleocin*).

- **Pelvic inflammatory disease (PID),** which is usually a complication of *Chlamydia* or gonorrhea, is treated with antibiotic combinations of two drugs—for example, cefotetan (*Cefotan*) and doxycycline (*Vibramycin*); clindamycin (*Cleocin*) and gentamicin (*Garamycin*); or cefoxitin (*Cefotan*) and doxycycline (*Vibramycin*).

- **Genital herpes infections** have no cure, but antiviral medications, such as acyclovir (*Zovirax*), famaciclovir (*Famvir*), and valacyclovir (*Valtrex*), can prevent or cut short outbreaks.

- **Syphilis** in its early stages requires a single dose of IM penicillin. If the infection has been present for more than a year, additional doses are required.

- **Human papilloma virus (HPV)** has 40 different types that infect the genital area. HPV can cause cervical cancer. There is no known treatment, but two vaccines are approved by the FDA. *Cervarix* protects against HPV types 16 and 18. *Gardasil* protects against types 6, 11, 16, and 18. Both protect against HPV types that cause 70% of cervical cancers, and *Gardasil* protects against HPV types that cause 90% of genital warts.

- **Human immunodeficiency virus (HIV) infections** have no cure. The aim of treatment is to maintain a good quality of life and prevent the development of **acquired immunodeficiency syndrome (AIDS).** Highly active antiretroviral therapy (**HAART**) is a combination of at least three drugs belonging to at least two types of **antiretroviral** agents. Without HAART, HIV infection progresses to AIDS in approximately 9 to 10 years.

The sexually transmitted diseases—chlamydia, trichomoniasis, gonorrhea, syphilis—are detailed in Lesson 8.1 of Chapter 8.

Abbreviations

AIDS	acquired immunodeficiency syndrome
HAART	highly active antiretroviral therapy
HIV	human immunodeficiency virus
HPV	human papilloma virus
PID	pelvic inflammatory disease
STD	sexually transmitted disease

WORD	PRONUNCIATION	ELEMENTS		DEFINITION
antiretroviral	**AN**-tee-**RET**-roh-vie-ral	S/ P/ P/ R/	**-al** *pertaining to* **anti-** *against* **-retro-** *back, backward* **-vir-** *virus*	An agent that inhibits or kills any virus of the family
retrovirus	**RET**-roh-vi-rus			A virus with RNA core genetic material
genital	**JEN**-it-al	S/ R/	**-al** *pertaining to* **genit-** *primary male or female sex organs*	Relating to the male or female sex organs
genitalia	**JEN**-ih-**TAY**-lee-ah	S/	**-ia** *condition*	External and internal organs of reproduction
vaginosis	vah-jih-**NOH**-sis	S/ R/	**-osis** *condition* **vagin-** *vagina*	Any disease of the vagina
vaginitis	vah-jih-**NIE**-tis	S/	**-itis** *inflammation*	Inflammation of the vagina

Exercises

A. Review what you learned in the earlier chapters about word elements. *Choose the correct answer for each question.* **LO 6.10, 6.A, 6.D**

1. What is most unusual about the term *antiretroviral*?

   a. it has two prefixes

   b. it does not have a root

   c. it has only one suffix

   d. it lacks a combining vowel

2. Vaginosis would be found in which body system?

   a. male

   b. female

3. Which of the following medications will not cure vaginal infections?

   a. *Cipro*

   b. *Flagyl*

   c. *Valtrex*

   d. *Tindamax*

B. Match the condition with the drug(s) used to treat it. *Choose the correct term in the second column.* **LO 6.10, 6.A, 6.F**

1. syphilis
2. HPV
3. PID
4. bacterial vaginosis
5. HIV

   a. antibiotic combination of two drugs

   b. HAART

   c. IM penicillin

   d. no known treatment

   e. *Flagyl*

LO 6.10 Urologic Drugs (continued)

Prostate Drugs

Prostatitis is usually an extension of an *E. coli* UTI. In the acute phase, antibiotics such as trimethoprim-sulfamethoxazole (*Bactrim, Septa*), fluoroquinolones (*Floxin, Cipro*), or doxycycline (*Vibramycin*) are given for 14 days. If the disease is chronic, the regimen is continued for 4 to 12 weeks.

Benign prostatic hypertrophy (BPH) can be treated with two main types of medication. **Alpha blockers,** such as doxazosin (*Cardura*) or alfuzosin (*Uroxatral*), relax smooth muscle at the bladder neck to allow a freer flow of urine. **5-alpha-reductase inhibitors,** such as finasteride (*Proscar, Propecia*) and dutasteride (*Avodart*), inhibit the production of dihydrotestosterone, which is believed to stimulate the prostate cells to grow.

Prostate cancer is treated primarily with surgery or radiation therapy. Other treatments such as hormonal or chemotherapy are not approved by the Federal Drug Administration (FDA).

Other Nonrenal Urinary Tract Drugs

Erectile dysfunction (ED) can be treated with drugs designed to improve the flow of blood to the penis. Examples include sildenafil (*Viagra*), tadalafil (*Cialis*), vardenafil (*Levitra*), and alprostadil (*Edex, Caverject*), which is injected into one of the corpus cavernosa of the penis. The latter drug is sometimes used for the treatment of **impotence.**

Urinary incontinence, which is any involuntary leakage of urine, almost always results from an underlying treatable medical condition. In an **overactive bladder,** which causes incontinence, drugs that relax the bladder muscle wall can alleviate the symptoms. They include tolterodine (*Detrol*), oxybutynin (*Ditropan*), trospium (*Sanctura*), solifenacin (*Vesicare*), darifenacin (*Enablex*), and an oxybutynin skin patch (*Oxytrol*).

WORD	PRONUNCIATION	ELEMENTS		DEFINITION
dysfunction	dis-**FUNK**-shun	P/ R/	**dys-** *difficult, painful* **-function** *perform*	Difficulty in performing
dysfunctional (adj)	dis-**FUNK**-shun-al	S/	**-al** *pertaining to*	Having difficulty in performing
impotence	**IM**-poh-tence		Latin *inability*	Inability to achieve an erection
overactive	**OH**-ver-**AK**-tiv	S/ P/ R/	**-ive** *function, connection* **over-** *above* **-act-** *process of doing*	An exaggerated response

Exercises

A. Match the condition with the drug(s) or other treatment types used to treat it. *Choose the correct term in the second column.* **LO 6.10, 6.A**

1. Prostate cancer

2. Erectile dysfunction

3. Prostatitis

4. Benign prostatic hypertrophy

5. Overactive bladder

a. solifenacin

b. Bactrim, Cipro

c. alpha blockers or alfuzosin

d. radiation therapy

e. sildenafil, tadalafil

B. Precision in communication involves correct spelling. *Select the pair of terms that is spelled incorrectly. Rewrite them as correct on the following lines.* **LO 6.A**

1. a. dysfunction

   b. inhibbitors

   c. erectile

   d. prostatitise

   e. genitalia

   overactive

   impotance

   cavernosa

   genital

   pelvic

2. Corrected first terms: _____

3. Corrected second terms: _____

Urinary System

Challenge Your Knowledge

A. System review. Understanding the structure and function of the urinary system will give you a better grasp of the terminology. Choose the correct answers to the following questions. **(LO 6.1, 6.2, 6.3)**

1. Where does waste-laden blood enter the kidney?

   a. the fascia   d. the renal vein

   b. the glomerulus   e. the portal vein

   c. the hilum

2. The medical term to describe urine being forced back up the ureter to the kidneys is

   a. reflux   d. absorption

   b. filtration   e. micturition

   c. excretion

3. What results if the kidney produces too much renin?

   a. hematuria   c. hypertension

   b. oliguria   d. anuria

4. What is the end product of nitrogen metabolism?

   a. ammonia   d. nitrates

   b. glycogen   e. renin

   c. lipid

5. What do urethritis, cystitis, pyelitis, and pyelonephritis all have in common?

   a. infection   d. fever

   b. skin rash   e. kidney

   c. bladder

6. Each kidney is the size of a(n)

   a. orange   d. bean

   b. golf ball   e. ping-pong ball

   c. clenched fist

7. All of the nephrons are located in the kidney's

   a. medulla   d. cortex

   b. calyces   e. hilum

   c. pelvis

8. The external opening of a passage is called a

   a. meatus   d. bladder

   b. urethra   e. hilum

   c. ureter

9. The glomerulus is encased in

   a. a blood vessel   d. the glomerular capsule

   b. a muscle   e. the urethra

   c. renal fascia

10. Nephrotic syndrome involves large amounts of

    _____ leaking out into the urine.

    a. protein   d. blood

    b. sugar   e. white blood cells

    c. red blood cells

11. *Muscular tube, about 10 inches long, that carries urine to the bladder.* This describes the

    a. ureter   c. renal vein

    b. urethra   d. nephron

12. Another name for a kidney stone is

    a. UTI   d. hematuria

    b. calculus   e. lithotripsy

    c. tumor

13. Water is returned to the blood by

    a. excretion   d. elimination

    b. filtration   e. respiration

    c. resorption

B. Abbreviations are not helpful if you do not understand their meaning and cannot use them to communicate safely and effectively. Demonstrate that you can put the appropriate abbreviation in the correct context. You will not use every abbreviation listed to fill in the blanks. **(LO 6.3, 6.7, 6.8, 6.F)**

ARF	ESWL	KUB	SPA
BUN	GRF	MRI	TNM
CRF	IV	PKD	UA
ESRD	IVP	SG	UTI

1. Dr. Lee ordered the _____ medication stat.

2. The patient informed me that there is a history of _____ in his family.

3. The patient with the kidney stone is scheduled for _____ early tomorrow morning.

4. The patient's renal carcinoma was staged using the _____ method.

5. The patient returns with her second _____ this month. Medication is prescribed.

C. Review. One or more roots or combining forms can have the same meaning. Demonstrate that you can use these elements correctly. *Remember: They are not interchangeable.* One particular root or combining form goes with a specific suffix. Fill in the blanks. **(LO 6.3, 6.9, 6.A, 6.C)**

-al	-in	-ic	-logist	-ectomy	-itis	-tomy	-logy

1. Having intermittent spasms or contractions   spasmod/ _____

2. Incision into the kidney   nephro/ _____

3. Pertaining to the kidney   ren/ _____

4. Removal of the kidney   nephr/ _____

5. Kidney enzyme that causes vasoconstriction   ren/ _____

6. Inflammation of the kidney   nephr/ _____

7. Study of the kidney   nephro/ _____

8. Specialist in kidney diseases   nephro/ _____

Urinary System

D. **Matching.** Confirm that your knowledge of the language of the urinary system and its functions is accurate. Match the statements in the first column to the correct answers in the second column. **(LO 6.7, 6.9)**

_____ 1. Outside the body

_____ 2. Pertaining to a disease of unknown cause

_____ 3. Donor organ to recipient

_____ 4. Reversal of normal flow

_____ 5. Hollow tube

_____ 6. Loss of bladder control

_____ 7. Disease state resulting from renal failure

_____ 8. Artificial kidney machine

a. uremia

b. idiopathic

c. catheter

d. extracorporeal

e. retrograde

f. dialyzer

g. transplant

h. incontinence

E. **Each of these diagnoses relates to a specific organ in the urinary system.** Fill in the chart. **(LO 6.1, 6.3, 6.5, 6.7)**

Diagnosis	Organ in the Urinary System
1. urethritis	
2. cystitis	
3. nephritis	
4. ureteritis	

F. **Tests and procedures.** Patients with urinary problems will be sent for various renal function tests and diagnostic procedures that may result in a surgical procedure. Any of the following procedures might be ordered for your patient. Do you know their purpose? Be prepared to discuss which terms are tests and which are procedures. **(LO 6.8, 6.9)**

_____ 1. Contrast material injected to locate stones

_____ 2. Collection of bladder sample in newborns

_____ 3. Incision for removal of kidney stone

_____ 4. Crushing renal stone by sound waves

_____ 5. Assess blood flow to the kidneys

_____ 6. Tissue bank matching of donor to recipient

_____ 7. Treatment for renal cell carcinoma

_____ 8. X-ray of the abdominal urinary organs

_____ 9. Viewing the bladder through a scope

_____ 10. Filtering blood through an artificial kidney machine

a. dialysis

b. transplant

c. KUB

d. retrograde pyelogram

e. cystoscopy

f. nephrolithotomy

g. nephrectomy

h. needle aspiration

i. renal angiogram

j. lithotripsy

G. **Patient documentation.** Answer the questions as they relate to the example of documentation presented below. Choose the correct answer for each question. (**LO 6.3, 6.8, 6.9, 6.A**)

Documentation

A 68-year-old female presents with hematuria, dysuria, and left-flank pain. I ordered a KUB and an IVP to ascertain the possibility or extent of obstruction. Test results indicate one large and several small calculi impacted in her left ureter just below the renal hilum. Patient would prefer ESWL, but surgical laparoscopy, I think, will offer better and quicker results to alleviate her pain. Patient will proceed with surgery tomorrow.

1. What are the patient's symptoms? (Choose all that apply.)

   a. KUB   **b.** calculi   **c.** hematuria   **d.** pain

2. What diagnostic tests were performed? (Choose all that apply.)

   a. KUB   **b.** calculi   **c.** ESWL   **d.** laparoscopy   **e.** hilum

3. What organs were checked in these tests? (Choose all that apply.)

   a. kidneys   **b.** ureters   **c.** bladder   **d.** urethra

4. What is a *laparoscopy*?

   a. removal of calculi   **c.** procedure to view the inside of the abdomen

   b. procedure to crush stones   **d.** surgical fixation of the urinary bladder

5. What is a preoperative diagnosis for this patient?

   a. urinary tract infection   **c.** renal calculi

   b. bladder cancer   **d.** acute renal failure

H. Roots and combining forms are the foundation of a medical term. Differentiate their meanings by analyzing the rest of the term. If the term does not have a particular word element, write n/a. Fill in the blanks. (**LO 6.3, 6.6, 6.7, 6.D**)

Medical Term	Meaning of Prefix	Meaning or Root/ Combining Form	Meaning of Suffix	Meaning of Term
anuria	1.	2.	3.	4.
dysuria	5.	6.	7.	8.
micturition	9.	10.	11.	12.
uremia	13.	14.	15.	16.
oliguria	17.	18.	19.	20.
interstitial	21.	22.	23.	24.

©2014 Nucleus Medical Media

The health professionals involved in the diagnosis and treatment of problems with the male reproductive system include:

- **Urologists**, who are specialists in the diagnosis and treatment of diseases of the urinary system.

- Health care professionals with training and expertise in providing urologic patient care, including **nurse practitioners, physicians' assistants,** and **technologists.**

Chapter Learning Outcomes

As you as an **EMT-P** in the Emergency Department set up the next stage of Joseph Davis's treatment, there are immediate decisions to be made. Joseph is in severe pain and could lose the function of his **testis** without immediate relief of the **torsion**. Also, you will need to communicate clearly with Dr. Helsinki and other health professionals and with Joseph and his mother. You must document his care. To be able to do all this effectively and efficiently, you must be able to:

LO 7.1 Identify and describe the structure and function of the organs of the male reproductive system and its accessory glands.

LO 7.2 Relate the structure of the testes and their spermatic cords to their functions.

LO 7.3 Describe the functions of testosterone.

LO 7.4 Explain spermatogenesis and the anatomy of a sperm.

LO 7.5 Discuss disorders of the testes.

LO 7.6 Define the structure and functions of the spermatic ducts.

LO 7.7 Relate the structures of the accessory glands to their functions.

LO 7.8 Explain disorders of the prostate gland.

LO 7.9 Discuss the causes and treatment of male infertility.

LO 7.10 Relate the structure of the penis to its functions.

LO 7.11 Describe disorders of the penis.

LO 7.12 Explain diagnostic procedures used in disorders of the male reproductive system

LO 7.13 Discuss therapeutic procedures used in disorders of the male reproductive system.

LO 7.14 Describe the medications used in disorders of the male reproductive system.

LO 7.A Use medical terms pertaining to the male reproductive system to communicate and document in writing accurately and precisely in any health care setting.

LO 7.B Use medical terms pertaining to the male reproductive system to communicate verbally with accuracy and precision in any health care setting.

LO 7.C Using word elements, construct medical terms associated with the male reproductive system.

LO 7.D Deconstruct medical terms associated with the male reproductive system into their word elements.

LO 7.E Identify health professionals involved in the care of patients with disorders of the male reproductive system.

LO 7.F Use approved abbreviations for medical reproductive terms correctly.

 ## Case Report (CR) 7.1

You are

. . . an EMT-P working in the Emergency Department at Fulwood Medical Center.

Your patient is

. . . Joseph Davis, a 17-year-old high school senior. He is brought in by his mother at 0400 hrs. He complains of **(c/o)** sudden onset of pain in his left **testicle** 3 hours earlier that woke him up. The pain is intense and has made him vomit. VS: T 99.2°F, P 88, R 15, BP 130/70. Examination reveals his left testicle to be enlarged, warm, and tender. His abdomen is normal to palpation.

At your request, Dr. Helinski, the emergency physician on duty, examines him immediately. He diagnoses a **torsion** of the patient's left testicle.

Lesson 7.1

MALE REPRODUCTIVE SYSTEM

Male Reproduction

Lesson Objectives

Unlike every other organ system, the reproductive system is not essential for an *individual human* to survive. However, without the reproductive system, the *human species* could not survive. The male reproductive system ensures the sexual maturation of each male; influences male behavior; and produces, maintains, and transports the male sex cells (sperm cells) to the female reproductive tract.

The information in this lesson will enable you to use correct medical terminology to:

7.1.1 Describe the anatomy and physiology of the primary and secondary male sex organs and their accessory glands.

7.1.2 Document the process of spermatogenesis.

7.1.3 List the functions of testosterone.

7.1.4 Discuss disorders of the testes.

Abbreviation

VS	vital signs, which include T (temperature), P (pulse rate), R (respiration rate), and BP (blood pressure).

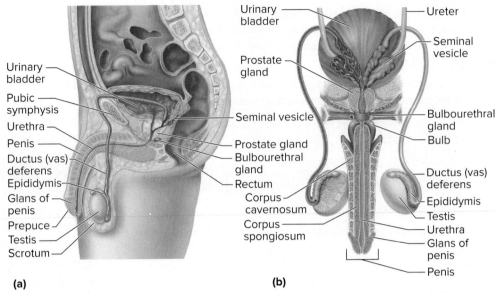

(a)   (b)

▲ **Figure 7.1** **Male Reproductive System.** [a] Male pelvic cavity: midsagittal section. [b] Male reproductive organs.

LO 7.1 Male Reproductive System

The male reproductive organ system *(Figure 7.1)* consists of

1. **Primary sex organs** or **gonads**: the **testes**

2. **Secondary sex organs:**
   a. **Penis**
   b. **Scrotum**
   c. **System of ducts**, including the **epididymis**, **ductus (vas) deferens**, and **urethra**

3. **Accessory glands:**
   a. **Prostate**
   b. **Seminal vesicles**
   c. **Bulbourethral (Cowper) glands**

Perineum

The **external genitalia** (the penis, scrotum, and testes) occupy the **perineum**, a diamond-shaped region between the thighs. Its border is at the pubic symphysis anteriorly and the coccyx posteriorly *(Figure 7.2)*. The anus is also in the perineum.

Scrotum

The **scrotum** is a skin-covered sac between the thighs. Its midline shows a distinct ridge called the **raphe**. It marks the position of the internal **median septum** that divides the scrotum into two compartments. Each compartment contains a testis.

The scrotum's function is to provide a cooler environment for the testes than that inside the body. This is because sperm are best produced and stored at a few degrees cooler than the internal body temperature.

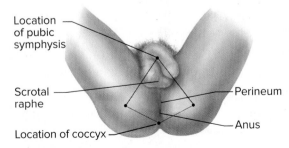

▲ **Figure 7.2** **Male Perineum.**

WORD	PRONUNCIATION	ELEMENTS		DEFINITION
bulbourethral	**BUL**-boh-you-**REE**-thral	S/ R/CF R/	-al *pertaining to* bulb/o- *bulb* -urethr- *urethra*	Pertaining to the bulbous penis and urethra
ductus deferens vas deferens (syn)	**DUK**-tus **DEH**-fuh-renz VAS **DEH**-fuh-renz		**ductus** Latin *to lead* **deferens** Latin *carry away* **vas** Latin *blood vessel, duct*	Tube that receives sperm from the epididymis
epididymis	**EP**-ih-**DID**-ih-miss	S/ P/ R/	-is *belonging to* epi- *above* -didym- *testis*	Coiled tube attached to the testis
genitalia	**JEN**-ih-**TAY**-lee-ah	S/ R/	-ia *condition* genit- *primary male or* *female sex organs*	External and internal organs of reproduction
genital	**JEN**-ih-tal	S/	-al *pertaining to*	Relating to reproduction or to the male or female sex organs
gonad gonads (pl)	**GOH**-nad **GOH**-nads		Greek *seed*	Testis or ovary
penis penile	**PEE**-nis **PEE**-nile	 S/ R/	Latin *tail* -ile *pertaining to* pen- *penis*	Conveys urine and semen to the outside Pertaining to the penis
perineum perineal	**PER**-ih-**NEE**-um **PER**-ih-**NEE**-al	 S/ R/CF	Greek *perineum* -al *pertaining to* perin/e- *perineum*	Area between thighs, extending from the coccyx to the pubis Pertaining to the perineum
raphe	**RAY**-fee		Greek *seam*	Line separating two symmetrical structures
scrotum scrotal (adj)	**SKROH**-tum **SKROH**-tal	 S/ R/	Latin *scrotum* -al *pertaining to* scrot- *scrotum*	Sac containing the testes Pertaining to the scrotum
semen seminal vesicle seminiferous	**SEE**-men **SEM**-in-al **VES**-ih-kull sem-ih-**NIF**-er-us	 S/ R/ S/ R/ S/ R/CF R/	Latin *seed* -al *pertaining to* semin- *semen* -le *small* vesic- *sac containing fluid* -ous *pertaining to* semin/i- *semen* -fer- *to bear*	Penile ejaculate containing sperm and seminal fluid Sac of ductus deferens that produces seminal fluid Pertaining to carrying semen
testicle (also called **testis**) testicular testis testes (pl)	**TES**-tih-kul tes-**TICK**-you-lar **TES**-tis **TES**-teez	 S/ R/	Latin *small testis* -ar *pertaining to* testicul- *testicle* Latin *testis*	One of the male reproductive glands Pertaining to the testicle A synonym for testicle

Exercises

A. In your own words. *You could be working in the Emergency Department when this patient comes in. Using the information presented in Case Report (CR) 7.1, document the case in the patient's record. Use the following terms to fill in the blanks. One term will be used more than once.* **LO 7.1, 7.A**

testicular   testes   testicle

This patient presented to the ED because of pain in his left **1.** _____ . Both **2.** _____ were examined, but the left **3.** _____ was enlarged, warm, and tender. The emergency physician on duty diagnosed **4.** _____ torsion. Patient will be scheduled for surgery immediately.

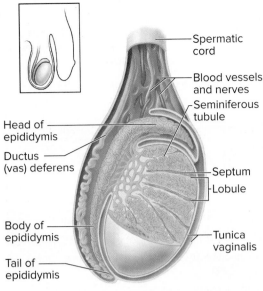

Spermatic cord

Blood vessels and nerves

Seminiferous tubule

Head of epididymis

Ductus (vas) deferens

Septum

Lobule

Body of epididymis

Tunica vaginalis

Tail of epididymis

▲ **Figure 7.3** **The Testis and Associated Structures.**

LO 7.2, 7.3 Testes, Testosterone, and Spermatic Cords

In the adult male, each testis is a small, oval organ about 2 inches (5 cm) long and ¾ inch (2 cm) wide (*Figure 7.3*). Each testis is covered by a serous membrane, the **tunica vaginalis**, which has an outer parietal layer and an inner visceral layer separated by serous fluid.

Inside the testis, thin septa subdivide the testis into some 250 lobules (*Figure 7.3*). Each lobule contains three or four **seminiferous tubules** in which several layers of germ cells are in the process of becoming sperm.

Between the seminiferous tubules are the interstitial cells. They produce hormones called **androgens**.

Testosterone

Testosterone is the major androgen produced by the interstitial cells of the testes. It has the following effects:

- **Sustains** the male reproductive tract throughout adulthood.
- **Stimulates spermatogenesis**; testosterone levels peak at age 20, and then decline steadily to one-third of that level at age 65.
- **Inhibits** the secretion of female hormones at age 65, and continues declining after that age.
- **Stimulates** the development of male secondary sex characteristics at **puberty**.
- **Enlarges** the **spermatic** ducts and accessory glands of the male reproductive system.
- **Stimulates** a burst of growth at puberty—including increased muscle mass, higher **basal metabolic rate (BMR)**, and larger larynx (this effect deepens the voice).
- **Stimulates** erythropoiesis, giving men a higher red blood cell (RBC) count than women.
- **Stimulates** the brain to increase **libido** (sex drive) in the male.

Spermatic Cord

The blood vessels and nerves to the testis arise in the abdominal cavity. They pass through the inguinal canal, where they join with connective tissue to form a spermatic cord that suspends each testis in the scrotum (*see Figure 7.3*). The left testis is suspended lower than the right. Within the cord are an artery, a plexus of veins, nerves, a thin muscle, and the ductus (vas) deferens (the passage into which sperm go when they leave the testis).

LO 7.4 Spermatogenesis

Spermatogenesis is the process in which the germ cells of the seminiferous tubules mature and divide **(mitosis)** and then undergo two divisions called **meiosis**. The four daughter cells differentiate into **spermatids** and then **spermatozoa (sperm)** (*Figure 7.4*). The germ cells have 23 pairs of chromosomes (a total of 46). Because of meiosis, each sperm has only 23 chromosomes that can combine at fertilization with the 23 chromosomes in a female **oocyte** (egg).

The mature sperm has a pear-shaped head and a long tail (*Figure 7.5*). The nucleus of the head contains 23 chromosomes.

The tail **(flagellum)** provides the movement as the sperm swims up the female reproductive tract.

Germ cell (46 chromosomes)

First meiotic division

Homologous chromosomes pairing

Spermatids (23 chromosomes)

Sperm cells

Head

Nucleus

Basal body

Mitochondria

Midpiece (body)

Principal piece

Tail

Endpiece

▲ **Figure 7.4** Spermatogenesis.

▲ **Figure 7.5** Mature Sperm.

WORD	PRONUNCIATION	ELEMENTS		DEFINITION
androgen	**AN**-droh-jen	S/ R/CF	-gen *form, create* andr/o- *masculine*	Hormone that promotes masculine characteristics
flagellum flagella (pl)	fla-**JELL**-um fla-**JELL**-ah		Latin *small whip*	Tail of a sperm
libido	li-**BEE**-doh		Latin *lust*	Sexual desire
meiosis	my-**OH**-sis	S/ R/	-osis *condition* mei- *lessening*	Two rapid cell divisions, resulting in half the number of chromosomes
mitosis	my-**TOH**-sis	S/ R/	-osis *condition* mit- *threadlike structure*	Cell division to create two identical cells, each with 46 chromosomes
puberty	**PYU**-ber-tee		Latin *grown up*	Process of maturing from child to young adult
seminiferous tubule	sem-ih-**NIF**-er-us **TU**-byul	S/ R/CF R/	-ous *pertaining to* semin/i- *semen* -fer- *to bear*	Coiled tubes in the testes that produce sperm
sperm (also called spermatozoon) spermatozoa (pl) spermatic (adj)	SPERM SPER-mat-oh-**ZOH**-ah SPER-mat-ik	S/ R/CF S/	Greek *seed* -zoa *animals* spermat/o- *sperm* -ic *pertaining to*	Mature male sex cell Sperm (plural of spermatozoon) Pertaining to sperm
spermatid spermatogenesis (*Note:* This term has no prefix or suffix.)	**SPER**-mah-tid **SPER**-mat-oh-**JEN**-eh-sis	S/ R/ R/CF R/	-id *having a particular quality* spermat- *sperm* spermat/o- *sperm* genesis *origin, creation*	A cell late in the development process of sperm The process by which male germ cells differentiate into sperm
testosterone	tes-**TOSS**-ter-ohn	S/ R/CF	-sterone *steroid* test/o- *testis*	Powerful androgen produced by the testes
tunica vaginalis	**TYU**-nih-kah vaj-ih-**NAHL**-iss	S/ R/	tunica Latin *coat* -alis *pertaining to* vagin- *sheath, vagina*	Covering, particularly of a tubular structure. The tunica vaginalis is the sheath of the testis and epididymis

Exercises

A. Deconstruction of medical terms is a tool for analyzing the meaning. *In the following chart, you are given a medical term. Deconstruct the term into its root (or combining form) and suffix. Note that none of these terms have prefixes, and not all of the terms have a suffix. Write the element in the appropriate column. The first one is done for you.* **LO 7.2, 7.3, 7.4, 7.D**

Term	Root/Combining Form	Suffix
androgen	*andro*	*-gen*
testosterone	1.	2.
meiosis	3.	4.
vaginalis	5.	6.

B. Define medical terms related to the male reproductive system. *Use the terms from Exercise A. Write the term the definition is describing. Fill in the blanks.* **LO 7.1, 7.2, 7.4**

1. A type of androgen: _____

2. Pertaining to a sheath: _____

3. Two rapid cell divisions, resulting in half the number of chromosomes: _____

4. Hormone that promotes masculine characteristics: _____

	Abbreviation
SET	self-examination of the testes
STD	sexually transmitted disease

Case Report (CR) 7.1 *(continued)*

In the opening scenario to this chapter, Joseph Davis presented with typical symptoms and signs of testicular torsion. The affected testis rapidly became painful, tender, swollen, and inflamed. Emergency surgery was performed, and the testis and cord were manually untwisted through an incision in the scrotum. The testis was stitched to surrounding tissues to prevent a recurrence.

Varicocele

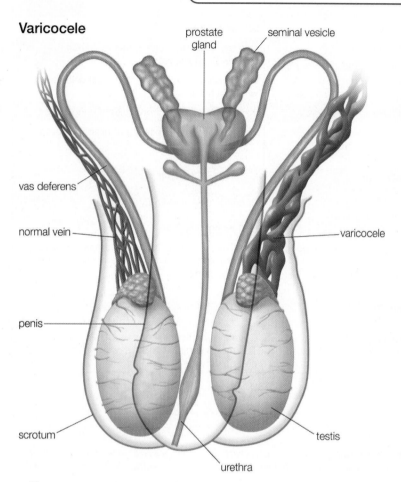

▲ **Figure 7.6** Illustration of Varicocele, Showing Varicose (Dliated) Veins of the Spermatic Cord in the Scrotum. ©Universal Images Group North America LLC/Alamy

Keynotes

- The testis in testicular torsion will die in some 6 hours unless the blood supply is restored.

- **Self-examination of the testes (SET)** for swelling or tenderness should be performed monthly by all men.

LO 7.5 Disorders of the Testes

Cryptorchism occurs when a testis fails to descend from the abdomen into the scrotum before the boy is 12 months old. In the **embryo**, the testes develop inside the abdomen at the level of the kidney. They must then migrate down the abdomen into the scrotum.

Testicular torsion is the twisting of a testis on its spermatic cord. As the testis twists, the spermatic cord has to twist because it is fixed in the abdomen. The testicular artery in the twisted cord becomes blocked, and the blood supply to the testis is cut off. The condition occurs in men between puberty and age 25. In half the cases, it starts in bed at night.

Varicocele *(Figure 7.6)* is a condition in which the veins in the spermatic cord become dilated and tortuous as varicose veins.

Hydrocele is a collection of excess fluid in the space between the visceral and parietal layers of the tunica vaginalis of the testis. It is most common after age 40. The diagnosis can be confirmed by transillumination, shining a bright light on the swelling to see the shape of the testis through the translucent excess fluid *(Figure 7.7)*. Surgical removal is performed for large hydroceles.

Spermatocele is a collection of sperm in a sac formed in the epididymis. It occurs in about 30% of men, is benign, and rarely causes symptoms. It does not require treatment unless it becomes bothersome.

Epididymitis and **epididymoorchitis** (**orchitis**) are both inflammatory diseases. Epididymitis is inflammation of the epididymis; epididymoorchitis is inflammation of the epididymis and testis. Orchitis is usually a consequence of epididymitis. They are most commonly caused by a bacterial infection spreading from a urinary tract infection or infection of the prostate. They also can be caused by **sexually transmitted diseases (STDs)**, such as gonorrhea or chlamydia *(see Chapter 6)*.

A viral cause of orchitis is mumps. In males past puberty who develop mumps, 30% will develop orchitis, and 30% of those will develop resulting testicular atrophy. If the testicular infection is bilateral, **infertility** can result. Mumps is avoidable by immunization during childhood.

Testicular cancer usually develops in men younger than 40.

Forty percent of testicular cancers are **seminomas**, made up of immature germ cells. Nonseminomas occur in different combinations of **choriocarcinoma**, **embryonal cell,** and **teratoma**. Lance Armstrong's cancer was 60% choriocarcinoma and 40% embryonal cell. The initial treatment for testicular cancer is surgical removal of the affected testis (orchiectomy), followed by chemotherapy and sometimes radiation therapy.

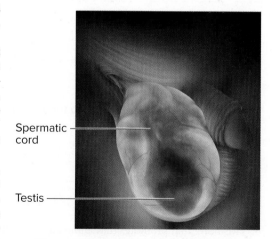

▲ **Figure 7.7** Transillumination of Hydrocele Showing Testis and Spermatic Cord. ©Brian Evans/Photo Researchers, Inc.

S = Suffix   P = Prefix   R = Root   R/CF = Combining Form

WORD	PRONUNCIATION	ELEMENTS		DEFINITION
choriocarcinoma	**KOH**-ree-oh-kar-sih-**NOH**-mah	S/ R/CF R/	-oma *tumor* chori/o- *membrane, chorion* -carcin- *cancer*	Highly malignant cancer in a testis or ovary
cryptorchism (syn: cryptorchidism)	krip-**TOR**-kizm	S/ P/ R/	-ism *condition* crypt- *hidden* -orch- *testicle*	Failure of one or both testes to descend into the scrotum
epididymitis	**EP**-ih-did-ih-**MY**-tis	S/ P/ R/	-itis *inflammation* epi- *above* -didym- *testis*	Inflammation of the epididymis
epididymoorchitis (syn: orchitis)	ep-ih-**DID**-ih-moh-or-**KIE**-tis	S/ P/ R/CF R/	-itis *inflammation* epi-*above* didym/o *testis* orch *testicle*	Inflammation of the epididymis and testicle
hydrocele	**HIGH**-droh-seal	S/ R/CF	-cele *cave* hydr/o- *water*	Collection of fluid in the space of the tunica vaginalis
infertility	in-fer-**TIL**-ih-tee	S/ P/ R/	-ity *condition* in- *not* -fertil- *able to conceive*	Failure to conceive
orchitis epididymoorchitis (syn)	or-**KIE**-tis	S/ R/	-itis *inflammation* orch/i- *testicle*	Inflammation of the testis
seminoma	sem-ih-**NOH**-mah	S/ R/	-oma *tumor, mass* semin- *scatter seed*	Neoplasm of germ cells of a testis
spermatocele	**SPER**-mat-oh-seal	S/ R/CF	-cele *cave, swelling* spermat/o- *sperm*	Cyst of the epididymis that contains sperm
teratoma	ter-ah-**TOH**-mah	S/ R/	-oma *tumor, mass* terat- *monster, malformed fetus*	Neoplasm of a testis or ovary containing multiple tissues from other sites in the body
torsion	**TOR**-shun		Latin *to twist*	The act or result of twisting
varicocele	**VAIR**-ih-koh-seal	S/ R/CF	-cele *cave, swelling* varic/o- *varicosity*	Varicose veins of the spermatic cord

Exercises

A. Construct medical terms using word elements. *Use the terms in the WAD above to complete the medical terms being described. Fill in the blanks.* **LO 7.4, 7.C**

1. Inflammation of the epididymis: epi/ _____ /its

2. Highly malignant cancer in the testis or ovary: chorio/ _____ /oma

3. Swelling containing water: _____ /cele

4. Neoplasm of the germ cells of the testis: semin/ _____

5. Inflammation of the testis: orch/ _____

6. Varicose veins of the spermatic cord: varico/ _____

Lesson 7.2

MALE REPRODUCTIVE SYSTEM

Spermatic Ducts and Accessory Glands

Lesson Objectives

The information provided in this lesson will enable you to:

7.2.1 Trace the pathway taken by a sperm cell from a testis to its ejaculation.

7.2.2 Identify the structure and functions of the prostate and other male accessory glands.

7.2.3 Describe the origins, composition, and functions of semen.

7.2.4 Discuss disorders of the prostate gland.

7.2.5 Identify the causes of male infertility.

Abbreviations

DRE	digital rectal examination
LCC-ST	Liaison Council on Certification for the Surgical Technologist

Case Report (CR) 7.2

You are

... a surgical technologist **(LCC-ST)** working with **urologist** Phillip Johnson, MD, in the **Urology** Clinic at Fulwood Medical Center.

Your patient is

... Mr. Ronald Detrick, a 60-year-old man who has been referred to the Urology Clinic c/o having to get out of bed to urinate four or five times at night.

Mr. Detrick has difficulty starting urination, has a weak stream, and feels he is not emptying his bladder completely. His symptoms have been gradually worsening over the past year. He has lost interest in sex. His physical examination is unremarkable except that **digital rectal examination (DRE)** reveals a diffusely enlarged prostate with no nodules.

LO 7.6 Spermatic Ducts

As the sperm cells mature in the testes over a 60-day period, they move down the seminiferous tubules and pass into a network of tubules called the **rete testis**. From here, they move into the epididymis, the ductus (vas) deferens, the ejaculatory duct, and finally the urethra to reach the outside of the body *(Figure 7.8)*.

The epididymis adheres to the posterior side of the testis. It is a single coiled duct in which the sperm are stored for 12 to 20 days until they mature and become **motile**. Stored sperm remain fertile for 40 to 60 days. If they become too old without being **ejaculated**, they disintegrate and are reabsorbed in the epididymis.

The ductus (vas) deferens is a muscular duct that travels up from the epididymis in the scrotum and through the inguinal canal *(see Chapter 5)* into the pelvic cavity *(see Figure 7.8)*. Here the ductus turns medially and passes behind the urinary bladder and widens into a terminal **ampulla**, which joins with the duct of the seminal **vesicle**.

The **ejaculatory duct,** formed by the ductus deferens and seminal vesicle, is a short (¾-inch or 2-cm) duct that passes through the prostate gland and empties its contents of sperm and seminal fluid (semen) into the urethra.

The male prostate and urethra have both **urologic** and **reproductive** functions, as the flow of urine and semen goes through both organs. Disorders of the prostate and urethra produce symptoms and signs that arise in both areas. This makes it essential to have knowledge of their anatomy, physiology, and terminology to be able to understand both functions.

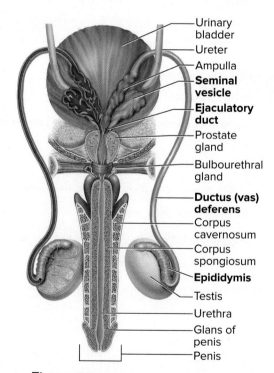

- Urinary bladder
- Ureter
- Ampulla
- **Seminal vesicle**
- **Ejaculatory duct**
- Prostate gland
- Bulbourethral gland
- **Ductus (vas) deferens**
- Corpus cavernosum
- Corpus spongiosum
- **Epididymis**
- Testis
- Urethra
- Glans of penis
- Penis

▲ **Figure 7.8** Components of Male Reproductive Ducts.

WORD	PRONUNCIATION	ELEMENTS		DEFINITION
ampulla	am-**PULL**-ah		Latin *two-handled bottle*	Dilated portion of a canal or duct
ejaculate (*Note:* This term can be a verb or noun.)	ee-**JACK**-you-late	S/ R/	-ate *composed of, pertaining to* ejacul- *shoot out*	To expel suddenly, or the semen expelled in ejaculation
ejaculation	ee-**JACK**-you-**LAY**-shun	S/	-ation *process*	Process of expelling semen
motile	**MOH**-til	S/ R/	-ile *capable* mot- *to move*	Capable of spontaneous movement
motility (noun)	moh-**TILL**-ih-tee	S/	-ility *condition, state of*	The ability for spontaneous movement
reproductive	ree-pro-**DUC**-tiv	S/ P/ R/	-ive *nature of, pertaining to* re- *again* -product- *lead forth*	Relating to the process by which organisms produce offspring
reproduction (noun)	ree-pro-**DUC**-shun	S/	-ion *action, process*	The process by which organisms produce offspring
rete testis	**REE**-teh **TES**-tis		**rete** Latin *net* **testis** Latin *testis*	Network of tubules between the seminiferous tubules and the epididymis
vesicle	**VES**-ih-kull		Latin *a blister*	Small sac containing liquid; for example, a blister or, in this case, semen

Exercises

A. Recall and review. *Become familiar with the terms relating to the spermatic ducts and accessory gland and how they relate clinical conditions related to the male reproductive system.*   **LO 7.6, 7.E, 7.F**

1. After leaving the testis, sperm are stored in the _____.

2. The ductus deferens widens at the _____ and then joins the ejaculatory duct.

3. The specialist treating the male reproductive system is a(n) _____.

4. What is the abbreviation for the procedure in which a finger is inserted into the rectum to evaluate the prostate gland? _____.

5. In the term *rete testis,* the word *rete* is Latin for the word _____.

Study Hint

"**SEVEN UP**" is used to remember the pathway of sperm.
S = seminiferous tubules
E = epididymis
V = vas deferens (now called ductus deferens)
E = ejaculatory duct
(N = nothing)
U = urethra
P = penis

Seminal fluid contains components produced by all three accessory glands *(Figure 7.9)*. The functions of seminal fluid are to:

- **Provide nutrients** to the sperm as they are in the urethra and female reproductive tract.
- **Neutralize acid secretions** of the vagina (in which sperm cannot survive).
- **Provide hormones (prostaglandins)** that widen the opening of the cervix to enable sperm to enter more easily.
- **Provide the fluid vehicle** in which sperm can swim.

The two seminal vesicles are located on the posterior surface of the urinary bladder. The wall of each vesicle contains mucosal folds. They produce a viscous, yellowish, alkaline fluid that contains fructose and prostaglandins. Fructose is a sugar that provides energy for the sperm.

The single **prostate gland** is located immediately below the bladder and anterior to the rectum and surrounds the urethra and the **ejaculatory** duct. It is composed of 30 to 50 glands that open directly into the urethra. The glands secrete a slightly milky fluid that contains:

- **Citric acid,** a nutrient for sperm.
- **An antibiotic** that combats **urinary tract infections (UTIs)** in males.
- **Clotting factors** that hold the sperm together in a sticky mass until **ejaculation**.
- **Prostate-specific antigen (PSA),** an enzyme that helps liquefy the sticky mass following ejaculation.

The two bulbourethral glands are located one on each side of the membranous urethra. Each gland has a short duct leading into the spongy (penile) urethra. The glands secrete a clear, slippery, alkaline mucus that protects the sperm as they pass through the urethra by neutralizing any residual acid urine. It also acts as a lubricant during sexual intercourse.

Semen is derived from the secretions of several glands:

- 5% comes from the testicles and epididymis.
- 50% to 80% comes from the seminal vesicles.
- 15% to 33% comes from the prostate gland.
- 2% to 5% comes from the bulbourethral glands.

(a)   LM 253   (b)   LM 803

▲ **Figure 7.9 Accessory Glands of the Male Reproductive System.** (a) Seminal vesicle. (b) Prostate gland. (a) ©Biophoto Associates/Photo Researchers, Inc. (b) ©McGraw-Hill Education/Dr. Alvin Tesler, photogrpaher.

WORD	PRONUNCIATION	ELEMENTS		DEFINITION
prostate	**PROS**-tate (*Note: not* **PROS**-trate.)		Greek *one standing before*	Organ surrounding the beginning of the urethra
prostatic (adj)	pros-**TAT**-ik	S/ R/	-tic *pertaining to* prosta- *prostate*	Pertaining to the prostate
prostaglandin	**PROS**-tah-**GLAN**-din	S/ R/ R/	-in *chemical* prosta- *prostate* -gland- *gland*	Hormone present in many tissues, but first isolated from the prostate gland
semen	**SEE**-men		Latin *seed*	Penile ejaculate containing sperm and seminal fluid

Exercises

A. Test your knowledge of the language of male reproduction. *Choose the best answer.* **LO 7.7, 7.D, 7.F**

1. PSA is
   a. an enzyme that liquefies semen
   b. an antibiotic that coats the urethra
   c. a diagnostic test for testicular torsion
   d. a hormone that dilates the cervix

2. The two bulbourethral glands are located
   a. near the ureters
   b. on each side of the membranous urethra
   c. behind the seminal vesicles
   d. on top of the prostate gland
   e. under the vas deferens

3. The suffix in the term **prostaglandin** tells you it is a
   a. hormone
   b. enzyme
   c. protein
   d. chemical
   e. blood cell

4. **Semen** is derived from the secretions of several glands:
   a. testicles, epididymis
   b. accessory glands
   c. thymus gland
   d. a, b, and c
   e. a and b only

5. The **prostate gland** is located
   a. below the bladder and posterior to the rectum
   b. beside the bladder and anterior to the rectum
   c. below the bladder and anterior to the rectum
   d. beside the bladder and posterior to the rectum
   e. between the bladder and the kidney

6. The root for **prostatic** is
   a. *adeno-*
   b. *prosta-*
   c. *gland-*
   d. *ren-*
   e. *nephro-*

7. What provides energy for sperm?
   a. citric acid
   b. prostaglandins
   c. fructose
   d. a and c
   e. none of these

8. What is a nutrient for sperm?
   a. alkaline mucus
   b. acid urine
   c. citric acid
   d. normal flora
   e. acid secretions of the vagina

9. In the abbreviation **PSA**, the "A" stands for
   a. antidiuretic
   b. antibiotic
   c. antigen
   d. antibody
   e. allergen

10. What is the fluid vehicle for sperm?
    a. bloodstream
    b. lymph system
    c. plasma
    d. aqueous humor
    e. seminal fluid

LO 7.8 Disorders of the Prostate Gland

By the age of 20, the prostate weighs about 20 grams. It remains at that weight until age 45 to 50, when it begins to grow again. By age 80, some 90% of men have **benign prostatic hyperplasia (BPH)** (*Figure 7.10*). This is a noncancerous enlargement that compresses the prostatic urethra to produce symptoms of:

- Difficulty starting and stopping the urine stream.
- **Nocturia**, **polyuria**, and **dysuria**.

Prostatic cancer affects more than 10% of men over the age of 50, and its incidence is increasing. It forms hard nodules in the periphery of the gland and is often asymptomatic in its early stages because it does not compress the urethra.

Several treatment options involving radiotherapy are available *(see Chapter 20)*. Sometimes, a **radical prostatectomy,** with complete surgical removal of the prostate and surrounding tissues, is performed.

Prostatitis is inflammation of the prostate gland. It occurs in three main types:

Type I—an acute bacterial infection with fever, chills, frequency, dysuria, and hematuria.

Type II—a chronic bacterial infection with less severe symptoms.

Type III—a chronic nonbacterial prostatitis in which the urinary symptoms are present, but no bacteria can be detected. This is the most common type. Its etiology is unknown, and treatment is difficult.

Normal Prostate Enlarged Prostate

▲ **Figure 7.10** Normal prostate and prostate with BPH.

LO 7.9 Male Infertility

Male infertility is the inability to conceive after at least one year of unprotected intercourse. The primary causes of infertility are:

1. Impaired sperm production:
    a. **Cryptorchism**
    b. **Anorchism** (absence of one or both testes)
    c. Testicular trauma
    d. Testicular cancer
    e. **Orchitis** after puberty
2. Impaired sperm delivery:
    a. Infections and blockage of spermatic ducts.
3. Testosterone deficiency **(hypogonadism):**
    a. Medications to treat hypertension and/or high cholesterol.
    b. Environmental endocrine disrupters that adversely affect the endocrine system; examples are phthalates in plastics and dioxins in paper production.

In the United States each year, 500,000 men choose to be made infertile **(sterile)** by having a **vasectomy.**

WORD	PRONUNCIATION	ELEMENTS		DEFINITION
anorchism	an-OR-kizm	S/ P/ R/	-ism *condition* an- *without, lack of* -orch- *testicle*	Absence of testes
dysuria	dis-YOU-ree-ah	S/ P/ R/	-ia *condition* dys- *difficult, painful* -ur- *urine*	Pain or difficulty when urinating
hyperplasia	high-per-PLAY-zee-ah	S/ P/ R/	-ia *condition* hyper- *excessive* -plas- *molding, formation*	Increase in the number of the cells in a tissue or organ
hypogonadism	HIGH-poh-GOH-nad-izm	S/ P/ R/	-ism *condition* hypo- *deficient* -gonad- *testes or ovaries*	Deficient gonad production of sperm, eggs, or hormones
nocturia	nok-TYU-ree-ah	S/ P/ R/	-ia *condition* noct- *night* -ur- *urine*	Excessive urination at night
polyuria	pol-ee-YOU-ree-ah	S/ P/ R/	-ia *condition* poly- *excessive* -ur- *urine*	Excessive production of urine
prostatitis	pross-tah-TIE-tis	S/ R/	-itis *inflammation* prostat- *prostate*	Inflammation of the prostate
sterile sterility	STER-ill steh-RIL-ih-tee	 S/ R/	Latin *barren* -ity *state, condition* steril- *barren*	Unable to fertilize or reproduce Inability to reproduce

Exercises

A. Recognition. *As you become more familiar with elements (especially suffixes), you will be able to recognize medical terms that are procedures and diagnoses. Practice with the terms in the above WAD. Choose the correct answer.* **LO 7.5, 7.8, 7.9, 7.D**

1. The root in the term **anorchism** means:

   a. hidden   **b.** testicle   **c.** reproductive   **d.** condition

2. In the term **hypogonadism,** the prefix means:

   a. below   **b.** above   **c.** deficient   **d.** excessive

3. The root in the term **hyperplasia** is:

   a. hyper   **b.** plas   **c.** ia

4. The meaning of the root in the term **hyperplasia** is:

   a. excessive   **b.** formation   **c.** condition   **d.** below

B. Matching. *Match the type of prostatitis with its correct description.* **LO 7.8**

Term		Meaning
_____	**1.** Type I	**a.** an acute bacterial infection with fever, chills, frequency, dysuria, and hematuria
_____	**2.** Type II	**b.** a chronic bacterial infection with less severe symptoms
_____	**3.** Type III	**c.** chronic nonbacterial prostatitis with urinary symptoms, but no bacteria can be detected

Lesson 7.3

The Penis and Its Disorders

Keynote

Erectile dysfunction (ED) occurs in some 20 million American men.

LO 7.10 Penis

The external, visible part of the penis comprises the **shaft** and the **glans** (*Figure 7.11a*), at the tip of which the external urethral meatus is located. The skin of the penis is very loosely attached to the shaft to permit expansion during erection. The skin continues over the glans as the **prepuce** (foreskin). A ventral fold of tissue, the **frenulum**, attaches the skin to the glans. The glans and facing prepuce contain sebaceous glands that produce a waxy secretion called **smegma**.

The shaft of the penis contains three **erectile** vascular bodies (*Figure 7.11b*):

- Paired **corpora cavernosa** are located dorsolaterally.
- A single **corpus spongiosum** is located inferiorly. It contains the urethra and goes on to form the glans.

The corpora cavernosa are composed of a network of venous sinuses surrounding a central artery. **Erection** occurs when the sinuses fill with blood, causing the erectile bodies to distend and become rigid. It is a parasympathetic nervous system response to stimulation.

Ejaculation occurs when the sympathetic nervous system stimulates the smooth muscle of the ductus deferens, ejaculatory ducts, and the prostate gland to contract. The seminal vesicles contract so that their fluids join to form semen. The internal urethral sphincter also contracts so that urine cannot enter the urethra and semen cannot enter the bladder.

Prepuce (Foreskin)

The functions of the prepuce (foreskin) (*see Figure 7.12*) are to cover and protect the glans and produce smegma, a lubricant containing lipids, cell debris, and some natural antibiotics.

Penile Urethra

The **penile urethra** passes through the single erectile body, the corpus spongiosum, to the external urethral meatus.

(a)

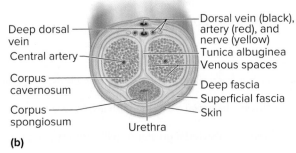

(b)

▲ **Figure 7.11** **Anatomy of Penis.** (a) External anatomy. (b) Cross-sectional view.

(a)   (b)

▲ **Figure 7.12** **Prepuce.** (a) Circumcised penis. (b) Uncircumcised penis.

WORD	PRONUNCIATION	ELEMENTS		DEFINITION
cavernosa	kav-er-**NOH**-sah	S/ R/	-osa *like* cavern- *cave*	Resembling a cave
corpus corpora (pl)	**KOR**-pus kor-**POR**-ah		Latin *body*	Major part of a structure
frenulum	**FREN**-you-lum		Latin *small bridle*	Fold of mucous membrane between the glans and prepuce
glans	GLANZ		Latin *acorn*	Head of the penis or clitoris
prepuce	**PREE**-puce		Latin *foreskin*	Fold of skin that covers the glans penis
smegma	**SMEG**-mah		Greek *ointment*	Oily material produced by the glans and prepuce
spongiosum	spun-jee-**OH**-sum	S/ R/	-um *structure* spongios- *sponge*	Spongelike tissue

Exercises

A. Many medical terms have Greek and Latin origins and cannot be deconstructed. *Match the term in the first column with its meaning in the second column.* **LO 7.10**

Term	Meaning
_____ 1. glans	**a.** acorn
_____ 2. corpora	**b.** small bridle
_____ 3. prepuce	**c.** body
_____ 4. smegma	**d.** foreskin
_____ 5. frenulum	**e.** ointment

LO 7.11 Disorders of the Penis

Disorders of the Penis

Trauma to the penis can vary from being caught in a pants zipper to a fracture of an erect penis during vigorous sexual intercourse.

Peyronie disease is a marked curvature of the erect penis caused by fibrous tissue. Its etiology is unknown, and there is no successful treatment.

Priapism is a persistent, painful **erection** when blood cannot escape from the erectile tissue. It can be caused by drugs (such as epinephrine), blood clots, or spinal cord injury.

Cancer of the penis occurs most commonly on the glans and is rare in circumcised men. Circumcision also offers some protection against HIV infection.

Syphilis can cause flat pink or gray growths called **condylomata** or a sore called a **chancre**.

Other **sexually transmitted diseases (STDs)** can produce small, firm genital warts called **condylomata acuminata** or firm, dimpled growths called **molluscum contagiosum**. The STDs are discussed in detail in *Chapter 6*.

Erectile dysfunction (impotence) is the inability to develop or maintain an erection of the penis during sexual activity. The problem can be caused by cardiovascular disease, diabetes, trauma from prostatectomy surgery, drug side effects, potassium deficiency, and psychological reasons.

Premature ejaculation occurs when a man ejaculates so quickly during intercourse that it causes embarrassment.

Disorders of the Prepuce

Disorders of the prepuce include:

- **Balanitis**—infection of the glans and foreskin with bacteria or yeast.
- **Phimosis**—a condition in which the foreskin is tight because of a small opening and cannot be retracted over the glans for cleaning (*Figure 7.13*). It can lead to balanitis.
- **Paraphimosis**—a condition in which the retracted foreskin cannot be pulled forward to cover the glans.

In all of these conditions, particularly if they are recurrent, circumcision as an adult may be necessary.

Disorders of the Penile Urethra

Urethritis is an inflammation of the urethra. It can be caused by:

- The same bacteria that cause UTIs (*see Chapter 6*).
- STDs such as chlamydia and gonorrhea (*see Chapter 8*).
- Herpes simplex virus and cytomegalovirus (*see Chapter 8*).
- Chemical irritants such as **spermicides** and **contraceptive** gels.

Urethritis presents with dysuria, increased frequency of urination, and discharge from the penis. After urine culture to identify the organism, antibiotics will clear a bacterial infection, usually without complications.

Urethral stricture is scarring that narrows the urethra. It results from infection or injury. It produces a less forceful stream of urine and can be a cause of UTI.

Hypospadias is a congenital defect in which the opening of the urethra is on the undersurface of the penis instead of at the head of the glans (*Figure 7.14*). It can be corrected surgically.

Epispadias is a congenital defect in which the opening of the urethra is on the **dorsum** of the penis. It can be corrected surgically.

▲ **Figure 7.13** Phimosis. ©Cardiff and Vale NHS Trust/Wellcome Images

▲ **Figure 7.14** Hypospadias. Source: Wellcome Library, London

Abbreviations	
ED	erectile dysfunction
STD	sexually transmitted disease

WORD	PRONUNCIATION		ELEMENTS	DEFINITION
acuminata	a-**KYU**-min-**AH**-ta	S/ R/	-ata *action, place* acumin- *to sharpen*	Tapering to a point
balanitis	bal-ah-**NIE**-tis	S/ R/	-itis *inflammation* balan- *glans penis*	Inflammation of the glans and prepuce of the penis
chancre	**SHAN**-ker		Latin *cancer*	Primary lesion of syphilis
condyloma condylomata (pl)	kon-dih-**LOH**-ma kon-dih-**LOH**-ma-tah		Greek *a knob*	Warty growth on external genitalia
contagiosum contagious (adj)	kon-**TAY**-jee-oh-sum kon-**TAY**-jus		Latin *to touch closely*	Infection spread from one person to another by direct contact Able to be transmitted, as infections transmitted from person to person or from person to air or surface to person
contraception	kon-trah-**SEP**-shun	S/ P/ R/	-ion *process, action* contra- *against* -cept- *to receive*	Prevention of conception
dorsum	**DOR**-sum		Latin *back*	Upper, posterior, or back surface
epispadias	ep-ih-**SPAY**-dee-as	S/ P/ R/	-ias *condition* epi- *above* -spad- *tear or cut*	Condition in which the urethral opening is on the dorsum of the penis
erection	ee-**REK**-shun	S/ R/	-ion *process, condition* erect- *straight, to set up*	Distended and rigid state of an organ
erectile	ee-**REK**-tile	S/	-ile *capable of*	Capable of erection or being distended with blood
hypospadias	high-poh-**SPAY**-dee-as	S/ P/ R/	-ias *condition* hypo- *below* -spad- *tear or cut*	Urethral opening more proximal than normal on the ventral surface of the penis
impotence	**IM**-poh-tence		Latin *inability*	Inability to achieve an erection
molluscum	moh-**LUS**-kum		Latin *soft*	Soft, round tumor of skin caused by a virus
paraphimosis	**PAR**-ah-fi-**MOH**-sis	S/ P/ R/	-osis *condition* para- *abnormal* -phim- *muzzle*	Condition in which a retracted prepuce cannot be pulled forward to cover the glans
phimosis	fi-**MOH**-sis			Condition in which the prepuce cannot be retracted
Peyronie disease	pay-**ROH**-nee diz-**EEZ**		François de la Peyronie, 1678–1747, French surgeon	Penile bending and pain on erection
priapism	**PRY**-ah-pizm		Priapus, mythical Roman god of procreation	Persistent erection of the penis
stricture	**STRICK**-shur		Latin *to draw tight*	Narrowing of a tube
syphilis	**SIF**-ih-lis		Possibly from the Latin poem "Syphilis sive Morbus Gallicus" by Fracastorius	Sexually transmitted disease caused by a spirochete
trauma traumatic	**TRAW**-mah traw-**MAT**-ik	S/ R/	Greek *wound* -tic *pertaining to* trauma- *injury*	A physical or mental injury Pertaining to or caused by trauma

Exercises

A. Latin and Greek terms stand alone and do not deconstruct into several elements the way other terms do. *Match the medical term in the first column to its definition in the second column.* **LO 7.11, 7.A**

_____ 1. trauma   **a.** warty growth on external genitalia

_____ 2. chancre   **b.** transmitted, as an infection spread from one person to another by direct contact

_____ 3. molluscum   **c.** inability to achieve an erection

_____ 4. condyloma   **d.** primary lesion of syphilis

_____ 5. impotence   **e.** soft, round tumor of skin caused by a virus

_____ 6. contagious   **f.** wound

Lesson 7.4

MALE REPRODUCTIVE SYSTEM

Procedures and Pharmacology

Keynote

- **Vasectomy** is almost 100% successful in producing male sterility.

- **Vasovasostomy** is a microsurgical procedure to suture back together **(anastomosis)** the cut ends of the ductus deferens if requested sometime after vasectomy.

Abbreviations

DRE	digital rectal examination
PDE5	phosphodiesterase type 5 inhibitor
PSA	prostate-specific antigen
TUIP	transurethral incision of the prostate
TURP	transurethral resection of the prostate

▲ **Figure 7.15** Vasectomy being performed. ©SPL/Photo Researchers, Inc.

LO 7.12 Diagnostic Procedures

A **digital rectal examination (DRE),** in which a lubricated, gloved finger is inserted into the rectum, is part of a routine physical examination in men and women. In men it is used to check for enlargement or other abnormalities of the prostate gland.

Prostate-specific antigen (PSA) is a protein produced by cells of the prostate gland, and the PSA test measures the level of PSA in a man's blood. The level is increased in cancer of the prostate, benign prostatic hyperplasia (BPH), and acute prostatitis.

Prostate biopsy is commonly performed under ultrasound guidance to remove samples of tissue for pathologic analysis. MRI-guided biopsies or a hybrid of MRI images with ultrasound also can be used.

LO 7.13 Therapeutic Procedures

Circumcision, the removal of the foreskin, can be indicated in an adult for pathological phimosis, **refactory** balanoposthitis, and chronic urinary tract infections. In many religions, circumcision is a ritual in the neonatal period or at varying ages before puberty. In the United States, 85% of all males are circumcised in the neonatal period. In Europe, less than 20% are circumcised.

Orchiopexy is a **surgical** procedure to move an undescended testicle (**cryptorchid**) from the abdomen into the scrotum and permanently fix it there.

Orchiectomy (orchidectomy) is the removal of one or both testicles performed for testicular cancer, sex reassignment surgery for transgender women, and advanced prostate cancer to stop the production of testosterone.

Urethrotomy is incision of the urethra to relieve stricture caused by injury or infection.

Benign prostatic hypertrophy (BPH) can be treated surgically by **transurethral resection of the prostate (TURP)**, in which a **resectoscope** is inserted through the penile urethra to remove prostate tissue obstructing the urethra; transurethral incision of the prostate (**TUIP),** in which the urethra is widened by incision in the neck of the bladder and in the prostate gland; laser surgery, which removes prostate tissue by **ablation** (melting) or **enucleation** (cutting) through insertion of a scope through the penile urethra; or open simple **prostatectomy**, in which the portion of the prostate gland blocking urine flow is removed through incisions or **laparoscopy** in the abdomen.

Cancer of the prostate can be treated with **active surveillance** for early-stage, asymptopmatic, slow-growing lesions; external beam **radiation therapy** or **brachytherapy**, in which many rice-sized radioactive seeds are implanted in the prostate; **cryosurgery**, in which small needles containing a very cold gas are inserted in the cancer using ultrasound images as guidance; **radical prostatectomy**, to remove the prostate gland, surrounding tissue, and lymph nodes surgically; and **chemotherapy.**

In a **vasectomy**, performed under local anesthesia, the ductus deferens is pulled through a small incision in the scrotum and cut in two places, a 1-centimeter segment is removed, and the ends are cauterized and tied (*Figure 7.15*). The procedure to reverse (repair) a vasectomy is called a vasovasostomy.

LO 7.14 Pharmacology

BPH can be treated medically with **alpha blockers** to relax the bladder neck muscles and muscle fibers in the prostate gland and/or **5-alpha reductase inhibitors,** which block hormones that spur the growth of the gland.

Prostate cancer can be treated with **hormone therapy** using medications that stop the body from producing testosterone, which prostate cancer cells need to grow, or **anti-androgens** that block testosterone from reaching the cancer cells.

Prostatitis is usually a bacterial infection and requires treatment with appropriate **antibiotics**.

Treatment of the underlying cause of **erectile dysfunction** can relieve the difficulty of maintaining an erection, and phosphodiesterase type 5 inhibitors (PDE5) such as *Viagra* and *Cialis* are now in common use. Less common treatments are a penile prosthesis or a penile pump.

WORD	PRONUNCIATION	ELEMENTS		DEFINITION
ablation	ab-**LAY**-shun	S/ P/ R/	-ion *action* ab- *away from* -lat- *to take*	Removal of tissue to destroy its function
brachytherapy	brah-kee-**THAIR**-ah-pee	P/ R/CF	brachy- *short* -therapy *treatment*	Radiation therapy in which the source of irradiation is implanted in the tissue to be treated
circumcision	ser-kum-**SIZH**-un	S/ P/ R/	-ion *process, action* circum- *around* -cis- *to cut*	To remove part or all of the prepuce
cryosurgery	cry-oh-**SUR**-jer-ee	S/ R/CF R/	-ery *process of* cry/o- *icy cold* -surg- *operate*	Use of liquid nitrogen or argon gas to freeze and kill abnormal tissue
digital	**DIJ**-ih-tal	S/ R/	-al *pertaining to* digit- *finger or toe*	Pertaining to a finger or toe
enucleation	ee-nu-klee-**A**-shun	S/ P/ R/	-ation *process* e- *out of, from* -nucle- *kernel*	Removal of an entire structure without rupture
orchiectomy (orchidectomy)	or-kee-**ECK**-toh-mee	S/ R/CF	-ectomy *surgical excision* orch/i- *testicle*	Removal of one testis or both testes
orchiopexy (**Note:** The letter "o" is added to make the word flow.)	**OR**-kee-oh-**PEK**-see	S/ R/CF	-pexy *surgical fixation* orch/i- *testicle*	Surgical fixation of a testis in the scrotum
prostatectomy	pross-tah-**TEK**-toh-mee	S/ R/	-ectomy *surgical excision* prostat- *prostate*	Surgical removal of the prostate
radical surgery	**RAD**-ih-kal **SUR**-jeh-ree	S/ R/	radical Latin *root* -ery *condition, process of* surg- *operate*	Surgical procedure in which the affected organ is removed along with the blood and lymph supply to that organ.
resection	ree-**SEK**-shun	S/ P/ R/	-ion *action* re- *back* -sect- *cut off*	Removal of a specific part of an organ or structure
surgical	**SUR**-jih-kal	S/ R/	-ical *pertaining to* surg- *operate*	Relating to surgery
urethrotomy	you-ree-**THROT**-oh-mee	S/ R/CF	-tomy *surgical incision* urethr/o- *urethra*	Incision of a stricture of the urethra
vasectomy	vah-**SEK**-toh-mee	S/ R/	-ectomy *surgical excision* vas- *duct*	Excision of a segment of the ductus (vas) deferens
vasovasostomy (also called **vasectomy reversal**)	**VAY**-soh-vay-**SOS**-toh-mee	S/ R/CF	-stomy *new opening* vas/o- *duct*	Reanastomosis of the ductus deferens to restore the flow of sperm

Exercises

A. Construct medical terms. *Recalling the meanings of word elements assists you in determining the meaning of a medical term. From the given definition, provide the missing word element. Fill in the blanks.* **LO 7.12, 7.13, 7.C**

1. Use of liquid nitrogen to freeze abnormal tissue.   _____ /o/surgery

2. Removal of a specific part of an organ or tissue.   re/_____ /ion

3. Excision of a section of the ductus deferens.   vas/_____

4. Surgical fixation of a testis in the scrotum   _____ /i/pexy

5. Pertaining to a finger or toe   _____ /al

6. Removal of tissue to destroy its function.   _____ /lat/ion

7. Removal of entire structure without rupture   e/_____ /ation

8. Radiation therapy for which the source of radiation is implanted into the tissue to be treated   _____ /therapy

Male Reproductive System

Challenge Your Knowledge

A. Language of male reproductive system. Every day on the job in the Urology Clinic, you will be asked to apply the language of urology to the anatomy and physiology of the male reproductive system. Select the correct choice. **(LO 7.1, 7.2)**

1. The prostate, seminal vesicles, and bulbourethral glands are

   a. gonads

   b. primary sex organs

   c. accessory glands

   d. secondary sex organs

   e. accessory vessels

2. The tube that carries the sperm from the epididymis:

   a. glans

   b. urethra

   c. vas (ductus) deferens

   d. raphe

   e. vesicle

3. A male secondary sex organ:

   a. prostate

   b. testis

   c. seminal vesicle

   d. bulbourethral glands

   e. penis

4. The final portion of the tubular system of the male reproductive system is the:

   a. testes

   b. urethra

   c. prostate

   d. penis

   e. scrotum

5. The skin-covered sac between the thighs of males:

   a. rete testis

   b. perineum

   c. median septum

   d. ductus deferens

   e. scrotum

B. Apply the language of urology to the anatomy and physiology of the male reproductive system. Select the correct choice. **(LO 7.1)**

1. Androgens are

    a. enzymes

    b. vitamins

    c. hormones

    d. special nerve cells

    e. flagella

2. The penis, scrotum, and testes collectively are known as

    a. primary sex organs

    b. accessory glands

    c. secondary sex organs

    d. external genitalia

    e. the perineum

3. The male gonads are the

    a. scrotum

    b. penis

    c. prostate

    d. ductus deferens

    e. testes

4. The medical term that refers to the area between the thighs is the

    a. perineum

    b. raphae

    c. spermatic cord

    d. genitalia

    e. varicocele

5. The distinct ridge in the scrotum is called the

    a. dartos

    b. raphe

    c. hydrocele

    d. epididymis

    e. cavernosa

©2014 Nucleus Medical Media

Male Reproductive System

C. **Explain spermatogenesis.** Demonstrate your knowledge of spermatogenesis by selecting the correct answer to the following questions. **(LO 7.2, 7.3, 7.4)**

1. The major androgen of the male reproductive system:

  a. estrogen

  b. testosterone

  c. semen

  d. cortisone

  e. spermatid

2. That which suspends each testis in the scrotum is the

  a. spermatic cord

  b. ductus deferens

  c. dartos muscle

  d. interstitial cells

  e. tunica

3. After meiosis, the four daughter cells differentiate into:

  a. spermatids

  b. spermatozoa

  c. germ cells

  d. flagella

  e. oocytes

4. How many chromosomes are found in a sperm cell?

  a. 15

  b. 20

  c. 23

  d. 35

  e. 43

5. The term that is the plural form of sperm:

  a. spermatic

  b. spermatozoon

  c. spermatid

  d. spermatogenesis

  e. spermatozoa

D. Roots. The following medical terms all share the same root/combining form. Employ your knowledge of the other elements to determine the correct term for the sentence. Use the provided terms to fill in the blanks. **(LO 7.5, 7.13, 7.A)**

cryptorchism   orchitis   epididymoorchitis   orchiopexy   orchiectomy   anorchism

1. Patient has inflammation of the epididymis and testicle on the right side. Diagnosis: _____

2. Patient was born without testes. Diagnosis: _____

3. Patient had one diseased testicle removed. Procedure: _____

4. Patient had testicular torsion repaired. Procedure: _____

5. Patient has inflammation of both testicles. Diagnosis: _____

6. Patient was born with an undescended right testicle. Diagnosis: _____

E. Proper documentation. Patients will explain procedures and conditions in common language. Can you interpret what they communicate into proper medical terminology? **(LO 7.5, 7.8, 7.13, 7.A)**

1. "I had a surgery so that I can't get a woman pregnant." His procedure was a _____.

2. "I have to get up a lot in the night to urinate." He is complaining of _____.

3. "I was unable to retract my foreskin." He had the condition _____.

4. "My husband had his entire prostate removed." His surgical procedure was a _____.

5. "My son was born with an undescended testicle." The child has _____.

F. Abbreviations are another form of precise communication. Demonstrate that you know the meanings of the abbreviations in this exercise. Select the best answer. **(LO 7.7, 7.11, 7.12, 7.F)**

1. Which of the following is a diagnosis for a type of prostate disease?

   a. BPH

   b. TURP

   c. PSA

   d. LCC-ST

2. Which of the following can produce *condylomata acuminata*?

   a. STD

   b. UTI

   c. ED

   d. TUIP

3. The abbreviation *DRE* relates to a:

   a. disorder of the penis

   b. structure of the male reproductive system

   c. diagnostic procedure

   d. medication to treat prostate cancer

Chapter 7 Review

©2014 Nucleus Medical Media

Male Reproductive System

G. Deconstruction. Deconstruction of medical terms is a tool for analyzing the meaning. In the following chart, you are given a medical term. Deconstruct the term into its prefix, root (or combining form) and suffix. Write the element and its meaning in the appropriate column and the meaning of the term in the last column. If the term does not have a word element, write n/a. The first one is done for you. **(LO 7.1, 7.8, 7.10, 7.D)**

Term	Prefix	Meaning of Prefix	Root/ Combining Form	Meaning of Root/Combing Form	Suffix	Meaning of Suffix	Meaning of Term
phimosis	1. n/a	2. n/a	3. phim	4. muzzle	5. -osis	6. condition	7. Condition in which the prepuce cannot be retracted
hyperplasia	8.	9.	10.	11.	12.	13.	14.
epididymis	15.	16.	17.	18.	19.	20.	21.
teratoma	22.	23.	24.	25.	26.	27.	28.
cavernosa	29.	30.	31.	32.	33.	34.	35.

H. Disorder or disease. Complete the diagnosis documentation for the following patients. Fill in the blanks with the correct medical term for the disorder or disease mentioned in each statement. **(LO 7.5, 7.8, 7.A, 7.C)**

1. Excess fluid has collected in the space between the visceral and parietal layers of the tunica vaginalis of the patient's right testis:

   hydro _____.

2. Noncancerous enlargement compressing the prostatic urethra is: benign _____ plasia.

3. Marked curvature of the erect penis caused by fibrous tissue is _____ disease.

4. Opening of the urethra is on the dorsum of the penis: _____ spadias.

5. Veins in the spermatic cord become tortuous and dilated: varico _____.

6. Opening of the urethra is on the undersurface of the penis instead of at the head of the glans:

   hypo _____.

7. Yeast infection of the glans and foreskin is _____ itis.

8. Foreskin is tight and cannot be retracted over the glans for cleaning: _____ sis.

9. Inflammation of the epididymis is _____ itis.

I. **Trace the pathway taken by a sperm cell from the testes to its ejaculation.** Number the following terms in the correct order. Fill in the blanks. *Remember your study hint!* (**LO 7.2, 7.10**)

_____ **a.** epididymis

_____ **b.** urethra

_____ **c.** testis

_____ **d.** seminiferous tubules

_____ **e.** ejaculatory duct

_____ **f.** ductus deferens

_____ **g.** penis

J. **Patient documentation.** Reread the Case Report 7.1 from the beginning of this chapter, shown as follows.

Case Report (CR) 7.1

You are

. . . an EMT-P working in the Emergency Department at Fulwood Medical Center.

Your patient is

. . . Joseph Davis, a 17-year-old high school senior.

He is brought in by his mother at 0400 hrs. He complains of (c/o) sudden onset of pain in his left testicle 3 hours earlier that woke him up. The pain is intense and has made him vomit. VS: T 99.2°F, P 88, R 15, BP 130/70. Examination reveals his left testicle to be enlarged, warm, and tender. His abdomen is normal to palpation.

At your request, Dr. Helinski, the emergency physician on duty, examines him immediately. He diagnoses a torsion of the patient's left testicle.

Joseph Davis presented with typical symptoms and signs of testicular torsion. The affected testis rapidly became painful, tender, swollen, and inflamed. Emergency surgery was performed, and the testis and cord were manually untwisted through an incision in the scrotum. The testis was stitched to surrounding tissues to prevent a recurrence.

Dr. Helinski, the emergency physician on duty, has referred Joseph Davis to a surgeon for repair of his condition, and it is your duty to obtain from the patient's insurance company preapproval for the surgery. You must be prepared to furnish answers to the following questions the insurance company will ask. Fill in the blanks. **LO 7.4, 7.13, 7.A**

1. What is the patient's diagnosis? _____

2. Is this condition the result of an accident? _____

3. What procedure is the surgeon going to perform? _____

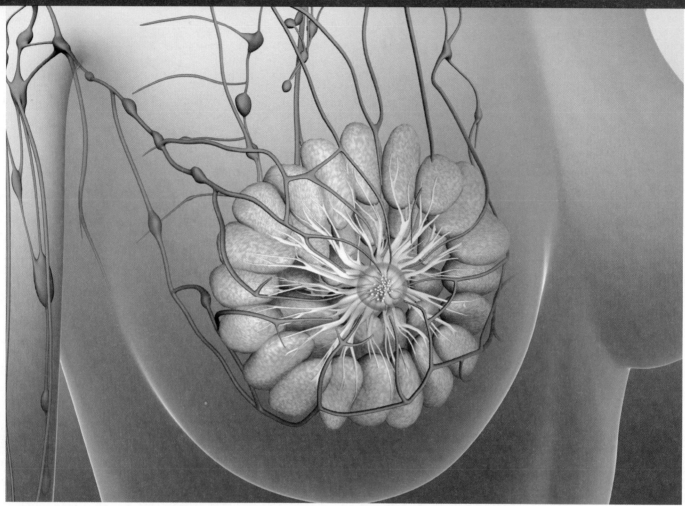

©2014 Nucleus Medical Media

The health professionals you will find involved in the care of women at different times in their lives include the following:

- **Gynecologists** are physicians who are specialists in diseases of the female reproductive tract.

- **Obstetricians** are physicians who are specialists in the care of women during pregnancy and childbirth.

- **Neonatologists** are physicians who are pediatric subspecialists in disorders of the newborn, particularly ill or premature infants.

- **Perinatologists** are physicians who are obstetric subspecialists in the care of mothers and fetuses at higher-than-normal risk for complications.

- **Certified midwives/nurse-midwives** are independent practitioners who provide care to mothers during pregnancy, delivery, and birth, and to mothers and newborn infants for 6 weeks after birth.

- **Obstetrical-gynecological nurse practitioners** are registered nurses who have acquired skills in the management of health and illness for women throughout their life cycle.

Chapter Learning Outcomes

In the adjoining Case Report 8.1, Mrs. Baker is clearly in need of urgent diagnosis and treatment. As you work with the nurse and physician to see her through this difficult time, you will find the need to be able to perform several of the following tasks:

LO 8.1 Describe the external genitalia and vagina.

LO 8.2 Discuss disorders of the external genitalia and vagina.

LO 8.3 Describe sexually transmitted diseases, their diagnosis, and their treatment.

LO 8.4 Relate the structure of the uterus, uterine tubes and ovaries to their functions.

LO 8.5 Discuss oogenesis and ovulation.

LO 8.6 Describe the ovarian hormones.

LO 8.7 Explain the female menstrual cycle.

LO 8.8 Describe disorders of the uterus, uterine tubes and ovaries.

LO 8.9 Discuss female infertility.

LO 8.10 Identify methods of contraception.

LO 8.11 Identify diagnostic and therapeutic procedures and medications used in gynecology.

LO 8.12 Describe fertilization of the egg to form a zygote and its implantation in the uterus.

LO 8.13 Relate the development of the placenta to that of the embryo and fetus.

LO 8.14 Explain the stages of pregnancy and childbirth.

LO 8.15 Discuss the disorders of pregnancy.

LO 8.16 Describe the disorders of childbirth.

LO 8.17 Identify diagnostic and therapeutic procedures and medications used in obstetrics.

LO 8.18 Relate the structure of the breast and mammary gland to their functions.

LO 8.19 Discuss disorders of the breast.

LO 8.20 Identify diagnostic and therapeutic procedures and medications used in disorders of the breast.

LO 8.A Use the medical terms of gynecology and obstetrics to communicate and document in writing accurately and precisely in any health care setting.

LO 8.B Use the medical terms of obstetrics and gynecology to communicate verbally with accuracy and precision in any health care setting.

LO 8.C Construct the medical terms of obstetrics and gynecology from their word elements.

LO 8.D Deconstruct the medical terms of obstetrics and gynecology into their word elements.

LO 8.E Identify the health professionals involved in gynecology and obstetrics.

LO 8.F Use approved abbreviations of medical terms in obstetrics and gynecology accurately.

 ## Case Report (CR) 8.1

You are

. . . a **registered nurse (RN)** working in the Emergency Department at Fulwood Medical Center.

Your patient is

. . . Ms. Lara Baker, a 32-year-old single mother who works in the billing department of the medical center. You have been asked to take her vital signs (VS). For the past couple of days, she has had muscle aches and a feeling of general uneasiness that she had thought were due to her heavy menstrual period. In the past 3 hours, she has developed a severe headache with nausea and vomiting. A diffuse rash over her trunk that looks like sunburn is now spreading to her upper arms and thighs.

VS: T 104.2°F, P 120 and irregular, R 20, BP 86/50. As you took her VS, you noted that she did not seem to understand where she was. She was unable to pass urine for a urine specimen.

For this patient, the treatment she receives in the next few minutes is vital for her survival. You have your supervising nurse and the emergency physician come to see her immediately. As you participate in this patient's care, clear communication among the team members is essential.

Lesson 8.1
FEMALE REPRODUCTIVE SYSTEM

External Genitalia and Vagina

Lesson Objectives

Both the female and male reproductive systems are dormant until puberty, when the gonads (ovaries in the female and testes in the male) begin to secrete significant quantities of sex hormones (estrogen and progesterone in the female, androgens in the male). In the female, the external genitalia become more prominent, pubic hair develops, the vagina becomes lubricated, and breast enlargement occurs. Understanding the anatomy and physiology of the mature external genitalia and vagina is an important introduction to the female reproductive system.

The information in this lesson will enable you to:

8.1.1 Identify the female external genitalia.

8.1.2 Detail the anatomy and physiology of the vagina.

8.1.3 Discuss the disorders of the vagina.

8.1.4 Describe common sexually transmitted diseases.

Abbreviations

GYN	gynecology
OB	obstetrics
RN	registered nurse

Keynote

- **Obstetrics (OB)** is the medical specialty for the care of women during pregnancy and the **postpartum** period.
- **Gynecology (GYN)** is the medical specialty for the care of the female reproductive system.

LO 8.1 External Genitalia

The area between the thighs extending from the coccyx to the **pubis** is called the **perineum**. The female external genitalia occupy most of the perineum and are collectively called the **vulva** *(Figure 8.1)*. The structures of the vulva include the:

- **Mons pubis**—a mound of skin and adipose tissue overlying the symphysis pubis. In **postpubescent** females, it is covered with **pubic** hair.
- **Labia majora**—a pair of thick folds of skin, connective tissue, and adipose tissue. In postpubescent females, their outer surface is covered with coarse hair, and the inner surface has numerous sweat and sebaceous glands.
- **Labia minora**—a pair of thin folds of hairless skin immediately internal to the labia majora. Sebaceous glands are present on these folds, together with melanocytes *(see Chapter 4)* that give the folds a dark melanin pigmentation. Anteriorly, the labia minora join together to form the prepuce (hood) of the clitoris. Posteriorly they merge with the labia majora.
- **Clitoris**—a small erectile body capped with a glans. It has two corpora cavernosa surrounded by connective tissue. The clitoris contains many sensory nerve receptors.

Deep to the labia majora on either side of the vaginal orifice is an erectile body called the **vestibular bulb** *(Figure 8.1b)*. The two bulbs become congested with blood and more sensitive during sexual arousal. Posterior to the vestibular bulbs on each side of the **vaginal** orifice is a pea-sized **greater vestibular gland (Bartholin gland).** These glands secrete mucin, which lubricates the vagina. Secretion is increased during sexual arousal and intercourse.

(a)

(b)

▲ **Figure 8.1** Female Perineum and Vulva. (a) Surface anatomy. (b) Subcutaneous structures.

WORD	PRONUNCIATION		ELEMENTS	DEFINITION
clitoris	**KLIT**-oh-ris		Greek *clitoris*	Erectile organ of the vulva
greater vestibular gland (also known as Bartholin gland)	**GRATE**-ur ves-**TIB**-you-lar GLAND		Casper Bartholin the Younger, 1655-1738, Danish anatomist	Pea-sized glands on the posterolateral walls of the vagina that secrete mucus.
gynecology	guy-nih-**KOL**-oh-jee	S/ R/CF	**-logy** *study of* **gynec/o-** *female*	Medical specialty for the care of the female reproductive system
gynecologist	guy-nih-**KOL**-oh-jist	S/	**-logist** *specialist*	Specialist in gynecology
labium labia (pl)	**LAY**-bee-um **LAY**-bee-ah		Greek *lip*	Fold of the vulva
majus majora (pl)	**MAY**-jus **MAY**-jor-ah		Latin *greater*	Bigger or greater; for example, labia majora
minus minora (pl)	**MY**-nus **MY**-nor-ah		Latin *smaller*	Smaller or lesser; for example, labia minora
mons pubis	MONZ **PYU**-bis		**mons** Latin *mountain* **pubis** Latin *pubic bone*	Fleshy pad with pubic hair, overlying the pubic bone
obstetrics (OB)	ob-**STET**-riks		Latin *a midwife*	Medical specialty for the care of women during pregnancy and the postpartum period
obstetrician	ob-steh-**TRISH**-un	S/ R/	**-ician** *expert, specialist* **obstetr-** *midwifery*	Medical specialist in obstetrics
perineum	**PER**-ih-**NEE**-um		Latin *perineum*	Area between the thighs, extending from the coccyx to the pubis
perineal (adj)	**PER**-ih-**NEE**-al	S/ R/	**-al** *pertaining to* **perine-** *perineum*	Pertaining to the perineum
postpubescent	post-pyu-**BESS**-ent	S/ P/ R/	**-ent** *pertaining to, end result* **post-** *after* **-pubesc-** *to reach puberty*	After the period of puberty
puberty	**PYU**-ber-tee	S/ R/	**-ty** *quality, state* **puber-** *growing up*	Process of maturing from child to young adult capable of reproducing
pubis pubic (adj)	**PYU**-bis **PYU**-bik	S/ R/	Latin *pubic bone* **-ic** *pertaining to* **pub-** *pubis*	Bony front arch of the pelvis of the hip; also called pubic bone Pertaining to the pubis
ruga rugae (pl)	**ROO**-gah **ROO**-jee		Latin *a wrinkle*	A fold, ridge, or crease
vestibule vestibular (adj)	**VES**-tih-byul ves-**TIB**-you-lar	S/ R/	Latin *entrance* **-ar** *pertaining to* **vestibul-** *vestibule*	Space at the entrance of a canal Pertaining to a vestibule
vestibular bulb	ves-**TIB**-you-lar BULB		Latin *bulb, onion*	Structure on each side of the entrance to the vagina
vulva	**VUL**-vah		Latin *a wrapper or covering*	Female external genitalia
vulvar (adj)		S/	**-ar** *pertaining to*	Pertaining to the vulva

Exercises

A. Latin and Greek terms cannot be further deconstructed into prefix, root, or suffix. *You must know them for what they are. Match the meaning in the left column with the correct medical term in the right column.* **LO 8.1**

_____ **1.** A covering or wrapper   **a.** labia

_____ **2.** Mountain   **b.** vulva

_____ **3.** Lesser   **c.** minora

_____ **4.** Lip   **d.** mons

Uterus
Urinary bladder
Pubic symphysis
Urethra

Uterine tube
Ovary
Cervix of uterus
Rectum
Vagina

Anterior   **Posterior**

▲ **Figure 8.2** Female Reproductive Organs.

LO 8.1 The Vagina

The **vagina**, or birth canal, is a fibromuscular tube, 4 to 5 inches (10 to 13 cm) in length *(Figure 8.2)*. It connects the vulva with the uterus. It has three main functions:

- Discharge of menstrual fluid
- Receipt of the penis and semen
- Birth of a baby

The vagina is located between the rectum and the urethra. The urethra is embedded in its anterior wall. In the wall of the vagina around the urethra are several small **paraurethral (Skene) glands** that open into the urethra.

At its posterior end, the vagina extends beyond the **cervix** of the uterus to form blind spaces called the anterior and posterior **fornices**. The lower end of the vagina contains numerous transverse folds, or rugae. A thin membranous fold, highly variable in appearance and thickness, stretches across the external opening of the vagina to form the **hymen**. The intact hymen contains one or two openings to allow the escape of menstrual fluid.

LO 8.2 Disorders of External Genitalia and Vagina

Bacterial vaginosis is the most common cause of **vaginitis** in women of childbearing age. In bacterial vaginosis, the different types of invading bacteria outnumber the normal bacteria of the vagina. The main symptom is an abnormal vaginal discharge with a fishlike odor. Diagnosis is made by laboratory examination of a specimen taken by vaginal swab.

Toxic shock syndrome is a life-threatening illness caused by toxins circulating in the bloodstream. Certain rare strains of bacteria produce these toxins. In the most common form of toxic shock syndrome, the bacteria are in the vagina of women, and their growth is encouraged by the presence of a superabsorbent **tampon** that is not changed frequently *(see Case Report (CR) 8.1)*.

Vulvovaginal candidiasis is a common cause of genital itching or burning, with a "cottage-cheese" **vaginal** discharge. It is caused by an overgrowth of the yeast fungus called *Candida* and can occur after taking antibiotics. Recent research has found that it is associated with vitamin D deficiency. Diagnosis is made by microscopic examination of a specimen taken by a vaginal swab.

Allergic and irritative causes of **vulvovaginitis** can be caused by vaginal hygiene products, spermicides, detergents, and synthetic underwear.

Vulvodynia is a chronic, lasting, severe pain around the vaginal orifice, which feels raw. Painful intercourse (**dyspareunia**) is common. The vulva may look normal or be slightly swollen. The etiology is unknown.

 Case Report (CR) 8.1 *(continued)*

In the opening Case Report to this chapter, Ms. Lara Baker presented to the Emergency Department with toxic shock syndrome. Because of her heavy period, she was using a superabsorbent tampon. She was admitted to intensive care. The **tampon** was removed and cultured, IV fluids and antibiotics were administered, and her kidney and liver functions were monitored. The causative organism was ***Staphylococcus aureus.*** She recovered well but had a second episode 6 months later.

WORD	PRONUNCIATION	ELEMENTS		DEFINITION
Candida candidiasis (also called **thrush**)	**KAN**-did-ah kan-dih-**DIE**-ah-sis	S/ R/	Latin *dazzling white* -iasis *state of, condition* candid- *Candida, a yeast*	A yeastlike fungus Infection with the yeastlike fungus *Candida*
fornix fornices (pl)	**FOR**-niks **FOR**-nih-seez		Latin *arch, vault*	Arch-shaped, blind-ended part of the vagina behind and around the cervix
dyspareunia	dis-pah-**RUE**-nee-ah	S/ P/ R/	-ia *condition* dys- *painful* -pareun- *lying beside, sexual intercourse*	Pain during sexual intercourse
hymen	**HIGH**-men		Greek *membrane*	Thin membrane partly occluding the vaginal orifice
paraurethral glands (also known as Skene glands)	**PAR**-ah-you-**REE**-thral GLANDZ SKEEN GLANDZ	S/ P/ R/	-al *pertaining to* para- *alongside* -urethr- *urethra* Alexander Skene, 1838–1900, New York gynecologist	Glands in the anterior wall of the vagina that secrete mucin to lubricate the vagina
vagina vaginal (adj)	vah-**JIE**-nah **VAJ**-in-al	S/ R/	Latin *a sheath* -al *pertaining to* vagin- *vagina*	Female genital canal extending from the uterus to the vulva Pertaining to the vagina
vaginosis vaginitis	vah-jih-**NOH**-sis vah-jih-**NIE**-tis	S/ R/ S/	-osis *condition* vagin- *vagina* -itis *inflammation*	Any disease of the vagina Inflammation of the vagina
vulvodynia	vul-voh-**DIN**-ee-uh	S/ R/CF	-dynia *pain* vulv/o- *vulva*	Chronic vulvar pain
vulvovaginal (adj)	**VUL**-voh-**VAJ**-ih-nal	S/ R/CF R/	-al *pertaining to* vulv/o- *vulva* -vagin- *vagina*	Pertaining to the vulva and vagina
vulvovaginitis	**VUL**-voh-vaj-ih-**NIE**-tis	S/ R/CF R/	-itis *inflammation* vulv/o- *vulva* -vagin- *vagina*	Inflammation of the vagina and vulva

Exercises

A. After reading *Case Report 8.1, answer the following questions. For multiple choice questions, select the correct answer. For the fill-in-the-blank questions, enter the correct term.* **LO 8.2, 8.A**

1. From Case Report 8.1, what was the diagnosis?

   a. vulvodynia

   b. toxic shock syndrome

   c. dyspareunia

2. Is the causative agent for the patient's condition bacterial or viral? _____

3. How would you classify her body temperature?

   a. high

   b. low

   c. normal

LO 8.3 Sexually Transmitted Diseases

Keynotes

- Infection with gonorrhea can be prevented by using a condom.
- A DNA probe is a diagnostic test where a sample of the affected area is taken with a cotton swab. The sample is then analyzed for the presence of the DNA of bacteria *Chlamydia trachomatis* and/or *N. gonorrhoeae*.

According to the **Centers for Disease Control and Prevention (CDC)**, 15 million cases of sexually transmitted diseases **(STDs)** are reported annually in the United States, with adolescents and young adults being at the greatest risk. Some of the common STDs are described as follows:

Chlamydia infection is known as the "silent" disease because infected women and men have no symptoms. When there are signs, a vaginal or penile discharge and irritation with dysuria are common.

Untreated, chlamydia can spread higher into the female reproductive tract and cause **pelvic inflammatory disease (PID)**. It can be passed on to a newborn during childbirth, causing eye infections or pneumonia. It is a reason why antibiotic eyedrops are given to newborns.

Gonorrhea is spread by unprotected sex and can be passed on to a baby in childbirth, causing a serious eye infection. This is another reason why newborns are given eyedrops. Symptoms in both male and female adults may not be present. In the female, they can include a vaginal discharge, bleeding, and dysuria. Gonorrhea is also a cause of PID.

Syphilis, caused by a **spirochete**, is transmitted sexually and can then spread through the bloodstream to every organ in the body. It is also transmitted among intravenous drug users who share needles. **Primary syphilis** begins 10 to 90 days after infection as an ulcer, a **chancre**, at the place of infection (*Figure 8.3*). Four to 10 weeks later, if the primary syphilis is not treated, **secondary syphilis** appears as a rash on the hands and soles of the feet, with swollen glands and muscle and joint pain. **Tertiary syphilis** can occur years after the primary infection and can cause permanent damage to the brain with dementia. Because primary syphilis is curable with penicillin or other antibiotics, tertiary syphilis is rarely seen today. A pregnant woman with untreated syphilis can transmit the infection to her fetus before birth.

Chancroid is an ulcerative disease (not caused by a spirochete) and is without systemwide effects, unlike syphilis. It develops as a chancre with swollen, tender lymph nodes in the groin.

Trichomoniasis ("trich") is caused by the parasite *Trichomonas vaginalis.* Men can carry the infection in their urethra and almost never have symptoms. The vagina is the common site of infection in women. It can produce a frothy yellow-green discharge with irritation and itching of the vulva. It is called a "ping-pong" infection because if both partners are not treated, the infection will be given back and forth to the partners.

Molluscum contagiosum is caused by a virus that can be sexually transmitted; the resulting tumors are small, shiny bumps that have a milky-white fluid inside (*Figure 8.4*). They can disappear and reappear anywhere on the body. Molluscum contagiosum is often seen in children and is not sexually transmitted in such cases.

▲ **Figure 8.3** Chancre of Primary Syphilis in Female.
©CNRI/Photo Researchers, Inc.

▲ **Figure 8.4** Molluscum Contagiosum. ©Biophoto Associates/Photo Researchers, Inc.

WORD	PRONUNCIATION		ELEMENTS	DEFINITION
chancre	**SHAN**-ker		Latin *cancer*	Primary lesion of syphilis
chancroid	**SHAN**-kroyd	S/ R	**-oid** *resembling* **chancr-** *chancre*	Infectious, painful, ulcerative STD not related to syphilis
chlamydia	klah-**MID**-ee-ah		Latin *cloak*	A species of bacteria causing an STD
gonorrhea	gon-oh-**REE**-ah	S/ R/CF	**-rrhea** *flow or discharge* **gon/o-** *seed*	Specific contagious sexually transmitted infection
molluscum contagiosum (**Note:** The "s" in contagiosum is added to make the word flow.)	moh-**LUS**-kum kon-**TAY**-jee-oh-sum	S/ R/ R/CF	**-um** *structure* **mollusc-** *soft* **contagi/o-** *transmissible by contact*	STD caused by a virus
spirochete	**SPY**-roh-keet	S/ R/CF	**-chete** *hair* **spir/o-** *spiral*	Spiral-shaped bacterium causing an STD (syphilis)
syphilis	**SIF**-ih-lis		Possibly from Latin poem "Syphilis Sive Morbus Gallicus," by Fracastorius Alteration	Sexually transmitted disease caused by a spirochete
Trichomonas trichomoniasis	trik-oh-**MOH**-nas **TRIK**-oh-moh-**NIE**-ah-sis	S/ R/CF R/	**-iasis** *condition* **trich/o-** *hair, flagellum* **-mon-** *single*	A parasite causing an STD Infection with *Trichomonas vaginalis*

Exercises

A. Disease. *Test your knowledge of diseases. Anyone working in a gynecology clinic or internal medicine practice will have patients diagnosed with sexually transmitted diseases. Make the correct association between the name of the STD and its description by matching the statement in the left column with the medical term in the right column.* **LO 8.3, 8.A**

_____ 1. "Silent disease"

_____ 2. Chancre appears at the place of infection

_____ 3. Female symptoms include dysuria and vaginal discharge

_____ 4. Chlamydia or gonorrhea can cause this

_____ 5. Can cause dementia if untreated

_____ 6. Appears as a rash with joint pain

_____ 7. "Ping-pong" infection

_____ 8. Ulcerative disease not caused by a spirochete

a. secondary syphilis

b. trichomoniasis

c. chlamydia

d. primary syphilis

e. pelvic inflammatory disease

f. tertiary syphilis

g. chancroid

h. gonorrhea

B. Sexually transmitted diseases have different causative agents. *Use the provided word bank to fill in the blanks.* **LO 8.3, 8.A**

| *trichomoniasis* | *molluscum contagiosum* | *syphilis* | *gonorrhea* |

1. This disease is caused by a spirochete. _____

2. A virus is responsible for causing this disease. _____

3. This disease is caused by a parasite. _____

4. This disease is caused by bacteria. _____

Vesicles

▲ **Figure 8.5** **Genital Herpes Simplex in Male.** ©Biophoto Associates/Photo Researchers, Inc.

Abbreviations

AIDS	acquired immu-nodeficiency syndrome
C-section	cesarean section
ELISA	enzyme-linked immunosorbent assay
HIV	human immunode-ficiency virus
HPV	human papilloma virus
HSV	herpes simplex virus
Pap	papanicolaou

LO 8.3 Sexually Transmitted Diseases (continued)

Genital herpes simplex is a disease caused by the virus **herpes simplex type 2 (HSV-2)** *(Figure 8.5)*. The sores are painful, and the disease can present with fever; joint pains; and enlarged, tender lymph nodes. The genital sores can recur throughout life. After the initial infection, the virus remains dormant in the dorsal root ganglia of nerves. Blisters around the mouth ("cold sores") are caused by a related virus, **herpes simplex type 1 (HSV-1)**.

Herpes of the newborn occurs when a pregnant woman with genital herpes sores delivers her baby vaginally and transmits the virus to the baby *(Figure 8.6)*. Because the baby's immune system is not well developed, the infection is destructive and can be fatal. If there is evidence of genital herpes lesions in the mother, the fetus should be delivered by cesarean section (C-section).

Human papilloma virus (HPV) causes genital warts in both men and women *(Figure 8.7)* and can also cause changes to the cells in the cervix. Some strains of the virus can increase a woman's risk for **cervical** cancer.

Medications such as podophyllin, trichloracetic acid, and *Aldara* cream can be applied to the warts, and cryotherapy or laser therapy also can be used. Because of the sites of the warts around the genitalia, condoms cannot provide complete protection.

Human immunodeficiency virus (HIV) is a virus that attacks the immune system and usually leads to **acquired immunodeficiency syndrome (AIDS)**. Because HIV is carried in body fluids, it is transmitted during unprotected sex. Sharing needles can spread the virus. The virus also can pass from an infected pregnant woman to her unborn child, and she must take medications to protect the baby.

Symptoms often do not appear until years after the initial infection. The initial symptoms of HIV are similar to the flu. A person is diagnosed HIV-positive using a blood test that identifies antibodies to the virus **(ELISA),** with a confirmatory western blot that identifies the specific antibody proteins. The CDC considers an HIV-infected person with a CD4 count below 200 to have AIDS, whether the person is sick or well; CD4 cells, also known as helper T cells, play key roles in the body's defense mechanisms.

HIV damages the immune system, so infections will develop that the body would normally cope with easily. These are **opportunistic infections** and include herpes simplex, candidiasis, syphilis, and tuberculosis.

▲ **Figure 8.7** HPV in the Female Vulva. Source: Joe Miller/Centers for Disease Control and Prevention

Herpes simplex vesicles

▲ **Figure 8.6** **Premature Baby Born with Herpes Simplex Infection.** ©Dr. M.A. Ansary/Photo Researchers, Inc.

WORD	PRONUNCIATION	ELEMENTS		DEFINITION
acquired immunodeficiency syndrome (AIDS)	ah-KWIRED IM-you-noh-de-FISH-en-see SIN-drome	S/ R/CF R/ P/ R/	**acquired** Latin *obtain* **-ency** *condition* **immun/o-** *immune response* **-defici-** *lacking, inadequate* **syn-** *together* **-drome** *running*	Infection with the HIV virus
herpes simplex virus (HSV)	HER-peez SIM-pleks VIE-rus	R/	**herpes** Greek *spreading skin eruption* **virus** *poison*	An infection that manifests with painful, watery blisters on the skin and mucous membranes
human immunodeficiency virus (HIV)	HYU-man IM-you-noh-dee-FISH-en-see VIE-rus	S/ R/CF R/ R/	**human** Latin *human being* **-ency** *condition* **immun/o-** *immune response* **-defici-** *lacking, inadequate* **virus** *poison*	Etiologic agent of AIDS
human papilloma virus (HPV)	HYU-man pap-ih-LOH-mah VIE-rus	S/ R/ R/	**human** Latin *human being* **-oma** *tumor* **papill-** *pimple* **virus** *poison*	An infection that causes warts on the skin and genitalia and can increase the risk for cervical cancer
opportunistic infection (*Note:* This term contains two suffixes.)	OP-or-tyu-NIS-tik in-FEK-shun	S/ S/ R/ S/ R/	**-ic** *pertaining to* **-ist-** *specialist in* **opportun-** *take advantage of* **-ion** *action, condition, process* **infect-** *corrupt, internal invasion, infection*	An infection that causes disease when the immune system is compromised for other reasons

Exercises

A. Disease. *Continue working with the medical terminology for sexually transmitted diseases. Make the correct association between the description of the disease in the left column and its medical term listed in the right column.* **LO 8.3, 8.F**

_____ 1. Causes cold sores around the mouth

_____ 2. Infection with this virus can lead to AIDS

_____ 3. Causes painful genital sores

_____ 4. Increases risk for cervical cancer

_____ 5. Infections that would not normally develop in healthy persons

_____ 6. Diagnosed when CD4 count is less than 200

_____ 7. Transmitted during vaginal delivery

a. herpes simplex type 2

b. AIDS

c. herpes of the newborn

d. HPV

e. herpes simplex type 1

f. opportunistic

g. HIV

Lesson 8.2

FEMALE REPRODUCTIVE SYSTEM

Ovaries, Uterine Tubes, and Uterus

Lesson Objectives

The female gonads, the primary sex organs, are the ovaries. The female internal accessory organs include a pair of uterine (fallopian) tubes, a uterus, and a vagina. Women are born with all the eggs (ova) that they will release, but it is not until puberty that the eggs mature and start to leave the ovary. The ovarian hormones, estrogen and progesterone, are involved in menstruation and pregnancy (PGY). The pituitary gland at the base of the brain produces other hormones that control the functions of the ovaries, uterus, and breast (see Chapter 17).

These complex interactions are the core of the human reproductive system and an essential part of understanding the human body. The information in this lesson will enable you to:

8.2.1 Describe the anatomy of an ovary, the fallopian tubes, and the uterus.

8.2.2 Identify the major events of oogenesis.

8.2.3 List the functions of estrogen and progesterone.

8.2.4 Explain the control of the pituitary gland over the female reproductive system.

8.2.5 Discuss the female menstrual cycle.

LO 8.4 Anatomy of the Female Reproductive Tract

Ovaries

Each **ovary** is an almond-shaped organ located in a shallow depression (ovarian fossa) in the lateral wall of the pelvic cavity *(Figure 8.8)*. The ovary is about 1 inch (2.5 cm) long and ½ inch (1.3 cm) in diameter. It is enclosed in a capsule called the *tunica albuginea*. Each ovary is held in place by ligaments that attach it to the pelvic wall and uterus.

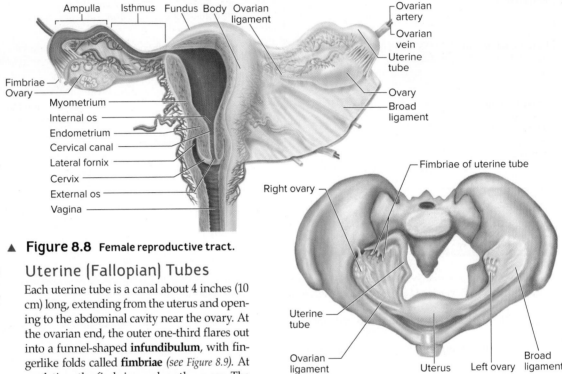

▲ **Figure 8.8** Female reproductive tract.

Uterine (Fallopian) Tubes

Each uterine tube is a canal about 4 inches (10 cm) long, extending from the uterus and opening to the abdominal cavity near the ovary. At the ovarian end, the outer one-third flares out into a funnel-shaped **infundibulum**, with fingerlike folds called **fimbriae** *(see Figure 8.9)*. At ovulation, the fimbriae enclose the ovary. The inner one-third of each tube approaching the uterus is called the **isthmus**. The tubes are supported by the broad ligament.

The wall of the tube has an inner layer of mucosal cells that secrete mucus. Some are ciliated. The cilia beat toward the uterus and transport the egg down the uterine tube with peristaltic contractions, a journey that takes three or four days.

The ovaries and uterine tubes are called the **adnexa** of the uterus.

▲ **Figure 8.9** Ovaries. The ovaries are located on each side against the lateral walls of the pelvic cavity. The right uterine tube is retracted to reveal the ovarian ligament.

Keynote

The wall of the uterus has three layers. From the outside, these are:

• The **perimetrium**—a continuation of the broad ligament.

• The **myometrium**—a thick layer of smooth muscle.

• The **endometrium**—the lining that sheds in menstruation.

Uterus

The uterus is a thick-walled, muscular organ in the pelvic cavity. It normally tilts forward **(anteverted)** over the urinary bladder. Anatomically, it is divided into three regions:

• **Fundus**—the broad, curved upper region between the lateral attachments of the uterine tubes.

• **Body**—the midportion.

• **Cervix**—the cylindrical inferior portion that projects into the vagina.

The cavity of the uterus is triangular, with its upper two corners receiving the openings of the uterine tubes. Its lower end communicates with the vagina through the **cervical canal,** which has an **internal os** from the lumen and an **external os** into the vagina (see Figure 8.8).

The cervical canal contains mucous glands; secretions of mucus help prevent the spread of infection from the vagina. The uterus is supported by the muscular floor of the pelvic outlet and by ligaments that extend to the pelvic wall from the uterus and cervix.

WORD	PRONUNCIATION		ELEMENTS	DEFINITION
adnexa (pl) adnexum (sing)	ad-**NEK**-sa ad-**NEK**-sum	S/ R/	Latin *connected parts* -**um** *structure* **adnex-** *connected parts*	Parts accessory to an organ or structure
adnexal (adj)	ad-**NEK**-sal	S/	-**al** *pertaining to*	Pertaining to accessory structures; for example, structures alongside the uterus, uterine tubes, and ovaries
anteverted	an-teh-**VERT**-ed	S/ P/ R/	-**ed** *pertaining to* **ante-** *before, forward* -**vert-** *to turn*	Tilted forward
anteversion	an-teh-**VER**-shun	S/	-**ion** *condition, process*	Forward tilting of the uterus
endometrium	en-doh-**MEE**-tree-um	S/ P/ R/	-**ium** *structure* **endo-** *within, inside* -**metr-** *uterus*	Inner lining of the uterus
endometrial (adj)	en-doh-**ME**-tree-al	S/	-**ial** *pertaining to*	Pertaining to the inner lining of the uterus
fimbria fimbriae (pl)	**FIM**-bree-ah **FIM**-bree-ee		Latin *fringe*	A fringe-like structure on the surface of a cell or a microorganism
fundus	**FUN**-dus		Latin *bottom*	Part farthest from the opening of a hollow organ
infundibulum infundibula (pl)	**IN**-fun-**DIB**-you-lum **IN**-fun-**DIB**-you-lah		Latin *funnel*	Funnel-shaped structure
isthmus	**IS**-mus		Greek *isthmus*	Part connecting two larger parts; in this case, the uterus to the uterine tube
myometrium	my-oh-**MEE**-tree-um	S/ R/CF R/	-**ium** *tissue* **my/o-** *muscle* -**metr-** *uterus*	Muscle wall of the uterus
os	OS		Latin *mouth*	Opening into a canal; for example, the cervix
ovary ovaries (pl)	**OH**-va-ree **OH**-vah-rees		Latin *egg*	One of the paired female egg-producing glands
ovarian (adj)	oh-**VAIR**-ee-an	S/ R/	-**an** *pertaining to* **ovari-** *ovary*	Pertaining to the ovary
perimetrium	per-ih-**MEE**-tree-um	S/ P/ R/	-**ium** *structure* **peri-** *around* -**metr-** *uterus*	The covering of the uterus; part of the peritoneum
uterus uterine (adj)	**YOU**-ter-us **YOU**-ter-ine	S/ R/	Latin *womb* -**ine** *pertaining to, substance* **uter-** *uterus*	Organ in which an egg develops into a fetus Pertaining to the uterus
uterine tubes (also called fallopian tubes)	**YOU**-ter-ine TUBES fah-**LOH**-pee-an TUBES			Tubes connected from the uterus to the abdominal cavity. Carry the ovum from the ovary to the uterus.

Exercises

A. Demonstrate your understanding of the language of *gynecology*. *Select the correct answer that completes each statement.* LO 8.4, 8.D

1. What is the "collective" (as a group) medical term for the ovaries and uterine tubes?

   a. infundibulum   **b.** fossa   **c.** os   **d.** adnexa

2. Another name for the uterine tube is the _____ tube.

   a. cervical   **b.** os   **c.** fallopian   **d.** ovarian

3. The fingerlike folds that envelope the ovary are the:

   a. os   **b.** adnexa   **c.** fimbriae   **d.** ampulla

4. The opening of a canal is the:

   a. os   **b.** cervix   **c.** infundibulum   **d.** fundus

5. In the term *anteversion,* the prefix means:

   a. to turn   **b.** before, forward   **c.** within   **d.** pertaining to

6. In the term *endometrium,* the prefix means:

   a. outer   **b.** inner   **c.** surrounding   **d.** structure   **e.** around

Developmental Sequence

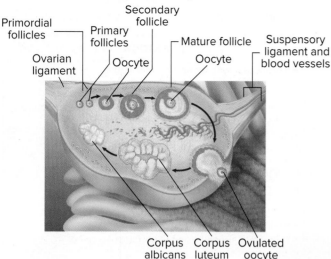

▲ Figure 8.10
Oogenesis. The development of the oocyte begins with the primordial follicles.

LO 8.5 Oogenesis and Ovulation

During **prenatal** development, small groups of cells within the female fetus's ovarian cortex form around 2 million **follicles**. In each group of cells, there is a single large cell, the primary **oocyte**, surrounded by a layer of **follicular cells.** Many of these follicular cells degenerate. Under normal circumstances, there are are no further changes within ovarian follicles until puberty.

At puberty, some 400,000 primary oocytes remain, each containing 23 pairs of chromosomes. They undergo meiosis to produce secondary oocytes, each containing 23 single chromosomes. As they mature, the follicular cells form a fluid-filled **primary follicle,** in which the oocyte is located *(Figure 8.10)*. **Oogenesis** begins in the fetal period and ends at menopause *(see Figure 8.11)*. Surrounding the oocyte (egg) and lining the fluid-filled **antrum** of the follicle are **granulosa cells** that secrete estrogen.

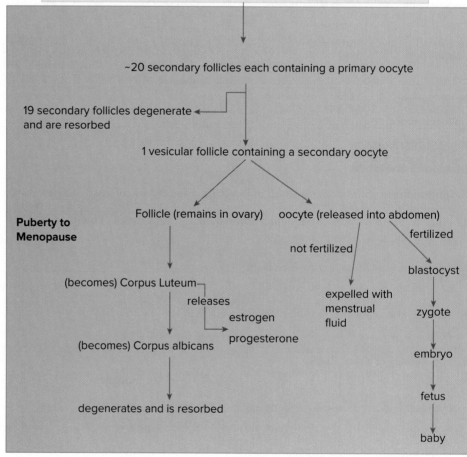

▲ Figure 8.11 Oogenesis from fetal period through menopause.

WORD	PRONUNCIATION	ELEMENTS		DEFINITION
antrum	**AN**-trum		Greek *cave*	A nearly closed cavity or chamber
corpus albicans	**KOR**-pus **AL**-bih-kanz		**albicans** Latin *white* **corpus** Latin *body*	An atrophied corpus luteum
corpus luteum	**KOR**-pus **LOO**-tee-um		**luteum** Latin *yellow*	Yellow structure formed at the site of a ruptured ovarian follicle
granulosa cell	gran-you-**LOH**-sah SELL	S/ R/	-osa *like* **granul-** *small grain*	Cell lining the ovarian follicle
menopause	**MEN**-oh-paws	R/CF R/	**men/o** *menses* **pause**, *cessation*	Permanent ending of menstrual periods.
oocyte	**OH**-oh-site	S/ R/CF	-cyte *cell* **o/o-** *egg*	Female egg cell
oogenesis Note: The *genesis* R/CF is used most often in a suffix position.	oh-oh-**JEN**-eh-sis	R/CF	-genesis *form, create*	Development of female egg cell
ovulation	**OV**-you-**LAY**-shun	S/ R/	-ation *process* **ovul-** *egg*	Release of an oocyte from a follicle
ovulate (verb)	**OV**-you-late	S/	-ate *composed of, pertaining to*	To release an oocyte from a follicle
prenatal	pree-**NAY**-tal	S/ P/ R/	-al *pertaining to* **pre-** *before* **-nat-** *born*	Before birth

Exercises

A. Apply your knowledge *of the female reproductive system by choosing the correct answer:* **LO 8.5, 8.7, 8.A**

1. The permanent ending of menstrual periods is:

   a. menopause   **b.** amennorhea   **c.** involution

2. The release of a female egg is called:

   a. oogenesis   **b.** ovulation   **c.** involution

3. Which is the correct spelling for the term?

   a. ooginesis   **b.** oogenisis   **c.** oogenesis

B. Describe the events and structures of oogenesis and ovulation. *Select the answer that correctly completes each statement.* **LO 8.5**

1. At which stage of human growth are follicles developed?

   a. puberty   **b.** menopause   **c.** fetal   **d.** childhood

2. Oocytes are contained in a:

   a. follicle   **b.** corpus albicans   **c.** corpus luteum   **d.** zygote

3. The fluid-filled area of the follicle is the:

   a. corpus luteum   **b.** antrum   **c.** oocyte   **d.** granulosum

Keynotes

- Menarche cannot occur until at least 17% of a girl's weight is body fat.
- High levels of estrogen and progesterone inhibit the secretion of GnRH. This is the basis for most forms of contraceptive medications.

Abbreviations

FSH	follicle-stimulating hormone
GnRH	gonadotropin-releasing hormone
LH	luteinizing hormone

LO 8.5 Ovulation

At the beginning of the menstrual cycle, as many as 20 primary follicles can start the maturing process, but only one develops fully. The remainder degenerate. By the midpoint of the menstrual cycle, the mature follicle bulges out on the surface of the ovary and ruptures **(ovulation)**. The oocyte and lining cells from the follicle can either be taken into the uterine tube or fall into the pelvic cavity and degenerate.

During the time that the follicles are developing and maturing, the endometrium is undergoing cyclical changes that are under the influence of hormones. The first phase occurs for 5 days and is the shedding of the endometrial lining. After this phase, the endometrial lining begins to rebuild in preparation to protect and nourish the fertilized egg. In the final phase, the endometrium becomes rich in blood supply and in the development of glands. If the ovum is unfertilized, then the uterine cycle starts over again, beginning with the shedding of the endometrium.

LO 8.6 Ovarian Hormones

The ovaries of the sexually mature female secrete **estrogens** and **progesterone**.

Estrogens are produced in the ovarian follicles. Their sexual functions are to:

1. Convert girls into sexually mature women through the onset of breast development, the growth of pubic hair, and the establishment of menstruation.
2. Participate in the menstrual cycle *(see Figure 8.12)*.
3. Participate in pregnancy when that occurs.

Progesterone is produced by the corpus luteum of the ovary and by the adrenal glands *(see Chapter 17)*. Its sexual functions are to:

1. Prepare the lining of the uterus for implantation of the egg *(see Figure 8.12)*.
2. Inhibit lactation during pregnancy.
3. Produce menstrual bleeding if pregnancy does not occur.

The synthesis and secretion of estrogen is stimulated by **follicle-stimulating hormone (FSH)** from the pituitary gland. FSH is controlled by the hypothalamic **gonadotropin-releasing hormone (GnRH)**. Progesterone production is stimulated by **luteinizing hormone (LH)** from the pituitary gland, which is also stimulated by GnRH.

The ovaries also secrete small amounts of androgens, male hormones.

LO 8.7 The Uterine (Menstrual) Cycle

The menstrual cycle averages 28 days in length. It begins with a 2-week follicular phase. The beginning of the cycle is recognized by physiologists as menstruation, which occurs during the first 3 to 5 days.

After menstruation ends, the uterus starts to replace the endometrial tissue lost during menstruation. The developing ovarian follicles mature, and one of them ovulates around day 14. Around this time, the fimbriae of the uterine tube envelope the ovaries and, in time with the mother's heartbeat, caress the released ovum to guide it into the uterine tube.

After ovulation, in the postovulatory phase, the endometrial lining continues to grow. The residual ovarian follicle becomes a **corpus luteum** containing **lutein** cells that are involved in progesterone production. Around day 24, the corpus luteum **involutes**. By day 26, it is an inactive scar called a **corpus albicans**. At this time, the arteries supplying the endometrium of the uterus contract. This leads to ischemia, tissue necrosis, and the start of menstruation.

▶ **Figure 8.12** Menstrual Cycle.

WORD	PRONUNCIATION	ELEMENTS		DEFINITION
estrogen	**ESS**-troh-gen	S/ R/CF	**-gen** *create, produce* **estr/o** *woman*	Generic term for hormones that stimulate female secondary sex characteristics
follicle	**FOLL**-ih-kull		Latin *small sac*	Spherical mass of cells containing a cavity, such as a hair follicle
follicular (adj)	fo-**LIK**-you-lar	S/ R/	**-ar** *pertaining to* **follicul-** *follicle*	Pertaining to a follicle
gonadotropin	**GO**-nad-oh-**TROH**-pin	S/ R/CF	**-tropin** *nourishing* **gonad/o-** *gonad*	Hormone capable of promoting gonad function
involution involute (verb)	in-voh-**LOO**-shun in-vol-**LUTE**	S/ P/ R/	**-ion** *process* **in-** *in* **-volut-** *shrink*	A decrease in size or vigor
menses menstruation	**MEN**-seez men-stru-**A**-shun	S/ R/CF	Latin *month* **-ation** *action* **menstr/u**	Monthly uterine bleeding Monthly uterine bleeding
menstruate menstrual	**MEN**-stru-ate **MEN**-stru-al	S/ S/	**-ate** *pertaining to* **-al** *pertaining to*	The act of menstruation Pertaining to menstruation
progesterone (**note:** two suffixes)	pro-**JESS**-ter-own	S/ S/ P/ R/	**-one** *hormone* **-er-** *agent* **pro-** *before* **-gest-** *pregnancy*	A steroid hormone released by the corpus luteum and involved in the menstrual cycle, pregnancy, and the development of an embryo

Exercises

A. Construct these medical terms. *Given the definition, fill in the blank with the missing word element.* **LO 8.5, 8.6, 8.C**

1. A decrease in size or vigor   in/ _____ /ion

2. Hormone that prepares the uterus for pregnancy   _____ /gest/er/one

3. The act of menstruation   menstru/ _____

4. Hormone that promotes female secondary sex characteristics   _____ /gen

5. Development of female egg cell   _____ /genesis

6. Pertaining to a follicle   follicul/ _____

Lesson 8.3

Disorders of the Female Reproductive Tract

Lesson Objectives

Use correct medical terminology to:

8.3.1 Describe disorders of the ovaries, uterus, and fallopian (uterine) tubes, and their effects on a woman's health.

8.3.2 Discuss the etiologies of infertility and modern treatments for the condition.

8.3.3 Identify modern methods of contraception and their rates of success.

Keynotes

- The peak incidence of ovarian cancer is in women in their fifties and sixties.
- Residual scarring of the uterine tubes from salpingitis is a common cause of infertility.

Abbreviations

CHES Certified Health Education Specialist
PCOS polycystic ovarian syndrome
PMS premenstrual syndrome
PGY pregnancy

Case Report (CR) 8.2

You are
. . . a certified health education specialist **(CHES)** employed by Fulwood Medical Center.

Your patient is
. . . Ms. Claire Marcos, a 21-year-old student referred to you by Anna Rusack, MD, a gynecologist.

Ms. Marcos has been diagnosed with **polycystic ovarian syndrome (PCOS),** and your task is to develop a program of self-care as part of her overall plan of therapy.

From her medical record, you see that she has presented with irregular, often missed menstrual periods since the beginning of puberty; persistent acne; patches of dark skin on the back of her neck and under her arms; loss of hair from the front of her scalp; and inability to control her weight. She is 5 feet 4 inches and weighs 150 pounds.

Her self-care program is to include exercise, diet, and regular use of birth control medication and metformin to lower insulin levels and help reduce her weight.

LO 8.8 Disorders of the Ovaries

Ovarian Cysts and Cancer

An ovarian cyst is a fluid-filled sac in the ovary. Most cysts are normal and are called *functional cysts.* They follow ovulation and disappear within 3 months.

Polycystic ovarian syndrome (PCOS), in which multiple follicular cysts form in both ovaries (*Figure 8.13*), is the disorder diagnosed in Ms. Marcos. Because of the repeated cyst formation, no egg matures and is released, ovulation does not occur, and progesterone is not produced. Without progesterone, her menstrual cycle is irregular or absent.

The cysts produce androgens, which prevent ovulation and produce acne, the male-pattern hair loss from the front of the scalp, and weight gain. In addition, women with PCOS make too much insulin, which interferes with normal fat metabolism and prevents it being used for energy. This leads to difficulty in losing weight and causes patches of dark skin. Metformin, a medication that affects glucose and insulin metabolism, can help with the weight problems associated with PCOS.

Women with PCOS are also at increased risk for endometrial cancer, type 2 diabetes, high blood cholesterol, hypertension, and heart disease.

Ovarian cancer is the second most common gynecologic cancer after endometrial cancer, but it accounts for more deaths than any other gynecologic malignancy. Symptoms develop late and are usually vague, making early diagnosis difficult. A mass in the abdomen may be detected during routine pelvic examination.

Treatment is to surgically remove the tumor and give chemotherapy. A majority of patients experience a recurrence. The 5-year survival rate is 45%.

LO 8.8 Disorders of the Uterus and Uterine Tubes

Primary amenorrhea occurs when a girl has not menstruated by age 16. This can occur with or without other signs of puberty. There are numerous possible causes: drastic weight loss from malnutrition; dieting; bulimia or anorexia nervosa (*see Chapter 18*); extreme exercise, as in some young gymnasts; extreme obesity; chronic illness; congenital abnormalities of the uterus or vagina; and congenital hormonal disorders. Treatment is directed to the basic cause.

Secondary amenorrhea occurs when a woman who has menstruated normally then misses three or more periods in a row and is not in her **menopause.** The causes include pregnancy (by far the most common cause); ovarian disorders such as PCOS; excessive weight loss; low body fat percentage; excessive exercise (e.g., in marathon runners); certain drugs, including antidepressants; and stress.

Primary dysmenorrhea, or **premenstrual syndrome (PMS),** refers to pain or discomfort associated with menstruation. The pain can begin 1 or 2 days before menses, peak on the first day of flow, and then slowly subside. The pain can be cramping or aching and be associated with headache, diarrhea or constipation, and urinary frequency. Treatment is with **nonsteroidal anti-inflammatory drugs (NSAIDs).** If these are ineffective, oral contraceptives are 80% to 90% effective.

Cysts   Cysts

▲ **Figure 8.13** Polycystic Ovary. ©Biophoto Associates/Photo Researchers, Inc.

WORD	PRONUNCIATION	ELEMENTS		DEFINITION
amenorrhea	a-men-oh-**REE**-ah	S/ P/ R/CF	-rrhea *flow or discharge* a- *without* -men/o- *month, menses*	Absence or abnormal cessation of menstrual flow
dysmenorrhea	dis-men-oh-**REE**-ah	S/ P/ R/CF	-rrhea *flow or discharge* dys- *painful or difficult* -men/o- *month, menses*	Painful and difficult menstruation
polycystic	pol-ee-**SIS**-tik	S/ P/ R/	-ic *pertaining to* poly- *many* -cyst- *cyst*	Composed of many cysts

Exercises

A. Apply your knowledge of the *language of gynecology* by choosing the correct answer to the following questions. *Choose the best answer.* **LO 8.8**

1. The *gynecologic malignancy* that accounts for the most deaths is

   a. cervical cancer   **b.** breast cancer   **c.** ovarian cancer

2. Secondary amenorrhea is a disorder in which

   a. a woman experiences painful menstruation

   b. a female has not had her first period by age 16

   c. the endometrium is implanted outside of the uterus

   d. a woman who has normally menstruated misses three periods in a row and is not in menopause

   e. the uterine tubes become infected and inflamed due to an infection that started in the vagina

B. Critical thinking. *Use Case Report (CR) 8.2 along with the reading to answer the following questions.* **LO 8.8, 8.F**

1. Ms. Marcos's ovaries were enlarged due to:

   a. cancer   **b.** endometriosis   **c.** cysts   **d.** testosterone

2. The abbreviation for her condition is:

   a. PMS   **b.** FSH   **c.** GnRH   **d.** PCOS

3. A consequence of her condition is that she does not:

   a. create oocytes   **b.** release oocytes   **c.** produce testosterone   **d.** have an appetite

4. Her condition is associated with what other condition?

   a. heart disease   **b.** peptic ulcer   **c.** decreased fat storage   **d.** hematuria

Secondary dysmenorrhea is pain associated with disorders such as infection in the genital tract or endometriosis.

Endometriosis is said to affect 1 in 10 American women of childbearing age. The endometrium becomes implanted outside the uterus on the fallopian (uterine) tubes, the ovaries, and the pelvic peritoneum. The displaced endometrium continues to go through its monthly cycle. It thickens and bleeds, but because there is nowhere for the blood to go, it leads to cysts and scar tissue and produces pain. The etiology of endometriosis is unknown.

Salpingitis is an inflammation of the uterine (fallopian) tubes and is part of pelvic inflammatory disease. A bacterial infection, often from an STD, spreads from the vagina through the cervix and uterus. Symptoms are lower abdominal pain, fever, and a vaginal discharge.

Uterine Prolapse

The uterus is normally supported by the muscles, ligaments, and connective tissue of the pelvic floor. Difficult childbirth can weaken these tissues, so the uterus can descend into the vaginal canal. Aging, obesity, lack of exercise, chronic coughing, and chronic constipation also are thought to play a role in the development of the **prolapse** *(Figure 8.14).*

If the uterus is tilted backward toward the rectum, its position would be **retroverted**, a condition found in 20% of women.

Uterine prolapse can be accompanied by prolapse of the bladder and anterior vaginal wall, called a **cystocele**, or of the rectum and posterior wall of the vagina, called a **rectocele**.

Uterine Fibroids

Fibroids are noncancerous growths of the uterus that appear during childbearing years. Three out of four women have them, but only one out of four women has symptoms from them.

The symptoms they can produce include:

- **Menorrhagia**—abnormally long, heavy menstrual bleeding.
- **Metrorrhagia**—irregular bleeding between menstrual periods.
- **Polymenorrhea**—too frequent periods (occur more often than every 21 days) and no ovulation in the cycle.
- **Pelvic pressure**—low-back pain, urinary incontinence, and frequency.

Uterine fibroids are also called **fibromyomas**, **leiomyomas**, or **myomas** *(Figure 8.15).* They arise in the myometrium, producing a pale, firm, rubbery mass separate from the surrounding tissue. They vary in size from seedlings to large masses that distort the uterus. They can protrude into the uterine cavity, causing menorrhagia, or project outside the uterus and press on the bladder or rectum to produce symptoms.

Other Causes of Uterine Bleeding

Dysfunctional uterine bleeding (DUB) is a term applied when no cause can be found for a patient's menorrhagia.

Endometrial polyps are benign extensions of the endometrium that can cause irregular and heavy bleeding. They can be removed by hysteroscopy or D&C.

Menopause

Menopause is diagnosed when a woman has not menstruated for a year and is not pregnant; she is in the "change of life." In this normal, natural, biological process of reproductive aging, levels of estrogen and progesterone start to decline around the age of 40. For most women, menstruation ceases between the ages of 45 and 55. Significant quantities of estrogen and progesterone are no longer secreted, so the endometrial lining of the uterus cannot grow and be shed as in a normal menstrual period.

Without estrogen and progesterone, the uterus, vagina, and breasts atrophy, and more bone is lost than is replaced. Blood vessels constrict and dilate in response to changing hormone levels and can cause hot flashes.

▲ **Figure 8.14** Complete prolapse of the uterus, which protrudes outside the vaginal canal. ©Scott Camazine/Sue Trainor/Photo Researchers, Inc.

Leiomyoma

▲ **Figure 8.15** Leiomyomas (Fibroids). In this sectioned uterus, a smaller rounded leiomyoma is present, causing a small, rounded bulge in the uterine wall. The larger mass at the top is another leiomyoma projecting from the surface into the uterine cavity. ©Zephyr/Photo Researchers, Inc.

WORD	PRONUNCIATION	ELEMENTS		DEFINITION
cystocele	**SIS**-toh-seal	S/ R/CF	-cele *swelling, hernia* cyst/o- *bladder*	Hernia of the bladder into the vagina
dysfunctional	dis-**FUNK**-shun-al	S/ P/ R/	-al *pertaining to* dys- *painful, difficult* -function- *perform*	Having difficulty in performing
endometriosis	**EN**-doh-mee-tree-**OH**-sis	S/ P/ R/CF	-osis *condition* endo- *within, inside* -metr/i- *uterus*	Endometrial tissue in the abdomen outside the uterus
fibroid	**FIE**-broyd	S/ R/	-oid *resembling* fibr- *fiber*	Uterine tumor resembling fibrous tissue
fibromyoma (also called **fibroid**)	**FIE**-broh-my-**OH**-mah	S/ R/CF R/	-oma *tumor, mass* fibr/o- *fiber* -my- *muscle*	Benign neoplasm derived from smooth muscle containing fibrous tissue
leiomyoma (also called **fibroid**)	**LIE**-oh-my-**OH**-mah	S/ R/CF R/	-oma *tumor, mass* lei/o- *smooth* -my- *muscle*	Benign neoplasm derived from smooth muscle
menopause (*Note:* This term has no suffix, only a combining form and a root.)	**MEN**-oh-paws	R/CF R/	men/o- *month, menses* -pause *cessation*	Permanent ending of menstrual periods
menopausal (adj)	men-oh-**PAWS**-al	S/	al *pertaining to*	Pertaining to menopause
menorrhagia	men-oh-**RAY**-jee-ah	S/ R/CF	-rrhagia *excessive flow, discharge* men/o- *menses*	Excessive menstrual bleeding
metrorrhagia	**MEH**-troh-**RAY**-jee-ah	S/ R/CF	-rrhagia *excessive flow, discharge* metr/o- *uterus*	Irregular uterine bleeding between menses
myoma	my-**OH**-mah	S/ R/	-oma *tumor, mass* my- *muscle*	Benign tumor of muscle
myomectomy	my-oh-**MEK**-toh-mee	S/ R/ R/	-ectomy *surgical excision* my- *muscle* -om- *tumor, body*	Surgical removal of a myoma (fibroid)
polymenorrhea	**POL**-ee-men-oh-**REE**-ah	S/ P/ R/CF	-rrhea *flow* poly- *many* men/o- *menses*	More than normal frequency of menses
prolapse	proh-**LAPS**		Latin *a falling*	The falling or slipping of a body part from its normal position
rectocele	**REK**-toh-seal	S/ R/CF	-cele *swelling, hernia* rect/o- *rectum*	Hernia of the rectum into the vagina
retroversion	reh-troh-**VER**-shun	S/ P/ R/	-ion *process, condition* retro- *backward* -vers- *turned*	The tipping backward of the uterus
retroverted	reh-troh-**VERT**-ed	S/	-ed *pertaining to*	Tilted backward
salpingitis	sal-pin-**JIE**-tis	S/ R/	-itis *inflammation* salping- *fallopian tube*	Inflammation of the uterine tube

Exercises

A. Build the *language of gynecology* by completing the medical term with the correct element. *Fill in the blanks.* **LO 8.8**

1. benign neoplasm derived from smooth muscle   lei/o/ _____ /oma

2. irregular bleeding between menses   metr/o/ _____

3. permanent ending of menstrual periods   _____ /o/pause

4. uterine tumor resembling fibrous tissue   _____ /oid

> 💡 **Study Hint**
>
> The combining form *metr/o* will be used to describe bleeding that is irregular.
> The combining form *men/o* will be used to describe bleeding that occurs at regular intervals.

Note: Although the suffix **-oma** *means tumor (or mass), it is not necessarily a malignancy. Fibromyomas, leiomyomas, and myomas are all benign neoplasms or tumors. This is an important distinction for coders especially to note.*

- Cervical cancer is extremely rare in women under 25 years.

- Approximately 20% of women now have their first child when they are aged 35 or older.

- In 20% to 30% of female infertility problems, no identifiable cause is found.

- The success rate for IVF is approximately 30% for each egg retrieval.

LO 8.8 Disorders of the Uterus and Uterine Tubes (continued)

Endometrial Cancer

Endometrial cancer is the fourth most common cancer in women (after lung, breast, and colon cancer). Forty thousand new cases are diagnosed each year, mostly in women between the ages of 60 and 70. The most common symptom is vaginal bleeding after menopause. It also can cause a vaginal discharge, pelvic pain, and dyspareunia. Higher levels than normal of estrogen are thought to be a risk factor for endometrial cancer.

Cervical Cancer

Cervical cancer is less common than endometrial cancer, but 50% of cases occur between ages 35 and 55. Some 10,000 new cases are diagnosed in the United States each year.

Early cervical cancer produces no symptoms or signs and may be found on a routine Pap test (see below). In the precancerous stage, abnormal cells **(dysplasia)** are found only in the outer layer of the cervix.

Thirteen types of human papilloma virus can convert these **dysplastic** cells to cancer cells. A vaccine has been developed that makes people immune to two of the most common types of HPV.

LO 8.9 Female Infertility

Infertility is the inability to become pregnant after 1 year of unprotected intercourse. It affects 10% to 15% of all couples. The causes of infertility are due to:

- The female factor alone in 35%
- The male factor alone in 30%
- Male and female factors in 20%
- Unknown factors in 15%

In women, fertility begins to decrease as early as age 30, and pregnancy rates are very low after age 44.

Causes of Infertility in the Female

- **Infrequent ovulation** is responsible in 20% of female infertility problems when both ovulation and menses occur at intervals of longer than 1 month. Bulimia, anorexia nervosa, rapid weight loss, excessive exercise training, low body weight, obesity, and polycystic ovarian syndrome are among the causes.

- **Scarring of the uterine tubes** is responsible for 30% of female infertility problems. Scarring can result from previous surgery, previous tubal pregnancy, pelvic inflammatory disease, or **endometriosis**. The scarring blocks the sperm from reaching the egg.

- **Structural abnormalities** of the uterus are responsible for 20% of female infertility problems. Fibroid tumors; uterine polyps; and scarring from infections, abortions, and miscarriages can all produce abnormalities of the uterus. These abnormalities also block the sperm from reaching the egg.

S = Suffix   P = Prefix   R = Root   R/CF = Combining Form

WORD	PRONUNCIATION	ELEMENTS		DEFINITION
dysplasia	dis-**PLAY**-zee-ah	S/ P/ R/	-ia *condition* **dys-** *painful, difficult* **-plas-** *molding*	Abnormal tissue formation
dysplastic (adj)	dis-**PLAS**-tic	S/	**-tic** *pertaining to*	Pertaining to abnormal tissue function
infertility infertile (adj)	in-fer-**TIL**-ih-tee in-**FER**-tile	S/ P/ R/	-ity *condition* **in-** *not* **-fertil-** *able to conceive*	Inability to conceive over a long period of time

Exercises

A. Proofread the following sentences for errors in documentation. *It may be an error of fact and/or spelling. Rewrite the correct form of the misspelled word. Fill in the blank.* **LO 8.8, 8.A**

1. Cervixal cancer is more common than endometrial cancer.

_____

2. The most common symptom of endometrial cancer is vaginal bleeding after mennopause.

_____

3. Displasia is abnormal tissue formation.

_____

4. A routine Pap test can detect the precancerus stage of cervical cancer.

_____

Precision is everything!

B. Discuss female infertility. *Select the best answer that completes each statement.* **LO 8.9**

1. Statistically speaking, the most common cause of infertility in the female is:

  a. scarring of the uterine tubes

  b. infrequent ovulation

  c. uterine polyps

  d. fibroid tumors

2. In order to be diagnosed with infertility, a female must be unable to conceive for a minimum of:

  a. 3 months

  b. 6 months

  c. 1 year

  d. 2 years

3. Infertility due to sperm being blocked from reaching the egg can result from:

  a. anorexia

  b. endometriosis

  c. excessive exercising

  d. bulimia

LO 8.10 Contraception

Contraception is the prevention of pregnancy. Common methods of contraception include the following.

Behavioral Methods

- **Abstinence** is reliable if followed consistently.
- **Rhythm method** avoids intercourse near the time of expected ovulation, which is difficult to determine. It has a 25% failure rate.
- **Coitus interruptus** involves the male withdrawing his penis before ejaculation. There is a 20% failure rate.

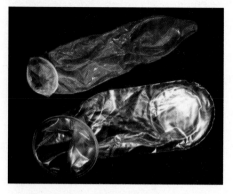

▲ **Figure 8.16** Male and female condoms. ©Scott Camazine/Photo Researchers, Inc.

Barrier Methods

- **Male condom**—a sheath of latex or rubber rolled on over the erect penis. There is a 14% to 15% failure rate for pregnancy.
- **Female condom**—a polyurethane sheath that fits into the vagina with a ring at one end to go over the cervix and a larger diameter at the other end to go over the vulva *(Figure 8.16)*. There is a 5% to 10% failure rate for pregnancy. Both male and female condoms help protect against STDs.
- **Diaphragm** *(Figure 8.17)* **and cervical cap**—a latex or rubber dome inserted into the vagina and placed over the cervix. When used with a **spermicide**, they have a 5% to 10% failure rate for pregnancy.
- **Spermicidal foam and gel**—inserted into the vagina. Used on their own, they have a 25% failure rate.
- **Sponge**—a spermicidal-coated polyurethane barrier placed in the vagina to inhibit sperm. It has a 10% failure rate.

Intrauterine Devices

Intrauterine devices (IUDs) are T-shaped flexible plastic or copper devices inserted into the uterus and left in place for 1 to 4 years. Failure rate is less than 3%.

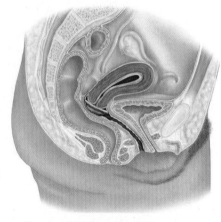

▲ **Figure 8.17** Diaphragm.

Hormonal Methods

- **Oral contraceptives** (birth control pills) utilize a mixture of estrogen and progesterone to prevent follicular development and ovulation *(Figure 8.18)*. They are taken orally and have a 5% failure rate, usually due to inconsistent pill taking.
- **Estrogen/progestin patches** deliver the hormones transdermally. Some are applied monthly, some weekly. Their failure rate is less than 1% when reapplied at the correct time.
- **Injected progestins,** such as *Depo-Provera,* are given by injection every 3 months. Their failure rate is less than 1%.
- **Implanted progestins,** such as *Implanon,* are contained in porous silicone tubes that are inserted under the skin and slowly release the progestin for up to 5 years. Their failure rate is less than 1%.
- **Morning-after pills,** such as Plan B, contain large doses of progestins to inhibit or delay ovulation. They are a backup when taken within 72 hours of unprotected intercourse. Their failure rate is around 10%.
- **Mifepristone (RU-486),** when taken with a prostaglandin, induces a miscarriage. It has an 8% failure rate.

Surgical Methods

- **Tubal ligation** ("getting your tubes tied") is performed with laparoscopy. Both uterine tubes are cut, a segment is removed, and the ends are tied off and cauterized shut. Failure rate is less than 1%. A **tubal anastomosis** is the procedure of rejoining the tubes if there is a subsequent change of mind.
- **Vasectomy** in the male is discussed in *Chapter 7.*

▲ **Figure 8.18** Oral Contraceptives. ©Getty Images RF

WORD	PRONUNCIATION	ELEMENTS		DEFINITION
abstinence	**AB**-stih-nens	S/	**-ence** *forming, quality of, state of*	Choosing to not participate in a behavior, in this case, sexual intercourse
		P/	**ab-** *away from*	
		R/	**-stin-** *partition*	
anastomosis anastomoses (pl)	ah-**NAS**-to-**MOH**-sis	S/	**-osis** *condition*	A surgically made union between two tubular structures
		R/	**anastom-** *join together*	
coitus	**KOH**-it-us		Latin *come together*	Sexual intercourse
condom	**KON**-dom		Old English *sheath or cover*	A sheath or cover for the penis or vagina to prevent conception and infection
contraception	kon-trah-**SEP**-shun	S/	**-ion** *process*	Prevention of pregnancy
		P/	**contra-** *against*	
		R/	**-cept** *receive*	
contraceptive	kon-trah-**SEP**-tiv	S/	**-ive** *quality of*	An agent that prevents conception
diaphragm (**Note:** Diaphragm also is the term for the muscle that separates the thoracic and abdominal cavities.)	**DIE**-ah-fram		Greek *partition or wall*	A ring and dome-shaped material inserted in the vagina to prevent pregnancy
intrauterine	**IN**-trah-**YOU**-ter-ine	S/	**-ine** *pertaining to*	Pertaining to the inside of the uterus.
		P/	**intra-** *inside, within*	
		R/	**uter-** *uterus*	
ligature ligation	**LIG**-ah-chur lie-**GAY**-shun	S/	Latin *band, tie* **-ion** *process*	Thread or wire tied around a tubal structure to close it Use of a tie to close a tube
		R/	**ligat-** *tie up*	
progestin	pro-**JESS**-tin	S/	**-in** *chemical compound*	A synthetic form of progesterone
		P/	**pro-** *before*	
		R/	**-gest-** *produce, pregnancy*	
spermicide	**SPER**-mih-side	S/	**-cide** *to kill*	Agent that destroys sperm
		R/CF	**sperm/i-** *sperm*	
spermicidal (adj)	**SPER**-mih-**SIDE**-al	S/	**-cidal** *pertaining to killing*	Pertaining to the destruction of sperm

Exercises

A. Review the medical terms relating to methods of contraception. *With critical thinking, you will be able to answer the following questions using these terms. Select the correct answer that completes each statement or answers each question.* **LO 8.10, 8.D, 8.F**

1. The prefix in the medical term **contraception** means:

   a. receive   **b.** process   **c.** against   **d.** before

2. The medical term that has a word element that means *chemical compound* is:

   a. spermicidal   **b.** coitus   **c.** progestin   **d.** diaphragm

3. Which of the following is considered to be a barrier method of contraception?

   a. intrauterine device   **b.** diaphragm   **c.** implanted progestins   **d.** birth control pill

4. A pill that induces miscarriage is:

   a. IUD   **b.** MRI   **c.** RU-486   **d.** PCOS

5. An agent that destroys sperm is a:

   a. progestin   **b.** spermicidal   **c.** spermicide   **d.** condom

Lesson 8.4

Gynecologic Diagnostic and Therapeutic Procedures and Pharmacology

Abbreviations

D and C	dilation and curettage
LEEP	loop electrosurgical excision procedure
Pap	Papanicolaou—a Greek gynecologist

LO 8.11 Gynecologic Diagnostic Procedures

Palpation is routinely used to feel the structures of the reproductive system.

Laparoscopy directly examines the uterus, fallopian tubes, and ovaries through a **laparoscope** inserted into the abdominal cavity through a small incision in the abdominal wall. Carbon dioxide can be pumped through the laparoscope to inflate the abdominal cavity so that the pelvic organs can be seen more clearly.

Cervical biopsy is a procedure to remove tissue from the cervix for pathological testing for precancerous lesions or cervical cancer.

Colposcopy uses an instrument with a magnifying lens and a light called a **colposcope** to examine the lining of the vagina and cervical canal. Both colposcopy and cervical biopsy are often performed because a Pap test result was abnormal.

Hysteroscopy is the examination of the inside of the uterus using a thin, flexible, lighted tube called a **hysteroscope** to look for abnormalities of the cervical canal and endometrium.

Hysterosalpingography is a procedure in which x-rays (**hysterosalpingograms**) are taken after a radiopaque dye is injected through the cervix into the uterus through a slender catheter to outline the interior of the uterus and fallopian tubes (*see Figure 8.19*). It can be used to help define the cause of female infertility or to confirm that a sterilization procedure to block the uterine tubes is successful.

Endometrial biopsy—biopsy of the lining of the uterus—is performed to determine the cause of abnormal uterine bleeding and to check the effects of hormones on the endometrium.

Dilation and curettage (D and C) is a surgical procedure in which the cervix is dilated so that the cervical canal and uterine endometrium can be scraped to remove abnormal tissues for pathological examination.

Loop electrosurgical excision procedure (LEEP) uses a wire loop heated by electricity to remove tissue from the vagina and cervix for pathological examination.

After a complete history and physical examination, including vagina and pelvic organs, other diagnostic tools to determine the cause(s) for infertility include:

- **Hormone blood levels** of progesterone, estrogens, and FSH.

- **Hysterosalpingogram,** in which x-rays of the uterus and uterine tubes are taken after dye is injected into the uterus through a slender catheter (*Figure 8.19*).

- **Ultrasound** of the abdomen, which can show the shape and size of the uterus, and vaginal ultrasound, which can show the shape and size of the ovaries.

- **Hysteroscopy,** which can visualize the inside of the uterus and be used to take an endometrial biopsy and remove polyps or fibroids.

- **Laparoscopy,** which allows inspection of the outside of the uterus and ovaries and removal of any scar tissue blocking tubes.

- **Postcoital testing,** in which the cervix is examined soon after unprotected intercourse to see if sperm can travel through into the uterus.

▲ **Figure 8.19** Hysterosalpingogram of a Normal Uterus, Uterine Tubes, and Ovaries. ©Du Cane Medical Imaging Ltd/Photo Researchers, Inc.

WORD	PRONUNCIATION	ELEMENTS		DEFINITION
biopsy Note: The "o" in the root *bio* is dropped from the spelling.	**BIE**-op-see	S/ R/CF	-opsy *to view* bio- *life*	Removal of living tissue for laboratory examination
colposcopy	kol-**POS**-koh-pee	S/ R/CF	-scopy *to view* colp/o- *vagina*	Examination of vagina and cervix with an endoscope
colposcope	**KOL**-poh-scope	S/	-scope *instrument for viewing*	Endoscope to view the vagina and cervix
conization	koh-nih-**ZAY**-shun	S/ R/	-ation *process* coniz- *cone*	Surgical excision of a cone-shaped piece of tissue
cryosurgery	cry-oh-**SUR**-jer-ee	S/ R/CF R/	-ery *process of* cry/o- *icy, cold* -surg- *operate*	Use of liquid nitrogen or argon gas to freeze and kill tissue
curette curettage	kyu-**RET** kyu-reh-**TAHZH**	S/ R/	French *cleanse* -age *related to* curett- *to cleanse*	Instrument with sharpened edges for scraping Scraping of the interior of a cavity
dilation	die-**LAY**-shun		Latin *to spread out*	Artificial enlargement of an opening or hollow structure
excision	eck-**SIZH**-un	S/ R/	-ion *action* excis- *cut out*	Surgical removal of part or all of a structure
hysterosalpingogram	**HIS**-ter-oh-sal-**PING**-oh-gram	S/ R/CF R/CF	-gram *a record* hyster/o- *uterus* -salping/o- *uterine tube*	Radiograph of uterus and uterine tubes after injection of contrast material
hysteroscope	**HIS**-ter-oh-skope	S/	-scope *instrument for viewing*	Endoscope to visually examine the uterine cavity
hysteroscopy	his-ter-**OS**-koh-pee	S/	-scopy *to view*	Visual examination of the uterine cavity
laparoscope	**LAP**-ah-roh-skope	S/ R/CF	-scope *instrument for viewing* lapar/o *abdomen*	Endoscope to view the contents of the abdomen
laparoscopy	lap-ah-**ROS**-koh-pee	S/	-scopy *to view*	Endoscopic examination of the contents of the abdomen
palpate (verb) palpation (noun)	**PAL**-pate pal-**PAY**-shun	S/ R/	Latin *to touch* -ion *process, action* palpat- *touch, stroke*	To examine with the fingers and hands Examination using the fingers and hands
postcoital	post-**KOH**-ih-tal	S/ P/ R/	-al *pertaining to* post- *after* -coit- *sexual intercourse*	After sexual intercourse

Exercises

A. Define gynecologic diagnostic procedures. *It is important to correctly use diagnostic terms when communicating verbally with health care professionals and documenting care of your patients. Choose the correct answer to complete each statement.* **LO 8.11, 8.A**

1. The term **palpate** means to:

   a. smell   **b.** touch   **c.** excise   **d.** incise

2. A diagnostic test for infertility in which the cervix is viewed after unprotected sexual intercourse:

   a. hysteroscopy   **b.** biopsy   **c.** postcoital testing   **d.** ultrasound

3. The injection of dye followed by an x-ray of the uterus and uterine tubes is termed:

   a. hysterosalpingography **b.** postcoital testing   **c.** mammography   **d.** endometrial biopsy

4. A **colposcope** is used to:

   a. view the vagina and cervical canal   **b.** x-ray the uterus   **c.** view the internal os of the cervix   **d.** remove cells from the uterus

▲ **Figure 8.20** **Pap Smear Being Performed.**

Normal cells   Dysplastic cells

▲ **Figure 8.21** **Abnormal Pap Smear with Dysplastic Cells.** ©Parviz M. Pour/Photo Researchers, Inc.

LO 8.11 Gynecologic Diagnostic Procedures (continued)

Pap Test

Pap test screens for cervical cancer. In a Pap test, the doctor brushes cells from the cervix *(Figure 8.20)*. The cells are smeared onto a slide or rinsed into a special liquid and sent to the laboratory for examination. This test enables abnormal cells (see *Figure 8.21*), precancerous or cancerous, to be detected. It is the most successful and accurate test for early detection of abnormalities. Current screening guidelines were last updated in March 2012 by the National Cancer Institute, the American Cancer Society, and other national organizations. According to the guidelines, a Pap test should be scheduled as follows:

- **Initial Pap test**—at age 21.

- **Age 21 to 29**—every 3 years.

- **Age 30 to 65**—Pap and HPV cotesting every 5 years or Pap alone every 3 years.

- **Age 65 onward**—continue screening if risk factors are present including HIV infection, **immunosuppression**, previous treatment for precancerous cervical lesion or cervical cancer. Schedule individually with your doctor.

- **Any abnormal result** at any age mandates working out the best schedule for follow-up testing with your doctor.

- A Pap test is best performed 10 to 20 days after the first day of the **last menstrual period (LMP).**

More than 90% of abnormal Papanicolaou **(Pap)** smears are caused by HPV infections. A vaccine is now available that can prevent lasting infections from the two HPV strains that cause 70% of cervical cancers and another two strains that cause 90% of genital warts.

Pelvic ultrasound uses sound waves to scan and picture the pelvic organs.

Swabs are used to determine the causative agents for infections. A sterile cotton swab is rubbed against the infected tissue to obtain a sample of the cells and secretions. The swab is then sent to the laboratory for testing.

DNA probes can be used to test for the presence of gonorrhea and chlamydia.

Diagnostic studies for fibroids include endometrial biopsy, **transabdominal ultrasound**, **transvaginal ultrasound**, **hysteroscopy**, computed tomography (CT), and magnetic resonance imaging (MRI).

WORD	PRONUNCIATION	ELEMENTS		DEFINITION
hysteroscopy	his-ter-**OS**-koh-pee	S/ R/CF	-scopy *view* hyster/o *uterus*	Visual inspection of the uterine cavity using an endoscope
cytologist	Sigh-**TOL**-oh-jist	S/ R/CF	-logist *specialist* cyt/o- *cell*	Specialist in the study of the anatomy, physiology and pathology of the cell
immunosuppression	**IM**-you-noh-suh-**PRESH**-un	S/ R/CF R/	-ion *process* immun/o- *immune response* -suppress *press under*	Suppression of the immune response by an outside agent, such as a drug
Pap test	PAP TEST		George Papanicolaou 1883-1962, Greek-US physisician and cytologist	Examination of cells taken from the cervix
swab	SWOB		Old English *to sweep*	Wad of cotton used to remove or apply something from/to a surface
ultrasound	**ULL**-trah-sound	P/ R/	ultra- *higher* -sound *noise*	Very high frequency sound waves

Exercises

A. The Pap test is an important diagnostic test for women. *Test your understanding of this diagnostic test by answering these questions. Select the correct answer for each question.* **LO 8.11**

1. How often should a 30-40 year old woman have a Pap test on its own?

   a. annually   **b.** biannually   **c.** every three years   **d.** every five years

2. What causes the majority of abnormal Pap smears?

   a. improper specimen collection

   b. poor hygiene

   c. infection by the human papilloma virus

   d. overgrowth of yeast in vagina

3. The optimal time to perform a Pap smear is _____ days after the last menstrual period.

   a. 2 - 3   **b.** 4 - 6   **c.** 8 - 12   **d.** 10 - 20

B. Construct medical terms. *Complete medical terms related to gynecologic diagnostic procedures. Be precise! Fill in the blanks.* **LO 8.11, 8.C**

  1. Use of very high frequency sound waves   _____ /sound

  2. Specialist in the study of the anatomy, physiology and pathology of the cell   cyt/o/ _____

  3. Visual inspection of the uterine cavity using an endoscope   hyster/o/ _____

Abbreviations

HRT	hormone replacement therapy
IVF	in vitro fertilization
LEEP	loop electrosurgical excision procedure

LO 8.11 Gynecologic Therapeutic Procedures

Hysterectomy—removal of the uterus—is performed because of uterine fibroids, uterine cancer, and endometriosis. **Subtotal hysterectomy** is removal of the upper uterus, leaving the cervix in place. **Total hysterectomy** is removal of the whole uterus and cervix. **Radical hysterectomy** removes the whole uterus, the cervix, and the top of the vagina; ovaries also may be removed. **Abdominal hysterectomy** is completed through an abdominal incision; **vaginal hysterectomy** through a vaginal incision; **laparoscopic hysterectomy** using a laparoscope and small abdominal incisions; **robot-assisted laparoscopic hysterectomy** using sophisticated robotic surgical tools through a laparoscope.

Oophorectomy is surgical removal of one or both ovaries.

Myomectomy removes fibroids surgically, leaving the uterus in place.

Endometrial ablation removes a thin layer of the uterine endometrium to reduce heavy menstrual bleeding in women who do not plan to have future children.

Tubal ligation prevents future pregnancies.

Sacral colpopexy treats pelvic organ prolapse by suspending the vaginal vault to the sacral promontory using a graft or surgical mesh. Treatment can be an individually fitted vaginal **pessary** inserted into the vagina to support the uterus. Surgical procedures such as **sacral colpopexy,** in which a mesh is inserted into the pelvic floor, or a **vaginal hysterectomy,** in which the uterus is removed through the vagina, achieve good results.

Colporrhaphy is surgical repair of a vaginal wall because of a **cystocele** (protrusion of the urinary bladder into the vagina) or a **rectocele** (protrusion of the rectum into the vagina).

Salpingitis is inflammation of the uterine tube. Treatment is with appropriate antibiotics. If a pelvic abscess has developed, it may be necessary to remove the damaged tube **(salpingectomy).**

Treatment options for fibroids are numerous and include:

- **Expectant management,** or watchful waiting.

- **Myomectomy**, removal of the fibroids surgically, leaving the uterus in place.

- **Hormone therapy,** which uses **GnRH agonists** to cause estrogen and progesterone levels to fall so that menstruation stops and fibroids shrink.

- **Hysterectomy**, major surgery that is performed by many gynecologists as a last resort.

Treatment for dysfunctional uterine bleeding (DUB) is with oral contraceptives. If that fails, **dilation and curettage (D&C)** may be effective. This procedure involves dilating the entrance to the uterus through the cervix so that a thin instrument can be inserted to scrape or suction away the lining of the uterus and take tissue samples. An alternative treatment is **endometrial ablation,** in which a heat-generating tool or a laser removes or destroys the lining of the uterus and prevents or reduces menstruation. Endometrial ablation and hysterectomy are used in women who have finished childbearing.

Endometrial cancer is staged at the time of any surgical procedure into four groups, depending on its localization to the uterus or its spread outside. Surgery is the most common treatment. It can be a total hysterectomy, in which the uterus and cervix are removed, or a radical hysterectomy, in which the uterine tubes and ovaries are removed and a pelvic lymph node dissection is also done. If the cancer has spread to other parts of the body, progesterone therapy, radiation therapy, and chemotherapy are used.

Treatment for cervical cancer depends on the stage of the cancer. In preinvasive cancer, when it is only in the outer layer of the lining of the cervix, treatment can include:

- **Conization.** A cone-shaped piece of tissue from around the abnormality is removed with a scalpel.

- **Loop electrosurgical excision procedure (LEEP).** A wire loop carries an electrical current to slice off cells from the mouth of the cervix.

- **Laser surgery.** A laser beam is used to kill precancerous and cancerous cells.

- **Cryosurgery.** Freezing is used to kill the precancerous and cancerous cells.

In an invasive stage when cancer has invaded the cervix and beyond, treatment can include total or radical hysterectomy, chemotherapy, and radiation therapy.

Infertility treatment is directed at the the underlying cause. If the cause of infertility is infrequent ovulation, the patient can be treated with hormones to stimulate release of the egg. These hormones include clomiphene citrate and injectable forms of FSH, LH, and GnRH.

Surgical procedures to initiate pregnancy include:

- **Intrauterine insemination.** Sperm are inserted directly into the uterus via a special catheter.

- **In vitro fertilization (IVF).** Eggs and sperm are combined in a laboratory dish, and two resulting embryos are placed inside the uterus. This can result in twins.

WORD	PRONUNCIATION	ELEMENTS		DEFINITION
ablation	ab-**LAY**-shun	S/ P/ R/	-ion *action* ab- *away from* -lat- *to take*	Removal of tissue to destroy its function
agonist	**AG**-on-ist		Greek *contest*	Agent that combines with receptors on cells to initiate drug actions
colpopexy	**KOL**-poh-pek-see	S/ R/CF	-pexy *surgical fixation* colp/o- *vagina*	Surgical fixation of the vagina
colporrhaphy	col-**POR**-ah-fee	R/CF R/	colp/o- *vagina* -rrhaphy *suture*	Suture of a rupture of the vagina
curettage	kyu-reh-**TAHZH**	S/ R/	-age *related to* curett- *to cleanse*	Scraping of the interior of a cavity
estrogen	**ES**-troh-jen	S/ R/CF	-gen *create* estr/o- *woman*	Generic term for hormones that stimulate secondary sex characteristics
estriol	**ESS**-tree-ol	R/CF S/	estr/i- *woman* -ol *chemical name*	One of the three main estrogens
hysterectomy	his-ter-**EK**-toh-mee	S/ R/	-ectomy *surgical excision* hyster- *uterus*	Surgical removal of the uterus
insemination	in-sem-ih-**NAY**-shun	S/ P/ R/	-ation *process* in- *in* -semin- *scatter seed*	Introduction of semen into the vagina
inseminate (verb)	in-**SEM**-ih-nate	R/	-ate *process*	semen into the vagina
in vitro fertilization (IVF)	IN **VEE**-troh **FER**-til-eye-**ZAY**-shun	 S/ R/	in vitro Latin *in glass* -ization *process of creating* fertil- *able to conceive*	Process of combining sperm and egg in a laboratory dish and placing the resulting embryos inside the uterus
myomectomy	my-oh-**MEK**-toh-mee	S/ R/ S/	-ectomy *surgical excision* my- *muscle* -om- *tumor*	Surgical removal of a fibroid
oophorectomy	**OH**-oh-for-**EK**-toh-mee	S/ R/	-ectomy *surgical excision* oophor- *ovary*	Surgical removal of the ovary(ies).
salpingectomy	sal-pin-**JEK**-toh-mee	S/ R/	-ectomy *surgical excision* salping- *uterine tube*	Surgical removal of uterine tube(s)

Exercises

A. Apply your knowledge of the language of gynecology. *Match the word element in the first column with its correct meaning in the second column.* **LO 8.11**

Term		Meaning
_____	**1.** *oophor-*	**a.** to cleanse
_____	**2.** *-ectomy*	**b.** uterine tube
_____	**3.** *hyster/o*	**c.** vagina
_____	**4.** *-pexy*	**d.** uterus
_____	**5.** *salping/o*	**e.** surgical removal
_____	**6.** *semin-*	**f.** surgical fixation
_____	**7.** *curette-*	**g.** scatter seed
_____	**8.** *colp/o*	**h.** ovary

LO 8.11 Gynecologic Pharmacology

Hormone replacement therapy (HRT)—medications to relieve menopausal symptoms by replacement of diminished circulating estrogen and progesterone hormones—have to be given in effective forms. **Estrogen** when taken orally is converted by the liver to estrone, a weaker estrogen. When estrogen, as **synthetic estradiol,** is used **transdermally** as a patch, gel, or vaginal **pessary,** it enters the bloodstream as a more effective **bioidentical** estrogen with fewer side effects. Similarly, **micronized** bioidentical progesterone is more effective and has fewer side effects than synthetic **progestin.** However, long-term **hormone therapy,** as it is now called, is no longer routinely recommended. When taken for more than a few years, it increases the risk of breast cancer.

Oral contraceptives usually contain the synthetic forms of the hormones progesterone (progestin) and estrogen (ethinyl estradiol). They work by (1) preventing ovulation, (2) thickening the cervical mucus to help prevent sperm from entering the uterus, and (3) making implantation in the uterine endometrium more difficult. They are taken for three weeks every month.

The **Minipill** contains only the synthetic progestin, and is taken every day, and functions in the same three ways as the oral contraceptives. It also stops the woman's menstrual period.

Depo-Provera is also a progestin-only drug given by intramuscular injection every three months.

Bacterial vaginosis is treated with antibiotics such as clindamycin. **Vulvovaginal candidiasis** can be treated by applying miconazole (*Monistat*) or clotrimazole (*Desenex*) vaginally, and, if necessary, taking fluconazole (*Diflucan*) orally.

Treatment for STDs

- **Trichomoniasis** infection of the vagina can be treated with a single oral dose of metronidazole (*Flagyl*). Because it is a "ping-pong" infection between partners, both individuals should be treated.

- Treatment for **chlamydia** is with oral antibiotics such as doxycycline, erythromycin, or azithromycin.

- **Gonorrhea** can be treated with a single dose of an antibiotic such as cefixime, but its causative agent, *Neisseria gonorrhoeae,* is developing resistance to antibiotics.

- Antibiotics such as azithromycin and ceftriaxone are effective in the treatment of **chancroid.**

- The lesions of **molluscum contagiosum** are treated with podophyllin ointment, or liquid nitrogen and laser surgery can be used.

Treatment for **vulvodynia** varies from local anesthetics and creams to biofeedback therapy with exercises to the muscles of the pelvic floor. Surgical removal of the affected area **(vestibulectomy)** has been tried with variable results.

There is no cure for genital herpes. Three antiviral medications can provide clinical benefit by limiting the **replication** of the virus. These are acyclovir (*Zovirax*), valacyclovir (*Valtrex*), and famcyclovir (*Famvir*). In people who have recurrent outbreaks, medication taken every day can reduce the recurrences by 70% to 80%.

Clomiphene (*Clomid*) is an oral medication used for stimulating ovulation by causing production of **gonadotrophins** by the pituitary gland (*see Chapter 17*).

The HPV vaccine (*Gardasil*) is offered to girls and women aged 9 to 26 and to boys and men of the same age group.

There is no cure for HIV or AIDS, but combinations of anti-HIV medications are taken to stop the replication of the virus in the cells of the body and stop the progression of the disease. Development of resistance to the drugs is a problem.

WORD	PRONUNCIATION	ELEMENTS		DEFINITION
estradiol	ess-trah-**DIE**-ol	S/ R/	-diol *chemical name* estra- *woman*	The most potent natural estrogen
pessary	**PESS**-ah-ree		Greek *an oval stone*	Appliance inserted into the vagina to support the uterus
synthetic	sin-**THET**-ik	S/ P/ R/	-ic *pertaining to* syn- *together* -thet- *arrange*	Built up or put together from simpler compounds
transdermal	trans-**DER**-mal	S/ P/ R/	-al *pertaining to* trans- *across* -derm- *skin*	Going across or through the skin
vestibulectomy	vess-tib-you-**LEK**-toe-me	S/ R/	-ectomy *surgical excision* vestibul- *entrance*	Surgical excision of the vulva

Exercises

A. Demonstrate your knowledge of gynecologic pharmacology. *Select the correct answer that completes the sentence or answers the question.* **LO 8.10, 8.11**

1. A pharmacologic method to treat vulvodynia is:

   a. transdermal estradiol   **b.** micronized bioidentical progesterone   **c.** topical anesthetic cream   **d.** *Gardasil injection*

2. A medication used to promote ovulation:

   a. clomiphene   **b.** podophyllin ointment   **c.** Minipill   **d.** acyclovir

3. Miconazole and clotrimazole are used to treat:

   a. chlamydia   **b.** vulvodynia   **c.** infertility   **d.** fungal infections

4. An increased risk of breast cancer is seen with which type of long-term pharmacologic therapy?

   a. pessary   **b.** antibiotic   **c.** hormone   **d.** antiviral

5. Which type of medication is used to reduce, not cure, herpes outbreaks?

   a. metronidazole   **b.** liquid nitrogen   **c.** valacyclovir   **d.** Gardasil

Lesson 8.5

FEMALE REPRODUCTIVE SYSTEM

Obstetrics: Pregnancy and Childbirth

LO 8.12 Conception

When released from the ovary, an egg takes 72 hours to reach the uterus, but it must be **fertilized** *(Figure 8.22)* within 12 to 24 hours to survive. Therefore, **fertilization** must normally take place in the distal third of the uterine tube.

Between 200 million and 600 million sperm are deposited in the vagina near the cervix. Many are destroyed by the acidity in the vagina or just drain out. Others fail to get through the cervical mucus. Approximately half the survivors will go up the wrong uterine tube. The journey through the uterus into the uterine tube takes about an hour. Some 2,000 to 3,000 sperm reach the egg. Several of these penetrate the outer layers of the egg and clear the path for the one sperm that will penetrate all the way into the egg cytoplasm to fertilize it *(see Figure 8.22).* and produce a **zygote**.

Sperm nucleus embedded in egg

Egg cytoplasm

▲ **Figure 8.22** Fertilization.

LO 8.12 Implantation

While still in the uterine tube, the **zygote** divides, producing a ball of cells called a **morula**. Within the morula, a fluid-filled cavity develops, and the morula becomes a **blastocyst**. A week after fertilization, the blastocyst enters the uterine cavity and burrows into the endometrium **(implantation)**. A group of cells in the blastocyst, the inner cell mass, differentiate into the germ layers and form the embryo. Other cells from the blastocyst, together with endometrial cells, form the **placenta**.

Twins (and other multiple births) can be produced in two ways:

- **Dizygotic** twins are produced when two eggs are released by the ovary and fertilized by two separate sperm. They can be of different sexes and are only as genetically similar as other siblings would be.

- **Monozygotic** twins are produced when a single egg is fertilized and later two inner cell masses form within a single blastocyst, each producing an embryo. These twins share a single placenta, are genetically identical, are the same sex, and look alike.

WORD	PRONUNCIATION	ELEMENTS		DEFINITION
blastocyst	**BLAS**-toh-sist	S/ R/CF	-cyst *bladder* blast/o- *germ cell*	The developing embryo during the first 2 weeks
conception	kon-**SEP**-shun		Latin *something received*	Fertilization of the egg by sperm to form a zygote
dizygotic	die-zie-**GOT**-ik	S/ P/ R/	-ic *pertaining to* di- *two* -zygot- *yoked together*	Twins from two separate zygotes
fertilize fertilization	**FER**-til-ize **FER**-til-eye-**ZAY**-shun	S/ R/	Latin *make fruitful* -ation *process* fertiliz- *make fruitful*	To penetrate an oocyte with a sperm so as to impregnate Union of a male sperm and a female egg
implantation	im-plan-**TAY**-shun	S/ P/ R/	-ation *process* im- *in* -plant- *to plant*	Attachment of a fertilized egg to the endometrium
monozygotic	**MON**-oh-zie-**GOT**-ik	S/ P/ R/	-ic *pertaining to* mono- *one* -zygot- *yoked together*	Twins from a single zygote
morula	**MOR**-you-lah		Latin *mulberry*	Ball of cells formed from divisions of a zygote
placenta	plah-**SEN**-tah		Latin *a cake*	Organ that allows metabolic interchange between the mother and fetus
placental (adj)	plah-**SEN**-tal	S/ R/	-al *pertaining to* placent- *placenta*	Pertaining to the placenta
zygote	**ZIE**-goht		Greek *joined together*	Cell resulting from the union of the sperm and egg

Exercises

A. Tracing the pathway of embryo implantation. *You are given the terminology—put it in the correct order of the implantation process.* **LO 8.12**

morula	embryo
blastocyst	zygote
fertilization	egg

1. _____

2. _____

3. _____

4. _____

5. _____

6. _____

B. Terminology challenge. *Fill in the blanks with the correct term being described.* **LO 8.12**

1. Cell resulting from the union of a sperm and an egg: _____.

2. Twins that originated from one fertilized egg: _____.

3. Twins that originated from two fertilized eggs: _____.

Maternal blood — **Developing placenta**
— Uterus
— Chorionic villus

Umbilical
blood vessels

Chorion —
— Yolk sac
— Amnion
— Amniotic cavity

▲ **Figure 8.23** Embryo at 4.5 Weeks.

Placenta —
— Umbilical
cord
— Yolk sac
— Amnion
— Lumen of
uterus

Uterine
wall
Amniotic
cavity

▲ **Figure 8.24** Embryo and Placenta at
13.5 Weeks.

▲ **Figure 8.25** Developing Fetus at 20
Weeks. ©BrandX Pictures/Punchstock RF

LO 8.13 Development of Embryo, Fetus, and Placenta

Embryo

From week 2 until week 8 is the **embryonic period,** in which most of the external structures and internal organs of the **embryo** are formed, together with the placenta, umbilical cord, **amnion, yolk sac,** and **chorion** (*Figure 8.23*). The amnion is a fluid-filled sac that protects the embryo. The yolk sac is a small sac arising from the ventral surface of the embryo. It contributes to the formation of the digestive tract and produces blood cells and future sex germ cells. The chorion forms the placenta by penetrating deeply into the endometrium. At the eighth week, all the organ systems are present; the embryo is just over 1 inch long and is now called a **fetus.**

The Placenta

The **placenta** is a disc of tissue that increases in size as pregnancy proceeds (*Figure 8.24*). The surface facing the fetus is smooth and gives rise to the **umbilical cord,** which contains two arteries and one vein. The surface attached to the uterine wall consists of treelike structures called **chorionic villi.** The cells of the **villi** keep the maternal and fetal circulations largely separate, but they are very thin and allow an exchange of gases, nutrients, and waste products to occur.

The functions of the placenta are to:

- **Transport nutrients** (such as glucose, amino acids, fatty acids, minerals) from mother to fetus.
- **Transport nitrogenous wastes** (such as ammonia, urea, creatinine) from fetus to mother, who can excrete them.
- **Transport oxygen** from mother to fetus and carbon dioxide from fetus to mother, who can excrete it.
- **Transport maternal antibodies** to the fetus.
- **Secrete hormones** (such as estrogen and progesterone) and allow maternal hormones to pass to the fetus.

Unfortunately, some undesirable items and many medications also can cross the placenta. These include the HIV and rubella viruses and the bacteria that cause syphilis. Alcohol, nicotine, carbon monoxide from smoking, and drugs (for example, heroin and cocaine) all have bad effects on the fetus.

Fetus

The **fetal period** lasts from the eighth week until birth. At the eighth week, the heart is beating. By the twelfth week, the bones have begun to calcify, and the external genitalia can be differentiated as male or female. In the fourth month, downy hair called **lanugo** appears over the body. In the fifth month, skeletal muscles become active, and the baby's movements are felt between 16 and 22 weeks of gestation (*Figure 8.25*). A protective substance called **vernix caseosa** covers the skin. In the sixth and seventh months, weight gain is increased, and body fat is deposited.

At 38 weeks, the baby is at full term and ready for birth.

The length of pregnancy, the gestation, is often considered to be 40 weeks, which is the time from a woman's last menstrual period to birth. However, the woman does not become pregnant until she ovulates 2 weeks after her last period, so gestation is really 38 weeks. Gestation is also divided into **trimesters.** The first trimester is up to week 12, the second from week 13 to 24, and the third from week 25 to birth.

A pregnant woman is described as a **gravida.** A woman in her first pregnancy is a **primigravida.** A woman in her second pregnancy is a gravida 2. **Parity** relates to outcome of the pregnancy: Deliveries after the twentieth week are numbered successively as **para** 1, 2, 3, and so on. **Abortus** refers to losses of pregnancy before the twentieth week. The total of abortus and paras equals a woman's gravidity.

WORD	PRONUNCIATION		ELEMENTS	DEFINITION
abortion	ah-**BOR**-shun	S/ R/	-ion *action, process* abort- *fail at onset*	Spontaneous or induced expulsion of an embryo or fetus from the uterus
abortus	ah-**BOR**-tus	S/	-us *pertaining to*	Product of abortion
amnion	**AM**-nee-on		Greek *membrane around fetus*	Membrane around the fetus that contains amniotic fluid
amniotic (adj)	am-nee-**OT**-ik	S/ R/CF	-tic *pertaining to* amni/o- *amnion*	Pertaining to the amnion
chorion	**KOH**-ree-on		Greek *membrane*	The fetal membrane that forms the placenta
chorionic (adj)	koh-ree-**ON**-ik	S/ R/	-ic *pertaining to* chorion- *chorion*	Pertaining to the chorion
chorionic villus	koh-ree-**ON**-ik **VILL**-us		villus Latin *shaggy hair*	Vascular process of the embryonic chorion to form the placenta
embryo	**EM**-bree-oh		Greek *a young one*	Developing organism from conception until the end of the second month
embryonic (adj)	em-bree-**ON**-ic	S/ R/CF	-nic *pertaining to* embry/o- *embryo*	Pertaining to the embryo
fetus	**FEE**-tus		Latin *offspring*	Human organism from the end of the eighth week after conception to birth
fetal (adj)	**FEE**-tal	S/ R/	-al *pertaining to* fet- *fetus*	Pertaining to the fetus
gravid (adj)	**GRAV**-id		Latin *pregnant*	Pregnant
gravida	**GRAV**-ih-dah		Latin *pregnant woman*	A pregnant woman
primigravida	pree-mih-**GRAV**-ih-dah	P/ R/	primi- *first* -gravida *pregnant woman*	First pregnancy
lanugo	la-**NYU**-go		Latin *wool*	Fine, soft hair on the fetal body
parity	**PAIR**-ih-tee		Latin *to bear*	Number of deliveries
para	**PAH**-rah		Latin *bring forth*	Abbreviation for number of deliveries
trimester	**TRY**-mes-ter		Latin *of 3 months' duration*	One-third of the length of a full-term pregnancy
umbilicus	um-**BIL**-ih-kus		Latin *navel*	Pit in the abdomen where the umbilical cord entered the fetus
umbilical (adj)	um-**BIL**-ih-kal	S/ R/	-al *pertaining to* umbilic- *umbilicus*	Pertaining to the umbilicus or the center of the abdomen
vernix caseosa	**VER**-niks kay-see-**OH**-sah		vernix Latin *varnish* caseosa Latin *cheese*	Cheesy substance covering skin of the fetus
villus	**VILL**-us		Latin *shaggy hair*	Thin, hairlike projection of a mucous membrane lining a cavity
villi (pl)	**VILL**-eye			
yolk sac	YOKE SACK		yolk Latin *yellow* sac Latin *pouch or bag*	Source of blood cells and future sex cells for the fetus

Exercises

A. Precision in documentation includes using the correct form (noun, verb, adjective) of the medical term. *Practice precision in this written **language of obstetrics**. Fill in the blanks.* **LO 8.13, 8.A**

amnion   amniotic

1. The _____ will be punctured in order to withdraw the _____ fluid.

embryo   embryonic

2. The _____ stage of gestation means the _____ has formed all major organ systems in the first 8 weeks of human development.

umbilical   umbilicus

3. The medical term for the navel is the _____. The _____ cord enters the fetus in the abdomen.

Maintain precision in spelling, please!

(a)   (b)   (c)   (d)

▲ **Figure 8.26** The Stages of Childbirth. (*a*) First stage: Early dilation of cervix. (*b*) First stage: Late dilation of cervix. (*c*) Second stage: Expulsion of the fetus. (*d*) Third stage: Expulsion of the placenta.

▲ **Figure 8.27** Delivery of Head. ©Photo Researchers, Inc.

LO 8.14 Pregnancy and Childbirth

Hormones of Pregnancy

Human chorionic gonadotropin (hCG) is secreted by the blastocyst and the placenta. Its presence in the mother's blood and urine is the basis for laboratory and home pregnancy tests. It can be detected as early as 9 or 10 days after conception. hCG stimulates the growth of the corpus luteum and its production of estrogen and progesterone.

Estrogen stimulates the mother's uterus to enlarge and her breasts to increase to twice their normal size. It makes the pelvic joints and ligaments more flexible so that the pelvic outlet widens for childbirth.

Progesterone is secreted by the corpus luteum and the placenta. It suppresses further ovulation, prevents menstruation, stimulates the proliferation of the endometrium to support the implantation, and inhibits contractions of the uterine muscle.

Follicle-stimulating hormone (FSH) and **luteinizing hormone (LH)** from the pituitary gland stimulate the maintenance of the corpus luteum and its estrogen and progesterone production.

Labor and Childbirth

Labor contractions begin about 30 minutes apart. They have to be intermittent because each contraction shuts down the maternal blood supply to the placenta and therefore shuts down the blood supply to the fetus. Labor pains are due to ischemia of the **myometrium**.

Labor is divided into three stages, each of which is usually longer in a **primipara** (first-time birth) than in a **multipara** (two or more births).

First Stage of Labor—Dilation of the Cervix

This is the longest stage. It can be a few hours in a multipara to more than 1 day in a primipara. **Dilation** is widening of the cervical canal to the same diameter as the baby's head (*Figure 8.26a and b*). At the same time, the wall of the cervix becomes thinner, a process called **effacement**. During dilation, the fetal membranes rupture, and the "waters break" as amniotic fluid is released.

Second Stage of Labor—Expulsion of the Fetus

As the uterus continues to contract, additional pain is generated by the stretching of the cervix and vagina by the baby's head. When the head reaches the vaginal opening and stretches the vulva, the head is said to be **crowning** (*Figure 8.27*). This process is sometimes helped by performing an **episiotomy**, an incision in the perineum to prevent tearing.

After the baby is delivered, the umbilical cord is clamped in two places and cut between the two clamps.

Third Stage of Labor—Expulsion of the Placenta

After the baby is delivered, the uterus continues to contract. It pushes the placenta off the uterine wall and expels it out of the vagina. This usually takes 5 to 15 minutes; after 30 minutes the placenta is said to be **retained** and may have to be removed manually by the obstetrician.

S = Suffix   P = Prefix   R = Root   R/CF = Combining Form

WORD	PRONUNCIATION	ELEMENTS		DEFINITION
autolysis	awe-**TOL**-ih-sis	P/ R/	**auto-** *self* **-lysis** *destruction*	Self-destruction of cells by enzymes within the cells
crowning	**KROWN**-ing	S/ R/	**-ing** *doing, quality of* **crown-** *crown*	During childbirth, when the maximum diameter of the baby's head comes through the vulvar ring
dilation	die-**LAY**-shun	S/ R/	**-ion** *process* **dilat-** *open out*	Stretching or enlarging of an opening
effacement	ee-**FACE**-ment	S/ R/	**-ment** *resulting state* **efface-** *wipe out*	Thinning of the cervix during labor
episiotomy	eh-peez-ee-**OT**-oh-mee	S/ R/CF	**-tomy** *surgical incision* **episi/o-** *vulva*	Surgical incision of the vulva
human chorionic gonadotropin	**HYU**-man koh-ree-**ON**-ik **GOH**-nad-oh-**TROH**-pin	 S/ R/ S/ R/CF	human Latin *human being* **-ic** *pertaining to* **chorion-** *chorion* **-tropin** *nourishing* **gonad/o-** *gonad*	Hormone secreted by the blastocyst and the placenta to maintain pregnancy
labor	**LAY**-bore		Latin *toil, suffering*	Process of expulsion of the fetus
lochia	**LOW**-kee-uh		Greek *relating to childbirth*	Vaginal discharge following childbirth
multipara	mul-**TIP**-ah-ruh	P/ S/	**multi-** *many* **-para** *to bring forth*	Woman who has given birth to two or more children
postpartum	post-**PAR**-tum	P/ R/	**post-** *after* **-partum** *childbirth*	After childbirth
primipara	pree-**MIP**-ah-ruh	P/ S/	**primi-** *first* **-para** *to bring forth*	Woman who has given birth for the first time
puerperium (**Note:** This term is composed only of roots.)	pyu-er-**PEE**-ree-um	R/ R/	**puer-** *child* **-perium** *bringing forth*	Six-week period after birth in which the uterus involutes

Exercises

A. Several of these elements you have seen before, and you will certainly see them again in other terms. *Learn each once, and recognize it all the time. Choose the best answer to the questions.* **LO 8.14, 8.A, 8.D**

1. The term that contains the prefix meaning *many* is
   a. primipara
   b. lochia
   c. multipara
   d. biopsy

2. The term that contains the suffix meaning *incision* is
   a. episiotomy
   b. curette
   c. dilation
   d. palpation

3. The term that contains the suffix meaning *to bring forth* is
   a. primipara
   b. involution
   c. effacement
   d. follicular

4. The term that contains the root meaning *child* is
   a. lochia
   b. multipara
   c. puerperium
   d. crowning

5. The term that contains the suffix meaning *process* is
   a. effacement
   b. episiotomy
   c. dilation
   d. coital

6. The term that contains the prefix meaning *first* is
   a. multipara
   b. puerperium
   c. primipara
   d. zygote

7. The term that contains the prefix meaning *self* is
   a. multipara
   b. autolysis
   c. lochia
   d. postpartum

8. The term that contains the prefix meaning *after* is
   a. primipara
   b. postpartum
   c. multipara
   d. lochia

B. Review the text regarding pregnancy and childbirth. *Select all answers that correctly complete each statement.* **LO 8.14, 8.F**

1. The hormones involved in pregnancy and childbirth are:
   a. FSH   b. LH   c. progesterone   d. BMT   e. MRI   f. HCG   g. estrogen   h. insulin

2. The first stage of labor:
   a. is dilation of the cervix.
   b. is the shortest stage of labor
   c. includes the process of effacement
   d. includes the rupture of the fetal membranes
   e. can be shorter in multipara and longer in primipara

Case Report (CR) 8.3

You are
. . . an obstetric assistant working with Garry Joiner, MD, an obstetrician at Fulwood Medical Center.

Your patient is
. . . Mrs. Gloria Maggay, a 29-year-old housekeeper.

Mrs. Maggay's last menstrual period (**LMP**) was 8 weeks ago, and she has a positive home pregnancy test. This is her first pregnancy. She has breast tenderness and mild nausea. For the past 2 days, she has had some cramping and right-sided, lower abdominal pain, and this morning she had vaginal spotting. Her VS are T 99°F, P 80, R 14, BP 130/70.

While you are waiting for Dr. Joiner to come and examine Mrs. Maggay, she complains of feeling faint and has a sharp, severe pain in her lower abdomen on the right side. Her pulse rate has increased to 92. You need to recognize what is happening. Mrs. Maggay's symptoms are those of an ectopic pregnancy. The sudden increase in the pain and the rise in pulse rate can indicate that the tube has ruptured and is hemorrhaging into the abdominal cavity. The gynecologist should see her immediately and, if necessary, take her to the **operating room (OR)** for laparoscopic surgery to stop the bleeding and evacuate the products of conception.

LO 8.15 Disorders of Pregnancy

Ectopic Pregnancy

If the uterine tube is obstructed, the fertilized egg will be prevented from moving into the uterus and will continue its development in the uterine tube. This is called an **ectopic pregnancy.** Tubal disorders that cause ectopic pregnancy include previous salpingitis, pelvic inflammatory disease (PID), and endometriosis.

Preeclampsia and Eclampsia

Preeclampsia is a sudden, abnormal increase in blood pressure after the 20th week of pregnancy, with proteinuria and edema.

Eclampsia is a life-threatening condition, characterized by the signs and symptoms of preeclampsia and with the addition of convulsions. Management involves immediate admission to the hospital with control of the mother's blood pressure. The baby is delivered as soon as the mother is stabilized, regardless of maturity.

Amniotic Fluid Abnormalities

Amniotic fluid abnormalities occur in the second trimester. Normally, the fetus breathes in and swallows amniotic fluid to promote development of the gastrointestinal tract and lungs.

- **Oligohydramnios** is too little amniotic fluid. It is associated with an increase in the risk of birth defects and poor fetal growth. Its etiology is unknown.
- **Polyhydramnios** is too much amniotic fluid. It causes abdominal discomfort and breathing difficulties for the mother. It also is associated with **preterm delivery,** placental problems, and fetal growth problems.

Gestational Diabetes Mellitus

In some pregnant women, the amount of insulin they can produce decreases. This leads to **gestational diabetes mellitus (GDM)** and increased risk of preeclampsia. For the neonate, it increases the risk of **perinatal mortality.** Later in life, both mother and child are at increased risk for developing type 2 diabetes and obesity.

Hyperemesis Gravidarum

Eighty percent of pregnant women experience some degree of "morning sickness." It is at its worst between 2 and 12 weeks and resolves in the second trimester. For a few women, nausea and vomiting persist. This is **hyperemesis gravidarum.** Severe cases may have to be admitted to the hospital for intravenous (IV) fluids.

WORD	PRONUNCIATION		ELEMENTS	DEFINITION
eclampsia	eh-**KLAMP**-see-uh		Greek *a shining forth*	Convulsions in a patient with preeclampsia
ectopic	ek-**TOP**-ik	S/ R/	**-ic** *pertaining to* **ectop-** *on the outside, displaced*	Out of place, not in a normal position
hyperemesis gravidarum	high-per-**EM**-eh-sis gra-vih-**DAR**-um	P/ R/	**hyper-** *excessive* **-emesis** *vomiting* **gravidarum** Latin *pregnant woman*	Excessive vomiting due to pregnancy
mortality	mor-**TAL**-ih-tee	S/ S/ R/	**-al-** *pertaining to* **-ity** *condition, state* **mort-** *death*	Fatal outcome or death rate
oligohydramnios	**OL**-ih-goh-high-**DRAM**-nee-os	P/ R/ R/	**oligo-** *too little, scanty* **-hydr-** *water* **-amnios** *amnion*	Too little amniotic fluid
polyhydramnios	**POL**-ee-high-**DRAM**-nee-os	P/	**poly-** *many*	Too much amniotic fluid
perinatal	per-ih-**NAY**-tal	S/ P/ R/	**-al** *pertaining to* **peri-** *around* **-nat-** *birth*	Around the time of birth
preeclampsia	pree-eh-**KLAMP**-see-uh	S/ P/ R/	**-ia** *condition* **pre-** *before* **-eclamps-** *shining forth*	Hypertension, edema, and proteinuria during pregnancy
preterm	**PREE**-term	P/ R/	**pre-** *before* **-term** *normal gestation*	Baby delivered before 37 weeks of gestation
premature (syn)	pree-mah-**TYUR**	R/	**-mature** *ripe, ready*	Occurring before the expected time; for example, an infant born before 37 weeks of gestation
teratogen	**TER**-ah-toh-jen	S/ R/CF	**-gen** *produce, create* **terat/o-** *monster, malformed fetus*	Agent that produces fetal deformities
teratogenesis teratogenic (adj)	**TER**-ah-toh-**JEN**-eh-sis **TER**-ah-toh-**JEN**-ik	R/CF S/	**-genesis** *form, create* **-ic** *pertaining to*	Process involved in producing fetal deformities Capable of producing fetal deformities

Exercises

A. After reading Case Report (CR) 8.3, answer the following questions. *Choose the best answer.* **LO 8.15**

1. Which of the following symptoms did Mrs. Maggay develop while she was in the office?

   a. decreased pulse rate   **b.** vaginal spotting   **c.** severe right-sided abdominal pain   **d.** mild nausea

2. Mrs. Maggay is most liking suffering from:

   a. fertilized egg implanted in a uterine tube   **b.** endometrial tissue occurring outside of the uterus

   c. prolapsed uterus   **d.** rupture of the appendix

B. Define the meaning of the word elements. *Select the correct answer that completes each statement.* **LO 8.15**

1. The word element that means **scanty**:
   a. *poly-*   **b.** *hyper-*   **c.** *oligo-*   **d.** *ectop-*   **e.** *-amnios*

2. The word element *terat-* means:
   a. four   **b.** condition of   **c.** death   **d.** monster   **e.** shining forth

3. The word element *-emesis* means:
   a. excessive   **b.** tension   **c.** vomiting   **d.** bleeding   **e.** nausea

▲ **Figure 8.28** Breech Presentation.

▲ **Figure 8.29** Postmature Infant. ©VisualDx

▲ **Figure 8.30** Placenta (Afterbirth).
©AzmanL/Getty Images RF

LO 8.16 Disorders of Childbirth

Fetal distress due to lack of oxygen is an uncommon complication of labor but is detrimental if not recognized.

Abnormal position of fetus occurs when the baby at the beginning of labor is not in a head-first **(vertex)** presentation facing rearward. Abnormal positions include:

- **Breech.** The buttocks present *(Figure 8.28)*.
- **Face.** The face instead of the top of the head presents.
- **Shoulder.** The shoulder and upper back are trying to exit the uterus first.

Nuchal cord is the condition of having the cord wrapped around the baby's neck during delivery. This occurs in 20% of deliveries.

Prolapsed umbilical cord occurs when the cord precedes the baby down the birth canal. Pressure on the cord can cut off the baby's blood supply, which is still being provided through the umbilical arteries.

Premature rupture of the membranes (PROM) occurs in 10% of normal pregnancies and increases the risk of infection of the uterus and fetus.

Gestational Classification

Every **neonate** (newborn) is one of the following:

- **Premature**—less than 37 weeks gestation.
- **Full-term**—between 37 and 42 weeks gestation.
- **Postmature**—longer than 42 weeks gestation *(Figure 8.29)*.

Prematurity occurs in about 8% of newborns. The earlier the baby is born, the more life-threatening problems occur.

Because their lungs are underdeveloped, premature babies can develop **respiratory distress syndrome (RDS),** also called **hyaline membrane disease**. The premature baby's lungs are not mature enough to produce **surfactant**, a mixture of lipids and proteins that keeps the alveoli from collapsing.

If their brains are underdeveloped, premature newborns can have inconsistent breathing with **apnea**. They are susceptible to bleeding into the brain. Their immune systems have low levels of antibodies to provide protection from infection.

An immature liver can impair the excretion of bilirubin *(see Chapter 5)*, and premature babies become jaundiced. High levels of bilirubin can produce **kernicterus**, in which deposits of bilirubin in the brain cause brain damage.

Postmaturity is much less common than prematurity. Its etiology is unknown, but the placenta begins to shrink and is less able to supply sufficient nutrients to the baby. This leads to hypoglycemia; loss of subcutaneous fat; dry, peeling skin; and, if oxygen is lacking, fetal distress. The baby can pass stools **(meconium)** into the amniotic fluid. In its distress, the baby can take deep gasping breaths and inhale the meconium fluid. This leads to **meconium aspiration syndrome (MAS)** and respiratory difficulty at birth.

Placental Disorders

Placenta abruptio is separation of the placenta from the uterine wall before delivery of the baby. The baby's oxygen supply is cut off, and fetal distress appears quickly. It is an obstetric (OB) emergency, and usually a C-section is indicated.

Placenta previa occurs when the placenta is positioned over the internal os of the cervix. The placenta may separate from the uterine wall during stage one of labor and the cervix starts to dilate.

Retained placenta is a low-lying placenta between the baby's head and the internal os of the cervix. It can cause severe bleeding during labor. The expulsion of the placenta *(Figure 8.30)* can happen naturally. The result of retained placenta is heavy uterine bleeding called **postpartum hemorrhage (PPH)**. Manual removal of the retained product may be necessary under spinal, epidural, or general anesthesia.

Abbreviations	
MAS	meconium aspiration syndrome
OB	obstetrics
PPH	postpartum hemorrhage
PROM	premature rupture of the membranes
RDS	respiratory distress syndrome

LO 8.16, 18.A
Word Analysis and Definition

S = Suffix   P = Prefix   R = Root   R/CF = Combining Form

WORD	PRONUNCIATION		ELEMENTS	DEFINITION
abruptio	ab-**RUP**-shee-oh		Latin *to break off*	Placenta abruptio is the premature detachment of the placenta
apnea	**AP**-nee-ah		Greek *lack of breath*	Absence of spontaneous respiration
breech	BREECH		Old English *trousers*	Buttocks-first presentation of fetus at delivery
distress	dis-**TRESS**		Latin *circumstance causing anxiety or hardship*	State that is causing pain or suffering
hyaline membrane disease	**HIGH**-ah-line **MEM**-brain diz-**EEZ**	P/ R/	**hyaline** Greek *glassy* **membrane** Latin *a skin* **dis-** *without* **-ease** *comfort*	Respiratory distress syndrome of the newborn
kernicterus	ker-**NIK**-ter-us	R/ R/	**kern-** *nucleus* **-icterus** *jaundice*	Bilirubin staining of the basal nuclei of the brain
meconium meconium aspiration syndrome	meh-**KOH**-nee-um meh-**KOH**-nee-um **AS**-pih-**RAY**-shun **SIN**-drome	S/ R/ P/ R/	Greek *a little poppy* **-ion** *process* **aspirat-** *to breathe* **syn-** *together* **-drome** *running*	The first bowel movement of the newborn Condition that occurs when the fetus passes the first bowel movement in the amniotic fluid and then inhales it into its lungs
neonate	**NEE**-oh-nate	P/ R/CF	**neo-** *new* **-nate** *born*	A newborn infant
neonatal	**NEE**-oh-**NAY**-tal	S/ R/	**-al** *new* **-nat-** *born*	Pertaining to the newborn infant or the newborn period
nuchal cord	**NYU**-kul KORD		French *the back (nape) of the neck*	Loop of umbilical cord around the fetal neck
postmature (adj)	post-mah-**TYUR**	P/ R/CF	**post-** *after* **matur/e** *ripe, ready*	Pertaining to an infant born after 42 weeks of gestation
postmaturity (noun)	post-mah-**TYUR**-ih-tee	S/	**-ity** *condition*	Condition of being postmature
premature (adj)	pree-mah-**TYUR**	P/ R/CF	**pre-** *before, in front of* **-mature** *ripe, ready*	Occurring before the expected time; for example, when an infant is born before 37 weeks of gestation
prematurity (noun) preemie (informal)	pree-mah-**TYUR**-ih-tee **PREE**-mee	S/	**-ity** *condition*	Condition of being premature Premature baby
previa	**PREE**-vee-ah	P/ R/	**pre-** *before, in front of* **-via** *the way*	Anything that blocks the fetus during its birth; for example, an abnormally situated placenta, placenta previa
vertex	**VER**-teks		Latin *whorl*	Topmost point of the vault of the skull

Exercises

A. Elements. *Real familiarity with obstetrical and reproductive terms means you can look at an element and identify it as either a prefix (P), root (R), or suffix (S). Identify each element by writing its type and meaning in the appropriate columns. The first one is done for you. Fill in the blanks.* **LO 8.16**

Element	Type	Meaning	Element	Type	Meaning
1. *post*	P	after	5. *mature*		
2. *ity*			6. *pre*		
3. *kern*			7. *dis*		
4. *via*					

B. Describe the disorders of childbirth. *Match the disorder in the first column with its correct description in the second column.* **LO 8.16**

	Term		Meaning
_____	1. prolapsed umbilical cord	a.	cord is wrapped around the baby's neck during delivery
_____	2. placenta previa	b.	cord comes before the baby during delivery
_____	3. kernicterus	c.	brain damage due to bilirubin deposits
_____	4. nuchal cord	d.	separation of the placenta from the uterine wall before delivery
_____	5. placenta abruptio	e.	placenta is positioned over the internal os of the cervix

LESSON 8.5 Obstetrics: Pregnancy and Childbirth   251

Lesson 8.6

Obstetrical Diagnostic and Therapeutic Procedures and Pharmacology

LO 8.17 Obstetric Diagnostic Procedures

Prenatal Screening Tests

These tests can help determine if the pregnancy is at a higher risk for the baby to have a specific problem; the test does not diagnose a problem, only whether it is more or less likely. There is no risk of miscarriage from these tests.

First trimester screening is done between the 11th and 13th weeks of pregnancy. It combines **maternal** blood testing for human **chorionic gonadotropin** (hCG) (the pregnancy hormone) and **pregnancy-associated plasma protein A (PAPP-A)** with an ultrasound measurement of the back of the baby's neck (**nuchal translucency—NT**). Women with higher than average NT measurements and/or higher or lower than average hCG or PAPP-A values *might* be at risk for having a baby with Down Syndrome or with another rare chromosomal problem, Trisomy 18.

Chorionic villus sampling (CVS) also uses ultrasound guidance to insert a needle through the abdomen or a catheter through the cervix to obtain a sample of placental tissue that can be tested for fetal chromosomal abnormalities. The main advantage of CVS is that it can be performed between 9 and 13 weeks of pregnancy, earlier than amniocentesis (*see below*).

Second trimester screening is done between the 15th and 18th weeks of gestation. Called the **quad screen,** it measures the levels of four substances in a pregnant woman's blood: **alpha-fetoprotein (AFP), hCG, unconjugated estriol,** and **dimeric inhibin.** These chemicals are made by the placenta and fetus. Women with high or low levels of these substances *may* be at risk for having a baby with Down Syndrome, Trisomy 18, a **neural tube defect** such as **spina bifida**, or an abdominal wall defect in which abdominal contents protrude through the abdominal wall.

Cystic fibrosis screening is a blood test to determine the presence of the gene that causes CF. Both parents have to be carriers of the gene for the baby to be at risk for CF.

Ultrasound can be used to show most of the organs and bones of the baby in utero. In addition to the screenings described above, ultrasound can be used between 18 and 20 weeks of pregnancy to provide a detailed picture of the baby's anatomy, its size, and growth. Ultrasound carries no known risks and is the most frequently used method of prenatal screening.

Diagnostic Tests

Diagnostic tests, as distinct from screening tests, can confirm the presence of the congenital anomaly suggested by the screening test.

Amniocentesis uses ultrasound guidance to insert a thin needle through the abdominal wall into the amniotic sac around the baby to remove a small amount of amniotic fluid. This fluid contains fetal skin fibroblasts that can be tested for abnormalities. Amniocentesis is performed between 15 and 20 weeks to diagnose chromosome abnormalities and neural tube defects.

Therapeutic Procedures

During labor, there is electronic fetal heart monitoring to determine whether the baby is in distress. Treatment is to give the mother oxygen or increase IV fluids. If distress persists, the baby is delivered as quickly as possible by **forceps extraction**, vacuum extractor, or **cesarean section (C-section)**.

WORD	PRONUNCIATION	ELEMENTS		DEFINITION
amniocentesis	AM-nee-oh-senTEE-sis	S/ R/CF	-centesis *puncture* amni/o- *amnion*	Removal of amniotic fluid for diagnostic purposes
cesarean section (C-section) (syn)	seh-ZAH-ree-an SEK-shun		Roman law under the Caesars required that pregnant women who died be cut open and the fetus extracted	Extraction of the fetus through an incision in the abdomen and uterine wall
chorion chorionic chorionic villus	KOH-ree-on koh-ree-ON-ik koh-ree-ON-ik VILL-us	S/ R/	Greek *membrane* -ic *pertaining to* chorion- *chorion* villus Latin *shaggy hair*	Outer fetal membrane that becomes the placenta Pertaining to the chorion Vascular process of the embryonic chorion to form the placenta
diagnostic	die-ag-NOS-tik	S/ P/ R/	-tic *pertaining to* dia- *complete* -gnos- *recognize an abnormal condition*	Pertaining to establishing the cause of a disease
forceps extraction	FOR-seps ek-STRAK-shun		forceps Latin *a pair of tongs* extraction Latin *to draw out*	Assisted delivery of the baby by an instrument that grasps the head of the baby
gonadotropin	GO-nad-oh-TROH-pin	S/ R/CF	-tropin *nourishing* gonad/o *gonad*	Hormone capable of promoting gonad function
maternal	mah-TER-nal	S/ R/	-al *pertaining to* matern- *mother*	Pertaining to, or derived from, the mother
neural neural tube	NYU-ral NYU-ral TYUB	S/ R/	-al *pertaining to* neur- *nerve*	Pertaining to any structure composed of nerve cells Embryologic tubelike structure that forms the brain and spinal cord
nuchal	NYU-kul		French *the back (nape) of the neck*	The back (nape) of the neck
screen screening	SKREEN SKREEN-ing	S/ R/	Middle English *screne* -ing *process* screen- *a system for separating*	A test to determine the presence or absence of a disease. A testing process that determines the presence or absence of a disease
translucent	tranz-LOO-sent	S/ P/ R/	-ent *pertaining to* trans- *across, through* -luc- *light*	Allowing light to pass through

Exercises

A. Describe the meaning of abbreviations related to obstetrical screening tests. *Given the abbreviation, choose its correct description.* **LO 8.17, 8.F**

1. PAPP-A is used to screen for:

   a. spina bifida   **b.** fetal alcohol syndrome   **c.** Down syndrome   **d.** cystic fibrosis

2. An abnormally high or low hCG level may indicate which disorder?

   a. nuchal translucency   **b.** spina bifida   **c.** fetal alcohol syndrome   **d.** cystic fibrosis

3. How is NT measured?

   a. maternal blood testing   **b.** fetal blood testing   **c.** amniocentesis   **d.** ultrasound

B. Construct medical terms related to obstetrics. *Given the definition, complete the described medical terms by inputting the correct word element.* **LO 8.17, 8.C**

1. Hormone capable of promoting gonad function: gonad/o/_____

2. To puncture the amniotic sac: amni/o/ _____

3. Pertaining to the mother: _____ /al

4. Allowing light to pass through: _____ /luc/ent

5. Pertaining to a nerve: _____ /al

Breast

LO 8.18 The Breast

Until the relatively recent introduction of bottles filled with liquid supplied by cows or soybeans, the milk produced by the female breast was essential for the survival of the human species. Nourishment of the infant remains the breast's major function.

Anatomy of the Breast

The breasts of males and females are identical until puberty, when ovarian hormones stimulate the development of the breast in females. Adult males still have main milk ducts in their breasts.

Each adult female breast has a **body** located over the pectoralis major muscle and an **axillary tail** extending toward the armpit. The **nipple** projects from the breast and contains multiple openings of the main milk ducts. The reddish-brown **areola** surrounds the nipple. The small bumps on its surface are **areolar glands.** These are sebaceous glands, the secretions of which prevent chapping and cracking during breastfeeding.

Internally, the breasts are supported by **suspensory ligaments** that extend from the skin to the fascia overlying the pectoralis major muscle *(Figure 8.31)*.

The **nonlactating breast** consists mostly of adipose and connective tissues. It has a system of ducts that branch through the connective tissue and converge on the nipple.

Mammary Gland

When the **mammary gland** develops during pregnancy, it is divided into 15 to 20 lobes that contain the secretory **alveoli** that produce milk. Each lobe is drained by the main milk ducts, called **lactiferous ducts** *(see Figure 8.34)*. Immediately before opening onto the nipple, each lactiferous duct dilates to form a **lactiferous sinus** in which milk is stored before being released from the nipple.

Keynotes

- There is no relationship between breast size and the ability to breastfeed.
- Breastfeeding is not a reliable means of contraception. It has a failure rate of around 10%.

Lactation

When the mammary gland develops during pregnancy, high estrogen levels cause the lactiferous ducts to grow and branch, and progesterone stimulates the budding of alveoli at the ends of the ducts. The alveoli are formed in grapelike clusters. The percentage of adipose and connective tissue diminishes.

In late pregnancy, the alveoli and ducts contain **colostrum**. This secretion contains more protein but less fat than human milk, but it also contains high levels of **immunoglobulins** *(see Chapter 12)* to give the newborn infant protection from infections. Colostrum is replaced by milk 2 or 3 days after the baby's birth, and this replacement is complete by day 5.

Milk production is mainly controlled by **prolactin**, a hormone from the pituitary gland. The other essential stimulus to milk production is the baby's sucking *(Figure 8.32)*, which stimulates prolactin production. In addition, the **sucking reflex** stimulates the pituitary gland to produce **oxytocin** *(see Chapter 17)*, which causes milk to be ejected from the alveoli into the duct system, and helps to form a bond between mother and child.

Rib

Adipose tissue

Intercostal muscles

Suspensory ligaments

Pectoralis major muscle

Lobe

Areola

Nipple

Lactiferous sinus

Lactiferous duct

Deep fascia

▲ **Figure 8.31** Anatomy of Lactating Breast.

▲ **Figure 8.32** Breastfeeding. ©Getty Images RF

WORD	PRONUNCIATION	ELEMENTS		DEFINITION
alveolus alveoli (pl)	al-VEE-oh-lus		Latin *small hollow or cavity*	Small empty sac or space
areola areolar (adj)	ah-**REE**-oh-luh	S/ R/	Latin *small area* -ar *pertaining to* areol- *area around the nipple*	Circular reddish area surrounding the nipple Pertaining to the areola
colostrum	koh-**LOSS**-trum		Latin *foremilk*	The first breast secretion at the end of pregnancy
duct	DUKT		Latin *to lead*	A tube to carry fluid or gas
lactation	lak-**TAY**-shun	S/ R/CF	-ation *process* lact/i- *milk*	Production of milk
lactiferous (adj) lactate (verb)	lak-**TIF**-er-us	S/ R/	-ous *pertaining to* -fer- *to bear, carry*	Pertaining to or yielding milk
mammary	**MAM**-ah-ree	S/ R/	-ary *pertaining to* mamm- *breast*	Relating to the lactating breast
nipple	**NIP**-el		Old English *small nose*	Projection from the breast into which the lactiferous ducts open
oxytocin	**OK**-see-**TOH**-sin	S/ R/CF R/	-in *chemical compound* ox/y- *oxygen* -toc- *labor, birth*	Pituitary hormone that stimulates the uterus to contract and causes breast milk to be ejected from the alveoli into the duct system
prolactin	pro-**LAK**-tin	S/ P/ R/	-in *chemical compound* pro- *before* -lact- *milk*	Pituitary hormone that stimulates production of milk

Exercises

A. Spelling your documentation correctly is a mark of an educated professional. *Read the following statements and insert the correctly spelled term in the blanks.* **LO 8.18, 8.A**

1. (Prolectin/Prolactin) _____ is the pituitary hormone that stimulates production of milk.

2. The circular, reddish area surrounding the nipple is the (aireola/areola) _____.

3. (Oxitocin/Oxytocin) _____ is the pituitary hormone that stimulates the uterus to contract.

4. The first breast secretion at the end of pregnancy is known as (colestrium/colostrum) _____.

5. The projection from the breast into which the milk ducts open is the (nippel/nipple) _____.

6. (Laktiferous/Lactiferous) _____ means *pertaining to or yielding milk.*

7. The areolar glands are (cebaceous/sebaceous) _____ glands.

B. Find the one false statement in the following choices. *Choose T if the statement is True. Choose F if the statement is False.* **LO 8.18, 8.A**

1. The lactiferous ducts produce milk.		T	F
2. In late pregnancy, the alveoli and ducts contain colostrum.		T	F
3. High levels of immunoglobulins are in breast milk.		T	F
4. Milk production is mainly controlled by prolactin.		T	F
5. The sucking reflex produces estrogen.		T	F
6. Milk flows from the lactiferous duct to the lactiferous sinus to the nipple.		T	F

LO 8.19 Disorders of the Breast

Mastitis, inflammation of the breast, can occur in association with breastfeeding if the nipple or areola is cracked or traumatized. It is usually segmental in one of the lobes of the breast and responds well to antibiotics. It is not an indication for stopping breastfeeding.

Mastalgia (breast pain) is the most common benign breast disorder. The pain can be associated with breast tenderness and be part of PMS.

Nipple discharge, particularly if it is from one breast and bloody, is an indication of an underlying disorder such as breast cancer and warrants investigation.

Fibroadenomas are circumscribed, small, benign tumors that can be either cystic or solid and can be multiple.

Fibrocystic disease of the breast presents as a dense, irregular cobblestone consistency of the breast, often with intermittent breast discomfort *(Figure 8.33)*. It occurs in over 60% of all women and is considered by many doctors as a normal variant.

Galactorrhea is the production of milk when a woman is not breastfeeding. Sometimes the cause cannot be found, but it can occur in association with hormone therapy, antidepressants, tumor of the pituitary gland *(see Chapter 17)*, and use of street drugs such as opiates and marijuana. In most cases, the milk production ceases with time.

Gynecomastia, enlargement of the breast, can be unilateral or bilateral and occur in both sexes. It is usually associated with either liver disease, marijuana, or drug therapy such as estrogens, calcium channel blockers, and antineoplastic drugs. It remits or disappears after the drug is withdrawn.

Breast cancer affects one in eight women in their lifetime. Risk factors include a family history, particularly if a woman carries either of the breast cancer **genes,** *BRCA1* or *BRCA2*; the use of postmenopausal estrogen therapy; and an early menarche and late menopause.

Jobs associated with the occurrence of breast cancer include automotive plastics manufacturing, metal working, food canning, agriculture, and bar/gambling. Women with a cosmetic breast implant have a 25% higher risk of being diagnosed with breast cancer when the disease has already advanced. Breast cancer occurs rarely in men.

Most breast cancers occur in the upper and outer quadrant of the breast, and symptoms include:

- A lump or thickening in the breast.
- Change in size, shape, or appearance of the breast.
- Dimpling of the skin of the breast.
- Pitting of the skin of the breast.
- Bloody discharge from the nipple.
- Peeling, flaking, redness, or scaling of the nipple and areola (**Paget's disease of the breast**).

Paget's disease of the breast *(see Figure 8.34)* occurs in 5% of breast cancers. The nipple and areola become scaly, red, flaky, and itchy due to cancer cells collecting there. The underlying cancer is usually found in the ducts of the nipple. The 19th-century British surgeon Sir James Paget first reported the relationship between the changes in the nipple and breast cancer.

Breast cancer can **metastasize** to lymph nodes, lungs, liver, bone, brain, and skin.

▲ **Figure 8.33** **Mammogram Showing Fibrocystic Disease of the Breast.** ©ALIX/ Phanie/Photo Researchers, Inc.

▲ **Figure 8.34** **Paget Disease of the Nipple Is Associated with Breast Cancer.** ©Wellcome Photo Library

S = Suffix   P = Prefix   R = Root   R/CF = Combining Form

WORD	PRONUNCIATION	ELEMENTS		DEFINITION
fibroadenoma	**FIE**-broh-ad-en-**OH**-mah	S/ R/CF R/	**-oma** *tumor* **fibr/o-** *fiber* **-aden-** *gland*	Benign tumor containing much fibrous tissue
fibrocystic disease	fie-broh-**SIS**-tik diz-**EEZ**	S/ R/CF R/	**-ic** *pertaining to* **fibr/o-** *fiber* **-cyst-** *cyst*	Benign breast disease with multiple tiny lumps and cysts
galactorrhea	gah-**LAK**-toh-**REE**-ah	S/ R/CF	**-rrhea** *flow* **galact/o-** *milk*	Abnormal flow of milk from the breasts
gynecomastia	**GUY**-nih-koh-**MAS**-tee-ah	S/ R/CF R/	**-ia** *condition* **gynec/o-** *female* **-mast-** *breast*	Enlargement of the breast
mastalgia	mass-**TAL**-jee-uh	S/ R/	**-algia** *pain* **mast-** *breast*	Pain in the breast
mastitis	mass-**TIE**-tis	S/ R/	**-itis** *inflammation* **mast-** *breast*	Inflammation of the breast
Paget's disease of the breast	**PA**-jet		Sir James Paget, 1814–1899, English surgeon	Changes in the nipple when associated with breast cancer

Exercises

A. Build your knowledge of suffixes, which always provide a big clue to the meaning of a medical term. *Review all the terms in the above WAD; then answer the following questions. All of these questions can be answered by analyzing the elements in each term. Fill in the blank.* **LO 8.19, 8.A**

1. Pain in the breast: _____

2. Inflammation of the breast: _____

3. A small, benign tumor of the breast: _____

4. Enlargement of the breast: _____

5. Benign breast disease with multiple tiny bumps and cysts: _____

B. Deconstruct medical terms to understand their meanings. *Fill in the blank.* **LO 8.19, LO 8.D**

1. The suffix in the term **galactorrhea** means: _____

2. The root in the term **mastalgia** means: _____

3. The combining form in the term **galactorrhea** means: _____

4. The suffix in the term **mastitis** means: _____

5. The suffix in the term **gynecomastia** means: _____

Diagnostic and Therapeutic Procedures and Pharmacology of Disorders of the Breast

▲ **Figure 8.35**
Mammogram showing breast cancer. ©UHB Trust/ Getty Images

Abbreviations

ACOG	American College of Obstetricians and Gynecologists
ACS	American College of Surgeons
AMA	American Medical Association
BSE	breast-self examination
ER-positive	Estrogen-receptor-positive
HER2	Human Growth Factor Receptor 2
NCI	National Cancer Institute
PEM	Positron emission mammography
SERM	selective estrogen receptor modulator
TNM	tumor, nodes, metastasis

LO 8.20 Diagnostic Procedures

Breast self-examination (BSE) on a monthly basis has been shown to be of questionable value. It is recommended by the American College of Obstetricians and Gynecologists (**ACOG**) and the American Medical Association (**AMA**) but neither recommended nor discouraged by the American Cancer Society (**ACS**), the National Cancer Institute (**NCI),** and other organizations.

However, many breast cancers are discovered as a lump by the patient during a self-examination. Another 40% are discovered on routine **mammogram** *(Figure 8.33)*. Routine **mammography** reduces breast cancer mortality by 25% to 30% *(Figure 8.35)*. However, it has a false positive rate of 7% and a false negative rate of 10%. 3D mammograms, ultrasound, magnetic resonance imaging (MRI), and **positron emission mammography (PEM)** are adjuncts to routine 2D mammography for further evaluation of suspicious lesions.

The pathology report on breast cancer cells will include results of a hormone receptor **assay.** A breast cancer is called **estrogen-receptor-positive (ER-positive)** if its cells have receptors for estrogen that promote their growth. A breast cancer is called **progesterone-receptor-positive** if its cells have receptors for progesterone that can promote their growth. Approximately two-thirds of breast cancers test positive for hormone receptors. The pathology report also will tell if the breast cancer cells have too many copies of the **gene HER2.** If the breast cancer cells are negative for both hormone receptors and HER2, it is called a **triple negative** breast cancer.

Stereotactic biopsy, a needle biopsy performed during mammography, and **excisional biopsy,** surgical removal of a tumor with a surrounding margin of normal breast tissue, provide material for a pathological diagnosis.

Staging of breast cancer (**TNM**) is based on the size of the tumor in the breast (T), the status of the lymph nodes in the axilla (N), and the metastatic spread to distant sites (M).

LO 8.20 Therapeutic Procedures

Surgical treatments for breast cancer include the following:

- **Lumpectomy** and **quadrantectomy** are breast-conserving surgical procedures.
- **Simple mastectomy** removes the whole breast.
- **Modified radical mastectomy** removes the whole breast and the axillary lymph nodes, but the muscle is left intact.
- **Radical mastectomy** is complete removal of all breast tissue, the underlying pectoralis major muscle, and all associated lymph nodes.

Radiation therapy uses high energy rays or particles to destroy cancer cells. **External beam radiation** is delivered from a machine outside the body. **Internal radiation (brachytherapy)** uses **radioactive** seeds or pellets placed inside the body for a short time at the site of the lesion.

Suction **lipectomy (liposuction)** is the insertion of a metal tube into an incision of the skin, and then suction is applied and fat tissue is aspirated and removed. This technique is used to treat excess breast tissue in **gynecomastia.** It also is used for other areas of the body not related to disorders of the breast.

LO 8.20 Pharmacology

Chemotherapy is a **systemic** therapy affecting the whole body by going through the bloodstream to destroy any cancer cells; unfortunately it also affects other body cells, producing side effects. Numerous standard chemotherapy regimens use combinations of the drugs *Adriamycin, Cytoxan, Fluorouracil, Taxotere,* and *Taxol.*

Selective estrogen receptor modulator (SERM) medications including tamoxifen and **aromatase inhibitors** such as letrozole block estrogen from attaching to the estrogen receptors of ER-positive breast cancer cells, either slowing the growth of or killing the cancer cells. These drugs are taken after surgery for 5 to 10 years.

For breast cancer cells that produce excessive amounts of HER2, *Herceptin* blocks this production, causing the cancer cells to die.

WORD	PRONUNCIATION		ELEMENTS	DEFINITION
assay	ASS-ay		French *to try*	Analysis of concentration of drugs or other biological markers
brachytherapy	brak-kee-**THAIR**-ah-pee	P/ R/	**brachy-** *short* **-therapy** *treatment*	Radiation therapy in which the source of irradiation is implanted in the tissue to be treated
chemotherapy	**KEE**-moh-**THAIR**-ah-pee	R/CF R/	**chem/o-** *chemical* **-therapy** *treatment*	Treatment using chemical agents
lipectomy	lip-**EK**-toh-mee	S/ R/	**-ectomy** *surgical excision* **lip-** *fatty tissue*	Surgical removal of adipose tissue
lumpectomy	lump-**EK**-toh-mee	S/ R/	**-ectomy** *surgical excision* **lump-** *piece*	Removal of a lesion with preservation of surrounding tissue
mammogram	**MAM**-oh-gram	S/ R/CF	**-gram** *a record* **mamm/o-** *breast*	The record produced by x-ray imaging of the breast
mammography	mah-**MOG**-rah-fee	S/	**-graphy** *process of recording*	Process of x-ray imaging of the breast
mastectomy	mass-**TEK**-toh-mee	S/ R/	**-ectomy** *surgical excision* **mast-** *breast*	Surgical excision of the breast
quadrantectomy	kwad-ran-**TEK**-toh-mee	S/ R/	**-ectomy** *surgical excision* **quadrant-** *quarter*	Surgical excision of a quadrant of the breast
radiation	ray-dee-**AY**-shun	S/ R/	**-ation** *process* **radi-** *radiation*	The sending forth of x-rays or other rays for treatment or diagnosis
radical	**RAD**-ih-kal		Latin *root*	Extensive or thorough
stereotactic	**STER**-ee-oh-**TAK**-tik	S/ R/CF R/	**-ic** *pertaining to* **stere/o-** *three-dimensional* **-tact-** *orderly arrangement*	Pertaining to a precise three-dimensional method to locate a lesion

Exercises

A. As a health care professional, you must know the proper use of each medical term. *Use the words provided below to correctly complete each sentence. Fill in the blanks.* **LO 8.20, 8.A**

mammography	mammogram	quadrantectomy	mastectomy

1. Mrs. Rivera makes a yearly checkup with her gynecologist to include a _____.

2. This year, the radiologist responsible for evaluating Mrs. Rivera's _____ tests noted an abnormal area in her right breast.

3. After several diagnostic tests, it was determined that Mrs. Rivera should have one-fourth of her breast removed, medically termed as a _____.

4. The pathologist reported her findings and the surgeon deemed it necessary to remove Mrs. Rivera's entire right breast along with the pectoralis major muscle and associated lymph nodes. Mrs. Rivera was advised to have a radical _____.

Female Reproductive System

Challenge Your Knowledge

A. **Language of gynecology.** Demonstrate your knowledge of gynecologic terminology by answering the following multiple-choice questions. Choose the correct answer. **(LO 8.1, 8.2, 8.A)**

1. The mons pubis, labia majora and minora, and clitoris are collectively called the

   a. prepuce

   b. hymen

   c. vulva

   d. vaginosis

   e. antrum

2. This procedure can be used to visualize the inside of the uterus, take a biopsy, and/or remove polyps or fibroids:

   a. cytoscopy

   b. hysteroscopy

   c. ureteroscopy

   d. bronchoscopy

   e. thoracoscopy

3. Painful intercourse is called

   a. salpingitis

   b. dyspnea

   c. hyperemesis

   d. dyspareunia

   e. candidiasis

4. The thin membrane that partially occludes the vagina is called the

   a. fornix

   b. mons

   c. vestibule

   d. hymen

   e. clitoris

5. Irregular bleeding between menstrual periods is called

   a. amenorrhea

   b. metrorrhagia

   c. polymenorrhea

   d. dysmenorrhea

   e. menorrhagia

6. The ovaries in the female and testes in the male can both be called

   a. adnexa

   b. ova

   c. fornices

   d. rugae

   e. gonads

7. Which of the following is an STD?

   a. toxic shock syndrome

   b. vulvovaginal candidiasis

   c. dyspareunia

   d. all of these

   e. none of these

8. Human immunodeficiency virus (HIV) damages the immune system, so infections will develop that the body would otherwise cope with easily. These infections are called

   a. bacterial

   b. staph

   c. opportunistic

   d. strep

   e. viral

9. Chronic, lasting, severe pain around the vaginal orifice is a condition called

   a. vulvitis

   b. vaginitis

   c. vulvodynia

   d. candidiasis

   e. endometriosis

10. Inflammation of the uterine tubes is called

    a. ureteritis

    b. uveitis

    c. hyperemesis

    d. endometriosis

    e. salpingitis

11. The process of egg formation is called

    a. oophorectomy

    b. ova

    c. oogenesis

    d. oophocentesis

    e. ovulation

12. Estrogen, progesterone, and androgen are all

    a. antigens

    b. enzymes

    c. hormones

    d. antibiotics

    e. vitamins

B. Latin and Greek terms cannot be further deconstructed into prefix, root, combining form, or suffix. You must know them for what they are. Test your knowledge of these terms with this exercise. Match the medical term in the first column with the correct meaning in the second column. **LO 8.1, 8.D**

_____ 1. fornix	**a.** fringe
_____ 2. menses	**b.** membrane
_____ 3. ruga	**c.** egg
_____ 4. chancre	**d.** month
_____ 5. os	**e.** sheath
_____ 6. hymen	**f.** neck
_____ 7. ovary	**g.** arch, vault
_____ 8. vagina	**h.** mouth
_____ 9. cervix	**i.** ridge or crease
_____ 10. fimbria	**j.** cancer

C. Deconstruction. Deconstruction of medical terms is a tool for analyzing the meaning. In the following chart, you are given a medical term. Deconstruct the term into its prefix, root (or combining form), and suffix. Write the element and its meaning in the appropriate column and the meaning of the term in the last column. If the term does not have a word element, write n/a. *The first one is done for you.* **LO 8.4, 8.13, 8.14, 8.16, 8.D**

Medical Term	Prefix	Meaning of Prefix	Root/ Combining Form	Meaning of Root/ Combining Form	Suffix	Meaning of Suffix	Meaning of Term
mammary	1. n/a	2. n/a	3. mamm	4. breast	5. ary	6. pertaining to	7. Pertaining to the breast
neonatal	8.	9.	10.	11.	12.	13.	14.
primigravida	15.	16.	17.	18.	19.	20.	21.
postpartum	22.	23.	24.	25.	26.	27.	28.
endometrium	29.	30.	31.	32.	33.	34.	35.

Female Reproductive System

D. Plurals of some medical terms can be difficult to convert from the singular because there are so many different rules for plurals. Practice makes perfect in your ability to form the correct plural of the term. Fill in the plural column. **LO 8.A**

Singular Term	Plural Term
cilium	1.
fimbria	2.
fornix	3.
infundibulum	4.
labium	5.
majus	6.
minus	7.
ovary	8.
ovum	9.
ruga	10.

E. Trace the pathway of conception. The following phrases describe the process of fertilization. Order the items A to H to indicate the correct order of their occurrence. **LO 8.12**

_____ **1.** Nuclei of male and female cells unite.

_____ **2.** Morula becomes a blastocyst.

_____ **3.** Inner cell mass differentiates and forms embryo.

_____ **4.** Zygote produces morula.

_____ **5.** Ovary releases egg.

_____ **6.** All organ systems are present; embryo becomes fetus.

_____ **7.** Blastocyst implants in the endometrium.

_____ **8.** Zygote is formed.

F. Language of obstetrics. Pregnancy has its own associated set of obstetric terms. Apply your knowledge of obstetric terms to answering the following questions. Circle the correct answer. **LO 8.14, 8.15, 8.16**

1. The *nuchal cord* is

   a. only present in ectopic pregnancy

   b. wrapped around the baby's neck during delivery

   c. a congenital malformation

   d. only present in breech births

   e. present in 50% of births

2. What keeps the maternal and fetal blood circulations separated?

   a. umbilical cord

   b. amnion

   c. yolk sac

   d. cells of the villi

   e. placenta

3. A test for chromosomal abnormalities and genetic birth defects is

   a. teratogenesis

   b. hyperemesis

   c. dilation

   d. labor

   e. amniocentesis

4. When the head is just starting to push out of the vaginal opening, it is said to be

   a. effacing

   b. crowning

   c. dilating

   d. ovulating

   e. none of these

5. Which undesirable item can cross the placenta into the fetus?

   a. rubella virus

   b. oxygen

   c. maternal antibodies

   d. glucose

   e. hormones

6. The pit in the abdomen where the umbilical cord enters the fetus is the

   a. meatus

   b. navel

   c. yolk sac

   d. a and b

   e. none of these

7. Postpartum vaginal discharge is called

   a. puerperium

   b. lochia

   c. polyhydramnios

   d. amniocentesis

   e. oligohydramnios

©2014 Nucleus Medical Media

Female Reproductive System

G. **Language of obstetrics.** Pregnancy has its own associated set of obstetric terms. Apply your knowledge of obstetric terms to answering the following questions. Circle the correct answer. **LO 8.12, 8.13, 8.14, 8.15**

1. Where does fertilization actually take place?

   a. left ovary

   b. distal third of the uterine tube

   c. right ovary

   d. proximal third of the uterine tube

   e. uterus

2. During the first stage of labor, what is the process in which the wall of the cervix becomes thinner?

   a. crowning

   b. effacement

   c. delivery

   d. autolysis

   e. involution

3. What is the term for a fertilized egg's development in the uterine tube instead of the uterus?

   a. preeclampsia

   b. postpartum

   c. eclampsia

   d. ectopic

   e. endometriosis

4. The protective layer covering the skin of the fetus in utero is the

   a. estrogen

   b. lanugo

   c. vernix caseosa

   d. chorion

   e. morula

5. A woman who has given birth for the first time is

   a. multipara

   b. gravidarum

   c. primipara

   d. postpartum

   e. puerperium

H. Patient documentation. The following mammogram report for a patient contains terminology you should understand after reading this chapter. Answer the questions about the report by filling in the blanks. **LO 8.20, 8.A**

Exam: Diagnostic bilateral mammogram

Reason for exam: Discomfort in both breasts

The glandular tissue is heterogeneously dense. There are scattered fibroglandular densities bilaterally. There is a benign-appearing curvilinear area of glandular tissue in the right lower inner breast. There are a few faint calcifications in the lower inner left breast and in the central left breast. Magnification views were performed of the left breast calcifications in two positions, and they have an appearance most consistent with benign process. There is no associated mass or distortion.

Impression: Heterogeneously dense glandular tissue with focal glandular density in the medial aspect of the right breast and faint calcifications in the left breast. Probably benign.

Recommendation: Comparison with prior films. If prior films are not available, recommend follow-up mammogram in 6 months. Findings were submitted to the patient in writing.

1. The term that means *pertaining to two sides:* _____

2. A density is found in the middle of the (right/left) breast: _____

3. Calcifications are found in the (right/left) breast. _____

4. Does this patient have signs of malignancies? _____

5. The medical term for discomfort in the breast: _____

I. Describe the events and structures of ovulation. Match the medical term in the first column with the correct meaning in the second column. **(LO 8.5)**

_____ 1. After menses ends, uterus replaces this	**a.** uterine cycle
_____ 2. Formed where ovarian follicle ruptures	**b.** fimbriae
_____ 3. Envelope the ovary	**c.** lutein
_____ 4. The first 14 days of menses	**d.** corpus albicans
_____ 5. Averages 28 days in length	**e.** follicular phase
_____ 6. Inactive scar	**f.** postovulatory phase
_____ 7. Mature ovarian follicle does this	**g.** corpus luteum
_____ 8. Cells involved in progesterone production	**h.** endometrial tissue
_____ 9. Period of time after ovulation	**i.** ruptures

NERVOUS SYSTEM
The Language of Neurology

©2014 Nucleus Medical Media

The health professionals involved in the diagnosis and treatment of patients with problems in the nervous system include:

- **Neurologists**, who are medical doctors who specialize in disorders of the nervous system.

- **Neurosurgeons**, who are medical doctors who perform surgical procedures on the nervous system.

- **Electroneurodiagnostic technicians** (also called EEG technicians), who are professionals who operate specialized equipment that measures the electrical activity of the brain, spinal cord, and peripheral nervous system.

Chapter Learning Outcomes

As a health professional technician working with Dr. Solis and his patient Mrs. Gaston, your roles are to communicate with other health professionals who will be involved in her care and to maintain, review, and document the progress and treatment of her epilepsy.
To be able to perform these roles, and to interact with other neurological patients, you must be able to:

LO 9.1 Specify the functions of the nervous system.

LO 9.2 Differentiate the different components of the structure of the nervous system.

LO 9.3 Define the structures and functions of the cells of the nervous system

LO 9.4 Discuss the structure and functions of the brain.

LO 9.5 Identify the functional brain regions.

LO 9.6 Describe the structure and functions of the cranial nerves.

LO 9.7 Define the structure and functions of the spinal cord and meninges.

LO 9.8 Explain disorders of the brain.

LO 9.9 Discuss disorders of the meninges.

LO 9.10 Describe disorders of the cranial nerves.

LO 9.11 Identify disorders of the myelin sheath.

LO 9.12 Explain disorders of the spinal cord.

LO 9.13 Discuss disorders of the peripheral nerves.

LO 9.14 Describe congenital anomalies of the nervous system.

LO 9.15 Explain the diagnostic procedures used in neurology.

LO 9.16 Discuss the therapeutic procedures used in neurology.

LO 9.17 Describe the pharmacologic agents used in neurology.

LO 9.18 Identify the different modalities of pain management.

LO 9.A Write the medical terms of neurology to communicate and document accurately and precisely in any health care setting.

LO 9.B Use the medical terms of neurology to communicate verbally with accuracy and precision in any health care setting.

LO 9.C Construct medical terms of neurology using their word elements.

LO 9.D Deconstruct medical terms of neurology into their word elements.

LO 9.E Identify health professionals involved in the care of patients with neurological problems.

LO 9.F Recognize approved abbreviations used in neurology.

 ## Case Report (CR) 9.1

You are

. . . an **electroneurodiagnostic technician** working with Gregory Solis, MD, a **neurosurgeon** at Fulwood Medical Center.

Your patient is

. . . Ms. Roberta Gaston, a 39-year-old woman, who has been referred by Raul Cardenas, MD, a **neurologist,** for evaluation for possible **neurosurgery**.

Ms. Gaston has had **epileptic seizures** since the age of 16. She has **generalized tonic-clonic seizures** occurring once a week. She also has daily minor spells when she stops interacting with her surroundings and blinks rhythmically for about 20 seconds, after which she returns to normal. Numerous **antiepileptic** drugs, including phenobarbital, valproic acid, and phenytoin, have been tried with no relief. She is not able to work and is cared for by her parents.

Her neurologic examination is normal. Her **EEG (electroencephalogram)** shows diffuse spike-and-wave discharges with a left-sided frontal predominance. Her **CT** (computed tomography) is normal. An **MRI** (magnetic resonance imaging) shows a 20-mm diameter mass adjacent to the anterior horn of her left **ventricle.** Continuous EEG/video monitoring shows **ictal** activity in the left frontal lobe.

Lesson 9.1

Functions and Structure of the Nervous System

Lesson Objectives

Every time you stop to smell the roses, touch a petal, bend down, cut a stem, carry it indoors, place it in a vase, and admire its color, a wide range of sensations and actions are interpreted and controlled by your nervous system. The trillions of cells in your body must communicate and work together for you to function effectively. All this is done through your nervous system, and it is essential that you understand how this system operates. You can then understand how your body functions and maintains its homeostasis to respond to changes in your internal and external environments.

In this lesson, you will learn to use correct medical terminology to:

9.1.1 Describe the specific functions of the nervous system.

9.1.2 Relate the specific functions of the nervous system to the structures of its components.

9.1.3 List the subdivisions of the nervous system.

9.1.4 Define the basic cells of the nervous system.

LO 9.F Abbreviations

CNS	central nervous system
CT	computed tomography
EEG	electroencephalogram
MRI	magnetic resonance imaging
PNS	peripheral nervous system

LO 9.1 Functions of the Nervous System

1. **Sensory input** to the brain comes from receptors all over the body at both the conscious and subconscious levels. Seeing the rose, touching it, smelling it, and noting your body position as you bend are external stimuli of which you are aware. Inside your body, internal stimuli about the amount of oxygen and carbon dioxide in your blood and other homeostatic variables are being continually processed at the subconscious level.

2. **Motor input** from the brain stimulates the skeletal muscles to contract and enables you to bend down, cut a stem, or move in any way. Smooth muscle in the walls of blood vessels contracts when stimulated by the nervous system. The production of sweat, saliva, and digestive enzymes is controlled by the nervous system.

3. **Evaluation and integration** occur in the brain to process the sensory input, initiate a motor response, and store the event in memory.

4. **Homeostasis** is maintained by the nervous system taking in internal sensory input and, for example, responding by stimulating the heart to deliver the correct volume of blood for oxygenation and removal of waste products.

5. **Mental activity** occurs in the brain so that you can think, feel, understand, respond, and remember.

Keynotes

- The brain and spinal cord are called the **central nervous system (CNS)** *(Figure 9.1)*.
- Nerves all over the body outside the CNS are called the **peripheral nervous system (PNS)** *(Figure 9.1)*.
- The medical specialty of disorders of the nervous system is called **neurology**.
- A specialist in neurology is called a **neurologist**, and a specialist who operates on the nervous system is a **neurosurgeon**.

Central nervous system (CNS)
- Brain
- Spinal cord

Peripheral nervous system (PNS)
- Nerves

▲ **Figure 9.1** The nervous system.

WORD	PRONUNCIATION	ELEMENTS		DEFINITION
antiepileptic	AN-tee-eh-pih-**LEP**-tik	S/	-tic *pertaining to*	A pharmacologic agent capable of preventing or arresting epilepsy
		P/	anti- *against*	
		R/	-epilep- *seizure*	
convulsion	kon-**VUL**-shun	S/	-ion *process*	Alternative name for seizure
		P/	con- *with, together*	
		R/	-vuls- *tear, pull*	
electroencephalogram (EEG)	ee-**LEK**-troh-en-**SEF**-ah-lohgram	S/	-gram *record*	Record of the electrical activity of the brain
		R/CF	electr/o- *electricity*	
		R/CF	-encephal/o- *brain*	
electroneurodiagnostic	ee-**LEK**-troh-**NYUR**-oh-die-ag-**NOS**-tik	S/	-tic *pertaining to*	Pertaining to the use of electricity in the diagnosis of a neurologic disorder
		R/CF	electr/o- *electricity*	
		R/CF	-neur/o- *nerve*	
		P/	-dia- *complete*	
		R/	-gnos- *knowledge*	
epilepsy epileptic (adj)	**EP**-ih-**LEP**-see **EP**-ih-**LEP**-tik		Greek *seizure*	Chronic brain disorder due to paroxysmal excessive neuronal discharges
		S/	-tic *pertaining to*	Pertaining to or suffering from seizures
		R/	epilep- *seizure*	
ictal	**IK**-tal	S/	-al *pertaining to*	Pertaining to, or condition caused by, a stroke or epilepsy
		R/	ict- *seizure*	
motor	**MOH**-tor		Latin *to move*	Pertaining to nerves that send impulses out to cause muscles to contract or glands to secrete
neurology	nyu-**ROL**-oh-jee	S/	-logy *study of*	Medical specialty of disorders of the nervous system
		R/CF	neur/o- *nerve*	
neurologist	nyu-**ROL**-oh-jist	S/	-logist *one who studies, specialist*	Medical specialist in disorders of the nervous system
neurologic (adj)	**NYUR**-oh-**LOJ**-ik	S/	-ic *pertaining to*	Pertaining to the nervous system
neurosurgeon	**NYU**-roh-**SUR**-jun	S/	-eon *one who does*	Specialist in operating on the nervous system
		R/CF	neur/o- *nerve*	
		R/	-surg- *operate*	
neurosurgery	**NYU**-roh-**SUR**-jer-ee	S/	-ery *process of*	Medical specialty in surgery of the nervous system
psychoactive	sigh-co-**AK**-tiv	S/	-active *agent of change*	An agent with the ability to alter mood, anxiety, behavior, cognitive processes, or mental tension
		R/CF	psych/o- *soul, mind*	
seizure	**SEE**-zhur	S/	-ure *process*	Event due to excessive electrical activity in the brain
		R/	seiz- *to grab, convulse*	
sensory	**SEN**-soh-ree	S/	-ory *having the function of*	Having the function of sensation; relating to structures of the nervous system that carry impulses to the brain
		R/	sens- *feel*	
tonic	**TON**-ik	S/	-ic *pertaining to*	In a state of muscular contraction
		R/	ton- *pressure, tension*	
tonic-clonic seizure	**TON**-ik-**KLON**-ik **SEE**-zhur	R/	clon- *violent action*	Generalized seizure due to epileptic activity in all or most of the brain

Exercises

A. Documentation. *Fill in the following paragraph with the appropriate language of neurology. There are some terms you will not need.* **LO 9.1, 9.A, 9.E**

electroneurodiagnostic electroencephalogram epilepsy neurologist neurosurgeon antiepileptic psychoactive

Ms. Roberta Gaston and her parents were sent to this office by her **(1)** _____. Dr. Solis has ordered some

(2) _____ tests because of her **(3)** _____. The process of doing this test is **(4)** _____.

Abbreviations	
ANS	autonomic nervous system
CNS	central nervous system
PNS	peripheral nervous system

LO 9.2 Divisions (Components) of the Nervous System

The nervous system has two major anatomical subdivisions (*Figure 9.2*):

1. The **central nervous system** (CNS), consisting of the brain and spinal cord.
2. The **peripheral nervous system** (PNS) consisting of all the **neurons**, **nerves**, **ganglia**, and **plexuses** outside the central nervous system. It includes 12 pairs of cranial nerves originating from the brain and 31 pairs of spinal nerves originating from the spinal cord.

The PNS, in turn, is further subdivided into

   a. **Sensory division,** in which sensory nerves (**afferent nerves**) carry messages toward the spinal cord and brain from sense organs (*Figure 9.3*). **Visceral nerves** carry signals from the viscera in the thoracic and abdominal cavities; for example, the heart and lungs and the stomach and intestines. **Somatic nerves** carry signals from the skin, muscles, bones, and joints.

   b. **Motor division,** in which motor nerves (**efferent nerves**) carry messages away from the brain and spinal cord to muscles and organs.

   i. The visceral motor division is called the **autonomic nervous system (ANS).** It carries signals to glands and to cardiac and smooth muscle. It operates at a subconscious level outside voluntary control. It has two subdivisions:

   (1) The **sympathetic division** arouses the body for action; for example, by increasing the heart and respiratory rates to increase oxygen supply to brain and muscles. At the same time, it slows digestion, so less blood flow is needed to the digestive system. Blood can be directed where it is needed more.

   (2) The **parasympathetic division** calms the body, slowing down the heartbeat but stimulating digestion.

   ii. The **somatic motor division** carries signals to the skeletal muscles and is under voluntary control.

Study Hint

Remember the acronym **SAME:** The **S**ensory nerves are **A**fferent (toward the brain) and the **M**otor nerves are **E**fferent (away from the brain or spinal cord).

Motor—**E**fferent SA**ME** (opposite of *afferent*)

Sensory—**A**fferent **SA**ME (opposite of *efferent*)

▲ **Figure 9.2** Components of the Nervous System.

▲ **Figure 9.3** Afferent and Efferent Neurons.

WORD	PRONUNCIATION	ELEMENTS		DEFINITION
afferent	**AF**-eh-rent		Latin *to bring to*	Conducting impulses inward *toward* the spinal cord or brain
autonomic	awe-toh-**NOM**-ik	S/ P/ R/	**-ic** *pertaining to* **auto-** *self* **-nom-** *law*	Not voluntary; pertaining to the self-governing visceral motor division of the peripheral nervous system
efferent	**EF**-eh-rent		Latin *to bring away from*	Conducting impulses outward *away from* the brain or spinal cord
ganglion ganglia (pl)	**GANG**-lee-on **GANG**-lee-ah		Greek *swelling*	Collection of nerve cell bodies outside the CNS
nerve nervous (adj)	NERV **NER**-vus	S/ R/	**-ous** *pertaining to* **nerv-** *nerve*	A cord of fibers in connective tissue that conduct impulses Pertaining to nerves
neuron	**NYUR**-on		Greek *nerve*	Technical term for a nerve cell; consists of the cell body with its dendrites and axons
parasympathetic (*Note:* This term has two prefixes.)	par-ah-sim-pah-**THET**-ik	S/ P/ P/ R/	**-ic** *pertaining to* **para-** *beside* **-sym-** *together* **-pathet-** *suffering*	Pertaining to division of autonomic nervous system; has opposite effects of the sympathetic division
peripheral	peh-**RIF**-er-al	S/ R/	**-al** *pertaining to* **peripher-** *outer part*	Pertaining to the periphery or external boundary
plexus plexuses (pl)	**PLEK**-sus **PLEK**-sus-ez		Latin *braid*	A weblike network of joined nerves
somatic	soh-**MAT**-ik	S/ R/	**-ic** *pertaining to* **somat-** *body*	Pertaining to a division of the peripheral nervous system serving the skeletal muscles
sympathetic	sim-pah-**THET**-ik	S/ P/ R/	**-ic** *pertaining to* **sym-** *together* **-pathet-** *suffering*	Pertaining to the part of the autonomic nervous system operating at the unconscious level
visceral	**VISS**-er-al	S/ R/	**-al** *pertaining to* **viscer-** *internal organs*	Pertaining to the internal organs

Exercises

A. The nervous system has two major anatomical subdivisions, each with specialized functions. *Keep in mind that there are systems and divisions of systems. Use the precise* **language of neurology** *to answer the following questions.* **LO 9.2**

1. This division carries signals to the skeletal muscles and is under voluntary control:

   a. somatic motor division   **b.** somatic sensory division   **c.** autonomic motor division   **d.** autonomic sensory division

2. This system consists of the brain and spinal cord:

   a. central nervous system   **b.** peripheral nervous system

3. This division carries messages to the brain from the sensory organs:

   a. somatic motor division   **b.** somatic sensory division   **c.** autonomic motor division   **d.** autonomic sensory division

4. The visceral motor division is also called the

   a. peripheral   **b.** somatic   **c.** autonomic   **d.** ganglionic

5. This division arouses the body for action:

   a. parasympathic   **b.** sympathetic   **c.** somatic

6. This system consists of neurons, nerves, ganglia, and plexuses:

   a. central nervous system   **b.** peripheral nervous system

7. This division calms the body and slows the heartbeat:

   a. parasympathic   **b.** sympathetic   **c.** somatic

8. This division has efferent nerves to carry messages from the brain to muscles and organs:

   a. motor   **b.** sensory

Direction of signal transmission toward the cell body

Dendrites

Cell body
Nucleus

Axon collateral

Axon

Direction of signal transmission away from cell body

Myelin sheath
Schwann cell

Synaptic terminals

▲ **Figure 9.4** Neuron.

Abbreviations	
C5	fifth cervical vertebra or nerve
T1	first thoracic vertebra or nerve

LO 9.3 Cells of the Nervous System

Neurons (nerve cells) receive stimuli and transmit impulses to other neurons or to receptors in other organs. Each neuron consists of a **cell body** and two types of processes or extensions, called **axons** and **dendrites** (Figure 9.4).

Dendrites are short, highly branched extensions of the neuron's cell body. They conduct impulses toward the cell body. The more dendrites a neuron has, the more impulses it can receive from other neurons.

A single axon, or nerve fiber, arises from the cell body and carries impulses away from the cell body. Each axon has a constant diameter but can range in length from a few millimeters to a meter. The axon is covered in a fatty **myelin** sheath that is covered by a membrane called the **neurilemma**. The myelin sheath, like the plastic covering of electrical wire, enables the nerve impulse to travel faster.

The axon terminates in a network of small branches. Each branch ends in a **synaptic terminal** that forms a **synapse** (junction) with a dendrite from another neuron or with a receptor on a muscle cell or gland cell (Figure 9.5). The synaptic terminals contain vesicles full of **neurotransmitters** that cross the synapse to stimulate or inhibit the receptor on a dendrite of another neuron or the cell of a muscle or gland. Examples of neurotransmitters are:

- **Acetylcholine**—stimulates muscle cells to contract.
- **Norepinephrine**—found in many areas of the brain and spinal cord; has a stimulatory effect that is increased by cocaine and amphetamines.
- **Serotonin**—found in many areas of the brain and spinal cord; is involved with mood, anxiety, and sleep.
- **Dopamine**—confined to small areas of the brain; plays a role in movement, memory, pleasurable reward, behavior and cognition, mood, and learning.
- **Endorphins**—found in areas around the brainstem; are the body's natural pain relievers.

Groups of cell bodies cluster together to form ganglia, and axons collect together to form nerves. Groups of nerves collect together to form a **plexus**, in which nerve fibers from different spinal nerves are sorted and recombined so that all the fibers (motor and sensory) going to a specific body part are located in a single nerve. The three plexuses are the **cervical plexus** to the neck, the **brachial plexus** to the arm, and the **lumbosacral plexus** to the pelvis and legs. Figure 9.6 shows an example of a plexus, the brachial plexus, in which spinal nerves **C5** to **T1** unite to form three **roots** that go on to supply the motor and sensory functions of the arm. The labeling of nerves is addressed in a later lesson in this chapter.

Dendrite

Cell Body

Presynaptic neuron

Axon

Direction of signal transmission

Synapses

Dendrite

Synaptic terminals at synapses

Postsynaptic neuron

Axon

Direction of signal transmission

▲ **Figure 9.5** Synapse.

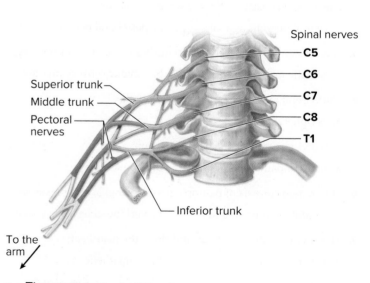

Spinal nerves

C5

C6

C7

C8

T1

Superior trunk
Middle trunk
Pectoral nerves

Inferior trunk

To the arm

▲ **Figure 9.6** Brachial Plexus.

WORD	PRONUNCIATION	ELEMENTS		DEFINITION
acetylcholine	**AS**-eh-til-**KOH**-leen	R/ R/	acetyl- *acetyl* -choline *choline*	Parasympathetic neurotransmitter
axon	**AK**-son		Greek *axis*	Single process of a nerve cell carrying nervous impulses away from the cell body
dendrite	**DEN**-dright		Greek *looking like a tree*	Branched extension of the nerve cell body that receives nervous stimuli
dopamine	**DOH**-pah-meen		Precursor of norepinephrine	Neurotransmitter in some specific small areas of the brain
endorphin (**Note:** The "m" of morphine is not used.)	en-**DOR**-fin	P/ R/	end- *within* -morphin *morphine*	Natural substance in the brain for pain relief
myelin	**MY**-eh-lin	S/ R/	-in *substance, chemical compound* myel- *spinal cord*	Material of the sheath around the axon of a nerve
neurilemma	nyu-ri-**LEM**-ah	S/ R/CF	-lemma *covering* neur/i- *nerve*	Covering of a nerve around the myelin sheath
neurotransmitter	**NYUR**-oh-trans-**MIT**-er	S/ P/ R/CF R/	-er *agent* -trans- *across* neur/o- *nerve* -mitt- *to send*	Chemical agent that relays messages from one nerve cell to the next
norepinephrine (**Note:** Two prefixes)	NOR-ep-ih-**NEFF**-rin	S/ P/ P/ R/	-ine *pertaining to* nor- *normal* -epi- *upon, above* -nephr- *kidney*	Parasympathetic neurotransmitter
serotonin	ser-oh-**TOH**-nin	S/ R/CF R/	-in *chemical compound* ser/o- *serum, serous* -ton- *tension*	Neurotransmitter in the central and peripheral nervous systems
synapse synaptic (adj)	**SIN**-aps sih-**NAP**-tik	P/ R/	syn- *together* -apse *clasp*	Junction between two nerve cells, or a nerve fiber and its target cell; where electrical impulses are transmitted between the cells

Exercises

A. Spelling is very important for every medical term. *Choose the correct spelling in the* **language of neurology.** LO 9.3

1. Junction between two nerve cells:

   a. synapses   b. sinapse   c. synapse

2. The material of the sheath around a nerve axon:

   a. myelin   b. myalin   c. myeline

3. Branched extension of the nerve cell body that receives an impulse:

   a. denderite   b. dendrite   c. dendryte

4. Chemical agent that relays messages:

   a. neutrontransmitter   b. neurontransmiter   c. neurotransmitter

5. Covering of a nerve around the sheath:

   a. neurelemma   b. neurilemmia   c. neurilemma

B. Using the terms relating to the cells of the nervous system, fill in the blanks in the following questions and statements. LO 9.3

1. The neurotransmitter that is a natural pain reliever. _____

2. Which part of the neuron carries impulses away from the cell body? _____

3. Which term comes from the Greek language meaning *looking like a tree*? _____

LO 9.3 Neuroglia

The trillion neurons in the nervous system are outnumbered 50 to 1 by the supportive **glial** cells (**neuroglia**). There are six types of neuroglia. Four are found in the CNS *(Figure 9.7)*:

1. **Astrocytes** are the most abundant glial cells. They are involved in the transportation of water and salts from capillaries to the neurons.

2. **Oligodendrocytes** form the myelin sheaths around axons in the brain and spinal cord. Axons that have myelin sheaths are called *myelinated axons.* Bundles of these axons appear white and create the **white matter** of the brain and spinal cord. Neuron cell bodies, dendrites, and synapses appear gray and create the **gray matter**.

3. **Microglia** phagocytose bacteria and cell debris.

4. **Ependymal cells** line the central canal of the spinal cord and the ventricles of the brain. They help regulate the composition of the **cerebrospinal fluid (CSF)**.

Two types of neuroglial cells are found in the PNS:

1. **Neurolemmocytes (Schwann cells)** form the myelin sheaths of the peripheral nerves that speed up signal conduction in the nerve fiber.

2. **Satellite cells** are found around the neuron cell bodies. Their function is unknown.

The **blood-brain barrier (BBB)** is a physical barrier between the capillaries that supply the CNS and most parts of the CNS. Astrocytes and the tight junctions between endothelial cells of the capillaries work together to prevent foreign substances, toxins, and infection from reaching the brain. Many medications are unable to pass this barrier, but alcohol gets through, producing its buzz and problems with coordination and **cognition**.

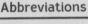

Abbreviations

BBB	blood-brain barrier
CSF	cerebrospinal fluid

▲ **Figure 9.7** Neuroglial Cells in the CNS.

WORD	PRONUNCIATION	ELEMENTS		DEFINITION
astrocyte	**ASS**-troh-site	S/ R/CF	-cyte *cell* astr/o- *star*	Star-shaped connective tissue cell in the nervous system
blood-brain barrier (BBB)	BLUD BRAYN **BAIR**-ee-er		**blood** Old English *fluid connective tissue* **brain** Old English *organ that controls the functions of the body* **barrier** Old French *obstacle, gatekeeper*	A selective mechanism that protects the brain from toxins and infections
cerebrospinal	**SER**-eh-broh-**SPY**-nal	S/ R/CF R/	-al *pertaining to* cerebr/o- *brain* -spin- *spinal cord*	Pertaining to the brain and spinal cord
cerebrospinal fluid (CSF)	**SER**-eh-broh-**SPY**-nal **FLU**-id	R/	fluid *flowing*	Fluid formed in the ventricles of the brain; surrounds the brain and spinal cord
ependyma ependymal (adj)	ep-**EN**-dih-mah ep-**EN**-dih-mal		Greek *garment*	Membrane lining the central canal of the spinal cord and the ventricles of the brain
glia glial (adj) microglia	**GLEE**-ah **GLEE**-al my-**KROH**-glee-ah	P/ R/	Greek *glue* micro- *small* -glia *glue, supportive tissue of the nervous system*	Connective tissue that holds a structure together Small nervous tissue cells that are phagocytes
neuroglia	nyu-**ROH**-glee-ah	R/CF	neur/o- *nerve*	Connective tissue holding nervous tissue together
gray matter	GRAY **MATT**-er		**gray** Old English *color between white and black* **matter** Latin *a physical substance*	Regions of the brain and spinal cord occupied by cell bodies and dendrites
neurolemmocyte (same as Schwann cell)	**NYU**-roh-**LEM**-oh-site SHWANN SELL	S/ R/CF R/CF	-cyte *cell* neur/o- *nerve* -lemm/o *rind, husk* Theodor Schwann, German anatomist, 1810–1882	Connective tissue cell of the peripheral nervous system that forms a myelin sheath
oligodendrocyte	**OL**-ih-goh-**DEN**- droh-site	S/ P/ R/CF	-cyte *cell* oligo- *scanty* -dendr/o- *treelike*	Connective tissue cell of the central nervous system that forms a myelin sheath
white matter	WITE **MATT**-er		**white** Old English *color opposite of black* **matter** Latin *a physical substance*	Regions of the brain and spinal cord occupied by bundles of axons

Exercises

A. Identify the correct meaning for each element. *Knowing the definitions of elements is your key to unlocking the meaning of medical terms. Match the element in the left column with its correct meaning in the right column.* **LO 9.3**

_____ **1.** *oligo*   **a.** cell

_____ **2.** *glia*   **b.** spinal cord

_____ **3.** *cerebro*   **c.** treelike

_____ **4.** *astro*   **d.** scanty

_____ **5.** *spin*   **e.** brain

_____ **6.** *cyte*   **f.** glue

_____ **7.** *dendro*   **g.** star

The Brain and Cranial Nerves

Lesson Objectives

Smelling the roses, seeing them, and touching them are recognized and interpreted in the brain, as are all sensations. The actions of bending down, cutting the rose stem, walking into the house, and placing it in a vase originate in the brain, as do all our voluntary actions. The integration of a sensory stimulus with a motor response occurs in the brain. The brain is the control center for many of the body's functions. The brain carries out the higher mental functions, such as reasoning, planning, forming ideas, and all aspects of memory.

The information in this lesson will enable you to:

9.2.1 Use correct medical terminology to describe the anatomy and physiology of the brain.

9.2.2 Identify the 12 pairs of cranial nerves and their functions.

9.2.3 Locate the major sensory and motor areas of the brain.

9.2.4 Describe how the brain is protected and supported.

9.2.5 Explain how common disorders of the brain and spinal cord affect health.

LO 9.4 Brain

The adult brain weighs about 3 pounds. Its size and weight are proportional to body size, not intelligence.

The brain is divided into three major regions: the **cerebrum**, the **brainstem**, and the **cerebellum**.

The cerebrum is about 80% of the brain and consists of two **cerebral hemispheres** that are anatomically mirror images of each other *(Figure 9.8)*. They are separated by a deep longitudinal fissure, at the bottom of which they are connected by a bridge of nerve fibers called the **corpus callosum**.

On the surface of the cerebrum, numerous ridges **(gyri)** are separated by grooves called **sulci**. Each cerebral hemisphere is divided into four **lobes** *(see Figure 9.8a)*:

1. The **frontal lobe** is located behind the forehead. It forms the anterior part of the hemisphere. It is responsible for memory, intellect, concentration, problem solving, emotion, and the planning and execution of behavior, including voluntary motor control of muscles.

2. The **parietal lobe**, located above the ear, is posterior to the frontal lobe. The parietal lobe receives and interprets sensations of pain, pressure, touch, temperature, and body part awareness.

3. The **temporal lobe**, located behind the ear, is below the frontal and parietal lobes. The temporal lobe is involved in interpreting sensory experiences, sounds, and spoken words.

4. The **occipital lobe**, located at the back of the head, forms the posterior part of the hemisphere. The occipital lobe interprets visual images and the written word.

The cerebral hemispheres are covered by a thin layer of gray matter (unmyelinated nerve fibers) called the **cerebral cortex**. It is folded into the gyri, sulci, and fissures and contains 70% of all the neurons in the nervous system. Below the cerebral cortex is a mass of white matter, in which bundles of myelinated nerve fibers connect the neurons of the cortex to the rest of the nervous system.

The **brain stem** relays sensory impulses from peripheral nerves to higher brain centers. It also controls vital cardiovascular and respiratory functions.

The **cerebellum**, the most posterior area of the brain, coordinates skeletal muscle activity to maintain the body's posture and balance.

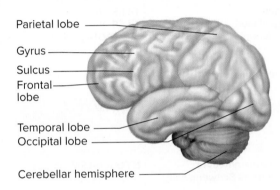

Parietal lobe

Gyrus

Sulcus

Frontal lobe

Temporal lobe

Occipital lobe

Cerebellar hemisphere

(a) View from left side

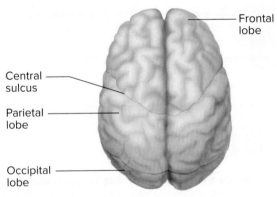

Frontal lobe

Central sulcus

Parietal lobe

Occipital lobe

(b) View from above

▲ **Figure 9.8** Brain.

WORD	PRONUNCIATION		ELEMENTS	DEFINITION
brainstem	BRAYN-stem		brain Old English *brain* stem Old English *support*	Region of the brain that includes the thalamus, pineal gland, pons, fourth ventricle, and medulla oblongata
cerebellum	ser-eh-BELL-um	S/ R/	-um *structure* cerebell- *little brain*	The most posterior area of the brain.
cerebrum cerebral (adj)	ser-EE-brum SER-eh-bral *or* ser-EE-bral	S/ R/	Latin *brain* -al *pertaining to* cerebr- *brain*	The major portion of the brain divided into two hemi-spheres (cerebral hemispheres) separated by a fissure Pertaining to the brain
corpus callosum	KOR-pus kah-LOH-sum	S/ R/	corpus Latin *body* -um *structure* callos- *thickening*	Bridge of nerve fibers connecting the two cerebral hemispheres
cortex cortical (adj)	KOR-teks KOR-ti-kal		Latin *shell*	Gray covering of cerebral hemispheres
frontal lobe	FRON-tal LOBE	S/ R/	-al *pertaining to* front- *forehead* lobe Greek *lobe*	Area of brain behind the forehead
gyrus gyri (pl)	JIE-rus JIE-ree		Greek *circle*	Rounded elevation on the surface of the cerebral hemispheres
occipital lobe	ok-SIP-it-al LOBE	S/ R/	-al *pertaining to* occipit- *back of head* lobe Greek *lobe*	Posterior area of cerebral hemispheres
parietal lobe	pah-RYE-eh-tal LOBE	S/ R/	-al *pertaining to* pariet- *wall* lobe Greek *lobe*	Area of brain above the ear
sulcus sulci (pl)	SUL-cuss SUL-sigh		Latin *furrow, ditch*	Groove on the surface of the cerebral hemispheres that separates gyri
temporal lobe	TEM-por-al LOBE	S/ R/	-al *pertaining to* tempor- *temple, side of head* lobe Greek *lobe*	Posterior two-thirds of cerebral hemispheres

Exercises

A. Roots. *The lobes of the cerebral hemispheres share a common suffix -al, meaning pertaining to. It is the root that describes the exact location of the lobe in the cerebral hemispheres. Use your knowledge of roots to understand the anatomical location of the lobes. Fill in the blanks.* **LO 9.4, 9.C**

1. The cerebral lobe located above the ear: _____/al   The root means _____.

2. The cerebral lobe located behind the forehead: _____/al. The root means _____.

3. The most posterior cerebral lobe: _____/al. The root means: _____.

B. Describe the structure of the cerebrum. *Identify the cerebral structures being described. Fill in the blanks.* **LO 9.4, 9.A**

1. Elevation or "wrinkle" of the cerebrum:

    singular form _____

    plural form _____.

2. Gray covering of the cerebrum: _____.

3. Shallow indention of the cerebrum:

    singular form _____

    plural form _____.

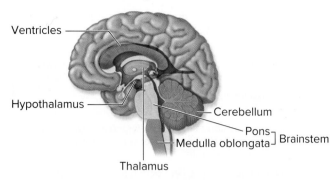

Midsagittal section

Ventricles
Hypothalamus
Cerebellum
Pons
Medulla oblongata — Brainstem
Thalamus

▲ **Figure 9.9** Lateral View of Functional Regions of Brain.

LO 9.5 Functional Brain Regions

Deep inside each cerebral hemisphere are spaces called **ventricles**. They contain the watery **cerebrospinal fluid (CSF)**, which circulates through the ventricles and around the brain and spinal cord. The CSF helps protect, cushion, and provide nutrition for the brain and spinal cord.

Underneath the cerebral hemispheres and the ventricles are important regions of the brain *(Figures 9.9 and 9.10)*:

1. **Thalamus**—receives all sensory impulses and channels them to the appropriate region of the cortex for interpretation. As the sensory fibers carrying impulses pass through the thalamus, they **decussate** (cross over) so that the impulses from the left side of the body go to the right brain, and impulses coming from the right side of the body go to the left brain. Similarly, motor impulses coming from the right brain decussate and supply the left side of the body, and motor impulses coming from the left brain decussate and supply the right side of the body. If a lesion caused by a stroke is in the right brain, the left side of the body will be affected, and vice versa.

2. The **hypothalamus** regulates
   a. Blood pressure
   b. Body temperature
   c. Water and electrolyte balance
   d. Hunger and body weight
   e. Sleep and wakefulness
   f. Movements and secretions of the digestive tract

3. The **basal nuclei** are collections of gray matter lateral to the thalamus that aid in controlling the amplitude of our voluntary muscular movements and posture, as well as playing a part in emotion and cognition.

4. The **limbic system** controls emotional experience, fear, anger, pleasure, and sadness.

5. The **brainstem** *(Figure 9.9)* contains two major areas:

   a. The **pons** *(Figure 9.9)*, which relays sensory impulses from peripheral nerves to higher brain centers.
   b. The **medulla oblongata** *(Figure 9.9)*, within which nuclei of gray matter form centers to control vital visceral activities, such as:
      i. **Cardiac center**—regulates heart rate.
      ii. **Respiratory center**—regulates breathing.
      iii. **Vasomotor center**—regulates vasoconstriction and vasodilation of blood vessels.
      iv. **Reticular formation**—responds to sensory impulses by arousing the cerebral cortex into wakefulness.

The most posterior area of the brain, the cerebellum *(Figures 9.9 and 9.10)*, coordinates skeletal muscle activity to maintain posture and balance.

Abbreviation	
CSF	cerebrospinal fluid

Motor areas involved with the control of voluntary muscles (precentral gyrus)
Concentration, planning, problem solving
Auditory area
Motor speech area (Broca area)
Interpretation of sensory experiences, memory of visual and auditory patterns
Sensory areas involved with cutaneous and other senses
Understanding speech, using words
General interpretative area (Wernicke area)
Combining visual images, visual recognition of objects
Visual area
Cerebellum
Brainstem

▲ **Figure 9.10** Cerebral Cortex, Functional Regions.

S = Suffix   P = Prefix   R = Root   R/CF = Combining Form

WORD	PRONUNCIATION		ELEMENTS	DEFINITION
brainstem	**BRAYN**-stem		**brain** Old English *brain* **stem** Old English *support*	Region of the brain that includes the thalamus, pineal gland, pons, fourth ventricle, and medulla oblongata
decussate	**DEE**-kuss-ate		Latin *to make in the form of a cross*	Cross over like the arms of an "X"
hypothalamus	high-poh-**THAL**-ah-muss	S/ P/ R/	**-us** *pertaining to* **hypo-** *below* **-thalam-** *thalamus*	Area of gray matter forming part of the walls and floor of the third ventricle
hypothalamic	high-poh-tha-**LAM**-ik	S/	**-ic** *pertaining to*	Pertaining to the hypothalamus
limbic	**LIM**-bic		Latin *border*	Pertaining to the limbic system, which controls vital functions of breathing, heart beat, and blood pressure
medulla oblongata	meh-**DULL**-ah ob-lon-**GAH**-tah	R/ S/ R/	**medulla** *middle* **-ata** *place* **oblong-** *elongated*	Most posterior subdivision of the brainstem, continuation of the spinal cord
pons	PONZ		Latin *bridge*	Relays sensory information from the peripheral nerves to different areas of the brain
reticulum	reh-**TIK**-you-lum	S/ R/	**-um** *structure* **reticul-** *fine net*	Fine network of cells in the medulla oblongata
reticular (adj)	reh-**TIK**-you-lar	S/	**-ar** *pertaining to*	Pertaining to the reticulum
thalamus	**THAL**-ah-mus		Greek *inner room*	Relays sensory information to the cerebral cortex
ventricle ventricular (adj)	**VEN**-trih-kel ven-**TRIK**-you-lar	S/ R/	Latin *belly* **-ar** *pertaining to* **ventricul-** *ventricle*	A cavity of the heart or brain Pertaining to a ventricle

Exercises

A. Latin and Greek terms cannot be deconstructed into prefix, root, and suffix. *You must know them for what they are. Test your knowledge of these terms with the following exercise. Match the terms in the left column to their correct meaning in the right column.* **LO 9.5, 9.A**

_____ **1.** thalamus

_____ **2.** decussate

_____ **3.** limbic

_____ **4.** pons

a. bridge

b. inner room

c. border

d. cross over

B. Recall from the lesson the correct medical terms that identify the appropriate answers to the questions. *Fill in the blanks.* **LO 9.5**

cardiac   respiratory   vasomotor   reticular formation   medulla oblongata

1. What is the center of the brain that controls vital and visceral activity?

_____

2. What part of the brain regulates heartbeat?

_____

3. What responds to sensory impulses by arousing the cerebral cortex into wakefulness?

_____

4. Where in the brain is breathing regulated?

_____

5. What regulates vasoconstriction and vasodilation of blood vessels?

_____

Table 9.1 Mnemonic for the Cranial Nerves

Oh	(olfactory–I)
once	(optic–II)
one	(oculomotor–III)
takes	(trochlear–IV)
the	(trigeminal–V)
anatomy	(abducens–VI)
final	(facial–VII)
very	(vestibulocochlear–VIII)
good	(glossopharyngeal–IX)
vacations	(vagus–X)
are	(accessory–XI)
heavenly!	(hypoglossal–XII)

LO 9.6 Cranial Nerves

To function, the brain must communicate with the rest of the body, and it does this through the spinal cord and the **cranial nerves.** Twelve pairs of cranial nerves arise from the base of the brain (*Figure 9.11*). A mnemonic to help you remember their names is in *Table 9.1.*

The two pairs of nerves for smell and vision contain only sensory fibers. The other 10 pairs are mixed nerves containing sensory, motor, and parasympathetic fibers. The cranial nerves have, from front to back, both names and numbers. The latter are always written in Roman numerals (*Table 9.2*).

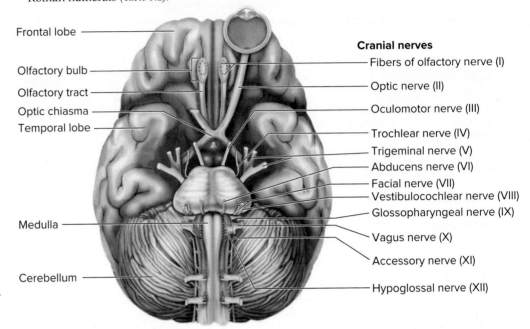

Cranial nerves
- Fibers of olfactory nerve (I)
- Optic nerve (II)
- Oculomotor nerve (III)
- Trochlear nerve (IV)
- Trigeminal nerve (V)
- Abducens nerve (VI)
- Facial nerve (VII)
- Vestibulocochlear nerve (VIII)
- Glossopharyngeal nerve (IX)
- Vagus nerve (X)
- Accessory nerve (XI)
- Hypoglossal nerve (XII)

(labels on left: Frontal lobe, Olfactory bulb, Olfactory tract, Optic chiasma, Temporal lobe, Medulla, Cerebellum)

Figure 9.11 Cranial Nerves. Base of brain showing origins of the 12 cranial nerves. ▶

Table 9.2 Cranial Nerves

Roman Numeral	Name	Description
I	**Olfactory** nerves	Sensory nerves for smell
II	**Optic** nerves	Sensory nerves for vision
III	**Oculomotor** nerves	Predominantly motor nerves for eye movement and pupil size
IV	**Trochlear** nerves	Predominantly motor nerves for eye movement
V	**Trigeminal** nerves	Sensory and motor nerves responsible for face, nose, and mouth sensations and for chewing
VI	**Abducens** nerves	Predominantly motor nerves responsible for eye movement
VII	**Facial** nerves	Mixed nerves associated with taste (sensory), facial expression (motor), and production of tears and saliva (parasympathetic fibers of motor nerves)
VIII	**Vestibulocochlear (auditory)** nerves	Predominantly sensory nerves associated with hearing and balance
IX	**Glossopharyngeal** nerves	Mixed nerves for sensation and swallowing in the pharynx
X	**Vagus** nerves	Mixed sensory and parasympathetic nerves supplying the pharynx, larynx (speech), and the viscera of the thorax and abdomen (*Figure 9.12*)
XI	**Accessory** nerves	Predominantly motor nerves supplying neck muscles, pharynx, and larynx
XII	**Hypoglossal** nerves	Predominantly motor nerves that move the tongue in speaking, chewing, and swallowing

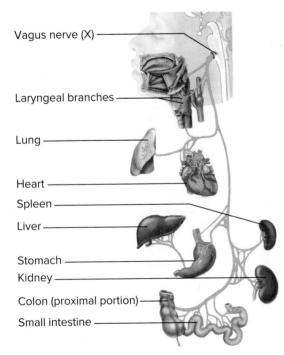

(labels: Vagus nerve (X), Laryngeal branches, Lung, Heart, Spleen, Liver, Stomach, Kidney, Colon (proximal portion), Small intestine)

▲ **Figure 9.12 Left Vagus Nerve.**

WORD	PRONUNCIATION	ELEMENTS		DEFINITION
abducens	ab-**DYU**-senz		Latin *abduct, draw away from*	Sixth (VI) cranial nerve; responsible for eye movement
accessory	ak-**SESS**-oh-ree		Latin *move toward*	Eleventh (XI) cranial nerve; supplying neck muscles, pharynx, and larynx
auditory	**AW**-dih-tor-ee	S/ R/	**-ory** *having the function of* **audit-** *hearing*	Pertaining to the sense of or the organs of hearing
cranial	**KRAY**-nee-al	S/ R/	**-al** *pertaining to* **crani-** *skull, cranium*	Pertaining to the skull
facial	**FAY**-shal		Latin *face*	Seventh (VII) cranial nerve; supplying the forehead, nose, eyes, mouth, and jaws
glossopharyngeal	**GLOSS**-oh-fah-**RIN**-jee-al	S/ R/CF R/	**-eal** *pertaining to* **gloss/o-** *tongue* **-pharyng-** *pharynx*	Ninth (IX) cranial nerve; supplying the tongue and pharynx
hypoglossal	high-poh-**GLOSS**-al	S/ P/ R/	**-al** *pertaining to* **hypo-** *below, under* **-gloss-** *tongue*	Twelfth (XII) cranial nerve; supplying muscles of the tongue
oculomotor	**OK**-you-loh-**MOH**-tor	S/ R/CF R/	**-or** *doer* **ocul/o-** *eye* **-mot-** *move*	Third (III) cranial nerve; moves the eye
olfactory	ol-**FAK**-toh-ree	S/ R/	**-ory** *having the function of* **olfact-** *smell*	First (I) cranial nerve; carries information related to the sense of smell
optic	**OP**-tik	S/ R/	**-ic** *pertaining to* **opt-** *eye*	Second (II) cranial nerve; carries visual information
trigeminal	try-**GEM**-in-al	S/ P/ R/	**-al** *pertaining to* **tri-** *three* **-gemin-** *double, twin*	Fifth (V) cranial nerve, with its three different branches supplying the face
trochlear	**TROHK**-lee-ar	S/ R/	**-ar** *pertaining to* **trochle-** *pulley*	Fourth (IV) cranial nerve; supplies one muscle of the eye
vagus	**VAY**-gus		Latin *to wander*	Tenth (X) cranial nerve; supplies many different organs throughout the body
vestibulocochlear (**Note:** This term starts with a combining form, not a prefix.)	ves-**TIB**-you-loh-**KOK**-lee-ar	S/ R/CF R/	**-ar** *pertaining to* **vestibul/o-** *vestibule of inner ear* **-cochle-** *cochlea*	Eighth (VIII) cranial nerve; carrying information for the senses of hearing and balance

Exercises

> **Study Hint**
> Note that some terms can start with a root or combining form instead of a prefix.

A. Elements. *Continue your work with elements to help build your knowledge of the language of neurology. One element in each of the following medical terms is set in bold. Identify the type of element (prefix, root, root/combining form, suffix) in the first column; then write the meaning of the element in the second column, and the function of the nerve: sensory, motor, or mixed (meaning both sensory and motor functions) in the right column. Fill in the chart.* **LO 9.6, 9.D**

Medical Term	Type of Element	Meaning of Element	Function
glosso**pharyng**eal	1.	2.	3.
tri**gemin**al	4.	5.	6.
auditory	7.	8.	9.
olfactory	10.	11.	12.

LO 9.7 Spinal Cord and Meninges

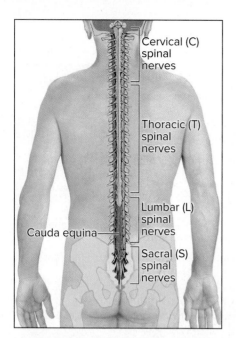

▲ **Figure 9.13** Spinal cord regions.

Abbreviations	
C1–C8	cervical spinal nerves
L1–L5	lumbar nerves
S1–S5	sacral nerves
T1–T12	thoracic spinal nerves

Spinal Cord

This part of the central nervous system consists of 31 segments, each of which gives rise to a pair of spinal nerves. These are the major link between the brain and the peripheral nervous system and are a pathway for sensory and motor impulses. The spinal cord occupies the upper two-thirds of the vertebral canal, extending from the base of the skull to the first lumbar vertebra. From here, a group of nerve fibers continues down the vertebral canal and is called the **cauda equina**. The spinal cord is divided into four regions (*Figure 9.13*):

1. The **cervical region** is continuous with the medulla oblongata. It contains the motor neurons that supply the neck, shoulders, and upper limbs through eight pairs of cervical spinal nerves (**C1–C8**).

2. The **thoracic region** contains the motor neurons that supply the thoracic cage, rib movement, vertebral column movement, and postural back muscles through 12 pairs of thoracic spinal nerves (**T1–T12**).

3. The **lumbar region** supplies the hips and front of the lower limbs through five pairs of lumbar nerves (**L1–L5**).

4. The **sacral region** supplies the buttocks, genitalia, and backs of the legs through five sacral nerves (**S1–S5**) and one coccygeal nerve.

A cross-section of the spinal cord (*Figure 9.14*) reveals that it has a core of gray matter shaped like a butterfly surrounded by white matter. In the center of the gray matter is the central canal that contains CSF. The gray matter contains the axons of sensory neurons bringing impulses into the cord and the neurons of motor nerves that send impulses out to skeletal muscles.

The white matter contains myelinated nerve fibers organized into **tracts** that conduct either sensory impulses up the cord to the brain or motor impulses down the cord from the brain.

All individual spinal nerves except C1 supply a specific segment of skin called a **dermatome**. Each spinal nerve, except for C1, exits and enters the spinal cord through an **intervertebral** space. Cervical nerve one passes between a space between the skull and the first vertebra.

Meninges

The brain and spinal cord are protected by the cranium and the vertebrae, cushioned by the CSF, and covered by the **meninges** (*Figure 9.15*). The meninges have three layers:

1. **Dura mater** —the outermost layer, composed of tough connective tissue attached to the inner surface of the cranium but separated from the vertebral canal by the **epidural space**, into which **epidural** injections are introduced.

2. **Arachnoid mater** —a thin web over the brain and spinal cord. The CSF is contained in the **subarachnoid space** between the arachnoid and pia mater.

3. **Pia mater** —the innermost layer of the meninges, attached to the surface of the brain and spinal cord. It supplies nerves and blood vessels that nourish the outer cells of the brain and spinal cord.

▲ **Figure 9.14** Cross-section of spinal cord.

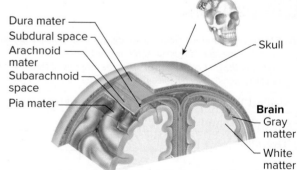

▲ **Figure 9.15** Meninges of the brain.

Word Analysis and Definition

S = Suffix   P = Prefix   R = Root   R/CF = Combining Form

WORD	PRONUNCIATION	ELEMENTS		DEFINITION
arachnoid mater	ah-**RAK**-noyd **MAY**-ter	S/ R/ R/	-oid *resembling* arachn- *cobweb, spider* mater *mother*	Weblike middle layer of the three meninges.
cauda equina (*Note:* Both these terms are stand-alone combining forms.)	**KAW**-dah eh-**KWIE**-nah	R/CF R/CF	caud/a *tail* equin/a *horse*	Bundle of spinal nerves in the vertebral canal below the ending of the spinal cord
cervical (*Note:* Cervical also is used to refer to a region of the uterus.)	**SER**-vih-kal	S/ R/	-al *pertaining to* cervic- *neck*	Pertaining to the neck region
dermatome	**DER**-mah-tome	S/ R/CF	-tome *instrument to cut* derm/a- *skin*	The area of skin supplied by a single spinal nerve; alternatively, an instrument used for cutting thin slices
dura mater (*Note:* Both terms are stand-alone roots.)	**DYU**-rah **MAY**-ter	R/CF R/	dur/a *hard* mater *mother*	Hard, fibrous outer layer of the meninges
epidural epidural space	ep-ih-**DYU**-ral ep-ih-**DYU**-ral SPASE	S/ P/ R/	-al *pertining to* epi- *above* -dur- *dura mater*	Above the dura Space between the dura mater and the wall of the vertebral canal or skull
intervertebral	**IN**-ter-**VER**-teh-bral	S/ P/ R/	-al *pertaining to* inter- *between* -vertebr- *vertebra*	The space between two vertebrae
lumbar	**LUM**-bar		Latin *loins*	Pertaining to the region in the back and sides between the ribs and pelvis
meninges	meh-**NIN**-jeez		Greek *membrane*	Three-layered covering of the brain and spinal cord
pia mater (*Note:* Both these terms are stand-alone roots.)	**PEE**-ah **MAY**-ter	R/ R/	pia *delicate* mater *mother*	Delicate inner layer of the meninges.
sacral	**SAY**-kral	S/ R/	-al *pertaining to* sacr-*sacrum*	In the neighborhood of the sacrum
subarachnoid space	sub-ah-**RAK**-noyd SPASE	S/ P/ R/	-oid *resembling* sub- *under* -arachn- *cobweb, spider*	Space between the pia mater and the arachnoid mater
thoracic	thor-**ASS**-ik	S/ R/	-ic *pertaining to* thorac-*chest*	Pertaining to the chest (thorax)
tract	TRAKT		Latin *draw out*	Bundle of nerve fibers with common origin and destination

Exercises

A. Place the meninges in order from superficial to deep. *Place a "1" in the blank for the most superficial layer and "3" for the deepest layer.*
   LO 9.7

_____ arachnoid mater

_____ pia mater

_____ dura mater

Lesson 9.3

Disorders of the Brain and Cranial Nerves

When patients communicate with you as a health professional, they will often enhance your continual, ongoing learning by informing you of and reinforcing your knowledge about a specific disorder.

Information in this lesson will enable you to:

9.3.1 Describe common disorders of the brain and cranial nerves.

9.3.2 Match common disorders of the brain and cranial nerves to normal and abnormal anatomy and physiology.

9.3.3 Use correct terminology to communicate about the brain and cranial nerves and their disorders with patients and other health professionals.

Case Report (CR) 9.2

You are

. . . a medical assistant working with Dr. Raoul Cardenas, a neurologist at Fulwood Medical Center.

Your patient is

. . . Mr. Lester Rood, a 75-year-old man who was diagnosed a year ago as having dementia.

Mr. Rood lives with his daughter, Judy, and she is with him today.

Patient Interview:

Mr. Lester Rood: "How am I feeling? Scared stiff. Sometimes I don't know where I am. I get so messed up. I can't cook anymore. I forget what I'm doing. I find myself in the street and don't know how I got there. Judy has to help me shower and remind me to go to the bathroom. And it's only going to get worse. I don't want to be a burden. I used to have 100 people work for me. Now, it's frustrating, so frightening. And the future . . . ."

LO 9.8 Disorders of the Brain

Dementia

Your **empathy** allowed Mr. Rood to talk without interruption. He reminded you that the symptoms of **dementia** include short-term memory loss, inability to solve problems, confusion, inappropriate behavior (such as wandering away), and impaired **cognitive** function that interferes with normal activities and relationships. In its early stages, it is a very frightening and frustrating situation for the patient. It requires a lot of **sympathy** and understanding from family and caregivers.

Dementia is *not* a normal part of aging and is *not* a specific disease. It is a term used for a collection of symptoms that can be caused by a number of disorders affecting the brain.

Alzheimer disease is the most common form of dementia. It affects 10% of the population over 65 and 50% of the population over 85. Nerve cells in the areas of the brain associated with memory and **cognition** are replaced by abnormal clumps and tangles of a protein *(Figure 9.16)*.

Vascular dementia is the second most common form of dementia. It can come on gradually when arteries supplying the brain become arteriosclerotic (narrowed or blocked), depriving the brain of oxygen, or can occur suddenly after a **stroke** *(see Chapter 7)*.

Confusion is used to describe people who cannot process information normally. For example, they cannot answer questions appropriately, understand where they are, or remember important facts. Confusion is often part of dementia or delirium.

Delirium is the sudden onset of disorientation, an inability to think clearly or pay attention. There is a change in the level of **consciousness**, varying from increased wakefulness to drowsiness. It is a mental state, not a disease. It can be part of dementia or a stroke.

Other conditions causing dementia are often treatable. They include:

- **Reactions to medications** (e.g., sedatives, antiarthritics). Remove or lower the dose of the medication.
- **Metabolic abnormalities** (e.g., hypoglycemia). Correct the metabolic abnormality.
- **Nutritional deficiencies** (e.g., vitamins B_1 and B_6). Remedy the nutritional deficiency.
- **Emotional problems** (e.g., depression in the elderly). Use behavioral therapy or antidepressives.
- **Infections** (e.g., AIDS, encephalitis). Treat the underlying infection.

(a)

(b)

▲ **Figure 9.16 Brain Sections.** (a) MRI scan of normal brain. (b) MRI scan of Alzheimer disease showing cerebral atrophy (yellow). ©Howard J Radzyner/ Diomedia/Medical Images RM

WORD	PRONUNCIATION	ELEMENTS		DEFINITION
Alzheimer disease	**AWLZ**-high-mer diz-**EEZ**		Alois Alzheimer, German neurologist, 1864–1915	Common form of dementia; brain tissue has protein clumps and tangles
cognition cognitive (adj)	kog-**NIH**-shun **KOG**-nih-tiv	S/ R/	Latin *knowledge* -ive *nature of, quality of pertaining to* cognit- *thinking*	Process of acquiring knowledge through thinking, learning, and memory Pertaining to the mental activities of thinking and learning
confusion	kon-**FEW**-zhun	S/ R/	-ion *action, condition* confus- *bewildered*	Mental state in which environmental stimuli are not processed appropriately
conscious consciousness unconscious	**KON**-shus **KON**-shus-ness un-**KON**-shus	 S/ R/ P/	Latin *to be aware* -ness *quality, state* conscious- *aware* un- *not*	Having present knowledge of oneself and one's surroundings The state of being aware of and responsive to the environment Not conscious, lacking awareness
delirium	de-**LIR**-ee-um	S/ R/	-um *structure* deliri- *confusion, disorientation*	Acute altered state of consciousness with agitation and disorientation; condition is reversible
dementia	dee-**MEN**-shee-ah	S/ P/ R/	-ia *condition* de- *without* -ment- *mind*	Chronic, progressive, irreversible loss of the mind's cognitive and intellectual functions
empathy	**EM**-pah-thee	P/ R/CF	em- *into* -pathy *disease*	Ability to place yourself into the feelings, emotions, and reactions of another person
sympathy	**SIM**-pa-thee	P/ R/CF	sym- *together* -pathy *disease*	Appreciation and concern for another person's mental and emotional state

Exercises

A. Deconstruct medical terms and define their meanings. *Multiple choice. Choose the letter that best completes each sentence.* **LO 9.8, 9.D**

1. The prefix in the term **sympathy** means:

   a. only   **b.** without   **c.** together   **d.** into

2. The suffix in the term **delirium** means:

   a. condition   **b.** structure   **c.** disease   **d.** aware

3. The root in the term **dementia** means:

   a. disease   **b.** without   **c.** mind   **d.** condition   **e.** confusion

B. Explain disorders of the brain. *Match each disorder with its correct description.* **LO 9.8**

_____	**1.** delirium	**a.** common form of dementia due to protein clumps and tangles
_____	**2.** Alzheimer disease	**b.** dementia due to decreased blood flow to the brain
_____	**3.** confusion	**c.** altered state of consciousness with agitation and disorientation
_____	**4.** vascular dementia	**d.** condition in which a person cannot properly process information

Atherosclerosis   Residual lumen of artery

(a)

Embolus

(b)

▲ **Figure 9.17 Causes of Ischemic Strokes.** (a) Atherosclerosis in a cerebral artery leaving a small, residual lumen. (b) Embolus blocking an artery. Healthy tissue is on the left (pink); blood-starved tissue is on the right (blue). ©Wellcome Photo Library ©R. Spencer Phippen/Diomedia/ Medical Images RM

Keynotes

- Risk factors for ischemic strokes are hypertension, diabetes mellitus, high cholesterol levels, cigarettes, and obesity.

- Risk factors for hemorrhagic strokes are hypertension, cerebral arteriovenous malformations, and cerebral aneurysms.

- More than 10% of people who have a TIA will have a stroke within 3 months.

Abbreviations

AVM	arteriovenous malformation
CVA	cerebrovascular accident
TIA	transient ischemic attack

LO 9.8 Cerebrovascular Accidents (CVAs) or Strokes

A **stroke** (also known as a **cerebrovascular accident,** or **CVA**) occurs when the blood supply to a part of the brain is suddenly interrupted and thus brain cells are deprived of oxygen (*see Chapter 10*). Some cells die; others are left badly damaged. With timely treatment, the damaged cells can be saved. There are two types of stroke:

1. **Ischemic strokes** account for 90% of all strokes and are caused by:

    a. **Atherosclerosis**—plaque in the wall of a cerebral artery (*Figure 9.17a*).

    b. **Embolism**—blood clot in a cerebral artery originating from elsewhere in the body (*Figure 9.17b*).

    c. **Microangiopathy**—occlusion of small cerebral arteries.

2. **Hemorrhagic strokes (intracranial hemorrhage)** occur when a blood vessel in the brain bursts or when a cerebral **aneurysm** or **arteriovenous malformation** (**AVM**) ruptures.

Symptoms of Strokes

The symptoms of a stroke can include the sudden onset of numbness or weakness, especially on one side of the body; difficulty in walking, balance, or coordination; trouble speaking or understanding speech; trouble seeing in one or both eyes; dizziness; confusion; and severe headache. A method to remember common warning signs of stroke is to use the acronym FAST:

Face—Ask the person to smile. Does one side of the face droop?

Arms—Ask the person to raise both arms. Does one arm drift downward?

Speech—Ask the person to repeat a simple phrase. Is his or her speech slurred or strange?

Time—If any of the previous signs is present, call 911 immediately.

Disability after Strokes

Although stroke is a disease of the brain, it can affect the whole body. A common residual disability is complete paralysis of one side of the body, called **hemiplegia**. If one side of the body is weak rather than paralyzed, the disability is called **hemiparesis**. Problems with forming and understanding speech and problems with awareness, attention, learning, judgment, and memory can remain after a stroke. Stroke patients may have difficulty controlling their emotions and may experience depression. All of these disabilities require well-planned rehabilitation.

Transient Ischemic Attack

Transient ischemic attacks **(TIAs)** are short-term, small strokes with symptoms lasting for less than 24 hours. If neurologic symptoms persist for more than 24 hours, then it is a full-blown stroke with brain cell damage and death.

The most frequent cause is a small **embolus** that occludes a small artery in the brain. Often, the embolus arises from a clot in the atrium in atrial fibrillation or from an atherosclerotic plaque in a carotid artery. If the impairment of blood supply lasts more than a few minutes, the affected nerve cells can die and cause permanent neurologic deficit.

WORD	PRONUNCIATION	ELEMENTS		DEFINITION
aneurysm aneurysmal (adj)	**AN**-yur-izm an-yur-**RIZ**-mal		Greek *dilation*	Circumscribed dilation of an artery or cardiac chamber
arteriovenous malformation	ar-**TEER**-ee-oh-**VEE**-nus mal-for-**MAY**-shun	S/ R/CF R/ S/ P/ R/	-ous *pertaining to* arteri/o *artery* -ven- *vein* -ion *process* mal- *bad* -format- *to form*	An abnormal communication between an artery and a vein
cerebrovascular accident (**Note:** also known as a stroke)	seh-**REE**-broh-**VAS**-cyoo-lar **AK**-si-dent STROHK	S/ R/CF R/	-ar *pertaining to* cerebr/o *brain* -vascul- *blood vessel* French *accident, what comes by chance*	Acute clinical event caused by an impaired cerebral circulation.
hemiparesis	**HEM**-ee-pah-**REE**-sis	P/ R/	hemi- *half* -paresis *weakness*	Weakness of one side of the body
hemiplegia hemiplegic (adj)	hem-ee-**PLEE**-jee-ah hem-ee-**PLEE**-jik	S/ P/ R/ S/	-ia *condition* hemi- *half* -pleg- *paralysis* -ic *pertaining to*	Paralysis of one side of the body Pertaining to or suffering from hemiplegia
microangiopathy	**MY**-kroh-an-jee-**OP**-ah-thee	S/ P/ R/CF	-pathy *disease* micro- *small* -angi/o- *blood vessel*	Disease of the very small blood vessels (capillaries)

Exercises

A. Use the terms related to cerebrovascular accidents to complete the clinic note presented below. *Replace the words in italics with the correct medical terms related to cerebrovascular accidents.* **LO 9.8, 9.A**

Mrs. Jacobson presents to the ED with her son. Her son was visiting when she began to slur her speech and the right side of her face appeared droopy. The physician suspects that Mrs. Jacobson has had a **(1)** *stroke*. Upon examination, the patient exhibits **(2)** *weakness* in her left hand grip as well as her left leg. A **(3)** *surgeon that specialized in treatment of disorders of the nervous system* is consulted. An MRI is performed and it is determined that the patient has an **(4)** *abnormal connection between a cerebral artery and vein* that has ruptured. She is immediately sent to surgery to place a clip on the ruptured vessel.

1. _____ .

2. Left-sided _____ .

3. _____ .

4. _____   _____ .

B. Deconstruct medical terms to decipher their meaning. *Being able to pick out the word elements and define them will help you determine the meaning of the entire medical term. Select the correct answer for each question.* **LO 9.8, 9.D**

1. The prefix in the term **hemiparesis** means:

   a. blood vessel   **b.** paralysis   **c.** weakness   **d.** half

2. The suffix in the term **malformation** means:

   a. process   **b.** structure   **c.** pertaining to   **d.** bad

3. The root in the term **arteriovenous** that means *vein* is:

   a. *arteri/o*   **b.** *ven/o*   **c.** *ven*   **d.** *ous*

4. The root/combining form in the term **cerebrovascular** that means *brain* is:

   a. *cerebr/o*   **b.** *vascul*   **c.** *vascul/a*   **d.** *ar*

LO 9.8 Cerebral Palsy

Definition

Cerebral palsy (CP) is the term used to describe the motor **impairment** resulting from brain damage in an infant or young child, regardless of the cause or the effect on the child. It is not hereditary. In congenital CP, the cause is often unknown but can be brain malformations or maternal use of cocaine; CP developed at birth or in the neonatal period is usually related to an incident causing hypoxia of the brain. Cerebral palsy causes delay in the development of normal milestones in infancy and childhood.

The medical terminology of the classification and effects of CP is important, and it is used in many other conditions, including the after effects of **strokes**. The technical terms that follow are labels used to describe the type and extent of a problem. They do not describe the individual.

Classification by Number of Limbs Impaired

- **Quadriplegia (tetraplegia).** All four limbs are involved *(Figure 9.18)*.
- **Diplegia.** Paralysis of corresponding parts (eg., both arms) on both sides of the body.
- **Hemiplegia.** The arm and leg of one side of the body are affected *(Figure 9.19)*.
- **Monoplegia.** Only one limb is affected, usually an arm *(Figure 9.20)*.
- **Paraplegia.** Both lower extremities are involved *(Figure 9.21)*.
- **Triplegia.** Three limbs are involved.

Classification by Movement Disorder

- **Spastic**—pertaining to tight muscles that are resistant to being stretched. They can become overactive when used and produce **clonic** movements.
- **Athetoid**—pertaining to difficulty in controlling and coordinating movements, leading to involuntary writhing movements in constant motion.
- **Ataxic**—pertaining to a poor sense of balance and depth perception, leading to a staggering walk and unsteady hands.

Combined Classifications

- The classifications of movement disorder and number of limbs involved are combined, for example, **spastic diplegia.**

▲ **Figure 9.18** **Quadriplegia.** ©Scott J. Ferrell/ Congressional Quarterly/Alamy Stock Photo

▲ **Figure 9.19** **Hemiplegia.** ©James Prince/ Photo Researchers, Inc.

▲ **Figure 9.20** **Monoplegia.** ©David Grossman/Photo Researchers, Inc.

▲ **Figure 9.21** **Paraplegia.** ©The Washington Post/Getty Images

WORD	PRONUNCIATION		ELEMENTS	DEFINITION
ataxia	a-**TAK**-see-ah	S/ P/ R/	-ia *condition* a- *without* -tax- *coordination*	Inability to coordinate muscle activity, leading to jerky movements
ataxic (adj)	a-**TAK**-sik	S/	-ic *pertaining to*	Pertaining to or suffering from ataxia
athetosis	ath-eh-**TOH**-sis **ATH**-eh-toyd	S/ R/	-osis *condition* athet- *uncontrolled,* *without position*	Slow, writhing involuntary movements
athetoid (adj)		S/	-oid *resembling*	Resembling athetosis
clonic	**KLON**-ik		Greek *turmoil*	Alternating muscular contraction and relaxation
diplegia	die-**PLEE**-jee-ah	S/ P/ R/	-ia *condition* di- *two* -pleg- *paralysis*	Paralysis of corresponding parts on both sides of the body (eg., both arms).
diplegic (adj)	die-**PLEE**-jik	S/	-ic *pertaining to*	Pertaining to or suffering from diplegia
impairment	im-**PAIR**-ment	S/ R/	-ment *action, state* impair- *worsen*	Diminishing of normal function
monoplegia	**MON**-oh-**PLEE**-jee-ah	S/ P/ R/	-ia *condition* mono- *one* -pleg- *paralysis*	Paralysis of one limb
monoplegic (adj)	**MON**-oh-**PLEE**-jik	S/	-ic *pertaining to*	Pertaining to or suffering from monoplegia
palsy	**PAWL**-zee		Latin *paralysis*	Paralysis or paresis from brain damage
paraplegia	par-ah-**PLEE**-jee-ah	S/ P/ R/	-ia *condition* para- *abnormal, beside* -pleg- *paralysis*	Paralysis of both lower extremities
paraplegic (adj)	par-ah-**PLEE**-jik	S/	-ic *pertaining to*	Pertaining to or suffering from paraplegia
quadriplegia	kwad-rih-**PLEE**-jee-ah	S/ P/ R/	-ia *condition* quadri- *four* -pleg- *paralysis*	Paralysis of all four limbs
quadriplegic (adj)	kwad-rih-**PLEE**-jik	S/	-ic *pertaining to*	Pertaining to or suffering from quadriplegia
spasm spastic (adj)	SPAZM **SPAS**-tik	S/ R/	Greek *spasm* -ic *pertaining to* spast- *tight*	Sudden involuntary contraction of a muscle group Increased muscle tone on movement Pertaining to or suffering from increased muscle tone on movement
stroke	STROHK		Old English *to strike*	Acute clinical event caused by an impaired cerebral circulation
tetraplegia	teh-trah-**PLEE**-jee-ah	S/ P/ R/	-ia *condition* tetra- *four* -pleg- *paralysis*	Paralysis of four limbs
tetraplegic (adj)	teh-trah-**PLEE**-jik	S/	-ic *pertaining to*	Pertaining to or suffering from tetraplegia
triplegia	try-**PLEE**-jee-ah	S/ P/ R/	-ia *condition* tri- *three* -pleg- *paralysis*	Paralysis of three limbs
triplegic (adj)	tri-**PLEE**-jik	S/	-ic *pertaining to*	Pertaining to or suffering from triplegia

Exercises

A. Deconstruct medical terms to determine their meaning. *Multiple choice. Choose the letter that best completes each sentence.* **LO 9.8, 9.D**

1. The prefix in the term **monoplegia** means:

   a. one   **b.** two   **c.** three   **d.** four   **e.** five

2. The root in the term **quadriplegia** means:

   a. two   **b.** four   **c.** paralysis   **d.** weakness

3. The suffix in the term **triplegia** means:

   a. one   **b.** three   **c.** pertaining to   **d.** condition of

Case Report (CR) 9.1 *(continued)*

For Ms. Roberta Gaston, who was seen in Dr. Solis' neurosurgery clinic, the EEG did not localize an epileptic source. Therefore, deep brain electrodes were inserted into the region of the suspicious mass that showed on MRI. Seizures were recorded as arising in the mass itself. Dr. Solis performed a surgical resection of the mass, which was a **glioma**. Ms. Gaston has been seizure-free since the surgery a year ago.

Epilepsy is a chronic disorder in which clusters of neurons in the brain discharge their electrical signals in an abnormal rhythm. This disturbed electrical activity (a seizure) can cause strange sensations and behavior, convulsions, and loss of consciousness.

The causes of epilepsy are numerous, from abnormal brain development to brain damage.

An accepted classification of seizures is from the **International League Against Epilepsy:**

1. **Partial seizures** occur when the epileptic activity is in one area of the brain only. For example, in a partial seizure the only symptom of an epileptic attack could be a series of involuntary jerking movements of a single limb.

2. **Generalized seizures:**

   a. **Absence seizures,** previously known as "**petit mal,**" are most common in children ages 4 to 14 but may continue through adult life. An absence seizure is a general onset seizure, meaning that it starts on both sizes of the brain. The child stares vacantly for less than 10 seconds, apparently out of contact with surroundings. The child may be accused of daydreaming. Recovery is quick.

   b. **Tonic-clonic seizures,** previously called "**grand mal,**" are dramatic. The person experiences a **loss of consciousness (LOC),** breathing stops, the muscles stiffen, and the jaw clenches. This "tonic" phase lasts for 30 to 60 seconds. It is followed by the "clonic" phase, in which the whole body shakes with a series of violent, rhythmic jerkings of the limbs. The seizures last for about one to three minutes, and consciousness returns.

   c. **Febrile seizures** are triggered by a high fever in infants age 6 months to 5 years. Very few of these infants go on to develop epilepsy.

Status epilepticus occurs when the brain is in a state of persistent seizure. It is defined as one continuous seizure lasting more than 10 minutes or three recurrent seizures without the person regaining consciousness between them. Many physicians believe that 5 minutes in this state is sufficient to damage neurons. Status epilepticus is a medical emergency and requires maintenance of the airway, breathing, and circulation and the **intravenous (IV)** administration of diazepam and anticonvulsant drugs.

Seizures may be followed by a period of diminished function in the area of the brain surrounding the seizure focus. This transient neurologic deficit is called a **postictal state.**

Most epileptic disorders respond to **antiepileptic** medication, but occasionally brain surgery is required. The first-aid treatment during a seizure is to place the person in a reclining position on his or her side and to cushion the head. Do not try to keep the limbs from moving.

Tourette syndrome (TS) and other **tic disorders** are characterized by episodes of involuntary, rapid, repetitive, fixed movements of individual muscle groups. They occur with varying frequency and are associated with meaningless vocal sounds or meaningful words and phrases. The tics are probably genetic. There is no cure, but they can be treated pharmacologically with haloperidol or clonidine.

Narcolepsy is a chronic disorder caused by the brain's inability to regulate the sleep-wake cycle. Patients fall asleep during the day for a few seconds or up to an hour. It is associated with **cataplexy,** the sudden loss of voluntary muscle tone with brief episodes of total paralysis and vivid hallucinations. There is no cure, but it can be treated pharmacologically with stimulants.

WORD	PRONUNCIATION	ELEMENTS		DEFINITION
absence seizure *Note:* Formerly referred to as "petit mal"	**AB**-sens **SEE**-zhur	P/ R/ S/ R/	ab- *away from* -sence *to feel* -ure *process* seiz- *to convulse*	A brief seizure characterized by absence of activity and occasionally clonic movements
cataplexy	**KAT**-ah-plek-see	P/ R/	cata- *down* -plexy *stroke*	Sudden loss of muscle tone with brief paralysis
epilepsy	**EP**-ih-**LEP**-see		Greek *seizure*	Chronic brain disorder due to paroxysmal excessive neuronal discharges
narcolepsy	**NAR**-coh-lep-see	S/ R/CF	-lepsy *seizure* narc/o- *stupor*	Condition with frequent incidents of sudden, involuntary deep sleep
postictal	post-**IK**-tal	S/ P/ R/	-al *pertaining to* post- *after* -ict- *seizure*	Occurring after a seizure
status epilepticus	**STAT**-us ep-ih-**LEP**-tik-us	S/ R/ S/ R/	-us *pertaining to* stat- *standing still* -ic- *pertaining to* epilept- *seizure*	A recurrent state of seizure activity lasting longer than a specific time frame (usually 30 minutes)
tic	TIK		French *tic*	Sudden, involuntary, repeated contraction of muscles
tonic-clonic seizure *Note:* Formerly referred to as "grand mal"	**TON**-ik-**KLON**-ik **SEE**-zhur	S/	-ic *pertaining to*	Generalized seizure due to epileptic activity in all or most of the brain
tonic **clonic** **seizure**	**TON**-ik **KLON**-ik **SEE**-zhur	R/ R/ S/ R/	ton- *pressure, tension* clon- *violent action* -ure *process* seiz- *to grab, convulse*	Muscular contraction in a continuous state Relating to muscle movements showing contraction and relaxation in rapid succession An epileptic attack
Tourette syndrome	tur-**ET SIN**-drome		Georges Gilles de la Tourette, French neurologist, 1857–1904	Disorder of multiple motor and vocal tics

Exercises

A. In practice, you will find that some people will use the new terms for seizures, and some will use the older traditional terms. It is important that you know both. *Fill in the blank with the correct term.* **LO 9.8**

1. A tonic-clonic seizure is traditionally known as a _____ mal seizure.

2. An absence seizure is traditionally known as a _____ mal seizure.

B. Match the signs of a brain disorder with their corresponding condition. LO 9.8, 9.A

_____ 1. sudden loss of muscle tone with brief paralysis   **a.** absence seizure

_____ 2. infant with high fever   **b.** narcolepsy

_____ 3. child appears to be daydreaming   **c.** febrile seizure

_____ 4. transient neurologic deficit after a seizure   **d.** Tourette syndrome

_____ 5. person suddenly falls asleep   **e.** cataplexy

_____ 6. a tic disorder   **f.** postictal state

LO 9.8 Other Brain Disorders

▲ **Figure 9.22** MRI Shows a Glioma (arrow). ©Simon Fraser/Photo Researchers, Inc.

Parkinson disease is caused by the degeneration of neurons in the basic ganglia that produce a neurotransmitter called **dopamine**. Motor symptoms of abnormal movements, **tremor** of the hands, rigidity, a shuffling or **festinant** (hastening, falling-forward) gait, and weak voice appear. The symptoms gradually increase in severity. The cause is unknown, and there is no cure.

Huntington disease (also known as **Huntington chorea**) is a hereditary disorder starting with mild personality changes between the ages of 30 and 50. Involuntary, irregular, jerky (**choreic**) movements and muscle weakness follow, and dementia occurs in the later stages. A gene defect is on chromosome 4, but there is no known cure.

Syncope (fainting or passing out) is a temporary loss of consciousness and posture. It is usually due to hypotension and the associated deficient oxygen supply (hypoxia) to the brain. This disorder is called **neurally mediated syncope (NMS)**. In adults, it may be associated with cardiac arrhythmias and other diseases. The first-aid treatment is to place the person in a reclining position.

Cerebral edema is excess accumulation of water in the intra- or extracellular spaces of the brain. It is associated with trauma, tumors, inflammation, toxins (such as aspirin in **Reye syndrome**), ischemia, and malignant hypertension.

Neoplasm

Brain tumors are most often secondary tumors that have metastasized from cancers in the lung, breast, skin, or kidney. **Primary brain tumors** arise from any of the glial cells and are called **gliomas** (*Figure 9.22*). The most malignant form of glioma is called **glioblastoma multiforme**.

Headaches

A headache (**cephalalgia**) is classified into either being primary or secondary. Secondary headaches occur for the first time in relation to another disorder.

Primary headaches include:

- **Migraine** produces an intense throbbing, pulsating pain usually in one area of the head, often with nausea and vomiting. It can be preceded by an **aura**, visual disturbances such as flashing lights, or temporary loss of vision. It occurs three times as often in women as men.

- **Tension-type** was previously known as a tension headache, ordinary headache, and muscle contraction headache. The exact cause of this type of headache is unknown. Patient will report increased tenderness with palpation of head and neck muscles.

- **Trigeminal autonomic cephalalgias** consist of **cluster headaches,** among other headache types, with intense unilateral pain in the supraorbital, orbital, and/or temporal regions. Attacks occur in series that may last for weeks or months (cluster periods).

- **Other primary headache disorders** are those that do not fit the previous categories and occur without a secondary cause. Examples of this category of headaches include headaches due to cough, exercise, or cold-stimulus.

Infections of the Brain

Brain abscess is most often a direct spread of infection from sinusitis, otitis media, or mastoiditis (*see Chapter 16*). It also can be a result of bloodborne pathogens from lung or dental infections. Abscesses are also formed by exotic fungal or protozoan organisms in immunosuppressive diseases like acquired immunodeficiency syndrome (AIDS) and **tuberculosis (TB).** Protozoa are single-celled organisms that like to live in the damp. An example, *Trichomonas*, is sexually transmitted (*see Chapter 8*).

Creutzfeldt-Jakob disease (CJD) produces a rapid deterioration of mental function with difficulty in coordination of muscle movement. Some cases are linked to the consumption of beef from cattle with **mad cow disease (bovine spongiform encephalopathy, or BSE).** Damage to the brain is thought to be caused by an abnormal infectious protein called a **prion**.

Encephalitis is inflammation of the **parenchyma** of the brain. It is usually caused by a virus such as human immunodeficiency virus (HIV), West Nile virus, herpes simplex, or the childhood diseases of measles, mumps, chickenpox, and rubella. It occurs most often in the elderly, those with compromised immune systems (*see Chapter 15*), and children.

Abbreviations	
BSE	bovine spongiform encephalopathy
CJD	Creutzfeldt-Jakob disease
NMS	neurally mediated syncope
TB	tuberculosis

Word Analysis and Definition

S = Suffix   P = Prefix   R = Root   R/CF = Combining Form

WORD	PRONUNCIATION	ELEMENTS		DEFINITION
aura	**AWE**-rah		Greek *breath of air*	Sensory experience preceding an epileptic seizure or a migraine headache
bovine spongiform encephalopathy (also called *mad cow disease*)	**BOH**-vine **SPON**-jee-form en-sef-ah-**LOP**-ah-thee	S/ R/ S/ R/CF S/ P/ R/	**-ine** *pertaining to* **bov-** *cattle* **-form** *appearance of* **spong/i-** *sponge* **-pathy** *disease* **en-** *in* **-cephal/o-** *head*	Disease of cattle (mad cow disease) that can be transmitted to humans, causing Creutzfeldt-Jakob disease
cephalalgia	sef-uh-**LAL**-jee-uh	S/ R/	**-algia** *pain* **cephal-** *head*	Pertaining to pain in the head
chorea choreic (adj)	kor-**EE**-ah kor-**EE**-ik	S/ R/	Greek *dance* **-ic** *pertaining to* **chore-** *dance*	Involuntary, irregular spasms of limb and facial muscles
Creutzfeldt-Jakob disease	**KROITS**-felt-**YAK**-op diz-**EEZ**		Hans Creutzfeldt, 1885–1964, and Alfons Jakob, 1884–1931, German neuropsychiatrists	Progressive incurable neurologic disease caused by infectious prions
festinant	**FES**-tih-nant		Latin *to hasten*	Shuffling, falling-forward gait
glioblastoma multiforme	**GLIE**-oh-blas-**TOH**-mah **MULL**-tih-**FOR**-mee	S/ R/CF R/ P/ S/	**-oma** *tumor* **gli/o-** *glue* **-blast-** *germ cell* **multi-** *many* **-forme** *appearance of*	A malignant form of brain cancer
glioma	glie-**OH**-mah	S/ R/	**-oma** *tumor, mass* **gli-** *glue*	Tumor arising in a glial cell
Huntington disease Huntington chorea (syn)	**HUN**-ting-ton diz-**EEZ** kor-**EE**-ah		George Huntington, U.S. physician, 1851–1916 chorea Greek *dance*	Progressive inherited, degenerative, incurable neurologic disease
migraine	**MY**-grain	P/ R/	**mi-** *derived from hemi; half* **-graine** *head pain*	Paroxysmal severe headache confined to one side of the head
parenchyma	pah-**RENG**-kih-mah		Greek *to pour in beside*	Characteristic functional cells of a gland or organ that are supported by the connective tissue framework
Parkinson disease	**PAR**-kin-son diz-**EEZ**		James Parkinson, British physician, 1755–1824	Disease of muscular rigidity, tremors, and a masklike facial expression
prion	**PREE**-on		derived from *protein-infectious particle*	Small infectious protein particle
Reye syndrome	RAY **SIN**-drome		R. Douglas Reye, 1912–1977, Australian pathologist	Encephalopathy and liver damage in children following an acute viral illness; linked to aspirin use
syncope	**SIN**-koh-peh		Greek *cutting short*	Temporary loss of consciousness and postural tone due to diminished cerebral blood flow
tremor	**TREM**-or		Latin *to shake*	Small, shaking, involuntary, repetitive movements of hands, extremities, neck, or jaw

Exercises

A. Based on the given scenario, determine the specific type of primary headache with which the patient is likely suffering.
Fill in the blanks. **LO 9.8, LO 9.A**

1. Patient complains of intense pain on only one side of the head. The patient states that the pain is mainly around and above her eye. She states that the headache occurs in a pattern in which it occurs for 2 weeks, stops for 1 week, and then repeats. _____ headache

2. Patient complains of a headache that occurs 5 minutes after he begins to run. Headache due to _____

3. Patient states she has been experiencing intense headaches that cause her nausea and vomiting. Just prior to the headache, she sees bright flashing lights. She has had three of these type headaches in the last two months. _____ headache

LO 9.8 Traumatic Brain Injury

Traumatic brain injury (TBI) causes damage to the brain. Over 1 million people are seen by medical doctors each year following a blow to the head. Of these, 50,000 to 100,000 will have prolonged problems affecting their work and their **activities of daily living (ADLs)**. These injuries can occur during combat situations, but they also occur in sports, such as boxing, ice hockey, and American football, which are all sports that often involve severe contact injuries to the head.

If you are driving your car at 50 miles per hour and are hit head-on, your brain goes from 50 miles per hour to zero instantly. Your soft brain tissue is propelled forward and squished against the front of your hard skull **(coup)**. Then the brain and the rest of your body rebound backward. The soft brain is then squished against the back of your rigid skull **(contrecoup)**. The squished front and back areas are at least bruised. This bruise is called a **contusion** *(Figure 9.23)*.

If the process is more severe, blood vessels tear and blood flows into the brain. In addition, the brain itself can tear and cut brain connections and signals. In any injury, brain swelling can occur. Because the skull is hard and rigid, it cannot expand to cope with this extra volume. So the soft brain tissue is compressed, and some areas can stop working.

A mild head injury is called a **concussion**. You may feel dazed or have a period of confusion during which you do not recall the event that caused the concussion. In more severe cases, you may lose consciousness for a brief period of time and have no memory of the event. Repeated concussions have a cumulative effect, with loss of mental ability (as in many American football players) and/or traumatically induced Parkinson disease (as happened with professional boxer Muhammad Ali).

In more severe TBIs, the symptoms will depend on the area of the brain damaged. Some symptoms, such as difficulty with memory or concentration, irritability, aggression, **insomnia**, or depression, can be long-term. Traumatic brain injury has become a signature wound of the wars in Iraq and Afghanistan.

Posttraumatic stress disorder (PTSD) arises after significant trauma like a life-threatening incident, loss of a loved one, abuse, or combat in war. Symptoms include re-experiencing the original trauma through flashbacks or nightmares, difficulty in sleeping, anger, and hypervigilance. The symptoms cause significant impairment in social, occupational, and family areas of functioning.

The residual effects of brain damage, whether due to trauma or stroke, have terminology:

- **Impairment** is a deviation from normal function; for example, not being able to control an unwanted muscle movement.
- **Disability** is a restriction in the ability to perform a normal activity of daily living (ADL), for example, a 3-year-old who cannot walk independently.
- **Handicap** is defined as having a disability that prevents a child or adult from achieving a normal role in society commensurate with age and sociocultural setting; for example, a 16-year-old who cannot take care of personal toiletry and hygienic needs.
- **Shaken baby syndrome (SBS)** is a type of TBI produced when a baby is violently shaken. The baby has weak neck muscles and a heavy head. Shaking makes the brain bounce back and forth in the skull, leading to severe brain damage. Other injuries include retinal hemorrhages, damage to the spinal cord, and fractures of the ribs and limb bones. This syndrome usually occurs in children younger than 2 years.

Abbreviations

ADLs	activities of daily living
PTSD	posttraumatic stress disorder
SBS	shaken baby syndrome
TBI	traumatic brain injury

Bruising (contusion)   Bruising   Bruising

1. Position prior to impact.   2. Impact from the front.   3. Contrecoup action.   4. Subsequent coup-contrecoup injury.

▲ **Figure 9.23** Contusions Caused by Back-and-Forth Movement of Brain in Skull.

WORD	PRONUNCIATION	ELEMENTS		DEFINITION
activities of daily living	ak-**TIV**-ih-teez of **DAY**-lee **LIV**-ing	S/ R/ S/ R/ S/ R/	-ity *condition, state* activ- *movement* -ly *every* dai- *day* -ing *quality of* liv- *life*	Daily routines for mobility and personal care: bathing, dressing, eating, and moving
concussion	kon-**KUSH**-un	S/ R/	-ion *action, condition* concuss- *shake violently*	Mild head injury
contusion	kon-**TOO**-zhun	S/ R/	-ion *action, condition* contus- *bruise*	Bruising of a tissue, including the brain
coup	KOO		French *a blow*	Injury to the brain occurring directly under the skull at the point of impact
contrecoup	**KON**-treh-koo		French *counterblow*	Injury to the brain at a point directly opposite the point of original contact
disability	dis-ah-**BILL**-ih-tee	P/ R/	dis- *away from* -ability *competence*	Diminished capacity to perform certain activities or functions
handicap	**HAND**-ee-cap		French *assess before a race*	Condition that interferes with a person's ability to function normally
insomnia	in-**SOM**-nee-ah	S/ P/ R/	-ia *condition* in- *not* -somn- *sleep*	Inability to sleep

Exercises

A. Write the abbreviation that is described in the following sentences. *Fill in the blanks.* **LO 9.8, 9.F**

1. An infant is brought to the emergency department after being shaken by the parent. The infant is very sleepy and does not respond to painful stimuli. The infant may be suffering from _____.

2. After suffering a stroke, the patient is no longer able to brush her hair or teeth. She has an injury that is affecting her _____.

3. The goal keeper for the high school soccer team slid into the goal post head first and lost consciousness. She will be sent to the emergency department to be evaluated for the presence of a _____.

B. Identify the correct definitions of common medical terms. *From the given definition, choose the correct term.* **LO 9.8**

1. A restriction in the ability to perform activities of daily living:
    a. disability   **b.** impairment   **c.** handicap   **d.** contusion

2. A deviation from normal function:
    a. disability   **b.** impairment   **c.** handicap   **d.** contusion

Figure 9.24 **Hematomas.** (a) CT scan of subdural hematoma compressing ventricles and pushing them laterally. (b) Epidural hematoma. ©Scott Camazine/Alamy Stock Photo ©ISM/Sovereign/ Diomedia/Medical Images

Ventricle
Ventricle
Subdural hematoma
Epidural hematoma
(a)
(b)

LO 9.9 Disorders of the Meninges

Subdural hematoma is bleeding into the subdural space outside the brain *(Figure 9.24a)*. Most subdural hematomas are associated with closed head injuries and bleeding from broken veins caused by violent rotational movement of the head. They have been seen following roller-coaster rides with high-speed turns that jerk and whip the head. Although the blood accumulation is slow, the bleeding must be stopped surgically.

Epidural hematoma is a pooling of blood in the epidural space outside the brain *(Figure 9.24b)*. Most are associated with a fractured skull and bleeding from an artery that lies in the meninges. If the bleeding is not stopped surgically by **ligating** (tying off) the blood vessel, brain compression with severe neurologic injury or death can occur.

Meningitis is inflammation of the meninges covering the brain and spinal cord. Viral meningitis is the most common form and occurs at all ages. Bacterial meningitis is more common in the very young or very old. **Meningococcal meningitis** is contagious, spread through droplet infection by coughing and sneezing and through close living conditions, as in college dormitories. Vaccines are available to prevent most causes of meningitis *(see Chapter 12)*.

Meningioma is a tumor originating in the arachnoid cells of the meninges, most commonly overlying the cerebral hemispheres. It is usually benign and produces a slow-growing, focal, spherical tumor. Symptoms can take years to develop. Surgical resection is usually curative.

▲ **Figure 9.25** Bell Palsy of Right Side of Face. ©Arlene Soodak/Diomedia/Medical Images RM

▲ **Figure 9.26** Horner Syndrome Showing Ptosis and Small Pupil of Left Eye. ©Science Photo Library RM/Diomedia/ Medical Images

LO 9.10 Disorders of the Cranial Nerves

Bell palsy is a disorder of the seventh cranial nerve (facial nerve), causing a sudden onset of weakness or paralysis of facial muscles on one side of the face *(Figure 9.25)*. Common symptoms are a **hemifacial** inability to smile, whistle, or grimace; drooping of the mouth with drooling of saliva; and inability to close the eye on the affected side. Early treatment with steroids and supportive measures is essential. The facial nerve also can be affected by trauma or tumors.

Trigeminal neuralgia (tic douloureux) is intermittent, shooting pain in the area of the face and head innervated by the fifth cranial nerve. The pain is abrupt (sudden), unilateral, and often severe, and can affect any area of the face from the crown of the head to the jaw. Chewing or touching the affected area causes pain.

Horner syndrome presents with a unilateral droopy eyelid (ptosis), small pupil, and decrease in perspiration on the face. It can occur in lung cancer and injuries to the head, neck, and cervical spinal cord *(Figure 9.26)*. The signs of Horner syndrome are due to the blocking of the sympathetic pathway to the eye.

WORD	PRONUNCIATION	ELEMENTS		DEFINITION
Bell palsy	BELL **PAWL**-zee		Charles Bell, 1774–1842, Scottish surgeon, anato-mist, and physiologist **palsy** Latin *paralysis*	Paresis or paralysis of one side of face
epidural	ep-ih-**DYU**-ral	S/ P/ R/	-al *pertaining to* epi- *above* -dur- *dura mater*	Above the dura
hematoma	hee-mah-**TOH**-mah	S/ R/	-oma *tumor, mass* hemat- *blood*	Collection of blood that has escaped from the blood vessels into tissue
hemifacial	hem-ee-**FAY**-shal	S/ P/ R/	-al *pertaining to* hemi- *half* -faci- *face*	Pertaining to one side of the face
Horner syndrome	**HOR**-ner **SIN**-drome	P/ R/	Johann Friedrich Horner, 1831–1886, Swiss ophthalmologist syn- *together* -drome *running*	Disorder of the sympathetic nerves to the face and eye Combination of symptoms and signs associated with a particular disease process
meningioma	meh-**NIN**-jee-**OH**-mah	S/ R/CF	-oma *tumor, mass* mening/i- *meninges*	Tumor arising from the arachnoid layer of the meninges
meningococcal	meh-nin-goh-**KOK**-al	S/ R/CF R/	-al *pertaining to* mening/i- *meninges* -cocc- *spherical bacterium*	Pertaining to the *meningococcus* bacterium
meningitis	men-in-**JIE**-tis	S/	-itis *infection*	Inflammation of the membranes surrounding the brain or spinal cord
neuralgia	nyu-**RAL**-jee-ah	S/ R/	-algia *pain* neur- *nerve*	Pain in the distribution of a nerve
subdural	sub-**DUR**-al	S/ P/ R/	-al *pertaining to* sub- *under* -dur- *dura mater*	Located in the space between the dura mater and arachnoid membrane
tic douloureux trigeminal neuralgia (syn)	TIK duh-luh-**RUE**		**douloureux** French *painful tic*	Painful, sudden, spasmodic, involuntary contractions of the facial muscles supplied by the trigeminal nerve

Exercises

A. Deconstruct the terms into their basic elements. LO 9.9, 9.10, 9.D

1. In the term **hematoma,** the meaning of the suffix is:

   a. meninges   **b.** spherical   **c.** mass   **d.** blood   **e.** bruise

2. In the term **hemifacial,** the prefix means:

   a. half   **b.** pertaining to   **c.** face   **d.** blood   **e.** nerve

3. In the term **meningitis,** the word part that means inflammation is the:

   a. prefix   **b.** root   **c.** suffix

B. Based on the given scenario, determine what disorder the person is likely to have. LO 9.10

1. Mr. Turner brings his 3-year-old son to the pediatrician. The father has noticed that his son's right eyelid is drooping and the pupil of the right eye remains small, even when the pupil of the left is large. The pediatrician may suspect that the child is suffering from:

   a. Huntington disease   **b.** Parkinson disease   **c.** Horner syndrome   **d.** Bell palsy

Lesson 9.4

NERVOUS SYSTEM

Disorders of the Spinal Cord and Peripheral Nerves

Lesson Objectives

There are many disorders of the nervous system that affect the spinal cord and the peripheral nerves without affecting the brain. In this lesson, the information will enable you to:

9.4.1 Discuss disorders of the spinal cord and peripheral nerves.

9.4.2 Distinguish between different diagnostic tests used for nervous system disorders.

9.4.3 Define methods by which nervous system medications influence disease processes.

9.4.4 Recognize common congenital disorders of the nervous system.

9.4.5 Use the correct terminology to communicate about the nervous system and its disorders with patients and other health professionals.

▲ **Figure 9.27** Multiple Sclerosis. Note areas of the spinal cord where myelin sheath has been destroyed (arrows). Normal spinal cord is yellow. ©James Cavallini/ Photo Researchers, Inc.

Abbreviations

MS	multiple sclerosis
VEP	visual evoked potential

 Case Report (CR) 9.3

You are

. . . Tanisha Colis, an electroneurodiagnostic technologist working with Raoul Cardenas, MD, a neurologist at Fulwood Medical Center.

Your patient is

. . . Mrs. Suzanne Kalish, a 42-year-old social worker employed by the medical center.

Mrs. Kalish has recently had an exacerbation of her symptoms due to **multiple sclerosis (MS).** She is going to have a **visual evoked potential (VEP)** test, followed by an MRI of her brain and spinal cord.

Patient Interview:

Tanisha: "Good morning, Mrs. Kalish, I'm Tanisha Colis, the technologist who'll be performing your visual evoked potential test. How are you feeling?"

Mrs. Kalish: "I've been doing OK for the last 4 or 5 years. Then, a few weeks ago, I started dragging my right foot like a wounded witch. I'm tired out, can't come to work. It's a struggle to walk the few yards just to pick up the mail."

Tanisha: "The MRI you are going to have today will give us a lot of information about what's going on."

Mrs. Kalish: "My mind is going 'wheelchair, wheelchair, wheelchair.' Especially since in the last couple of days the vision in my right eye has got all blurred."

Tanisha: "That's the reason you are having the visual evoked potential test."

Mrs. Kalish: "I hate this disease. If I had cancer, I'd have a chance. I'd fight it to the end, whatever that would be."

Tanisha: "Let me help you up, and we'll go get this test done."

Mrs. Kalish: "I can manage on my own, thank you."

LO 9.11 Disorders of the Myelin Sheath of Nerve Fibers

When the myelin sheath surrounding nerve fibers is damaged, nerves do not conduct impulses normally. **Demyelination**, the destruction of an area of the myelin sheath, can occur in the PNS caused by inflammation, vitamin B$_{12}$ deficiency, poisons, and some medications.

Guillain-Barré syndrome is a disorder of the peripheral nerves in which the body makes antibodies against myelin, leading to loss of nerve conduction, muscle weakness, and **paresthesias** (changes in sensation). Treatment is with corticosteroids, and recovery of neurologic function is slow.

Demyelination of nerve fibers in the brain, spinal cord, and optic nerves also can occur. **Multiple sclerosis (MS)** is the most common of these demyelination disorders. As you can tell from Mrs. Kalish's story in CR 9.3, MS is a chronic, progressive disorder. **Intermittent** myelin damage and scarring slow nerve impulses (*Figure 9.27*). This leads to muscle weakness, pain, numbness, and vision loss. Because different nerve fibers are affected at different times, MS symptoms often worsen (**exacerbations**) or show partial or complete reduction (**remissions**). Mrs. Kalish is now in an exacerbation.

MS has an average age of onset between 18 and 35 years and is more common in women. Its cause is unknown, but it is thought to be an autoimmune disease.

Other causes of demyelination in the CNS are injury, ischemia, toxic agents such as chemotherapy or radiotherapy, and congenital disorders such as **Tay-Sachs disease.** After viral infections or vaccinations, **postinfectious encephalomyelitis** is a demyelination process, as is **HIV encephalitis**, which is seen in up to 30% of patients with AIDS.

WORD	PRONUNCIATION	ELEMENTS		DEFINITION
demyelination	dee-**MY**-eh-lin-**A**-shun	S/ P/ R/	-ation *process* de- *away from, without* -myelin- *myelin*	Process of losing the myelin sheath of a nerve fiber
encephalitis encephalomyelitis	en-**SEF**-ah-**LIE**-tis en-**SEF**-ah-loh-**MY**-eh-**LIE**-tis	S/ R/ R/CF R/	-itis *inflammation* encephal- *brain* encephal/o- *brain* -myel- *spinal cord*	Inflammation of brain cells and tissues Inflammation of the brain and spinal cord
exacerbation (contrast remission)	ek-zas-er-**BAY**-shun	S/ R/	-ation *process* exacerb- *increase, aggravate*	Period when there is an increase in the severity of a disease
Guillain-Barré syndrome	**GEE**-yan-bah- **RAY SIN**-drome		Georges Guillain, 1876– 1961, and Jean-Alexandre Barré, 1880–1967, French neurologists	Disorder in which the body makes antibodies against myelin, disrupting nerve conduction
intermittent	**IN**-ter-**MIT**-ent	S/ P/ R/	-ent *end result* inter- *between* -mitt- *send*	Alternately ceasing and beginning again
paresthesia paresthesias (pl)	par-es-**THEE**-ze-ah	S/ P/ R/	-ia *condition* par(a)- *abnormal* -esthes- *sensation, feeling*	Abnormal sensation; for example, tingling, burning, prickling
remission (contrast exacerbation)	ree-**MISH**-un	S/ P/ R/	-ion *action, condition* re- *back* -miss- *send*	Period when there is a lessening or absence of the symptoms of a disease

Exercises

A. Test yourself on the elements and terms related to disorders of the myelin sheath of nerve fibers. *Choose the best answer.* **LO 9.11, 9.A, 9.D**

1. **Guillain-Barré syndrome** disrupts
   a. nerve conduction   b. blood flow   c. metabolism

2. In the term **paresthesia,** the prefix means
   a. between   b. abnormal   c. many

3. **Remission** is the opposite of
   a. intermittence   b. exacerbation   c. demyelination

4. To **modify** something is to
   a. dispose of it   b. change it   c. renew it

5. In the term **demyelination,** the prefix means
   a. away from   b. in front of   c. in between

6. **Encephalomyelitis** is inflammation of the
   a. brain   b. spinal cord   c. brain and spinal cord

LO 9.12 Disorders of the Spinal Cord

Trauma

The spinal cord is injured in three ways (*Figure 9.28*):

1. **Severed.**

2. **Contused.**

3. **Compressed,** by a broken or dislocated vertebra, bleeding, or swelling.

Because of its anatomy with nerve fibers and tracts going up and down, to and from the brain, injury to the spinal cord results in loss of function *below the injury.* For example, if the cord is injured in the thoracic region, the arms function normally, but the legs can be **paralyzed**. Both muscle control and sensation are lost.

If the spinal cord is severed, the loss is permanent. Contusions can cause temporary loss lasting days, weeks, or months. Compression injuries may require surgical intervention to relieve the pressure. Compression also can be due to a **herniated** disc.

The first goal of treatment is to prevent further damage, which is why you see football players being carried off the field strapped to a board and carefully padded to prevent even slight shifting of the spine.

Approximately half a million people in the United States have **spinal cord injuries (SCIs)**. About 17,000 new injuries occur each year; 80% involve males. Quadriplegia is slightly more common than paraplegia (*see definitions on page 289*).

Compression of the cord also can occur slowly from a tumor in the cord or spine. Cancer or osteoporosis can cause a vertebra to collapse and compress the cord.

- **Cervical spondylosis** is a disorder in which the discs and vertebrae in the neck degenerate, narrow the spinal canal, and compress the spinal cord and/or the spinal nerve roots.

- In **syringomyelia**, fluid-filled cavities grow in the spinal cord and compress nerves that detect pain and temperature. There is no specific cure.

Other Disorders

Acute transverse myelitis is a localized disorder of the spinal cord that blocks transmission of impulses up and down the spinal cord. People who have **Lyme disease**, **syphilis**, or **tuberculosis** or those who inject heroin or amphetamines intravenously are at risk of developing this disorder. The disorder causes loss of sensation, muscle **paralysis**, and loss of bladder and bowel control. There is no specific treatment. Most people recover completely.

Subacute combined degeneration of the spinal cord is due to a deficiency of vitamin B_{12}. The sensory nerve fibers in the spinal cord degenerate, producing weakness, clumsiness, tingling, and loss of the position sense as to where limbs are. Treatment is injections of vitamin B_{12}.

Poliomyelitis (polio) is an acute infectious disease, occurring mostly in children, that is caused by the poliovirus. The virus can be asymptomatic in the nasopharynx and **gastrointestinal (GI)** tract. When it spreads to the nervous system, it replicates in the spinal cord and destroys motor neurons. Symptoms are progressive muscle **paralysis**. Poliomyelitis is preventable by vaccination and has almost been eradicated in the world.

Postpolio syndrome (PPS), in which people develop tired, painful, and weak muscles many years after recovery from polio, is classified as a motor neuron disorder.

Motor neuron disorders occur when motor nerves in the spinal cord and brain progressively deteriorate. This leads to muscle weakness that can progress to paralysis. **Amyotrophic lateral sclerosis (ALS,** or Lou Gehrig disease) and its variants, **progressive muscular atrophy** and **primary lateral sclerosis,** are examples. There is no cure.

Severed spinal cord

(a) Fracture-dislocation of vertebra

(b) Fractured vertebra

▲ **Figure 9.28** Spinal Cord Injuries. (*a*) Severed spinal cord from fracture-dislocation of vertebra. (*b*) Compressed spinal cord with vertebral fracture.

©Wellcome Photo Library ©Simon Fraser/ Newcastle Hospitals NHS/Science Photo Library/ Photo Researchers, Inc.

WORD	PRONUNCIATION	ELEMENTS		DEFINITION
amyotrophic	a-my-oh-**TROH**-fik	S/ P/ R/ R/	-ic *pertaining to* a- *without* -my/o *muscle* -troph- *nourishment,* *development*	Pertaining to muscular atrophy
atrophy	**AT**-roh-fee	P/ R/	a- *without* -trophy *nourishment,* *development*	Wasting or diminished volume of a tissue or organ
compression	kom-**PRESH**-un	S/ P/ R/	-ion *action* com- *together* -press- *squeeze*	A squeezing together so as to increase density and/or decrease a dimension of a structure
hernia (noun)	**HER**-nee-ah		Latin *rupture*	Protrusion of a structure through the tissue that normally contains it.
herniation	**HER**-nee-**AY**-shun	S/ R	-ation *process* herni- *rupture*	Protrusion of an anatomical structure from its normal location
herniate (verb)	**HER**-nee-ate	S/	-ate *composed of*	To protrude
Lyme disease	LIME diz-**EEZ**		Named in 1977 after a group of children in Lyme, Connecticut who acquired the disease.	Disease transmitted by the bite of an infected deer tick
myelitis	**MY**-eh-**LIE**-tis	S/ R/	-itis *inflammation* myel- *spinal cord*	Inflammation of the spinal cord
paralyze	**PAR**-ah-lize	P/ R/	para- *abnormal* -lyze *destroy*	To make incapable of movement
paralysis	pah-**RAL**-ih-sis	S/	-lysis *destruction*	Loss of voluntary movement
paralytic	par-ah-**LYT**-ic	S/	-lytic *loosen*	Pertaining to or suffering from paralysis
poliomyelitis polio (abbrev)	**POH**-lee-oh-**MY**-eh-**LIE**-tis	S/ P/ R/	-itis *inflammation* polio- *gray matter* -myel- *spinal cord*	Inflammation of the gray matter of the spinal cord, leading to paralysis of the limbs and muscles of respiration
postpolio syndrome	post-**POH**-lee-oh **SIN**-drome	P/ P/ R/	post- *after* syn- *together* -drome *running*	Progressive muscle weakness in a person previously affected by polio
spondylosis	spon-dih-**LOH**-sis	S/ R/	-osis *condition* spondyl- *vertebra*	Degenerative osteoarthritis of the spine
syringomyelia	sih-**RING**-oh-my-**EE**-lee-ah	S/ R/CF R/	-ia *condition* syring/o- *tube, pipe* -myel- *spinal cord*	Abnormal longitudinal cavities in the spinal cord that cause paresthesias and muscle weakness

Exercises

A. Identify the meaning of the basic word elements. *Match the word element in the first column to its correct meaning in the second column.* **LO 9.12**

_____ **1.** *a-*

_____ **2.** *-ic*

_____ **3.** *my/o*

_____ **4.** *spondyl-*

_____ **5.** *-ia*

_____ **6.** *-lysis*

_____ **7.** *para-*

a. abnormal

b. destruction

c. pertaining to

d. without

e. vertebra

f. condition of

g. muscle

> **Study Hint**
>
> The word element *para-* has different meanings. To determine its particular meaning, you need to interpret its meaning within its context.
> *Para-* can mean around or near, as in *parasympathetic.* It can be used to describe a woman that has given birth, as in *primipara.*
> It can mean abnormal, as in *paraplegia.*

LO 9.13 Disorders of the Peripheral Nerves

The term **neuropathy** is used here as any disorder affecting one or more peripheral nerves.

Mononeuropathy is damage to a single peripheral nerve. Prolonged pressure on a nerve that runs close to the surface over a bony prominence is a common cause. Examples are:

- **Carpal tunnel syndrome.** The median nerve at the wrist is compressed between the wrist bones and a strong overlying ligament. Numbness, pain, and tingling of the thumb side of the hand are the symptoms. Incision of the ligament relieves the pressure.

- **Ulnar nerve palsy.** Nerve damage occurs as the ulnar nerve crosses too close to the surface over the humerus at the back of the elbow. Pins-and-needles sensation and weakness in the hand result. Hitting the ulnar nerve is the cause of pain when you hit your "funny bone."

- **Peroneal nerve palsy.** Nerve damage occurs as the peroneal nerve passes too close to the surface near the back of the knee. Compression of the nerve occurs in people who are bedridden or strapped in a wheelchair.

Polyneuropathy is damage to, and the simultaneous malfunction of, many peripheral nerves throughout the body.

Symptoms of acute polyneuropathy include muscle weakness and a pins-and-needles sensation or loss of sensation. The symptoms begin suddenly in the legs and work upward to the arms.

In **diabetic chronic polyneuropathy,** only sensation is affected, most commonly in the feet. Pins and needles, numbness, and a burning sensation are prominent.

When people with a neuropathy are unable to sense pain, they can injure a joint many times without feeling it. The joint malfunctions and can progress to being permanently destroyed. Joints involved in this **neuropathic joint disease** are called **Charcot joints**.

Herpes zoster (shingles) is an infection of peripheral nerves arising from a reactivation of the primary virus infection in childhood with **chickenpox (varicella).** During the primary infection of chickenpox, the virus gains entry into sensory dorsal root ganglia. Later in life, for unknown reasons, the virus can produce the painful, unilateral **dermatome** rash of shingles *(Figure 9.29).*

Postherpetic neuralgia is acute dermatome pain persisting after the acute rash of shingles has subsided. It is debilitating and very difficult to treat.

Neuromuscular junction disorders occur where nerves connect with muscle fibers and interfere with the **neurotransmitter acetylcholine.** Examples are:

- **Myasthenia gravis,** in which the immune system produces antibodies that attack the acetylcholine receptors on the muscle cells. The common symptoms are drooping eyelids; weak eye muscles, causing double vision; difficulty talking and swallowing; and muscle weakness in the limbs.

- **Botulism,** a rare, life-threatening food poisoning caused by toxins from the bacterium **Clostridium botulinum.** These **neurotoxins** paralyze the muscles. Botulism can develop from ingesting food containing the toxin or from a wound infected with *Clostridium botulinum.*

- Certain **insecticides (organophosphates)** and nerve gases used in chemical warfare that act on neuromuscular junctions.

- Nerve **compression** occurring when the space around a nerve is constricted. The pinched nerve becomes **edematous** and later fibrotic and produces pain and **paresthesias.** Examples are **sciatica,** when the **sciatic** nerve is compressed in the lower spine, and **carpal tunnel syndrome,** when the median nerve is compressed at the wrist.

▲ **Figure 9.29** Herpes Zoster (Shingles).
©Bob Tapper/Diomedia/Medical Images RM

Keynote

Herpes zoster occurs in people with depressed immune responses, HIV infection, or cancer and those on chemotherapy and/or radiation therapy, as well as for no apparent reason.

WORD	PRONUNCIATION		ELEMENTS	DEFINITION
botulism	**BOT**-you-lizm		Latin *sausage*	Caused by the neurotoxin produced by *Clostridium botulinum*
carpal	**KAR**-pal	S/ R/	-al *pertaining to* carp- *wrist*	Pertaining to the wrist
carpal tunnel syndrome	**KAR**-pal **TON**-nell **SIN**-drome	P/ R/	**tunnel** English *tube, pipe* syn- *together* -drome *running*	Compression of the median nerve in the wrist causing numbness, pain and tingling in the fingers and thumb
Charcot joint	**SHAR**-koh JOYNT		Jean-Martin Charcot, 1825–1893, French neurologist	Bone and joint destruction secondary to a neuropathy and loss of sensation
chickenpox varicella (syn)	**CHICK**-en-pocks **VAIR**-uh-**SELL**-uh		Disease originally considered a "chicken" (not dangerous) version of smallpox	Acute, contagious viral disease
Clostridium botulinum	klos-**TRID**-ee-um bot-you-**LIE**-num			Bacterium that causes botulism
herpes zoster shingles (syn)	**HER**-pees **ZOS**-ter **SHING**-guls		**herpes** Greek *spreading skin eruption* **zoster** Greek *girdle*	Painful eruption of vesicles that follows a dermatome or nerve root on one side of the body
myasthenia gravis	my-as-**THEE**-nee-ah **GRA**-vis	S/ R/ P/ R/ R/	-ia *condition* **my-** *muscle* **-a-** *without* -sthen- *strength* gravis *serious*	Disorder of fluctuating muscle weakness
neuralgia	nyu-**RAL**-jee-ah	S/ R/	-algia *pain* neu r- *nerve*	Pain in the distribution of a nerve.
neuromuscular	**NYUR**-oh-**MUSS**-kyu-lar	S/ R/CF R/	-ar *pertaining to* neur/o- *nerve* -muscul- *muscle*	Pertaining to both nerves and muscles
neuropathy	nyu-**ROP**-ah-thee	S/ R/CF	-pathy *disease* neur/o- *nerve*	Any disease of the nervous system
neuropathic (adj) mononeuropathy polyneuropathy	nyur-oh-**PATH**-ik **MON**-oh-nyu-**ROP**-ah-thee **POL**-ee-nyu-**ROP**-ah-thee	S/ P/ P/	-ic *pertaining to* mono- *one* poly- *many*	Pertaining to a disease of the nervous system Disorder affecting a single nerve Disorder affecting many nerves
neurotoxin	**NYUR**-oh-tock-sin	R/CF R/	neur/o- *nerve* -toxin *poison*	Agent that poisons the nervous system
peroneal	pair-uh-**NEE**-al	S/ R/	-eal *pertaining to* peron- *fibula*	Pertaining to the lateral part (fibula) of the lower leg, or the nerve named after it
postherpetic	**POST**-her-**PET**-ik	S/ P/ R/	-ic *pertaining to* post- *after* -herpet- *herpes*	Pertaining to after herpes infection.
sciatica sciatic (adj)	sigh-**AT**-ih-kah sigh-**AT**-ik		Greek *related to the hip joint*	Pain from compression of L5 or S1 nerve roots Pertaining to the sciatic nerve or sciatica
ulnar	**UL**-nar	S/ R/	-ar *pertaining to* uln- *ulna*	Pertaining to the ulna (medial forearm bone) or any of the structures (artery, vein, nerve) named after it

Exercises

A. Complete the definition with the correct medical language. *Review the above WAD for the elements you need to construct the term. Fill in the blanks.* **LO 9.13, 9.C**

1. Disorder affecting the nervous system   neur/o/ _____

2. Agent that poisons the nervous system   neur/o/ _____

3. Disorder affecting a single nerve   _____ /neur/o/pathy

4. Pertaining to the lateral side of the lower leg   _____ /eal

▲ **Figure 9.30** **Newborn with Anencephaly.** ©McGraw-Hill Education

▲ **Figure 9.31** **Infant with Hydrocephalus.** ©Bob Tapper/Diomedia/ Medical Images RM

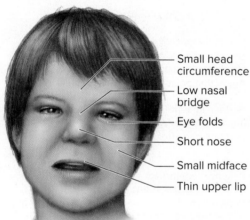

- Small head circumference
- Low nasal bridge
- Eye folds
- Short nose
- Small midface
- Thin upper lip

▲ **Figure 9.32** **Fetal Alcohol Syndrome.**

Abbreviation	
FAS	fetal alcohol syndrome

LO 9.14 Congenital Anomalies of the Nervous System

Some of the most devastating **congenital neurologic anomalies** develop in the first 8 to 10 weeks of gestation, when the nervous system is in its early stages of formation. These malformations can be detected by using ultrasonography and amniocentesis (*see Chapter 8*). Many can be prevented by the mother taking 4 mg/day of **folic acid** before conception and during early pregnancy.

A **teratogen** is an agent that can cause malformations of an embryo or fetus (*see Chapter 8*). It can be a chemical, virus, or radiation. Some teratogens are encountered in the workplace and include textile dyes, photographic chemicals, semiconductor materials, lead, mercury, and cadmium. One of the early uses of the drug thalidomide was to control morning sickness in pregnancy, but it caused severe limb and other deformities in the baby.

Anencephaly is absence of the cerebral hemispheres and is always fatal (*Figure 9.30*).

Microcephaly, decreased head size, is associated with small cerebral hemispheres and with moderate to severe motor and mental retardation. One cause of microcephaly is an infection during pregnancy with the Zika virus. This virus is carried by an aggressive mosquito that can bite in the daytime or at night, and also can be passed from an infected person to another person during sex.

Hydrocephalus, ventricular enlargement in the cerebral hemispheres with excessive CSF, is usually due to an obstruction that prevents the CSF from exiting the ventricles to circulate around the spinal cord (*Figure 9.31*). A **shunt** can be placed to drain the excess CSF from the ventricles to either the peritoneal cavity or an atrium of the heart.

Fetal alcohol syndrome (FAS) can occur when a pregnant woman drinks alcohol. The child born with FAS has a small head, narrow eyes, and a flat face and nose (*Figure 9.32*). Intellect and growth are **impaired.** Fetal alcohol syndrome is a cause of mental retardation.

Spina bifida occurs mostly in the lumbar and sacral regions (*Figure 9.33*). It is very variable in its presentation and symptoms. **Spina bifida occulta** presents with a small partial defect in the vertebral arch. The spinal cord or meninges do not protrude. Often the only sign is a tuft of hair on the skin overlying the defect. In **spina bifida cystica**, no vertebral arch is formed. The spinal cord and meninges protrude through the opening and may or may not be covered with a thin layer of skin (*see Figure 9.33a and b*). Protrusion of the meninges only is called a **meningocele**; protrusion of the meninges and spinal cord is called a **meningomyelocele**. Paralysis of the lower limbs may be present. The defect must be closed promptly to preserve spinal cord function and prevent infection. The cause of spina bifida is not known.

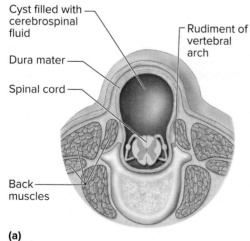

- Cyst filled with cerebrospinal fluid
- Dura mater
- Spinal cord
- Rudiment of vertebral arch
- Back muscles

(a)

(b)

▲ **Figure 9.33** **Spina Bifida Cystica.** (*a*) cross section of spinal cord in spina bifida cystica. (*b*) Child with spina bifida cystica. ©Biophoto Associates/Photo Researchers, Inc.

LO 9.14 Word Analysis and Definition

S = Suffix   P = Prefix   R = Root   R/CF = Combining Form

WORD	PRONUNCIATION	ELEMENTS		DEFINITION
anencephaly	**AN**-en-**SEF**-ah-lee	S/ P/ R/	-y *condition* an- *without* -encephal- *brain*	Born without cerebral hemispheres
anomaly	ah-**NOM**-ah-lee		Greek *abnormality*	A structural abnormality
hydrocephalus	**HIGH**-droh-**SEF**-ah-lus	S/ R/CF R/	-us *pertaining to* hydr/o- *water* -cephal- *head*	Enlarged head due to excess CSF in the cerebral ventricles
meningocele	meh-**NING**-oh-seal	S/ R/CF	-cele *hernia* mening/o- *meninges*	Protrusion of the meninges from the spinal cord or brain through a defect in the vertebral column or cranium
meningomyelocele (Note: also referred to as *myelomeningocele*)	meh-**NING**-oh-**MY**-el-oh-seal	R/CF	-myel/o- *spinal cord*	Protrusion of the spinal cord and meninges through a defect in the vertebral arch of one or more vertebrae
microcephaly	**MY**-kroh-**SEF**-ah-lee	S/ P/ R/	-y *condition* micro- *small* -cephal- *head*	An abnormally small head
shunt	SHUNT		**Middle English** *divert*	A bypass or diversion of fluid
spina bifida	**SPY**-nah **BIH**-fih-dah	R/CF P/ R/	spin/a *spine* bi- *two* -fida *split*	Failure of one or more vertebral arches to close during fetal development
spina bifida cystica	**SPY**-nah **BIH**-fih-dah **SIS**-tik-ah	S/ R/	-ica *pertaining to* cyst- *cyst*	Meninges and spinal cord protrude through the absent vertebral arch and have the appearance of a cyst
spina bifida occulta	**SPY**-nah **BIH**-fih-dah oh-**KUL**-tah	R/	occulta *hidden*	The deformity of the vertebral arch is not apparent from the skin surface
teratogen	**TER**-ah-toh-jen	S/ R/CF	-gen *produce, create* terat/o- *monster, malformed fetus*	Agent that produces fetal deformities
teratogenic (adj) (**Note:** Has two suffixes.)	**TER**-ah-toh-jen-ik	S/	-ic *pertaining to*	Capable of producing fetal deformities

Exercises

A. Search and find the correct term for the element you are given. *Choose the best answer.* **LO 9.14, 9.D**

1. Find the term with the prefix meaning *without:*
   a. hydrocephalus   **b.** anencephaly   **c.** impairment

2. Find the term with the root meaning *cyst:*
   a. meningocele   **b.** cystica   **c.** teratogen

3. Find the term with the root meaning *monster:*
   a. teratogen   **b.** spina   **c.** myelomeningocele

4. Find the term with the root meaning *split:*
   a. bifida   **b.** occulta   **c.** cystica

5. Find the term with the root meaning *head:*
   a. anomaly   **b.** hydrocephalus   **c.** meningocele

6. Find the term with the root meaning *hidden:*
   a. spina bifida   **b.** spina bifida cystica   **c.** spina bifida occulta

7. Find the term with the combining form meaning *water:*
   a. teratogenic   **b.** hydrocephalus   **c.** myelomeningocele

8. Find the term with the suffix meaning *hernia:*
   a. meningocele   **b.** hydrocephalus   **c.** anomaly

9. Find the term with the combining form meaning *spinal cord:*
   a. meningomyelocele   **b.** cystocele   **c.** meningocele

10. Find the term with the prefix meaning *small:*
    a. anencephaly   **b.** teratogenic   **c.** microcephaly

LESSON 9.4 Disorders of the Spinal Cord and Peripheral Nerves   305

Procedures and Pharmacology

Abbreviations

CT	computed tomography
EMG	electromyography
LP	lumbar puncture
MRI	magnetic resonance imaging
PET	positron emission tomography

LO 9.15 Diagnostic Procedures in Neurology

To obtain a specimen of CSF, a **lumbar puncture (LP)** or **spinal tap** is performed *(Figure 9.34)*. A needle is inserted through the skin, back muscles, spinal ligaments of an intervertebral space, epidural space, dura mater, and arachnoid mater into the subarachnoid space. The CSF is then aspirated. Laboratory examination of the CSF that shows white blood cells suggests meningitis. High protein levels indicate meningitis or damage to the brain or spinal cord. Blood suggests a brain hemorrhage or a traumatic tap.

Electroencephalography records the brain's electrical activity and helps identify seizure disorders, sleep disturbances, degenerative brain disorders, and brain damage *(Figure 9.35)*.

Computed tomography (CT), a computer-enhanced x-ray technique, generates images of slices of the brain and can detect a wide range of brain and spinal cord disorders, including tumors, areas of dead brain tissue due to stroke, and birth defects.

Magnetic resonance imaging (MRI) produces highly detailed anatomical images of most neurologic disorders, including strokes, brain tumors, and myelin sheath damage *(Figure 9.36)*.

Magnetic resonance angiography uses an injection of a radiopaque dye to produce images of blood vessels of the head and neck during MRI.

Cerebral angiography is an invasive procedure in which a radiopaque dye is injected into the blood vessels of the neck and brain. It can detect blood vessels that are partially or completely blocked, aneurysms, or arteriovenous malformations.

Cerebral arteriography can determine the site of bleeding in hemorrhagic strokes.

Color Doppler ultrasonography uses high-frequency sound (ultrasound) waves to show different rates of blood flow through the arteries of the neck or the base of the brain. This evaluates TIAs and the risk of a full-blown stroke.

Echoencephalography uses ultrasound waves to produce an image of the brain in children under the age of 2 because their skulls are thin enough for the waves to pass through them.

Positron emission tomography (PET) involves attaching radioactive molecules onto a substance necessary for brain function (for example, the sugar glucose). As the molecules circulate in the brain, the radioactive labels give off positively charged signals that can be recorded *(Figure 9.35)*.

Myelography is the use of x-rays of the spinal cord that are taken after a radiopaque dye has been injected into the CSF by spinal tap. It has been replaced by MRI when that is available.

Evoked responses are a procedure in which stimuli for vision, sound, and touch are used to activate specific areas of the brain and their responses are measured with EEG or PET scans. This provides information about how that specific area of the brain is functioning in disorders such as MS.

Electromyography (EMG) involves placing small needles into a muscle to record its electrical activity at rest and during contraction. It is used to provide information in disorders of muscles, peripheral nerves, and the **neuromuscular** junction.

Nerve conduction studies measure the speed at which motor or sensory nerves conduct impulses. The studies exclude disorders of the brain, spinal cord, and muscles and focus on the peripheral nerves.

Intervertebral space
Lumbar puncture needle
Subarachnoid space
L3
L4
Vertebral canal

▲ **Figure 9.34** Lumbar puncture (spinal tap).

Primary motor cortex

▲ **Figure 9.35** PET Scan of the Brain Showing the Motor Cortex. ©Marcus E. Raichle

WORD	PRONUNCIATION	ELEMENTS		DEFINITION
angiography	an-jee-**OG**-rah-fee	S/	-**graphy** *process of recording*	Process of recording the image of blood vessels after injection of contrast material
		R/CF	**angi/o-** *blood vessel*	
arteriography	ar-teer-ee-**OG**-rah-fee	S/	-**graphy** *process of recording*	X-ray visualization of an artery after injection of contrast material
		R/CF	**arteri/o-** *artery*	
Doppler	**DOP**-ler		Johann Christian Doppler, 1803–1853, Austrian mathematician and physicist	Diagnostic instrument that sends an ultrasonic beam into the body
Doppler ultrasonography	**DOP**-ler **UL**-trah-soh-**NOG**-rah-fee	S/	-**graphy** *process of recording*	Imaging that detects direction, velocity, and turbulence of blood flow; used in workup of stroke patients
		P/	**ultra-** *beyond*	
		R/CF	-**son/o-** *sound*	
color Doppler ultrasonography				Computer-generated color image to show directions of blood flow
echoencephalography	**EK**-oh-en-sef-ah-**LOG**-rah-fee	S/	-**graphy** *process of recording*	Use of ultrasound in the diagnosis of intracranial lesions
		R/CF	**ech/o-** *sound wave*	
		R/CF	-**encephal/o-** *brain*	
electroencephalogram (EEG)	ee-**LEK**-troh-en-**SEF**-ah-loh-gram	S/	-**gram** *recording*	Record of the electrical activity of the brain
		R/CF	**electr/o-** *electricity*	
		R/CF	-**encephal/o-** *brain*	
electroencephalograph	ee-**LEK**-troh-en-**SEF**-ah-loh-graf	S/	-**graph** *to write, record*	Device used to record the electrical activity of the brain
electroencephalography	ee-**LEK**-troh-en-**SEF**-ah-**LOG**-rah-fee	S/	-**graphy** *process of recording*	The process of recording the electrical activity of the brain
electromyography	ee-**LEK**-troh-my-**OG**-rah-fee	S/	-**graphy** *process of recording*	Recording of electrical activity in muscle
		R/CF	**electr/o-** *electricity*	
		R/CF	-**my/o-** *muscle*	
myelography	my-eh-**LOG**-rah-fee	S/	-**graphy** *process of recording*	Radiography of the spinal cord and nerve roots after injection of contrast medium into the subarachnoid space
		R/CF	**myel/o-** *spinal cord*	
nerve conduction study	NERV kon-**DUK**-shun **STUD**-ee	R/	**nerve** *nerve*	Procedure to measure the speed at which an electrical impulse travels along a nerve
		S/	-**ion** *action*	
		P/	**con-** *with, together*	
		R/	-**duct-** *lead*	
		R/	**study** *inquiry*	

Exercises

A. Create medical terms common to diagnostic procedures in neurology. *Given the definition, complete the medical term it is defining using word elements related to diagnostic terms in neurology. Fill in the blanks.* **LO 9.15, 9.C**

1. The machine that creates the record of the electrical activity of the brain. electr/o/encephal/o/_____

2. The process of recording arteries. arteri/o/ _____

3. The use of high-fequency sound waves to view blood flow. Doppler ultra/_____ /o/graphy

4. Process of recording the spinal cord. _____ /o/graphy

5. Process of recording the electrical activity of the muscle. electr/o/_____ /o/graphy

LO 9.16 Therapeutic Procedures

Craniotomy is the surgical removal of part of a skull bone (the bone flap) to expose the brain for surgery.

Cranioplasty is the repair of a bone defect in the skull, often the result of craniotomy.

Deep brain stimulation is the surgical placement of electrodes deep into specific areas of the brain to deliver electrical stimulations to treat the tremors of Parkinson disease, essential tremor, or multiple sclerosis.

Endoscopic pituitary surgery utilizes an approach through the inside of the nose to remove pituitary tumors.

Endovascular coiling blocks the blood flow to an aneurysm.

Flow diversion uses **stents** placed via a catheter to maintain blood flow through a blood vessel where blockage or an aneurysm has occurred.

Treatment of many acute ischemic strokes is by **thrombolysis** using clotbusters such as **tissue plasminogen activator (tPA)** within 4½ hours of the stroke, with supportive measures followed by rehabilitation.

Treatment for TIA is directed at the underlying cause. **Carotid endarterectomy** may be necessary if a carotid artery is significantly occluded with plaque.

Treatment of Cerebral Palsy

A multidisciplinary team of health professionals is required to develop an individualized treatment plan and to involve the patients, families, teachers, and caregivers in decision making and planning.

Physical therapy is designed to prevent muscles from becoming weak or rigidly fixed with **contractures**, to improve motor development, and to facilitate independence. Speech therapy and psychotherapy complement physical therapy.

Muscle relaxants, such as diazepam, can reduce **spasticity** for short periods of time, and a variety of devices and mechanical aids ranging from muscle braces to motorized wheelchairs help overcome physical limitations.

Treatment of Gliomas

Treatment is a combination of surgery, radiotherapy, and chemotherapy. The combination is necessary because even if you remove 99% of a tumor, there will be up to 1 billion cells remaining. A more recent therapy, **brachytherapy**, implants small radioactive pellets directly into the tumor. The radiation is released over time.

WORD	PRONUNCIATION	ELEMENTS		DEFINITION
Botox	**BOH**-tox		Botulinum toxin	Neurotoxin injected into muscles to prevent the muscles from contracting
brachytherapy	brah-kee-**THAIR**-ah-pee	P/ R/	**brachy-** *short* **-therapy** *medical treatment*	Radiation therapy in which the source of irradiation is implanted in the tissue to be treated
cranium	**KRAY**-nee-um		Greek *skull*	The bony container of the brain, excluding the face
cranioplasty	**KRAY**-nee-oh-**PLASTY**	S/ R/CF	**-plasty** *surgical repair* **crani/o-** *skull*	Repair of a bone defect in the skull
craniotomy	**KRAY**-nee-**OT**-oh-mee	S/	**-tomy** *surgical incision*	Surgical removal of part of a skull bone to expose the brain for surgery
endovascular	**END**-oh-**VAS**-kyu-lar	S/ P/ R/	**-ar** *pertaining to* **endo-** *inside* **-vascul-** *blood vessel*	Relating to the inside of a blood vessel

Exercise

A. Demonstrate understanding of word elements in medical terms. *This will make short work of answer questions in this course and interpreting patient medical records in clinical practice. This exercise uses layman's terms and asks you to replace those words the medical term they are describing. Fill in the blanks* **LO 9.16, 9.A, 9.E**

A 27 year old male is brought to the emergency department by paramedics. The male is unconscious. The paramedics report that he was involved in an altercation at a bar when he was struck in the head with a barstool. He was immediately brought to the operating room where the (1) *surgical expert in the treatment of neurological conditions* performed a (2) *procedure in which part of the skull was removed*. A large clot was removed from the subdural space. The wound was closed and the patient was admitted to the surgical ICU. The injury to skull shattered several areas of the (3) *bones that cover the brain*, and therefore the patient will require a (4) *repair of defect of the skull* at a later date when he becomes medically stable

1. The medical term that replaces the italicized words: _____

2. The medical term that replaces the italicized words: _____

3. The medical term that replaces the italicized words: _____

4. The medical term that replaces the italicized words: _____

Abbreviations

LSD	lysergic acid diethylamide
MDMA	methylenedioxymeth-amphetamine (ecstasy)
PCP	phencyclidine (angel dust)
THC	tetrahydrocannabinol (marijuana)

LO 9.17 Pharmacology of the Nervous System

The transmission of impulses from one neuron to another and from a neuron to a cell is achieved by neurotransmitters at synaptic connections. Drugs that affect the nervous system, called *psychoactive drugs,* target this synaptic mechanism.

Psychoactive drugs are able to change mood, behavior, cognition, and anxiety. They can be classified into several families:

1. **Stimulants**—caffeine, nicotine, amphetamines, and cocaine—enhance the **stimulation** provided by the sympathetic nervous system. They cause the level of dopamine to rise in the synapses, leading to the pleasurable effects associated with these drugs.

2. **Sedatives**—ethanol (beverage alcohol), barbiturates, and meprobamate—decrease the sensitivity of the postsynaptic neurons to quiet the nervous excitement. They also act on the sleep centers to induce sleep.

3. Inhaled anesthetics such as isoflurane act similarly to, but are more powerful than, sedatives.

4. Opiates—morphine, codeine, heroin, methadone, and oxycodone—depress nerve transmission in the synapses of sensory pathways of the brain and spinal cord. They also inhibit centers in the brain controlling coughing, breathing, and intestinal motility. Codeine is used in cough medicines. Constipation is a side effect of all these drugs. Opiates are **addictive** because they produce tolerance and physical dependence.

5. Opiate **antagonists**, such as naloxone and naltrexone, prevent opiates from acting in the synapses. They can be used in drug overdoses and to help recovering heroin addicts stay drug-free.

6. **Tranquilizers**, such as chlorpromazine, haloperidol, and the benzodiazepines (*Librium, Valium, Xanax*), act like sedatives but without their sleep-inducing effect.

7. Antidepressants all increase the amount of serotonin at the synapses, where it is a neurotransmitter. *Zoloft* and *Prozac* are examples.

8. **Antiepileptics** act in different ways on the synaptic junction to keep stimuli from passing across the synapse. Phenytoin and carbamazepine are examples.

9. **Psychedelics** distort sensory perceptions, particularly sight and sound. They can be natural plant products, such as mescaline, psilocybin, and dimethyltryptamine. They also can be synthetic, such as **lysergic acid diethylamide (LSD), methylenedioxymethamphetamine** (MDMA or "ecstasy"), and **phencyclidine** (PCP or "angel dust"). They increase the amount of serotonin in the synaptic junctions, and some have an additional amphetamine stimulation.

10. **Marijuana** has the active ingredient **tetrahydrocannabinol (THC).** It produces the drowsiness of sedatives like alcohol, the dulling of pain like opiates, and, in high doses, the perception distortions of the psychedelics. Unlike the case with opiates or sedatives, **tolerance** does not occur.

WORD	PRONUNCIATION	ELEMENTS		DEFINITION
addict	**AD**-ikt	P/	**ad-** *to*	Person with a psychologic or physical dependence on a substance or practice
addiction	ah-**DIK**-shun	R/	**-dict** *consent, surrender*	Habitual psychologic and physiologic dependence on a substance or practice
		S/	**-ion** *condition, action*	
addictive	ah-**DIK**-tiv	S/	**-ive** *quality of, pertaining to*	Pertaining to or causing addiction
antagonism	an-**TAG**-oh-nizm	S/	**-ism** *process, action*	Situation of opposing
		P/	**ant-** *against*	
		R/	**-agon-** *contest against*	
antagonist	an-**TAG**-oh-nist	S/	**-ist** *agent*	An opposing structure, agent, disease, or process
antiepileptic	**AN**-tee-eh-pih-**LEP**-tik	S/	**-tic** *pertaining to*	A pharmacologic agent capable of preventing or arresting epilepsy
		P/	**anti-** *against*	
		R/	**-epilep-** *seizure*	
psychedelic	sigh-keh-**DEL**-ik	S/	**-ic** *pertaining to*	Agent that intensifies sensory perception
		R/CF	**psych/e-** *mind, soul*	
		R/	**-del-** *visible*	
psychoactive	sigh-koh-**AK**-tiv	S/	**-ive** *quality of, pertaining to*	Able to alter mood, behavior, and/or cognition
		R/CF	**psych/o-** *mind, soul*	
		R/	**-act-** *to do*	
sedative	**SED**-ah-tiv	S/	**-ive** *quality of, pertaining to*	Agent that calms nervous excitement
		R/	**sedat-** *to calm*	
sedation	seh-**DAY**-shun	S/	**-ion** *condition, action*	State of being calmed
stimulant	**STIM**-you-lant	S/	**-ant** *forming*	Agent that excites or strengthens functional activity
stimulate (verb)	**STIM**-you-late	R/	**stimul-** *excite, strengthen*	
stimulation	stim-you-**LAY**-shun	S/	**-ation** *process*	Arousal to increased functional activity
tolerance	**TOL**-er-ants	S/	**-ance** *state of, condition*	The capacity to become accustomed to a stimulus or drug
		R/	**toler-** *endure*	
tranquilizer	**TRANG**-kwih-lie-zer	S/	**-izer** *affects in a particular way*	Agent that calms without sedating or depressing
		R/	**tranquil-** *calm*	

Exercises

A. Deconstruct this *language of neurology* into its basic elements to help understand the meaning of the term. *Write the elements between the slashes. A combining vowel will have a space to enter it in. The first one is done for you. Every term does not need every element, so you will have some blanks.* **LO 9.16, 9.17, 9.D**

1. antagonist   _____ant_____ / _____agon_____ / _____ist_____

2. addict   _____ / _____ / _____

3. tranquilizer   _____ / _____ / _____

4. stimulant   _____ / _____ / _____

5. psychedelic   _____ / _____ / _____ / _____

6. tolerance   _____ / _____ / _____

7. psychoactive   _____ / _____ / _____ / _____

LO 9.18 Pain Management

Pain persisting longer than 3 months is said to be **chronic**. It can be caused by cancer, arthritis, fibromyalgia, low-back or neck problems, headache, or injuries that have not healed. Normal activities can be restricted or be impossible.

Among Americans, 6 million to 10 million are affected by fibromyalgia, 5 million are disabled by back problems, 8 million experience chronic neck and facial pain, and 40 million suffer from chronic recurrent headaches. In modern health care, chronic pain management has become essential and often uses a multidisciplinary approach. Pain management is now a board-certified subspecialty for **anesthesiologists**.

Medications are the cornerstone of pain management, and the following can be used depending on the severity of the pain:

- Mild pain. **Analgesics**, such as acetaminophen, and **nonsteroidal anti-inflammatory drugs (NSAIDs),** such as ibuprofen, are used. A study published in 2017 of 28,947 Danish patients showed that patients taking NSAIDs had a 31% increased risk of having cardiac arrest.

- Moderate pain. **Opiate** medications in combination with acetaminophen or NSAIDs are used. Some opiates used in combination medications are codeine, hydrocodone, and oxycodone. Examples are hydrocodone/acetaminophen (*Vicodin*), oxycodone/acetaminophen (*Percocet*), and oxycodone/aspirin (*Percodan*). These opiate medications are addictive, and are frequently abused and sold on the street.

- Severe pain. Higher doses of opiates are used, often not as combination products. These include **morphine**, fentanyl, and oxy- and hydromorphone. The opiates can be taken orally, by patch, sublingually, by intravenous (IV) infusion, or by continuous delivery systems. These oral opiates are also addictive and are sold on the street.

- **Buprenorphine**—the most commonly prescribed medication to treat opioid addiction—is an important strategy to combat the opioid addiction epidemic occurring in the United States. It is a controlled substance (*see Chapter 22*) and there are strict federal regulations on the qualifications of physicians allowed to prescribe it.

Central sensitization pain is a new concept describing how neurons in the spinal cord sending messages to the brain become excitable. They exaggerate the pain response in tissues they supply. The input can be somatic from skeletal muscles (as in fibromyalgia) or visceral (as in irritable bowel syndrome).

Interventional pain management, particularly for pain originating in the spine and spinal nerves, is being increasingly used. Examples are:

- **Epidural or facet nerve blocks.** Anesthetic or anti-inflammatory agents are injected into an area surrounding the pain-generating nerve.

- **Radiofrequency (RF) nerve ablation.** A probe heats the area around a pain-generating spinal nerve and temporarily deactivates it.

- **Spinal infusion pump.** Pain medications such as morphine are delivered through an indwelling catheter into the **intrathecal** CSF surrounding the spinal cord. A pump delivery device is inserted under the skin of the abdomen.

Phantom limb pain occurs following the amputation of a limb or part of a limb. Any stimulation of the remaining intact portion of the sensory pathway coming originally from the limb is interpreted by the brain as coming from the original limb. The pain can be severe and debilitating or just an insatiable urge to scratch an itch.

Referred pain occurs when pain in the viscera is felt in the skin or other superficial sites (*Figure 9.36*). An example is the pain of a heart attack felt along the front of the left shoulder and down the underside of the left arm. This is because spinal cord segments T1 to T5 receive sensory input from the heart, as well as from the skin of the shoulder and arm. This input is transmitted to the brain. The brain cannot distinguish the true source of the pain. It assumes it is coming from the skin, which has more pain receptors than the heart and is injured more often.

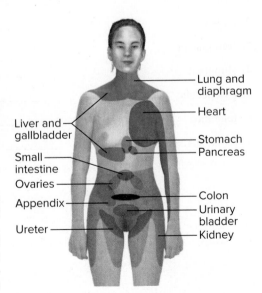

▲ **Figure 9.36** Referred Pain.

WORD	PRONUNCIATION	ELEMENTS		DEFINITION
ablation	ab-**LAY**-shun	S/ P/ R/	-ion *action, condition* ab- *away from* -lat- *to take*	Removal of tissue to destroy its function
analgesia	an-al-**JEE**-zee-ah	S/ P/ R/	-ia *condition* an- *without* -alges- *sensation of pain*	State in which pain is reduced
analgesic	an-al-**JEE**-zik	S/	-ic *pertaining to*	Substance that produces analgesia
anesthesia	an-es-**THEE**-zee-ah	P/ R/CF	an- *without* -esthesi/a *sensation, feeling*	Complete loss of sensation
anesthesiologist	**AN**-es-thee-zee-**OL**-oh-jist	S/ P/ R/CF	-logist *one who studies,* *specialist* an- *without* -esthesi/o- *feeling, sensation*	Medical specialist in anesthesia
anesthesiology	**AN**-es-thee-zee-**OL**-oh-jee	S/	-logy *study of*	Medical specialty of anesthesia
anesthetic	an-es-**THET**-ik	S/ P/ R/	-ic *pertaining to* an- *without* -esthet- *sensation, perception*	An agent that causes absence of feeling or sensation
facet	**FAS**-et		French *little face*	Small area, in this case around a pain-generating nerve
intrathecal	**IN**-trah-**THEE**-kal	S/ P/ R/	-al *pertaining to* intra- *within* -thec- *sheath*	Within the subarachnoid or subdural space
morphine	**MOR**-feen		Latin *god dreams*	Derivative of opium used as an analgesic or sedative
opiate	**OH**-pee-ate		Latin *bringing sleep*	A drug derived from opium

Exercises

A. Deconstruct the following *language of neurology*. *Write the meaning of each element to see how it will aid you in understanding the meaning of the complete term. Fill in the blank.* **LO 9.18, 9.D**

1. *an-* _____.

2. *intra-* _____.

3. *thec-* _____.

4. *-ia* _____.

5. *ab-* _____.

B. The language of pain management is specific. *It is important to use medical terms related to pain management correctly. Choose the correct answer for each question.* **LO 9.18, 9.E**

1. A medical specialist in area of pain management is a(n):

  a. neurologist   **b.** anesthesiologist   **c.** analgesic   **d.** urologist

2. A medication indicated for *moderate* pain is:

  a. codeine   **b.** ibuprofen   **c.** morphine   **d.** fentanyl

3. A medication that blocks all sensation, including pain:

  a. analgesic   **b.** anesthetic

4. A medication that blocks pain but allows other sensations to be felt:

  a. analgesic   **b.** anesthetic

Nervous System

Challenge Your Knowledge

A. Construct the proper medical terms for the statements. You have an assortment of prefixes, roots, combining forms, and suffixes with which to construct your terms. Fill in the blanks. **(LO 9.8, 9.10, 9.18, 9.A, 9.C)**

hydro	lepsy	esthesia
narco	lysis	a
algia	occulta	para
neur/o	itis	post
an	trophy	

1. Recurring episodes of falling asleep during the day: _____

2. Complete loss of sensation: _____

3. Pain in the distribution of a nerve: _____

4. Wasting away of tissue: _____

5. Derived from a word meaning *hidden:* _____

B. Similar but different. The following medical terms contain a similar root, but the suffixes change the meaning of the terms. Use the correct form of these terms in the following sentences. Fill in the blanks. **(LO 9.A, 9.C, 9.E)**

neurosurgery   neurologic   neurologist   neurosurgeon   neurology

The _____ from the Fulwood _____ Department referred the patient to

a _____ for surgical consultation. The patient's _____ condition was deteriorating

rapidly, and she would probably need _____.

C. Identify the elements in each medical term and unlock the meaning of the word. Fill in the chart. If the word does not have a particular word element, write n/a. **(LO 9.4, 9.8, 9.12, 9.18, 9.D)**

Medical Term	Meaning of Prefix	Meaning of Root/Combining Form	Meaning of Suffix	Meaning of the Term
dementia	1.	2.	3.	4.
sympathy	5.	6.	7.	8.
confusion	9.	10.	11.	12.
hemiparesis	13.	14.	15.	16.
hypothalamic	17.	18.	19.	20.
anesthetic	21.	22.	23.	24.
cataplexy	25.	26.	27.	28.

D. Diseases and disorders. The Fulwood Neurology Clinic treats patients with varied diseases and disorders of the nervous system. Are you familiar enough with their terminology and symptoms to match the correct disease or disorder with the appropriate statement for each patient? Select the correct choice. **(LO 9.8, 9.10, 9.13)**

1. Patient has had a hemorrhagic stroke. Another name for this is:

   a. intercranial hemorrhage   **b.** intercerebral hemorrhage   **c.** intracranial hemorrhage

2. Patient bumped head on low doorway:

   a. concussion   **b.** seizure   **c.** convulsion

3. Patient has inflammation of the parenchyma of the brain:

   a. meningitis   **b.** encephalitis   **c.** vasculitis

4. Infection of the peripheral nerves arising from a reactivation of the chickenpox (varicella) virus is:

   a. herpes simplex   **b.** shingles   **c.** post herpetic neuralgia

5. Infant has motor impairment resulting from brain damage at birth:

   a. Bell palsy   **b.** cerebral palsy   **c.** palsy

6. Patient had very bad dental infection that resulted in bloodborne pathogens lodging in her brain:

   a. brain tumor   **b.** brain abscess   **c.** brain hematoma

7. Patient complains of intermittent, shooting pain in the area of the face and head:

   a. trigeminal neuralgia   **b.** peripheral neuropathy   **c.** neuritis

E. Abbreviations are helpful only if you know what they are meant to communicate. Write the correct abbreviation for each described condition, structure, or procedure. **(LO 9.2, 9.8, 9.15, 9.F)**

1. This system is composed of the brain and the spinal cord.

   _____

   _____

2. The neurologist ordered a test to evaluate the electrical activity of the brain.

   _____

   _____

3. The infant's condition of monoplegia was due to a reduction of oxygen delivered to her brain during her birth.

   _____

   _____

F. Plurals. Refresh your memory on the rules for plurals. Precision in communication depends on this. The singular form is given; circle the best answer for the plural form. **(LO 9.2, 9.3, 9.A, 9.B)**

1. **ganglion:**   **a.** ganglius   **b.** ganglia   **c.** gangli

2. **plexus:**   **a.** plexuses   **b.** plexuia   **c.** plexui

3. **sulcus:**   **a.** sulces   **b.** sulci   **c.** sulcia

4. **gyrus:**   **a.** gyri   **b.** gryia   **c.** gryuses

©2014 Nucleus Medical Media

Nervous System

G. **Roots and combining forms remain the core of a medical term.** Reinforce your knowledge of these elements with this exercise. Match the correct root or combining form in the left column to its meaning in the right column. **(LO 9.4, 9.8, 9.12, 9.13)**

_____ 1. *pathy*　　　　　　　　　　a. hearing

_____ 2. *cephalo*　　　　　　　　　b. muscle

_____ 3. *algesia*　　　　　　　　　c. sleep

_____ 4. *syringo*　　　　　　　　　d. blood vessel

_____ 5. *audit*　　　　　　　　　　e. tube, pipe

_____ 6. *trophy*　　　　　　　　　f. disease

_____ 7. *my*　　　　　　　　　　　g. development

_____ 8. *pleg*　　　　　　　　　　h. head

_____ 9. *somn*　　　　　　　　　　i. sensation of pain

_____ 10. *angio*　　　　　　　　　j. paralysis

H. **Medical language.** The nervous system is a complicated one and has a large range of vocabulary. Assess your knowledge of the nervous system by selecting the correct answer in the following questions. **(LO 9.3, 9.4)**

1. The area of the brain that controls emotional experience, fear, anger, pleasure, and sadness:

 a. cerebral cortex　　　**b.** corpus callosum　　　**c.** central sulcus　　　**d.** limbic system

2. Astrocytes, oligodendrocytes, microglia, ependymal, Schwann, and satellite are all terms relating to:

 a. capillaries　　　**b.** tumors　　　**c.** hematomas　　　**d.** neuroglia　　　**e.** ganglia

3. Body temperature is regulated by the:

 a. thalamus　　　**b.** hypothalamus　　　**c.** limbic system　　　**d.** pons　　　**e.** cerebellum

4. Centers that control vital visceral activities are located in the:

 a. pons　　　**b.** corpus　　　**c.** medulla oblongata　　　**d.** hypothalamus　　　**e.** CSF

I. **Latin and Greek terms do not deconstruct like some medical terms.** Test your knowledge of these terms with this exercise. Match the terms in the left column to their correct meaning in the right column. **(LO 9.4)**

_____ 1. gyrus　　　　　　　　　a. bridge

_____ 2. sulcus　　　　　　　　　b. circle

_____ 3. efferent　　　　　　　　c. brain

_____ 4. cerebrum　　　　　　　d. ditch, furrow

_____ 5. pons　　　　　　　　　e. away from

J. **Medical language.** The nervous system is a complicated one and has a large range of vocabulary. Assess your knowledge of the nervous system by selecting the correct answer to the following questions. **(LO 9.1, 9.2, 9.3, 9.8, 9.12, 9.14, 9.17, 9.D, 9.F)**

1. An agent capable of preventing or arresting epilepsy is called an:

 a. antidiuretic　　　**b.** antibiotic　　　**c.** antiepileptic　　　**d.** antidepressant　　　**e.** antibody

2. Administration of tPA is for:

 a. ALS　　　**b.** thrombolysis　　　**c.** seizures　　　**d.** dementia　　　**e.** meningitis

3. Hypoglossal refers to structures that can be found under the:

a. diaphragm　　　b. tongue　　　c. jawbone　　　d. bronchus　　　e. alveoli

4. In simple terms, a **synapse** is a:

a. malformation　　b. birth defect　　c. junction　　d. seizure　　e. vesicle

5. Implantation of radioactive pellets directly into a tumor is called:

a. bradytherapy　　b. bradycardia　　c. brachytherapy　　d. brachial plexus　　e. none of the above

6. A condition a child is born with that was caused by his/her mother's consumption of alcohol. The child has a small head, narrow eyes, and a flat face and nose.

a. MDMA　　b. LOC　　c. NMS　　d. VEP　　e. FAS

7. The groove that separates gyri is called:

a. gyrus　　b. cortex　　c. fissure　　d. sulcus　　e. dermatome

8. The cerebral hemispheres are covered by a thin layer of gray matter called the:

a. basal ganglia　　b. corpus callosum　　c. frontal lobe　　d. cerebral cortex　　e. cerebellum

9. The abbreviation for a short-term, small stroke is:

a. EEG　　b. HACE　　c. TIA　　d. PET　　e. SBS

10. The medical term that means *pertaining to or caused by a seizure* is:

a. clonic　　b. ictal　　c. tonic　　d. visceral　　e. synaptic

K. Test-taking strategy practice. Use your knowledge of medical terminology to insert the correct term in the appropriate statement. Not all answers will be used, and no answer will be used more than once. **(LO 9.1, 9.8, 9.14, 9.A)**

hemiplegia	**somatic**	**afferent**
meningitis	**meningioma**	**quadriplegia**
festinant	**microcephaly**	**visceral**
neurotransmitters	**dendrite**	**dementia**

> **Study Hint**
>
> Start by answering the questions for which you are sure of the correct answer. Cross off the answer in the column after you insert it in the statement, and then answer the rest of the questions from the choices you have left. You will then be working with a smaller and smaller group of choices, which will make it easier to spot the correct answer.

1. _____ nerves carry signals from major organs such as the heart, lungs, stomach, and intestines.

2. An abnormally small head: _____

3. A process or extension of a neuron: _____

4. Shuffling gait: _____

5. Loss of the mind's cognitive functions: _____

6. Paralysis of all four limbs: _____

7. Chemicals that cross the synapse to another neuron: _____

8. _____ nerves carry signals from the skin, muscles, bones, and joints.

©2014 Nucleus Medical Media

Nervous System

L. Analyze the following diagnostic procedures on the basis of their elements alone; then answer the questions. Fill in the blanks. **(LO 9.15, 9.D, 9.A)**

   1. echoencephalography

      The combining form _____ tells me this is a diagnostic procedure on the _____.

   2. electromyography

      The combining form _____ tells me this is a diagnostic procedure on the _____.

   3. myelography

      The combining form _____ tells me this is a diagnostic procedure on the _____.

   4. electroencephalography

      The combining form _____ tells me this is a diagnostic procedure on the _____.

   5. Each of the four procedures listed previously ends with the suffix _____, which means

      _____.

Use the terms in questions 1 to 5 to identify (define) the statements in questions 6 through 8. (Hint: In some cases you are asked for the *record,* and in some cases you are asked for the *recording.*) Be precise! Fill in the blanks.

   6. Recording of electrical activity in muscle: _____

   7. Radiography of the spinal cord and nerve roots after injection of contrast medium into the subarachnoid space:

      _____

   8. Record of the electrical activity of the brain: _____

M. Diagnostic testing. You are responsible for scheduling diagnostic procedures for patients in the Neurology Clinic at Fulwood Medical Center. Practice your *language of neurology* by scheduling these patients appropriately, using the following procedures. **(LO 9.16)**

CT scan   angiography

myelography   magnetic resonance imaging

evoked responses   nerve conduction studies

electromyography   electroencephalogram

lumbar puncture or spinal tap   magnetic resonance angiography

Patient Needs/Symptoms:	Schedule Patient for:
1. Dr. Solis would like to measure the speed at which a patient's motor nerves conduct impulses.	
2. Doctor has ordered a recording of the electrical activity of the patient's brain.	
3. Dr. Solis suspects a tumor and needs to see a highly detailed anatomical image of the brain.	
4. Patient needs x-rays of the spinal cord taken after dye has been injected into it.	
5. Dr. Solis wants a sample of the patient's CSF.	
6. Patient has to schedule a study with contrast to image the cerebral blood vessels.	
7. Patient has a blocked carotid artery.	
8. Patient has possibly had a stroke; study will be looking for areas of dead brain tissue.	
9. Sensory stimuli will be used to activate specific areas of the brain and measure responses with EEG.	
10. Doctor wants to test and record the electrical activity of a patient's muscle at rest and during contractions.	

N. **Review this chapter's Case Report 9.1.** *Utilize the language of neurology and previous chapters to correctly answer each question. Fill in the blanks.* (**LO 9.8, 9.15, 9.17, 9.E**)

 Case Report (CR) 9.1

You are

. . . an **electroneurodiagnostic technician** working with Gregory Solis, MD, a **neurosurgeon** at Fulwood Medical Center.

Your patient is

. . . Ms. Roberta Gaston, a 39-year-old woman, who has been referred by Raul Cardenas, MD, a **neurologist,** for evaluation for possible **neurosurgery.**

Ms. Gaston has had **epileptic seizures** since the age of 16. She has **generalized tonic-clonic seizures** occurring once a week. She also has daily minor spells when she stops interacting with her surroundings and blinks rhythmically for about 20 seconds, after which she returns to normal. Numerous **antiepileptic** drugs, including phenobarbital, valproic acid, and phenytoin, have been tried with no relief. She is not able to work and is cared for by her parents.

Her neurologic examination is normal. Her **EEG** (electroencephalogram) shows diffuse spike-and-wave discharges with a left-sided frontal predominance. Her **CT** (computed tomography) is normal. An **MRI** (magnetic resonance imaging) shows a 20-mm diameter mass adjacent to the anterior horn of her left **ventricle.** Continuous EEG/video monitoring shows **ictal** activity in the left frontal lobe.

1. Which diagnostic test revealed the cause of Ms. Gaston's seizures? (write the abbreviation, not the term)

   _____

2. Which specialist will treat the cause of the seizures? _____

3. What is causing the seizures? _____

4. Of all of the diagnostic tests, which ones did you administer? _____

5. Were the medications effective in controlling the seizures? _____

©2014 Nucleus Medical Media

The health professionals involved in the diagnosis and treatment of cardiovascular problems include:

- **Cardiologists,** medical doctors who specialize in disorders of the cardiovascular system.

- **Cardiovascular surgeons,** medical doctors who specialize in surgery of the heart and peripheral blood vessels.

- **Cardiovascular nurses,** who have extensive additional training and experience in treating patients with heart disease and often work in intensive care units, cardiovascular surgery, and cardiac clinics.

- **Cardiovascular technologists** and **technicians,** who assist physicians in the diagnosis and treatment of cardiovascular disorders.

- **Cardiac sonographers** or **echocardiographers,** who are technologists who use **ultrasound** to observe the heart chambers, valves, and blood vessels.

- **Phlebotomists,** who assist physicians by drawing patient blood samples for laboratory testing.

Chapter Learning Outcomes

The heart and blood vessels together comprise the **cardiovascular** system. In any health care discipline and setting, the condition of the patient's cardiovascular system will always be a factor in diagnosis and treatment. In order to understand and communicate that information, it is essential to know the medical terminology involved and be able to:

LO 10.1 Describe the position of the heart.

LO 10.2 Relate the structure of the heart to its functions.

LO 10.3 Describe the blood flow through the heart.

LO 10.4 Discuss the cardiac cycle.

LO 10.5 Explain disorders of the heart.

LO 10.6 Identify the circulatory systems.

LO 10.7 Relate the structure of the blood vessels to their functions.

LO 10.8 Explain disorders of the circulatory systems.

LO 10.9 Identify diagnostic procedures used in cardiovascular disorders.

LO 10.10 Discuss therapeutic procedures used in cardiovascular disorders.

LO 10.11 Describe pharmacologic agents used in the treatment of cardiovascular disorders.

LO 10.A Use the medical terms of cardiology to communicate and document in writing accurately and precisely in any health care setting.

LO 10.B Use the medical terms of cardiology to communicate verbally with accuracy and precision in any health care setting.

LO 10.C Using word elements, construct medical terms associated with cardiology.

LO 10.D Deconstruct medical terms associated with cardiology into their word elements.

LO 10.E Use correctly the approved abbreviations for cardiac terms.

LO 10.F Identify the health professionals involved in the care of cardiac patients.

 ## Case Report (CR) 10.1

You are

. . . a **cardiovascular technologist** (**CVT**) employed by the **Cardiology** Department at Fulwood Medical Center. You have been called to the Emergency Department immediately (**STAT**) to take an **electrocardiogram** (**ECG** or **EKG**).

Your patient is

. . . Mr. Hank Johnson. From his medical records, you see that he is the 64-year-old owner of a printing company.

Eight months ago, Mr. Johnson had a left total hip replacement. In the past 3 months, he has returned to his daily workouts. This morning, while riding his exercise bike, he felt tightness in his chest. He kept on cycling and developed pain in the center of his chest radiating down his left arm and up into his jaw. He became **diaphoretic**. His personal trainer called 911.

You perform the ECG, and the automatic report describes abnormalities in the chest leads.

As you remove the electrodes, Mr. Johnson complains that he is feeling faint and has shortness of breath (**SOB**). You are the only person in the room.

Lesson 10.1

CARDIOVASCULAR SYSTEM

Heart

If you have a healthy heart rate of 60 beats per minute and you live to be 80 years old, your heart will beat (contract and relax) at least 2,522,880,000 times. Your heart pumps approximately 2,000 gallons of blood each day. In 80 years of life, it will have pumped a total of 58,400,000 gallons of blood. If your heart is unable to maintain this ability to pump blood for just a few minutes, your life is in danger.

The information in this lesson will enable you to use correct medical terminology to:

10.1.1 Describe the location of the heart and its relation to other structures.

10.1.2 Discuss the functions of the heart.

10.1.3 Identify the chambers of the heart and the pathway blood takes through them.

10.1.4 Explain the causes of the sounds of the heartbeat heard through a stethoscope.

10.1.5 Identify the blood supply to the heart muscle.

10.1.6 Distinguish between contraction and relaxation during the heart cycle.

10.1.7 Describe the electrical properties of the heart.

Abbreviations

CPR	cardiopulmonary resuscitation
CVT	cardiovascular technician
ECG	electrocardiogram
EKG	electrocardiogram
SOB	shortness of breath
STAT	immediately

LO 10.1 Position of the Heart

Location of the Heart

The heart is roughly the size of a fist and weighs around 10 ounces. It is a blunt cone that points down and to the left. The heart lies obliquely between the lungs, with one-third of its mass behind the **sternum** and two-thirds to the left of the sternum (*Figure 10.1a*). The **apex** can normally be palpated in the fifth **intercostal** space, between the fifth and sixth ribs. The base of the heart lies behind the sternum and the second intercostal space, between the second and third ribs. The region of the thoracic cavity in which the heart lies is called the **mediastinum** (*Figure 10.1b*).

It is important to know the position of the heart so that you can perform effective **cardiopulmonary resuscitation** (CPR), position a **stethoscope** to hear heart sounds, or position the **electrodes** correctly for an ECG.

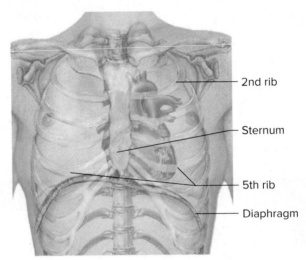

- 2nd rib
- Sternum
- 5th rib
- Diaphragm

(a) Relationship of heart to sternum

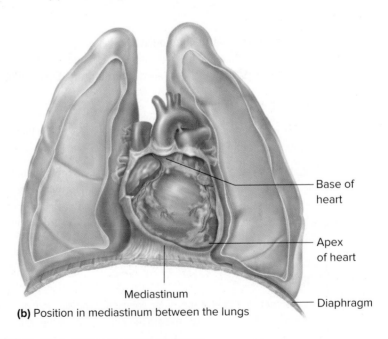

- Base of heart
- Apex of heart
- Mediastinum
- Diaphragm

(b) Position in mediastinum between the lungs

▲ **Figure 10.1** **Position of Heart in Thoracic Cavity.**

LO 10.1, 10.A, 10.F
Word Analysis and Definition

S = Suffix   P = Prefix   R = Root   R/CF = Combining Form

WORD	PRONUNCIATION		ELEMENTS	DEFINITION
apex	**AY**-peks		Latin *summit or tip*	Tip or end of cone-shaped structure, such as the heart
cardiac	**KAR**-dee-ak	S/ R/	-ac *pertaining to* cardi- *heart*	Pertaining to the heart
cardiologist	kar-dee-**OL**-oh-jist	S/ R/CF	-logist *specialist* cardi/o- *heart*	A medical specialist in diagnosis and treatment of the heart (cardiology)
cardiology	kar-dee-**OL**-oh-jee	S/	-logy *study of*	Medical specialty of diseases of the heart
cardiopulmonary resuscitation	**KAR**-dee-oh-**PUL**-moh-nair-ee ree-sus-ih-**TAY**-shun	S/ R/CF R/ S/ R/	-ary *pertaining to* cardi/o- *heart* -pulmon- *lung* -ation *process* resuscit- *revival from apparent death*	The attempt to restore cardiac and pulmonary function
cardiovascular	**KAR**-dee-oh-**VAS**-kyu-lar	S/ R/CF R/	-ar *pertaining to* cardi/o- *heart* -vascul- *blood vessel*	Pertaining to the heart and blood vessels
intercostal	**IN**-ter-**KOS**-tal	S/ P/ R/	-al *pertaining to* inter- *between* -cost- *rib*	The space between two ribs
mediastinum	**MEE**-dee-ass-**TIE**-num	S/ P/ R/	-um *structure* media- *middle* -stin- *partition*	Area between the lungs containing the heart, aorta, venae cavae, esophagus, and trachea
sternum	**STIR**-num		Latin *chest*	Long, flat bone forming the center of the anterior wall of the chest

Exercises

A. Build your *language of cardiology* by completing the following documentation. *There is only one best answer for each blank.*
LO 10.1, 10.A, 10.F

cardiology   cardiovascular   cardiologist   cardiac

The **(1)** _____ Department sent a specialist to examine the patient in the Emergency Room. The

(2) _____ ordered a cardiac catheterization, which showed three obstructed arteries in

the patient's heart, so the **(3)** _____ surgeon was notified immediately to perform

(4) _____ surgery.

B. Describe the health care professionals specific to the care of the heart. *Match the health care professional in the first column with its correct description in the second column.* **LO 10.A, 10.F**

Term		Meaning
_____ 1. echocardiographer		**a.** medical doctor specializing in surgery of the heart and peripheral blood vessels
_____ 2. phlebotomist		**b.** technician who uses ultrasound to observe the structures of the heart
_____ 3. cardiologist		**c.** assists physicians in the diagnosis and treatment of cardiovascular disorders
_____ 4. cardiovascular surgeon		**d.** draws patient blood samples for laboratory testing
_____ 5. cardiovascular technician		**e.** medical doctor specializing in disorders of the cardiovascular system

LESSON 10.1 Heart   323

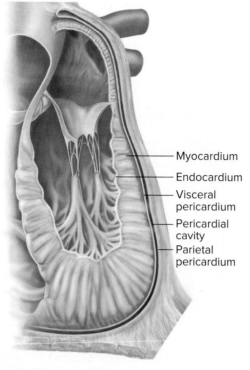

▲ **Figure 10.2** Heart Wall.

Myocardium
Endocardium
Visceral pericardium
Pericardial cavity
Parietal pericardium

▲ **Figure 10.3** Coronary Arterial Circulation.

Superior vena cava
Aortic arch
Left coronary artery
Circumflex artery
Right coronary artery
Left ventricle
Right ventricle

LO 10.2 Functions and Structure of the Heart

Functions of the Heart

1. **Pumping blood.** Contractions of the heart generate the pressure to produce movement of blood through the blood vessels.
2. **Routing blood.** The heart can be described as two pumps. A pump on the right side of the heart sends blood through the **pulmonary** circulation of the lungs and back to the pump on the left side, which sends blood through the **systemic** circulation of the body. The valves of the heart ensure this one-way flow of blood.
3. **Regulating blood supply.** The changing metabolic needs of tissues and organs (for example, when you exercise) are met by changes in the rate and force of the heart's contraction.

Structure of the Heart

The heart wall consists of three layers *(Figure 10.2):*

1. **Endocardium**—a single layer of cells over a thin layer of connective tissue lining the heart.
2. **Myocardium**—cardiac muscle cells that enable the heart to contract.
3. **Epicardium**—a thin serous membrane that is the inner layer of the pericardium.

The **pericardium** is a connective tissue sac that surrounds and protects the heart. It consists of an inner **visceral** layer **(epicardium)** and outer **parietal** layer, between which is the **pericardial** cavity. This cavity contains a lubricant fluid that allows the heart to beat with very little friction around it.

Blood Supply to Heart Muscle

Because the heart beats continually and strongly, it requires an abundant supply of oxygen and nutrients. To meet this need, the cardiac muscle has its own blood circulation, the **coronary circulation** *(Figure 10.3)*.

Immediately above the aortic valve in the root of the aorta, the right and left **coronary arteries** exit from the aorta and divide into branches to begin the coronary circulation.

After the blood has flowed through the arteries into the capillaries of the myocardium, 80% drains into veins that flow into the right atrium and 20% flows into the right ventricle. There, the deoxygenated blood mixes with the deoxygenated blood from the rest of the body.

Abbreviation	
MI	myocardial infarction ("heart attack")

📁🩺 Case Report (CR) 10.1 *(continued)*

Changes on Mr. Johnson's ECG show he was having an **MI**. Cardiac muscle cells have very limited capability to replicate, and the repair of muscle cell death is mainly by **fibrosis**. This limits cardiac function; Mr. Johnson's heart muscle will have a diminished capacity to contract normally after he recovers from the heart attack.

WORD	PRONUNCIATION	ELEMENTS		DEFINITION
coronary circulation	**KOR**-oh-nair-ee **SER**-kyu-**LAY**-shun	S/ R/	-ary *pertaining to* coron- *crown* Latin *to encircle*	Blood flow through the vessels supplying the heart
endocardium	**EN**-doh-**KAR**-dee-um	S/ P/ R/	-um *structure* endo- *inside* -cardi- *heart*	The inside lining of the heart
endocardial (adj)	**EN**-doh-**KAR**-dee-al	S/	-al *pertaining to*	Pertaining to the endocardium
epicardium	**EP**-ih-**KAR**-dee-um	S/ P/ R/	-um *structure* epi- *upon, above* -cardi- *heart*	The outer layer of the heart wall
myocardium	**MY**-oh-**KAR**-dee-um	S/ R/CF R/	-um *structure* my/o- *muscle* -cardi- *heart*	All the heart muscle
myocardial (adj)	**MY**-oh-**KAR**-dee-al	S/	-al *pertaining to*	Pertaining to the myocardium
parietal	pah-**RYE**-eh-tal	S/ R/	-al *pertaining to* pariet- *wall*	Pertaining to the outer layer of the pericardium and other body cavities
pericardium	per-ih-**KAR**-dee-um	S/ P/ R/	-um *structure* peri- *around* -cardi- *heart*	Structure around the heart
pericardial (adj)	per-ih-**KAR**-dee-al	S/	-al *pertaining to*	Pertaining to the pericardium
pulmonary	**PULL**-moh-**NAIR**-ee	S/ R/	-ary *pertaining to* pulmon- *lung*	Pertaining to the lungs and their blood supply
systemic	sis-**TEM**-ik	S/ R/	-ic *pertaining to* system- *body as a whole*	Relating to the entire organism
visceral	**VISS**-er-al	S/ R/	-al *pertaining to* viscer- *an organ*	Pertaining to the internal organs

Exercises

A. Define the words in bold using the correct medical term. *Use the terms related to the function and structure of the heart to correctly answer the questions. Fill in the blanks.* **LO 10.2, 10.A**

1. With the exception of the cranial and spinal cavities, all other cavities are lined with a double-walled serous membrane. The inner layer touches the **organ,** the outer layer forms the **wall** of the cavity.

   Which medical term means pertaining to an *organ*? _____.

   Which medical term means pertaining to a *wall*? _____.

2. The right side of the heart pumps blood through arteries to the **lungs** to pick up oxygen. The left side of the heart pumps blood through arteries to deliver oxygenated blood to the organs of each body **system.**

   The right side of the heart pumps blood to the _____ circulation.

   The left side of the heart pumps blood to the _____ circulation.

B. Construct medical terms. *Provide the correct prefix to the term to correctly complete each sentence.* **LO 10.2, 10.C**

1. The **inside** of the heart is termed the _____ /cardium.

2. The **muscular** part of the heart is termed the _____ /cardium.

3. The **outer** layer of the heart is termed the _____ /cardium.

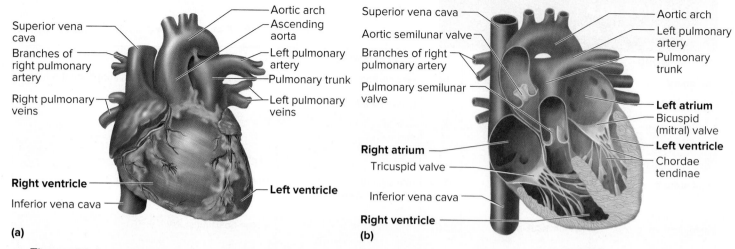

Labels for figure (a), External Anatomy:
- Superior vena cava
- Branches of right pulmonary artery
- Right pulmonary veins
- Aortic arch
- Ascending aorta
- Left pulmonary artery
- Pulmonary trunk
- Left pulmonary veins
- **Right ventricle**
- Inferior vena cava
- **Left ventricle**

(a)

Labels for figure (b), Internal Anatomy:
- Superior vena cava
- Aortic semilunar valve
- Branches of right pulmonary artery
- Pulmonary semilunar valve
- **Right atrium**
- Tricuspid valve
- Inferior vena cava
- **Right ventricle**
- Aortic arch
- Left pulmonary artery
- Pulmonary trunk
- **Left atrium**
- Bicuspid (mitral) valve
- **Left ventricle**
- Chordae tendinae

(b)

▲ **Figure 10.4** External (a) and Internal (b) Anatomy of the Heart: Frontal View.

▲ **Figure 10.5** General Schematic of the Cardiovascular Circulation. ©Sergey Ryzhov/ Shutterstock.com RF

Keynote

The pulmonary circulation is the only place in the body where deoxygenated blood is carried in arteries and oxygenated blood is carried in veins.

LO 10.3 Blood Flow through the Heart

The heart has four chambers (*Figure 10.4b*):

1. Right **atrium**
2. Right **ventricle**
3. Left atrium
4. Left ventricle

The right and left sides of the heart are separated by the cardiac **septum**, which can be described in two sections:

- The right and left atria are separated by a thin muscle wall called the **interatrial** septum.
- The right and left ventricles are separated by a thicker muscle wall called the **interventricular** septum.

In addition, the **atrioventricular (AV)** septum is located between and behind the right atrium and left ventricle.

Blood circulates around the body (through the systemic circulation) to unload oxygen and nutrients and pick up carbon dioxide and metabolic waste products. This deoxygenated blood returns to the heart via the **superior and inferior venae cavae**. These large veins open into the right atrium. When the right atrium contracts, the blood flows through the **tricuspid valve** into the right ventricle. The tricuspid valve then shuts so when the right ventricle contracts, blood cannot flow back into the atrium.

When the right ventricle contracts, the blood is pushed out through the **semilunar pulmonary valve** into the **pulmonary trunk** (*Figure 10.4a and b*) to begin the pulmonary circulation. The pulmonary valve then shuts to prevent blood flowing back into the ventricle. The pulmonary trunk divides into two arteries; the right pulmonary artery goes to the right lung and the left pulmonary artery goes to the left lung. In the lungs, carbon dioxide is unloaded, and oxygen is picked up from the air by the blood. The oxygen-rich blood is returned to the heart by the pulmonary veins (*Figure 10.4a and b*).

The blood from the pulmonary veins flows into the left atrium. When the atrium contracts, the blood flows through the **mitral** (or **bicuspid**) valve into the left ventricle. The bicuspid valve then shuts so that blood cannot flow back into the left atrium when the ventricle contracts. The bicuspid and tricuspid valves are anchored to the floor of the ventricles by stringlike **chordae tendineae** (*see Figure 10.4b*).

When the left ventricle contracts, the oxygenated blood is forced out under pressure through the **aortic** semilunar valve into the **aorta**, to return to circulating round the body in the systemic circulation (*Figure 10.5*). The aortic valve then shuts so blood cannot flow back into the left ventricle. The four valves all allow the blood to flow only in one direction.

WORD	PRONUNCIATION	ELEMENTS		DEFINITION
aorta aortic (adj)	ay-**OR**-tuh ay-**OR**-tic	S/ R/	Greek *lift up* -ic *pertaining to* aort- *aorta*	Main trunk of the systemic arterial system Pertaining to the aorta
atrioventricular (AV)	**AY**-tree-oh-ven-**TRIK**-you-lar	S/ R/CF R/	-ar *pertaining to* atri/o- *entrance, atrium* -ventricul- *ventricle*	Pertaining to both the atrium and the ventricle
atrium atria (pl) atrial (adj)	**AY**-tree-um **AY**-tree-ah **AY**-tree-al	S/ R/	Latin *entrance* -al *pertaining to* atri- *entrance, atrium*	Chamber where blood enters the heart on both right and left sides Pertaining to the atrium
bicuspid	by-**KUSS**-pid	S/ P/ R/	-id *having a particular quality* bi- *two* -cusp- *point*	Having two points; a bicuspid heart valve has two flaps
chordae tendineae (pl)	**KOR**-dee ten-**DIN**-ee		chorda Latin *cord* tendinea Latin *tendons*	Tendinous cords attaching the bicuspid and tricuspid valves to the heart wall
interatrial	**IN**-ter-**AY**-tree-al	S/ P/ R/	-al *pertaining to* inter- *between* -atri- *atrium, entrance*	Between the atria of the heart
interventricular	**IN**-ter-ven-**TRIK**-you-lar	S/ P/ R/	-ar *pertaining to* inter- *between* -ventricul- *ventricle*	Between the ventricles of the heart
mitral	**MY**-tral		Latin *turban*	Shaped like the headdress of a Catholic bishop
semilunar	sem-ee-**LOO**-nar	S/ P/ R/	-ar *pertaining to* semi- *half* -lun- *moon*	Appears like a half moon
septum septa (pl)	**SEP**-tum **SEP**-tah		Latin *partition*	A wall dividing two cavities
tricuspid	try-**KUSS**-pid	S/ P/ R/	-id *having a particular quality* tri- *three* -cusp- *point*	Having three points; a tricuspid heart valve has three flaps
vena cava venae cavae (pl)	**VEE**-nah **KAY**-vah **VEE**-nee **KAY**-vee	R/CF R/	ven/a *vein* cava *cave*	One of the two largest veins in the body
ventricle	**VEN**-trih-kel		Latin *small belly*	Chamber of the heart or brain

Exercises

A. Plurals of medical terms follow certain established rules. *Apply these rules and change the singular forms into plurals.* **LO 10.2, 10.3, 10.A, 10.C**

1. Singular: **atrium** Plural: _____

2. Singular: **septum** Plural: _____

3. Singular: **vena cava** Plural: _____

4. Singular: **ventricle** Plural: _____

> ### Study Hint
> Blood flow through the heart and vessels follows an A-V-A-V pattern. Blood flows from atrium to ventricle, to artery, (to organ) to vein, and then into the atrium to repeat the process.

B. Describe the blood flow through the heart. *Given the name of the blood vessel, describe how it interacts with the heart chambers. Match the term in the first column with its proper description in the second column.* **LO 10.3**

Blood Vessel

_____ 1. aorta

_____ 2. venae cavae

_____ 3. pulmonary arteries

_____ 4. pulmonary veins

Interaction with the Heart

a. receives blood from the right ventricle

b. receives blood from the left ventricle

c. empties blood into the left atrium

d. empties blood into the right atrium

LO 10.4 The Cardiac Cycle

The action of the four heart chambers is coordinated. When the atria contract (atrial **systole**), the ventricles relax (ventricular **diastole**, or ventricular filling). When the atria relax (atrial diastole), the ventricles contract (ventricular systole). Then the atria and ventricles all relax briefly. This series of events is a complete cardiac cycle, or heartbeat.

The "*lub*-dub, *lub*-dub" sounds heard through the **stethoscope** are made by the snap of the heart valves as they close.

Electrical Properties of the Heart

As the cardiac muscles contract, they generate a small electrical current. Because the muscle cells are coupled together electrically, they stimulate their neighbor cells so that the myocardium of the atria, and that of the ventricles, each acts as a *single* unit.

To keep the heart beating in a rhythm, a **conduction system** is in place. It consists of five components *(Figure 10.6)*:

1. A small region of specialized muscle cells in the right atrium initiates the electrical current and, therefore, the heartbeat. This area is called the **sinoatrial (SA) node**. It is the **pacemaker** of heart rhythm.

2. Electrical signals from the SA node spread out through the atria and then come back together at the **atrioventricular (AV) node.** This is the electrical gateway to the ventricles, and normally electrical currents cannot get to the ventricles by any other route. The AV node delays impulses to ensure that the atria have ejected their blood into the ventricles before the ventricles contract.

3. Electrical signals leave the AV node to reach the ventricles through the **AV bundle (bundle of His)**.

4. This AV bundle divides into the right and left **bundle branches,** which supply the two ventricles.

5. From the two bundle branches, **Purkinje fibers** spread through the ventricular myocardium and distribute the electrical stimuli to cause contraction of the ventricular myocardium.

Keynote

The normal heartbeat with normal electrical conduction through the heart leading to a ventricular rate of around 60 to 90 beats per minute is called **sinus rhythm**.

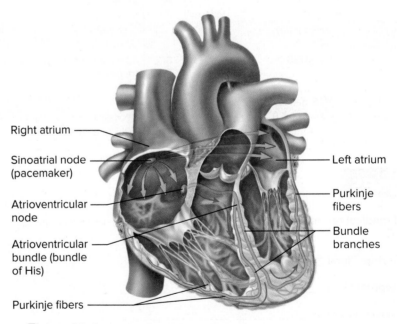

Right atrium

Sinoatrial node (pacemaker)

Atrioventricular node

Atrioventricular bundle (bundle of His)

Purkinje fibers

Left atrium

Purkinje fibers

Bundle branches

▲ **Figure 10.6** Cardiac Conduction System.

WORD	PRONUNCIATION	ELEMENTS		DEFINITION
atrioventricular	**AY**-tree-oh-ven-**TRIK**-you-lar	S/ R/CF R/	-ar *pertaining to* atri/o- *entrance, atrium* -ventricul- *ventricle*	Pertaining to both the atrium and ventricle
AV bundle bundle of His (syn) **AV node**	**AY-VEE BUN**-del **BUN**-del OV HISS **AY-VEE** NODE		(bundle) Old English *to bind* (His) Wilhelm His Jr., 1863–1934, Swiss cardiologist and anatomist	Pathway for electrical signals to be transmitted to the ventricles Part of the heart's conduction system that receives the electrical impulse that traveled from the atria, delays it, and then sends it to AV bundle
conduction	kon-**DUCK**-shun	S/ P/ R/	-ion *process* con- *together, with* -duct- *lead*	Process of transmitting energy
diastole	die-**AS**-toh-lee		Greek *dilation*	Relaxation of heart cavities, during which they fill with blood
diastolic (adj)	die-as-**TOL**-ik	S/ R/	-ic *pertaining to* diastol- *dilate*	Pertaining to relaxation of the heart cavities
pacemaker	**PACE**-may-ker	S/ R/	-maker *one who makes* pace- *step, pace*	Device that regulates cardiac electrical activity
Purkinje fibers	per-**KIN**-jee **FIE**-bers		Johannes von Purkinje, 1787–1869, Bohemian anatomist and physiologist	Network of nerve fibers in the myocardium
sinoatrial node	sigh-noh-**AY**-tree-al NODE	S/ R/CF R/	-al *pertaining to* sin/o- *sinus* -atri- *entrance, atrium*	The center of modified cardiac muscle fibers in the wall of the right atrium that acts as the pacemaker for the heart rhythm
sinus rhythm	**SIGH**-nus **RITH**-um		**sinus** Latin *channel, cavity* **rhythm** Greek *to flow*	The normal (optimal) heart rhythm arising from the sinoatrial node
systole systolic (adj)	**SIS**-toh-lee sis-**TOL**-ik	S/ R/	Greek *contraction* -ic *pertaining to* systol- *contract*	Contraction of the heart muscle Pertaining to contraction of the heart muscle

Exercises

A. Place in order the electrical events of the heart. *In the list below, number the events as they normally occur in the heart. Start with 1 for the first event, through 5 for the last event.* **LO 10.4**

_____ AV bundle

_____ SA node

_____ Purkinje fibers

_____ AV node

_____ bundle branches

B. Define the events of the cardiac cycle. *From the provided definition, give the correct term it is describing. Fill in the blanks.* **LO 10.4, 10.A**

1. Period of time when the heart chamber is contracting. _____

2. Period of time when the heart chamber is filling with blood. _____

Lesson 10.2

CARDIOVASCULAR SYSTEM

Disorders of the Heart

Every different structure within the heart may not function properly. In this lesson, you will learn the common disorders of the heart and the medical terminology to describe them.

10.2.1 Describe common types of cardiac arrhythmias

10.2.2 Explain common disorders of the heart valves.

10.2.3 Discuss common disorders of the heart wall and its blood supply.

10.2.4 Describe hypertensive heart disease and congestive heart failure.

10.2.5 Discuss congenital heart disease.

Abbreviations

A-fib	atrial fibrillation
PAT	paroxysmal atrial tachycardia
PVC	premature ventricular contraction
V-fib	ventricular fibrillation

LO 10.5 Disorders of the Heart

Abnormal Heart Rhythms

When the heart is beating outside of normal sinus rhythm, the condition is termed **arrhythmia** or **dysrhythmia** (these two terms are synonyms). The normal rate of heartbeat is 60 to 100 beats per minute. A heart rate slower than 60 is called **bradycardia** *(Figure 10.7)*. A heart rate faster than 100 is called **tachycardia** *(Figure 10.8)*.

There are four common types of **arrhythmias (dysrhythmias),** abnormal or irregular heartbeats:

1. **Premature beats** may originate in either the atrium or the ventricle, or both. They may occur in individuals of all ages and could be associated with caffeine and stress.

2. **Atrial fibrillation (A-fib)** occurs when the two atria quiver rather than contract in an organized fashion to pump blood into the ventricle. This causes blood to pool in the atria and sometimes clot. **Paroxysmal atrial tachycardia (PAT)** presents with periods of rapid, regular heartbeats that originate in the atrium. The episodes begin and end abruptly. The heart rate speeds up to 160 to 200 beats per minute.

3. **Ventricular arrhythmias** consist of several types. **Ventricular tachycardia** is a rapid heartbeat arising in the ventricles. **Premature ventricular contractions (PVCs)** occur when extra impulses arise from a ventricle. **Ventricular fibrillation (V-fib)** is characterized by erratic ventricular contractions. The ventricles quiver and beat ineffectively instead of pumping.

4. **Heart block** occurs when interference in cardiac electrical conduction causes the contractions of the atria to fail to coordinate with the contractions of the ventricles.

Palpitations are unpleasant sensations of a rapid or irregular heartbeat that last a few seconds or minutes. They can be brought on by exercise, anxiety, and stimulants like caffeine. Occasionally, they can be caused by an arrhythmia.

▲ **Figure 10.7** Bradycardia.

▲ **Figure 10.8** Tachycardia.

WORD	PRONUNCIATION	ELEMENTS		DEFINITION
arrhythmia (note the double "rr")	ah-**RITH**-mee-ah	S/ P/ R/	-ia *condition* a- *without* -rrhythm- *rhythm*	An abnormal heart rhythm
bradycardia	brad-ee-**KAR**-dee-ah	S/ P/ R/	-ia *condition* brady- *slow* -card- *heart*	Slow heart rate (below 60 beats per minute)
dysrhythmia	dis-**RITH**-mee-ah	S/ P/ R/	-ia *condition* dys- *bad* -rhythm- *rhythm*	An abnormal heart rhythm.
fibrillation	fih-brih-**LAY**-shun	S/ R/	-ation *process* fibrill- *small fiber*	Uncontrolled quivering or twitching of the heart muscle
palpitation	pal-pih-**TAY**-shun	S/ R/	-ation *process* palpit- *throb*	Forcible, rapid beat of the heart felt by the patient
paroxysmal	par-ok-**SIZ**-mal	S/ R/	-al *pertaining to* paroxysm- *irritation*	Occurring in sharp, spasmodic episodes
tachycardia	tak-ih-**KAR**-dee-ah	S/ P/ R/	-ia *condition* tachy- *rapid* -card- *heart*	Rapid heart rate (above 100 beats per minute)

Exercises

A. The definitions for the medical terms relating to abnormal heart rhythms are given to you—construct each term by providing the missing word element. *Fill in the blanks with the missing prefix or root.* **LO 10.5, 10.A, 10.C**

1. Forcible, rapid beat of the heart: _____ /ation

2. Uncontrolled heart muscle twitching: _____ /ation

3. Sharp, spasmodic episode: _____ /al

4. Rapid heart rate (greater than 100 beats per minute): _____ /card/ia

5. Slow heart rate (less than 60 beats per minute): _____ /card/ia

6. Abnormal heart rhythm: _____ /rrhythm/ia

LO 10.5 Disorders of the Heart (continued)

Disorders of the Heart Valves

Heart valves can **malfunction** in two basic ways:

1. **Stenosis** occurs when the valve does not open fully, and its opening is narrowed (constricted). Blood cannot flow freely through the valve and accumulates behind the valve.

2. **Incompetence** or **insufficiency** occurs when the valve cannot close fully, and blood can **regurgitate** (flow back) through the valve to the chamber from which it started.

   Mitral valve stenosis can occur following rheumatic fever. Because the blood cannot flow freely through the valve, the left atrium becomes dilated. Eventually, **chronic heart failure** results. (*Figure 10.9* enables you to review the locations of the valves and chambers.)

   Mitral valve incompetence occurs when there is leakage back through the valve as the left ventricle contracts. The left atrium becomes dilated. Again, chronic heart failure results.

   Mitral valve prolapse (**MVP**) occurs when the cusps of the valve bulge back into the left atrium when the left ventricle contracts, thus allowing blood to flow back into the atrium.

   Aortic valve stenosis is common in the elderly when the valves become calcified due to **atherosclerosis**. Blood flow into the systemic circuit is diminished, leading to dizziness and fainting. The left ventricle dilates, hypertrophies, and ultimately fails.

   Aortic valve incompetence initially produces few symptoms other than a murmur, but eventually the left ventricle fails.

   Rheumatic fever is an inflammatory disease. If a sore throat caused by group A beta-hemolytic streptococcus (*see Chapter 13*) is not treated with a complete course of antibiotics, antibodies to the bacteria can develop and attack normal tissue. Multiple joints are inflamed, and endocarditis can affect the function of the heart valves—particularly the mitral and aortic valves.

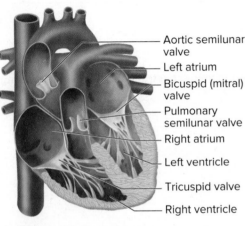

- Aortic semilunar valve
- Left atrium
- Bicuspid (mitral) valve
- Pulmonary semilunar valve
- Right atrium
- Left ventricle
- Tricuspid valve
- Right ventricle

▲ **Figure 10.9** Heart Valves.

Disorders of the Heart Wall

Endocarditis is inflammation of the lining of the heart. It is usually secondary to an infection elsewhere. Intravenous drug users and people with damaged heart valves are at high risk for endocarditis.

Myocarditis is inflammation of the heart muscle. It can be bacterial, viral, or fungal in origin or a complication of other diseases, such as influenza.

Pericarditis is inflammation of the covering of the heart. The inflammation causes an **exudate** (pericardial **effusion**) to be released into the pericardial space. This interferes with the heart's ability to contract and expand normally, and cardiac output falls—a condition called **cardiac tamponade**.

Cardiomyopathy is a weakening of the heart muscle that causes it to pump inadequately. The etiology can be viral, idiopathic (when the cause is unknown), or alcoholic. It causes **cardiomegaly** and heart failure.

WORD	PRONUNCIATION		ELEMENTS	DEFINITION
cardiomegaly	KAR-dee-oh-MEG-ah-lee	S/ R/CF	-megaly *enlargement* cardi/o- *heart*	Enlargement of the heart
cardiomyopathy	KAR-dee-oh-my-OP-ah-thee	S/ R/CF R/CF	-pathy *disease* cardi/o- *heart* my/o- *muscle*	Disease of heart muscle, the myocardium
cor pulmonale	KOR pul-moh-NAH-lee	R/ S/ R/	cor *heart* -ale *pertaining to* pulmon- *lung*	Right-sided heart failure arising from chronic lung disease
effusion	eh-FYU-shun		Latin *pouring out*	Collection of fluid that has escaped from blood vessels into a cavity or tissues
endocarditis	EN-doh-kar-DIE-tis	S/ P/ R/	-itis *inflammation* endo- *within* -card- *heart*	Inflammation of the lining of the heart
exudate	EKS-you-date	S/ P/ R/	-ate *process, composed of* ex- *out of* -ud- *sweat*	Fluid that has come out of a tissue or its capillaries because of inflammation or injury
incompetence	in-KOM-peh-tense	S/ P/ R/	-ence *quality of* in- *not* -compet- *strive together*	Failure of valves to close completely
insufficiency	in-suh-FISH-en-see	S/ P/ R/CF	-ency *quality of* in- *not* -suffic/i- *enough*	Lack of completeness of function; in the heart, failure of a valve to close properly
malfunction	mal-FUNK-shun	S/ P/ R/	-ion *action, condition* mal- *bad, inadequate* -funct- *perform*	Inadequate or abnormal function
myocarditis	MY-oh-kar-DIE-tis	S/ R/CF R/	-itis *inflammation* my/o- *muscle* -card- *heart*	Inflammation of the heart muscle
pericarditis	PER-ih-kar-DIE-tis	S/ P/ R/	-itis *inflammation* peri- *around* -card- *heart*	Inflammation of the pericardium, the covering of the heart
prolapse	proh-LAPS		Latin *a falling*	The falling or slipping of a body part from its normal position
regurgitate	ree-GUR-jih-tate	S/ P/ R/	-ate *pertaining to* re- *back* -gurgit- *flood*	To flow backward; in this case, through a heart valve
stenosis	steh-NOH-sis	S/ R/CF	-sis *abnormal condition* sten/o- *narrow*	Narrowing of a canal or passage, as in the narrowing of a heart valve
tamponade	tam-poh-NAID	S/ R/	-ade *process* tampon- *plug*	Pathologic compression of an organ such as the heart

Exercises

A. Use your knowledge of the *language of cardiology* to match the description in the left column with the correct medical term in the right column. *Match the term to its correct meaning.* **LO 10.5, 10.A**

_____ 1. Weakening of heart muscle

_____ 2. Inflammation that causes exudates

_____ 3. Cusps of valve bulge back into atrium

_____ 4. Constricted valve opening

_____ 5. Failure of right ventricle to pump properly

_____ 6. Cardiomyopathy can be the cause

_____ 7. Causes valve regurgitation

_____ 8. Inflammatory disease that affects the heart

a. incompetence

b. cardiomegaly

c. cor pulmonale

d. pericarditis

e. rheumatic fever

f. cardiomyopathy

g. prolapse

h. stenosis

All of the following risk factors can be reduced by changes in lifestyle.

Risk factors for CAD include:

- Obesity
- Lack of exercise (**sedentary**)
- Tobacco
- Diabetes mellitus
- High BP (**hypertension**)
- Elevated serum cholesterol
- Stress

Cardiac arrest is the sudden cessation of cardiac activity resulting from **anoxia**. The ECG shows a flat line, **asystole** (Figure 10.11).

Abbreviations

ASHD	arteriosclerotic heart disease
BP	blood pressure
CAD	coronary artery disease
MI	myocardial infarction

Case Report (CR) 10.1 (continued)

In the Emergency Room, the ECG indicated that Mr. Johnson was having a myocardial **infarction** (**MI**) affecting the anterior wall of his left ventricle. The cardiovascular technologist did not want to leave Mr. Johnson, so he used the call system to summon help.

LO 10.5 Disorders of the Heart (continued)

Coronary Artery Disease (CAD)

The arteries supplying the myocardium become narrowed by atherosclerotic **plaques**, called **atheroma**. As the atheroma increases, the lumen of the artery becomes increasingly narrow (*compare Figure 10.10a and b*). The blood supplied to the cardiac muscle by the artery is reduced. Platelet aggregation can occur on the plaque to form a blood clot (**coronary thrombosis**). **Atherosclerosis** is the most common form of **arteriosclerosis** (hardening of the arteries) and can lead to **arteriosclerotic heart disease (ASHD)**.

    Angina pectoris, pain in the chest on exertion, is often the first symptom of reduced oxygen supply to the myocardium.

    When blood flow in any of the coronary arteries is blocked (**occluded**), **myocardial ischemia** occurs. If ischemia is not reversed within 4 to 6 hours, the myocardial cells die, resulting in a condition called **myocardial infarction.** The area of **necrosis** becomes **fibrotic** (stiff), which decreases the ability of the heart to pump blood.

    Cardiogenic shock occurs when the heart fails to pump effectively and organs and tissues are **perfused** inadequately. The pulse is weak and rapid, and **blood pressure** (**BP**) drops. The patient becomes pale, cold, sweaty, and anxious.

    The other form of circulatory shock is **hypovolemic shock,** in which there is a loss of blood volume, often from hemorrhage or dehydration.

    Death is recorded by a flat ECG line as in **asystole** (*Figure 10.11*)

(a)   Lumen⎯   � Artery wall

(b)   Lumen⎤   ⎣Plaque   ⎣Artery wall

▲ **Figure 10.10** Arterial Structure. (a) Normal coronary artery. (b) Advanced atherosclerosis with narrowed lumen. ©Ed Reschke/Getty Images

▲ **Figure 10.11** Electrocardiogram (ECG) Showing Asystole. ©Pasieka/SPL/Photo Researchers, Inc.

WORD	PRONUNCIATION		ELEMENTS	DEFINITION
angina pectoris	an-**JUH**-nuh **PEK**-tor-iss		**angina** Greek *strangling* **pectoris** Latin *chest*	Condition of severe pain in the chest due to coronary heart disease
anoxia	an-**OK**-see-ah	S/ P/ R/	-ia *condition* an- *without* -ox- *oxygen*	Without oxygen
anoxic (adj)	an-**OK**-sik	S/	-ic *pertaining to*	Pertaining to or suffering from a lack of oxygen
arteriosclerosis	ar-**TEER**-ee-oh-skler-**OH**-sis	S/ R/CF R/CF	-sis *abnormal condition* arteri/o- *artery* -scler/o- *hardness*	Hardening of the arteries
arteriosclerotic (adj)	ar-**TEER**-ee-oh-skler-**OT**-ik	S/	-tic *pertaining to*	Pertaining to or suffering from arteriosclerosis
asystole	ay-**SIS**-toh-lee	P/ R/	a- *without* -systole *contraction*	Absence of contractions of the heart
atheroma	ath-er-**ROH**-mah	S/ R/	-oma *tumor* ather- *porridge, gruel*	Lipid deposit in the lining of an artery
atherosclerosis	**ATH**-er-oh-skler-**OH**-sis	S/ R/CF R/CF	-sis *abnormal condition* ather/o *porridge, gruel* -scler/o- *hardness*	Atheroma in arteries
cardiogenic	**KAR**-dee-oh-**JEN**-ik	S/ R/CF R/	-ic *pertaining to* cardi/o- *heart* -gen- *produce, create*	Of cardiac origin
fibrosis	fie-**BROH**-sis	S/ R/CF	-sis *condition* fibr/o- *fiber*	Repair of dead tissue cells by formation of fibrous tissue
fibrotic (adj)	fie-**BROT**-ik	S/	-tic *pertaining to*	Pertaining to fibrosis
hypovolemic	**HIGH**-poh-voh-**LEE**-mik	S/ P/ R/	-emic *in the blood* hypo- *below* -vol- *volume*	Having decreased blood volume in the body
infarct	in-**FARKT**	P/ R/	in- *in* -farct *stuff*	Area of cell death resulting from an infarction
infarction	in-**FARK**-shun	S/	-ion *process*	Sudden blockage of an artery
ischemia	is-**KEE**-mee-ah	S/ R/	-emia *blood condition* isch- *to keep back*	Lack of blood supply to a tissue
ischemic (adj)	is-**KEE**-mik	S/	-emic *in the blood*	Pertaining to or affected by ischemia
necrosis	neh-**KROH**-sis	S/ R/	-osis *condition* necr- *death*	Pathologic death of tissue or cells
necrotic (adj)	neh-**KROT**-ik	S/ R/CF	-tic *pertaining to* necr/o- *death*	Affected by necrosis
occlude (verb)	ok-**KLUDE**		Latin *to close*	To close, plug, or completely obstruct
occlusion (noun)	ok-**KLU**-zhun	S/ R/	-ion *process* occlus- *to close*	A complete obstruction
perfuse	per-**FYUSE**		Latin *to pour*	To force blood to flow through a lumen or a vascular bed
perfusion (noun)	per-**FYU**-shun	S/ R/	-ion *action, condition* perfus- *to pour*	The act of perfusing
plaque	PLAK		French *a plate*	Patch of abnormal tissue
sedentary	sed-en-**TAIR**-ee	S/ R/	-ary *pertaining to* sedent- *sitting*	Accustomed to little exercise or movement
thrombosis	throm-**BOH**-sis	S/ R/	-osis *abnormal condition* thromb- *clot*	Formation of a clot (thrombus)

Exercises

A. Consult the text content related to coronary artery disease for the best medical terms to complete the following sentences in patient documentation. *Fill in the blank with the correct term. Use the words in parentheses as a hint to the correct medical term to use.* **LO 10.5, 10.A**

1. His _____ (little exercise or movement) lifestyle, coupled with obesity, increases his risk factors for a heart attack.

2. After the myocardial infarction, the area of the myocardium became _____ (stiff).

3. _____ (absence of heart contractions) occurred at 2251 hrs, and the patient was pronounced dead.

4. Angioplasty showed a large clot _____ (complete obstruction) her left coronary artery.

5. The prolonged period of ischemia led to tissue _____ (death).

6. Cardiogenic shock occurred, and the patient's tissues were not _____ (forcing blood through a vascular bed or lumen) adequately.

LO 10.5 Disorders of the Heart (continued)

Hypertensive Heart Disease

Hypertension (HTN) is the most common cardiovascular disorder in this country, affecting more than 20% of the adult population. It results from a prolonged elevated blood pressure (BP) throughout the vascular system. The high pressure forces the ventricles to work harder to pump blood. Eventually, the myocardium becomes strained and less efficient. It is the major cause of heart failure, stroke, and kidney failure.

High BP is currently defined as a BP reading at or above 120/80 mm **Hg** (mercury). A normal BP is below 120/80 mm Hg. The first number, or **systolic** reading, reflects the BP when the heart is contracting. The second number, or **diastolic** reading, reflects BP when the heart is relaxed between contractions.

Primary (essential) hypertension is the most common type of hypertension. Its etiology is unknown. Its risk factors are:

- Being overweight
- Stress
- Lack of exercise
- Using tobacco
- Using alcohol

Secondary hypertension results from other diseases, such as kidney disease, atherosclerosis, and hyperthyroidism.

Malignant hypertension is a rare, severe, life-threatening form of hypertension in which the BP reading can be greater than 200/120 mm Hg. Aggressive intervention is indicated to reduce the blood pressure.

Prehypertension, with a systolic pressure between 120 and 139 mm Hg and a diastolic pressure between 80 and 90 mm Hg, may indicate an increased risk for cardiovascular disease.

Congestive Heart Failure (CHF)

Congestive heart failure occurs with the inability of the heart to supply enough cardiac output to meet the body's metabolic needs. The patient shows **shortness of breath (SOB)** and **orthopnea**.

The most common conditions leading to CHF are:

- Cardiac **ischemia**
- Cardiomyopathy
- Chronic lung disease
- Valvular **regurgitation**
- Severe hypertension
- Aortic **stenosis**

Congenital Heart Disease (CHD)

Congenital heart disease is the result of abnormal development of the heart in the fetus.

Common congenital defects include:

- **Atrial septal defect (ASD).** A hole in the interatrial septum allows blood to **shunt** from the higher-pressure left atrium to the lower-pressure right atrium *(Figure 10.12)*.
- **Ventricular septal defect (VSD).** A hole in the interventricular septum allows blood to shunt from the higher-pressure left ventricle to the lower-pressure right ventricle *(see Figure 10.12)*.
- **Patent ductus arteriosus (PDA).** The ductus arteriosus is a normal blood vessel in the fetus that usually closes within 24 hours of birth. When the artery remains open (patent), blood can shunt from the aorta to the pulmonary artery, and the higher pressure causes damage to the lungs.
- **Coarctation of the aorta.** This is a narrowing of the aorta shortly after the artery to the left arm branches from the aorta. It causes **hypertension** in the arms behind the narrowing and **hypotension** in the lower limbs and organs like the kidney below the narrowing.
- **Tetralogy of Fallot (TOF).** This is a **syndrome** with four congenital heart defects. All these congenital abnormalities can be surgically repaired.

▲ **Figure 10.12** Atrial and Ventricular Septal Defects.

Abbreviations

ASD	atrial septal defect
CHD	congenital heart disease
CHF	congestive heart failure
HTN	hypertension
PDA	patent ductus arteriosus
SOB	shortness of breath
TOF	tetralogy of Fallot
VSD	ventricular septal defect

WORD	PRONUNCIATION	ELEMENTS		DEFINITION
coarctation	koh-ark-**TAY**-shun	S/ R/	-ation *process* coarct- *press together*	Constriction stenosis, particularly of the aorta
congenital	kon-**JEN**-ih-tal	S/ P/ R/	-al *pertaining to* con- *together, with* -genit- *bring forth*	Present at birth, either inherited or due to an event during gestation up to the moment of birth
defect	**DEE**-fect		Latin *to lack*	An absence, malformation, or imperfection
hypertension	**HIGH**-per-**TEN**-shun	S/ P/ R/	-ion *action, condition* hyper- *excessive* -tens- *pressure*	Persistent high arterial blood pressure
hypertensive (adj) hypotension prehypertension	**HIGH**-per-**TEN**-siv **HIGH**-poh-**TEN**-shun pree-**HIGH**-per-**TEN**-shun	S/ P/ P/	-ive *quality of* hypo- *low, below* pre- *before*	Suffering from hypertension Persistent low arterial blood pressure Precursor to hypertension
orthopnea orthopneic (adj)	or-**THOP**-nee-ah or-**THOP**-nee-ik	S/ R/CF S/	-pnea *breathe* orth/o- *straight* -ic *pertaining to*	Difficulty in breathing when lying flat Pertaining to or affected by orthopnea
patent ductus arteriosus	**PAY**-tent **DUK**-tus ar-**TEER**-ee-oh-sus		patent Latin *lie open* ductus Latin *leading* arteriosus Latin *like an artery*	An open, direct channel between the aorta and the pulmonary artery
shunt	SHUNT		Middle English *divert*	A bypass or diversion of fluid; in this case, blood
syndrome	**SIN**-drohm	P/ R/	syn- *together* -drome *running*	Combination of signs and symptoms associated with a particular disease process
tetralogy of Fallot (TOF)	teh-**TRAL**-oh-jee OV fah-**LOH**	S/ P/	-logy *study of* tetra- *four* Etienne-Louis Fallot, 1850–1911, French physician	Set of four congenital heart defects occurring together

Exercises

A. Abbreviations need to be used carefully so that you communicate exactly what is necessary. *Match the abbreviation to the correct condition described.* **LO 10.5, 10.E**

1. ASD

2. TOF

3. VSD

4. PDA

5. CHF

6. BP

7. HTN

a. force of blood pushing on the vessel walls

b. artery remains open instead of normally closing after birth

c. chronic elevated blood pressure

d. congenital heart defect that is made up of four congenital abnormalities

e. abnormal opening between the atria

f. abnormal opening between the ventricles

g. heart is unable to pump enough blood to meet the body's needs

Lesson 10.3

Circulatory Systems

Lesson Objectives

To understand the etiologies and effects of Mrs. Jones's problems (see CR 10.2) and communicate with her and Dr. Bannerjee about them, you need to have the medical terminology and knowledge to be able to:

10.3.1 Explain the functions of the peripheral circulation.

10.3.2 Identify the major arteries and veins in the body.

10.3.3 Match the structure of the different blood vessels to their functions.

10.3.4 Explain the dynamics and control of blood flow in the circulatory systems.

10.3.5 Describe the effects of common disorders of the circulatory systems on health.

Keynote

The peripheral circulation

- Transports oxygen, nutrients, hormones, and enzymes to the cells and carries carbon dioxide and waste products to the lungs, liver, and kidney for excretion.

- Maintains homeostasis by enabling cells to meet their metabolic needs and maintains a steady flow of blood and blood pressure in the tissues.

Case Report (CR) 10.2

You are

. . . a medical assistant working for Dr. Lokesh Bannerjee, a cardiologist in Fulwood Medical Center.

Your patient is

. . . Mrs. Martha Jones. You are documenting her medical record after Dr. Bannerjee has interviewed, examined, and reported his findings back to Dr. Susan Lee, who referred Mrs. Jones to Dr. Bannerjee.

Documentation:

Fulwood Medical Center
Consultation Request and Report Form

Patient's Name: Jones, MARTHA   Age: 52
To: Dr. LOKESH BANNERJEE   Department: Cardiology
From: Dr. Susan Lee   Department: Primary Care
Patient's Location: FULWOOD MEDICAL CENTER
Type of Consultation Desired:
　　☐ Consultation Only
　　☐ Consulation and follow Jointly
　　☒ Accept in Transfer
Referring Diagnoses: CLAUDICATION, POSSIBLE DVT
Reason for Consultation: Severe pain in both legs on walking

Signature: _____   Date: 12/K4/12   Time 1105 hrs
Consultation Report: by Lokesh Bannerjee
Chief complaint: Pt. c/o severe pain in both legs on walking about 100 yards or climbing a flight of stairs. Pain is so severe she must stop and wait 5 mins. before she can go on. For the past two weeks she has noticed soreness and hardness along a vein in her left calf.
Past medical history: Known type 2 diabetic with hypertension, CAD, diabetic retinopathy, and OA of her hips and knees. Several episodes of ketoacidosis and one of pulmonary edema. Bariatric surgery performed 8 months prior at 275 lbs.
Medications: metformin, verapamil, propanolol, Mevacor
Allergies: NKA
Physical examination: Ht: 5'2" Wt: 190 lbs. BP: 170/100 sitting, P: 80, regular. Both feet show slight pitting edema and skin is pale, cold, and dry. Small ulcer on lateral margin of each big toe. Varicosities, both legs. Tender cord in superficial vein of left calf. Flexion of left foot produces pain in left calf. Chest clear. Heart sounds unremarkable. No loss of sensation in legs or feet.
Impression: 1. varicose veins, both legs.
　　　　　　2. severe claudication, both legs.
　　　　　　3. probable deep vein thrombosis, left leg
　　　　　　4. possible peripheral neuropathy
　　　　　　5. H/o diabetes type 2, CAD, hypertension, retinopathy, OA
Plan: Admit patient to cardiology unit stat for IV heparin and conversion to oral anticoagulant therapy with Coumadin. Doppler studies, venogram, and angiogram have been ordered.

Signature: _____   Date 12/K4/12   Time 1250 hrs

WORD	PRONUNCIATION		ELEMENTS	DEFINITION
artery	**AR**-ter-ee		Greek *artery*	Thick-walled blood vessel carrying blood away from the heart
brachiocephalic	**BRAY**-kee-oh-seh-**FAL**-ik	S/ R/CF R/	**-ic** *pertaining to* **brachi/o-** *arm* **-cephal-** *head*	Pertaining to the head and arm, as an artery supplying blood to both
carotid	kah-**ROT**-id		Greek *carotid artery*	Main artery of the neck
circulation	**SER**-kyu-**LAY**-shun		Latin *to encircle*	Continuous movement of blood through the heart and blood vessels
peripheral	peh-**RIF**-er-al	S/ R/	**-al** *pertaining to* **peripher-** *outer part*	Pertaining to a part of the body away from a central point. For example, the peripheral circulation is away from the heart
popliteal	pop-**LIT**-ee-al	S/ R/CF	**-al** *pertaining to* **poplit/e-** *back of knee*	Pertaining to the back of the knee
pulmonary	**PULL**-moh-**NAIR**-ee	S/ R/	**-ary** *pertaining to* **pulmon-** *lung*	Pertaining to the lungs and their blood supply
subclavian	sub-**CLAY**-vee-an	S/ P/ R/	**-ian** *one who does* **sub-** *under* **-clav-** *clavicle*	Underneath the clavicle

Exercises

A. Proper pronunciation of terms is key to verbal communication. *Choose the answer that correctly completes each statement.* **LO 10.B**

1. In the combining form *brachi/o*, the vowel *i* is pronounced like the vowel in:

    a. key   **b.** eye   **c.** sick   **d.** rate

2. When pronouncing the term *popliteal*, emphasis is put on the syllable:

    a. pop   **b.** lit   **c.** ee   **d.** al

3. The first syllable in the term *carotid* sounds like the first syllable in the term:

    a. cat   **b.** carrot   **c.** cousin   **d.** cake

B. Blood travels through the body in a system of connected tubes called blood vessels. *Below are sentences that describe this system. Use the words provided to correctly fill in the blanks.* **LO 10.6, 10.A**

    circulation   peripheral   artery   pulmonary

The body has a system that moves blood to all of the organs. This system that delivers blood to the body's organs is called the systemic (1)_____. This circulation delivers oxygen-rich blood to the (2) _____ organs which include the arms and legs. The (3) _____ system delivers blood to the lungs to pick up oxygen and get rid of carbon dioxide. Any vessel that carries blood away from the heart is called an (4) _____.

LO 10.6 Blood Circulation Systems

There are two major **circulations**: the **pulmonary** and the **systemic**.

Pulmonary Circulation

Deoxygenated blood from the body flows into the right atrium of the heart and then into the right ventricle, which pumps it out into the pulmonary trunk *(Figure 10.13)*. This trunk branches into the right pulmonary **artery** to the right lung and the left pulmonary artery to the left lung. Gas exchange occurs between the air in the lungs and blood *(see Chapter 13)*. Carbon dioxide is removed from the blood and excreted into the air. Oxygen is taken into the blood from the air in the lungs.

The blood exits each lung through two pulmonary veins. All four pulmonary veins take blood into the left atrium of the heart.

Systemic Arterial Circulation

The systemic circulation *(Figures 10.13 and 10.14)* refers to the process wherein oxygenated blood enters the left side of the heart from the pulmonary veins. The blood passes through the left atrium into the left ventricle. The ventricle pumps it out into the **aorta**, which takes the blood to all areas of the body. The **coronary circulation** takes blood to and away from the myocardium. The **peripheral** vessels are those that carry blood to and from the other body tissues.

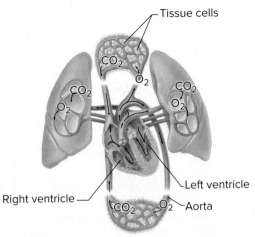

Tissue cells

Right ventricle

Left ventricle

Aorta

▲ **Figure 10.13** Systemic and Pulmonary Circulations.

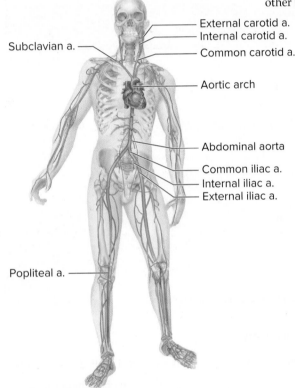

- External carotid a.
- Internal carotid a.
- Common carotid a.
- Subclavian a.
- Aortic arch
- Abdominal aorta
- Common iliac a.
- Internal iliac a.
- External iliac a.
- Popliteal a.

▲ **Figure 10.14** The Major Systemic Arteries.
(a. = artery)

The aorta is described in four parts:

1. **Ascending aorta,** which gives rise to the coronary circulation. Right and left coronary arteries branch from it to supply the myocardium.

2. **Aortic arch** *(Figure 10.14)*, which has three main branches:
   a. **Brachiocephalic artery,** a short artery that divides into two arteries:
      i. **Right common carotid artery,** which supplies the right side of the head, brain, and neck.
      ii. **Right subclavian artery,** which supplies the right upper limb.
   b. **Left common carotid artery,** which supplies the left side of the head, brain, and neck. The right and left common carotid arteries divide into two branches:
      i. The **internal carotid** artery, which enters the cranial cavity through a foramen in the base of the skull and supplies the brain.
      ii. The **external carotid** artery, which supplies the neck and face.
   c. **Left subclavian artery,** which supplies the left upper limb.

3. **Thoracic aorta,** which has two major groups of branches:
   a. **Visceral** branches—small **bronchial arteries** that supply the bronchi and bronchioles *(see Chapter 13)*, the esophagus, and the pericardium.
   b. **Parietal** branches—**intercostal arteries** that supply the chest wall and a **phrenic artery** that supplies the diaphragm.

4. **Abdominal aorta,** which has two major groups of branches:
   a. **Visceral branches** that supply the abdominal organs:
      i **Celiac trunk,** which supplies the stomach, liver, gallbladder, pancreas, and spleen.
      ii. **Superior mesenteric artery,** which supplies the small intestine and part of the large intestine.
      iii. **Inferior mesenteric artery,** which supplies the remainder of the large intestine.
      iv. Paired **renal arteries,** which supply the kidneys and adrenal glands.
      v. Paired **gonadal arteries,** which supply the testes or ovaries.
   b. Four pairs of **lumbar** arteries that supply the abdominal wall.

At the level of the fifth lumbar vertebra (at the top of the pelvis), the aorta divides into the right and left **common iliac arteries.** Visceral branches from these arteries supply the urinary bladder, uterus, and vagina. The common iliac arteries give off an internal iliac artery to supply the pelvis. The common iliac artery becomes the external iliac artery and then the femoral artery as it goes down the thigh and supplies the lower limb. The pulse that can be felt in the back of the knee is from the **popliteal artery.**

WORD	PRONUNCIATION	ELEMENTS		DEFINITION
bronchus bronchi (pl)	**BRONG**-kus		Latin *windpipe*	One of the two subdivisions of the trachea
bronchial	**BRONG**-key-al	S/ R/CF	**al** *pertaining to* **bronch/i** *bronchus*	Pertaining to the bronchi
gonad gonadal (adj)	**GO**-nad go-**NAD**-al		Greek *seed*	Testis or ovary Pertaining to a testis or ovary
iliac	**ILL**-ee-ak		Latin *groin, flank*	Pertaining to, or near, the ilium (pelvic bone)
lumbar	**LUM**-bar		Latin *loin*	Relating to the region in the back and sides between the ribs and pelvis
mesentery	**MESS**-en-ter-ee	P/ R/	**mes-** *middle* **-entery** *intestine*	A double layer peritoneum enclosing the abdominal viscera
mesenteric (adj)	**MESS**-enter-ree	S/	**-ic** *pertaining to*	Pertaining to the mesentery
renal	**REE**-nal	S/ R/	**-al** *pertaining to* **ren-** *kidney*	Pertaining to the kidney
subclavian	sub-**CLAY**-vee-an	S/ P/ R/	**-ian** *one who does* **sub-** *under* **-clav-** *clavicle*	Underneath and behind the clavicle
visceral	**VISS**-er-al	S/ R/	**-al** *pertaining to* **viscer-** *an organ*	Pertaining to the internal organs

Exercises

A. Use the medical terminology of the circulatory system. *Select the correct answer to complete each statement.* **LO 10.6, 10.A**

1. The blood exits each lung through the
   a. vena cava   b. pulmonary veins   c. aorta   d. pulmonary arteries

2. The *coronary circulation* arises in the
   a. thoracic aorta   b. carotid arteries   c. ascending aorta   d. subclavian arteries

3. *Carbon dioxide* is removed from the blood and excreted through
   a. dehydration   b. inspiration   c. inhalation   d. expiration

4. *Deoxygenated blood* from the body flows into the
   a. right atrium   b. right ventricle   c. left atrium   d. left ventricle

5. *Gas exchange* occurs between the air in the lungs and the
   a. heart   b. blood   c. ventricles   d. windpipe

6. The pulse that can be felt at the back of the knee is from the
   a. aorta   b. popliteal vein   c. carotid artery   d. popliteal artery

7. The _____ arteries supply the chest wall.
   a. phrenic   b. visceral   c. intercostal   d. mesenteric

8. This circulation takes blood to all areas of the body
   a. coronary   b. pulmonary   c. cardiovascular   d. systemic

9. The *subclavian* artery is located
   a. above the heart   b. below the stomach   c. above the neck   d. below the collarbone

10. The _____ circulation takes blood to the lungs to become oxygenated.
    a. systemic   b. pulmonary   c. coronary   d. carotid

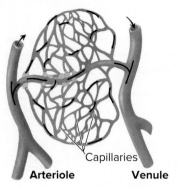

Capillaries

Arteriole   **Venule**

▲ **Figure 10.15** Capillary Bed.

LO 10.7 Blood Vessels in the Circulations

Arterioles, Capillaries, and Venules

As the arteries branch farther away from the heart and distribute blood to specific organs, they become smaller, muscular vessels called **arterioles**. By contracting and relaxing, these arterioles are the primary controllers by which the body directs the relative amounts of blood that organs and structures receive.

From there, the blood flows into **capillaries** and **capillary beds** *(Figure 10.15)*. There are approximately 10 billion capillaries in the body. Each capillary consists of only a single layer of **endothelium** supported by a thin connective tissue basement membrane. Between the overlapping **endothelial** cells are thin slits through which larger water-soluble substances can pass. Red blood cells flow through the small capillaries in single file.

From the capillaries, tiny **venules** accept the blood and merge to form **veins**. The veins form reservoirs for blood; at any moment 60% to 70% of the total blood volume is contained in the venules and veins.

The circulatory system exists to serve the capillaries because capillaries are the only place where water and materials are exchanged between the blood and tissue fluids.

Diffusion is the means by which this capillary exchange occurs. Nutrients and oxygen diffuse from a higher concentration in the capillaries to a lower concentration in the **interstitial** fluid around the cells. Waste products diffuse from a higher concentration in the interstitial fluid to a lower concentration in the capillaries.

External jugular v.
Internal jugular v.
Subclavian v.
Brachiocephalic v.

Brachial v.
Superior vena cava

Inferior vena cava

Common iliac v.

Femoral v.

Great saphenous v.

▲ **Figure 10.16** The Major Systemic Veins. (*v.* = vein)

Systemic Venous Circulation

There are three major types of veins *(Figure 10.16)*:

1. **Superficial**—such as those you can see under the skin of your arms and hands.
2. **Deep**—running parallel to arteries and draining the same tissues that the arteries supply.
3. **Venous sinuses**—in the head and heart and having specific functions.

In the lower limb, the superficial veins merge to form the **saphenous vein.** The deep veins form the **femoral vein.** They join together with veins from the pelvis to form the **common iliac vein.** The right and left common iliac veins form the **inferior vena cava (IVC).**

Veins draining the abdominal organs merge into the **hepatic portal vein,** which delivers nutrients from the stomach and intestines to the liver. Within the liver, the nutrients are either stored or converted into chemicals that can be used by other cells in the body. The blood leaves the liver in **hepatic veins** that drain into the IVC.

In the upper limb, the superficial veins merge to form the **axillary vein.** The deep veins alongside the limb arteries empty into the **brachial veins.** These also flow into the axillary vein.

As the axillary vein passes behind the clavicle, its name changes to the **subclavian vein.**

In the head and neck, the superficial veins outside the skull drain into the right and left **external jugular veins.** Inside the cranial cavity, **venous sinuses** around the brain drain into the right and left **internal jugular veins.**

The external jugular veins empty into the subclavian veins. The internal jugular veins join with the subclavian veins on each side to form the **brachiocephalic veins.** The right and left brachiocephalic veins join together to form the **superior vena cava (SVC).** The SVC empties into the right atrium.

Abbreviations	
IVC	inferior vena cava
SVC	superior vena cava

S = Suffix   P = Prefix   R = Root   R/CF = Combining Form

WORD	PRONUNCIATION	ELEMENTS		DEFINITION
arteriole	ar-**TEER**-ee-ole	S/ R/	-ole *small* arteri- *artery*	Small terminal artery leading into the capillary network
axilla axillary (adj)	**AK**-sill-ah **AK**-sil-air-ee	S/ R/	Latin *armpit* -ary *pertaining to* axill- *armpit*	Medical name for the armpit Pertaining to the axilla
brachial	**BRAY**-kee-al	S/ R/	-al *pertaining to* brachi- *arm*	Pertaining to the arm
capillary	**KAP**-ih-lair-ee	S/ R/	-ary *pertaining to* capill- *hairlike structure*	Minute blood vessel between the arterial and venous systems
endothelial	en-doh-**THEE**-lee-al	S/ P/ R/	-al *pertaining to* endo- *inside, within* -theli- *lining*	A type of epithelial cell that lines the inside of blood vessels, lymphatic vessels, and the heart
endothelium	en-doh-**THEE**-lee-um	S/	-um *structure*	Tissue found lining the inside of blood vessels and lymphatic vessels
femoral	**FEM**-oh-ral	S/ R/	-al *pertaining to* femor- *femur*	Pertaining to the femur
interstitial	in-ter-**STISH**-al	S/ R/	-ial *pertaining to* interstit- *spaces within tissues*	Pertaining to spaces between cells in a tissue or organ
jugular	**JUG**-you-lar	S/ R/	-ar *pertaining to* jugul- *throat*	Pertaining to the throat
saphenous	**SAF**-ih-nus		Arabic *hidden, concealed*	Relating to the saphenous vein in the thigh
vein venous (adj)	VANE **VEE**-nuss	S/ R/	Latin *vein* -ous *pertaining to* ven- *vein*	Blood vessel carrying blood toward the heart Pertaining to venous blood or the venous circulation
venule	**VEN**-yule	S/	-ule *small*	Small vein leading from the capillary network

Exercises

A. Identify the meanings of the word elements. *Choose the correct answer that relates to the definitions of word elements.* **LO 10.7, 10.D**

1. Identify a suffix listed below that means *small*:

   a. -ary   **b.** -ial   **c.** -ery   **d.** -ule

2. In the term **femoral,** the root is

   a. -al   **b.** fem-   **c.** fem/o   **d.** femor-   **e.** -oral

3. The root *jugul-* means

   a. neck   **b.** head   **c.** throat   **d.** large

B. Identify the medical term for each of the following descriptions. *Fill in the blanks.* **LO 10.6, 10.7, 10.A**

1. Write the term that means *small vein:* _____.

2. Write the term that means *small artery:* _____.

3. The only type of vessel where diffusion of gases between tissues and blood takes place (singular): _____.

4. The two large veins in the neck are the _____ veins.

Endothelium of
tunica interna

Middle layer
(tunica media)

Lumen

Lumen

Outer layer
(tunica externa)

(a)   (b)

▲ **Figure 10.17** Anatomy of an Artery and Vein.

(a) Artery. (b) Vein. ©CNRI/Photo Researchers, Inc.

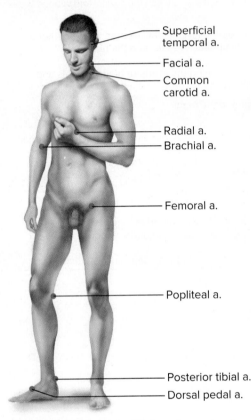

Superficial
temporal a.

Facial a.

Common
carotid a.

Radial a.

Brachial a.

Femoral a.

Popliteal a.

Posterior tibial a.

Dorsal pedal a.

▲ **Figure 10.18** Arterial Pulses. (a. = artery)

LO 10.7 Blood Vessel Function Related to Structure

Except for the capillaries and venules, all the blood vessel walls show a basic structure of three layers *(Figure 10.17)*:

1. **Tunica intima** (interna)—the innermost layer of endothelial cells, with thin layers of fibrous and elastic connective tissue supporting them.

2. Tunica **media**—a middle layer of smooth muscle cells arranged circularly around the blood vessel. A membrane of elastic tissue separates the tunica media from the outer layer of the wall.

3. Tunica **adventitia** (externa)—an outer connective tissue layer of varying density and thickness.

The larger arteries near the heart, the aorta and its major branches, have to cope with large quantities of blood and fluctuating pressures between systole and diastole. Therefore, these arteries have a large number of elastic fibers and a relatively small number of muscle fibers.

The functions of the medium-sized and smaller arteries are to regulate the blood supply to the different regions of the body and to ensure that the blood pressure in the arteries is at an appropriate level. The tunica media of these arteries contains 25 to 40 layers of smooth muscle to enable the muscles to contract (**vasoconstriction**) and to relax (**vasodilation**) to increase flow.

The function of the veins is to return the blood from the periphery to the heart in a low-pressure system. For example, by the time blood reaches the venules, its pressure has dropped from the 120 mm Hg of systole to around 15 mm Hg. By the time the blood is in the venae cavae, the **central venous pressure (CVP)** is down to around 4 to 5 mm Hg.

Veins have a much thinner tunica media than arteries, with few muscle cells and elastic fibers *(Figure 10.17)*. They have a larger lumen and a thick tunica adventitia that merges with the connective tissue of surrounding structures. In the limbs, the veins are surrounded and massaged by muscles to squeeze the blood along the veins. One-way valves in the veins allow the blood to flow toward the heart but not away from the heart. They are shaped like and function like the semilunar valves of the heart.

Space Medicine

Normally, gravity helps the blood circulate in the lower limbs. When astronauts are weightless for long periods of time, blood pools in the central and upper areas of the body, and there appears to be an excess blood volume. The kidney compensates by excreting more fluid, leading to a 10% to 20% decrease in blood volume and a low blood pressure. Astronauts compensate for this by wearing lower-body suction suits, which apply a vacuum force to draw blood into the lower limbs.

Arterial Pulses

The pulse is always part of a clinical examination because it can show heart rate, rhythm, and the state of the arterial wall by **palpation**. There are nine locations on each side of the body where large arteries are close to the surface and can be palpated *(Figure 10.18)*.

The most easily accessible is the **radial artery** at the wrist, where the pulse is usually taken. The **brachial artery** at the elbow is also used for taking blood pressure readings. All the pulse sites can be used as **pressure points** to temporarily reduce arterial bleeding in an emergency.

The two pulses that can be palpated in the feet are the **pedal** pulses, one in each foot.

Blood Pressure

Blood pressure (BP) is the force the blood exerts on arterial walls as it is pumped around the circulatory system by the left ventricle.

WORD	PRONUNCIATION		ELEMENTS	DEFINITION
adventitia	ad-ven-**TISH**-ah		Latin *from outside*	Outer layer of connective tissue covering blood vessels or organs
intima	**IN**-tih-ma		Latin *inmost*	Inner layer of a structure, particularly a blood vessel
media	**MEE**-dee-ah		Latin *middle*	Middle layer of a structure, particularly a blood vessel
pedal	**PEED**-al	S/ R/	**-al** *pertaining to* **ped-** *foot*	Pertaining to the foot
radial	**RAY**-dee-al	S/ R/	**-al** *pertaining to* **radi-** *radius (forearm bone)*	Pertaining to the forearm
tunica	**TYU**-nih-kah		Latin *coat*	A layer in the wall of a blood vessel or other tubular structure
vasoconstriction	**VAY**-soh-con-**STRIK**-shun	S/ R/CF R/	**-ion** *process* **vas/o-** *blood vessel* **-constrict-** *narrow*	Reduction in diameter of a blood vessel
vasodilation	**VAY**-soh-die-**LAY**-shun	S/ R/CF R/	**-ion** *process* **vas/o-** *blood vessel* **-dilat-** *open up*	Increase in diameter of a blood vessel
vital signs	**VIE**-tal SIGNS		**vital** Latin *life* **signs** Latin *mark*	A procedure during a physical examination in which temperature, pulse rate, respiration rate, and blood pressure are measured to assess general health and cardiorespiratory function

Exercises

A. Match the definition in the left column with the correct medical term in the right column. LO 10.7

_____ 1. Pertaining to the forearm

_____ 2. Reduction in diameter of a blood vessel

_____ 3. Inner layer of a structure

_____ 4. Latin for *coat*

_____ 5. Outer tissue covering of an organ

_____ 6. Middle layer of a structure

_____ 7. Pertaining to the foot

_____ 8. Increase in diameter of a blood vessel

a. radial

b. vasodilation

c. adventitia

d. pedal

e. vasoconstriction

f. media

g. intima

h. tunica

Case Report (CR) 10.2 *(continued)*

Mrs. Martha Jones, who had been referred to Dr. Bannerjee's cardiovascular clinic, has several circulatory problems related to her diabetes and obesity. She was diagnosed previously with hypertension, CAD, and diabetic retinopathy. She now has severe pain in her legs when walking.

Her **ankle/brachial index (ABI),** which measures the ratio of the blood pressure in her ankle to that in her arm, showed significant blockage of blood flow. Doppler studies confirmed this. This blockage produces the pain when walking (intermittent **claudication**). It is due to arteriosclerosis of the large arteries in her legs. Angiograms showed several atherosclerotic areas in her popliteal artery.

The ulcers on the edges of her big toes result from thickening of the walls of her capillaries and arterioles and the resulting poor circulation to her feet. Again, this is due to her diabetes.

In the venous system of her legs, the tender cordlike lesion is due to **thrombophlebitis** of a superficial vein in her left leg.

Pain in the calf on flexion of the ankle (Homans sign) indicates that she may have **deep vein thrombosis (DVT).** A venogram confirmed this diagnosis.

▲ Figure 10.19 Varicose Veins of Leg.
©Dr. P. Marazzi/Photo Researchers, Inc.

Abbreviations

ABI	ankle/brachial index
DVT	deep vein thrombosis
PVD	peripheral vascular disease

LO 10.8 Circulatory Disorders

Disorders of Veins

Phlebitis is an inflammation of a vein. There are many causes for phlebitis, including venous infections and the presence of an intravenous (IV) catheter.

Thrombophlebitis is an inflammation of the lining of a vein (tunica intima), allowing clots (thrombi) to form.

Deep vein thrombosis (DVT) is thrombus formation in a deep vein, often due to reduced blood flow. Risk factors include immobility, surgery, prolonged travel, and contraception (estrogen). The increased pressure in the capillaries due to back pressure from the blocked blood flow in the veins causes an increase in the flow of fluid from the capillaries to the interstitial spaces. The collection of fluid is called **edema**.

A major complication of thrombus formation is that a piece of the clot can break off and be carried in the bloodstream to lodge in a blood vessel in another organ and block blood flow. The piece that breaks off is called an **embolus** or **thromboembolism**. It often lodges in the lungs, producing pulmonary embolus *(see Chapter 13).*

Varicose veins are superficial veins that have lost their elasticity and appear swollen and tortuous *(Figure 10.19).* Their valves become incompetent, and blood flows backward and pools. Smaller, more superficial varicose veins are called **spider veins**. Varicose veins are associated with a family history, obesity, and prolonged standing. **Collateral** circulations develop to take the blood through alternative routes.

LO 10.8 Disorders of Arteries

Peripheral vascular disease (PVD) is a general term describing all the disorders of the systemic arterial and venous systems.

An **aneurysm** is a localized dilation of an artery as a result of a localized weakness of the vessel wall. Common sites occur along the aorta, mostly the abdominal aorta. They can rupture, leading to severe bleeding and hypovolemic shock.

Intracranial aneurysms, particularly at the base of the brain, are an important cause of bleeds into the cranial cavity *(see Chapter 9).*

Thromboangiitis obliterans (Buerger disease) is an inflammatory disease of the arteries with clot formation, usually in the legs. The occlusion of arteries and impaired circulation leads to intermittent claudication.

Carotid artery disease affects the two major arteries supplying the brain. They can be involved in **arteriosclerosis** and the deposition of plaque, which puts the patient at risk for a stroke.

WORD	PRONUNCIATION		ELEMENTS	DEFINITION
aneurysm	**AN**-yur-izm		Greek *dilation*	Circumscribed dilation of an artery or cardiac chamber
claudication	klaw-dih-**KAY**-shun	S/ R/	**-ation** *process* **claudic-** *limping*	Intermittent leg pain and limping
collateral	koh-**LAT**-er-al	S/ P/ R/	**-al** *pertaining to* **col-** *before* **-later-** *at the side*	Situated at the side, often to bypass an obstruction
edema edematous (adj) pitting edema	ee-**DEE**-mah ee-**DEM**-ah-tus **PIT**-ing ee-**DEE**-mah	S/ R/	Greek *swelling* **-tous** *pertaining to* **edema-** *swelling, edema*	Excessive accumulation of fluid in cells and tissues Pertaining to or marked by edema Edema that maintains indentations made by applying pressure to the area for a time
embolus emboli (pl)	**EM**-boh-lus		Greek *plug, stopped*	Detached piece of thrombus, a mass of bacteria, quantity of air, or foreign body that blocks a blood vessel
peripheral	peh-**RIF**-er-al	S/ R/	**-al** *pertaining to* **peripher-** *outer part*	Pertaining to the periphery or an external boundary
phlebitis	fleh-**BIE**-tis	S/ R/	**-itis** *inflammation* **phleb-** *vein*	Inflammation of a vein
thromboembolism	**THROM**-boh-**EM**-boh-lizm	S/ R/CF R/	**-ism** *condition* **thromb/o-** *clot* **-embol-** *plug*	A piece of detached blood clot (embolus) blocking a distant blood vessel
thrombophlebitis	**THROM**-boh-fleh-**BIE**-tis	S/ R/CF R/	**-itis** *inflammation* **thromb/o-** *clot* **-phleb-** *vein*	Inflammation of a vein with clot formation
thrombus thrombosis	**THROM**-bus throm-**BOH**-sis	S/ R/ S/	**-us** *pertaining to* **thromb-** *clot* **-osis** *condition*	A clot attached to a diseased blood vessel or heart lining Formation of a thrombus

Exercises

A. Apply the language of the cardiovascular system. *Select the best answer to complete each statement.* **LO 10.7, 10.8, 10.D**

1. The suffix tells you that **thrombophlebitis** is a(n)
   a. puncture   **b.** inflammation   **c.** excision   **d.** vein

2. Collateral means
   a. at the front   **b.** in the middle   **c.** at the side

3. The combining form *phleb/o-* means
   a. artery   **b.** vein   **c.** capillary

4. The combining form *scler/o-* describes a
   a. softening   **b.** clotting   **c.** hardening   **d.** constriction

5. The symptom of **edema** is a
   a. rash   **b.** swelling   **c.** lesion

6. Aneurysm describes a blood vessel that is
   a. dilated   **b.** constricted   **c.** collapsed   **d.** obstructed

7. The roots tell you that **thromboembolism** is a(n)
   a. clot or plug   **b.** tear or rupture   **c.** swelling or lesion   **d.** vein or artery

8. The combining form *thromb/o-* means
   a. clot   **b.** lump   **c.** plug   **d.** vein

Cardiovascular Procedures and Pharmacology

LO 10.9 Cardiovascular Diagnostic Tests

Blood Tests

Lipid profile helps determine the risk of CAD and comprises:

- **Total cholesterol**
- **High-density lipoprotein (HDL)** ("good cholesterol")
- **Low-density lipoprotein (LDL)** ("bad cholesterol")
- **Triglycerides**

The following are chemical indicators used as risk factors in the diagnosis and monitoring of cardiovascular diseases:

- **B-type natriuretic peptide (BNP),** a brain hormone, is used to diagnose and monitor congestive heart failure and to predict the course of end-stage heart failure.

- **C-reactive protein (CRP),** produced by the endothelial cells of arteries, when elevated, has been identified as a risk factor for atherosclerosis and CAD.

- **Homocysteine** is an amino acid in the blood. Elevated levels are related to a higher risk of CAD, stroke, and peripheral vascular disease.

- **Creatine kinase (CK)** is an enzyme released into the blood by dead myocardial cells in MI.

- **Troponin I and T** are part of a protein complex in muscle that is released into the blood during myocardial injury. Troponin I is found in heart muscle but not in skeletal muscle. Its presence in blood is therefore a highly sensitive indicator of a recent MI. Both CK and Troponin I and T are used to confirm a suspected MI.

WORD	PRONUNCIATION	ELEMENTS		DEFINITION
cholesterol	koh-**LESS**-ter-ol	S/ R/CF	-sterol *steroid* chol/e- *bile*	Steroid formed in liver cells which circulates in the plasma
creatine kinase	**KREE**-ah-teen **KI**-nase	S/ R/ S/ R/	-ine *pertaining to* creat- *flesh* -ase *enzyme* kin- *motion*	Enzyme elevated in the plasma following heart muscle damage
electrode	ee-**LEK**-trode	S/ R/	-ode *way, road* electr- *electricity*	A device for conducting electricity
homocysteine	ho-moh-**SIS**-teen	P/ R/	homo- *same* cysteine *an amino acid*	An amino acid similar to cysteine
lipid	**LIP**-id		**Greek** *fat*	General term for all types of fatty compounds
lipoprotein	**LIE**-poh-pro-teen	R/CF R/	lip/o- *fat* -protein *protein*	Molecules made of combinations of fat and protein
natriuretic peptide	**NAH**-tree-you-**RET**-ik **PEP**-tide	S/ R/CF R/ S/ R/	-ic *pertaining to* natr/i *sodium* -uret- *ureter* -ide *particular quality* pept- *amino acid*	Protein that increases the excretion of sodium by the kidney
profile	**PRO**-file	S/ R/	pro- *forward* -file *contour, line*	A set of characteristics which determine the structure of a group
triglyceride	try-**GLISS**-eh-ride	S/ P/ R/	-ide *having a particular quality* tri- *three* -glycer- *glycerol*	Any of a group of fats containing three fatty acids
troponin	**TROH**-po-nin	S/ R/	-onin *chemical substance* trop(h)- *nourishment*	A protein complex found in myocardial muscle fibers and released into the blood within 4 hours of myocardial damage

Exercises

A. Describe blood tests that aid in the diagnosis of heart disease. *Match the term in the first column with its correct description in the second column.* **LO 10.9, 10.E**

Term

_____ 1. CK

_____ 2. HDL

_____ 3. LDL

_____ 4. BNP

_____ 5. CRP

Meaning

a. "good" cholesterol

b. "bad" cholesterol

c. used to diagnose and monitor congestive heart failure

d. produced by the endothelial cells of the arteries

e. enzyme released by dead myocardial cells.

LO 10.9 Diagnostic Tests

1. **Auscultation** via a **stethoscope** is used to listen to the sounds of the heart during the cardiac cycle. A **murmur** can be heard when blood flows against a restriction, such as a stenosed or incompetent valve. A **bruit** can be auscultated over an area of restricted blood flow, such as a plaque in an artery.

2. Arterial blood pressure is measured with a **sphygomanometer** and a stethoscope.

3. An instrument called an **electrocardiograph** picks up the electrical changes in the heart muscle and amplifies them to record an **electrocardiogram (ECG or EKG)** in the form of five waves *[Figure 10.20]*. The waves are labeled P, Q, R, S, and T.

4. **Cardiac stress testing** is an exercise tolerance test to raise your heart rate and monitor the effect on cardiac function. **Nuclear imaging** of the heart, using an injection of a radioactive substance, can be used with the stress test.

5. A **Holter monitor** is a continuous ECG recorded on a digital recording device as you work, play, and rest for 24 to 48 hours. The patient keeps a diary of all symptoms and activities so that the data on the monitor can be correlated with symptoms and activities.

6. **Persantine/thallium exercise testing** is used for people unable to engage in physical exercise. It combines nuclear imaging with a drug that increases the demand on the heart.

7. **Echocardiography** uses ultrasound waves to study cardiac function at rest. The test is performed by a **sonographer**, who places a **transducer** on the patient's chest. A stress echocardiogram is performed after the patient has exercised on a treadmill.

8. **Transesophageal echocardiography (TEE)** involves insertion of a small probe into the esophagus to record the anatomy and function of heart valves.

9. An **event monitor** is used for patients whose symptoms occur sporadically. A monitor is held over the chest when an event occurs. The data are stored and transmitted by telephone to a monitoring station.

10. An **ambulatory blood pressure monitor** provides a record of your BP over a 24-hour period as you go about your daily activities.

11. **Electron beam tomography (EBT)** is a scan that identifies calcium deposits in arteries.

12. **Cardiac catheterization** detects patterns of pressures and blood flows in the heart. A thin tube is guided into the heart under x-ray guidance after being inserted into a vein or artery.

13. **Coronary angiogram** *[Figure 10.21]* uses a contrast dye injected during cardiac catheterization to identify coronary artery blockages.

14. A **venogram** is a radiograph (x-ray record) of a vein. It is used to view the blood flow through the veins.

15. **Color Doppler ultrasonography** uses high-frequency sound (ultrasound) waves to show different rates of blood flow through the heart and blood vessels.

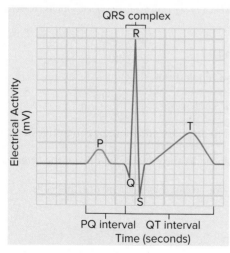

▲ **Figure 10.20** Normal Electrocardiogram.

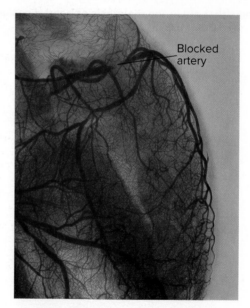

▲ **Figure 10.21** Coronary angiogram showing blocked artery. ©SPL/Photo Researchers, Inc.

WORD	PRONUNCIATION		ELEMENTS	DEFINITION
angiogram	**AN**-jee-oh-gram	S/ R/CF	**-gram** *a record* **angio-** *blood vessel*	Radiograph obtained after injection of radiopaque contrast material into blood vessels
auscultation	aws-kul-**TAY**-shun	S/ R/	**-ation** *process* **auscult-** *listen to*	Diagnostic method of listening to body sounds with a stethoscope
catheter	**KATH**-eh-ter		**Greek** *to send down*	Hollow tube that allows passage of fluid into or out of a body cavity, organ or blood vessel
catheterize (verb) catheterization (**Note:** 3 suffixes)	**KATH**-eh-ter-**RIZE**	S/ S/ R/ S/	**-ize** *action* **-er-** *agent* **cathet-** *catheter* **-ation** *process*	To introduce a catheter Introduction of a catheter
Doppler	**DOP**-ler		Johann Christian Doppler, 1803–1853 Austrian physicist	Diagnostic instrument that sends an ultrasonic beam into the body
ultrasonography	**ULL**-trah-soh-**NOG**-rah-fee	S/ P/ R/CF	**-graphy** *process of recording* **ultra-** *beyond* **-son/o** *sound*	ImagingR that detects direction, velocity and turbulence of blood flow
electrocardiogram	ee-**LEK**-troh-**KAR**-dee-oh-gram	S/ R/CF R/CF	**-gram** *record* **electro-** *electricity* **-cardi/o-** *heart*	Record of the electrical signals of the heart.
electrocardiograph	ee-**LEK**-troh-**KAR**-dee-oh-graph	S/	**-graph-** *to record*	Machine that makes the electrocardiogram
electrocardiography	ee-**LEK**-troh-**KAR**-dee-**OG**-rah-fee	S/	**-graphy** *process of recording*	The process of making an electrocardiogram
echocardiogram	**ECK**-oh-**KAR**-dee-oh-gram	S/ R/CF R/CF	**-gram** *record* **ech/o-** *sound wave* **-cardi/o** *heart*	Ultrasound recording of heart function
murmur	**MUR**-mur		**Latin** *low voice*	Abnormal sound heard on auscultation of the heart or blood vessels
sphygmomanometer	**SFIG**-moh-mah-**NOM**-ih-ter	S/ R/CF R/CF	**-meter** *instrument to measure* **sphygmo-** *pulse* **-man/o-** *pressure*	Instrument to measure arterial blood pressure
tomography	toe-**MOG**-rah-fee	S/ R/CF	**-graphy** *process of recording* **tom/o** *section, slice*	Radiographic image of a selected slice of tissue
venogram	**VEE**-no-gram	S/ R/CF	**-gram** *a record* **ven/o-** *vein*	Radiograph of vein after injection of radiopaque image

Exercises

A. Build your language of cardiology by completing the following documentation. *There is only one best answer for each blank.*
Fill in the blanks. **LO 10.9, 10.A, 10.E**

electrode   electrocardiogram   electrocardiograph   electrocardiography

The patient was scheduled for (1) _____ today. The CVT attached the (2) _____ to the patient's chest
and proceeded to turn on the (3) _____. Unfortunately, a malfunction of the machine prevented him from obtaining
the (4) _____. This study will have to be rescheduled for the patient.

B. Build your language of cardiology by completing the following documentation. *There is only one best answer for each blank. Fill in the blanks.*

catheter   catheterization   catheterize

The cardiologist performed coronary artery (1) _____ to determine if the patient had any coronary artery blockage.

A cardiac (2) _____ was inserted into the patient's left coronary artery. The cardiologist will also

(3) _____ right coronary artery to determine if a blockage exists there.

LO 10.10 Cardiovascular Treatment Procedures

The most immediate need in the treatment of MI is to provide perfusion to get blood and oxygen to the affected myocardium. This can be attempted in several ways:

1. **Clot-busting drugs (thrombolysis)**. Streptokinase or tissue plasminogen activator **(tPA)** are injected within a few hours of the MI to dissolve the thrombus.

2. **Artery-cleaning angioplasty** also called **percutaneous transluminal coronary angioplasty** (PTCA). A balloon-tipped catheter is guided to the site of the blockage and inflated to expand the artery from the inside by compressing the plaque against the walls of the artery.

3. **Stent placement.** To reduce the likelihood that the artery will close up again (occlude), a wire mesh tube, or stent *(Figure 10.22)*, is placed inside the vessel. Some stents (**drug-eluting** stents) are covered with a special medication to help keep the artery open.

▲ **Figure 10.22** Stent.
©Clouds Hill Imaging Ltd./Photo Researchers, Inc.

4. **Coronary artery bypass graft (CABG).** In this procedure, mostly used for people with extensive disease in several arteries, healthy blood vessels harvested from the leg, chest, or arm detour blood around blocked coronary arteries. The procedure is performed by using a heart-lung machine that pumps the recipient's blood through the machine to oxygenate it while surgery is performed. More recently, the procedure is being performed "off-pump" with the heart still beating.

5. **Rotational atherectomy.** A high-speed rotational device is used to "sand" away plaque. This procedure has limited acceptance.

6. **Heart transplant,** in which the heart of a recently deceased person (donor) is transplanted to the recipient after the recipient's diseased heart has been removed. The immune characteristics of the donor and recipient have to be a close match.

Procedures used in cardiology to treat arrhythmias:

- **Cardioversion**, which uses a therapeutic dose of electrical current to the heart synchronized to a specific moment in the electrical cycle (at the QRS complex) to convert an abnormally fast heart rate or cardiac arrhythmia to a normal rhythm.

▲ **Figure 10.23**
Automated External Defibrillator (AED).
©McGraw-Hill Education/Rick Brady, photographer.

- **Defibrillation**, which uses a nonsynchronized electrical shock to terminate ventricular fibrillation or pulseless ventricular tachycardia and revert to a normal rhythm. It is not effective for asystole.

- **Radiofrequency ablation**, which uses a catheter with an electrode in its tip guided into the heart to destroy the cells from which abnormal cardiac rhythms are originating.

- **Artificial pacemakers,** which consist of a battery, electronic circuits, and computer memory to generate electronic signals. The signals are carried along thin, insulated wires to the heart muscle. The most common need for a pacemaker is a very slow heart rate (bradycardia).

- **Implantable cardioverter/defibrillator (ICD),** which senses abnormal rhythms and gives the heart a small electrical shock to return the rhythm to normal.

- **Automated external defibrillators (AEDs)** *(Figure 10.23),* which send an electrical shock to the heart to restore a normal contraction rhythm.

A prolapsed or incompetent heart valve can often be repaired. There are two valve replacement options:

1. **A mechanical (prosthetic) valve.** Various models and designs are made from different metal alloys and plastics.

2. **Tissue valves.** This can come from a pig (porcine) or cow (bovine). Occasionally, a tissue valve can come from a human donor, or a valve can be constructed of tissue from the patient's own pericardium.

Treatments for Peripheral Vascular Disorders

1. **Varicose veins** can be treated with laser technology and **sclerotherapy**, where solutions that scar (**sclerose**) the veins are injected into them.

2. **Peripheral angioplasty** is the use of a balloon to open a peripheral artery in the leg or abdomen and is often used with stenting. It is occasionally used to treat venous stenosis.

3. **Lifestyle changes** to treat or prevent peripheral vascular disease include stopping smoking, regular exercise, healthy diet, and maintaining a healthy weight.

Abbreviations

AED	automated external defibrillator
CABG	coronary artery bypass graft
ICD	implantable cardioverter/defibrillator
PTCA	percutaneous transluminal coronary angioplasty
tPA	tissue plasminogen activator

WORD	PRONUNCIATION	ELEMENTS		DEFINITION
ablation	ab-**LAY**-shun	S/ R/	-ion *process* ablat- *take away*	Removal of a tissue to destroy its function
angioplasty	**AN**-jee-oh-**PLAS**-tee	S/ R/CF	-plasty *surgical repair* angi/o- *blood vessel*	Recanalization of a blood vessel by surgery
atherectomy	ath-er-**EK**-toh-mee	S/ R/	-ectomy *excision* ather- *porridge, gruel*	Surgical removal of the atheroma
cardioversion	**KAR**-dee-oh-**VER**-shun	S/ R/CF R/	-ion *action, process* cardi/o- *heart* -vers- *turn*	Restoration of a normal heart rhythm by electrical shock
cardioverter	**KAR**-dee-oh-**VER**-ter	R/	-verter *that which turns*	Device used to generate the electrical shock to the heart
defibrillation	dee-fib-rih-**LAY**-shun	S/ P/ R/	-ation *process* de- *without, away from* -fibrill- *small fiber*	Restoration of uncontrolled twitching of cardiac muscle fibers to normal rhythm
defibrillator	dee-**FIB**-rih-lay-tor	S/	-ator *instrument*	Instrument for defibrillation
implantable	im-**PLAN**-tah-bul	S/ P/ R/	-able *capable of* im- *in* -plant- *insert*	Able to be inserted into tissues
prosthesis	**PROS**-thee-sis		Greek *an addition*	A manufactured substitute for a missing or diseased part of the body
prosthetic (adj)	pros-**THET**-ik	S/ R/	-ic *pertaining to* prosthet- *addition*	Pertaining to a prosthesis
sclerotherapy	**SKLAIR**-oh-**THAIR**-ah-pee	R/CF R/	scler/o- *hardness* -therapy *treatment*	To collapse a vein by injecting a solution into it to harden it
sclerose (verb)	skleh-**ROZE**	S/	-ose *full of*	To harden or thicken
sclerosis (noun)	skleh-**ROH**-sis	S/	-osis *condition*	Thickening or hardening of a tissue
stent	STENT		Charles Stent, 1807–1885, English dentist	Wire mesh tube used to keep arteries open
thrombolysis	throm-**BOL**-eye-sis	S/ R/CF	- lysis *dissolve* thromb/o-	Dissolving a thrombus (clot)

Exercises

A. Determine the treatment for the condition. *From the given information, determine the treatment that would be appropriate to treat the cardiovascular disease.* **LO 10.10**

1. A person suffers a cardiac arrest at a college. The students use a device that shocks the heart. What is the device they will use?

   a. Automated external defibrillator   **b.** Stent placement   **c.** Radiofrequency ablation   **d.** Pacemaker

2. Mr. Rosares arrives at the emergency department with chest pain. When asked, he states that the chest pain started one hour ago. The cardiologist determines that he has a clot occluding one of his coronary arteries. Which procedure will the cardiologist likely choose?

   a. Defibrillation   **b.** Heart transplant   **c.** Thrombolysis   **d.** Cardioversion

B. Determine the type of condition that is treated with a particular procedure. *Choose the primary condition that the procedure would be used to treat.* **LO 10.10**

1. Coronary artery bypass grafting

   a. Arrhythmia   **b.** Occluded coronary artery

2. Radiofrequency ablation

   a. Arrhythmia   **b.** Occluded coronary artery

3. Cardioversion

   a. Arrhythmia   **b.** Occluded coronary artery

Abbreviations	
ACE	angiotensin converting enzyme
ARB	angiotensin receptor blocker
AV	atrioventricular
CCB	calcium channel blocker
FDA	Food and Drug Administration
tPA	tissue plasminogen activator

Keynotes

Diuretics indirectly affect the heart by acting on the kidneys to stimulate urinary fluid loss, thus lessening the amount of fluid the heart must cope with; chloro-thiazide (*Diuril*), furosemide (*Lasix*), and spironolactone (*Aldactone*) are examples of diuretics.

LO 10.11 Cardiovascular Drugs

Beta Blockers

Beta blockers diminish the effects of **epinephrine** and other stress hormones (*see Chapter 17*). All beta blockers are approved for the treatment of hypertension. Specific beta blockers are approved for treatment of:

- angina
- atrial arrhythmias
- coronary artery disease
- heart failure
- hypertension
- early posttraumatic stress disorder (*see Chapter 9*)

Beta blockers are also sometimes used in the prevention of migraines. There are some 20 different beta-blocking agents altogether, including propanolol (*Inderal*), atenolol (*Tenormin*), metoprolol (*Lopressor*), pinidolol (*Visken*), labetalol (*Normodyne*), and carvedilol (*Coreg*).

The **renin-angiotensin** system is a complex biological system between the heart, brain, blood vessels, and kidneys. It plays an important role in the pathology of hypertension, cardiovascular disease, chronic kidney disease, and diabetic nephropathy (*see Chapter 17*). The potent chemical angiotensin II is formed in the blood from angiotensin I by the angiotensin converting enzyme (**ACE**). Angiotensin II causes blood vessels to contract and narrow, leading to hypertension.

ACE inhibitors inhibit, or slow, the activity of the angiotensin converting enzyme (ACE). This action decreases the formation of angiotensin II, so blood vessels dilate more and blood pressure falls. Some 10 different ACE inhibitors have been approved to control hypertension, treat heart failure, prevent strokes, and improve survival rates after heart attacks.

Angiotensin receptor blockers (**ARBs**) block the interaction between angiotensin and the angiotensin receptors on the muscles in the wall of blood vessels, allowing blood vessels to dilate. They are used when patients are unable to tolerate ACE inhibitors because of persistent cough or, more rarely, angioedema.

Calcium channel blockers (**CCBs**) inhibit the flow of calcium through channels in cardiac muscles and in the muscles in the walls of blood vessels. This leads to a decrease in muscle contraction and dilation of the blood vessels. More than 20 CCBs have been approved to treat hypertension (particularly in elderly patients), angina, arrhythmias, and Raynaud disease. A high mortality rate has been reported among people who take the drugs over an extended dosage period.

Statins

Statins are a class of drugs that block the enzyme in the liver that is responsible for making **cholesterol**, an essential component in all cell membranes that is necessary for the production of bile acids, steroid hormones, and Vitamin D. However, the body's production of cholesterol also contributes to the development of atherosclerosis. Seven statins are approved by the **FDA** for use; they vary in their potency to decrease cholesterol levels. Examples include atorvastatin (*Lipitor*), lovastatin (*Mevacor*), rosuvastatin (*Crestor*), simvastatin (*Zocor*), and pravastatin (*Pravachol*).

One new drug, omega-3-acid esters (*Lovaza*), lowers very high triglyceride levels. Another new drug, evolocumab (*Repatha, Praluent*), when taken with statins, in a study published in 2017 markedly reduced LDL cholesterol levels and achieved a 15% reduction in the combined risk of having a heart attack or stroke or dying from cardiovascular disease. However, the drug is given by injection and has a list price of almost $15,000.

Other Cardiovascular Drugs

Chronotropic drugs alter the heart rate. Epinephrine (adrenaline), norepinephrine (noradrenaline), and atropine increase the heart rate. Quinidine (*Quinidex*), procainamide (*Pronestyl*), lidocaine (*Xylocaine*), and propranolol (*Inderal*) slow the heart.

Inotropic drugs alter the contractions of the myocardium. Digitalis and its derivatives, digoxin and digitoxin, increase the strength of contractions of the myocardium, thus leading to increased cardiac output.

Dromotropic drugs affect the conduction speed in the atrioventricular (**AV**) node and subsequently the rate of conduction of electrical impulses in the heart. A calcium channel blocker, such as verapamil, slows the speed of conduction through the cardiac neural system and has a negative dromotropic effect.

Anticoagulants reduce susceptibility to thrombus formation. These include aspirin, warfarin (*Coumadin*), heparin and a low molecular weight heparin named dalteparin (*Fragmin*), and new thrombin inhibitors (*see Chapter 11*) such as dabigatran etexilate (*Pradaxa*) and rivaroxaban (*Xarelto*).

- **Streptokinase**, which is derived from hemolytic streptococci, dissolves the fibrin in blood clots. If administered intravenously within 3 to 4 hours of a heart attack caused by a clot, it can be effective in dissolving the clot.
- **Tissue plasminogen activator (tPA)** binds strongly to fibrin and dissolves clots that have caused heart attacks. It is similar in effect and use to streptokinase. Reteplase (*Retavase*) and urokinase (*Abbokinase*) are forms of tPA.

WORD	PRONUNCIATION	ELEMENTS		DEFINITION
beta blocker	**BAY**-tah **BLOK**-er	S/ R/	**beta** Greek *second letter in Greek alphabet* **-er** *agent* **block-** *to obstruct*	A beta-adrenergic blocking agent used in the treatment of cardiac arrhythmias, hypertension, and other diseases
chronotropic	**KRONE**-oh-**TROH**-pik	S/ R/CF	**-tropic** *change* **chron/o-** *time*	Affecting the heart rate
diuretic	die-you-**RET**-ik	S/ P/ R/	**-ic** *pertaining to* **di-** *from* **dia-** *throughout* **-uret-** *urine, urination*	Agent that acts on the kidney to increase urine output
dromotropic	**DROH**-moh-**TROH**-pik	S/ R/CF	**-tropic** *change* **drom/o-** *race, a running*	Affecting the rate of conduction in the AV node, and subsequently the heart rate
inhibit	in-**HIB**-it		Latin *to keep back*	To curb or restrain
inotropic	**IN**-oh-**TROH**-pik	S/ R/CF	**-tropic** *change* **in/o-** *sinew*	Affecting the contractility of cardiac muscle
statin	**STAT**-in		Latin *condition, state*	A drug used to lower cholesterol in the bloodstream

Exercises

A. Abbreviations are commonly used in verbal communication and written documentation. *From the definition, identify the correct abbreviation. Use the provided abbreviations below. Fill in the blanks.* **LO 10.11, 10.E**

ACE   ARB   AV   CCB   FDA   tPA

1. The organization responsible for approving drugs for use in the United States: _____

2. The medication that dissolves clots: _____

3. Dromotropic medications work by affecting the _____ node.

4. This medication reduces blood pressure by blocking an enzyme from functioning: _____

5. The medication _____ blocks angiotensin receptors on muscles, thus reducing blood pressure.

6. A reduction in heart muscle contractility can be achieved through the use of _____.

B. Construct terms using word elements. *The roots/combining forms are important when describing the effects of cardiac medications. Given the definition, provide the missing combining form element. Enter it as one term, for example: sclero* **LO 10.11, 10.C**

1. A medication that slows down the rate of conduction through the heart. _____/tropic

2. A medication that affects the heart rate: _____/tropic

3. A medication that affects the contractility of the heart: _____/tropic

Cardiovascular System

Challenge Your Knowledge

A. Diagnostic tests may yield results that indicate a procedure should be performed. Match up the following cardiac procedures. **(LO 10.10, 10.11, 10.E)**

1. to reduce occlusion of an artery, this may be inserted

2. donor to recipient

3. arrhythmia is converted back to normal rhythm

4. clot-busting drug therapy

5. surgical removal of the lipid deposit in an artery

6. catheter with electrode destroys abnormal cells

7. healthy blood vessels are harvested to detour blood around blocked vessels

8. high-speed rotational device "sands away" plaque

9. artery-cleaning angioplasty

a. radiofrequency ablation

b. rotational atherectomy

c. atherectomy

d. stent

e. transplant

f. CABG

g. defibrillation

h. PTCA

i. thrombolysis

B. Choose the professional whose primary job is described. Write the term described. **(LO 10.F)**

cardiologist   cardiovascular technician   phlebotomist   sonographer

1. obtain venous blood used for diagnostic testing: _____

2. diagnose and treat heart conditions: _____

3. perform cardiac tests ordered by physicians: _____

4. person who specializes in obtaining ultrasounds of body structures: _____

C. Abbreviations are present throughout medical documentation, and you must be absolutely certain you are interpreting them correctly. Fill in the correct abbreviation in the following patient documentation. All of the abbreviations contain some combination of the following letters. You will have to use some letters more than once. **(LO 10.E)**

A   C   D   F   H   I   M   P   S   V   O

1. Studies show that the patient has a hole in the interventricular septum, allowing blood to shunt from the higher-pressure left ventricle to the lower-pressure right ventricle. The abbreviation for the diagnosis is _____.

2. The pediatric cardiologist was called to the Neonatal Unit because the baby's fetal blood vessel had not closed normally. The baby was diagnosed with _____.

3. The patient's arterial vessels have become dangerously narrowed due to his _____, and an angioplasty will be scheduled.

4. Due to her sedentary lifestyle, obesity, hypertension, and smoking history, the patient is at great risk for _____.

5. This patient's left ventricle is failing because it cannot pump out the blood it receives. He is going into _____.

6. An infant male was born with tetralogy of Fallot (_____). This is a form of _____.

7. This patient's ischemic attack resulted in occlusion of her coronary artery, and a (surgical procedure) _____ followed.

D. Translate from layman's language to medical terminology. Provide a medical term for every underlined word or phrase. Fill in the blanks. **(LO 10.5, 10.8)**

1. If any of the <u>heart</u> (_____) arteries become <u>blocked</u> (_____), the blood supply to a part of the <u>heart muscle</u> (_____) is cut off and the cells supplied by that artery are <u>dead</u> (_____) within minutes.

2. Aortic valve <u>narrowing</u> (_____) is common in the elderly and may need to be replaced with a <u>mechanical</u> (_____) valve. This often occurs as a consequence of <u>lipid deposits in the lining of an artery</u> (_____).

3. The <u>cause</u> (_____) of weakening of the <u>heart muscle</u> (_____) can be viral, <u>unknown</u> (_____), or alcoholic.

4. <u>Inflammation of the lining of a vein</u> (_____) allows <u>clots</u> (_____) to form.

E. The cardiac cycle can be heard through the stethoscope. Apply the correct terms in the appropriate place to describe what happens in the chambers of the heart during the cardiac cycle. One term you will use twice. Three terms you will not use at all. **(LO 10.4)**

atrial diastole	relax	heartbeat	atrial systole	ventricular systole
atria	ventricular diastole	contraction	contract	murmur

1. When the atria _____, called _____ (atrial emptying), the ventricles _____, called _____ (or ventricular filling).

2. When the atria relax, called _____, the ventricles _____, called _____.

3. Then the atria and ventricles all relax briefly. This series of events is the complete cardiac cycle or _____.

Cardiovascular System

F. Build your knowledge of the heart's location and function by selecting the correct answers to the following questions: (LO 10.1, 10.2)

1. Which of the following is *NOT* a function of the heart?

   a. pulmonary circulation

   b. maintaining respiration

   c. systemic circulation

   d. regulating blood supply

   e. pumping blood

2. The heart lies in the thoracic cavity between the lungs in an area called the

   a. sternum

   b. mediastinum

   c. ventricle

   d. atrium

   e. vena cava

3. If the *base* of the heart is the upper end of the heart, what is the tip (or other end) of the heart called?

   a. tricuspid

   b. atrium

   c. aorta

   d. semilunar

   e. apex

4. What is responsible for ensuring the one-way flow of blood in the heart?

   a. blood vessels

   b. pulmonary circulation

   c. coronary circulation

   d. valves

   e. blood pressure

G. Test your knowledge of the cardiovascular system by selecting the correct answer. (LO 10.1, 10.2, 10.3, 10.E)

1. The long, flat bone forming the center of the anterior wall of the chest is the

   a. mediastinum

   b. sternum

   c. myocardium

   d. apex

   e. pericardium

2. The area of cell death caused by the sudden blockage of a blood vessel is termed

   a. fibrosis

   b. infarct

   c. coronary

   d. sinus

   e. visceral

3. The term **sinus rhythm** refers to

   a. the AV node

   b. normal heartbeat

   c. dysrhythmias

   d. arrthythmias

   e. a pacemaker

4. Pathologic compression of the heart is known as

   a. endocarditis

   b. prolapse

   c. tamponade

   d. regurgitation

   e. effusion

5. The abbreviations that represent cardiac diagnoses are

   a. SOB and EKG

   b. MI and PAT

   c. CPR and CVT

   d. STAT and SA

   e. AED and ID

6. What is the purpose of the four valves in the heart?

   a. Blood flows in only one direction.

   b. Blood gets oxygenated.

   c. The heart muscle can rest between beats.

   d. They prevent infection.

   e. They are the gateway to the heart.

7. In the term **cardioversion,** the suffix *-ion* means

   a. a structure

   b. a process

   c. to pour

   d. pertaining to

   e. small

Cardiovascular System

H. Test your knowledge of the cardiovascular system with the following questions. (LO 1.2, 10.9, 10.19, 10.E)

1. Tissue for heart valves can come from

   a. rabbits

   b. monkeys

   c. occasionally humans

   d. dogs

   e. horses

2. Abnormality in valve closure produces

   a. exudate

   b. infarct

   c. murmur

   d. necrosis

   e. fibrillation

3. The cordlike tendons that anchor the mitral and tricuspid heart valves to the floor of the ventricles are

   a. semilunar

   b. intraventricular

   c. mesenteric

   d. chordae tendinae

   e. fibrotic

4. The pacemaker of heart rhythm is the

   a. AV node

   b. bundle branch

   c. SA node

   d. coronary sinus

   e. PVC

5. Vessels that take blood away from the heart are termed

   a. veins

   b. capillaries

   c. arteries

   d. tendons

   e. muscles

6. Which of the following terms does NOT apply to blood vessels?

   a. arterioles

   b. venules

   c. hilum

   d. veins

   e. arteries

7. The term **visceral** pertains to

   a. an artery

   b. a vein

   c. a capillary

   d. the aorta

   e. an internal organ

8. Capillary exchange occurs by

   a. infusion

   b. transfusion

   c. perfusion

   d. diffusion

   e. effusion

9. The circulatory system that takes blood to the lungs to pick up oxygen and get rid of carbon dioxide is the

   a. coronary

   b. pulmonary

   c. systemic

I. Challenge your knowledge of medical terminology and provide the correct answers to the following questions. (LO 10.5, 10.7, 10.10, 10.11, 10.E)

1. A *flat line* on an ECG is called _____.

2. *Death of tissue* is _____.

3. *Arrhythmia* is another term for _____.

4. An *abnormal sound* in the closure of a heart valve is a _____.

5. A medication that *affects the heart rate* is called a _____.

6. *Medications that lower cholesterol* are also called _____.

7. A *bypass* or diversion of fluid is _____.

8. A *hollow tube* that allows passage of fluid into or out of a body cavity is _____.

9. An agent that *increases* urine output is a _____.

10. *The main artery* in the neck is the _____.

J. Form medical terms to fill in the blanks. (LO 10.6, 10.8, 10.9, 10.A, 10.E, 10.F)

1. A _____ is a specialist in the study of the heart.

2. In the abbreviation CPR, the "C" stands for _____.

3. The abbreviation ECG stands for _____.

4. The study of the heart is the specialty called _____.

5. The term that means *pertaining to the heart and blood vessels* is _____.

6. The instrument used for taking an ECG is _____.

7. The device that measures blood pressure is _____.

K. The following procedures could all be performed by a cardiovascular surgeon. Deconstruct each medical term into its elements. Fill in the blanks. (LO 10.10, 10.D)

1. ablation: _____ / _____ / _____
                      P   R/CF   S

2. angioplasty: _____ / _____ / _____
                         P   R/CF   S

3. defibrillation: _____ / _____ / _____
                            P   R/CF   S

4. sclerotherapy: _____ / _____ / _____
                           P   R/CF   S

5. atherectomy: _____ / _____ / _____
                         P   R/CF   S

©2014 Nucleus Medical Media

Cardiovascular System

L. Use your knowledge of cardiac pharmacology and insert the correct medical term for the drugs defined.
Fill in the blanks with the class of drugs being described. **(LO 10.11)**

1. class of drugs that block the enzyme in the liver responsible for making cholesterol: _____

2. alter the contractions of the myocardium: _____

3. reduce susceptibility to clot formation: _____

4. stimulate urinary fluid loss to lessen fluid volume the heart has to cope with: _____

5. alter the heart rate: _____

M. Using your knowledge of the terminology in the following report, choose the correct answer for the following questions. (LO 10.1, 10.6)

CHEST X-RAY REPORT

The left ventricle is slightly enlarged. Right atrium and right ventricle appear to be dilated. There is tortuosity of the thoracic aorta, with arteriosclerosis. The hilar and interstitial structures are somewhat accentuated. There are large pericardial fat pads. Tricuspid and pulmonic valves appear normal but are not well seen. Mitral valve appears grossly normal for age. Aortic valve appears grossly normal for age.

1. Where are the pericardial fat pads?

   a. in the heart
   b. around the heart
   c. below the heart
   d. beside the heart
   e. above the heart

2. Which two heart chambers have a somewhat similar appearance?

   a. right and left ventricle
   b. right and left atrium
   c. left atrium and right ventricle
   d. right atrium and left ventricle
   e. right atrium and right ventricle

3. What is another spelling and pronunciation for *dilation?*

   a. dillation
   b. dilatation
   c. dillatation
   d. diletation
   e. dilletation

4. **Interstitial** means

   a. space between the cells of a structure or organ
   b. cavity between the cells of a structure or organ
   c. fluid between the cells of a structure or organ
   d. membrane between the cells of a structure or organ
   e. wall between the cells of a structure or organ

N. Procedures. You have passed your certification examination and have been hired as the coder for the Cardiology Department at Fulwood Medical Center. You are coding the claims for the following tests performed in the department. How much do you know about cardiology testing? Match the letter to the numbered blank. **(LO 10.9, 10.10)**

_____ 1. Thallium testing

_____ 2. EKG, also known as

_____ 3. Continuous ECG recorded digitally

_____ 4. Cardiac stress testing

_____ 5. TEE

_____ 6. Helps determine risk of CAD

_____ 7. Event tracker

_____ 8. Sound waves study heart function

_____ 9. Electron beam CT

_____ 10. Cardiac catheterization

_____ 11. Radioactive substance injected

_____ 12. X-ray record of a vein

_____ 13. Dye injected to find heart blockage

a. venogram

b. through esophagus to record heart valves

c. echocardiography

d. detects patterns of pressure in the heart

e. used when people are unable to do physical exercise

f. coronary angiogram

g. exercise tolerance test

h. sporadic symptoms

i. lipid profile

j. ECG

k. Holter monitor

l. identifies calcium in arteries

m. nuclear imaging

O. Identify the elements in each medical term and unlock the meaning of the word. Fill in the chart. If the word does not have a particular word element, write n/a. **(LO 10.D)**

Medical Term	Meaning of Prefix	Meaning of Root/ Combining Form	Meaning of Suffix	Meaning of the Term
incompetence	1.	2.	3.	4.
dysrhythmia	5.	6.	7.	8.
arteriole	9.	10.	11.	12.
mediastinum	13.	14.	15.	16.
venogram	17.	18.	19.	20.
inotropic	21.	22.	23.	24.
chronotropic	25.	26.	27.	28.

©2014 Nucleus Medical Media

Laboratory Report

Luisa Sosin, ID # 7248412

Blood smear: Red blood cells are **microcytic**, **hypochromic**, and **poikilocytic**.

Red Blood Cell **Index**	Patient's Result	Reference Range
Hemoglobin Concentration	10.4 g/dL	12–16 g/**dL** (grams per deciliter)
Mean **Corpuscular** Volume (**MCV**)	71 fL	86–98 **fL** (femtoliters)
Mean Corpuscular Hemoglobin (**MCH**)	21.5 pg/cell	26–32 **pg**/cell (picograms per cell)
Mean Corpuscular Hemoglobin Concentration (**MCHC**)	27.5%	32%–36%
Serum Iron	35 mcg/100 mL	50–150 **mcg**/100 mL (micrograms per 100 milliliters)
Serum Ferritin	20 mcg/100 mL	5–280 mcg/100 mL
Total Iron-Binding Capacity (**TIBC**)	500 mcg/100 mL	250–410 mcg/100 mL

The reference range is the usual range of test values for a healthy population.

Chapter Learning Outcomes

To understand Case Report 11.1, to be able to communicate intelligently and clearly with Dr. Lee about the patient, and to document Mrs. Sosin's medical care and progress, it is essential to have knowledge of the anatomy, physiology, and medical terminology of **hematology**. This chapter provides information that will enable you to:

LO 11.1 Identify the components of blood.

LO 11.2 Discuss the functions of blood.

LO 11.3 Relate the structure of red blood cells (RBCs) to their function.

LO 11.4 Describe disorders of RBCs.

LO 11.5 Identify the types of white blood cells (WBCs) and their functions.

LO 11.6 Discuss disorders of WBCs.

LO 11.7 Explain hemostasis.

LO 11.8 Identify and explain disorders of coagulation (coagulopathies).

LO 11.9 Differentiate red cell antigens and their functions.

LO 11.10 Discuss the diagnostic procedures used for hematologic disorders.

LO 11.11 Explain the therapeutic procedures used for hematologic disorders.

LO 11.12 Describe the pharmacologic agents used in the treatment of hematologic disorders.

LO 11.A Use the medical terms of hematology to communicate in writing and document accurately and precisely in any health care setting.

LO 11.B Use the medical terms of hematology to communicate verbally with accuracy and precision in any health care setting.

LO 11.C Construct medical terms of hematology from their word elements.

LO 11.D Deconstruct medical terms of hematology into their word elements.

LO 11.E Identify the health care professionals involved in the care of hematologic patients.

LO 11.F Use approved abbreviations of terms used in hematology correctly.

 ## Case Report (CR) 11.1

You are

. . . a medical assistant working with Susan Lee, MD, a primary care physician at Fulwood Medical Center.

Your patient is

. . . Mrs. Luisa Sosin, a 47-year-old woman who presented a week ago with fatigue, lethargy, and muscle weakness. Physical examination revealed **pallor** of her skin, a pulse rate of 100, and a respiratory rate of 20. Dr. Lee referred her for extensive blood work. Dr. Lee also determined that the patient had been taking aspirin and other **nonsteroidal anti-inflammatory drugs (NSAIDs)** for the past 6 months for low-back pain.

You are responsible for documenting her investigation and care. She is your next patient, and you are reviewing the laboratory report above.

Components of Blood

The information in this lesson relates to the composition, functions, and uses of blood and will enable you to use correct medical terminology to:

11.1.1 Identify the components of blood.

11.1.2 Describe plasma and its functions.

11.1.3 Explain the functions of blood.

LO 11.1 Components of Blood

Blood is a type of connective tissue and consists of cells contained in a liquid matrix.

Blood volume varies with body size and the amount of adipose tissue. An average-size adult has about 5 L (liters) (10 pints) of blood, which represents some 8% of body weight.

If a specimen of blood is collected in a tube and centrifuged, the cells of the blood are packed into the bottom of the tube *(Figure 11.1)*. These cells are called the formed elements of blood and consist of 99% red blood cells (**RBCs**), together with white blood cells (**WBCs**) and platelets. The blood sample is normally about 45% formed elements.

The **hematocrit (Hct)** is the percentage of total blood volume composed of red blood cells. The red blood cells can account for 40% to 54% of the total blood volume in normal males and 38% to 47% in females.

Plasma is the remaining 55% of the blood sample. It is a clear, yellowish liquid that is 91% water. Plasma is the fluid noncellular part of blood. Plasma is a **colloid**, a liquid that contains suspended particles, most of which are the plasma proteins named:

- **Albumin**—makes up 58% of the proteins.

- **Globulin**—makes up 38% of the plasma proteins. Antibodies are globulins *(see Chapter 12)*.

- **Fibrinogen**—makes up 4% of the plasma proteins and is part of the mechanism for blood clotting *(see Lesson 11.4)*.

Nutrients, **waste products, hormones**, and **enzymes** are dissolved in plasma for transportation.

When blood is allowed to clot and the solid clot is removed, **serum** is left. Serum is identical to plasma except for the absence of clotting proteins.

dL	deciliter; one-tenth of a liter
fL	femtoliter; one-quadrillionth of a liter
Hct	hematocrit
L	liter
MCH	mean corpuscular hemoglobin; the average amount of hemoglobin in the average red blood cell
MCHC	mean corpuscular hemoglobin concentration; the average concentration of hemoglobin in a given volume of red blood cells
MCV	mean corpuscular volume; the average volume of a red blood cell
mcg	microgram; one-millionth of a gram; sometimes written as mg
NSAID	nonsteroidal anti-inflammatory drug
pg	picogram; one-trillionth of a gram
RBC	red blood cell
TIBC	total iron-binding capacity; the amount of iron needed to saturate transferrin, the protein that transports iron in the blood
WBC	white blood cell

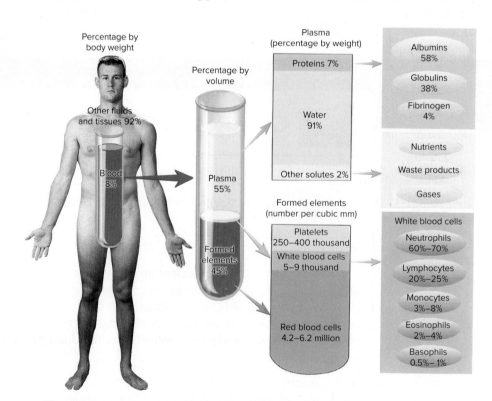

▲ **Figure 11.1 Components of Blood** ©McGraw-Hill Education/Joe DeGrandis, photographer.

WORD	PRONUNCIATION	ELEMENTS		DEFINITION
albumin	al-**BYU**-min		Latin *white of an egg*	Simple, soluble protein
colloid	**COLL**-oyd	S/ R/	**-oid** *appearance of* **coll-** *glue*	Liquid containing suspended particles
fibrin fibrinogen	**FIE**-brin fie-**BRIN**-oh-jen	S/ R/CF	Latin *fiber* **-gen** *create, produce* **fibrin/o-** *fibrin*	Stringy protein fiber that is a component of a blood clot Precursor of fibrin in blood-clotting process
globulin	**GLOB**-you-lin		Latin *globule*	Family of blood proteins
hematocrit	hee-**MAT**-oh-krit	S/ R/CF	**-crit** *to separate* **hemat/o-** *blood*	Percentage of red blood cells in the blood
hemoglobin	**HEE**-moh-**GLOH**-bin	R/CF R/	**hem/o-** *blood* **globin** *protein*	Red-pigmented protein that is the main component of red blood cells
index indices (pl)	**IN**-deks **IN**-dih-seez		Latin *one that points out*	A standard indicator of measurement relating one component to another
microcytic	my-kroh-**SIT**-ik	S/ P/ R/	**-ic** *pertaining to* **micro-** *small* **-cyt-** *cell*	Pertaining to a small cell
plasma	**PLAZ**-mah		Greek *something formed*	Fluid, noncellular component of blood
serum	**SEER**-um		Latin *whey*	Fluid remaining after removal of cells and fibrin clot

Exercises

A. Know your elements—they will increase your medical vocabulary! *This exercise consists of elements taken from the above WAD. Match the element to its correct meaning.* **LO 11.1, 11.A, 11.C**

_____ **1.** oid

_____ **2.** gen

_____ **3.** hem

_____ **4.** crit

_____ **5.** coll

_____ **6.** globin

a. protein

b. blood

c. glue

d. create, produce

e. appearance of

f. to separate

LO 11.2 Functions of Blood

The functions of blood are to:

1. **Maintain the body's homeostasis** *(see Chapter 4).*

2. **Maintain body temperature.** Warm blood is transported from the interior of the body to its surface, where heat is released from the blood.

3. **Transport nutrients, vitamins, and minerals** from the digestive system and storage areas to organs and cells where they are needed. Examples of nutrients are glucose and amino acids *(see Chapter 5).*

4. **Transport waste products** from cells and organs to the liver and kidneys for detoxification and excretion. Examples are **creatinine**, **urea**, bilirubin, and lactic acid *(see Chapter 5).*

5. **Transport hormones** from endocrine glands to the target cells. Examples are insulin and thyroxin *(see Chapter 17).*

6. **Transport gases** to and from the lungs and cells. Examples are oxygen and carbon dioxide *(see Chapter 13).*

7. **Protect against foreign substances.** Cells and chemicals in the blood are an important part of the immune system for dealing with microorganisms and toxins *(see Chapter 12).*

8. **Form clots.** Clots provide protection against blood loss and are the first step in tissue repair and restoration of normal function.

9. **Regulate pH and osmosis.**

Hydrogen ion concentration is measured by using a **pH** scale to show the balance between **acid** and **alkaline** in any solution. Pure water is the neutral solution and has a pH of 7.0. Solutions with a pH less than 7.0 are acidic. Solutions with a pH greater than 7.0 are alkaline (or basic). Blood has a pH between 7.35 and 7.45 and must be maintained within that range for life to continue. **Buffer** systems in the blood are used to maintain the correct pH range. Examples of buffer systems are bicarbonate and phosphate.

Osmosis is the passage of water through a selectively permeable membrane, such as a cell membrane, from the "more watery" side to the "less watery" side. All cells exchange water by osmosis, and red blood cells exchange 100 times their own volume across the cell membrane every second.

Viscosity, the resistance of a fluid to flow, is an important element that affects the blood's ability to flow through blood vessels. Whole blood is five times as **viscous** as water. If the viscosity decreases because red blood cells are deficient (as in **anemia**), blood flows more easily and puts a strain on the heart because of the increased amount of blood being returned to it in a unit of time.

Abbreviation

pH	hydrogen ion concentration

WORD	PRONUNCIATION	ELEMENTS		DEFINITION
acid	**ASS**-id		Latin *sour*	Substance with a pH below 7.0
alkaline (basic (syn))	**AL**-kah-line	S/ R/	**-ine** *pertaining to, substance* **alkal-** *base*	Substance with a pH above 7.0
buffer	**BUFF**-er		Latin *cushion*	Substance that resists a change in pH
creatinine	kree-**AT**-ih-neen	S/ R/	**-ine** *pertaining to, substance* **creatin-** *creatine*	Breakdown product of the skeletal muscle protein creatine
homeostasis	hoh-mee-oh-**STAY**-sis	S/ R/CF	**-stasis** *control* **home/o-** *the same*	Stability or equilibrium of a system or the body's internal environment
osmosis	oz-**MOH**-sis	S/ R/	**-sis** *process* **osmo-** *push*	The passage of water across a cell membrane
urea	you-**REE**-ah		Greek *urine*	End product of nitrogen metabolism
viscous viscosity	**VISS**-kus vis-**KOS**-ih-tee	S/ R/CF	Latin *sticky* **-sity** *condition, state* **visc/o** *resistance to flow*	Sticky; resistant to flowing The resistance of a fluid to flow

Exercises

A. Identify the medical term being described below. *Fill in the blanks.* **LO 11.1, LO 11.2**

1. A substance that resists a change in pH _____.

2. A substance with a pH greater than 7.0 _____.

3. A substance with a pH less than 7.0 _____.

4. Movement of water across a cell membrane _____.

5. Resistance of a fluid to flow _____.

B. Deconstruct medical terms to decipher their meaning. *Identify where the slash would occur to deconstruct terms into their word elements. Choose the correct answer for each term.* **LO 11.D**

1. viscosity

   a. vis/co/sity   **b.** visc/osity   **c.** visc/o/sity   **d.** viscos/ity

2. alkaline

   a. alkal/ine   **b.** al/ka/line   **c.** alkl/aline   **d.** al/kal/ine

3. osmosis

   a. o/sm/o/sis   **b.** os/mo/sis   **c.** osm/o/sis   **d.** osmo/sis

4. homeostasis

   a. homeo/stas/is   **b.** home/o/stasis   **c.** homeo/sta/sis   **d.** ho/meo/stas/is

Lesson 11.2

BLOOD

Red Blood Cells (Erythrocytes)

Top view

(a)   (b)

▲ **Figure 11.2** RBCs. ©Bill Longcore/Photo Researchers, Inc.

LO 11.3 Structure and Function of Red Blood Cells

Structure of Red Blood Cells

Each RBC is a **biconcave** disc with edges that are thicker than the center *(Figure 11.2)*. This biconcave shape gives the disc a larger surface area than if it were a sphere. The biconcave surface area enables a more rapid flow of gases into and out of the RBC.

The main component of RBCs is **hemoglobin (Hb)**, which gives the cell its red color. Hemoglobin occupies about one-third of the total cell volume and is composed of the iron-containing pigment **heme** bound to a protein called globin. The rest of the red blood cell consists of the cell membrane, water, electrolytes, and enzymes. Mature RBCs do not have a nucleus.

RBCs are unable to move themselves and are dependent on the heart and blood to move them around the body.

Function of Red Blood Cells

The functions of the RBCs are to

1. **Transport oxygen (O_2)** from the lungs to cells all over the body. Oxygen is transported in combination with hemoglobin (**oxyhemoglobin**).

2. **Transport carbon dioxide (CO_2)** from the tissue cells to the lungs for excretion.

3. **Transport nitric oxide (NO),** a gas produced by cells lining the blood vessels that signals smooth muscle to relax and is also a transmitter of signals between nerve cells.

Life History of Red Blood Cells

Red blood cell formation (**erythropoiesis**) occurs in the spaces in bones filled with red bone marrow. **Hematopoietic stem cells** become nucleated **erythroblasts** and then nonnucleated **reticulocytes,** which are released into the bloodstream. In approximately five days, the reticulocytes mature into **erythrocytes**.

A hormone, **erythropoietin**, produced by the kidneys and liver, controls the rate of RBC production. A lack of oxygen in the blood triggers the release of erythropoietin, which travels in the blood to the red bone marrow to stimulate RBC production.

RBC production is also influenced by the availability of iron, the B vitamins B_{12} and folic acid, and amino acids through absorption from the digestive tract *(Figure 11.3)*.

The average life span of an RBC is 120 days, during which time the cell has circulated through the body about 75,000 times. With age, the cells become more fragile, and squeezing through tiny capillaries ruptures them. **Macrophages** in the liver and spleen take up the hemoglobin that is released and break it down into its components heme and globin. The heme is broken down into iron and into a rust-colored pigment called bilirubin.

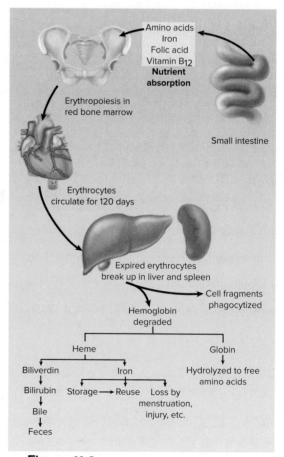

▲ **Figure 11.3** Life and Death of RBCs

WORD	PRONUNCIATION	ELEMENTS		DEFINITION
biconcave	BIE-kon-KAVE	P/ R/	bi- *two, double* -concave *arched, hollow*	Having a hollowed surface on both sides of a structure
erythroblast	eh-RITH-roh-blast	S/ R/CF	-blast *germ cell* erythr/o- *red*	Precursor to a red blood cell
erythrocyte	eh-RITH-roh-site	S/ R/CF	-cyte *cell* erythr/o- *red*	Another name for a red blood cell
erythropoiesis	eh-RITH-roh-poy-EE-sis	S/ R/CF	-poiesis *to make* erythr/o- *red*	The formation of red blood cells
erythropoietin	eh-RITH-roh-POY-ee-tin	S/	-poietin *the maker*	Protein secreted by the kidney that stimulates red blood cell production
hematopoietic	HEE-mah-toh-poy-ET-ik	S/ S/ R/CF	-ic *pertaining to* -poiet- *the making* hemat/o- *blood*	Pertaining to the making of red blood cells
heme	HEEM		Greek *blood*	The iron-based component of hemoglobin that carries oxygen
macrophage	MAK-roh-fayj	P/ R/CF	macro- *large* -phag/e *to eat*	Large white blood cell that removes bacteria, foreign particles, and dead cells
oxyhemoglobin	OK-see-HEE-moh-GLOH-bin	R/CF R/CF R/	ox/y- *oxygen* -hem/o- *blood* -globin *protein*	Hemoglobin in combination with oxygen
reticulocyte	ri-TIK-you-loh-site	S/ R/CF	-cyte *cell* reticul/o- *netlike*	Immature red blood cell

Exercises

A. Given the definition, identify the word element. *One word in the definition is in bold; find the element in the term that has the same meaning. The first one is done for you. Fill in the blanks.* **LO 11.3**

1. **macrophage:**   Element _____*macro*_____ = _____*large*_____

   Definition: **large** white blood cell that removes bacteria and dead cells

2. **erythroblast:**   Element _____ = _____

   Definition: **precursor** to red blood cell

3. **biconcave:**   Element _____ = _____

   Definition: having a hollowed surface on **both** sides of a structure

4. **erythropoiesis:**   Element _____ = _____

   Definition: the **formation** of red blood cells

5. **reticulocyte:**   Element _____ = _____

   Definition: immature red blood **cell**

6. **erythropoietin:**   Element _____ = _____

   Definition: protein that is secreted by kidney and stimulates **red blood cell** production

7. **hematopoietic:**   Element _____ = _____

   Definition: **pertaining to** the making of red blood cells

(a)   1200×

(b)   1000×

▲ **Figure 11.4** **Red Blood Cells.** (a) Normal RBCs. (b) Hypochromic RBCs. ©Ed Reschke

Abbreviations

PA	pernicious anemia
SOB	shortness of breath
MCH	mean corpuscular hemoglobin
MCV	mean corpuscular volume

Keynote

- Anemia reduces the oxygen-carrying capacity of blood.
- Hemolysis liberates hemoglobin from red blood cells.

Normal RBC

Sickle cell

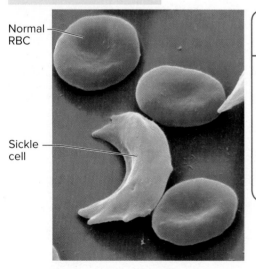

▲ **Figure 11.5** **Sickle Cell Anemia.** ©Meckes/ Ottawa/Photo Researchers, Inc.

LO 11.4 Disorders of Red Blood Cells

Anemia is a reduction in the number of RBCs or in the amount of hemoglobin each RBC contains *(Figure 11.4)*. Both of these conditions reduce the oxygen-carrying capacity of the blood and produce the symptoms of shortness of breath (**SOB**) and fatigue. They also produce **pallor** (paleness of the skin) because of the deficiency of the red-colored oxyhemoglobin, the combination of oxygen and hemoglobin, and the red blood cells are **hypochromic** *(Figure 11.4b)*

There are several types of anemia:

- **Iron-deficiency anemia** is the diagnosis for Mrs. Luisa Sosin. In her case, the cause was chronic bleeding from her gastrointestinal tract due to the aspirin and other painkillers she was taking. Her stools were positive for occult blood. Other causes can be heavy menstrual bleeding or a diet deficient in iron.

- **Pernicious anemia (PA)** is due to vitamin B_{12} deficiency. This is caused by a shortage of *intrinsic factor (see Chapter 5)*, which is normally secreted by cells in the lining of the stomach and binds with vitamin B_{12}; this complex is absorbed into the bloodstream. Without vitamin B_{12}, hemoglobin cannot be formed. The RBCs decrease in number and in hemoglobin concentration and increase in size (**macrocytic**).

- **Sickle cell anemia** (also called *sickle cell disease*) is a genetic disorder found most commonly in African Americans, Africans, and some Mediterranean populations. It results from the production of an abnormal hemoglobin that causes the RBCs to form a rigid sickle cell shape *(Figure 11.5)*. The abnormal cells are sticky, clump together (**agglutinate**), and block small capillaries. This causes intense pain in the **hypoxic** tissues (a sickle cell crisis) and can cause stroke and kidney and heart failure.

There is a minor form of the disease, sickle cell trait, in which symptoms rarely occur and do not progress to the full-blown disease.

- **Hemolytic anemia** is due to excessive destruction of normal and abnormal RBCs. **Hemolysis** can be caused by such toxic substances as snake and spider venoms, mushroom toxins, and drug reactions. Trauma to RBCs by hemodialysis or heart-lung machines can produce a hemolytic anemia.

- **Aplastic anemia** is a condition in which the bone marrow is unable to produce sufficient new cells of all types—red cells, white cells, and platelets. It can be associated with exposure to radiation, benzene, and certain drugs.

- **Hemoglobinopathies**, such as sickle cell disease and **thalassemia**, with their inherited abnormal hemoglobins, also cause hemolysis of RBCs. Hemolysis also can occur through **incompatible** blood transfusions or maternal-fetal incompatibilities *(see Lesson 11.5)*. Jaundice is a complication.

- **Polycythemia vera** is an overproduction of RBCs and WBCs due to an unknown cause.

- **Poikilocytosis** is a categorical term referring to the presence of irregular-shaped red blood cells. Examples include **spherocytes** and sickle cells.

📁 Case Report (CR) 11.1 *(continued)*

Because Mrs. Luisa Sosin was deficient in iron and hemoglobin, her RBCs were small (microcytic) and lacked the red color of oxyhemoglobin (hypochromic; *Figure 11.4*), and some were irregular-shaped (poikilocytic) rather than the normal, round shape. The volume of each cell, mean corpuscular volume (MCV), and the amount of hemoglobin in each cell, mean corpuscular hemoglobin (MCH), were decreased. The amount of iron in her blood (serum iron) and the amount of ferritin in her serum were decreased. Her total iron-binding capacity was raised because the shortage of iron resulted in an increased availability of the protein to which iron is bound in the bloodstream.

LO 11.4, 11.A
Word Analysis and Definition

S = Suffix   P = Prefix   R = Root   R/CF = Combining Form

WORD	PRONUNCIATION		ELEMENTS	DEFINITION
agglutinate	ah-**GLUE**-tin-ate	S/ P/ R/	-ate *composed of, pertaining to* ag- *to* -glutin- *stick together, glue*	Stick together to form clumps
aplastic anemia	ay-**PLAS**-tik ah-**NEE**-mee-ah	S/ P/ R/ R/ P/	-tic *pertaining to* a- *without* -plas- *formation* emia *blood* an- *without, lack of*	Condition in which the bone marrow is unable to produce sufficient red cells, white cells, and platelets
hemoglobinopathy	**HEE**-moh-**GLOH**-bih-**NOP**-ah-thee	S/ R/CF R/CF	-pathy *disease* hem/o- *blood* -globin/o- *protein*	Disease caused by the presence of an abnormal hemoglobin in the red blood cells
hemolysis	hee-**MOL**-ih-sis	S/ R/CF	-lysis *destruction* hem/o- *blood*	Destruction of red blood cells so that hemoglobin is liberated
hemolytic (adj)	hee-moh-**LIT**-ik	S/ R/	-ic *pertaining to* -lyt- *destroy*	Pertaining to the process of destruction of red blood cells
hypochromic	high-poh-**CROH**-mik	S/ P/ R/	-ic *pertaining to* hypo- *deficient, below* -chrom- *color*	Pale in color, as in RBCs when hemoglobin is deficient
hypoxia (**Note:** The surplus "o" is not used.)	high-**POK**-see-ah	S/ P/ R/	-ia *condition* hypo- *deficient* -ox- *oxygen*	Below normal levels of oxygen in tissues, gases, or blood
hypoxic	high-**POK**-sik	S/	-ic *pertaining to*	Deficient in oxygen
incompatible	in-kom-**PAT**-ih-bul	S/ P/ R/	-ible *can do* in- *not* -compat- *tolerate*	Substances that interfere with each other physiologically
macrocyte	**MAK**-roh-site	R/CF P/	cyt/e *cell* macro- *large*	Large red blood cell
macrocytic (adj)	mak-roh-**SIT**-ik	S/ R/	-ic *pertaining to* -cyt- *cell*	Pertaining to macrocytes
microcytic	my-kroh-**SIT**-ik	P/	micro- *small*	Pertaining to a small cell
pallor	**PAL**-or		Latin *paleness*	Paleness of the skin or a red blood cell
pernicious anemia (PA)	per-**NISH**-us ah-**NEE**-mee-ah	R/ P/	**pernicious** Latin *destructive* emia *blood* an- *without, lack of*	Chronic anemia due to lack of vitamin B$_{12}$
poikilocytic	**POY**-kee-loh-**SIT**-ik	S/ P/ R/	-ic *pertaining to* poikilo- *irregular* -cyt- *cell*	Pertaining to an irregular-shaped red blood cell
poikilocytosis	**POY**-kee-loh-sigh-**TOH**-sis	S/	-osis *condition*	A condition of irregular-shaped red blood cells
polycythemia vera	**POL**-ee-sigh-**THEE**-mee-ah **VEH**-rah	S/ P/ R/	-hemia *blood condition* poly- *many, much* -cyt- *cell* **vera** Latin *truth*	Chronic disease with bone marrow hyperplasia and increase in number of red blood cells and in blood volume
spherocyte	**SFEER**-oh-site	S/ R/CF	-cyte *cell* spher/o- *sphere*	A spherical cell
spherocytosis	**SFEER**-oh-sigh-**TOH**-sis	S/ R/	-osis *condition* -cyt- *cell*	Presence of spherocytes in blood
thalassemia	thal-ah-**SEE**-mee-ah	S/ R/	-emia *blood condition* thalass- *sea*	Group of inherited blood disorders that produce a hemolytic anemia and occur in people living around the Mediterranean Sea.

Exercises

A. Use Case Report 11.1 (continued) to answer the following questions. LO 11.4, 11.A, 11.F

1. If a term means *deficient in,* what element would it start with? _____

2. What is the opposite of *microcytic*? _____

3. The condition in which the bone marrow is unable to produce sufficient red cells, white cells, and platelets is _____

4. Mrs. Sosin's pallor is due to an abnormality in which type of blood cell? (use the 3-letter abbreviation) _____

White Blood Cells (Leukocytes)

Lesson Objectives

The information in this lesson will enable you to use correct medical terminology to:

11.3.1 Distinguish the different types of WBCs.

11.3.2 Describe the functions of the different types of WBCs.

11.3.3 Explain white blood cell counts and differential WBC counts.

11.3.4 Discuss the effect of common disorders of WBCs on health.

Abbreviation	
PMNL	polymorphonuclear leukocyte

Case Report (CR) 11.2

You are

... a laboratory technician reviewing a peripheral blood smear.

Your patient is

... Mrs. Latisha Masters, a 27-year-old student.

Mrs. Masters presented with a 5-day history of fatigue, low-grade fever, and sore throat. Physical examination showed tonsillitis with bilateral, enlarged, tender cervical lymph nodes and an enlarged spleen.

The WBC count you performed showed 9,200 cells per cubic millimeter. The peripheral smear you are looking at is reported as showing the presence of atypical mononuclear cells with abundant cytoplasm.

LO 11.5 Types of White Blood Cells

Granulocytes

1. **Neutrophils** *(Figure 11.6)* are normally 50% to 70% of the total WBC count. They are also called **polymorphonuclear leukocytes (PMNLs).** These cells phagocytize bacteria, fungi, and some viruses and secrete a group of enzymes called lysozymes, which destroy some bacteria.

2. **Eosinophils** *(Figure 11.7)* are normally 2% to 4% of the total WBC count. They are mobile cells that leave the bloodstream to enter tissue undergoing an allergic response.

3. **Basophils** *(Figure 11.8)* are normally less than 1% of the total WBC count. Basophils migrate to damaged tissues, where they release histamine (which increases blood flow) and **heparin** (which prevents blood clotting).

Because of their granular cytoplasm surrounding a nucleus, the above three types of WBCs are called **granulocytes.** Their granules are the sites for production of enzymes and chemicals.

▲ **Figure 11.6** Neutrophils Are Granulocytes. ©Ed Reschke/Getty Images

▲ **Figure 11.7** Eosinophils Are Granulocytes. ©Ed Reschke

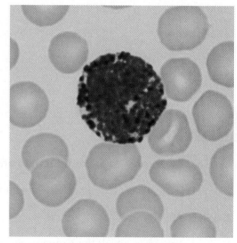

▲ **Figure 11.8** Basophils Are Granulocytes. ©Ed Reschke/Getty Images

WORD	PRONUNCIATION	ELEMENTS		DEFINITION
basophil	**BAY**-so-fill	S/ R/CF	-phil *attraction* bas/o- *base*	A basophil's granules attract a basic blue stain in the laboratory
eosinophil	ee-oh-**SIN**-oh-fill	S/ R/CF	-phil *attraction* eosin/o- *dawn*	An eosinophil's granules attract a rosy-red color on staining
granulocyte	**GRAN**-you-loh-site	S/ R/CF	-cyte *cell* granul/o- *small grain*	A white blood cell that contains multiple small granules in its cytoplasm
heparin	**HEP**-ah-rin	S/ R/	-in *chemical* hepar- *liver*	An anticoagulant secreted particularly by liver cells
leukocyte (Note: alternative spelling **leucocyte**)	**LOO**-koh-site	S/ R/CF	-cyte *cell* leuk/o- *white*	Another term for a white blood cell
neutrophil	**NEW**-troh-fill	S/ R/CF	-phil *attraction* neutr/o- *neutral*	A neutrophil's granules take up purple stain equally whether the stain is acid or alkaline
polymorphonuclear	**POL**-ee-more-foh-**NEW**-klee-ar	S/ P/ R/CF R/	-ar *pertaining to* poly- *many* -morph/o- *shape* -nucle- *nucleus*	White blood cell with a multilobed nucleus

Exercises

A. Define the meaning of word elements related to the functions of white blood cells. *Fill in the blanks with the correct definition.*
LO 11.5

1. The root in the medical term **heparin** means _____.

2. The suffix that means *attraction* is _____.

3. The prefix that means *many* is _____.

B. Using the medical terms related to the functions of white blood cells, match the correct term in column one to its meaning in column two. LO 11.5

_____ **1.** eosinophil	**a.** anticoagulant secreted by liver cells
_____ **2.** leucocyte	**b.** white blood cell with a multilobed nucleus
_____ **3.** basophil	**c.** white blood cell
_____ **4.** heparin	**d.** releases histamine in damaged tissues
_____ **5.** polymorphonuclear	**e.** involved in an allergic response

LO 11.5 Types of White Blood Cells (continued)

Agranulocytes

Because monocytes and lymphocytes have no granules in their cytoplasm, they are called **agranulocytes**.

1. **Monocytes** *(Figure 11.9)* are the largest blood cell and are normally 3% to 8% of the total WBC count. Monocytes leave the bloodstream and become macrophages that phagocytize bacteria, dead neutrophils, and dead cells in the tissues.

2. **Lymphocytes** *(Figure 11.10)* are normally 25% to 35% of the total WBC count. They are the smallest type of WBC. Lymphocytes are produced in red bone marrow and migrate through the bloodstream to lymphatic tissues—lymph nodes, tonsils, spleen, and thymus—where they proliferate.

There are two main types of lymphocyte:

a. **B cells** that differentiate into plasma cells. These are stimulated by bacteria or toxins to produce **antibodies**, or **immunoglobulins (Igs)**.

b. **T cells** that attach directly to foreign antigen-bearing cells such as bacteria, which they kill with toxins they secrete.

▲ **Figure 11.9** Monocytes Are Agranulocytes.
©Ed Reschke/Getty Images

▲ **Figure 11.10** Lymphocytes Are Agranulocytes.
©Ed Reschke/Getty Images

WORD	PRONUNCIATION	ELEMENTS		DEFINITION
agranulocyte	ay-**GRAN**-you-loh-site	S/ P/ R/CF	**-cyte** *cell* **a-** *without, not* **-granul/o-** *granule*	A white blood cell without any granules in its cytoplasm
antibody **antibodies (pl)**	**AN**-tih-body	P/ R/	**anti-** *against* **-body** *substance*	Protein produced in response to an antigen
immunoglobulin	**IM**-you-noh-**GLOB**-you-lin	S/ R/CF R/	**-in** *chemical* **immun/o-** *immune response* **-globul-** *protein*	Specific protein evoked by an antigen; all antibodies are immunoglobulins
lymphocyte	**LIM**-foh-site	S/ R/CF	**-cyte** *cell* **lymph/o** *lymph*	Small white blood cell with a large nucleus

Exercises

A. Use the medical terminology learned in this lesson to answer the questions. *Select the correct answer to correctly complete each statement.* **LO 11.5, 11.D**

1. In the term **agranulocyte,** there is an element meaning
   a. within
   b. alongside
   c. under
   d. without, not
   e. beside

2. In the term **agranulocyte,** there is a term meaning
   a. blue
   b. behind
   c. cell
   d. against
   e. deficient

3. In the term **immunoglobulin,** there is an element meaning
   a. protein
   b. many
   c. against
   d. liquid
   e. black

4. The correct plural of **antibody** is
   a. antibodys
   b. antibodies
   c. antibodyies
   d. antebodyies
   e. antybodies

B. True or False. *Choose T if the statement is true. Choose F if the statement is false.* **LO 11.5**

1. Because monocytes and lymphocytes have no granules in their cytoplasm, they are called *agranulocytes.*   T   F

2. Monocytes are the largest blood cell.   T   F

3. A lymphocyte is a white blood cell.   T   F

4. B cells and T cells are types of monocytes.   T   F

5. Lymphocytes are the smallest type of white blood cell.   T   F

Abbreviations

ALL	acute lymphoblastic leukemia
EBV	Epstein-Barr virus
mm³	cubic millimeter

 Case Report (CR) 11.2 *(continued)*

Latisha Masters' blood smear indicated a diagnosis of **infectious mononucleosis** caused by the **Epstein-Barr virus (EBV)**. This virus infects white blood cells. A positive **heterophile reaction (Monospot test)** was present. Infectious mononucleosis occurs in the 15- to 25-year-old population. Its cause, the EBV, is a very common virus, a member of the herpes virus family. The EBV is transmitted by exchange of saliva, as in kissing. In patients with symptoms compatible with infectious mononucleosis, a positive Monospot test is diagnostic.

Keynotes

- Leukocytosis is the presence of too many white blood cells.
- Leukopenia is the presence of too few white blood cells.
- **Pancytopenia** is the presence of too few red blood cells, white blood cells, and platelets.
- Acute lymphoblastic leukemia is the most common leukemia in children.

LO 11.6 Disorders of White Blood Cells

Normally a cubic millimeter (**mm³**) of blood contains 5,000 to 10,000 white blood cells. **Leukocytosis** is defined as a total WBC count of normal cells exceeding 10,000/mm³ due to any cause.

Causes of leukocytosis are:

- **Neutrophilia**, an increase in the number and percentage of neutrophils. This can be due to bacterial infections, for example, appendicitis or bacterial pneumonia.

- **Eosinophilia**, an increase in the number of eosinophils. This occurs with allergic reactions or parasitic infection.

- **Basophilia**, which occurs when there is an increase in basophils. Basophilia can be caused by allergic reactions or infection due to tuberculosis, chicken pox, and influenza.

Leukopenia results when the WBC count drops below 5,000 cells/mm³ of blood. Leukopenia is most often associated with **neutropenia**, but it also can be associated with decreases in the other white blood cells. This condition reduces the body's ability to fight infection.

Monocytosis is a condition in which there is an increase in monocytes. This condition occurs in cases of chronic infection and autoimmune diseases. **Monocytopenia** is a decrease in monocytes, which can arise from chemotherapy.

Lymphocytosis is an increase in the number of lymphocytes. This condition can can be caused by infection, HIV/AIDs, and **mononucleosis.** AIDS also can lead to **lymphocytopenia,** as can hepatitis, influenza, and tuberculosis.

Leukemia is cancer of the hematopoietic tissues and produces a high number of leukocytes and their **precursors** in the WBC count. As the **leukemic** cells proliferate, they take over the bone marrow and cause a deficiency of normal RBCs, WBCs, and **platelets**. This makes the patient anemic and vulnerable to infection and bleeding.

Myeloid leukemia is characterized by uncontrolled production of granulocytes and their precursors *(Figure 11.11)* and starts in the bone marrow. It can be in an acute or chronic form.

Lymphoid leukemia is characterized by uncontrolled production of lymphocytes. It can be in an acute or chronic form. **Acute lymphoblastic leukemia (ALL)** is the most common form of childhood cancer and is curable with modern treatments, such as chemotherapy and bone marrow and umbilical cord **stem cell** transplants.

Pancytopenia occurs when the erythrocytes (RBCs), leukocytes (WBCs), and thrombocytes (**platelets**) in the circulating blood are all markedly reduced. This can occur with cancer chemotherapy.

▲ **Figure 11.11** Myeloid Leukemia.
©Andrew Syred/SPL/Photo Researchers, Inc.

WORD	PRONUNCIATION	ELEMENTS		DEFINITION
basophilia	**BAY**-so-**FILL**-ee-ah	S/ R/CF	-**philia** *attraction* bas/o- base	Condition of increased basophil cells
eosinophilia	ee-oh-**SIN**-o-**FILL**-ee-ah	S/ R/CF	-**philia** *attraction* eosin/o- *dawn*	Condition of increased eosinophil cells
leukemia	loo-**KEE**-mee-ah	S/ R/	-**emia** *blood condition* leuk- *white*	Disease in which the blood is taken over by white blood cells and their precursors
leukemic (adj)	loo-**KEE**-mik	S/	-**emic** *in the bood*	Pertaining to having the characteristics of leukemia
leukocytosis	**LOO**-koh-sigh-**TOH**-sis	S/ R/CF R/	-**osis** *condition* leuk/o- *white* -cyt- *cell*	An excessive number of white blood cells
lymphocytopenia	**LIM**-foh-sigh-toh-**PEE**-nee-ah	S/ R/CF R/CF	-**penia** *deficiency* lymph/o- *lymph* -cyt/o- *cell*	Condition of decreased lymphocytes in the blood
lymphocytosis	**LIM**-foh-sigh-**TOH**-sis	S/ R/CF R/	-**osis** *condition* lymph/o- *lymph* -cyt- *cell*	Condition of increased lymphocytes in the blood.
lymphoid	**LIM**-foyd	S/ R/	-**oid** *resembling* lymph- *lymph*	Resembling lymphatic tissue
lymphoid leukemia	**LIM**-foyd loo-**KEE**-mee-ah	S/ R/	-**emia** *blood condition* leuk- *white*	Malignant disease marked by an uncontrolled production of lymphocytes
monocytosis	**MON**-oh-sigh-**TOH**-sis	S/ P/ R/CF	-**osis** *condition* mono- *single* -cyt/o- *cell*	Increased number of monocytes in the blood
monocytopenia	**MON**-oh-sigh-toh-**PEE**-nee-ah	S/	-**penia** *deficiency*	Decreased number of monocytes in the blood
mononucleosis	**MON**-oh-nyu-klee-**OH**-sis	S/ P/ R/	-**osis** *condition* mono- *single* -nucle- *nucleus*	Presence of large numbers of mononuclear leukocytes
myeloid	**MY**-eh-loyd	S/ R/	-**oid** *resembling* myel- *bone marrow*	Resembling cells derived from bone marrow
myeloid leukemia	**MY**-eh-loyd loo-**KEE**-mee-ah	S/ R/	-**emia** *blood condition* leuk- *white*	Leukemia that begins with cells in the bone marrow and moves into the blood
neutrophilia	**NEW**-troh-**FILL**-ee-ah	S/ R/CF	-**philia** *attraction* neutr/o- *neutral*	An excess number of neutrophils
neutropenia	**NEW**-troh-**PEE**-nee-ah	S/	-**penia** *deficiency*	A deficiency of neutrophils
pancytopenia	**PAN**-sigh-toh-**PEE**-nee-ah	S/ P/ R/CF	-**penia** *deficiency* pan- *all* -cyt/o- *cell*	Deficiency of all types of blood cells
platelet	**PLAYT**-let	S/ R/	-**let** *small* plate- *flat*	Cell fragment involved in clotting process
thrombocyte (syn)	**THROM**-boh-site	S/ R/CF	-**cyte** *cell* thromb/o- *blood clot, clot*	
precursor	pree-**KUR**-sir	P/ R/	pre- *before, in front of* -cursor *run*	Cell or substance formed earlier in the development of the cell or substance
stem cell	STEM SELL		**stem** Old English *stalk of a plant*	Undifferentiated cell found in a differentiated tissue that can divide to yield the specialized cells in that tissue

Exercises

A. Define word elements pertaining to hematology. *If you can remember the meaning of word elements, you can define the medical term.* **LO 11.6, 11.D**

1. The suffix that means *attraction* is:

    a. *-osis*   **b.** *-penia*   **c.** *-ic*   **d.** *-philia*

2. The combining form that means *white* is:

    a. *neutr/o*   **b.** *leuk/o*   **c.** *cyt/o*   **d.** *bas/o*

3. The suffix *–penia* means:

    a. deficiency   **b.** excessive   **c.** one   **d.** white

Lesson 11.4

Hemostasis

When you are employed in any clinical area in health care—in an office, in a hospital, or out in the field—at many times in your career, you will be faced with a patient who is bleeding.

Before you can take blood for laboratory examination, you need to have an awareness of the medical terminology for possible diagnoses and the appropriate tests that will be performed. In this lesson, information will be available for you to use correct medical terminology to:

11.4.1 Identify the functions of platelets.

11.4.2 Discuss the body's mechanisms for controlling bleeding.

11.4.3 Describe the methods of producing blood clots.

11.4.4 Explain some disorders of blood clotting.

Abbreviations

EMT	emergency medical technician
vWD	von Willebrand disease
vWF	von Willebrand factor

Tissue factors, clotting factors, platelets

↓ That convert

Prothrombin

↓ To

Thrombin

↓ That converts

Fibrinogen

↓ To

Fibrin Clot

▲ **Figure 11.12** Blood Coagulation.

Case Report (CR) 11.3

You are
... an **emergency medical technician (EMT)** employed in the Fulwood Medical Center Emergency Department.

Your patient is
... Janis Tierney, a 17-year-old high school student.

Ms. Tierney presents with fainting at school. She is pale. Her pulse is 90. Blood pressure (BP) is 100/60. She tells you that she is having a menstrual period with excessive bleeding. Her physical examination is otherwise unremarkable. She has a history of easy bruising and recurrent nosebleeds and an episode of severe bleeding after a tooth extraction. Laboratory tests reveal that she has a deficiency of **von Willebrand factor (vWF).** Her platelets are unable to stick together or adhere to the wall of an injured blood vessel, and a platelet plug cannot form in the lining of her uterus to help end her menstrual flow.

Von Willebrand disease (vWD) is the most common hereditary bleeding disorder. It affects at least 1% of the population and both sexes equally.

LO 11.7 Hemostasis

Hemostasis, the control of bleeding, is a vital issue in maintaining homeostasis, the state of equilibrium of the body. Uncontrolled bleeding can take the body out of balance by decreasing blood volume and lowering blood pressure, leading to death.

Platelets (also called **thrombocytes**) play a key role in hemostasis. They are minute fragments of large bone marrow cells called **megakaryocytes.** They have no nucleus. Platelet granules secrete chemicals that are critical to hemostasis:

- **Coagulation factors**—proteins and enzymes—that initiate the process.
- **Vasoconstrictors** that cause constriction in injured blood vessels.
- **Chemicals** that attract neutrophils and monocytes to sites of inflammation.

Hemostasis is achieved through a three-step mechanism:

1. **Vascular spasm**—an immediate but temporary constriction of the injured blood vessel.

2. **Platelet plug formation**—an accumulation of platelets that bind themselves together and adhere to surrounding tissues. The binding and adhesion of platelets is mediated through **von Willebrand factor (vWF),** a protein produced by the cells lining blood vessels.

3. **Blood coagulation**—the process beginning with the production of molecules that make **prothrombin** and **thrombin** and finishing with the formation of a blood clot that traps blood cells, platelets, and tissue fluid in a network of fibrin *(Figures 11.12).*

After a blood clot forms, platelets adhere to strands of fibrin and contract to pull the fibers closer together. As the blood clot shrinks, it pulls the edges of the broken blood vessel together. **Fibroblasts** invade the clot to produce a fibrous connective tissue that seals the blood vessel.

380   CHAPTER 11 Blood The Language of Hematology

WORD	PRONUNCIATION	ELEMENTS		DEFINITION
anticoagulant	**AN**-tee-koh-**AG**-you-lant	S/ P/ R/	-ant *forming* anti- *against* -coagul- *clump*	Substance that prevents clotting
coagulant coagulation	koh-**AG**-you-lant koh-ag-you-**LAY**-shun	S/ S/	-ant *forming* -ation *process*	Substance that induces clotting The process of blood clotting
fibroblast	**FIE**-broh-blast	S/ R/CF	-blast *immature cell* fibr/o- *fiber*	Cell that forms collagen fibers
hemostasis (***Note:*** Homeostasis has a very different meaning.)	hee-moh-**STAY**-sis	S/ R/CF	-stasis *control, stop* hem/o- *blood*	Controlling or stopping bleeding
megakaryocyte	**MEG**-ah-**KAIR**-ee-oh-site	S/ P/ R/CF	-cyte *cell* mega- *enormous* -kary/o- *nucleus*	Large cell with large nucleus. Parts of the cytoplasm break off to form platelets
platelet thrombocyte (syn)	**PLAYT**-let	S/ R/	-let *small* plate- *flat*	Cell fragment involved in the clotting process
prothrombin	proh-**THROM**-bin	S/ P/ R/	-in *substance* pro- *before* -thromb- *clot*	Protein formed by the liver and converted to thrombin in the blood-clotting mechanism
thrombin thrombocyte (also called **platelet**) thrombus	**THROM**-bin **THROM**-boh-site **THROM**-bus	S/ R/CF	Greek *clot* -cyte *cell* thromb/o- *clot*	Enzyme that forms fibrin Another name for a platelet A clot attached to a blood vessel or heart lining
thrombosis	throm-**BOH**-sis	S/ R/	-osis *condition* thromb- *clot*	Formation of a thrombus

Exercises

A. Refer to Case Report 11.3 along with the other text material to answer the following questions. *Select the answer that correctly completes each statement.* **LO 11.7, 11.A, 11.F**

1. Because Ms. Tierney has a deficiency in vWF, she is unable to:

   a. produce fibrinogen   **b.** coagulate her blood   **c.** form a platelet plug   **d.** create a vascular spasm

2. Her excessive loss of blood is causing her heart rate to:

   a. stay within normal limits   **b.** increase   **c.** decrease

3. Her abnormal blood pressure is related to:

   a. stress   **b.** recurrent nose bleeds   **c.** loss of blood   **d.** her tooth extraction

B. Place the steps of hemostasis in the correct order. *There are three steps to hemostasis. Place them in order, with the first step being "1" and the last step being "3."* **LO 11.7**

_____ platelet plug

_____ vascular spasm

_____ blood coagulation

C. Use the language of hematology to answer the following questions. *Fill in each blank with the correct medical term relating to hemostasis.* **LO 11.1, 11.7**

1. A cell that forms collagen fibers: _____.

2. A platelet is a fragment of a _____.

3. The process of forming a clot: _____

LO 11.8 Disorders of Coagulation (Coagulopathies)

Hemophilia in its classical form (hemophilia A) is a disease males inherit from their mothers and is due to a deficiency of a coagulation factor, called factor VIII. The disorder causes painful bleeding into skin, joints, and muscles. Concentrated factor VIII is given intravenously to reduce the symptoms.

Von Willebrand disease (vWD) is a deficiency of a specific protein of the factor VIII complex that is different from the part involved in hemophilia.

Disseminated intravascular coagulation (DIC) occurs when the clotting mechanism is activated simultaneously throughout the cardiovascular system. The trigger is usually a severe bacterial infection. Small clots form and obstruct blood flow into tissues and organs, particularly the kidney, leading to renal failure. As the clotting mechanisms are overwhelmed, severe bleeding occurs.

Thrombus formation (**thrombosis**) is a clot that attaches to diseased or damaged areas on the walls of blood vessels or the heart. If part of the thrombus breaks loose and moves through the circulation, it is called an **embolus**.

Thrombocytopenia is a low platelet count (below 100,000/mm^3 of blood). It occurs when bone marrow is destroyed by radiation, chemotherapy, or leukemia. Small capillary hemorrhages called **petechiae** and bruises can be seen in the skin. **Idiopathic (immunologic) thrombocytopenic purpura (ITP)** is an acute self-limiting form of the disease usually seen in children.

Thrombotic thrombocytopenic purpura (TTP) and **hemolytic-uremic syndrome (HUS)** are acute, potentially fatal disorders in which loose strands of fibrin are deposited in numerous small blood vessels. This causes damage to platelets and RBCs, causing thrombocytopenia and hemolytic anemia.

Henoch-Schönlein purpura (anaphylactoid purpura) is a disorder involving purpura, joint pain, and **glomerulonephritis** *(see Chapter 6)*. The etiology is unknown. Most cases resolve spontaneously.

Purpura is bleeding into the skin from small arterioles that produces a larger individual lesion than petechiae from capillary bleeding *(Figure 11.13)*. **Bruises** (or **hematomas**) are **extravasations** of blood from all types of blood vessels.

(a)

(b)

(c)

▲ **Figure 11.13** **Subsurface Bleeding.** (a) Purpura. (b) Pinpoint petechiae. (c) Bruises.
©Medical-on-line/Alamy Stock Photo ©Dr. P. Marazzi/Science Photo Library/Photo Researchers, Inc.
©Paul Cox/Alamy Stock Photo

WORD	PRONUNCIATION	ELEMENTS		DEFINITION
coagulopathy coagulopathies (pl)	koh-ag-you-**LOP**-ah-thee	S/ R/CF	-pathy *disease* coagul/o- *clotting*	Disorder of blood clotting
disseminate	dih-**SEM**-in-ate	S/ P/ R/	-ate *composed of, pertaining to* dis- *apart* -semin- *scatter seed*	Widely scatter throughout the body or an organ
embolus	**EM**-boh-lus		Greek *plug, stopper*	Detached piece of thrombus, a mass of bacteria, quantity of air, or foreign body that blocks a blood vessel
extravasate	eks-**TRAV**-ah-sate	S/ P/ R/	-ate *composed of, pertaining to* extra- *out of, outside* -vas- *blood vessel*	To ooze out from a vessel into the tissues
hematoma bruise (syn)	hee-mah-**TOH**-mah BROOZ	S/ R/	-oma *mass, tumor* hemat- *blood* Old English *to bruise*	Collection of blood that has escaped from the blood vessels into tissue
hemophilia	hee-moh-**FILL**-ee-ah	S/ R/CF	-philia *attraction* hem/o- *blood*	An inherited disease from a deficiency of clotting factor VIII
petechia petechiae (pl)	peh-**TEE**-kee-ah peh-**TEE**-kee-ee		Latin *spot on the skin*	Pinpoint capillary hemorrhagic spot in the skin
purpura	**PUR**-pyu-rah		Greek *purple*	Skin hemorrhages that are red initially and then turn purple
thrombocytopenia	**THROM**-boh-sigh-toh-**PEE**-nee-ah	S/ R/CF R/CF	-penia *deficiency* thromb/o- *clot* -cyt/o- *cell*	Deficiency of platelets in circulating blood

Exercises

A. Fill in the blank with the correct medical term related to disorders of coagulation. LO 11.8

1. A decrease in the number of thrombocytes in the circulating blood: _____.

2. A thrombus that has detached and lodged in another blood vessel: _____.

3. A pinpoint hemorrhage: _____.

B. Match the term in the first column to its correct definition in the second column. LO 11.8

_____ 1. hematoma

_____ 2. extravasate

_____ 3. petechia

_____ 4. purpura

_____ 5. disseminate

a. widely scatter throughout the body

b. bleeding into the skin from arterioles

c. escape from a blood vessel

d. collection of blood that has escaped from a blood vessel

e. small capillary hemorrhage

C. Choose the correct abbreviation. *From the given description, choose the correct abbreviation of the described conditions.* **LO 11.8, 11.F**

1. Loose strands of fibrin are deposited in numerous small blood vessels:

   a. DIC   b. ITP   c. TTP   d. vWD

2. Deficiency of factor VIII:

   a. DIC   b. ITP   c. TTP   d. vWD

Lesson 11.5

BLOOD

Blood Groups

Lesson Objectives

To make an appropriate decision, it is critical that you are able to use correct medical terminology to:

11.5.1 List the different blood groups.

11.5.2 Explain what determines a person's ABO blood type and how this relates to transfusion compatibility.

11.5.3 Describe the effect of an incompatibility between mother and fetus in the rhesus (Rh) blood type.

(a) Type A blood

(b) Type B blood

(c) Type AB blood

(d) Type O blood

▲ **Figure 11.14** ABO Blood Types.

Keynotes

- All blood groups are inherited.
- Rh factor is an antigen on the surface of a red blood cell.

📁 Case Report (CR) 11.4

You are

... an emergency medical technician–paramedic (EMT-P) working in the Level One Trauma Unit at Fulwood Medical Center.

Your patient is

... Ms. Joanne Rodi, an 18-year-old student.

Ms. Rodi has been admitted to the unit from the operating room after surgery for multiple fractures in a car accident. She is receiving a blood transfusion. You document that her temperature has risen to 102°F and her respirations to 24 per minute and she has chills. You take her BP; it has fallen to 90/60. What should you do?

LO 11.9 Red Cell Antigens

On the surfaces of red blood cells are molecules called **antigens**. In the plasma, antibodies are present. Each antibody can combine with only a specific antigen. If the plasma antibodies combine with a red cell antigen, bridges are formed that connect the red cells together. This is called **agglutination**, or clumping, of the cells. Hemolysis (rupture) of the cells also occurs.

The antigens on the surfaces of the cells have been categorized into groups, of which two are the most important. These are the ABO and Rhesus (Rh) blood groups.

ABO Blood Group

Figure 11.14 shows the different combinations of antigens and antibodies in the different blood types. The two major antigens on the cell surface are antigen A and antigen B.

A person with only antigen A has *type A* blood.

A person with only antigen B has *type B* blood.

A person with both antigen A and antigen B has *type AB* blood and is a universal recipient who can receive blood from any other type in the ABO system.

A person with neither antigen has *type O* blood and is a universal donor, able to give blood to any other person no matter what that person's blood type is.

📁 Case Report 11.4 *(continued)*

In Miss Rodi's case, she has type A blood and, by mistake, received type AB blood, which agglutinated in the presence of her anti-B antibodies. Your immediate response is to stop the transfusion, replace it with a saline **infusion**, call your supervisor, and notify the doctor.

WORD	PRONUNCIATION	ELEMENTS		DEFINITION
agglutination	ah-glue-tih-**NAY**-shun	S/ P/ R/	-ation *process* ag- *to* -glutin- *glue*	Process by which cells or other particles adhere to each other to form clumps
antibody	**AN**-tih-body	P/ R/	**anti-** *against* **-body** *substance*	Protein produced in response to an antigen
antigen	**AN**-tih-jen	P/ R/	**anti-** *against* **-gen** *to produce*	Any substance that can trigger an immune response
infusion	in-**FYU**-zhun	P/ R/	**in-** *in* **-fusion** *to pour*	Introduction intravenously of a substance other than blood

Exercises

A. Review the elements in the above WAD before starting this exercise. *Match the elements in the first column with the correct meanings in the second column.* **LO 11.9**

_____ **1.** *anti*

_____ **2.** *fusion*

_____ **3.** *glutin*

_____ **4.** *ation*

_____ **5.** *osis*

_____ **6.** *in*

a. condition

b. in

c. to pour

d. glue

e. against

f. process

B. Identify the components of blood typing. *Choose the correct term in the parentheses that completes each statement.* **LO 11.9**

1. It is the (antigen/antibody) on the erythrocyte that determines a person's blood type.

2. It is the (red blood cells/plasma) that contains antibodies that seek out antigens.

3. A person with type B blood has B (antigens/antibodies).

4. A person with type A blood has anti-B (antigens/antibodies).

5. A person with type O blood has no (anti-A antibodies/antigens).

LO 11.9 Red Cell Antigens (Continued)

Rhesus (Rh) Blood Group

If an **Rh** antigen is present on an RBC surface, the blood is said to be Rh-positive (Rh$^+$). If there is no Rh antigen on the surface, the blood is Rh-negative (Rh$^-$). The presence or absence of Rh antigen is inherited. The antigen is named the **Rhesus factor** because it was first found on the red blood cell of a rhesus monkey.

If an Rh-negative person receives a transfusion of Rh-positive blood, anti-Rh antibodies will be produced. This can cause RBC agglutination and hemolysis.

If an Rh-negative woman and an Rh-positive man conceive an Rh-positive child *(Figure 11.15a)*, the placenta normally prevents maternal and fetal blood from mixing. However, at birth or during a miscarriage, fetal cells can enter the mother's bloodstream. These Rh-positive cells stimulate the mother's tissues to produce Rh-antibodies *(Figure 11.15b)*.

If the mother becomes pregnant with a second Rh-positive fetus, her Rh-antibodies can cross the placenta and agglutinate and hemolyze the fetal RBCs *(Figure 11.15c)*. This causes hemolytic disease of the newborn (**HDN,** or **erythroblastosis fetalis**).

Hemolytic disease of the newborn due to Rh-incompatibility can be prevented. The Rh-negative mother should be given Rh immune globulin (RhoGAM) during pregnancy, or soon after giving birth to an Rh-positive child.

Other causes of hemolytic disease of the newborn include ABO incompatibility, incompatibility in other blood group systems, hereditary **spherocytosis**, and some infections acquired before birth.

Abbreviations	
HDN	hemolytic disease of the newborn (erythroblastosis fetalis)
Rh	rhesus
RhoGAM	rhesus immune globulin

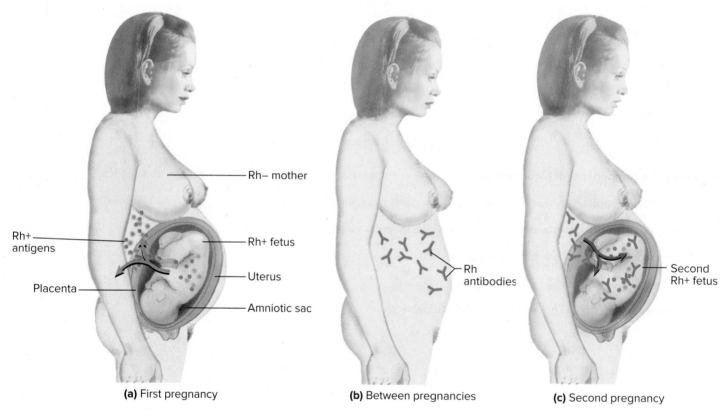

(a) First pregnancy (b) Between pregnancies (c) Second pregnancy

▲ **Figure 11.15** Hemolytic Disease of the Newborn.

WORD	PRONUNCIATION	ELEMENTS		DEFINITION
erythroblastosis fetalis	eh-**RITH**-ro-blas-**TOH**-sis fee-**TAH**-lis	S/ R/CF R/ S/ S/ R/	-osis *condition* erythr/o- *red* -blast- *germ cell, immature cell* -is *belonging to* -al- *pertaining to* fet- *fetus*	Hemolytic disease of the newborn due to Rh incompatibility
Rhesus factor	**REE**-sus **FAK**-tor	R/	**Rhesus** Greek *mythical king of Thrace* factor *maker*	Antigen on red blood cells of Rh-positive (Rh⁺) individuals. It was first identified in the blood of a rhesus monkey
spherocytosis	**SFEER**-oh-sigh-**TOH**-sis	S/ R/CF R/	-osis *condition* spher/o *sphere* -cyt- *cell*	Presence of spherocytes in blood

Exercises

A. Deconstruct medical terms to determine their meanings. *Using the terms relating to rhesus factor, identify the meanings of the word elements.* **LO 11.9, 11.D**

1. In the medical term **erythroblastosis fetalis,** the condition affects which component of the blood?

   a. white blood cells   **b.** plasma   **c.** coagulation   **d.** red blood cells

2. In the medical condition **erythroblastosis fetalis,** who is harmed: the mother or the baby?

   a. mother   **b.** baby

B. Explain the disorder erythroblastosis fetalis. *Choose the correct answer for each question regarding this condition.* **LO 11.9**

1. In order for this disorder to occur, the mother must have blood that is:

   a. type A   **b.** type B   **c.** type O   **d.** Rh–   **e.** Rh+

2. The trigger for this condition to occur is a baby with blood that is:

   a. type A   **b.** type B   **c.** type O   **d.** Rh–   **e.** Rh+

3. It is impossible for the first child to have this condition.

   a. True   **b.** False

Lesson 11.6

BLOOD

Procedures and Pharmacology

Lesson Objectives

The information in this lesson will enable you to use medical terminology to:

11.6.1 Explain the diagnostic procedures used for hematologic disorders.

11.6.2 Discuss the therapeutic disorders used for hematologic disorders.

11.6.3 Describe the pharmacologic agents used in the treatment of hematologic disorders.

Abbreviations

CBC	complete blood count
ESR	erythrocyte sedimentation rate
INR	International Normalized Ratio
MCH	mean corpuscular hemoglobin
MCHC	mean corpuscular hemoglobin concentration
MCV	mean corpuscular volume
PT	prothrombin time
PTT	partial thromboplastin time

LO 11.10 Diagnostic Procedures

A **complete blood count (CBC)** measures the following:

- The number of red blood cells (RBC count)
- The amount of hemoglobin in the blood
- The percentage of the blood composed of red blood cells (hematocrit)
- Average red blood cell size **(MCV)**
- Hemoglobin amount per red blood cell **(MCH)**
- Amount of hemoglobin relative to the size of the red blood cell **(MCHC)**
- The number of white blood cells (WBC count)
- The types of white blood cells (WBC differential)
- Platelet count

Serum iron is the amount of iron in the blood.

Serum ferritin is the amount in the blood of the iron-protein complex that regulates iron storage and transport.

Erythrocyte sedimentation rate (ESR) is a nonspecific measure of inflammation.

Bone marrow is found inside the larger bones and contains cells that produce RBCs, WBCs, and platelets. **Bone marrow biopsy** and **aspiration** are performed in the investigation of anemias, polycythemia, cancers (to determine if the cancer has spread to the bones), and bone marrow diseases.

Prothrombin time (PT), partial thromboplastin time (PTT), and **International Normalized Ratio (INR)** are used to evaluate bleeding and clotting disorders and to monitor anticoagulation therapies *(see Lesson 11.4).*

A **Monospot test** is used to diagnose infectious mononucleosis caused by the Epstein-Barr virus. It detects the presence of antibodies that the body developed in response to external antigens.

LO 11.11 Therapeutic Procedures

A **transfusion** of blood or packed red blood cells *(Figure 11.16)* replaces lost red blood cells to restore the blood's oxygen-carrying capacity. During **autologous** donation and transfusion, people donate their own blood ahead of time to be given to them if necessary during a surgical procedure.

Bone marrow transplant is the transfer of bone marrow from a healthy, compatible bone marrow donor to a patient with aplastic anemia, leukemia, lymphoma, multiple myeloma, or other disease.

Hematopoietic stem cells are found in the bone marrow and are capable of generating all our blood cells such as red cells, white cells, and platelets. In hematology, clinical trials to treat hemophilia and thalassemia with **gene therapy** are underway using **allogenic** cells from a **compatible** donor.

Gene therapy is an experimental technique to treat or prevent disease by replacing a **mutated** gene with a healthy copy, by inactivating a mutated gene that is functioning improperly, or by introducing a new gene into the body.

▲ **Figure 11.16** Patient receiving blood transfusion.
©Dave Moyer

WORD	PRONUNCIATION		ELEMENTS	DEFINITION
allogen	**AL**-oh-jen	P/ R/	**allo-** *different* **-gen** *to produce*	Antigen from someone else in the same species
allogenic (adj)	al-oh-**JEN**-ik	S/	**-ic** *pertaining to*	Pertaining to an allogen
aspiration	**AS**-pih-**RAY**-shun	S/ R/	**-ion** *process* **aspirat-** *to breathe*	Removal by suction of fluid or gas from a body cavity.
autologous	awe-**TOL**-oh-gus	P/ R/	**auto-** *self, same* **-logous** *relation*	Blood transfusion with the same person as donor and recipient
compatible	kom-**PAT**-ih-bul	S/ P/ R/	**-ible** *able to* **com-** *with* **-pat-** *lie together*	Able to exist together with something else
corpuscle	**KOR**-pus-ul	S/ R/	**-cle** *small (can also be cule)* **corpus-** *body*	A blood cell
corpuscular	kor-**PUS**-kyu-lar	S/ S/	**-ar** *pertaining to* **-cul-** *small*	Pertaining to corpuscle
ferritin	**FER**-ih-tin	S/ R/	**-in** *chemical* **ferrit-** *iron*	Iron-protein complex that regulates iron storage and transport
gene	JEEN		Greek *birth*	Functional unit of heredity
Monospot test (Trade name)	**MON**-oh-spot TEST			Detects heterophile antibodies in infectious mononucleosis
mutate mutation	**MYU**-tayt myu-**TAY**-shun	S/ R/	Latin *to change* **-ion** *action, condition, process* **mutat-** *change*	Change the chemistry of a gene Change in the chemistry of a gene
transfusion	trans-**FYU**-zhun	P/ R/	**trans-** *across* **-fusion** *to pour*	Transfer of blood or a blood component from donor to recipient
transplant	**TRANZ**-plant	P/ R/	**trans-** *across* **-plant** *plant*	The tissue or organ used or the act of transferring tissue from one person to another

Exercises

A. Identify the meaning of the word parts as they relate to hematology. *Select the answer that correctly completes each statement.*
LO 11.10, 11.11, 11.C

1. The word element that means **different:**

   a. *allo-*   **b.** *trans-*   **c.** *corpus-*   **d.** *-gen*

2. The word part *ferrit-* means:

   a. blood   **b.** cell   **c.** iron   **d.** protein

B. Interpret abbreviations. *Given the abbreviation, choose what the diagnostic test is measuring.* **LO 11.10, 11.F**

1. WBC differential

   a. number of leukocytes   **c.** types of leukocytes

   b. measure of inflammation   **d.** average red blood cell size

2. PT

   a. evaluates bleeding and clotting disorders   **c.** counts the number of platelets

   b. hemoglobin amount per erythrocyte   **d.** determines presence of bone cancer

3. MCH

   a. measures amount of iron in the blood   **c.** measures the various blood cell components

   b. determines amount of hemoglobin per erythrocyte   **d.** used to monitor anticoagulation therapies

LO 11.12 Pharmacology

Anticoagulants used to reduce or prevent blood clotting include:

- **Aspirin,** which reduces platelet **adherence** and is used in small 81 mg doses to reduce the incidence of heart attack.

- **Heparin,** which prevents prothrombin and fibrin formation and is given **parenterally**; its dose is monitored by **activated partial thromboplastin time** (aPTT).

- **Warfarin** *(Coumadin),* which inhibits the synthesis of prothrombin and others to act as an anticoagulant. It is given by mouth and its dose is monitored by **prothrombin times** (PTs), which are reported as an **International Normalized Ratio** (INR).

- **Dabigatran etexilate** *(Pradaxa)* and **rivaroxaban** *(Xarelto),* which inhibit the **synthesis** of thrombin and are given by mouth to reduce the risk of **embolism** and stroke in patients with nonvalvular atrial fibrillation *(see Chapter 10).* **Idarucizumab** *(Praxbind injection)* is available for patients using *Pradaxa* when reversal of its anticoagulant effects is needed for emergency surgery, for urgent procedures, or in life-threatening or uncontrolled bleeding.

- **Streptokinase,** derived from hemolytic streptococci, which dissolves the fibrin in blood clots. Given intravenously within 3 to 4 hours of a heart attack, it is often effective in dissolving a clot that has caused the heart attack.

Recombinant Factor VIII, developed through **recombinant DNA** technology, is the main medication used to treat hemophilia A. It is given intravenously through a vein in the arm or a port in the chest. **Desmopressin acetate** *(DDAVP)* is a synthetic version of **vasopressin** that helps stop bleeding in patients with mild hemophilia.

Pernicious anemia is treated initially with injections of vitamin B_{12}, and then the vitamin B_{12} can be given through a nasal gel.

Eltrombopag *(Promacta)* is available for pediatric patients with idiopathic thrombocytopenic purpura (ITP) who have not responded to corticosteroids, immunoglobulins, or splenectomy.

Most **leukemias** in both adults and children are treated with **chemotherapy**, often with added radiation therapy and a stem cell transplant.

WORD	PRONUNCIATION	ELEMENTS		DEFINITION
adhere adherence	add-**HEER** add-**HEER**-ents	S/ R/	Latin *to stick to* **-ence** *forming, quality of* **adher-** *stick to*	To stick to something The act of sticking to something
chemotherapy	**KEE**-moh-**THAIR**-ah-pee	R/CF R/	**chem/o-** *chemical* **therapy** *treatment*	Treatment using chemical agents
embolism	**EM**-boh-lizm		Greek *a plug or patch*	A plug of tissue or air from afar that obstructs a blood vessel
parenteral	pah-**REN**-ter-al	S/ P/ R/	**-al** *pertaining to* **par-** *abnormal* **-enter-** *intestine*	Administering medication by any means other than the GI tract
recombinant DNA	ree-**KOM**-bin-ant **DEE**-en-a	S/ P/ R/	**-ant** *forming* **re-** *again* **-combin-** *combine*	Deoxyribonucleic acid (DNA) altered by inserting a new sequence of DNA into the chain
streptokinase	strep-toh-**KIE**-nase	P/ R/	**strepto-** *curved* **-kinase** *enzyme*	An enzyme that dissolves clots
vasopressin (also called antidiuretic hormone)	vay-soh-**PRESS**-in	S/ R/CF R/	**-in** *chemical compound* **vas/o** *blood vessel* **-press-** *close, press*	Pituitary hormone that constricts blood vessels and decreases urinary output

Exercises

A. Describe the action of medications as they relate to hematology. *Place the anticoagulant with the action it uses to prevent or reduce the formation of clots.* **LO 11.12, 11.A**

Pradaxa   aspirin   *Coumadin*   streptokinase   *Xarelto*   **heparin (has two actions, use the term twice)**

Dissolves fibrin in blood clots	Decreases platelet adherence	Inhibits synthesis of prothrombin	Inhibits synthesis of thrombin
1.	2.	3.	5.
		4.	6.
			7.

B. Match the therapy In the first column to the disorder it treats in the second column. LO 11.12

_____ **1.** Vitamin B$_{12}$

_____ **2.** *Promacta* (eltrombopag)

_____ **3.** desmopressin acetate

_____ **4.** Recombinant Factor VIII

a. idiopathic thrombocytopenic purpura

b. mild hemophilia

c. pernicious anemia

d. hemophilia A

Blood

Challenge Your Knowledge

A. **True or false.** The following statements about blood are either true or false. *Choose T if the statement is true. Choose F if the statement is false.* (**LO 11.1, 11.2**)

1. The formed elements of blood are RBCs, WBCs, platelets, and serum.   T   F

2. Buffer systems in the blood maintain the correct pH range.   T   F

3. Serum is identical to plasma except for the absence of clotting proteins.   T   F

4. Sickle cell anemia is a genetic disorder.   T   F

5. All cells exchange water by thrombosis.   T   F

6. Plasma is the fluid, noncellular part of blood.   T   F

7. The bloodstream is a liquid transport system.   T   F

8. Whole blood is less viscous than water.   T   F

9. Monocytes are the largest blood cells.   T   F

10. Erythropoiesis occurs in bone spaces filled with red bone marrow.   T   F

B. **Medical terms may be similar in appearance.** You need to use your knowledge of prefixes, roots, and suffixes to help determine the difference between similar terms. Using the following terms, correctly insert them into the following paragraph. Use the italicized words as a hint as to which term goes into the blank. (**LO 11.3, 11.4**)

erythrocyte   erythroblast   erythroblastosis   erythropoiesis   erythropoietin

The *immature RBC* (1) (_____) undergoes *the process of formation* (2) (_____) in the red bone marrow.

Too many immature cells result in a condition known as (3) _____. A mature RBC is called an (4) _____.

The hormone (5) _____ controls the rate of RBC production.

C. **Pharmacology of blood clotting.** Anyone working with patients must know about prescribed drugs and their function. Match the drug action in the first column with the correct drug in the second column. (**LO 11.12**)

_____ 1. Dissolves fibrin in blood clots   **a.** heparin

_____ 2. Reduces platelet adherence   **b.** Xarelto

_____ 3. Prevents prothrombin and fibrin formation   **c.** Coumadin

_____ 4. Inhibits formation of prothrombin   **d.** streptokinase

_____ 5. Inhibits synthesis of thrombin   **e.** aspirin

D. How well do you understand what you read? First, read the paragraph aloud to check your pronunciation. Enter the term found in the paragraph in the left column of the chart next to its correct meaning. **(LO 11.A, 11.B)**

When a lab tech takes a blood sample, he spins it in a centrifuge. Formed elements are separated from the colloidal suspension and are packed into the bottom of the tube. The patient's hematocrit can be determined from this test. Whole blood contains all the formed elements. Transfusions can be done with either whole blood or only certain portions of the formed elements—only transfusing RBCs or platelets, for instance. The remaining part (55%) of a blood sample is the plasma, which is mostly water. Plasma provides the fluid transport for the formed elements as well as nutrients, hormones, and enzymes for body cells. Waste cell products dissolve in plasma and are excreted through the kidneys and liver.

Term	Meaning
1.	percentage of RBCs in the blood
2.	liquid containing particles that do not settle
3.	introduction of blood or a blood component into a vein
4.	something life sustaining
5.	blood clotting cell
6.	instrument for separating a blood sample
7.	stimulates function of an organ or tissue
8.	erythrocyte
9.	liquid transport system
10.	induces chemical changes in other substances

E. List the different blood types in the ABO blood group. Be sure to note which type is the "universal donor" and which type is the "universal recipient." Fill in the blanks. **(LO 11.9)**

The two major antigens on the cell surface are antigen A and antigen B.

1. A person with only antigen A has type _____ blood.

2. A person with only antigen B has type _____ blood.

3. A person with *both* antigen A and antigen B has type _____ blood.

4. A person with *neither* antigen A nor antigen B has type _____ blood.

5. Because the blood type in question 4 has *neither* antigen, it is compatible with any blood type; therefore, it is the universal (donor/recipient) _____.

6. Because the blood type in question 3 has *both* antigens, it is the universal (donor/recipient) _____.

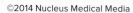
Blood

F. Build medical terms from the following group of elements. The definition is given to you; fill in the medical term. You will not use every element, and some you may use twice. Fill in the blanks. **(LO 11.A, LO 11.C)**

Use a combination of these elements to complete the terms:

ic	micro	auto	osis	hypo	crit	ox
ary	cyte	thrombo	macro	ar	erythro	cyt

1. Another name for an RBC   erythro/_____

2. Pertaining to a small cell   _____/cyt/_____

3. Blood transfusion with the same person as both donor and recipient   _____/logous

4. Large RBC   _____/cyte

5. Percentage of RBCs in blood   hemato/_____

6. Same as a platelet   _____/cyte

7. Formation of a clot   thromb/_____

G. Test your knowledge of blood, blood groups, and Rh factor by choosing the correct answer to the following questions. Select the answer that correctly completes each sentence. **(LO 11.9)**

1. A person with both antigen A and antigen B will have

   a. blood type O

   b. blood type A

   c. blood type B

   d. blood type AB

   e. blood type B–

2. Where are antibodies synthesized after birth?

   a. in the heart

   b. in the blood

   c. in the arteries

   d. in the plasma

   e. in the veins

3. What normally prevents maternal and fetal blood from mixing during pregnancy?

   a. cell membranes

   b. the peritoneum

   c. the placenta

   d. the amniotic sac

   e. the matrix

4. Blood is said to be Rh-positive if

   a. the Rh antigen is present on the RBC surface

   b. the Rh antibody is present in the blood type

   c. the Rh antibody is present in the plasma

   d. the Rh antigen is present on the WBCs

   e. the blood type is AB

5. **Agglutination** occurs when

   a. you have not been vaccinated

   b. you are given the wrong blood type

   c. your antibodies are low

   d. your hematocrit is high

   e. you are Rh-positive

6. The term **transfusion** is used only for

   a. plasma

   b. whole blood

   c. blood or a blood component

   d. saline solution

   e. intravenous (IV) antibiotics

H. Multiple choice. Use the *language of hematology* to answer the following questions. Remember that in the case of multiple choice, there is only one best answer. **(LO 11.1, 11.2, 11.5, 11.6, 11.10, 11.11 11.D)**

1. Blood volume varies with

    a. your body size

    b. your weight

    c. the amount of your connective tissue

    d. the amount of your erythrocytes

    e. your height

2. The percentage of erythrocytes in a blood sample is called the

    a. hemoglobin

    b. hematocrit

    c. hematemesis

    d. hemolysis

    e. hemostasis

3. In the term **hypochromic,** the root means

    a. blood

    b. center

    c. color

    d. glue

    e. air

4. How many types of leukocytes also qualify as granulocytes?

    a. one

    b. two

    c. three

    d. four

    e. five

5. **Myeloid leukemia** is a disorder of

    a. erythrocytes

    b. leukocytes

    c. platelets

    d. plasma

    e. hemoglobin

6. In the term **erythrocyte,** the combining form means

    a. yellow

    b. red

    c. white

    d. black

    e. blue

7. **Heparin** is an

    a. antidepressant

    b. antihistamine

    c. antibody

    d. anticoagulant

    e. antibiotic

8. Which of these terms cannot be connected with blood?

    a. liquid matrix

    b. complete blood count

    c. formed elements

    d. infusion

    e. transfusion

9. The largest leukocyte is

    a. monocyte

    b. macrophage

    c. eosinophil

    d. basophil

    e. neutrophil

10. What is plasma minus its protein fibrinogen?

    a. hemoglobin

    b. antithrombin

    c. plasmin

    d. serum

    e. a formed element

Blood

I. **There are many diseases associated with the various components of blood.** Select the correct answer in the following descriptions; then, on the blanks, write in which blood component is associated with the disease you circled. Use RBC, WBC, and P (for platelet) for blood component notations. **(LO 11.4, 11.6, 11.8, 11.F)**

Blood Component

1. Chronic bleeding from the gastrointestinal tract can cause

   a. iron-deficiency anemia   **b.** pernicious anemia   **c.** sickle cell anemia   _____

2. A deficiency of a specific protein of the factor VIII complex is

   a. thrombus   **b.** von Willenbrand disease   **c.** iron-deficiency anemia   _____

3. Cancer of the hematopoietic tissues is called

   a. leukemia   **b.** lukemia   **c.** lukemmia   _____

4. A disease resulting from vitamin B_{12} deficiency is

   a. pernicious anemia   **b.** hemolytic anemia   **c.** polycythemia vera   _____

5. A disease males inherit from their mothers is

   a. hemmaphilia   **b.** hemophilia   **c.** hemmophilia   _____

6. A hereditary disease found mostly in people of African descent is

   a. sickle cell anemia   **b.** iron-deficiency anemia   **c.** polycythemia vera   _____

7. In this disease, numerous small clots form and obstruct blood flow into organs:

   a. DIC   **b.** vWD   **c.** EBV   _____

8. This is seen in viral infections such as influenza:

   a. leukopenia   **b.** leukocytosis   **c.** leukemia   _____

9. Low blood cell count that produces a tendency to bleed is

   a. thrombocitopenia   **b.** thrombocytopenia   **c.** thrombocytopennia   _____

10. Destruction of blood cells by toxic substances is

   a. polycythemia vera   **b.** hemolytic anemia   **c.** pernicious anemia   _____

J. **Demonstrate your knowledge of word elements by deconstructing the following medical terms.** Place each word element from the medical term to its correct type. If the term does not have a particular element, write n/a. **(LO 11.D)**

Term	Prefix	Root/Combining Form	Suffix
agranulocyte	1.	2.	3.
hypochromic	4.	5.	6.
monocytosis	7.	8.	9.
poikilocytic	10.	11.	12.
precursor	13.	14.	15.
microcytic	16.	17.	18.
pancytopenia	19.	20.	21.

K. **Write the terms next to the appropriate statement that follows.** Fill in the blanks. **LO 11.3, 11.4, 11.6, 11.12**

1. That which comes before something _____

2. Pertaining to a small cell _____

3. Decreased number of erythrocytes _____

4. Pigmented protein in erythrocytes _____

5. Excessively high leukocyte count _____

6. Deficiency of all formed elements in the blood _____

7. Increase in the number of monocytes in the blood _____

8. Pertaining to an erythrocyte of irregular shape _____

L. With the possible exception of the appendix, everything in the body has a function. The functions are listed as follows. Assign each a letter for the blood component that performs the function. **(LO 11.2, 11.3, 11.5, 11.7)**

Functions

    a. A function of an erythrocyte

    b. A function of a leukocyte

    c. A function of a platelet

    d. A function of plasma

Assign one of the previous functions to each of the following statements: Fill in the blank with the correct letter that corresponds to each function.

    1. Transport oxygen   _____

    2. Help maintain hemostasis   _____

    3. Migrate to damaged tissues and release histamine   _____

    4. Carry nutrients, hormones, and enzymes to cells   _____

    5. Dissolve cellular waste products   _____

    6. Secrete lysozymes   _____

    7. Transport carbon dioxide   _____

    8. Seal off injury and hemorrhage   _____

    9. Provide fluid environment to formed elements   _____

    10. Transport nitric oxide   _____

M. After rereading Case Report 11.4, answer the following questions. **(LO 11.3, 11.4, 11.11, 11.A)**

Case Report (CR) 11.4

You are

. . . an emergency medical technician–paramedic (EMT-P) working in the Level One Trauma Unit at Fulwood Medical Center.

Your patient is

. . . Ms. Joanne Rodi, an 18-year-old student.

Ms. Rodi has been admitted to the unit from the operating room after surgery for multiple fractures in a car accident. She is receiving a blood transfusion. You document that her temperature has risen to 102°F and her respirations to 24 per minute and she has chills. You take her BP; it has fallen to 90/60. What should you do?

In Miss Rodi's case, she has type A blood and, by mistake, received type AB blood, which agglutinated. Your immediate response is to stop the transfusion, replace it with a saline infusion, call your supervisor, and notify the doctor.

---

    1. What does it mean when blood has *agglutinated*? _____

    2. What specific antigen did Miss Rodi's type A blood react to? _____

    3. Is her blood pressure within normal limits, too high, or too low? _____

    4. What medical term describes her blood pressure condition? _____

    5. What is the difference between a *transfusion* and an *infusion*? _____

©2014 Nucleus Medical Media

The health professionals involved in the diagnosis and treatment of problems with the lymphatic and immune systems include:

- **Immunologists** and **allergists,** who are physicians who specialize in immune system disorders, such as allergies, asthma, and immunodeficiency and autoimmune diseases.

- **Epidemiologists,** who are medical scientists involved in the study of epidemic diseases and how they are transmitted and controlled.

- **Medical** or **laboratory technicians,** who perform testing procedures on blood, body fluids, and other tissues using microscopes, computers, and other equipment.

Chapter Learning Outcomes

The lymphatic and immune systems are the major defenders of the body against disease. The content of this chapter is designed to enable you to:

LO 12.1 Describe the anatomy and flow of the lymphatic system.

LO 12.2 Relate the structure of the lymph nodes, tissues, and cells to their functions.

LO 12.3 Explain the structure and functions of the lymphatic organs.

LO 12.4 Discuss disorders of the lymphatic system.

LO 12.5 Define the characteristics of the immune system.

LO 12.6 Explain immunity.

LO 12.7 Describe disorders of the immune system and transplantation.

LO 12.8 Discuss HIV and AIDS infections.

LO 12.9 Identify diagnostic and therapeutic procedures and medications used in disorders of the lymphatic and immune systems.

LO 12.A Use the medical terms of immunology to communicate and document in writing accurately and precisely in any health care setting.

LO 12.B Use the medical terms of immunology to communicate verbally with accuracy and precision in any health care setting.

LO 12.C Construct the medical terms of immunology from their word elements.

LO 12.D Deconstruct the medical terms of immunology into their word elements.

LO 12.E Identify health professionals involved in the care of patients with immune disorders.

LO 12.F Use approved abbreviations of terms used in immunology correctly.

Case Report (CR) 12.1

You are

. . . a medical assistant working with Susan Lee, MD, in her primary care clinic at Fulwood Medical Center.

Your patient is

. . . Ms. Anna Clemons, a 20-year-old waitress, who is a new patient. She has noticed a lump in her right neck. On questioning, you find that she has lost about 8 pounds in weight in the past couple of months, has felt tired, and has had some night sweats.

Her vital signs (VS) are normal. There are two firm, enlarged lymph nodes in her right neck. Physical examination is otherwise unremarkable, and there is no evidence of infection in her head, throat, or upper respiratory tract.

Lesson 12.1

LYMPHATIC AND IMMUNE SYSTEMS

Lymphatic System

LO 12.1 Lymphatic System

The body has three lines of defense mechanisms against foreign organisms **(pathogens)**, cells **(cancer)**, and molecules **(pollutants** and **allergens)**:

1. **Physical mechanisms**—the skin and mucous membranes, chemicals in perspiration, saliva and tears, hairs in the nostrils, cilia and mucus to protect the lungs. These are described in the individual body system chapters.

2. **Cellular mechanisms**—based on defensive cells **(lymphocytes)** that directly attack suspicious cells such as cancer cells, transplanted tissue cells, or cells infected with viruses or **parasites.** This is the basis for the lymphatic system.

3. **Humoral defense mechanisms**—based on **antibodies** that are found in body fluids and bind to bacteria, **toxins,** and extracellular viruses, tagging them for destruction. This is the basis for the **immune** system.

The lymphatic system *(Figure 12.1)* **has three components:**

1. A network of thin **lymphatic capillaries and vessels,** similar to blood vessels, that penetrates into the interstitial spaces of nearly every tissue in the body except cartilage, bone, red bone marrow, and the central nervous system (CNS).

2. A group of tissues and organs that produce **immune cells.**

3. **Lymph**, a clear colorless fluid similar to blood plasma but whose composition varies from place to place in the body. It flows through the network of lymphatic capillaries and vessels.

The lymphatic system has three functions:

1. To **absorb** excess interstitial fluid and return it to the bloodstream.

2. To **remove** foreign chemicals, cells, and debris from the tissues.

3. To **absorb** dietary lipids from the small intestine *(see Chapter 5).*

The lymphatic network begins with **lymphatic capillaries,** which are closed-ended tubes nestled among blood capillary networks *(Figure 12.2).* The lymphatic capillaries are designed to let interstitial fluid enter, and the interstitial fluid becomes lymph. In addition, bacteria, viruses, cellular debris, and traveling cancer cells can enter the lymphatic capillaries with the interstitial fluid. The lymphatic capillaries converge to form the larger lymphatic collecting vessels. These resemble small veins and have one-way valves in their lumen. They travel alongside veins and arteries.

The larger lymphatic collecting vessels merge into **lymphatic trunks** that drain lymph from a major body region. In turn, these lymphatic trunks merge into two large **lymphatic ducts:**

1. The **right lymphatic duct** receives lymph from the right arm, right side of the thorax, and right side of the head and drains into the **right subclavian vein** *(Figure 12.1).*

2. The **thoracic duct** on the left, the largest lymphatic vessel, receives lymph from both sides of the body below the diaphragm and from the left arm, left side of the head, and left thorax. It begins in the abdomen at the level of the second lumbar vertebra (L2) and passes up through the diaphragm and mediastinum to empty into the **left subclavian vein** *(Figure 12.1).*

Lesson Objectives

As part of your defense mechanisms, the lymphatic system and its fluid provide surveillance and protection against foreign materials.

In this lesson, the information provided will enable you to use correct medical terminology to:

12.1.1 Describe the anatomy and flow of the lymphatic system.

12.1.2 List the functions of the lymphatic system.

12.1.3 Identify the major cells of the lymphatic system and their functions.

12.1.4 Detail the anatomy and functions of the lymph nodes, tonsils, thymus gland, and spleen.

12.1.5 Explain the effects of common disorders of the lymphatic system on health.

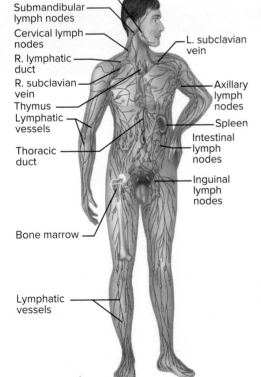

▲ **Figure 12.1** **The Lymphatic System.**
(R. = right; L. = left)

Palatine tonsil
Submandibular lymph nodes
Cervical lymph nodes
R. lymphatic duct
R. subclavian vein
Thymus
Lymphatic vessels
Thoracic duct
Bone marrow
Lymphatic vessels
L. subclavian vein
Axillary lymph nodes
Spleen
Intestinal lymph nodes
Inguinal lymph nodes

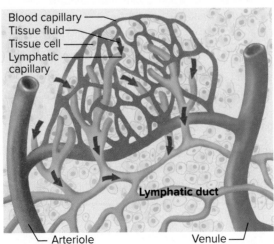

Blood capillary
Tissue fluid
Tissue cell
Lymphatic capillary
Lymphatic duct
Arteriole
Venule

▲ **Figure 12.2** **Lymphatic Flow.**

WORD	PRONUNCIATION	ELEMENTS		DEFINITION
allergen (*Note:* The duplicate letter "g" is deleted to better form the word.)	**AL**-er-jen	S/ R/ R/	-gen *to produce* all- *different, strange* -erg- *work*	Substance producing a hypersensitivity (allergic) reaction
allergic	ah-**LER**-jic	S/	-ic *pertaining to*	Pertaining to or suffering from an allergy
allergy	**AL**-er-jee	S/	-ergy *process of working*	Hypersensitivity to a particular allergen
antibody antibodies (pl)	**AN**-tih-body **AN**-tih-bod-ees	P/ R/	anti- *against* -body *substance, body*	Protein produced in response to an antigen
humoral	**HYU**-mor-al	S/ R/	-al *pertaining to* humor- *fluid*	Defense mechanism arising from antibodies in the blood
immune	im-**YUNE**		Latin *protected from*	Protected from an infectious disease
immunity	im-**YOU**-nih-tee	S/ R/	-ity *condition* immun- *immune response*	State of being protected
immunology	im-you-**NOL**-oh-jee	S/ R/CF	-logy *study of* immun/o- *immune response*	The science and practice of immunity and allergy
immunologist	im-you-**NOL**-oh-jist	S/	-logist *one who studies, specialist*	Medical specialist in immunology
immunize	**IM**-you-nize	S/ R/	-ize *affect in a specific way* immun- *immune response*	Make resistant to an infectious disease
immunization	im-you-nih-**ZAY**-shun	S/	-ization *process of affecting in a specific way*	Administration of an agent to provide immunity
immunoglobulin	**IM**-you-noh-**GLOB**-you-lin	S/ R/CF R/	-in *chemical compound* immun/o- *immune response* -globul- *protein*	Specific protein evoked by an antigen; all antibodies are immunoglobulins
lymph	LIMF		Latin *clear spring water*	A clear fluid collected from tissues and transported by lymph vessels to the venous circulation
lymphatic	lim-**FAT**-ik	S/ R/	-atic *pertaining to* lymph- *lymph*	Pertaining to lymph or the lymphatic system
lymphocyte	**LIM**-foh-site	S/ R/CF	-cyte *cell* lymph/o- *lymph*	Small white blood cell with a nucleus
node	NOHD		Latin *a knot*	A circumscribed mass of tissue
parasite	**PAR**-ah-site		Greek *a guest*	An organism that attaches itself to, lives on or in, and derives its nutrition from another species
pathogen	**PATH**-oh-jen	S/ R/CF	-gen *to produce* path/o- *disease*	A disease-causing microorganism
pollutant	poh-**LOO**-tant	S/ R/	-ant *pertaining to* pollut- *unclean*	Substance that makes an environment unclean or impure
toxin	**TOK**-sin		Greek *poison*	Poisonous substance formed by a cell or organism
toxic (adj)	**TOK**-sick	S/ R/	-ic *pertaining to* tox- *poison*	Pertaining to a toxin, poisonous
toxicity (contains two suffixes)	toks-**ISS**-ih-tee	S/	-ity *state, condition*	The state of being poisonous

Exercises

A. Build the correct medical terms that match the definitions given. *If the term does not have a particular word element, leave it empty.*
Fill in the blanks. **LO 12.1, 12.D**

1. substance that makes the environment unclean or impure:

_____/_____/_____
P   R/CF   S

2. make resistant to infectious disease:

_____/_____/_____
P   R/CF   S

3. the basis of humoral defense mechanisms:

_____/_____/_____
P   R/CF   S

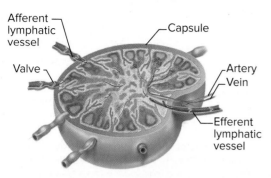

Afferent lymphatic vessel

Capsule

Valve

Artery

Vein

Efferent lymphatic vessel

▲ **Figure 12.3** Lymph Node.

LO 12.2 Lymphatic Nodes, Tissues, and Cells

Lymph Nodes

At irregular intervals, the lymphatic collecting vessels enter into the part of the lymphatic network called **lymph nodes** *(Figure 12.3)*. There are hundreds of lymph nodes stationed all over the body. They are especially concentrated in the neck, axilla, and groin. Their functions are to filter impurities from the lymph and alert the immune system to the presence of pathogens.

The lymph moves slowly through the node *(Figure 12.3)*, which filters the lymph and removes any foreign matter. On its journey back to the bloodstream, lymph passes through several nodes and becomes cleansed of most foreign matter. **Macrophages** in the lymph nodes ingest and break down the foreign matter and display fragments of it to **T cells** *(see the following section)*. This alerts the immune system to the presence of an invader. Lymph leaves the nodes again when it enters into the efferent collecting vessels. All these lymph vessels move lymph toward the thoracic cavity.

Lymphatic Tissues and Cells

Many organs have a sprinkling of lymphocytes in their connective tissues and mucous membranes, particularly in passages that open to the exterior—the respiratory, digestive, urinary, and reproductive tracts—where invaders have access to the body.

In some organs, lymphocytes and other cells form dense clusters called **lymphatic follicles.** These are constant features in the tonsils, the adenoids, and the ileum.

Lymphatic tissues are composed of a variety of cells that include:

1. **T lymphocytes (T cells).** The "T" stands for *thymus,* where they mature.
   T lymphocytes make up 75% to 85% of body lymphocytes. There are several types of T cells:

   a. **Cytotoxic or "killer" T cells** destroy target cells. Their cell membrane holds a **coreceptor** that can recognize a specific antigen. Coreceptors are named with the letters "**CD**" **(cluster of differentiation)** followed by a number, for these cells, CD8.

   b. **Helper T cells** contain the CD4 coreceptor and are called CD4 cells. They begin the defensive response against a specific antigen.

   c. **Memory T cells** arise from cytotoxic T lymphocytes that have previously destroyed a foreign cell. If they encounter the same antigen, they can now quickly kill it without initiation by a helper T cell.

   d. **Suppressor T cells** suppress activation of the immune system. Failure of these cells to function properly may result in autoimmune diseases.

2. **B lymphocytes (B cells).** These cells mature in the bone marrow. B lymphocytes make up 15% to 25% of lymphocytes. They are activated by helper T cells, respond to a specific antigen, and cause the production of antibodies called **immunoglobulins (Ig).** The mature B cells are called **plasma cells** and secrete large quantities of antibodies that immobilize, neutralize, and prepare the specific antigen for destruction.

3. **Null cells.** These are large granular lymphocytes that are natural killer cells but lack the specific surface markers of the T and B lymphocytes.

4. **Macrophages.** These cells develop from monocytes *(see Chapter 11)* that have migrated from blood. They ingest and destroy tissue debris, bacteria, and other foreign matter **(phagocytosis).**

Keynotes

- **Tissues** that are the first line of defense against pathogens—for example, the airway passages—have lymphatic tissue in the submucous layers to help protect against invasion.

- T cells (or T lymphocytes) mature in the thymus and make up 75% to 85% of the body's lymphocytes.

- B cells (or B lymphocytes) mature in the bone marrow and make up 15% to 25% of the body's lymphocytes.

- Macrophages are produced and stored in the spleen.

Abbreviations

B cells	B lymphocytes
CD	cluster of differentiation
Ig	immunoglobulin
T cells	T lymphocytes

WORD	PRONUNCIATION	ELEMENTS		DEFINITION
coreceptor	koh-ree-**SEP**-tor	S/ P/ R/	**-or** *a doer* **co-** *with, together* **-recept-** *receive*	Cell surface protein to enhance the sensitivity of an antigen receptor
cytotoxic (adj)	sigh-toh-**TOK**-sik	S/ R/CF	**-toxic** *able to kill* **cyt/o-** *cell*	Agent able to destroy cells
follicle	**FOLL**-ih-kull		Latin *a small sac*	Spherical mass of cells containing a cavity, or a small cul-de-sac such as a hair follicle
macrophage	**MAK**-roh-fayj	R/CF P/	**-phag/e** *to eat* **macro-** *large*	Large white blood cell (WBC) that removes bacteria, foreign particles, and dead cells
null cells	NULL SELLS		**null** Latin *none*	Lymphocytes with no surface markers, unlike T cells or B cells
phagocyte	**FAG**-oh-site	S/ R/CF	**-cyte** *cell* **phag/o-** *to eat*	Blood cell that ingests and destroys foreign particles and cells
phagocytize (verb)	**FAG**-oh-site-ize	S/ R/	**-ize** *action* **-cyt-** *cell*	Ingest foreign particles and cells
phagocytosis phagocytic (adj)	**FAG**-oh-sigh-**TOH**-sis fag-oh-**SIT**-ik	S/ S/	**-osis** *condition* **-ic** *pertaining to*	Process of ingestion and destruction of foreign particles and cells Pertaining to phagocytes or phagocytosis
plasma cell	**PLAZ**-mah SELL		**plasma** Greek *something formed*	Cell derived from B lymphocytes and active in formation of antibodies

Exercises

A. Elements. *Knowledge of elements is your best key to understanding medical terminology. Reinforce that knowledge with this exercise. Select the best choice.* **LO 12.2, 12.A**

1. In the term **cytotoxic,** one element means

   a. to eat   **b.** able to kill   **c.** large

2. The prefix in **macrophage** identifies

   a. color   **b.** location   **c.** size

3. The suffix in **phagocyte** means

   a. cyst   **b.** cell   **c.** mass

4. The prefix *co-* means

   a. next to   **b.** with   **c.** under

5. The suffix *-phage* means

   a. flow   **b.** eat   **c.** produce

6. This suffix means condition:

   a. *-osis*   **b.** *-ize*   **c.** *-ic*

▲ **Figure 12.4** **Position of Spleen.** ©McGraw-Hill Education/Dennis Strete, photographer

(Labels in figure: Diaphragm (cut), **Spleen**, Splenic artery, Pancreas, Kidney, Inferior vena cava, Aorta)

LO 12.3 Lymphatic Organs

Spleen

The **spleen**, a highly vascular and spongy organ, is the largest lymphatic organ. It is located in the left upper quadrant of the abdomen below the diaphragm and lateral to the kidney *(Figure 12.4)*. It is the only organ the body can live without.

The spleen contains two basic types of tissue:

1. **White pulp**—which is a part of the immune system that produces T cells, B cells, and macrophages. The blood passing through the spleen is monitored for antigens. Antibodies are produced, and the foreign matter is removed.

2. **Red pulp**—which acts as a **reservoir** for erythrocytes, platelets, and macrophages that remove old and defective erythrocytes.

Thus, the functions of the spleen are to:

· **Produce** T cells, B cells, and macrophages.

· **Phagocytize** bacteria and other foreign materials.

· **Initiate an immune response** to produce antibodies when antigens are found in the blood.

· **Phagocytize** old, defective erythrocytes and platelets (hemolysis).

· **Serve as a reservoir** for erythrocytes and platelets.

Tonsils

The **tonsils** *(see Chapter 13)* are two masses of lymphatic tissue located at the entrance to the oropharynx, where they entrap inhaled and ingested pathogens. **Adenoids** are similar tissue on the posterior wall of the nasopharynx *(see Chapter 13)*. The tonsils and adenoids form lymphocytes and antibodies, trap bacteria and viruses, and drain them into the tonsillar lymph nodes for elimination. They can become infected themselves.

Thymus Gland

The thymus gland has both endocrine *(see Chapter 17)* and lymphatic functions. T cells develop and mature in it and are released into the bloodstream. The thymus is largest in infancy and childhood *(Figure 12.5a and b)* and reaches its maximum size at puberty. It then regresses into a small structure in the adult *(Figure 12.5 (b))* and is eventually replaced by fibrous and adipose tissue.

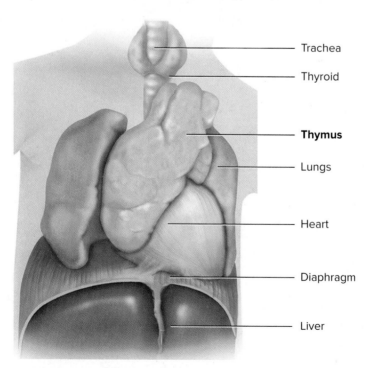

▲ **Figure 12.5(a)** Large Thymus in an Infant.

(Labels: Trachea, Thyroid, **Thymus**, Lungs, Heart, Diaphragm, Liver)

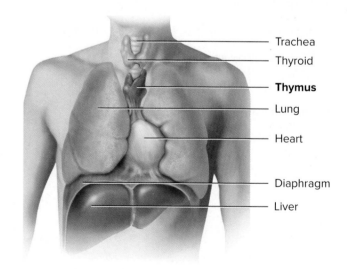

▲ **Figure 12.5(b)** Adult Thymus.

(Labels: Trachea, Thyroid, **Thymus**, Lung, Heart, Diaphragm, Liver)

S = Suffix   P = Prefix   R = Root   R/CF = Combining Form

WORD	PRONUNCIATION	ELEMENTS		DEFINITION
adenoid	ADD-eh-noyd	S/ R/	-oid *resemble* aden- *gland*	Single mass of lymphoid tissue in the midline at the back of the throat
spleen	SPLEEN		Greek *spleen*	Vascular, lymphatic organ in the left upper quadrant of the abdomen
splenectomy (*Note:* The "ee" in spleen becomes "e" for easier pronunciation.)	spleh-NEK-toh-mee	S/ R/	-ectomy *surgical excision* splen- *spleen*	Surgical removal of the spleen
splenomegaly	spleh-noh-MEG-ah-lee	S/ R/CF	-megaly *enlargement* splen/o- *spleen*	Enlarged spleen
tonsil	TON-sill		Latin *tonsil*	Mass of lymphoid tissue on either side of the throat at the back of the tongue
tonsillectomy	ton-sih-LEK-toh-mee	S/ R/	-ectomy *surgical excision* tonsill- *tonsil*	Surgical removal of the tonsils
tonsillitis	ton-sih-LIE-tis	S/	-itis *inflammation*	Inflammation of the tonsils

Exercises

A. Identify the correct answer that contains all the lymphatic organs. *Select the best choice.* **LO 12.3, 12.A**

1. Which of the following is a list of only lymphatic organs?

   a. liver, spleen, thyroid gland

   b. spleen, lungs, kidney

   c. tonsils, spleen, parathyroid gland

   d. thymus gland, spleen, lymph vessels and nodes

   e. gallbladder, spleen, thyroid gland

B. The spleen is a very important organ in the body. *Select T if the statement is True. Select F if the statement is False.* **LO 12.3**

   1. The spleen is a highly vascular and spongy organ.   T   F

   2. The spleen is the largest of the lymphatic organs.   T   F

   3. The spleen is located in the right upper quadrant of the body.   T   F

   4. The spleen contains white pulp and red pulp.   T   F

   5. The spleen serves as a reservoir for RBCs and platelets.   T   F

C. This exercise describes the "where" of lymphatic tissue—you need to supply the term that is the "what." "*What am I?*" *Identify the correct medical term for each of the following questions.* **LO 12.3, 12.A**

1. I am located below the diaphragm and lateral to the kidney. _____

2. I am located at the entrance to the oropharynx, where I trap pathogens. _____

3. I am located on the posterior wall of the nasopharynx. _____

4. I am located in the chest cavity. _____

Case Report (CR) 12.1 *(continued)*

Ms. Clemons has cancerous nodes in her neck. They were not caused by metastatic cancer but by a cancer of the lymph nodes called **Hodgkin lymphoma**.

▲ **Figure 12.6** Hodgkin Lymphoma.
The lymphatic tissues in Hodgkin disease contain specific cells called Reed-Sternberg cells that are not found in any other cancerous lymphomas or cancers. ©James Cavallini/Photo Researchers, Inc.

▲ **Figure 12.7** Tonsillitis.
Open mouth and throat of a 15-year-old girl with inflamed tonsils. They are flecked with infected white patches due to tonsillitis, an infection usually caused by streptococci bacteria. ©Dr. P. Marazzi/Science Photo Library, Photo Researchers, Inc.

LO 12.4 Disorders of the Lymphatic System

Physicians routinely palpate accessible lymph nodes in the neck **(cervical nodes)**, axillae **(axillary nodes)**, and groin **(inguinal nodes)** for enlargement and tenderness. Their presence indicates disease in the tissues drained by the lymph nodes. Cancerous lymph nodes are enlarged, firm, and usually painless.

Infections in the lymph nodes cause them to be swollen and tender to the touch, a condition called **lymphadenitis.** All lymph node enlargements are collectively called **lymphadenopathy.** When lymph nodes are removed, it is called **lymphadenectomy.**

Lymphoma is a malignant neoplasm of the lymphatic organs, usually the lymph nodes. The disorder usually presents as an enlarged, nontender lymph node, often in the neck or axilla.

Lymphomas are grouped into two categories:

1. **Hodgkin lymphoma**—characterized by the presence of abnormal, cancerous B cells called **Reed-Sternberg cells.** These are large cells with two nuclei resembling the eyes of an owl *(Figure 12.6)*. The cancer spreads in an orderly manner to adjoining lymph nodes. This enables the disease to be staged, depending on how far it has spread. Diagnostic procedures include biopsy of an enlarged node to look for Reed-Sternberg cells, x-rays, computed tomography (CT) and magnetic resonance imaging (MRI) scans, **lymphangiogram**, and bone marrow biopsy. Treatment options include radiation, chemotherapy, and an autologous bone marrow transplant.

2. **Non-Hodgkin lymphomas**—occur much more frequently than Hodgkin lymphoma. They include some 30 different disease entities in 10 different subtypes. Treatment depends on the rate of growth of the disease and varies from careful observation to chemotherapy and radiation to bone marrow transplantation.

Tonsillitis, inflammation of the tonsils and adenoids, occurs mostly in the first years of life. The infection can be viral or bacterial (usually streptococcal). It produces enlarged, tender lymph nodes under the jaw *(Figure 12.7)*. A rapid strep test can determine if *Streptococcus* is the cause, in which case a full course of antibiotics is indicated. The infection can be recurrent, and **tonsillectomy** is sometimes performed.

Splenomegaly, an enlarged spleen, is not a disease in itself but the result of an underlying disorder. However, when the spleen enlarges, it traps and removes an excessive number of blood cells and platelets **(hypersplenism)** and reduces the number of blood cells and platelets in the bloodstream.

The potential causes of splenomegaly are numerous and include infections such as infectious mononucleosis, lymphomas, anemias such as sickle cell anemia, and storage diseases such as Gaucher disease.

Diagnosis and treatment focus on the underlying cause. Occasionally, **splenectomy** is necessary.

Ruptured spleen is a common complication from car accidents or other trauma when the abdomen and rib cage are damaged. Intra-abdominal bleeding from the ruptured spleen can be extensive, with a dramatic fall in blood pressure (BP), and is a surgical emergency requiring splenectomy. After splenectomy, patients are very susceptible to infection but function very well.

Lymphedema is localized, nonpitting fluid retention caused by a compromised lymphatic system, often after surgery or radiation therapy. It also can be primary, where the cause is unknown.

S = Suffix   P = Prefix   R = Root   R/CF = Combining Form

WORD	PRONUNCIATION		ELEMENTS	DEFINITION
Hodgkin lymphoma	HOJ-kin lim-FOH-muh	S/ R/	Thomas Hodgkin, 1798–1866, British physician -oma *tumor, mass* lymph- *lymph*	Disease marked by chronic enlargement of lymph nodes spreading to other nodes in an orderly way
hypersplenism (Note the one "e.")	high-per-SPLEN-izm	S/ P/ R/	-ism *condition, process* hyper- *excessive* -splen- *spleen*	Condition in which the spleen removes blood components at an excessive rate
lymphadenectomy lymphadenitis lymphadenopathy	lim-FAD-eh-NEK-toh-mee lim-FAD-eh-NIE-tis lim-FAD-eh-NOP-ah-thee	S/ R/ S/ S/ R/CF	-ectomy *surgical excision* lymphaden- *lymph node* -itis *inflammation* -pathy *disease* lymphaden/o *lymph node*	Surgical excision of a lymph node Inflammation of a lymph node Any disease process affecting a lymph node
lymphangiogram	lim-FAN-jee-oh-gram	S/ R/CF	-gram *recording* lymphangi/o- *lymphatic vessels*	Radiographic images of lymph vessels and nodes following injection of contrast material
lymphedema	LIMF-eh-DEE-mah	R/ R/	lymph- *lymph* -edema *edema*	Tissue swelling due to lymphatic obstruction
lymphoma	lim-FOH-mah	S/ R/	-oma *tumor* lymph- *lymph*	Any neoplasm of lymphatic tissue
splenectomy (Note: The "ee" in spleen becomes "e" for easier pronunciation.) splenomegaly	sple-NEK-toh-mee sple-noh-MEG-ah-lee	S/ R/ S/ R/CF	-ectomy *surgical excision* splen- *spleen* -megaly *enlargement* splen/o- *spleen*	Surgical removal of the spleen Enlarged spleen
tonsillectomy tonsillitis	ton-sih-LEK-toh-mee ton-sih-LIE-tis	S/ R/ S/	-ectomy *surgical excision* tonsill- *tonsil* -itis *inflammation*	Surgical removal of the tonsils Inflammation of the tonsils

Exercises

A. Deconstruct medical terms into their elements. *Deconstruct each term using the slashed lines.* **LO 12.4, 12.A, 12.D**

1. splenectomy: _____ / _____
                       R   S

2. tonsillitis: _____ / _____
                R   S

3. lymphadenitis: _____ / _____
                   R   S

4. hypersplenism: _____ / _____ / _____
                     P   R   S

B. Use the terms related to disorders of the lymphatic system above that is described by each statement. LO 12.4, 12.A

1. Write the term that means *tumor of lymphatic tissue*: _____

2. Write the term that means *removal of the tonsils*: _____

3. The term that means *tissue swelling that occurs as a result of obstructed lymphatics*: _____

4. The term that means *inflammation of a lymph node*: _____

Lesson 12.2
LYMPHATIC AND IMMUNE SYSTEMS

Immune System

Lesson Objectives

The study of the immune system is called immunology. The medical specialist involved in the study and research of the immune system and in treating disorders of the immune system is called an immunologist. The information in this lesson will enable you to use correct medical terminology to:

12.1.1 Define the immune system and its specific reactions to stimulation.

12.1.2 Contrast cellular and humoral immunity.

12.1.3 Describe the life histories of B cells and T cells.

12.1.4 Explain the structure and actions of antibodies.

12.1.5 Discuss some common disorders of the immune system, including human immunodeficiency virus (HIV) and acquired immune deficiency syndrome (AIDS).

Keynotes

• The immune system is not an organ system but a group of specialized cells.

• Receptors on the surface of T cells and B cells recognize specific nonself (foreign) antigens.

• Antigens are molecules that trigger an immune response. Each antigen has a unique structure that is recognized by the immune system.

• **Haptens** are small, foreign molecules that attach themselves to host molecules to form large, unique complexes that the immune system can recognize as foreign. Haptens are found in cosmetics, detergents, industrial chemicals, poison ivy, and animal dander.

 Case Report (CR) 12.2

You are

. . . a laboratory technician working the night shift at Fulwood Medical Center.

Your patient is

. . . Mr. Michael Cowan, a 40-year-old homeless man and drug addict, who has presented to the Emergency Department with a high fever for which no cause is obvious on clinical examination.

You are called to the Emergency Room to take blood from Mr. Cowan. You have inserted the needle into an antecubital vein, and he starts jerking his arm around and trying to get off the gurney. In the struggle, the needle comes out of the vein and pricks your hand through your glove.

As you immediately *flush* and *clean* the wound, *report* the incident, seek *immediate medical attention,* and go through your *initial medical evaluation,* it is essential that you have knowledge about your immune system and its response to the potential infection. Then you can make *informed decisions* about your treatment and future employment.

LO 12.5 The Immune System

The immune system is a group of specialized cells in different parts of the body that recognize foreign substances and neutralize them. It is the third line of defense listed at the beginning of this chapter. When the immune system is functioning correctly, it protects the body against bacteria, viruses, cancer cells, and foreign substances. When the immune system is weak, it allows pathogens (including the viruses that cause common colds and "flu") and cancer cells to successfully invade the body.

Three characteristics distinguish immunity from the first two lines of defense:

1. **Specificity.** The immune response is directed against a particular pathogen. Immunity to one pathogen does not confer immunity to others. Specificity has one disadvantage. If a virus or a bacterium changes a component of its genetic code, it will lead to a change in the structure and/or physiology of the microorganism, which then is no longer recognized by the immune system. This **mutation** occurs, for example, in bacteria in response to antibiotics and in HIV's response to anti-HIV drugs (development of **resistance**).

2. **Memory.** When exposure to the same identical pathogen occurs again, the immune system recognizes the pathogen and has its responses ready to act quickly.

3. **Discrimination.** The immune system learns to recognize agents **(antigens)** that represent **"self"** and agents that are **"nonself"** (foreign). Most of this recognition is developed prior to birth. A variety of disorders occur when this discrimination breaks down. They are known as **autoimmune** disorders.

Word Analysis and Definition

S = Suffix   P = Prefix   R = Root   R/CF = Combining Form

WORD	PRONUNCIATION		ELEMENTS	DEFINITION
antigen	**AN**-tih-jen	P/ R/	**anti-** *against* **-gen** *produce, create*	Substance capable of triggering an immune response
autoimmune	aw-toh-im-**YUNE**	P/ R/	**auto-** *self, same* **-immune** *immune response*	Immune reaction directed against a person's own tissue
discrimination	**DIS**-krim-ih-**NAY**-shun	S/ P/ R/	**-ation** *process* **dis-** *away from, apart* **-crimin-** *distinguish*	Ability to distinguish between different things
hapten	**HAP**-ten		Greek *to fasten or bind*	Small molecule that has to bind to a larger molecule to form an antigen
mutate mutation	**MYU**-tayt myu-**TAY**-shun	S/ R/	Latin *to change* **-ion** *action, condition, process* **mutat-** *change*	To make a change in the chemistry of a gene Change in the chemistry of a gene
resistance resistant	ree-**ZIS**-tants ree-**ZIS**-tant	S/ R/ S/	**-ance** *state of, condition* **resist-** *to withstand* **-ant** *pertaining to*	Ability of an organism to withstand the effects of an antagonistic agent Able to resist
specific specificity (*Note:* two suffixes)	speh-**SIF**-ik spes-ih-**FIS**-ih-tee	S/ R/ S/	**-ic** *pertaining to* **specif-** *species* **-ity** *condition, state*	Relating to a particular entity State of having a fixed relation to a particular entity

Exercises

A. Build your knowledge of elements and their meaning by matching the element in the left column with the definition in the right column. LO 12.5

_____ 1. *crimin*

_____ 2. *ity*

_____ 3. *specif*

_____ 4. *anti*

_____ 5. *dis*

_____ 6. *ation*

_____ 7. *ic*

_____ 8. *gen*

a. species

b. away from

c. distinguish

d. process

e. pertaining to

f. condition, state

g. produce, create

h. against

B. Analyze Case Report 12.2, then answer the following questions. LO 12.5, 12.A

1. What is the purpose of flushing the wound?

  a. Hydrate the skin

  b. Replace any lost blood

  c. Remove pathogens from the wound

  d. Water is a natural antibiotic

2. Mr. Cowan's high fever is most likely due to:

  a. an infection   **b.** heatstroke   **c.** an allergic reaction   **d.** cardiac arrest

3. If you have been exposed to a pathogen, your body will react to it by creating:

  a. haptens   **b.** erythrocytes   **c.** mutations   **d.** antibodies

Abbreviations

IgA	immunoglobulin A
IgD	immunoglobulin D
IgE	immunoglobulin E
IgG	immunoglobulin G
IgM	immunoglobulin M

Keynotes

- The immune system is thought to be able to produce some 2 million different antibodies.
- Antibodies do not actively destroy an antigen. They render it harmless and mark it for destruction by phagocytes.
- Antibodies can be produced naturally in response to an antigen or artificially in response to immunizations and vaccines.

LO 12.6 Immunity

Immunity is classified biologically into two types, though both mechanisms often respond to the same antigen:

1. **Cellular (cell-mediated) immunity** is a direct form of defense based on the actions of lymphocytes to attack foreign and diseased cells and destroy them.

   The many different types of T cells, B cells, and macrophages described in the previous lesson of this chapter are involved in this style of attack.

2. **Humoral (antibody-mediated) immunity** is an indirect form of attack that employs antibodies produced by plasma cells, which have been developed from B cells. The antibodies bind to an antigen and thus tag them for destruction.

These antibodies are called **immunoglobulins (Igs),** defensive gamma globulins in the blood plasma and body secretions. There are five classes of antibodies (immunoglobulins):

- **IgG** makes up about 80% of the antibodies. It is found in plasma and tissue fluids. It crosses the placenta to give the fetus some immunity.
- **IgA** makes up about 13% of the antibodies. It is found in exocrine secretions such as breast milk, tears, saliva, nasal secretions, intestinal juices, bile, and urine.
- **IgM** makes up about 6% of antibodies. It develops in response to antigens in food or bacteria.
- **IgD** is found on the surface of B cells and acts as a receptor for antigens.
- **IgE** is found in exocrine secretions along with IgA and also in the serum.

Once released by plasma cells, the antibodies function in several ways to make antigens harmless, including:

- **Neutralization.** An antibody binds to the antigen and masks it.
- **Agglutination.** An antibody binds to two or more bacteria to prevent them from spreading through the tissues.
- **Precipitation.** Antibodies create an antigen-antibody complex that is too heavy to stay in solution. The complex precipitates (drops out of solution) and can be ingested and destroyed by phagocytes.
- **Complement fixation.** The complement system is a group of 20 or more proteins continually present in blood plasma; IgG and IgM bind to foreign cells, initiating the **binding of complement** to the cell and leading to its destruction. Complement fixation is the major defense mechanism against bacteria and mismatched blood cells.

Based on the production or acquisition of antibodies, four classes of immunity can be described:

1. **Natural active immunity**—the production of your own antibodies as a result of normal maturation, pregnancy, or an infection.
2. **Artificial active immunity**—the production of your own antibodies as a result of **vaccination** or **immunization**. A **vaccine** consists of either killed or **attenuated** (weakened) pathogens (antigens).
3. **Natural passive immunity**—a temporary immunity that results from acquiring antibodies from another individual. This occurs for the fetus through the placenta (IgG) or for the infant through breast milk (IgA).
4. **Artificial passive immunity**—a temporary immunity that results from the injection of an **immune serum** from another individual or an animal. Immune serum is used to treat snakebite, tetanus, and rabies.

Definition of Terms

- **Immunity** is protection from an infectious disease. If you are immune to a disease, you can be exposed to it without becoming infected.
- A **vaccine** is a product that stimulates a person's immune system to produce immunity to a specific disease, protecting that person from that disease. Vaccines are administered through needle injections, by mouth, or by nasal spray.
- **Vaccination** is the act of introducing a vaccine into the body to produce immunity to a specific disease.
- **Immunization** is the process by which a person becomes protected against a disease through vaccination. This term is often used interchangeably with vaccination or **inoculation.**

   These definitions are provided by the U.S. Centers for Disease Control and Protection.

WORD	PRONUNCIATION	ELEMENTS		DEFINITION
agglutination	ah-glue-tih-**NAY**-shun	S/ R/	-ation *process* agglutin- *sticking together, clumping*	Process by which cells or other particles adhere to each other to form clumps
agglutinate (verb)	ah-**GLUE**-tin-ate	S/	-ate *composed of, pertaining to*	Stick together to form clumps
attenuate	ah-**TEN**-you-ate	S/ R/	-ate *composed of, pertaining to* attenu- *to weaken*	Weaken the ability of an organism to produce disease
attenuated (adj)	ah-**TEN**-you-ay-ted	S/	-ated *process*	Weakened
complement	**KOM**-pleh-ment		Latin *that which completes*	Group of proteins in serum that finish off the work of antibodies to destroy bacteria and other cells
humoral immunity	**HYU**-mor-al im-**YOU**-nih-tee	S/ R/ S/ R/	-al *pertaining to* humor- *fluid* -ity *condition* immun- *immune response*	Defense mechanism arising from antibodies in the blood
immune serum (also called **antiserum**)	im-**YUNE SEER**-um		**immune** Latin *protected from* **serum** Latin *whey*	Serum taken from another human or animal that has antibodies to a disease
vaccine vaccinate (verb)	vak-**SEEN** **VAK**-sin-ate	S/ R/	Latin *relating to a cow* -ate *composed of, pertaining to* vaccin- *giving a vaccine*	Preparation to generate active immunity To administer a vaccine
vaccination	vak-sih-**NAY**-shun	S/	-ation *process*	Administration of a vaccine

Exercises

A. Identify the meanings of the word elements. *Knowing the meanings of the word elements will help you to define medical terms. Select the answer that correctly completes each statement.* **LO 12.5, 12.6**

1. The root *attenu-* means:

   a. clumping   **b.** inject   **c.** fluid   **d.** weaken

2. The suffix *-ity* means:

   a. source   **b.** process   **c.** condition   **d.** pertaining to

B. Relate the name of the four classes of immunity to how it creates an immunity. *Select the answer that correctly completes each statement.* **LO 12.6**

1. If the source of the immunity originates with an injection or a fluid that is inhaled or swallowed, then it is termed to be:

   a. natural   **b.** artificial

2. If the person creates his or her antibodies after exposure, then the immunity is termed:

   a. active   **b.** passive

3. If the source of the immunity originates within a person's own body or from a mother to her baby, then the immunity is termed:

   a. natural   **b.** artificial

4. If a person is given antibodies, then the immunity is termed:

   a. active   **b.** passive

▲ **Figure 12.8** Sun Allergy. ©BSIP/Photo Researchers, Inc.

LO 12.7 Disorders of the Immune System

Hypersensitivity is an excessive immune response to an antigen that would normally be tolerated. Hypersensitivity includes:

- **Allergies,** which are reactions to environmental antigens such as pollens, molds, and dusts; to foods such as peanuts, shellfish, and eggs; to plants such as poison ivy; to sunlight *(Figure 12.8);* and to drugs such as penicillin, as well as asthmatic reactions to inhaled antigens (see following text).

- Abnormal reactions to your *own* tissues **(autoimmune disorders).**

- Reactions to tissues **transplanted** from *another* person **(alloimmune disorders).**

In most allergic (hypersensitivity) reactions, **allergens** (antigens) bind to IgE on the membranes of basophils and mast cells *(see Chapter 11)* and, within seconds of exposure, stimulate the cells to produce **histamine.** This triggers vasodilation, increased capillary permeability, and smooth muscle spasms. The symptoms produced by these changes include edema; mucus hypersecretion and congestion; watery eyes; hives **(urticaria);** and sometimes cramps, diarrhea, and vomiting.

Anaphylaxis is an acute, immediate, and severe allergic reaction. It can be relieved by antihistamines.

Anaphylactic shock is more severe and is characterized by dyspnea due to bronchiole constriction, circulatory shock, and sometimes death. It is a life-threatening medical emergency and requires immediate epinephrine and circulatory support.

Asthma is triggered by allergens (as listed earlier) and by air pollutants, drugs, and emotions. These all stimulate plasma cells to secrete IgE, which binds to cells in the respiratory mucosa and releases a mixture of histamine and interleukins. Within minutes, the bronchioles constrict spasmodically (bronchospasm), leading to the wheezing and coughing of asthma.

Autoimmune disorders are an overvigorous response of the immune system in which the immune system fails to distinguish self-antigens from foreign antigens. These self-antigens produce autoantibodies that attack the body's own tissues. This type of response occurs, for example, in lupus erythematosus, type 1 diabetes, multiple sclerosis, rheumatoid arthritis, and psoriasis.

Immunodeficiency disorders are a deficient response of the immune system in which it fails to respond vigorously enough. They are in three categories:

1. **Congenital** (inborn)—caused by a genetic abnormality that is often sex-linked, with boys affected more often than girls. An example from among the 20 or more congenital immunodeficiency diseases is **inherited combined immunodeficiency disease,** in which there is an absence of both T cells and B cells. Affected children are very susceptible to opportunistic infections and must live in protective sterile enclosures.

2. **Immunosuppression**—a common side effect of corticosteroids in treatment to prevent transplant rejection and in chemotherapy treatment for cancer. These drugs reduce the numbers of all lymphocytes, making it possible for opportunistic infections to invade the body.

3. **Acquired immunodeficiency**—a result of diseases such as acquired immunodeficiency syndrome (AIDS) that involve a severely depressed immune system from infection with the human immunodeficiency virus (HIV).

LO 12.7 Immunology of Transplantation

The success of any organ **transplantation** is based on control of the recipient's immune system to prevent rejection of the **allograft,** tissue from another individual of the same species.

Transplant immunity is designed to cause rejection, and both cellular and humoral defense mechanisms are involved. To try to prevent this, the recipient and donor must match at both the human lymphocyte antigen (HLA) and blood group system (ABO) *(see Chapter 11)* types. A combination of immunosuppressive drugs is used to control graft rejection, but the drugs have adverse side effects on the recipient. One combination is corticosteroids with cyclosporine or FK506. Other drugs are in clinical trials.

WORD	PRONUNCIATION	ELEMENTS		DEFINITION
allogen	**AL**-oh-jen	P/ R/	allo- *strange, different* -gen *producing*	Antigen from someone else in the same species
allogenic (adj) allograft	al-oh-**JEN**-ik **AL**-oh-graft	S/ R/	-ic *pertaining to* -graft *tissue for transplant*	Pertaining to allogen Tissue graft from another person or cadaver
alloimmune	**AL**-oh-im-**YUNE**	P/ R/	allo- *strange, different* -immune *immune response*	Reaction directed against foreign tissue
anaphylaxis	**AN**-ah-fih-**LAK**-sis	P/ R/	ana- *away from* -phylaxis *protection*	Immediate severe allergic response
anaphylactic (adj)	**AN**-ah-fih-**LAK**-tik	S/ R/	-tic *pertaining to* -phylac- *protect*	Pertaining to anaphylaxis
histamine	**HISS**-tah-meen	S/ R/	-amine *nitrogen containing* hist- *derived from histidine*	Compound liberated in tissues as a result of injury or an allergic response
antihistamine	an-tee-**HISS**-tah-meen	P/	anti- *against*	Drug used to treat allergic symptoms because of its action antagonistic to histamine
hypersensitivity	**HIGH**-per-sen-sih-**TIV**-ih-tee	S/ P/ R/	-ity *condition* hyper- *excessive* -sensitiv- *feeling*	Exaggerated abnormal reaction to an allergen
immunodeficiency	**IM**-you-noh-dee-**FISH**-en-see	S/ R/CF R/	-ency *quality* immun/o- *immune response* -defici- *failure*	Failure of the immune system
immunosuppression	**IM**-you-noh-suh-**PRESH**-un	S/ R/CF R/	-ion *process* immun/o- *immune response* -suppress- *pressed under*	Suppression of the immune response by an outside agent, such as a drug
transplant	**TRANZ**-plant	P/ R/	trans- *across* -plant *plant*	The tissue or organ used, or the act of transferring tissue from one person to another
transplantation	**TRANZ**-plan-**TAY**-shun	S/	-ation *process, action*	The moving of tissue or an organ from one person or place to another
urticaria	ur-tih-**KARE**-ee-ah		Latin *nettle*	Rash of itchy wheals (hives)

Exercises

A. Build more medical vocabulary for immunology. *Complete the construction of the medical term by using the following elements to fill in the blanks.* **LO 12.7, 12.C**

hyper	defici	phylaxis	auto	suppress	graft
ion	anti	sensitiv	trans	allo	gen

1. Exaggerated, abnormal reaction to an antigen   _____/_____/ity

2. Suppression of the immune response caused by an outside agent   immuno/_____/_____

3. Immediate, severe, allergic response   ana/_____

4. Skin from another person or cadaver   allo/_____

5. Failure of the immune system   immuno/_____/ency

6. Transferring tissue or an organ from one person to another   _____/plant

7. Antigen from someone else in the same species   allo/_____

8. Reaction against foreign tissue   _____/immune

9. Drug used to treat allergic symptoms   _____/histamine

Case Report (CR) 12.3

You are

. . . a medical assistant working with Henry Vandenberg, MD, in the AIDS Clinic at Fulwood Medical Center.

Your patient is

. . . Mr. Eugene Holman, a 40-year-old male who is known to be **HIV-positive (HIV+)** and has been receiving treatment with efavirenz, zidovudine, and lamivudine.

In the past couple of months, Mr. Holman has not been taking his medication regularly. In the previous week, he has noticed a progressive shortness of breath and a nonproductive cough. Vital signs are T 102°, P 120, R 32, BP 110/60. He is anxious and dyspneic but not cyanotic. His breath sounds are clear, with no rales or rhonchi heard. You have called Dr. Vandenberg to see him.

Mr. Holman's chest x-ray shows bilateral, diffuse, fluffy infiltrates spreading out from the hila. Bronchial **lavage** with laboratory examination shows *Pneumocystis jiroveci*. His CD4 count is 140. Mr. Holman has developed an **opportunistic** infection, which is probably due to *Pneumocystis jiroveci*.

▲ **Figure 12.9** **Lesions of Kaposi Sarcoma.** ©SPL/Photo Researchers, Inc.

LO 12.8 HIV and AIDS

Human immunodeficiency virus (HIV) is one of a group of **viruses** known as **retroviruses**. Like other viruses, it can replicate only inside a living host cell; HIV invades helper T (CD4) cells and cells in the upper respiratory tract and CNS. Inside the cell, the virus generates new deoxyribonucleic acid (DNA) and can stay **dormant** in the cell for months or years. When it is activated, the new viruses emerge from the dying host cell and attack more CD4 cells. This dormant phase **(incubation)** can range from a few months to 12 years.

The CD4 cells are the central coordinators for the immune response. As the virus destroys more and more cells, the CD4 count falls, and antibodies cannot be produced. Symptoms appear, including chills, fever, night sweats, fatigue, weight loss, and lymphadenitis.

When CD4 cells are very low, **opportunistic infections** by bacteria, viruses, and fungi can occur. These infections include toxoplasmosis, pneumocystis, tuberculosis, herpes simplex, cytomegalovirus, and candidiasis. If human immunodeficiency virus (HIV) invades the brain, it causes dementia. Cancers also can invade, and a form of malignancy called **Kaposi sarcoma** *(Figure 12.9)* is often seen in association with autoimmune deficiency syndrome (AIDS).

HIV is found in blood, semen, vaginal secretions, saliva, tears, and the breast milk of infected mothers. The most common means of transmission of HIV are:

- **Sexual intercourse** (vaginal, oral, anal).
- **Sharing of needles** for drug use.
- **Contaminated blood products.** (All donated blood is now tested for HIV.)
- **Transplacental** (from an infected mother to her fetus).

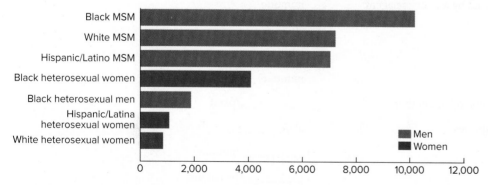

The virus survives poorly outside the human body. It is destroyed by laundering, dishwashing, chlorination, disinfectants, alcohol, and germicidal skin cleansers.

In the United States, the number of new HIV diagnoses declined about 19% from 2005 to 2014, but diagnoses have increased among certain groups and in certain geographical regions so new infections continue to occur *(Figure 12.10)*.

▲ **Figure 12.10** **HIV Diagnoses.** New HIV diagnoses in the United States for the most-affected subpopulations, 2015. (MSM, men who have sex with men.)

LO 12.8, 12.A
Word Analysis and Definition

S = Suffix   P = Prefix   R = Root   R/CF = Combining Form

WORD	PRONUNCIATION	ELEMENTS		DEFINITION
dormant	**DOR**-mant	S/ R/	-ant *forming* **dorm**- *sleep*	Inactive
incubation	in-kyu-**BAY**-shun	S/ R/	-ation *process* **incub**- *sit on, hatch*	Process to develop an infection
opportunistic	**OP**-or-tyu-**NIS**-tik	S/ S/ R/	-ic *pertaining to* -ist- *agent* **opportun**- *take advantage of*	An organism or a disease in a host with lowered resistance
retrovirus	**REH**-troh-**VIE**-rus	P/ R/	**retro**- *backward* -virus *poison*	Virus that replicates in a host cell by converting its ribonucleic acid (RNA) core into deoxyribonucleic acid (DNA)
sarcoma	sar-**KOH**-mah	S/ R/	-oma *tumor, mass* **sarc**- *flesh*	A malignant tumor originating in connective tissue
Kaposi sarcoma	ka-**POH**-see sar-**KOH**-mah		Moritz Kaposi, 1837–1902, Hungarian dermatologist	A malignancy often seen in AIDS patients
virus	**VIE**-rus		Latin *poison*	Group of infectious agents that require living cells for growth and reproduction
viral (adj)	**VIE**-ral	S/ R/	-al *pertaining to* **vir**- *virus*	Pertaining to or caused by a virus

Exercises

A. Analyze Case Report 12.3 and then answer the following questions. *Select the answer that correctly completes each statement.* **LO 12.8**

1. Mr. Holman developed an opportunistic infection because:

    a. the pathogen is potent   **c.** he forgets to take his medication

    b. he is homeless   **d.** his immune system is compromised

2. The diagnostic test that determined the reason for the infection was:

    a. breath sounds   **b.** bronchial lavage   **c.** CD4 count   **d.** chest x-ray

B. Identify the meaning of the word elements. *Given the term, identify the correct definition of the indicated word element.* **LO 12.8**

1. In the term **viral,** the root means:

    a. pertaining to   **b.** cancer   **c.** process   **d.** virus

2. In the term **sarcoma,** the root means:

    a. cancer   **b.** flesh   **c.** tumor   **d.** inflammation

3. In the term **dormant,** the suffix means:

    a. forming   **b.** take advantage   **c.** pertaining to   **d.** sleep

Procedures and Pharmacology

Immunoassays rely on the ability of an antibody to recognize and bind to a specific antigen and produce a measurable response. In some cases they can use an antigen to detect for the presence of antibodies, and again produce a measurable response. A wide range of medical tests are immunoassays:

12.3.1 Identify immunodiagnostic tests that involve an antigen-antibody reaction.

12.3.2 Define the mechanism of agglutination tests.

12.3.3 Recognize diagnostic tests used for allergies.

LO 12.9 Diagnostic Procedures

Immunodiagnostics uses an antigen-antibody reaction as a diagnostic tool; an antigen is used to detect antibodies to a **pathogen;** an antibody is used to detect an antigen of a pathogen in a patient's specimen. Very small amounts of biochemical substances can be detected when antibodies specific for a desired antigen are **conjugated** with a radiolabel, fluorescent label, or a color-forming enzyme and used as a "probe" to detect it.

Applications include pregnancy testing, dipsticks, and **enzyme-linked immunosorbent assay (ELISA).** ELISA uses antibodies and enzymes linked to color-changing dyes to detect specific antibodies and chemicals. ELISA is used to diagnose HIV, West Nile virus, malaria, tuberculosis, and rotavirus in feces, as well as in drug screening.

In **agglutination tests,** a particle such as a latex bead or a **bacterium** is coupled to a **reagent** antigen or antibody and the resulting particle **complex** is mixed with the specimen (e.g., serum or CSF). If the target antibody or antigen is present in the specimen, it attaches to the particle complex and produces agglutination.

A **complement fixation** test measures the amount of an antibody in the serum or CSF to viral and fungal infections such as **coccidioidomycosis.**

Diagnostic tests for allergies include:

- **nasal smears** to check the amount of eosinophils in the nose.

- **skin tests** to measure the level of IgE antibodies in response to allergens that are injected under the skin or applied with a small scratch. A reaction appears as a small red area.

- **blood tests** measure IgE antibodies to specific allergens in the blood. A **radioallergosorbent test (RAST)** uses a **radioimmunoassay** to detect the specific IgE antibodies, but is now little used.

- **Challenge testing** is performed by an allergist, who administers a very small amount of an allergen orally or by inhalation and monitors its effect.

High blood levels of IgA are found in multiple myeloma, autoimmune diseases such as rheumatoid arthritis and systemic lupus erythematosus *(see Chapter 15),* and cirrhosis of the liver *(see Chapter 5).* Low levels of IgA occur in some types of leukemia *(see Chapter 11)* and in nephrotic syndrome *(see Chapter 6).*

High blood levels of IgG can indicate a chronic infection, such as HIV and in chronic hepatitis and multiple sclerosis. Low levels are found in some types of leukemia and in nephrotic syndrome.

High blood levels of IgE are also found in patients with parasitic infections.

WORD	PRONUNCIATION	ELEMENTS		DEFINITION
bacterium bacteria (pl)	bak-**TEER**-ee-um bak-**TEER**-ee-ah		Greek *a staff*	A unicellular microorganism that multiplies by cell division
complex	**KOM**-pleks		Latin *woven together*	A stable combination of two or more compounds in the body
conjugate	**KON**-joo-gate	S/ P/ R/	-ate *composed of, pertaining to* con- *together* jug- *yoke*	To join together, usually in pairs.
immunoassay	**IM**-you-no-**ASS**-ay	R/CF R/	immun/o- *immune* -assay *evaluate*	Biochemical test that uses the reaction of an antibody to its antigen to measure the amount of a substance in a liquid
immunodiagnostics	**IM**-you-no-die-ag-**NOSS**-tiks	S/ R/CF R/	-ics *pertaining to* immun/o- *immune* -diagnost- *decision*	A diagnostic process using antigen-antibody reactions
radioallergosorbent	**RAY**-dee-oh-ah-**LUR**-go-**SOAR**-bent	S/ R/CF R/CF R/	-ent *end result* radi/o- *radiation* -allerg/o- *allergy* -sorb- *suck in*	A radioimmunoassay to detect IgE-bound allergens responsible for tissue hypersensitivity
radioimmunoassay	**RAY**-dee-oh-im-you-no-**ASS**-ay	R/CF R/	-immun/o *immune* -assay *evaluate*	Immunoassay of a substance that has been radioactively labeled

Exercises

A. Immunoglobulin (Ig) levels are used to support the diagnosis of lymphatic system disorders. *Match the Ig levels in the first column with the condition it is associated with in the second column.* **LO 12.9**

_____ 1. increased IgE antibodies

_____ 2. increased IgG antibodies

_____ 3. decreased IgG antibodies

a. HIV infection

b. leukemia

c. parasitic infections

B. Choose the correct test used in the diagnosis of conditions caused by immune system disorders. LO 12.9, 12.F

1. The test used to detect the presence of HIV infection:

   a. ELISA   b. RAST   c. challenge testing   d. Ig levels

2. Patient inhales allergens to see if they cause an allergic reaction:

   a. skin test   b. blood test   c. challenge testing   d. agglutination testing

3. Measures the amount of antibody present in cerebrospinal fluid or serum:

   a. RAST   b. complement fixation test   c. ELISA   d. challenge testing

LO 12.9 Therapeutic Procedures and Drugs for the Immune System

Immunotherapy, also called **biologic therapy,** is designed to boost the body's natural defenses against cancer by using substances either made in the laboratory or made by the body to enhance or restore immune system function. This form of therapy can stop or slow the growth of cancer cells, and stop cancer from metastasizing.

The types of immunotherapy include:

- **Monoclonal antibodies,** made in the laboratory, can attach to cancer cells to flag them so that macrophages in the body's immune system can recognize and destroy them. Two pathways inside cells that cancers use to evade the immune system have been identified and named PD-1/PD-L1 and CTLA-4. These pathways can be blocked with antibodies called **immune checkpoint inhibitors** to allow the body's immune system to respond to the cancer. Immune checkpoint inhibitors ipilimumab *(Yervoy),* nivolumab *(Opdivo),* and pembrolizumab *(Keytruda)* have been shown to improve overall patient survival in advanced melanoma.

- **Interferons** are a nonspecific immunotherapy mostly given at the same time as other cancer treatments such as chemotherapy or radiation therapy. An interferon called **interferon alpha** made in a laboratory is the most common type of interferon used in cancer treatment.

- **Interleukins** are also a nonspecific immunotherapy used to treat kidney and skin cancers, including melanoma.

Human immunoglobulins are given by injection to confer passive (temporary) immunity that provides immediate protection lasting several weeks. There are two types:

- **Human normal immunoglobulin (HNIG)** made from the plasma of about 1,000 unselected donors to provide antibodies against hepatitis A, rubella, measles, and other viruses found in the general population.

- **Hyperimmune specific immunoglobulins** are made from selected donors and provide antibodies individually against hepatitis B, varicella zoster, rabies, tetanus, and cytomegalovirus.

Immunosuppressant Drugs

Immunosuppressant drugs inhibit or prevent activity of the immune system and are used to prevent the rejection of transplanted organs and tissues, treat autoimmune diseases, and help control long-term allergic asthma. There are four main types of immunosuppressant drugs:

- **Glucocorticoids,** which suppress cell-mediated immunity and protect through T-cells and macrophages, and by stimulating cells to secrete **cytokines.**

- **Cytostatics,** which inhibit cell division. Cyclophosphamide *(Cytoxan),* a nitrogen mustard **alkylating** agent, is probably the most potent immunosuppressant. Methotrexate, an **antimetabolite,** interferes with the **synthesis** of nucleic acids and is used in the treatment of autoimmune diseases. Azathioprine **(***Imuran***)** is the main immunosuppressive **cytotoxic** substance and is used to control transplant rejection reactions.

- **Antibodies** can be used as quick immunosuppressive therapy and are described above in sections on monoclonal antibodies and immunoglobulins.

- **Calcineurin** is a phosphatase that stimulates the growth and differentiation of T cells. **Calcineurin inhibitors** such as ciclosporin *(Sandimmune),* tacrolimus *(Prograf),* and sirolimus *(Rapamune)* are used in the prevention and treatment of transplant rejection reactions.

Alcohol, marijuana, and illicit drugs have been shown to depress the immune system.

WORD	PRONUNCIATION	ELEMENTS		DEFINITION
alkylation	al-kih-**LAY**-shun	S/ R/	-ation *process* alkyl- *alkali*	Introduction of a side chain into a compound
antimetabolite	**AN**-tih-meh-**TAB**- oh-lite	S/ P/ R/	-ite *resembling* anti- *against* -metabol- *change*	A substance that antagonizes another substance
biologic	**BI**-oh-**LOJ**-ik	S/ R/CF R/	-ic *pertaining to* bio- *life* -log- *study of*	Pertaining to the study of life and living organisms
calcineurin	kal-see-**NYUR**-in	S/ R/CF R/	-in *chemical* calc/i *calcium* -neur- *nerve*	A chemical that stimulates the growth and differentiation of T-cells
cytokine	**SIGH**-toh-kine	S/ R/CF	-kine *movement* cyt/o- *cell*	A hormone-like protein that regulates the intensity of an immune response
cytostatic	**SIGH**-toh-**STAT**-ik	S/ R/CF R/	-ic *pertaining to* cyt/o *cell* -stat- *stop*	Inhibiting cell division
cytotoxic	**SIGH**-toh-**TOK**-sik	S/	-toxic *able to kill*	Destructive to cells
immunoglobulin	**IM**-you-noh-**GLOB**-you-lin	S/ R/CF R/	-in *chemical* immun/o *immune response* -globul- *protein*	Specific protein (antibody) generated by an antigen
immunotherapy	**IM**-you-noh-**THAIR**-ah-pee	R/ R/CF	immun/o *immune response* -therapy *treatment*	Treatment to boost immune system function
inhibitor	in-**HIB**-ih-tor	S/ R/	-or *that which does* inhibit- *restrain*	An agent that restrains a chemical action
interferon	in-ter-**FEER**-on	S/ P/ R/	-on *on* inter- *between* -fer- *to strike*	A small protein produced by T-cells in response to infection
interleukin	**IN**-ter-**LOO**-kin	S/ P/ R/	-in *chemical* inter- *between* leuk- *white*	A group of cytokines synthesized by white blood cells
monoclonal	**MON**-oh-**KLOH**-nal	S/ P/ R/	-al *pertaining to* mono- *one* -clon- *cutting used for propagation*	Derived in the laboratory from a protein from a single colony of cells

Exercises

A. Identify the action of the drug based on a word element that it contains. *Being able to pick out and define word elements can help you determine the meaning of the word. Select the answer that correctly completes each statement.* **LO 12.9**

1. A medication that would provide antibodies to persons to prevent viral infections:

   a. cytostatic   **b.** glucocorticoid   **c.** human normal immunoglobulin   **d.** monoclonal antibodies

2. A medication that would inhibit cell division:

   a. cytostatic   **b.** calcineurin   **c.** interleukin   **d.** interferon

B. Categorize medications of immunotherapy. *Match the medication in the first column with the disorder it is used to treat in the second column.* **LO 12.9**

_____ **1.** interleukin   **a.** treat kidney and skin cancers

_____ **2.** interferons   **b.** flag cancer cells for macrophages

_____ **3.** monoclonal antibodies   **c.** given alongside chemotherapy and radiation therapy

C. Categorize immunosuppressant drugs. *Match the medication in the first column with the disorder it is used to treat in the second column.* **LO 12.9**

_____ **1.** methotrexate   **a.** interferes with nucleic acids as a means to treat autoimmune diseases

_____ **2.** tacrolimus (*Prograf*)   **b.** inhibits cell division

_____ **3.** glucocorticoid   **c.** suppresses cell-mediated immunity

_____ **4.** cyclophosphamide (*Cytoxan*)   **d.** prevents and treats transplant rejection reactions

Lymphatic and Immune Systems

Challenge Your Knowledge

A. **Latin and Greek elements cannot be deconstructed into prefix, root, or suffix.** You must know them for what they are. Test your knowledge of these elements with this exercise. Match the meaning in the left column with the correct medical term in the right column. **(LO 12.1, 12.D)**

_____ **1.** Protected from   **a.** conjugate

_____ **2.** That which completes   **b.** hapten

_____ **3.** None   **c.** lymph

_____ **4.** To fasten or bind   **d.** assay

_____ **5.** To join   **e.** mutate

_____ **6.** A knot   **f.** complement

_____ **7.** To change   **g.** edema

_____ **8.** To evaluate   **h.** immune

_____ **9.** Swelling   **i.** null

_____ **10.** Clear fluid   **j.** node

B. Language of immunology. Challenge your knowledge of the immune system and employ the *language of immunology* to answer the following questions. Choose the correct answer. **(LO 12.1, 12.3, 12.4, 12.7, 12.A)**

1. Choose the correct pair of spellings:

   a. tonsel   tonselectomy

   b. tonsil   tonsillectomy

   c. tonssil   tonsilectomy

   d. tonsill   tonsilectomy

   e. tonnsil   tonsillectomy

2. This triggers vasodilation in an allergic response:

   a. interferon

   b. complement fixation

   c. histamine

   d. hormones

   e. antihistamine

3. The largest lymphatic vessel is the

   a. thoracic duct

   b. lymph node

   c. spleen

   d. lymphatic duct

   e. aorta

4. Kaposi sarcoma is a form of

   a. lymphadenitis

   b. malignancy

   c. lymphadenopathy

   d. lung cancer

   e. lymphoma

5. Ingestion and destruction of tissue debris and bacteria is called

   a. lymphadenitis

   b. phagocytosis

   c. lymphadenopathy

   d. agglutination

   e. osmosis

6. A life-threatening medical emergency that cannot be relieved by antihistamines is

   a. asthma

   b. Kaposi sarcoma

   c. anaphylactic shock

   d. urticaria

   e. lymphadenitis

7. An allergic reaction is one of

   a. hypoglycemia

   b. hypersensitivity

   c. hypotension

   d. hyperglycemia

   e. hypertension

8. White pulp and red pulp can be found in the

   a. lymph nodes

   b. spleen

   c. lymph vessels

   d. kidney

   e. thymus

©2014 Nucleus Medical Media

Lymphatic and Immune Systems

C. Language of immunology. Challenge your knowledge of the immune system and employ the *language of immunology* to answer the following questions. Circle the correct choice. **(LO 12.4, 12.7, 12.9)**

1. Which disease is likely to cause enlarged lymph nodes under the jaw?

   a. tonsillitis

   b. lymphoma

   c. hypersplenism

   d. asthma

   e. urticaria

2. Abnormal, cancerous B cells are known as

   a. macrophages   d. killer cells

   b. osteoblasts   e. phagocytes

   c. Reed-Sternberg cells

3. Lymph nodes accessible for palpation are in the

   a. neck   d. all of these

   b. axilla   e. only A and C

   c. groin

4. Immunosuppressive drugs are given after

   a. organ transplant

   b. anaphylactic shock

   c. retrovirus

   d. opportunistic infection

   e. viral load count

5. Serum used to treat a snake bite is an example of

   a. natural active immunity

   b. artificial active immunity

   c. natural passive immunity

   d. artificial passive immunity

D. Correct spelling of medical terms is *always important*. Listed below are two examples of medical terms for which a variation of the term is not always spelled the same as the original term. Fill in the blanks with the correctly spelled medical terms. **(LO 12.1, 12.4, 12.9, 12.A)**

Example 1:

Lymphatic organ in LUQ of abdomen   1. _____

Excision/removal of this organ   2. _____

Enlargement of this organ due to an underlying disorder   3. _____

Example 2:

Lymphoid tissue on either side of the throat   4. _____

Inflammation of this tissue   5. _____

Removal of this tissue   6. _____

E. Construct the entire term by entering the prefix *on* the line, write the meaning of the prefix *under* the line. Fill in the blanks. **(LO 12.1, 12.C)**

1. Reaction directed against foreign tissue   _____/immune

2. Substance produced in response to an antigen   _____/body

3. Surface protein that enhances sensitivity of antigen receptor   _____/recept/or

4. Spleen removes blood components at an excessive rate   _____splen/ism

5. Virus that converts its RNA core to DNA in a host cell   _____/virus

F. **Suffixes.** Construct new terms using your knowledge of word elements from this and previous chapters. Take a basic root/combining form, add a variety of suffixes, and change the meaning different ways to form six new terms. Fill in the chart, then fill in the blanks. **(LO 12.1, 12.2, 12.4, 12.C)**

Root/Combining Form	Suffix	Meaning of Term
lymph	1.	Neoplasm of lymphatic tissue
lymphaden	2.	Inflammation of a lymph node
lympho	3.	Small white blood cell with large nucleus
lymphaden	4.	Removal of a lymph node
lymph	5.	Pertaining to lymph
lymphadeno	6.	Any disease process affecting a lymph node

7. Which of the previous terms would be found in a surgeon's dictation? _____

8. Which of the previous terms would a pathologist use? _____

9. Which of the previous terms would an oncologist use in dictation? _____

Lymphatic and Immune Systems

G. **Immune system.** Build your knowledge of the immune system and its components by correctly matching the definition in the left column with the medical term in the right column. Fill in the blanks. **(LO 12.4, 12.7, 12.9)**

_____ 1. Molecule that triggers an immune response	**a.** mutation
_____ 2. Major defense mechanism against bacteria	**b.** agglutination
_____ 3. Preparation for active development of antibodies	**c.** hapten
_____ 4. Weakened ability to produce disease	**d.** hypersensitivity
_____ 5. Change in the chemistry of a gene	**e.** immunoglobulins
_____ 6. Often appears after surgery or radiation therapy	**f.** antigen
_____ 7. Excessive immune response to an antigen	**g.** lymphedema
_____ 8. Small molecule has to bind to a larger molecule	**h.** attenuate
_____ 9. Cells clumping together	**i.** vaccine
_____ 10. Antibodies produced by humoral immunity	**j.** complement fixation

H. **Elements.** With the exception of Greek and Latin terms that do not deconstruct, most medical terms from any body system can typically be reduced into their basic elements for analysis. Deconstruct the following medical terms into their basic elements to analyze the meanings for the *language of immunology*. The first one is done for you. Fill in the table. **(LO 12.3, 12.D)**

Medical Term	Prefix	Root/ Combining Form	Suffix
coreceptor	*co*	*recept*	*or*
interleukin	1.	2.	3.
dormant		4.	5.
hypersplenism	6.	7.	8.
tonsillitis		9.	10.
anaphylaxis	11.	12.	13.
retrovirus	14.	15.	16.

I. Read Case Report 12.1 and answer the following questions. (LO 12.A)

Case Report (CR) 12.1

You are

. . . a medical assistant working with Susan Lee, MD, in her primary care clinic at Fulwood Medical Center.

Your patient is

. . . Ms. Anna Clemons, a 20-year-old waitress, who is a new patient. She has noticed a lump in her right neck. On questioning, you elicit that she has lost about 8 pounds in weight in the past couple of months, has felt tired, and has had some night sweats.

Her vital signs (VS) are normal. There are two firm, enlarged lymph nodes in her right neck. Physical examination is otherwise unremarkable, and there is no evidence of infection in her head, throat, or upper respiratory tract.

Ms. Clemons has cancerous nodes in her neck. They were not caused by metastatic cancer but by a cancer of the lymph nodes called Hodgkin lymphoma.

1. What outward sign does the patient have?

   a. infection

   b. cancerous nodes

   c. weight loss

   d. tachycardia

2. What is the patient's chief complaint?

   a. feeling tired

   b. shortness of breath

   c. fever

   d. headache

3. Did the patient present with an increased body temperature?

   a. yes

   b. no

4. What is the medical term for enlarged lymph nodes?

   a. immunosuppression

   b. lymphadenopathy

   c. lymphedema

   d. cytokine

5. What findings were present on physical examination?

   a. hypertension

   b. pain

   c. swelling

   d. enlarged cervical lymph nodes

   e. edema

6. The cancerous nodes were not caused by *metastatic cancer.* What does this mean?

   a. it started at the nodes

   b. the cancer is congenital

   c. the cancer spread from another location

   d. it is incurable

7. What are some of the diagnostic tests used to confirm this disease? (Choose all correct answers)

   a. lymph node biopsy

   b. lymphangiogram

   c. chemotherapy

   d. radiation

8. What is the surgical procedure to remove malignant lymph nodes? _____

©2014 Nucleus Medical Media

Health professionals involved in the diagnosis and treatment of respiratory problems include:

- **Pulmonologists,** physicians who specialize in the diagnosis and treatment of respiratory disorders.

- **Thoracic surgeons,** physicians who specialize in the surgical treatment of lung/pulmonary problems.

- **Registered respiratory therapists (RRTs)** or **respiratory care practitioners,** who exercise independent clinical judgment in evaluating, treating, and caring for patients who have respiratory disorders. They also supervise RTs.

- **Respiratory therapy technicians (RTs),** who assist physicians and RRTs in evaluating, monitoring, and treating patients with respiratory disorders.

Chapter Learning Outcomes

To provide optimal care to Mr. Jacobs (Case Report 13.1), to determine what is causing his symptoms and signs, to be involved in his future care, and to communicate with the doctors and other health professionals involved in his care, you need to be able to:

LO 13.1 Relate the structure of the respiratory system to its functions.

LO 13.2 Describe the structure and functions of the nose.

LO 13.3 Discuss the disorders of the nose.

LO 13.4 Integrate the functions of the pharynx with its structure.

LO 13.5 Explain the disorders of the pharynx.

LO 13.6 Describe the structure and functions of the larynx.

LO 13.7 Discuss the disorders of the larynx.

LO 13.8 Describe the functions of the trachea.

LO 13.9 Explain the structure of the lungs.

LO 13.10 Relate the structure of the pleura to its functions.

LO 13.11 Describe the structure of the bronchi.

LO 13.12 Integrate the structure of the bronchioles and alveoli with their functions.

LO 13.13 Discuss the mechanics of respiration.

LO 13.14 Describe the symptoms and signs of respiratory disorders.

LO 13.15 Discuss disorders of the lower respiratory tract.

LO 13.16 Explain the diagnostic procedures used for disorders of the respiratory system.

LO 13.17 Discuss the therapeutic procedures used for disorders of the respiratory system.

LO 13.18 Describe the pharmacologic agents used in the treatment of respiratory disorders.

LO 13.A Use the medical terms of pulmonology to communicate and document in writing accurately and precisely in any health care setting.

LO 13.B Use the medical terms of pulmonology to communicate verbally with accuracy and precision in any health care setting.

LO 13.C Construct the medical terms of pulmonology from their word elements.

LO 13.D Deconstruct the medical terms of pulmonology into their word elements.

LO 13.E Identify the health professionals involved in the care of respiratory patients.

LO 13.F Use correctly the approved abbreviations of medical terms in pulmonology.

Case Report (CR) 13.1

You are

. . . an advanced-level **registered respiratory therapist (RRT)** working in the Acute Respiratory Care Unit of Fulwood Medical Center with **pulmonologist** Tavis Senko, MD.

Your patient is

. . . Mr. Jude Jacobs, a 68-year-old retired mail carrier, who is known to have **chronic obstructive pulmonary disease (COPD)** and is on continual oxygen by nasal prongs (**cannulae**). He has smoked two packs per day for all his adult life.

Last night, he was unable to sleep because of increased **shortness of breath (SOB)** and cough. His cough is productive of yellow **sputum**. He had to sit upright in bed to be able to breathe.

Vital signs (**VS**) are temperature (**T**) 101.6°F, pulse (**P**) 98, respirations (**R**) 36, blood pressure (**BP**) 150/90.

On examination, he is cyanotic and frightened and has nasal prongs with oxygen. Air entry is diminished in both lungs, and there are **rales** (crackles) at both bases.

You have been ordered to draw blood for arterial blood gases (**ABGs**) and to measure the amount of air entering and leaving his lungs by using **spirometry**.

Lesson 13.1
RESPIRATORY SYSTEM

Respiratory System

Lesson Objectives

It sounds like a good scheme. Humans and animals can breathe in oxygen (O_2) and breathe out carbon dioxide (CO_2); plants and trees can breathe in CO_2 and breathe out O_2 and nature stays in balance. Unfortunately, we humans have generated increasing amounts of CO_2 in the air by burning coal, oil, and natural gas and cutting down forests to disturb the balance. In addition, we have created organic and inorganic chemicals and small particles of solid matter in the air that can damage our respiratory tract and be taken into our bodies to cause cancer, brain damage, and birth defects. These materials are called pollutants. This lesson will start the process of understanding how we breathe and will:

13.1.1 Define the six connected elements of the respiratory tract.

13.1.2 Explain the four components of respiration.

13.1.3 Discuss the five functions of the respiratory system.

Abbreviations

ABG	arterial blood gas
BP	blood pressure
CO₂	carbon dioxide
COPD	chronic obstructive pulmonary disease
O₂	oxygen
P	pulse
R	respiration
RRT	registered respiratory therapists
RT	respiratory therapy technicians
SOB	shortness of breath
T	temperature
VS	vital signs

LO 13.1 Structure and Functions of the Respiratory System

The **respiratory tract** (*Figure 13.1*) has six connected elements:

1. Nose
2. Pharynx
3. Larynx
4. Trachea
5. Bronchi and bronchioles
6. Alveoli

Respiration is the exchange of gases. Respiration is the transport of O_2 from the outside air to tissue cells and the transport of CO_2 in the opposite direction.

Respiration has four components:

1. **Ventilation,** which is the movement of air and its gases into and out of the lungs (inspiration and expiration).

2. **Pulmonary exchange of gases** between air in the alveoli and pulmonary capillaries (external respiration).

3. **Gas transport** from the pulmonary capillaries through the arterial system to the peripheral capillaries in tissues and the transport of gases back to the lung capillaries through the venous system.

4. **Peripheral gas exchange** between tissue capillaries and tissue cells for use in cellular metabolism (internal respiration) *(see Chapter 3).*

The five **functions** of the respiratory system are:

1. **Exchange of gases.** All the body cells need O_2 and produce CO_2. The respiratory system allows O_2 from the air to enter the blood and CO_2 to leave the blood and enter the air.

2. **Regulation of blood pH.** This is accomplished by changing blood CO_2 levels *(see Chapter 3).*

3. **Protection.** The respiratory system uses nasal hair, cilia lining the airways, and mucus formed throughout the system to protect against foreign bodies and against some microorganisms.

4. **Voice production.** Movement of air across the vocal cords makes speech and other sounds possible.

5. **Olfaction.** The 12 million receptor cells for smell are in a patch of epithelium the size of a quarter that is in the extreme superior region of the nasal cavity, the **olfactory region** (*Figure 13.2*). Each cell has 10 to 20 hairlike structures called **cilia** that project into the nasal cavity covered in a thin mucous film. Because the olfactory region is right at the top of the nose, you often have to sniff the air right up there to stimulate the sense of smell. A dog has 4 billion receptor cells, which is why dogs can be trained to sniff for drugs, explosives, and dead bodies.

Many of your sensations of taste are influenced by your sense of smell. For example, without its aroma, coffee tastes only bitter. The same is true for peppermint. This is why, when you have a cold, much of your sense of taste is lost.

▲ **Figure 13.1** The Respiratory System.

(Labels: Nasal cavity, Hard palate, Nostril, Pharynx, Larynx, Trachea, Right lung, Pleural cavity, Bronchiole, Soft palate, Epiglottis, Left lung, Left primary bronchus, Secondary bronchus, Tertiary bronchus)

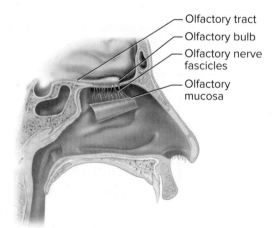

▲ **Figure 13.2** Olfactory Region of Nose.

(Labels: Olfactory tract, Olfactory bulb, Olfactory nerve fascicles, Olfactory mucosa)

WORD	PRONUNCIATION	ELEMENTS		DEFINITION
alveolus alveoli (pl) alveolar (adj)	al-**VEE**-oh-lus al-**VEE**-oh-lee al-**VEE**-oh-lar	 S/ R/	Latin *hollow sac* -ar *pertaining to* alveol- *alveolus*	Tiny air sac terminal element of the respiratory tract Pertaining to the alveoli
bronchus bronchi (pl) bronchiole	**BRONG**-kuss **BRONG**-key **BRONG**-key-ole	 S/ R/	Greek *windpipe* -ole *small* bronchi- *bronchus*	One of two subdivisions of the trachea Increasingly smaller subdivisions of bronchi
cannula cannulae (pl)	**Kan**-you-lah **Kan**-you-lee		Latin *reed*	Tube inserted into a blood vessel as a channel for fluids or gases
cilium cilia (pl)	**SILL**-ee-um **SILL**-ee-ah		Latin *eyelash*	Hairlike motile projection from the surface of a cell
larynx laryngeal (adj)	**LAIR**-inks lah-**RIN**-jee-al	 S/ R/	Greek *larynx* -eal *pertaining to* laryng- *larynx*	Organ of voice production Pertaining to the larynx.
olfaction olfactory (adj)	ol-**FAK**-shun ol-**FAK**-toh-ree	S/ R/ S/	-ion *action, process* olfact- *smell* -ory *having the function of*	Sense of smell Carries information related to the sense of smell
pharynx pharyngeal (adj)	**FAIR**-inks fah-**RIN**-jee-al	 S/ R/	Greek *throat* -eal *pertaining to* pharyng- *pharynx*	Air tube from the back of the nose to the larynx Pertaining to the pharynx
pulmonary (adj) pulmonology pulmonologist	**PULL**-moh-**NAIR**-ee **PULL**-moh-**NOL**-oh-jee **PULL**-moh-**NOL**-oh-jist	S/ R/ S/ R/CF S/	-ary *pertaining to* pulmon- *lung* -logy *study of* pulmon/o- *lung* -logist *one who studies, specialist*	Pertaining to the lungs and their blood supply Study of the lungs, or the medical specialty of disorders of the respiratory tract Medical specialist in pulmonary disorders
respiration respiratory (adj)	**RES**-pih-**RAY**-shun **RES**-pir-ah-**TOR**-ee	S/ P/ R/ S/	-ation *process* re- *again* -spir- *to breathe* -atory *pertaining to*	Fundamental process of life used to exchange oxygen and carbon dioxide Pertaining to respiration
sputum	**SPYU**-tum		Latin *to spit*	Matter coughed up and spat out by individuals with respiratory disorders
thorax thoracic (adj)	**THOR**-acks thor-**ASS**-ik	 S/ R/	Greek *breastplate* -ic *pertaining to* thorac- *chest*	The trunk between the abdomen and neck Pertaining to the thorax
trachea	**TRAY**-kee-ah		Greek *windpipe*	Air tube from the larynx to the bronchi
ventilation	ven-tih-**LAY**-shun	S/ R/	-ation *process* ventil- *wind*	Movement of gases into and out of the lungs

Exercises

A. Identify the basic structures and functions of the respiratory system. *Match each term on the left with its definition on the right.* **LO 13.1**

_____ 1. ventilation

_____ 2. respiration

_____ 3. olfaction

_____ 4. pharynx

_____ 5. larynx

_____ 6. trachea

a. organ that produces the voice

b. organ that connects the mouth with the larynx

c. sense of smell

d. movement of gases in and out of the lungs

e. organ that connects the larynx to the bronchi

f. exchange of gases

Lesson 13.2

RESPIRATORY SYSTEM

Upper Respiratory Tract

The upper respiratory tract consists of the nose, pharynx, and larynx. It is the first site that brings air and its pollutants inside your body. As a health professional, you must understand the roles of the upper respiratory tract in trying to protect you, as well as enabling you to live by transporting O_2 into and CO_2 out of your body.

The information in this lesson will enable you to use correct medical terminology to:

13.2.1 Trace the flow of air from the nose through the pharynx and larynx.

13.2.2 Relate the function of each segment of the upper airway to its structure.

13.2.3 Define the protective mechanisms of the upper respiratory tract.

13.2.4 Describe how sound is produced.

13.2.5 Explain how smells are recognized.

13.2.6 Describe common disorders of the upper respiratory tract.

Keynotes

- Your nose is the first line of defense against pollutants.
- In a deviated nasal septum, the partition between the two nostrils is pushed to one side, leading to a partially obstructed airway in one nostril.
- **Rhinoplasty** is a surgical procedure to alter the size and/or shape of the nose.

Abbreviation

URI	upper respiratory infection

LO 13.2 Structure and Functions of the Nose

When you breathe in air through your nose, the air goes through the nostrils (**nares**) into the **vestibule** of the **nasal cavity**. The nares are guarded by internal (guard) hairs to prevent the entry of large particles.

The nasal cavity is divided by the nasal **septum** into right and left compartments. On the medial wall of each nasal cavity, three bony ridges called **conchae (turbinate bones)** stick out into each cavity. Beneath each concha is a passageway called a **meatus** *(Figure 13.3)*. The palate *(see Chapter 14)* forms the floor of the nose.

The nasal cavity is lined with a mucous membrane (mucosa) containing goblet cells that secrete mucus. Mucus forms a protective layer that can trap particles of dust and solid pollutants.

The **paranasal**, frontal, and maxillary **sinuses** open into the nose. Because they are hollow, the functions of these sinuses are to reduce the weight of the skull and to act as resonating chambers for the sounds of the voice. If your sinuses are congested, your voice loses its normal quality.

The following are functions of the nose:

- **Passageway for air.** The palate is the floor of the nasal cavity that separates it from the mouth and enables you to breathe even with food in your mouth.
- **Air cleanser.** The hairs in the vestibule trap some of the large particles in the air.
- **Air moisturizer.** Moisture from nasal mucus and from tears that drain into the cavity through the nasolacrimal duct *(see Chapter 16)* is added to the air.
- **Air warmer.** The blood flowing through the nasal cavity beneath the mucous membrane also warms the air. This prevents damage from the cold to the more fragile lower respiratory passages.
- **Sense of smell (olfaction).** The olfactory region recognizes some 4,000 separate smells.

LO 13.3 Disorders of the Nose

The **common cold** is a viral **upper respiratory infection (URI)**. It is contagious, being transmitted from person to person in airborne droplets from coughing and sneezing. There is no proven effective treatment.

Rhinitis is an inflammation of the nasal mucosa, usually viral in origin. It is also called **coryza**.

Allergic rhinitis affects 15% to 20% of the population. There is swelling of the mucous membranes of the nose, pharynx, and sinuses, with a clear watery discharge.

Sinusitis is an infection of the paranasal sinuses, often following a cold. The infection can be bacterial, producing a **mucopurulent** discharge from the nose. Treatment with **antibiotics** and **decongestants** may be indicated.

Epistaxis is bleeding from the septum of the nose, usually from trauma. If pinching the nose or packing the nostril with gauze does not stop the bleeding, **cautery** (burning and scarring) with silver nitrate or electrical cautery is indicated.

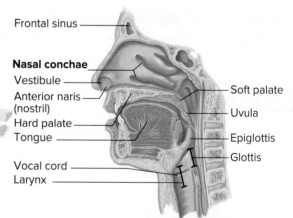

▲ **Figure 13.3** Upper Respiratory Tract.

WORD	PRONUNCIATION		ELEMENTS	DEFINITION
cautery	KAW-ter-ee		Greek *a branding iron*	Agent or device used to burn or scar a tissue
concha conchae (pl)	KON-kah KON-kee		Latin *shell*	Shell-shaped bone on the lateral wall of the nasal cavity
coryza *rhinitis* (syn)	koh-RYE-zah		Greek *catarrh*	Viral inflammation of the mucous membrane of the nose
epistaxis	ep-ih-STAK-sis	S/ P/ R/	-is *condition* epi- *above, over* -stax- *fall in drops*	Nosebleed
meatus	mee-AY-tus		Latin *a passage*	Passage or channel; also used to denote the external opening of a passage
mucopurulent	myu-koh-PYUR-you-lent	S/ R/CF R/	-ent *forming* muc/o- *mucus* -purul- *pus*	Mixture of pus and mucus
naris nares (pl) nasal paranasal	NAH-ris NAH-reez NAY-zal PAR-ah-NAY-zal	 S/ R/ P/	Latin *nostril* -al *pertaining to* nas- *nose* para- *adjacent to*	Nostril Pertaining to the nose Adjacent to the nose
rhinitis *coryza* (syn) rhinoplasty	rye-NIE-tis RYE-noh-plas-tee	S/ R/ S/ R/CF	-itis *inflammation* rhin- *nose* -plasty *surgical repair* rhin/o- *nose*	Inflammation of the nasal mucosa Surgical procedure to change the size or shape of the nose
sinus sinusitis	SIGH-nus sigh-nuh-SIGH-tis	 S/ R/	Latin *cavity* -itis *inflammation* sinus- *sinus*	Cavity or hollow space in a bone or other tissue Inflammation of the lining of a sinus
turbinate	TUR-bin-ate		Latin *shaped like a top*	Another name for the nasal conchae on the medial walls of the nasal cavity

Exercises

A. Elements. *Work with elements to build your knowledge of the language of pulmonology.* **LO 13.2, 13.3, 13.A**

1. The root in the term **rhinitis** means:

   a. shell   **b.** inflammation   **c.** cavity   **d.** nose

2. The suffix in the term **epistaxis** means:

   a. above   **b.** condition of   **c.** bleeding   **d.** nasal

3. The prefix in the term **paranasal** means:

   a. above   **b.** nose   **c.** adjacent to   **d.** pertaining to

B. Greek and Latin terms. *Not all terms can be deconstructed into word parts. Identify the definitions of the following terms related to the language of pulmonology.* **LO 13.2, 13.A**

_____   1. concha   **a.** a passage

_____   2. sinus   **b.** shell

_____   3. coryza   **c.** nostril

_____   4. meatus   **d.** catarrh

_____   5. naris   **e.** cavity

Case Report (CR) 13.2

You are

. . . a sleep technologist in the Sleep Disorders Clinic at Fulwood Medical Center. You are about to position the electrodes on your patient for an overnight **polysomnography** (sleep study).

Your patient is

. . . Mr. Tye Gawlinski, a 29-year-old professional football player.

Mr. Gawlinski's wife states that he snores loudly and has 40 or 50 periods in the night when he stops breathing. The snoring is so loud that she cannot sleep even in the adjoining bedroom. Mr. Gawlinski complains of being tired all day and not having the energy he needs for his job. The sleep study is being performed to confirm a diagnosis of **obstructive sleep apnea**.

Abbreviation	
OSA	obstructive sleep apnea

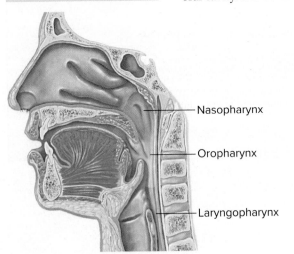

▲ **Figure 13.4** Regions of Pharynx.

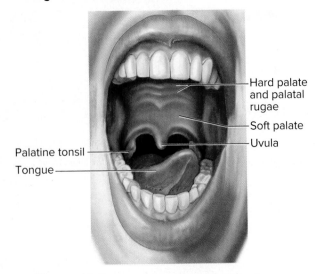

▲ **Figure 13.5** Soft Tissues at Back of Mouth.

LO 13.4 Structure and Functions of the Pharynx

The **pharynx** is a muscular funnel that receives air from the nasal cavity and food and drink from the oral cavity. It is divided into three regions *(Figure 13.4):*

1. **Nasopharynx**—located at the back of the nose, above the soft palate and uvula. It is lined with a mucous membrane that includes goblet cells, which produce mucus. Mucus, including any trapped debris, is moved from the nasal cavity through the nasopharynx and swallowed. The posterior surface contains the **pharyngeal tonsil (adenoid).** Only air moves through this region.

2. **Oropharynx**—located below the soft palate and above the epiglottis. It contains two sets of tonsils called the *palatine* and *lingual* tonsils. Air, food, and drink all pass through this region.

3. **Laryngopharynx**—located below the tip of the epiglottis. This is the pathway to the esophagus. During swallowing, the epiglottis shuts off the trachea so that food cannot enter it. Only food and drink pass through the laryngopharynx.

LO 13.5 Disorders of the Pharynx

Twenty-five percent of normal adults are habitual snorers. The condition is most frequent in overweight males, and it becomes worse with age. The noises of **snoring** are made at the back of the mouth and nose where the tongue and upper pharynx meet the soft palate and uvula *(Figure 13.5).* When there is obstruction to the free flow of air, these structures hit each other, and the vibration produces the sounds of snoring.

Obstructive sleep apnea (OSA) is the condition Mr. Gawlinski has. He has bulky neck tissue from his football training regimen. Obstructive sleep apnea occurs when obstruction by the soft tissues at the back of the nose and mouth causes frequent episodes of gasping for breath followed by complete cessation of breathing (**apnea**). These episodes of apnea can last for 10 to 30 seconds and occur many times every hour of sleep. The episodes reduce the level of O_2 in the blood (**hypoxemia**), causing the heart to pump harder. After several years with this problem, hypertension and cardiac enlargement can occur.

Pharyngitis is an acute or chronic infection involving the pharynx, tonsils, and uvula. It is usually of viral origin in children.

Tonsillitis is an infection of the tonsils in the oropharynx by a virus or, in less than 20% of cases, a streptococcus.

Nasopharyngeal carcinoma is a rare form of cancer that occurs mostly in males between the ages of 50 and 60.

WORD	PRONUNCIATION	ELEMENTS		DEFINITION
adenoid	**ADD**-eh-noyd	S/ R/	-oid *resembling* aden- *gland*	Single mass of lymphoid tissue in midline at the back of the throat
apnea	**AP**-nee-ah	P/ R/	a- *without* -pnea *breathe*	Absence of spontaneous respiration
hypoxemia	**HIGH**-pok-**SEE**-mee-ah	S/ P/ R/	-emia *blood condition* hyp(o)- *below* -ox- *oxygen*	Decreased levels of oxygen in the blood
anoxia	an-**OK**-see-ah	S/ P/	-ia *condition* an- *without*	Complete deprivation of oxygen supply
laryngopharynx	lah-**RING**-oh-**FAIR**-inks	R/CF R/	laryng/o- *larynx* -pharynx *pharynx*	Region of the pharynx below the epiglottis that includes the larynx
nasopharynx	**NAY**-zoh-**FAIR**-inks	R/CF R/	nas/o- *nose* -pharynx *pharynx*	Region of the pharynx at the back of the nose above the soft palate
nasopharyngeal (adj)	**NAY**-zoh-fair-**IN**-jee-al	S/ R/	-eal *pertaining to* -pharyng- *pharynx*	Pertaining to the nasopharynx
oropharynx	**OR**-oh-**FAIR**-inks	R/CF R/	or/o- *mouth* -pharynx *pharynx*	Region at the back of the mouth between the soft palate and the tip of the epiglottis
oropharyngeal (adj)	**OR**-oh-fair-**IN**-jee-al	S/ R/	-eal *pertaining to* -pharyng- *pharynx*	Pertaining to the oropharynx
pharynx pharyngitis	**FAIR**-inks fair-in-**JIE**-tis	S/ R/	Greek *throat* -itis *inflammation* pharyng- *pharynx*	Air tube from the back of the nose to the larynx Inflammation of the pharynx
pharyngeal (adj)	fair-**IN**-jee-al	S/	-eal *pertaining to*	Pertaining to the pharynx
polysomnography	pol-ee-som-**NOG**-rah-fee	S/ P/ R/CF	-graphy *process of recording* poly- *many* -somn/o- *sleep*	Test to monitor brain waves, muscle tension, eye movement, and oxygen levels in the blood as the patient sleeps
snore	SNOR		Old English *snore*	Noise produced by vibrations in the structures of the nasopharynx
tonsil	**TON**-sill		Latin *tonsil*	Mass of lymphoid tissue on either side of the throat at the back of the tongue
tonsillitis (note the double "ll")	ton-sih-**LIE**-tis	S/ R/	-itis *inflammation* tonsill- *tonsil*	Inflammation of the tonsils

Exercises

A. After reading Case Report 13.2, answer the following questions. LO 13.4, 13.5

1. What are Mr. Gawlinski's symptoms? (Choose all that apply)

   a. daytime sleepiness   **b.** sore throat   **c.** lack of energy   **d.** runny nose

2. Mr. Gawlinski underwent the diagnostic procedure of:

   a. tonsillectomy   **b.** endoscopy   **c.** polysomnography   **d.** sonogram

3. If left untreated, his chronic obstructive sleep apnea could cause:

   a. sinus infection   **b.** hypertension   **c.** cardiac arrest   **d.** lymphedema

4. What causes Mr. Gawlinski's obstructive sleep apnea to occur?

   a. smoking   **b.** carcinoma   **c.** increased neck tissue   **d.** hypoxemia

5. Why is *polysomnography* done overnight?

   a. The test requires at least 8 hours of monitoring.   **b.** The technicians are only hired for the night shift.

   c. Sleep apnea only occurs in the nighttime hours.   **d.** The test requires monitoring of a typical night's sleep.

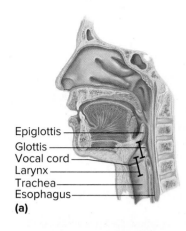

Epiglottis —
Glottis —
Vocal cord —
Larynx —
Trachea —
Esophagus —

(a)

Epiglottis
False vocal cord
Thyroid cartilage
Glottis
True vocal cord
Trachea
Cricoid cartilage

(b)

▲ **Figure 13.6** Larynx.
(a) Location. (b) Structure.

Abbreviation

LTB laryngotracheobronchitis

LO 13.6 Structure and Functions of the Larynx

The flow of inhaled air moves on from the pharynx to the **larynx** *(Figure 13.6a)*, an enlargement of the airway located between the oropharynx and the trachea. The upper opening into it from the oropharynx is called the **glottis**.

The larynx has an outer casing of nine **cartilages** connected to one another by muscles and ligaments. The uppermost cartilage, the leaf-shaped **epiglottis**, guards the glottis. During the swallowing of food, the epiglottis is pushed down by the tongue to close the glottis and direct food into the esophagus that lies behind it.

The **thyroid cartilage,** or "Adam's apple," is the largest cartilage in the body and forms the anterior and lateral walls of the larynx. Below the thyroid cartilage the ring-shaped **cricoid** cartilage connects the larynx to the trachea *(Figure 13.6b)*.

Inside the larynx are the **true vocal cords** *(Figure 13.6b)*. **Intrinsic** muscles control the cords.

Functions of the Larynx

- The thyroid and cricoid cartilages maintain an open passage for the movement of air to and from the trachea.

- The epiglottis and vestibular folds prevent food and drink from entering the larynx *(Figure 13.6b)*.

- The vocal cords *(Figure 13.6a)* are the source of sound production.

Sound Production

Air moving past the vocal cords makes them vibrate to produce sound. The force of the air moving past the vocal cords determines the loudness of the sound. The intrinsic muscles of the cords pull them closer together with varying degrees of tautness. A high-pitched sound is produced by taut cords *(Figure 13.7b)* and a lower pitch by more relaxed cords *(Figure 13.7a)*.

The male vocal cords are longer and thicker than the female, vibrate more slowly, and produce lower-pitched sounds.

The crude sounds produced by the larynx are transformed into words by the actions of the pharynx, tongue, teeth, and lips.

LO 13.7 Disorders of the Larynx

Laryngitis is inflammation of the mucosal lining of the larynx, producing hoarseness and sometimes progressing to loss of voice **(aphonia)**.

Epiglottitis is inflammation of the epiglottis. **Acute epiglottitis** is seen most commonly in children between ages 2 and 7 years and is caused by *Haemophilus influenzae type b* bacteria. Swelling in the epiglottis can cause acute airway obstruction. It is preventable with an available vaccine.

Laryngotracheobronchitis (LTB), commonly referred to as **croup**, is a viral respiratory infection in children aged 3 months to 5 years. It causes inflammation and obstruction of the upper airway. It produces a characteristic cough that sounds like a seal barking. In severe cases, the child makes a high-pitched, squeaky inspiratory noise called **stridor**. Humidity is the initial treatment.

Papillomas or laryngeal **polyps** are benign tumors of the larynx that result from overuse or irritation and are treated by surgical excision using a **laryngoscope**.

Carcinoma of the larynx produces a persistent hoarseness. Its incidence peaks in smokers in their fifties and sixties. Treatment can be surgery, radiation, and/or chemotherapy.

Abbreviation

LTB	laryngotracheobronchitis

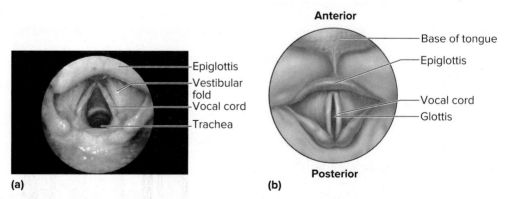

Anterior

Base of tongue
Epiglottis
Vocal cord
Glottis

Posterior

Epiglottis
Vestibular fold
Vocal cord
Trachea

(a)   **(b)**

▲ **Figure 13.7** View of Larynx. (a) Using laryngoscope. (b) Vocal cords pulled close and taut.
©CAMAL/ISM/Diomedia/Medical Images

S = Suffix   P = Prefix   R = Root   R/CF = Combining Form

WORD	PRONUNCIATION	ELEMENTS		DEFINITION
aphonia	ay-**FOH**-nee-ah	S/ P/ R/	-ia *condition* a- *without* -phon- *voice*	Loss of voice
cricoid	**CRY**-koyd		Latin *a ring*	Ring-shaped cartilage in the larynx
glottis	**GLOT**-is	S/	Greek *opening of larynx* -is *pertaining to*	The opening from the oropharynx into the larynx
epiglottis	ep-ih-**GLOT**-is	P/ R/	epi- *above* -glott- *opening of larynx*	Leaf-shaped plate of cartilage that shuts off the larynx during swallowing
epiglottitis	ep-ih-glot-**TIE**-tis	S/	-itis *inflammation*	Inflammation of the epiglottis
intrinsic	in-**TRIN**-sik		Latin *on the inside*	Any muscle whose origin and insertion are entirely within the structure under consideration; for example, inside the vocal cords or the eye
larynx laryngitis	**LAIR**-inks lair-in-**JIE**-tis	S/ R/	Greek *larynx* -itis *inflammation* laryng- *larynx*	Organ of voice production Inflammation of the larynx
laryngoscope	lah-**RING**-oh-skope	S/	-scope *instrument for viewing*	Hollow tube with a light and camera used to visualize or operate on the larynx
laryngotracheobronchitis croup (syn)	lah-**RING**-oh-**TRAY**-kee-oh-brong-**KIE**-tis	R/CF R/CF R/	laryng/o- *larynx* -trache/o- *trachea* -bronch- *bronchus*	Inflammation of the larynx, trachea, and bronchi
thyroid	**THIGH**-royd		Greek *an oblong shield*	Gland in the neck, or a cartilage of the larynx
vocal	**VOH**-kal	S/ R/	-al *pertaining to* voc- *voice*	Pertaining to the voice

Exercises

Study Hint

Whether the term is 24 letters long or 5 letters long, the principle is the same. Know the meaning of the elements, and you will know the meaning of the term!

A. Deconstruct. *For long or short medical terms, deconstruction into word elements is your key to solving the meaning of the term. If there is no particular element, leave the space blank.* **LO 13.6, 13.7, 13.D**

1. **laryngoscope**

   Rewrite this term, and slash all its elements:

   _____/ _____/ _____

              P   R/CF   S

2. **epiglottitis**

   Rewrite this term, and slash all its elements:

   _____/ _____/ _____

              P   R/CF   S

3. **aphonia**

   Rewrite this term, and slash all its elements:

   _____/ _____/ _____

              P   R/CF   S

B. Define disorders of the larynx. *It is important to discriminate between the different disorders of the larynx. Given the definition, write the condition it is describing.* **LO 13.7**

1. Viral infection of the larynx, trachea, and bronchi. Another term for the condition called *croup:* _____

2. Inflammation of the larynx: _____

3. Bacterial infection of the epiglottis: _____

Lesson 13.3

RESPIRATORY SYSTEM

Lower Respiratory Tract

Lesson Objectives

Once the air you inhale has passed through the upper airway and many of the pollutants and impurities have been filtered out and swallowed into the digestive system, there still remain the major needs of getting O_2 into the blood and removing CO_2 from the blood. To do these, the inhaled air passes down the trachea, through the bronchi and bronchioles, and into the alveoli of the lungs, where these exchanges can occur. These structures form the lower respiratory tract.

In this lesson, you will learn to use correct medical terminology to:

13.3.1 Trace the passage of air from the larynx into the alveoli and back.

13.3.2 Explain the exchange of O_2 from the air into the blood.

13.3.3 Explain the exchange of CO_2 from the blood into the air.

13.3.4 Describe the mechanics of ventilation.

13.3.5 Match the functions of the different elements of the lower airway with their structure.

13.3.6 Discuss the effects of common disorders of the lungs on overall health.

LO 13.8 Trachea

The flow of inhaled air now moves into the **trachea** (windpipe). This is a rigid tube that descends from the larynx to divide into the two main bronchi *(Figure 13.8a)*. The rigidity of the trachea is produced by 16 to 20 C-shaped rings of cartilage that form its anterior and lateral walls *(Figure 13.8b)*. The open part of the "C" faces posteriorly and is closed by the **trachealis** muscle. The trachea divides into the two primary (main) bronchi for the right and left lungs *(Figure 13.8a)*.

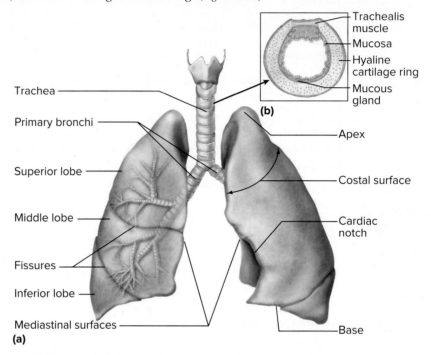

▲ **Figure 13.8** **Lower Respiratory Tract.** (*a*) Gross anatomy. (*b*) Cross-section of the trachea to show the C-shaped tracheal cartilage.

LO 13.9 Structure of the Lungs

The two lungs are the main organs of respiration and are located in the thoracic cavity. Each lung is a soft, spongy, conical organ with its base resting on the **diaphragm**. Its apex lies above and behind the clavicle. Its outer, convex costal surface presses against the rib cage. Its inner, concave surface lies alongside the **mediastinum**.

The right lung has three **lobes**: superior, middle, and inferior. The left lung has two lobes: superior and inferior *(see Figure 13.8a)*. The lobes are separated from each other by **fissures**. The heart makes a concave impression in the left lung, known as the *cardiac notch*.

Each lung receives its bronchus, blood vessels, lymphatic vessels, and nerves through its **hilum** *(Figure 13.9)*. The lung's specific functional cells are called the lung **parenchyma** and are supported by a thin connective tissue framework called the **stroma**. This consists mostly of collagen and elastic fibers, and its elasticity is a factor in the lung's recoil after inhalation.

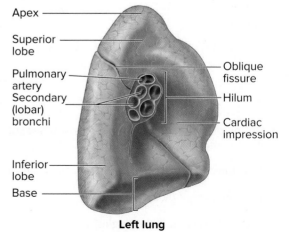

Left lung

▲ **Figure 13.9** **Left Lung Hilum: Medial Surface.**

Word Analysis and Definition

S = Suffix   P = Prefix   R = Root   R/CF = Combining Form

WORD	PRONUNCIATION		ELEMENTS	DEFINITION
diaphragm	**DIE**-ah-fram		Greek *diaphragm*	Musculoligamentous partition separating the abdominal and thoracic cavities
diaphragmatic (adj)	**DIE**-ah-frag-**MAT**-ic	S/ R/	**-atic** *pertaining to* **diaphragm-** *diaphragm*	Pertaining to the diaphragm
fissure fissures (pl)	**FISH**-ur	S/ R/	**-ure** *result of* **fiss-** *split*	Deep furrow or cleft
hilum hila (pl)	**HIGH**-lum **HIGH**-lah		Latin *small area*	The site where the nerves and blood vessels enter and leave an organ
lobe lobar (adj)	LOBE **LOH**-bar	S/ R/	Greek *lobe* **-ar** *pertaining to* **lob-** *lobe*	Subdivision of an organ or other part Pertaining to or part of a lobe
mediastinum	**MEE**-dee-ah-**STIE**-num	S/ P/ R/	**-um** *tissue, structure* **media-** *middle* **-stin-** *partition*	Area between the lungs containing the heart, aorta, venae cavae, esophagus, and trachea
mediastinal (adj)	**MEE**-dee-ah-**STIE**-nal	S/	**-al** *pertaining to*	Pertaining to or part of the mediastinum
parenchyma	pah-**RENG**-kih-mah		Greek *to pour in beside*	Characteristic functional cells of a gland or organ that are supported by the connective tissue framework
stroma	**STROH**-mah		Greek *bed*	Connective tissue framework that supports the parenchyma of an organ or gland
trachealis	tray-kee-**AY**-lis	S/ R/	**-alis** *pertaining to* **trache-** *trachea*	Pertaining to the trachea

Exercises

A. Precision in communication means using the correct form of the medical term, as well as the correct spelling. *Test your knowledge of plurals, adjectives, and spelling with this exercise. Select the correct choice.* **LO 13.8, 13.9**

1. The area between the lungs containing the heart, aorta, venae cavae, esophagus, and trachea is the
   a. mediastenum   **b.** medisternum   **c.** mediastinum   **d.** midiasternum

2. The patient was diagnosed with _____ pneumonia.
   a. lobe   **b.** lobular   **c.** lobar   **d.** lumbar

3. _____ is the term for the functional cells of an organ.
   a. Perenchyma   **b.** Parenchyma   **c.** Perinchkima   **d.** Perenkima

4. Because there is a hilum in each lung, collectively they are referred to as the
   a. hilla   **b.** hila   **c.** hilia   **d.** hilea

5. The muscle separating the abdominal and thoracic cavities is the
   a. diaphram   **b.** diaphragm   **c.** diahragm   **d.** diapragm

6. Removal of a lobe of a lung would be a
   a. lobotomy   **b.** lobectomy   **c.** lobarectomy   **d.** lobarotomy

B. Select the correct pronunciation of the following two terms. **LO 13.9, 13.B**

1. stroma
   a. STROM a
   b. STRO mah
   c. STROH mah
   d. STROH ma
   e. STROM ah

2. diaphragm
   a. DIE a fram
   b. DI a frame
   c. DI ah fram
   d. DIE ah fram
   e. DE a fram

(a)

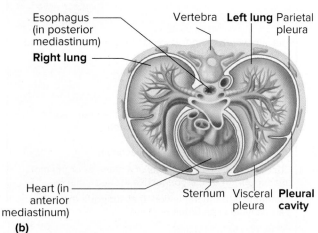

Esophagus
(in posterior
mediastinum)

Vertebra   **Left lung** Parietal
                                pleura

Right lung

Heart (in
anterior
mediastinum)

Sternum   Visceral   **Pleural
                 pleura   cavity**

(b)

▲ **Figure 13.10** **Pleural Cavity and Membranes.** (*a*) Site
of cross-section of superior view. (*b*) Pleural cavity and
membranes in the superior view.

LO 13.10 Structure and Functions of Pleura

The surface of each lung is covered with a serous membrane called the
visceral pleura (*Figure 13.10*). At the hilum, the visceral pleura turns back
on itself to form the **parietal pleura,** which lines the rib cage. The space
between the visceral and parietal pleurae is called the **pleural cavity,**
which contains a thin film of lubricant called the **pleural fluid.**

The functions of the **pleurae** and pleural fluid are to:

1. **Reduce friction.** The lubricant quality of the pleural fluid enables the
    lungs to expand (**inspiration**) and contract (**expiration**) with minimal
    friction.

2. **Assist in inspiration.** The pressure in the pleural cavity is lower than
    the pressure of the atmospheric air in the lungs. This assists the
    inflation of the lungs on inspiration.

3. **Separation.** The **pleurae, mediastinum**, and **pericardium** protect the
    organs inside them to prevent infections from spreading easily from
    one organ to another.

LO 13.11 Structure of Bronchi

As the inhaled air continues down the respiratory tract, the trachea
divides and air flows into the right and left main (primary) bronchi,
which enter each lung at the hilum.

In turn, the main bronchi divide into a secondary (lobar) bronchus for
each lobe. There are three secondary bronchi in the right lung and two in
the left lung. Each secondary bronchus divides into tertiary bronchi that
supply segments of each lobe (*Figure 13.11*).

LO 13.12 Structure and Functions of Bronchioles and Alveoli

The tertiary bronchi divide into **bronchioles**, which in turn divide into **terminal bronchioles** and then
smaller respiratory bronchioles (*Figure 13.12*). None of these bronchioles has cartilage in the walls, but
smooth muscle enables them to dilate or constrict. These bronchioles in turn divide into thin-walled
alveoli.

Each alveolus is a thin-walled sac with its cells supported by a thin **respiratory membrane** that
allows the exchange of gases with the surrounding pulmonary capillary network (*Figure 13.12*). About
5% of the alveolar cells secrete a detergent-like substance called **surfactant** that keeps the alveolar sacs
from collapsing. There are approximately 300 million alveoli in the two lungs.

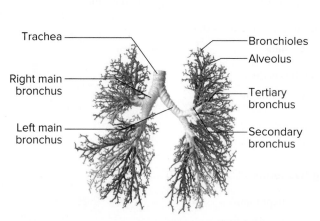

Trachea

Right main
bronchus

Left main
bronchus

Bronchioles

Alveolus

Tertiary
bronchus

Secondary
bronchus

▲ **Figure 13.11** Latex Cast of Tracheobronchial Tree.
©Dave King/Dorling Kindersley/Photo Researchers, Inc.

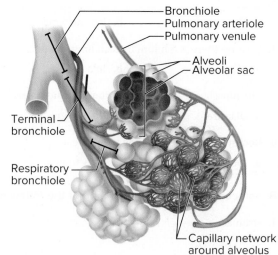

Bronchiole
Pulmonary arteriole
Pulmonary venule

Alveoli
Alveolar sac

Terminal
bronchiole

Respiratory
bronchiole

Capillary network
around alveolus

▲ **Figure 13.12** Bronchioles and Alveoli.

WORD	PRONUNCIATION	ELEMENTS		DEFINITION
exhale	**EKS**-hail	P/	**ex-** *out*	Breathe out
		R/	**-hale** *breathe*	
expiration	**EKS**-pih-**RAY**-shun	S/	**-ation** *process*	The process of breathing out
(opposite of inspiration)		P/	**ex-** *out*	
(*Note:* The "s" is deleted from the root *spir-* because the prefix *ex-* already has the "s" sound.)		R/	**-(s)pir-** *to breathe*	
inflate (verb)	in-**FLAYT**		Latin *blow up*	Expand with air
inflation (noun)	in-**FLAY**-shun	S/	**-ation** *process*	Process of expanding with air
(same as inspiration)		P/	**in-** *into*	
		R/	**-flat-** *blow up*	
inhale	**IN**-hail	P/	**in-** *in*	Breathe in
		R/	**-hale** *breathe*	
inspiration	in-spih-**RAY**-shun	S/	**-ation** *process*	The process of breathing in
(opposite of expiration)		P/	**in-** *into*	
		R/	**-spir-** *to breathe*	
parietal	pah-**RYE**-eh-tal	S/	**-al** *pertaining to*	Pertaining to the outer layer of the serous membrane lining the thoracic and other body cavities
		R/	**pariet-** *wall*	
pleura	**PLUR**-ah		Greek *rib, side*	Membrane covering the lungs and lining the ribs in the thoracic cavity
pleurae (pl)	**PLUR**-ee			
pleural (adj)	**PLUR**-al	S/	**-al** *pertaining to*	Pertaining to the pleura
		R/	**pleur-** *pleura*	
surfactant	ser-**FAK**-tant	S/	**-ant** *pertaining to*	A protein and fat compound that creates surface tension to hold lung alveolar walls apart
		R/	**surf-** *surface*	
		R/	**-act-** *to do, perform*	

Exercises

A. Define the meanings of the word elements. *Select the correct word element being described.* **LO 13.D**

1. The word element that means *out* is:

   a. *-ation*   **b.** *spir-*   **c.** *in-*   **d.** *ex-*

2. The word element that means *blow up:*

   a. *flat-*   **b.** *-itic*   **c.** *pleur-*   **d.** *in-*

3. The word element *spir-* means:

   a. surface   **b.** to breathe   **c.** process   **d.** wall

B. Define structure and functions of the pleura, bronchi, bronchioles, and alveoli. *The structures are distinct and have a distinct purpose. It is important to be able to differentiate these structures and functions.* **LO 13.10, 13.11, 13.12**

1. The substance that lines the alveoli to help keep them open: _____

2. The smallest of the airways that do not participate in gas exchange: _____

3. The serous membrane that covers the lungs: _____ pleura

4. The fluid that reduces friction between the lungs and the thoracic cavity: _____ fluid

5. The large airway that enters each lung at the hilum: _____

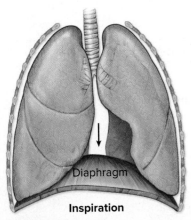

Inspiration

Diaphragm contracts; vertical dimensions of thoracic cavity increase.

(a)

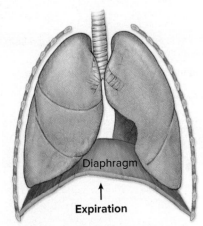

Expiration

Diaphragm relaxes; vertical dimensions of thoracic cavity decrease.

(b)

▲ **Figure 13.13** Inspiration and expiration.

Keynotes

• **Hiccups** are reflex spasms of the diaphragm, causing an involuntary inhalation followed by a sudden closure of the glottis that produces an audible sound—the "hic." The etiology is unknown, and there is no specific medical cure.

• **Yawning** is a reflex that originates in the brainstem in response to hypoxia, boredom, or sleepiness. The exact mechanisms are not known.

LO 13.13 Mechanics of Respiration

A resting adult breathes 10 to 15 times per minute, **inhales** about 500 mL of air during inspiration *(Figure 13.13 (a))*, and **exhales** it during expiration *(Figure 13.13 (b))*. The mission is to get air into and out of the alveoli so that O_2 can get into the blood and CO_2 can get out of the blood.

The diaphragm does most of the work. In inspiration it drops down and flattens to expand the volume of the thoracic cavity and reduce the pressure in the airways *(Figure 13.13a)*. In addition, the external intercostal muscles lift the chest wall up and out to further expand the thoracic cavity.

Expiration is a passive process of letting go. The diaphragm and intercostal muscles relax, and the thoracic cavity springs back to its orginal volume *(Figure 13.13 (b))*.

LO 13.14 Common Signs and Symptoms of Respiratory Disorders

1. **Coughing** is triggered by irritants in the respiratory tract. You close the glottis and contract the muscles of expiration to develop high pressure in the lower tract. Then you suddenly open the glottis to release an explosive blast of air.

   The irritants can be cigarette smoke (as with Mr. Jacobs), infection, or tumors (as in lung cancer). A productive cough produces sputum that can be swallowed or **expectorated**. Bloody sputum is called **hemoptysis**. Thick, yellow (purulent) sputum indicates infection. A nonproductive cough is dry and hacking. Abnormal amounts of expectorated clear mucus are called **phlegm**.

2. **Dyspnea**, or shortness of breath (SOB), can be on exertion or, in severe disorders, at rest when all the respiratory muscles can exchange only a small volume of air.

   Dyspnea can result from airway obstruction. Wheezing associated with dyspnea is the sound of air being forced through constricted airways, as in asthma. Dyspnea also can be produced by fibrosis of lung tissues, when the lungs' **compliance** is reduced. Compliance is the ability of the lungs to expand on inspiration.

3. **Cyanosis** is seen when the blood has increased levels of **unoxygenated hemoglobin,** which has a characteristic dark gray–blue color. The color is best seen in the lips, mucous membranes, and nail beds where there is no skin pigmentation to mask it.

   • **Peripheral cyanosis** occurs when there is peripheral vasoconstriction. The reduced flow allows hemoglobin to yield more of its O_2, leading to increased unoxygenated hemoglobin.

   • **Central cyanosis** occurs with inadequate blood oxygenation in the lungs as a result of impaired airflow or impaired blood flow through the lungs. Central cyanosis is detected by examining the color of the lips, gums, and tongue.

4. **Changes in rate of breathing. Eupnea** is the normal, easy, automatic respiration—around 15 breaths per minute in a resting adult. Both **tachypnea** (rapid rate of breathing) and **hyperpnea** (breathing deeper and more rapidly than normal) are signs of respiratory difficulty, as is **bradypnea** (slow breathing).

5. **Sneezing** is caused by irritants in the nasal cavity. The glottis stays open while the soft palate and tongue block the flow of air from getting out. Then they suddenly release to let air burst out through the nose.

WORD	PRONUNCIATION	ELEMENTS		DEFINITION
bradypnea (opposite of tachypnea)	brad-ip-**NEE**-ah	S/ P/	-pnea *breathe* brady- *slow*	Slow breathing
compliance	kom-**PLY**-ance	S/ R/	-ance *state of, condition* compli- *fulfill*	Measure of the capacity of a chamber or hollow viscus to expand, in this case, the lungs
cyanosis	sigh-ah-**NOH**-sis	S/ R/	-osis *condition* cyan- *blue*	Blue discoloration of the skin, lips, and nail beds due to low levels of oxygen in the blood
cyanotic (adj)	sigh-ah-**NOT**-ik	S/ R/CF	-tic *pertaining to* cyan/o- *blue*	Marked by cyanosis
dyspnea	disp-**NEE**-ah	R/ P/	-pnea *breathe* dys *difficult*	Difficulty breathing
eupnea	yoop-**NEE**-ah	R/ P/	-pnea *breathe* eup- *normal*	Normal breathing
expectorate	ek-**SPEC**-toh-rate	S/ P/ R/	-ate *process* ex- *out* -pector- *chest*	Cough up and spit out mucus from the respiratory tract
hemoptysis	hee-**MOP**-tih-sis	R/CF R/	hem/o- *blood* -ptysis *spit*	Bloody sputum
hyperpnea	high-perp-**NEE**-ah	R/ P/	-pnea *breathe* hyper- *excessive*	Deeper and more rapid breathing than normal
phlegm	FLEM		Greek *flame*	Abnormal amounts of mucus expectorated from the respiratory tract
pleurisy	**PLUR**-ih-see	S/ R/	-isy *inflammation* pleur- *pleura*	Inflammation of the pleura
pleuritic (adj)	plur-**IT**-ik	S/	-itic *pertaining to*	Pertaining to pleurisy
tachypnea (opposite of bradypnea)	tak-ip-**NEE**-ah	R/ P/	-pnea *breathe* tachy- *rapid*	Rapid breathing

Exercises

A. Build terms. *Knowing just one element will enable you to build more terms with the addition of other elements. Practice building your pulmonology terms with the following root and various prefixes. Fill in the blanks.* **LO 13.14, 13.C**

1. The suffix *-pnea* means _____.

Add the following prefixes to -pnea to form new terms for questions 2 through 6.

> **Study Hint**
> Remember the prefixes in the preceding WAD—they can be applied to many other roots for new terms.

| tachy | brady | dys | eu | hyper |

2. Difficult breathing   _____pnea

3. Deeper breathing than normal   _____pnea

4. Slow breathing   _____pnea

5. Normal breathing   _____pnea

6. Rapid breathing   _____pnea

LO 13.15 Disorders of the Lower Respiratory Tract

Acute bronchitis can be viral or bacterial, leading to the production of excess mucus with some obstruction of airflow. A single episode resolves without significant residual damage to the airway.

Chronic bronchitis is the most common obstructive disease, due to cigarette smoking or repeated episodes of acute bronchitis. In addition to excess mucus production, cilia are destroyed. A pattern develops, involving chronic cough, sputum production, dyspnea, and recurrent acute infections.

In advanced chronic bronchitis, **hypoxia** and **hypercapnia** develop, and heart failure follows.

Bronchiolitis, inflammation of the small airway bronchioles, occurs in the adult as the early and often unrecognized beginning of airway changes in cigarette smokers or those exposed to "secondhand smoke," inhaling the smoke produced by other peoples' cigarettes.

Bronchiolitis affects children under the age of 2 because their small airways become blocked very easily. The disease is viral and in severe cases can cause marked respiratory distress, with drawing in of the neck and intercostal spaces of the chest with each breath (known as **retractions**).

Pulmonary emphysema is a disease of the respiratory bronchioles and alveoli. These airways become enlarged, and the septa between the alveoli are destroyed, forming large sacs **(bullae).** There is a loss of surface area for gas exchange. Because the septa contain elastic tissue that assists the lungs' recoil in exhalation, recoil becomes more difficult, and air is trapped in the bullae. This leads to **hyperinflation** of the lungs and the enlarged "barrel chest" shown by many patients with emphysema.

Chronic airway obstruction (CAO) is also called **chronic obstructive pulmonary disease (COPD).** This is a progressive disease, as Mr. Jacobs' history shows. It involves both chronic bronchitis and emphysema. A history of heavy cigarette smoking, with chronic cough and sputum production, is followed by exertional dyspnea. By the time Mr. Jacobs' dyspnea was severe, irreversible lung damage *(Figure 13.14)* had led to emphysema, recurrent infections, and episodes of respiratory insufficiency. The insufficiency became permanent, and supplementary O_2 is now necessary round the clock. Right-sided heart failure **(cor pulmonale)** is the end-result of pulmonary hypertension and blood backing up into the right ventricle *(see Chapter 10).*

Bronchiectasis is the abnormal dilatation of the small bronchioles due to repeated infections. The damaged, dilated bronchi are unable to clear secretions, so additional infections and more damage can occur.

Bronchial asthma is a disorder with recurrent acute episodes of bronchial obstruction as a result of constriction of bronchioles **(bronchoconstriction), hypersecretion** of mucus, and inflammatory swelling of the bronchiolar lining. The airflow obstruction these produce is mainly during expiration, and the wheezing exhalation heard in asthma is the result of forcing air out of the lungs through constricted, swollen bronchioles. Between attacks, breathing can be normal. The **etiology** of asthma is an allergic response to substances such as pollen, animal dander, or the feces of house dust mites.

Cystic fibrosis (CF) is caused by an increased viscosity of secretions from the pancreas, salivary glands, liver, intestine, and lungs. In the lungs, a particularly thick mucus obstructs the airways and causes repeated infections. Respiratory failure is the cause of death, often before the age of 30. The disorder is genetic.

Pulmonary edema is the collection of fluid in the lung tissues and alveoli. It is most frequently the result of left ventricular failure or mitral valve disease with **congestive heart failure (CHF).** Noncardiogenic pulmonary edema can result from sepsis, renal failure, disseminated intravascular coagulation (DIC) *(see Chapter 11),* and opiate or barbiturate poisoning.

(a)

(b)

▲ **Figure 13.14** **Whole Lungs.**
(*a*) Nonsmoker's lungs. (*b*) Smoker's lungs.
©Pixologic Studio/Photo Researchers, Inc. ©Ingo Schulz/imageBROKER RM/Diomedia/Medical Images

Abbreviations

CAO	chronic airway obstruction
CF	cystic fibrosis
CHF	congestive heart failure
COPD	chronic obstructive pulmonary disease

WORD	PRONUNCIATION		ELEMENTS	DEFINITION
asthma	**AZ**-mah		Greek *asthma*	Episodes of breathing difficulty due to narrowed or obstructed airways
asthmatic (adj)	az-**MAT**-ic	S/ R/	**-tic** *pertaining to* **asthma-** *asthma*	Pertaining to, or suffering from, asthma
bronchiectasis	brong-kee-**EK**-tah-sis	S/ R/CF	**-ectasis** *dilation* **bronch/i** *bronchus*	Chronic dilation of the bronchi following inflammatory disease and obstruction
bronchiolitis	brong-kee-oh-**LIE**-tis	S/ R/	**-itis** *inflammation* **bronchiol-** *small bronchus*	Inflammation of the small bronchioles
bronchoconstriction	**BRONG**-koh-kon-**STRIK**-shun	S/ R/CF R/	**-ion** *process* **bronch/o-** *bronchus* **-constrict-** *to narrow*	Reduction in diameter of a bronchus
bulla bullae (pl)	**BULL**-ah **BULL**-ee		Latin *bubble*	Bubble-like dilated structure
cor pulmonale	KOR pul-moh-**NAH**-lee	S/ R/	**cor** Latin *heart* **-ale** *pertaining to* **pulmon-** *lung*	Right-sided heart failure arising from chronic lung disease
cystic fibrosis (CF)	**SIS**-tik fie-**BROH**-sis	S/ R/ S/ R/	**-ic** *pertaining to* **cyst-** *cyst* **-osis** *condition* **fibr-** *fiber*	Genetic disease in which excessive viscid mucus obstructs passages, including bronchi
emphysema	em-fih-**SEE**-mah	P/ R/	**em-** *in, into* **-physema** *blowing*	Dilation of respiratory bronchioles and alveoli
hypercapnia	**HIGH**-per-**KAP**-nee-ah	S/ P/ R/	**-ia** *condition* **hyper-** *excessive* **-capn-** *carbon dioxide*	Abnormal increase of carbon dioxide in the arterial bloodstream
hyperinflation	**HIGH**-per-in-**FLAY**-shun	S/ P/ P/ R/	**-ion** *process* **hyper-** *excessive* **-in-** *in* **-flat-** *blow up*	Overdistension of pulmonary alveoli with air resulting from airway obstruction
hypersecretion	**HIGH**-per-seh-**KREE**-shun	S/ P/ R/	**-ion** *process* **hyper-** *excessive* **-secret-** *secrete*	Excessive secretion of mucus (or enzymes or waste products)
hypoxia	high-**POK**-see-ah	S/ P/ R/	**-ia** *condition* **hyp(o)-** *deficient, below* **-ox-** *oxygen*	Decrease below normal levels of oxygen in tissues, gases, or blood
hypoxic (adj)	high-**POK**-sik	S/	**-ic** *pertaining to*	Deficient in oxygen
retraction	ree-**TRAK**-shun	S/ P/ R/	**-ion** *process* **re-** *back* **-tract-** *pull*	A pulling back, as a pulling back of the intercostal spaces and the neck above the clavicle

Exercises

A. These elements all appear in the language of pulmonology. *Challenge your knowledge of these elements, and make the correct match. Fill in the blanks.* **LO 13.15**

_____	**1.** *re*	**a.**	to narrow
_____	**2.** *em*	**b.**	process
_____	**3.** *capn*	**c.**	pull
_____	**4.** *ole*	**d.**	dilation
_____	**5.** *osis*	**e.**	back
_____	**6.** *constrict*	**f.**	CO_2
_____	**7.** *ion*	**g.**	into
_____	**8.** *tract*	**h.**	bronchus
_____	**9.** *ectasis*	**i.**	small
_____	**10.** *bronchi*	**j.**	condition

▲ **Figure 13.15** Chest X-Ray of Patient with Pneumonia in the Left Lung. A normal lung appears as mostly black space but with some lung markings on an x-ray because its spongy structure is filled with air. In contrast, a pneumonic lung appears white or opaque on an x-ray as a result of accumulation of fluid and cells in the alveoli. ©Giancarlo Zuccotto/Diomedia/Medical Images RM

▲ **Figure 13.16** Left Pneumothorax. There are no lung markings seen in the area of the pneumothorax. ©Wellcome Photo Library

Abbreviations

ARDS	acute respiratory distress syndrome
ARF	acute respiratory failure
CHF	congestive heart failure
NRDS	neonatal respiratory distress syndrome

LO 13.15 Disorders of the Lower Respiratory Tract (Continued)

Pneumonia is an acute infection affecting the alveoli and lung parenchyma (*Figure 13.15*). Bacterial infections focus on the alveoli; viral infections, on the parenchyma. **Lobar pneumonia** is an infection limited to one lung lobe. **Bronchopneumonia** is used to describe an infection in the bronchioles that spreads to the alveoli.

When an area of the lung (**segment**) or a lobe becomes airless as a result of the infection, the lung is **consolidated.** When an area of the lung collapses as a result of bronchial obstruction, the condition is called **atelectasis.**

Pleurisy, an inflammation of the pleurae, can be a complication of pneumonia. This condition is very painful on breathing. The inflammation often leads to an exudate accumulating in the pleural cavity—a **pleural effusion.** If the pleural effusion contains pus, it is called **empyema (pyothorax).** If it contains blood, it is called **hemothorax.**

Lung abscess can be a complication of bacterial pneumonia or cancer. Long-term antibiotics are used, and surgical resection of the abscess may be required.

Pneumothorax is the entry of air into the pleural cavity (*Figure 13.16*). The cause can be unknown (**spontaneous pneumothorax**), but it often results from trauma when a fractured rib, knife blade, or bullet lacerates the parietal pleura.

Thromboembolism is caused by an embolus, usually arising in the deep vein of the calf and lodging in a branch of the pulmonary artery. The symptoms are chest pain, dyspnea, tachypnea (increased respiratory rate), and a reduction in blood O_2 levels.

Acute respiratory distress syndrome (ARDS) is sudden life-threatening lung failure caused by a variety of underlying conditions, from major trauma to sepsis. The alveoli fill with fluid and collapse, and gas exchange is shut down. Hypoxia results. Mechanical ventilation has to be provided. The mortality is from 35% to 50%.

Neonatal respiratory distress syndrome (NRDS) is seen in premature babies whose lungs have not matured enough to produce surfactant. The alveoli collapse, and mechanical ventilation is needed to keep them open.

Chronic infections of the lung parenchyma are the result of prolonged exposure to infection or to occupational irritant dusts or droplets. These disorders are called **pneumoconioses.** Levels of dust inhalation overwhelm the airways' particle-clearing abilities; the dust particles accumulate in the alveoli and parenchyma, leading to fibrosis. **Asbestosis** from inhaling asbestos particles can lead to a cancer (**mesothelioma**) in the pleura. **Silicosis** from inhaling silica particles is called *stone mason's lung.* **Anthracosis** from inhaling coal dust particles is called *coal miners' lung.* **Sarcoidosis** is an **idiopathic** fibrotic disorder of the lung parenchyma.

Pulmonary tuberculosis is a chronic, infectious disease of the lungs.

Lung cancer, related to tobacco use, used to be a male disease, but now fatalities in women from lung cancer exceed those from breast cancer. Ninety percent of lung cancers arise in the mucous membranes of the larger bronchi and are called **bronchogenic carcinomas.** The tumor obstructs the bronchus, spreads into the surrounding lung tissues, and metastasizes to lymph nodes, liver, brain, and bone.

Acute respiratory failure (ARF) is abnormal respiratory function resulting in inadequate tissue oxygenation or CO_2 elimination that is severe enough to impair vital organ functions. Causes of ARF include congestive heart failure (CHF), chronic obstructive pulmonary disease (COPD,) chest trauma with resultant **flail chest,** spinal cord injury, and neuromuscular disorders in which the muscles of respiration are weak or paralyzed.

WORD	PRONUNCIATION	ELEMENTS		DEFINITION
anthracosis	an-thra-**KOH**-sis	S/ R/	-osis *condition* anthrac- *coal*	Lung disease caused by the inhalation of coal dust
asbestosis	as-bes-**TOH**-sis	S/ R/	-osis *condition* asbest- *asbestos*	Lung disease caused by the inhalation of asbestos particles
atelectasis	at-el-**EK**-tah-sis	P/ R/	atel- *incomplete* -ectasis *dilation*	Collapse of part of a lung
bronchogenic	brong-koh-**JEN**-ik	S/ R/CF	-genic *creation* bronch/o- *bronchus*	Arising from a bronchus
bronchopneumonia	**BRONG**-koh-new-**MOH**-nee-ah	S/ R/CF R/	-ia *condition* bronch/o- *bronchus* -pneumon- *air, lung*	Acute inflammation of the walls of smaller bronchioles with spread to lung parenchyma
effusion	eh-**FYU**-shun		Latin *pouring out*	Collection of fluid that has escaped from blood vessels into a cavity or tissues
empyema	**EM**-pie-**EE**-mah	S/ P/ R/	-ema *result* em- *in* -py- *pus*	Pus in a body cavity, particularly in the pleural cavity
pyothorax (syn)		S/ R/CF	-thorax *chest* py/o *pus*	Empyema in a pleural cavity
flail chest	FLAIL CHEST		**flail** Old English *flapping* **chest** Greek *basket, hamper*	Condition in which three or more consecutive ribs have been fractured, resulting in uncontrolled movement of that segment of the chest
hemothorax	hee-moh-**THOR**-aks	R/ R/	thorax *chest* hem/o- *blood*	Blood in the pleural cavity
idiopathic	**ID**-ih-oh-**PATH**-ik	S/ R/CF R/	-ic *pertaining to* idi/o- *personal, distinct, unknown* -path- *disease*	Pertaining to a disease of unknown etiology
mesothelioma	**MEEZ**-oh-thee-lee-**OH**-mah	S/ P/ R/CF	-oma *tumor, mass* meso- *middle* -thel/i- *lining*	Cancer arising from the cells lining the pleura or peritoneum
pleurisy	**PLUR**-is-see	S/ R/	-isy *inflammation* pleur- *pleura*	Inflammation of the pleura
pneumoconiosis	new-moh-koh-nee-**OH**-sis	S/ R/CF R/	-osis *condition* pneum/o- *air, lung* -coni- *dust*	Fibrotic lung disease caused by the inhalation of different dusts
pneumonia	new-**MOH**-nee-ah	S/ R/	-ia *condition* pneumon- *air, lung*	Inflammation of the lung parenchyma
pneumonitis (syn)	new-moh-**NIE**-tis	S/	-itis *inflammation*	
pneumothorax	new-moh-**THOR**-aks	S/ R/CF	-thorax *chest* pneum/o- *air, lung*	Air in the pleural cavity
sarcoidosis (*Note*: Two suffixes.)	sar-koy-**DOH**-sis	S/ S/ R/	-osis *condition* -oid- *resembling* sarc- *sarcoma*	Granulomatous lesions of lungs and other organs; cause is unknown
silicosis	sil-ih-**KOH**-sis	S/ R/	-osis *condition* silic- *silicon*	Fibrotic lung disease from inhaling silica particles
thromboembolism	**THROM**-boh-**EM**- boh-lizm	S/ R/CF R/	-ism *condition* thromb/o- *blood clot* -embol- *plug*	A piece of detached blood clot (embolus) blocking a distant blood vessel
tuberculosis	too-**BER**-kyu-**LOH**-sis	S/ R/	-osis *condition* tubercul- *nodule, tuberculosis*	Infectious disease that can infect any organ or tissue

Exercises

A. Differentiate between the types of conditions of the pleura. *Word elements indicate major differences in conditions and thus the approach to care of patients. Identify the meanings of the following terms as they relate to abnormal contents of the pleural cavity.* **LO 13.15**

1. Abnormal contents of the pleural cavity often contain the suffix:

   a. *osis*   **b.** *pulmon/o*   **c.** *pleur*   **d.** *thorax*

2. An abnormal collection of blood in the pleural cavity contains the root:

   a. *hem/o*   **b.** *pleur/o*   **c.** *idi/o*   **d.** *purul/o*

Lesson 13.4

RESPIRATORY SYSTEM

Procedures and Pharmacology

Lesson Objectives

Many of the diagnostic and therapeutic procedures used in the diagnosis and treatment of respiratory disorders are performed by technicians under the orders of the physicians and it is important to understand the medical language used to order, perform, and document these procedures. This lesson will enable you to:

LO 13.4.1 Explain diagnostic procedures used for pulmonary disorders.

LO 13.4.2 Discuss therapeutic procedures used for pulmonary disorders.

LO 13.4.3 Describe pharmacologic agents used to treat pulmonary disorders.

Keynotes

Measure pulmonary function with spirometers, peak flow meters, and ABGs.

A PFT value that is less than 70% of the predicted value is considered abnormal.

Abbreviations

ABGs	arterial blood gas
FEV$_1$	forced expiratory volume in 1 second
FVC	forced vital capacity
msec	millisecond
PEFR	peak expiratory flow rate
PFT	pulmonary function test

Case Report 13.1 *(continued)*

Mr. Jacobs' FEV$_1$ was only 40% of the predicted value for a man of his age, height, and weight. Mr. Jacobs' FVC also was reduced because of the fibrotic effects of repeated infections on his lung tissues reducing the volume in his airways. When he was off O$_2$, Mr. Jacobs' O$_2$ levels were below 50% of normal. Even with nasal prongs and the administration of O$_2$, his blood O$_2$ levels were only 75% of normal.

LO 13.16 Pulmonary Diagnostic Procedures

Pulmonary Function Tests

A **spirometer** is a device used to measure the **volume** of air that moves in and out of the respiratory system *(Figure 13.17)*. You ask the patient to breathe in as deeply as possible and then breathe out as rapidly and completely as possible through the spirometer. The volume of air expired at the end of this **pulmonary function test (PFT)** is the patient's **forced vital capacity (FVC).**

The spirometer also measures **flow rates.** The **forced expiratory volume in 1 second (FEV$_1$)** is the amount of air expired in the first second of the test.

In obstructive lung disorders such as asthma or COPD, the lumina of the airways are constricted and resistant to airflow. This will cause a reduction in the FEV$_1$.

In restrictive lung disorders in which the lung tissue is fibrotic or scarred and resists expansion, there will be a reduction in the FVC.

A **peak flow meter** records the greatest flow of air that can be sustained for 10 milliseconds **(msec)** on forced expiration, the **peak expiratory flow rate (PEFR).** It is of value in following the course of asthma and, in postoperative care, in monitoring the return of lung function after anesthesia.

Arterial blood gases (ABGs), the measurement of the levels of O$_2$ and CO$_2$ in the blood, are good indicators of respiratory function.

▲ **Figure 13.17** Spirometer. ©Garo/Photo Researchers, Inc.

Auscultation

The stethoscope is used to detect normal **(vesicular)** and abnormal **(adventitious)** breath sounds. Abnormal breath sounds are categorized as:

- **Wheezes (rhonchi):** musical quality; associated with bronchoconstriction found with asthma. Wheezes are characteristic of asthma.
- **Crackles** (formally known as **rales**): nonmusical, explosive sounds; attributed to the popping opening of the airways with or without the movement of air through secretions in larger airways. Crackles can be auscultated with pneumonia, pulmonary edema, and atelectasis.
- **Pleural rub:** nonmusical sound, often described as a grating or creaking sound. It is caused by the inflamed visceral and parietal pleurae rubbing together, which can occur with pleurisy.
- **Stridor**: loud, high-pitched sound with a musical quality. Associated with constriction of the airways of the upper respiratory tract such as croup.

WORD	PRONUNCIATION		ELEMENTS	DEFINITION
crackle rale (syn) rales (pl)	KRAK-el RAHL RAHLS		To crack French *rattle*	Explosive popping sound due to the sudden opening of small airways or air moving through secretions
pleural rub	PLUR-al RUB	S/ R/	-al *pertaining to* pleur- *pleura* rub East Frisian *to rub, scrape*	Grating sound due to pleural membranes rubbing against each other
rhonchus rhonchi (pl) *wheeze* (syn)	RONG-kuss RONG-key		Greek *snoring*	Wheezing sound heard on auscultation of the lungs, made by air passing through a constricted lumen
spirometer	spy-ROM-eh-ter	R/CF R/	spir/o- *to breathe* -meter *measure*	An instrument used to measure respiratory volumes
stridor	STRIE-door		Latin *a harsh, creaking sound*	High-pitched noise made when there is respiratory obstruction in the larynx or trachea
wheeze wheezes (pl)	WEEZ		Old English *action of blowing*	Musical sound of the airways associated with asthma

Exercises

A. Define components of pulmonary function testing (PFT). *Given the description of the PFT result, choose the PFT that it used to help diagnose the respiratory disorder.* **LO 13.16, 13.A, 13.F**

1. The measurement used in the evaluation of asthma.

    a. forced vital capacity

    b. peak expiratory flow rate

    c. forced expiratory volume in 1 second

2. If this value is less than 70% of predicted, it indicates the presence of COPD.

    a. forced vital capacity

    b. peak expiratory flow rate

    c. forced expiratory volume in 1 second

3. If this value is less than 70% of predicted, it indicates the presence of restrictive lung disease.

    a. forced vital capacity

    b. peak expiratory flow rate

    c. forced expiratory volume in 1 second

B. Define adventitious breath sounds. *Breath sounds can be used to indicate the presence of disease. Match the adventitious breath sound with its correct description.* **LO 13.16**

_____ 1. musical sound, indicating narrowing of the lower airways

_____ 2. grating sound

_____ 3. explosive, popping sound

_____ 4. high-pitch sound associated with constricted upper airway

a. stridor

b. crackle

c. pleural rub

d. wheeze

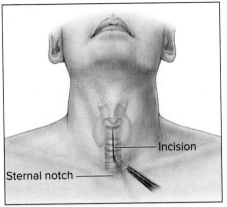

(1) Tracheotomy incision is made superior to sternal notch.

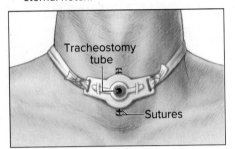

(2) A tracheostomy tube is inserted, and the remaining incision is sutured closed.

▲ **Figure 13.18** Tracheostomy Procedure.

Abbreviations

AP	anteroposterior
ARDS	adult respiratory distress syndrome
CPAP	continuous positive airway pressure
CT	computed tomography
CXR	chest x-ray
MRA	magnetic resonance angiography
NRDS	neonatal respiratory distress syndrome
PA	posteroanterior
PDT	postural drainage therapy
PEEP	positive end-expiratory pressure
PET	positron emission tomography

Keynotes

- **Pulmonary resection** is the surgical removal of lung tissue.
- **Wedge resection** is the removal of a small localized area of diseased lung.
- **Segmentectomy** is the removal of lung tissue attached to a bronchus.
- **Lobectomy** is the removal of a lobe.
- **Pneumonectomy** is the removal of an entire lung.

LO 13.16 Diagnostic Procedures (continued)

Chest x-ray (CXR) is a radiograph image of the chest taken in **anteroposterior (AP)**, **posteroanterior (PA)**, lateral, and sometimes oblique and lateral decubitus positions.

Computed tomography (CT), **angiography** of the pulmonary circulation using contrast materials, **magnetic resonance angiography (MRA)** to define emboli in the pulmonary arteries, and **ultrasonography** of the pleural space are chest imaging techniques in current use. **Positron emission tomography (PET)** can sometimes distinguish benign from malignant lesions.

Bronchoscopy is the insertion of a fiber-optic endoscope (called a **bronchoscope**) into the bronchial tree to visually examine it, take a tissue biopsy, or take a wash for secretions.

Mediastinoscopy is used to stage lung cancer and diagnose mediastinal masses. The mediastinoscope is inserted through an incision in the sternal notch.

Tracheal aspiration uses a soft catheter that allows brushings and washings to be performed to remove cells and secretions from the trachea and main bronchi. It can be passed through a tracheostomy, **endotracheal** tube, or the mouth or nose.

Thoracentesis is the insertion of a needle through an intercostal space to remove fluid from a pleural effusion for laboratory study or to relieve pressure. It is also called a **pleural tap.**

Thoracotomy is used to obtain an open biopsy of tissue from the lung, hilum, pleura, or mediastinum. It is performed through an intercostal incision under general anesthesia.

In many disorders of the lower respiratory tract, during **auscultation** of the chest, the air bubbling through abnormal fluid in the alveoli and small bronchioles (as in pulmonary edema) produces a noise called **rales**. When the bronchi are partly obstructed and air is being forced past an obstruction, a high-pitched noise called a **rhonchus** is heard.

LO 13.17 Therapeutic Procedures

Rhinoplasty is a surgical procedure to alter the size and/or shape of the nose.

Pulmonary rehabilitation includes education, breathing retraining, exercises for the upper and lower extremities, and psychosocial support.

Nutritional support is critical for patients who have difficulty breathing or who lose a lot of weight.

Immunizations are available against influenza and the pneumococcus bacterium, the most common cause of bacterial pneumonia.

Postural drainage therapy (PDT) uses gravity to promote drainage of secretions from lung segments by positioning and tilting the patient. Chest percussion (tapping) can help loosen, mobilize, and drain the retained secretions.

Continuous positive airway pressure (CPAP) is an attempt to keep the airway open by maintaining a positive pressure. A mask is fitted over the nose and mouth and attached to a ventilator. This can be used at night when a person is sleeping for sleep apnea or in acute situations for COPD.

Positive end-expiratory pressure (PEEP) is a technique in ventilation to keep the alveoli from collapsing in conditions such as **adult respiratory distress syndrome (ARDS)** and **neonatal respiratory distress syndrome (NRDS)**.

Intubation uses an oropharyngeal airway in the unconscious patient during bag-and-mask ventilation to maintain an open airway. A tube is inserted to prevent the tongue from falling back to obstruct the airway and facilitates suctioning the airway.

Endotracheal intubation involves the placement of a tube into the trachea. This allows patients to be placed on a ventilator and their breathing controlled. Endotracheal intubation and mechanical ventilation are used when the patient is unable to adequately ventilate on his or her own, such as when the patient is paralyzed, has ARDS, has a significant lung infection, or has a COPD or asthma exacerbation.

Tracheotomy is an incision made into the trachea (windpipe) so that a temporary or permanent opening into the windpipe, called a **tracheostomy**, can be created (*Figure 13.18*). A tracheostomy tube is placed into the opening to provide an airway. A tracheostomy is used to maintain an airway when there is obstruction or paralysis in the respiratory structures above it and for long-term ventilation.

Mechanical ventilation is a process by which gases are moved into and out of the lungs via a device that is set to meet the respiratory requirements of the patient. It requires that a tracheostomy tube or endotracheal tube be attached to the mechanical device (respirator, ventilator). It can augment or replace the patient's own ventilatory efforts.

S = Suffix   P = Prefix   R = Root   R/CF = Combining Form

WORD	PRONUNCIATION	ELEMENTS		DEFINITION
bronchoscope	**BRONG**-koh-skope	S/	**-scope** *instrument for viewing*	Endoscope used for bronchoscopy
bronchoscopy	brong-**KOS**-koh-pee	R/CF S/	**bronch/o-** *bronchus* **-scopy** *to examine*	Examination of the interior of the tracheobronchial tree with an endoscope
endotracheal	en-doh-**TRAY**-kee-al	S/ P/ R/	**-al** *pertaining to* **endo-** *inside* **-trache-** *trachea*	Pertaining to being inside the trachea
lobectomy	loh-**BEK**-toh-mee	S/ R/	**-ectomy** *surgical excision* **lob-** *lobe*	Surgical removal of a lobe of the lungs
mediastinoscopy	**MEE**-dee-ass-tih-**NOS**-koh-pee	S/ P/ R/CF	**-scopy** *to examine* **media-** *middle* **stin/o-** *partition*	Examination of the mediastinum using an endoscope
pneumonectomy	**NEW**-moh-**NEK**-toh-mee	S/ R/	**-ectomy** *surgical excision* **pneumon-** *lung, air*	Surgical removal of a lung
resection	ree-**SEK**-shun	S/ P/ R/	**-ion** *action* **re-** *back* **-sect-** *cut off*	Removal of a specific part of an organ or structure
resect (verb)	ree-**SEKT**			
segmentectomy	seg-men-**TEK**-toh-mee	S/ R/	**-ectomy** *surgical excision* **segment-** *a section*	Surgical excision of a segment of a tissue or organ
thoracentesis pleural tap (syn)	**THOR**-ah-sen-**TEE**-sis	S/ R/	**-centesis** *to puncture* **thora-** *chest*	Insertion of a needle into the pleural cavity to withdraw fluid or air
thoracotomy	thor-ah-**KOT**-oh-mee	S/ R/CF	**-tomy** *surgical incision* **thorac/o-** *chest*	Incision through the chest wall
tomography	toh-**MOG**-rah-fee	S/ R/CF	**-graphy** *process of recording* **tom/o-** *section*	Radiographic image of a selected slice or section of tissue
tracheostomy	tray-kee-**OST**-oh-mee	S/ R/CF	**-stomy** *new opening* **trache/o-** *trachea*	Surgical opening into the windpipe, through which a tube can be inserted to assist breathing
tracheotomy	tray-kee-**OT**-oh-mee	S/	**-tomy** *surgical incision*	Incision made into the trachea to create a tracheostomy
ultrasonography	**UL**-trah-soh-**NOG**-rah-fee	S/ P/ R/CF	**-graphy** *process of recording* **ultra-** *beyond* **-son/o-** *sound*	Delineation of deep structures using sound waves

Exercises

A. Put the following elements into the right combinations to form medical terms for the definitions provided. *Some elements you will use more than once; some elements you will not use at all. Fill in the blanks.* **LO 13.16, 13.17, 13.C**

endo-	-ectomy	trans-	bronch/o-	-trache/o-	-ion
lob-	-al	-ator	pharyng/e-	pneumon-	immuniz-
-ation	-son/o-	-tomy	-trache-	in-	-scopy
-sect-	ultra-	re-	thorac/o-	-stomy	ventil-
-graphy	-ic	-stomy	hyper-	tom/o	

1. Surgical removal of a lung _____

2. Examination of a bronchus _____

3. Radiographic image of a selected slice of tissue _____

4. Image of deep structures using sound waves _____

5. Pertaining to being inside the trachea _____

6. Removal of a specific part of an organ _____

7. Incision through the chest wall _____

8. New opening in the neck to the trachea _____

Abbreviations

COPD	chronic obstructive pulmonary disease
DPI	dry powder inhaler
LABA	long-acting $\beta 2$-receptor agonist
MDI	metered dose inhaler
SABA	short-acting $\beta 2$-receptor agonist

LO 13.18 Respiratory Drugs

Bronchodilators dilate the bronchi and bronchioles by altering smooth muscle tone. This decreases resistance in the airway, increases airflow to the lungs, and increases the forced expiratory volume in one second (FEV_1). Three types of bronchodilators are in clinical use:

- **$\beta 2$-receptor agonists** can be **short acting** (**SABAs**) to provide quick, temporary relief of bronchoconstriction (e.g., for asthma) or long acting for up to 12 hours to control and prevent bronchoconstriction (e.g., for **COPD**). Short-acting $\beta 2$ receptor agonists include **albuterol** (salbutamol, *Proventil,* or *Ventolin*), available as an **aerosol inhaler,** tablet, or IV or IM applications. **Long-acting $\beta 2$-receptor agonists** (**LABAs**) include **salmeterol** (*Serevent*), a powder **inhaler** that provides maintenance and prevention of COPD symptoms for up to 12 hours, and **formoterol** (*Foradil, Performist*), a dry powder inhaler (**DPI**) or **inhalation** solution that controls symptoms of COPD and asthma for up to 12 hours.

- **Anticholinergics** act as bronchodilators to improve lung function and the quality of life for COPD patients. **Ipratropium bromide** (*Atrovent*) opens up the medium and large airways by causing smooth muscles to relax. It is administered by inhalation through an **inhaler** or **nebulizer**. Its effect begins within 30 minutes and lasts three or four hours. **Tiotropium** (*Spiriva*) is a dry powder inhalation formulated for once-daily dosing providing 24-hour bronchodilation.

Glucocorticosteroids reduce airway inflammation in asthma, providing improvement in symptoms. These medications can be inhaled into the nose to decrease swelling due to allergies. Oral inhalation is the means by which these medications are inhaled into the lungs to treat conditions such as COPD and asthma. In COPD the response is poor, but is improved when given with a long-acting $\beta 2$-receptor agonist. *Symbicort* and *Advair* are examples of medications that are combinations of LABAs and **glucocorticosteroids.** These formulations are available for oral inhalation into the lungs.

For asthma, the first new drug in 20 years is in the late stages of clinical trials. **Fevipiprant** has significantly decreased the symptoms of asthma, improved lung function, reduced inflammation, and repaired the lining of airways, and should soon be given FDA approval for clinical use.

Expectorants increase the amount of hydration of bronchial secretions and as a byproduct lubricate an irritated respiratory tract. **Guaifenesin** is an expectorant available in many cough syrups, tablets, and caplets.

Decongestants are used to relieve nasal congestion by producing local vasoconstriction. The active ingredient is either **pseudoephedrine** or **phenylephrine.**

Mucolytics break down the chemical structure of mucus molecules so that the mucus becomes thinner and can be removed more easily by coughing. There are several mucolytic agents: **erdosteine** (*Erdostin, Mucotec*), **acetylcysteine** (*Mucomyst, Bronkyl, Fluimucil*), **bromheksin** (*Bisolvon*), and **carbocysteine** (*Mucodyne*).

Aerosol therapy is the administration of a mist to be breathed into the airway. Nasal pumps deliver aerosol to the nasal passages and sinuses. For inhalation into the lungs, aerosol can be delivered via DPI, MDI, or nebulizer. A DPI allows for the patient to inhale a dry medicated powder into the lungs. An MDI delivers a premeasured puff of medicated mist for oral inhalation. A nebulizer creates an aerosol mist via compressed air. The mist may contain medication or can be composed of sterile water, which can be administered to soothe the upper airway, as in the treatment of croup.

Oxygen is used in hypoxia and can be given by nasal **cannula** or by mask. Patients with severe COPD can be attached to a portable oxygen cylinder.

WORD	PRONUNCIATION		ELEMENTS	DEFINITION
aerosol	**AIR**-oh-sol	S/ R/CF	**-sol** solution **aer/o** air	Stable liquid suspension intended for use by inhalation
agonist	**AG**-on-ist		Greek contest	Agent that combines with receptors on cells to initiate drug actions
anticholinergic	**AN**-tee-kohl-ih-**NER**-jik	S/ P/ R/ R/	**-ic** pertaining to **anti-** against **-cholin-** choline **-erg-** work	Antagonistic to the action of parasympathetic nerve fibers
cannula cannulae (pl)	**KAN**-you-lah **KAN**-you-lee			Latin reed Tube inserted into a cavity or blood vessel as a channel for fluid or gases
decongestant	dee-con-**JESS**-tant	S/ P/ R/	**-ant** pertaining to **de-** take away **-congest-** accumulation of fluid	Agent that reduces the swelling and fluid in the nose and sinuses
glucocorticosteroid	**GLU**-koh- **KOR**-tih-koh-**STER**-oyd	S/ R/CF R/CF R/	**-oid** resemble **gluc/o** sugar **-cortic/o** cortex **-ster-** solid	Hormone of the adrenal cortex that influences glycogen metabolism and exerts an anti-inflammatory effect
inhalation	in-hah-**LAY**-shun	S/ P/ R/	**-ation** process **in-** in **-hal-** breathe	The act of breathing in—inspiration
inhaler	in-**HALE**-er	S/	**-er** agent	Instrument for delivering medication by inhalation
mucolytic	**MYU**-koh-**LIT**-ik	S/ R/CF R/	**-ic** pertaining to **muc/o** mucus **-lyt-** dissolve	Agent capable of dissolving or liquefying mucus
nebulizer	**NEB**-you-lize-er	S/ R/	**-izer** line of action **nebul-** cloud	Device used to deliver liquid medicine in a fine mist for inhalation

Exercises

A. Medications used in the treatment of respiratory diseases have different mechanisms of action. *Respiratory medications act by increasing the internal size of the airway or by helping to clear mucus from the body. Identify the mechanism of action of the following medications. Some questions have more than one correct answer as indicated. Answers can be used more than once.* **LO 13.18**

decongestant   anticholinergic   β **agonist**   mucolytic   glucocorticoid

1. Thins the mucus. _____

2. Relaxes bronchial smooth muscles. (choose 2 answers) _____

3. Reduces swelling in the upper and lower airways. _____

4. Used to treat swelling in the nose and sinuses. (choose 2 answers) _____

B. Identify the devices that deliver medications to the respiratory airways. *Match the devices on the left with their correct description on the right.* **LO 13.18, 13.F**

1. nasal pump

2. MDI

3. nebulizer

4. DPI

a. delivers mist via compressed air

b. creates a dry powder for inhalation

c. generates a premeasured puff of wet aerosol for oral inhalation

d. used to administer aerosol to the nasal airways and sinuses

©2014 Nucleus Medical Media

Respiratory System
Challenge Your Knowledge

A. Plurals. Refresh your memory for the rules of plurals with this exercise. Fill in the chart with the plural. **(LO 13.A)**

Medical Term	Plural
1. alveolus	
2. cilium	
3. bronchus	
4. concha	
5. naris	

B. Spelling. The following terms come directly from Latin and Greek. Choose the correct spelling based on the definition following the numbers. Select the best answer. **(LO 13.A)**

1. reed   **a.** cannula   **b.** canula   **c.** canulla

2. passage   **a.** miatus   **b.** meatis   **c.** meatus

3. shell   **a.** conca   **b.** conka   **c.** concha

4. branding iron   **a.** cautiry   **b.** cautery   **c.** cautary

5. lack of breath   **a.** apenea   **b.** apnea   **c.** apnia

6. throat   **a.** pharynix   **b.** parynix   **c.** pharynx

7. ring   **a.** cricoid   **b.** crickoid   **c.** crecoid

8. creaking sound   **a.** strideor   **b.** stridore   **c.** stridor

9. oblong shield   **a.** thyrhoid   **b.** thiroyd   **c.** thyroid

10. nerves enter and leave this area   **a.** hylum   **b.** hilum   **c.** hylim

C. Pharmacology. For any body system, it is important to know the various types of medications and when they might be prescribed. Demonstrate your knowledge of pharmacology for the respiratory system by assigning the correct drug category in the right column to the statements in the left column. *Answers may be used more than once.* The first one has been done for you. **(LO 13.18)**

__d__	1. Example: penicillin	**a.** bronchodilators
_____	2. Relax smooth muscles of the bronchioles	**b.** anti-inflammatories
_____	3. Corticosteroids	**c.** mucolytics
_____	4. Used in hypoxia	**d.** antibiotics
_____	5. Used when a bacterial infection is present	**e.** O_2
_____	6. Best given by inhalation	
_____	7. Administered by nasal cannula	
_____	8. Breaks up mucus	

D. **Interpretation.** Use your knowledge of the **language of pulmonology** to understand the Case Report and answer the following questions. **(LO 13.14, 13.17, 13.A, 13.E, 13.F)**

 Case Report 13.1

You are

. . . an advanced-level RRT working in the Acute Respiratory Care Unit of Fulwood Medical Center with pulmonologist Tavis Senko, MD.

Your patient is

. . . Mr. Jude Jacobs, a 68-year-old white retired mail carrier, who is known to have COPD and is on continual oxygen by nasal prongs. He has smoked two packs a day for his adult life. Last night, he was unable to sleep because of increased shortness of breath and cough. His cough produced yellow sputum. He had to sit upright in bed to be able to breathe.

VS are T 101.6°F, P 98, R 36, BP 150/90. On examination, he is cyanotic and frightened and has nasal prongs in his nose. Air entry is diminished in both lungs, and there are crackles at both bases. You have been ordered to draw blood for ABGs and to measure the amount of air entering and leaving his lungs by using spirometry.

1. What is your profession?

   a. nurse

   b. physical therapist

   c. physician

   d. respiratory therapist

2. What is another name for nasal "prongs"?

   a. cannula

   b. ventilator

   c. respirator

   d. intubation

3. The medical term for "shortness of breath" is

   a. tachypnea

   b. apnea

   c. dyspnea

   d. eupnea

4. The yellow sputum is indicative of

   a. asthma

   b. bacterial infection

   c. atelectasis

   d. pleurisy

5. Cyanosis may indicate

   a. decreased oxygen in the blood

   b. he has a barrel chest

   c. increased heart rate

   d. increased carbon dioxide in the blood

6. An ABG comes from

   a. pleural fluid

   b. exhaled air

   c. arterial blood

   d. sputum analysis

Respiratory System

E. **Language of pulmonology.** You are a new student in the Respiratory Therapy program. The following questions contain terminology you will use every day on the job. Select the answer that correctly completes each statement. **(LO 13.2, 13.13, 13.14, 13.17)**

1. **Cyanosis** signals deficient oxygenation of blood and will turn nail beds

   a. yellow

   b. red

   c. black

   d. white

   e. blue

2. A shell-shaped bone in the nose is the

   a. meatus

   b. concha

   c. nares

   d. vestibule

   e. choana

3. Which of the following medical terms can be associated with mucopurulent discharge?

   a. pleurisy

   b. sinusitis

   c. epistaxis

   d. pneumonia

   e. nasal polyps

4. A segment of the chest wall separates from the rest of the thoracic cage in

   a. pneumoconiosis

   b. epiglottitis

   c. flail chest

   d. thoracentesis

   e. ARF

5. Surgical repair of the nose is

   a. rhinoplasty

   b. thoracentesis

   c. tracheostomy

   d. lobectomy

F. **Construct terms.** The suffix -itis is one that you will meet over and over again in this book. Build the correct medical term to match its definition. Fill in the blanks. **(LO 13.5, 13.7, 13.15, 13.C)**

1. inflammation of the bronchus _____itis

2. inflammation of the organ of voice production _____itis

3. inflammation of the tonsils _____itis

4. inflammation of the throat _____itis

5. inflammation of the nose _____itis

6. inflammation of the epiglottis _____itis

7. croup _____itis

8. inflammation of the small bronchioles _____itis

9. inflammation of the lung parenchyma _____itis

G. Analyze. Knowledge of medical terms includes choosing the correct term for the meaning you want to convey either verbally or in documentation. Analyze the suffixes to help you choose the term. Use the following medical terms to fill in the statements, all relating to the bronchus. Fill in the blanks. **(LO 13.9, 13.15, 13.16, 13.17, 13.18)**

bronchogenic	bronchi	bronchopneumonia	bronchioles	bronchiolitis
bronchus	bronchial asthma	bronchial	bronchitis	bronchiectasis

1. Greek word for *windpipe:* _____

2. Plural of the word bronchus: _____

3. Pertaining to the windpipe: _____

4. Tertiary bronchi divide into these: _____

5. Inflammation of the bronchus: _____

6. Abnormal dilation of bronchioles due to repeated infections: _____

7. Infection in the bronchioles that usually spreads to the alveoli: _____

8. Inflammation of the bronchioles: _____

9. Recurrent acute episodes of bronchial obstruction due to constriction: _____

10. Arising from a bronchus: _____

Now, using the word elements that follow, build new terms relating to the bronchus. Your root or combining form will still be bronch/o-.

malacia	stenosis	plasty
scope	pathy	pulmonary
dilation	scopy	dilator
		gram

> **Study Hint**
>
> In the term **bronchopneumonia**, the combining form is used, and it is one word. In the term **bronchial asthma**, the suffix -*al* makes it an adjective, and the two words are separated.

11. An instrument used to see into the bronchus: _____

12. Drug meant to open bronchial passages: _____

13. A softening or deficiency in the wall of a bronchus: _____

14. Surgical procedure for plastic repair on a bronchus: _____

15. Any disease of a bronchus: _____

16. Pertaining to the bronchus and the lung: _____

17. Widening the area of the bronchus: _____

18. The procedure of looking into the bronchus: _____

19. Constriction or narrowing of the bronchus: _____

20. The record obtained by bronchography: _____

Respiratory System

H. **Deconstruct the following terms, and then answer the following questions.** (LO 13.14, 13.15, 13.D)

Medical Term	Prefix	Root/Combining Form	Suffix
empyema	1.	2.	3.
mesothelioma	4.	5.	6.
expectorate	7.	8.	9.

Choose the correct preceding terms to complete the following sentences. Use the terms that you deconstructed above.

10. Cancer arising from the cells lining the pleura _____.

11. Pleural effusion containing pus is also termed _____.

12. To cough up and spit out mucus _____.

I. **Trace the pathway.** The tracheobronchial tree begins with the trachea, which starts air on its pathway all the way down to the alveoli, where gas exchange can occur. Trace this path by sequentially lettering the following choices A through H. (LO 13.8, 13.11)

1. Each secondary bronchus divides into tertiary bronchi. _____

2. Terminal bronchioles divide into several alveoli. _____

3. Bronchi enter the lung at the hilum. _____

4. Bronchioles divide into terminal bronchioles. _____

5. Main bronchi divide into a secondary bronchus for each lobe. _____

6. Tertiary bronchi divide into bronchioles. _____

7. At the carina, the trachea divides into right and left main bronchi. _____

8. The trachea starts air on the pathway to the alveoli _____

J. **Test-taking skills.** Employ your test-taking skills when you answer multiple-choice questions. Start by reading the question and ALL the answers. Immediately eliminate answers you know to be incorrect. With the choices you have left, one answer will clearly be the *best* choice. Select the answer that correctly completes the statement or answers the question. **(LO 13.2, 13.9, 13.16)**

1. The hairlike structures in the nasal cavity are called

    a. polyps

    b. cilia

    c. adenoids

    d. bullae

    e. trachealis

2. What is the total number of lobes in *both* lungs?

    a. 4

    b. 5

    c. 6

    d. 2

    e. 3

3. What exactly is a lobe?

    a. an opening into an organ

    b. an exit from an organ

    c. a subdivision of an organ

    d. a blood reservoir in an organ

    e. a pathway through an organ

4. An instrument used to measure breathing volume is called

    a. bronchoscope

    b. spirometer

    c. endoscope

    d. tenometer

    e. sphygmomanometer

5. What is surfactant?

    a. creates surface tension

    b. a mucous membrane

    c. keeps a muscle from collapsing

    d. a subcutaneous lesion

    e. a place where two bones meet to make a joint

Respiratory System

K. **Use your knowledge of the language of respiration to answer the following questions.** Select the answer that correctly completes the statement or answers the question. **(LO 13.1, 13.2, 13.3, 13.7, 13.15, 13.16)**

1. The measure of the capacity of a chamber or hollow viscus to expand is called

   a. expectorate

   b. idiopathic

   c. compliance

   d. postural drainage

   e. consolidation

2. Which of the following is another name for the nasal **conchae** on the lateral wall of each nasal cavity?

   a. meatus

   b. choana

   c. nares

   d. turbinates

   e. septum

3. A bubblelike structure is called a

   a. bronchiole

   b. barbiturate

   c. bulla

   d. bronchus

   e. bradypnea

4. The sense of smell is

   a. external respiration

   b. aspiration

   c. internal respiration

   d. exhalation

   e. olfaction

5. Which of the following is another term for heart failure?

   a. cyanosis

   b. conchae

   c. choana

   d. cor pulmonale

   e. chordae tendinae

6. Laryngeal polyps are

   a. benign tumors of the larynx

   b. localized infection of the larynx

   c. papillomas

   d. malignant tumors of the trachea

   e. verucca in the larynx

7. The medical term for the nostrils is

   a. nares

   b. adenoids

   c. polyps

   d. tonsils

   e. papillomas

L. **Define abbreviations that relate to the respiratory system.** Match the definition in the first column to the correct abbreviation in the second column (**LO 13.F**)

Disease

_____ 1. common cold

_____ 2. dyspnea

_____ 3. CAO is also called

_____ 4. condition is inherited

_____ 5. sudden, life-threatening lung failure

Abbreviation

a. COPD

b. CF

c. SOB

d. ARF

e. URI

M. **Diagnostic and therapeutic procedures are performed for different reasons.** Use the language of pulmonology to identify their medical terminology. Select letter **a** if the term is a diagnostic procedure; letter **b** if the term is a therapeutic procedure. (**LO 13.16, 13.17, 13.F**)

1. intubation

   a. diagnostic

   b. therapeutic

2. PDT

   a. diagnostic

   b. therapeutic

3. tracheotomy

   a. diagnostic

   b. therapeutic

4. CXR

   a. diagnostic

   b. therapeutic

5. mediastinoscopy

   a. diagnostic

   b. therapeutic

6. CT

   a. diagnostic

   b. therapeutic

7. bronchoscopy

   a. diagnostic

   b. therapeutic

©2014 Nucleus Medical Media

The health professionals involved in the diagnosis and treatment of problems of the **skeletal** system include:

- **Orthopedic surgeons (orthopedists),** medical doctors (**MDs**) who deal with the prevention, correction, disorders, and injuries of the skeletal system.

- **Osteopathic physicians,** who have earned a doctorate in **osteopathy** (**DO**) and receive additional training in the skeletal system and how it affects the whole body.

- **Physiatrists,** who are physicians specializing in physical medicine and rehabilitation.

- **Chiropractors (DCs),** who focus on the manual adjustments of joints—particularly the spine—to maintain and restore health.

- **Physical therapists,** who evaluate and treat pain, disease, or injury by physical therapeutic measures as opposed to medical and surgical measures.

- **Physical therapist assistants,** who work under the direction of a physical therapist to assist patients with their physical therapy.

- **Orthopedic technologists** and **technicians,** who assist orthopedic surgeons in treating patients.

- **Podiatrists,** who are practitioners in the diagnosis and treatment of disorders and injuries of the foot.

- **Orthotists,** who make and fit orthopedic appliances (**orthotics**).

Chapter Learning Outcomes

This chapter will review the whole musculoskeletal system and will enable you to:

LO 14.1 Identify the components of the skeletal system and the functions of the bones.

LO 14.2 Discuss the growth and structure of bones.

LO 14.3 Describe diseases of bones.

LO 14.4 Explain the different types of bone fractures and their healing process.

LO 14.5 Describe the components of joints and classify joints based on the amount of movement they allow.

LO 14.6 Differentiate the movements of joints.

LO 14.7 Explain the diseases of joints.

LO 14.8 Identify the components and functions of the axial skeleton.

LO 14.9 Identify the components of the vertebral column.

LO 14.10 Describe common disorders of the vertebral column.

LO 14.11 Describe the skull and facial skeleton.

LO 14.12 Relate the structure of the shoulder girdle to its functions.

LO 14.13 Explain common disorders of the shoulder joint.

LO 14.14 Identify the components of the upper arm and elbow joint.

LO 14.15 Describe common disorders of the elbow joint.

LO 14.16 Explain the structure of the forearm and wrist.

LO 14.17 Discuss common disorders of the wrist.

LO 14.18 Relate the structure of the hand to its functions.

LO 14.19 Describe disorders of the hand.

LO 14.20 Relate the structure of the pelvic girdle to its functions.

LO 14.21 Explain disorders of the pelvic girdle.

LO 14.22 Identify the bones and joints of the hip and thigh.

LO 14.23 Describe disorders of the hip joint.

LO 14.24 Discuss the bones and joints of the knee and thigh.

LO 14.25 Understand disorders of the knee joint.

LO 14.26 Describe the bones and joints of the lower leg, ankle, and foot.

LO 14.27 Explain disorders of the ankle and foot.

LO 14.28 Discuss diagnostic procedures for disorders of the skeletal system.

LO 14.29 Explain therapeutic procedures for disorders of the skeletal system.

LO 14.30 Describe pharmacologic agents used in the treatment of disorders of the musculoskeletal system.

LO 14.A Use the medical terms of the skeletal system to communicate in writing and document accurately and precisely in any health care setting.

LO 14.B Use the medical terms of the skeletal system to communicate verbally with accuracy and precision in any health care setting.

LO 14.C Using word elements, construct medical terms associated with the skeletal system.

LO 14.D Deconstruct medical terms into their word elements (roots, combining forms, prefixes, and suffixes).

LO 14.E Identify health professionals involved in the care of patients with skeletal disorders.

LO 14.F Identify abbreviations as they relate to the words they abbreviate and use them in context to medical care.

 ## Case Report (CR) 14.1

You are

... an **orthopedic technologist** working with Kevin Stannard, MD, an **orthopedist** in the Fulwood Medical Group.

Your patient is

... Mrs. Amy Vargas, a 70-year-old housewife, who tripped going down the front steps from her house. She has severe pain in her right hip and is unable to stand. An x-ray shows a hip fracture and marked **osteoporosis**. Dr. Stannard examined her in the Emergency Department and has admitted her for a hip replacement.

For you to work with Dr. Stannard to give optimal care to Mrs. Vargas and help her and her family understand the significance of her bone disorder and injury, you will need to be familiar with the terminology of bone structure and function and bone disorders.

Lesson 14.1

SKELETAL SYSTEM

Functions of the Skeletal System

LO 14.1 Functions of the Skeletal System

The four components of the skeletal system *(Figure 14.1)* are

1. *Bones*
2. *Cartilage*
3. *Tendons*
4. *Ligaments*

The bones provide the following functions:

- **Support.** The bones of your vertebral column, pelvis, and legs hold up your body. The jawbone supports your teeth. **Cartilage** supports your nose, ears, and ribs. **Tendons** support and attach your muscles to bone. **Ligaments** support and hold your bones together.

- **Protection.** The skull protects your brain. The vertebral column protects your spinal cord. The rib cage protects your heart and lungs.

- **Movement. Muscles** could not function without their attachments to skeletal bones, and muscles are responsible for your movements.

- **Blood formation.** Bone marrow in many bones is the major producer of blood cells, including most of those in your immune system *(see Chapter 12).*

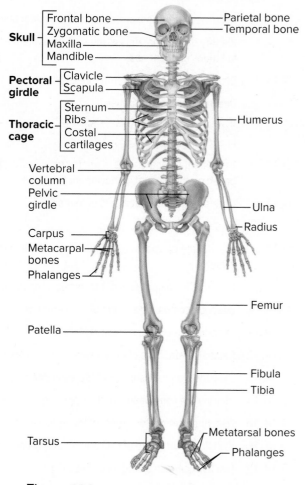

▲ **Figure 14.1** **Adult Skeleton: Anterior View.**

- **Mineral storage and balance.** The skeletal system stores calcium and phosphorus. These are released when your body needs them for other purposes. For example, calcium is needed for muscle contraction, communication between neurons *(see Chapter 9),* and blood clotting *(see Chapter 11).*

- **Detoxification.** Bones remove metals such as lead and radium from your blood, store them, and slowly release them for excretion.

Lesson Objectives

If you didn't have a skeleton, you'd be like a rag doll, shapeless and unable to move. Your skeleton provides support, protects many organ systems, and is the landmark for much of medical terminology. For example, the radial artery you use for taking a pulse is so named because it travels beside the radial bone of the forearm.

In addition, the surface anatomy of bones and their markings enable you to describe and document the sites of symptoms, signs, and clinical, diagnostic, and therapeutic procedures.

The information in this lesson will enable you to use correct medical terminology to:

14.1.1 Recognize the different health professionals involved in the diagnosis and treatment of skeletal problems.

14.1.2 Identify the tissues that form the skeletal system.

14.1.3 Discuss the structures and functions of the skeletal system.

14.1.4 Explain the structure and functions of bones.

14.1.5 Describe the major problems and diseases that oocur in the skeletal system.

Abbreviations

DC	doctor of chiropractic
DO	doctor of osteopathy
MD	doctor of medicine

Keynote

Bones are divided into four classes based on their shape: long, short, flat, and irregular.

WORD	PRONUNCIATION		ELEMENTS	DEFINITION
cartilage	**KAR**-tih-lij		Latin *gristle*	Nonvascular, firm connective tissue found mostly in joints
chiropractic	kie-roh-**PRAK**-tik	S/ R/CF R/	-ic *pertaining to* chir/o- *hand* -pract- *efficient*	Diagnosis, treatment, and prevention of mechanical disorders of the musculoskeletal system
chiropractor	kie-roh-**PRAK**-tor	S/	-or *a doer*	Practitioner of chiropractic
detoxification	dee-**TOKS**-ih-fih-**KAY**-shun	S/ P/ R/CF	-fication *remove* de- *from, out of* tox/i- *poison*	Removal of poison from a tissue or substance
ligament	**LIG**-ah-ment		Latin *band, sheet*	Band of fibrous tissue connecting two structures
muscle musculoskeletal	**MUSS**-el **MUSS**-kyu-loh-**SKEL**-eh-tal	S/ R/CF R/	Latin *muscle* -al *pertaining to* muscul/o- *muscle* -skelet- *skeleton*	Tissue consisting of contractile cells Pertaining to the muscles and the bony skeleton
orthopedic (also spelled orthopaedic) orthopedist	or-thoh-**PEE**-dik or-thoh-**PEE**-dist	S/ R/CF R/ S/	-ic *pertaining to* orth/o- *straight* -ped- *child* -ist *specialist*	Pertaining to the correction and cure of deformities and diseases of the musculoskeletal system; originally, most of the deformities treated were in children Specialist in orthopedics
osteopath osteopathy	**OS**-tee-oh-path **OS**-tee-**OP**-ah-thee	R/ R/CF S/	-path *disease* oste/o- *bone* -pathy *disease*	Practitioner of osteopathy Medical practice based on maintaining the structural integrity of the musculoskeletal system
tendon	**TEN**-dun		Latin *sinew*	Fibrous band that connects muscle to bone

Exercises

A. Identify the components of the skeletal system and the functions of the bones. *Choose the correct organ or tissue being described.* **LO 14.1**

1. Band of strong tissue that connects two structures (such as bone to bone).

   a. muscle   **b.** ligament   **c.** tendon   **d.** cartilage

2. Tissue containing contractile cells.

   a. muscle   **b.** ligament   **c.** tendon   **d.** cartilage

3. Firm connective tissue found mostly in joints.

   a. muscle   **b.** ligament   **c.** tendon   **d.** cartilage

4. Fibrous band that connects muscle to bone.

   a. muscle   **b.** ligament   **c.** tendon   **d.** cartilage

B. Identify the professionals related to the skeletal system. *Many professionals specialize in different aspects of the care of the skeletal system. It is important to understand their specialty. Refer to the Introduction section of this chapter to assist you in matching the specialty in the first column with its correct description in the second column.* **LO 14.A, 14.E**

Term	Meaning
_____ **1.** orthopedist	**a.** treats pain by physical therapeutic measures.
_____ **2.** chiropractor	**b.** treats mechanical disorders of the musculoskeletal system.
_____ **3.** podiatrist	**c.** makes and fits orthopedic devices
_____ **4.** physical therapist	**d.** specialist in the treatment of the skeletal system
_____ **5.** orthotist	**e.** specialist in the treatment of disorders and injuries of the feet

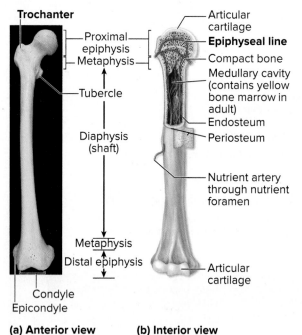

Trochanter

Proximal epiphysis
Metaphysis
Tubercle
Diaphysis (shaft)
Metaphysis
Distal epiphysis
Condyle
Epicondyle

Articular cartilage
Epiphyseal line
Compact bone
Medullary cavity (contains yellow bone marrow in adult)
Endosteum
Periosteum
Nutrient artery through nutrient foramen
Articular cartilage

(a) Anterior view   **(b) Interior view**

▲ **Figure 14.2** Femur: Long Bone of the Thigh.

(a) ©McGraw-Hill Education/Christine Eckel, photographer.

LO 14.2 Bone Growth and Structure

Bone Growth

Factors that affect bone growth include:

1. **Genes.** Genes determine the size and shape of bones and the ultimate adult height.

2. **Nutrition.** Calcium and phosphorus are needed to develop good bone density.

3. **Exercise.** Exercise increases bone density and total bone mass.

4. **Mineral deposition.** Calcium and phosphate are taken from plasma and deposited in bone.

5. **Mineral resorption.** Calcium and phosphate are released from bone back into the plasma when they are needed elsewhere. For example, calcium is needed for muscle contraction, communication between neurons, and blood clotting. Phosphate is a component of deoxyribonucleic acid (DNA) and ribonucleic acid (RNA).

6. **Vitamins.** Vitamin A activates **osteoblasts**; vitamin C is essential for collagen synthesis; vitamin D stimulates absorption of calcium and phosphate, its transport, and its deposition into bones.

7. **Hormones.** For example, growth hormone stimulates the epiphyseal plate to calcify, and estrogen and testosterone accelerate bone growth after puberty and maintain bone density *(see Chapter 17)*.

Structure of Bones

Long bones are the most common type of bone in the body *(Figure 14.2a)*.

The shaft of a long bone is called the **diaphysis**. Each end of the bone is called the **epiphysis** and is expanded to provide extra surface area for the attachment of ligaments and tendons.

Sandwiched between the diaphysis and epiphysis is a thin area called the **metaphysis**. Thin layers of cartilage cells in the **epiphyseal plate** enable the diaphysis (bone shaft) to grow in length. When growth stops, compact bone grows into the epiphyseal plate and forms the **epiphyseal line** *(Figure 14.2b)*.

A tough connective tissue sheath called **periosteum** covers the outer surface of all bones and is attached to the compact or **cortical** bone by tough collagen fibers. The periosteum protects the bone and anchors blood vessels and nerves to the surface of the bone.

The hollow cylinder inside the diaphysis is called the **medullary cavity**. It contains bone **marrow** and is lined by a thin membrane called the **endosteum**. The marrow is a fatty tissue that contains blood cells in different stages of development *(see Chapter 11)*.

The endosteum and periosteum contain **osteoblasts**, cells that produce the matrix of new bone tissue. This process is called **osteogenesis**. Bone **matrix** consists of cells, collagen fibers, a gel that supports and suspends the fibers, and calcium phosphate crystals that give bone its hardness.

When osteoblasts are incorporated into the new bone, they become **osteocytes**. These cells, which maintain the matrix, reside in small spaces in the matrix called **lacunae**.

Osteoclasts are produced by the bone marrow. They dissolve calcium, phosphorus, and the organic components of the bone matrix. There is a continual balancing act going on as osteoclasts remove matrix and osteoblasts produce matrix. If osteoclasts outperform the osteoblasts, then **osteoporosis** occurs, as with Mrs. Vargas.

All bones are well supplied with blood *(Figure 14.3)*. The blood vessels travel through the bone in a system of small **central (haversian) canals**. Because of its good blood supply, bone heals.

Nerve
Vein   Artery
Osteocyte
Haversian canal
Bone matrix

▲ **Figure 14.3** Blood Supply to Bone.

Keynote

Minerals are deposited in bone when the supply is ample and released when they are needed elsewhere.

WORD	PRONUNCIATION		ELEMENTS	DEFINITION
cortex cortical (adj)	**KOR**-teks **KOR**-tih-kal	S/ R/	Latin *bark* -al *pertaining to* cortic- *cortex*	Outer portion of an organ, such as bone Pertaining to the cortex
diaphysis	die-**AF**-ih-sis		Greek *growing between*	The shaft of a long bone
endosteum	en-**DOSS**-tee-um	S/ P/ R/	-um *tissue, structure* end- *within* -oste- *bone*	A membrane of tissue lining the inner (medullary) cavity of a long bone
epiphysis	eh-**PIF**-ih-sis	P/ R/	epi- *upon, above* -physis *growth*	Expanded area at the proximal and distal ends of a long bone that provides increased surface area for attachment of ligaments and tendons
epiphyseal plate	eh-pih-**FIZ**-ee-al PLATE	S/ R/	-eal *pertaining to* -phys- *growth* plate Greek *broad, flat*	Layer of cartilage between epiphysis and metaphysis where bone growth occurs
haversian canals (also called **central canals**)	hah-**VER**-shan ka-**NALS**		Clopton Havers, 1655–1702, English physician	Vascular canals in bone
lacuna lacunae (pl)	la-**KOO**-nah la-**KOO**-nee		Latin *a pit, lake*	Small space or cavity within the matrix of bone
marrow	**MAH**-roh		Old English *marrow*	Fatty, blood-forming tissue in the cavities of long bones
matrix	**MAY**-triks		Latin *mother, womb*	Substance that surrounds cells, is manufactured by cells, and holds them together
medulla medullary (adj)	meh-**DULL**-ah **MED**-ul-ah-ree	S/ R/	Latin *marrow* -ary *pertaining to* medulla- *middle*	Central portion of a structure surrounded by cortex Pertaining to the medulla
metaphysis	meh-**TAF**-ih-sis	P/ R/	meta- *beyond, after, subsequent to* -physis *growth*	Region between the diaphysis and the epiphysis where bone growth occurs
osteoblast	**OS**-tee-oh-blast	S/ R/CF	-blast *germ cell* oste/o- *bone*	Bone-forming cell
osteoclast	**OS**-tee-oh-klast	S/ R/CF	-clast *break down* oste/o- *bone*	Bone-removing cell
osteocyte	**OS**-tee-oh-site	S/ R/CF	-cyte *cell* oste/o- *bone*	Bone-maintaining cell
osteogenesis osteogenic (adj)	**OS**-tee-oh-**JEN**-eh-sis **OS**-tee-oh-**JEN**-ik	S/ R/CF S/	-genesis *creation* oste/o- *bone* -genic *producing*	Creation of new bone Relating to the creation of new bone
osteoporosis	**OS**-tee-oh-poh-**ROH**-sis	S/ R/CF R/	-osis *condition* oste/o- *bone* -por- *opening*	Condition in which the bones become more porous, brittle, and fragile, and are more likely to fracture
periosteum periosteal (adj)	**PER**-ee-**OSS**-tee-um **PER**-ee-**OSS**-tee-al	S/ P/ R/ S/	-um *tissue, structure* peri- *around* -oste- *bone* -al *pertaining to*	Strong membrane surrounding a bone Pertaining to the periosteum

Exercises

A. The combining form oste/o means "bone" and is the main element in each of the following terms. *You choose the correct suffix to complete the term. Fill in the blanks.* **LO 14.1, 14.2, 14.C**

blast   cyte   genesis   clast   genic   porosis

The osteo_____ process begins with osteo_____, which produce the matrix of new bone tissue. Osteo_____ has begun. Once these cells incorporate into new bone, they are termed osteo_____. These cells maintain matrix. Osteo_____ are produced by bone marrow. A delicate balance must be maintained between cells that remove matrix and cells that produce matrix. If more matrix is removed than produced, osteo_____ will result.

Case Report (CR) 14.1 *(continued)*

On questioning, Mrs. Vargas demonstrated many of the risk factors for osteoporosis, including a family history, lack of exercise, cigarette smoking, inadequate diet, postmenopause, and increasing age.

Normal bone   Osteoporotic bone

LM 5×

▲ **Figure 14.4** **Normal Bone and Osteoporotic Bone.** ©Dr. Michael Klein/Getty Images

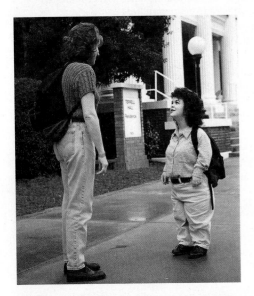

▲ **Figure 14.5** **Achondroplastic Dwarf with College Roommate.** ©McGraw-Hill Education/Joe DeGrandis, photographer.

LO 14.3 Diseases of Bone

Osteoporosis results from a loss of bone density *(Figure 14.4)* when the rate of bone **resorption** exceeds the rate of bone formation. It is more common in women than in men, and its incidence increases with age. Ten million people in the United States already have osteoporosis, and 18 million more have low bone density (**osteopenia**) and are at risk for developing osteoporosis.

In women, production of the hormone estrogen decreases after menopause, and its protection against osteoclast activity is lost. This leads to fragile, brittle bones. In men, reduction in testosterone has a similar but less marked effect.

Osteomyelitis is an inflammation of an area of bone due to bacterial infection, usually with a staphylococcus. Untreated tuberculosis can spread from its original infection in the lungs to bones via the bloodstream to produce tuberculous osteomyelitis.

Osteomalacia, known as **rickets** in children, is a disease caused by vitamin D deficiency. When bones lack calcium, they become soft and flexible. They are not strong enough to bear weight, and become bowed. Osteomalacia occurs in some developing nations and occasionally in this country when children drink soft drinks instead of milk fortified with vitamin D.

Achondroplasia occurs when the long bones stop growing in childhood but the bones of the axial skeleton are not affected *(Figure 14.5)*. This leads to short-stature individuals who are about 4 feet tall. Intelligence and life span are normal. It is caused by a spontaneous gene mutation that then becomes a dominant gene for succeeding generations.

Osteogenic sarcoma is the most common malignant bone tumor. Peak incidence is between 10 and 15 years of age; the tumor often occurs around the knee joint.

Osteogenesis imperfecta is a rare genetic disorder, producing very brittle bones that are easily fractured, often in utero (while inside the uterus).

WORD	PRONUNCIATION	ELEMENTS		DEFINITION
achondroplasia	ay-kon-droh-PLAY-zee-ah	S/ P/ R/CF	-plasia *formation* a- *without* -chondr/o- *cartilage*	Condition with abnormal conversion of cartilage into bone, leading to dwarfism
osteogenesis imperfecta	OS-tee-oh-JEN-eh-sis im-per-FEK-tah	S/ R/CF	-genesis *creation* oste/o- *bone* imperfecta Latin *unfinished*	Inherited condition in which bone formation is incomplete, leading to fragile, easily broken bones
osteomalacia	OS-tee-oh-mah-LAY-shee-ah	S/ R/CF	-malacia *abnormal softness* oste/o- *bone*	Soft, flexible bones lacking in calcium
osteomyelitis	OS-tee-oh-my-eh-LIE-tis	S/ R/CF R/	-itis *inflammation* oste/o- *bone* -myel- *bone marrow*	Inflammation of bone tissue
osteopenia	OS-tee-oh-PEE-nee-ah	S/ R/CF	-penia *deficient* oste/o- *bone*	Decreased calcification of bone
resorption	ree-SORP-shun		Latin *to suck back*	Loss of substance, such as bone
rickets	RIK-ets		Old English *to twist*	Disease in children due to vitamin D deficiency, producing soft, flexible bones
sarcoma	sar-KOH-mah	S/ R/	-oma *tumor, mass* sarc- *flesh*	A malignant tumor originating in connective tissue
osteogenic sarcoma	OS-tee-oh-JEN-ik sar-KOH-mah	S/ R/CF	-genic *creation* oste/o- *bone*	Malignant tumor originating in bone-producing cells

Exercises

A. Bone diseases can strike at any age. *Refer to the text regarding diseases of the bone for the correct terminology to identify each disease. Fill in the blanks.* **LO 14.3**

1. Inflammation of an area of bone, usually due to staph infection _____

2. Bone disease in children caused by vitamin D deficiency _____

3. Leads to short stature (height) _____

4. Rare, genetic disorder causing brittle bones _____

5. Decreased calcification of bone _____

6. Most common malignant bone tumor _____

7. Also known as *rickets* in children _____

8. When bone resorption exceeds bone formation, _____ results.

B. Critical thinking: *Fill in the blanks.* **LO 14.3**

1. What organic element and vitamin are critical in bone health? _____ and vitamin _____ encourage bone health.

▲ **Figure 14.6** Bone Fractures.

▲ **Figure 14.7** Healing of Bone Fracture.

LO 14.4 Bone Fractures

A fracture is a break of a bone and can have a traumatic or pathological reason for occurring. The types of bone fractures are shown in *Figure 14.6* and described in *Table 14.1).*

Healing of Fractures

Uncomplicated fractures take 8 to 12 weeks to heal.

Step 1: When a bone is fractured, blood vessels bleed into the fracture site, forming a **hematoma** *(Figure 14.7a).*

Step 2: A few days after the fracture **(Fx)**, osteoblasts move into the hematoma and start to produce new bone. This is called a **callus** *(Figure 14.7b).*

Step 3: Osteoblasts produce immature, lacy, **cancellous** (spongy) bone that replaces the callus *(Figure 14.7c).*

Step 4: Osteoblasts continue to produce bone cells. They produce compact bone and fuse the bone segments together *(Figure 14.7d).*

Abbreviation	
Fx	fracture

Table 14.1 Classification of Bone Fractures

Name	Description	Reference
Closed	A bone is broken, but the skin is not broken.	*Figure 14.6b, c, d, f, and g*
Open	A fragment of the fractured bone breaks the skin, or a wound extends to the site of the fracture.	*Figure 14.6e*
Displaced	The fractured bone parts are out of alignment.	*Figure 14.6e*
Complete	A bone is broken into at least two fragments.	*Figure 14.6a*
Incomplete	The fracture does not extend completely across the bone; it can be **hairline** (as in a stress fracture in the foot when there is no separation of the two fragments).	*Figure 14.6a*
Comminuted	The bone breaks into several pieces, usually two major pieces and several smaller fragments.	*Figure 14.6b*
Transverse	The fracture is at a right angle to the long axis of the bone.	*Figure 14.6b*
Impacted	One bone fragment is driven into the other, with resulting shortening of a limb.	*Figure 14.6c*
Spiral	The fracture spirals around the long axis of the bone.	*Figure 14.6d*
Oblique	A diagonal fracture runs across the long axis of the bone.	*Figure 14.6d*
Linear	The fracture runs parallel to the long axis of the bone.	*Figure 14.6f*
Greenstick (closed)	This is a partial fracture: one side breaks, the other bends.	*Figure 14.6g*
Pathologic	The fracture occurs in an area of bone weakened by disease (such as cancer). Also called stress fracture.	—
Compression	The fracture occurs in a vertebra from trauma or pathology, leading to the vertebra being crushed.	—

WORD	PRONUNCIATION		ELEMENTS	DEFINITION
callus (Note: Callous is a nonmedical word meaning *insensitive*.)	KAL-us		Latin *hard skin*	The mass of fibrous connective tissue that forms at a fracture site and becomes the foundation for the formation of new bone
cancellous	KAN-sell-us		Latin *lattice*	Bone that has a spongy or lattice-like structure
closed fracture (opposite of open)	KLOHZD **FRAK**-chur	S/ R/	**closed** Latin *intact* -ure *result of* **fract-** *break*	A bone is broken but the skin over it is intact
comminuted fracture	KOM-ih-nyu-ted	S/ R/	-ed *pertaining to* **comminut-** *break into small pieces*	A fracture in which the bone is broken into pieces
complete fracture	kom-**PLEET**		Latin *fill up*	A bone is fractured into two separate pieces
compression fracture	kom-**PRESH**-un	S/ R/	-ion *condition, action* **compress-** *press together*	Fracture of a vertebra causing loss of height of the vertebra
displaced fracture	dis-**PLAYSD**	P/ R/	**dis-** *apart, away from* -placed *in an area*	A fracture in which the fragments are separated and are not in alignment
greenstick fracture	**GREEN**-stik	R/ R/	**green-** *green* -stick *branch, twig*	A fracture in which one side of the bone is partially broken and the other side is bent. Occurs mostly in children
hairline fracture	**HAIR**-line		**hair** Old English *hair* **line** Latin *a mark*	A fracture without separation of the fragments
hematoma	hee-mah-**TOH**-mah	S/ R/	-oma *tumor, mass* **hemat-** *blood*	Collection of blood that has escaped from the blood vessels into tissue
impacted fracture	im-**PAK**-ted	S/ P/ R/	-ed *pertaining to* **im-** *in* -pact- *driven in*	A fracture in which one bone fragment is driven into the other
incomplete fracture	in-kom-**PLEET**	P/ R/	**in-** *not* -complete *fill in*	A fracture that does not extend across the bone, as in a hairline fracture
linear fracture	**LIN**-ee-ar	S/ R/	-ar *pertaining to* **line-** *a mark*	A fracture running parallel to the length of the bone
oblique fracture	ob-**LEEK**		Latin *slanting*	A diagonal fracture across the long axis of the bone
open fracture	**OH**-pen		Old English *not enclosed*	The skin over the fracture is broken
pathologic fracture	path-oh-**LOJ**-ik	S/ R/CF R/	-ic *pertaining to* **path/o-** *disease* -log- *to study*	Fracture occurring at a site already weakened by a disease process, such as cancer. Also called stress fracture
spiral fracture	**SPY**-ral	S/ R/	-al *pertaining to* **spir-** *a coil*	A fracture in the shape of a coil
transverse fracture	trans-**VERS**	P/ R/	**trans-** *across* -verse *travel*	A fracture perpendicular to the long axis of the bone

Exercises

A. Fractures. You are working as the new radiology technician in the Radiology Department at the hospital. *You are attempting to identify the types of fractures with the pictures you see on the film. Match the description of the fracture on the left to its correct fracture on the right. Refer to Table 14.1.* **LO 14.4**

Fracture Seen on the Film

_____ 1. Fracture at a right angle to the long axis of the radius

_____ 2. Femur broken into two clean pieces

_____ 3. Cancer patient with vertebral fracture

_____ 4. Broken ankle but no broken skin

_____ 5. Diagonal fracture across the long axis of the femur

_____ 6. Fractured hand with bone fragments sticking out of the skin

Type of Fracture

a. open fracture

b. oblique fracture

c. closed fracture

d. transverse fracture

e. pathologic fracture

f. displaced fracture

Lesson 14.2

Joints

Lesson Objectives

Without joints you would be a statue. Joints allow you to move, but movable parts that rub together can wear out. Damage or disease in a joint can make movement very difficult and painful. The structure of any joint, or articulation, is directly related to its mobility and function. To understand, describe, and document your patient's joint problems, you need to be able to use correct medical terminology to:

14.2.1 Classify the different types of joints.

14.2.2 Identify the tissues that form the different joints.

14.2.3 Match structures to functions in the different joints.

14.2.4 Describe the major problems and diseases that occur in joints.

Case Report (CR) 14.2

You are

. . . an orthopedic technologist working for orthopedic surgeon Kenneth Stannard, MD, at Fulwood Medical Center.

Your patient is

. . . Mr. Hank Johnson, a 63-year-old white male. Mr. Johnson has been active all his life.

In his youth, Mr. Johnson played football and baseball. As an adult, he has played racquetball weekly and jogged 3 to 4 miles most mornings on the streets of his neighborhood. For the past year, he has had lower-back stiffness and pain, particularly in the mornings. Six months ago, while out hiking, he slid down a mountain on his left side for about 100 feet. He is now having pain in his left groin and thigh, with difficulty walking and climbing stairs.

You are responsible for documenting the doctor's diagnostic procedures and treatment and for making sure that Mr. Johnson understands the significance of the diagnostic findings and the recommendations for his treatment.

LO 14.5 Classes of Joints

Joints are classified structurally into three types:

1. **Fibrous** joints are two bones tightly bound together by bands of fibrous tissue with no joint space. They come in three varieties:

   a. **Sutures** occur between the bones of the skull (*Figure 14.8*); the two opposing bones have interlocking processes to add stability to the joint. The **periosteum** on each of the the outer and inner surfaces of the two bones is continuous and holds the joint together.

   b. **Syndesmosis** is a joining of two bones with fibrous ligaments. Their movement is minimal. An example is the joint above the ankle where the tibia and fibula are attached.

   c. **Gomphoses** are pegs that fit into sockets and are held in place by fine collagen fibers. Examples are the joints between teeth and their sockets.

2. **Cartilaginous** joints join two bones with cartilage:

   a. **Synchondroses** join two bones with **hyaline** cartilage, which allows little or no movement between them, as between your ribs and costal cartilages.

   b. **Symphyses** join two bones with **fibrocartilage**. An example is the symphysis pubis, where your two pubic bones meet at the front of your pelvis.

3. **Synovial** joints contain synovial fluid as a lubricant and allow considerable movement (*Figure 14.9*). Most joints in the legs and arms are synovial joints. The ends of the bones are covered with hyaline **articular** cartilage. In some joints, an additional plate of fibrocartilage is located between the two bones. In the knee, this plate is incomplete and is called a **meniscus**.

A **bursa** is an extension of the synovial joint that forms a cushion between structures that otherwise would rub against each other; for example, in the knee joint between the patellar tendon and the patellar and tibial bones (*Figure 14.9*).

Anterior

Frontal bone
Coronal suture
Parietal bone
Sagittal suture
Lambdoid suture
Occipital bone

Posterior

▲ **Figure 14.8** Sutures of Skull: Superior View.

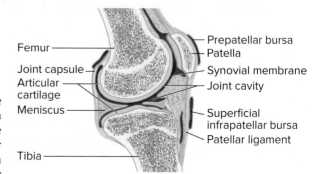

Femur
Joint capsule
Articular cartilage
Meniscus
Tibia

Prepatellar bursa
Patella
Synovial membrane
Joint cavity
Superficial infrapatellar bursa
Patellar ligament

▲ **Figure 14.9** Synovial Joint.

WORD	PRONUNCIATION	ELEMENTS		DEFINITION
articulation	ar-tik-you-**LAY**-shun	S/ R/	-ation *process* articul- *joint*	A joint
articulate (verb) articular (adj)	ar-**TIK**-you-late ar-**TIK**-you-lar	S/ S/	-ate *pertaining to* -ar *pertaining to*	Joint movement Pertaining to a joint
bursa	**BURR**-sah		Latin *purse*	A closed sac containing synovial fluid
fibrocartilage	fie-broh-**KAR**-til-ij	R/CF R/CF	fibr/o- *fiber* -cartilag/e *cartilage*	Cartilage containing collagen fibers
gomphosis gomphoses (pl)	gom-**FOH**-sis gom-**FOH**-sees	S/ R/	-osis *condition* gomph- *bolt, nail*	Joint formed by a peg and socket
hyaline	**HIGH**-ah-line		Greek *glass*	Cartilage that looks like frosted glass and contains fine collagen fibers
meniscus menisci (pl)	meh-**NISS**-kuss meh-**NISS**-kee		Greek *crescent*	Disc of connective tissue cartilage between the bones of a joint; for example, in the knee joint
suture sutures (pl)	**SOO**-chur **SOO**-churs		Latin *a seam*	Place where two bones are joined together by a fibrous band continuous with their periosteum, as in the skull. Also means to unite two surfaces by sewing; the material used in the sewing together; and the seam formed by the sewing together
symphysis symphyses (pl)	**SIM**-feh-sis **SIM**-feh-sees		Greek *growing together*	Two bones joined by fibrocartilage
synchondrosis synchondroses (pl)	sin-kon-**DROH**-sis sin-kon-**DROH**-sees	S/ P/ R/	-osis *condition* syn- *together* -chondr- *cartilage*	A rigid articulation (joint) formed by cartilage
syndesmosis syndesmoses (pl)	sin-dez-**MOH**-sis sin-dez-**MOH**-sees	S/ P/ R/	-osis *condition* syn- *together* desm- *bind*	An articulation (joint) formed by ligaments
synovial	sih-**NOH**-vee-al	S/ P/ R/CF	-al *pertaining to* syn- *together* -ov/i- *egg*	Pertaining to synovial fluid and synovial membrane

Exercises

A. It is important to recognize the singular and plural versions of medical terms. *Identify the word as being singular or plural. Select the correct choice.* **LO 14.5, 14.A**

1. syndesmoses

    a. singular   **b.** plural

2. suture

    a. singular   **b.** plural

3. gomphosis

    a. singular   **b.** plural

4. menisci

    a. singular   **b.** plural

B. Identify the word elements that compose medical terms. *Knowing the meaning of the word elements helps you to quickly define medical terms. Select the answer that correctly completes each sentence.* **LO 14.5, 14.D**

1. The root in the term *synchondroses* means:

    a. egg   **b.** joint   **c.** cartilage   **d.** seam

2. The prefix in the term *synchondroses* means:

    a. condition   **b.** together   **c.** crescent   **d.** pertaining to

3. The root in the term *syndesmoses* means:

    a. pertaining to   **b.** egg   **c.** bind together   **d.** bolt

4. The root in the term *gomphosis* means:

    a. pertaining to   **b.** egg   **c.** bind together   **d.** bolt

▲ **Figure 14.11** Movement of the Limbs. (*a*) Abduction and adduction of the upper limb. (*b*) Abduction and adduction of the fingers. (*c*) Medial and lateral rotation of the arm. (*d*) Circumduction. (*e*) Pronation and supination of the hand. (*f*) Eversion and inversion of the foot. (a-f) ©McGraw-Hill Education/Eric Wise, photographer

Keynotes

- **Circumduction of Joints.** **Circumduction** of the shoulder is moving it in a circular movement so that it forms a cone, with the shoulder joint as the apex of the cone (*Figure 14.11d*).

- **Inversion and Eversion.** When you turn your ankle so that the sole of your foot faces toward the opposite foot, that is supination or **inversion**. When you turn your ankle so that the sole of the foot faces laterally away from the other foot, that is pronation or **eversion** (*Figure 14.11f*).

▲ **Figure 14.10** Joint Flexion and Extension. (*a*) Flexion of the elbow. (*b*) Extension of the elbow. (*c*) Extension of the wrist. (*d*) Neutral position of the wrist. (*e*) Flexion of the wrist. (*f*) Flexion of the spine. (*g*) Flexion of the shoulder. (*h*) Extension of the shoulder. (a-h) ©McGraw-Hill Education/Tim Vacula, photographer

LO 14.6 Joint Movement

Flexion and Extension of Joints

The following figures show **flexion** (bending) and **extension** (straightening) in the elbow joint (*Figure 14.10a and b*), in the wrist joint (*Figure 14.10c, d, and e*), and in the shoulder joint (*Figure 14.10g and h*). When standing in anatomic position, every joint except the ankle is in extension.

For most of the rest of the body, flexion is movement of a body part *anterior* to the **coronal plane** (see Chapter 3). Extension is movement *posterior* to the coronal plane. For example, when you bend your trunk forward, that is flexion (*Figure 14.10f*). When you bend your trunk backward, that is extension (*see Figure 14.10g*). When you bend your trunk sideways to the right or left, that is called *lateral flexion*.

Abduction and Adduction of Joints

Abduction is movement away from the midline. **Adduction** is movement toward the midline. Abduction of your arm is moving it sideways away from your trunk. Adduction is bringing it back to the side of your trunk (*Figure 14.11a*). Abduction of your fingers is spreading them apart, away from the middle finger. Adduction is bringing them back together (*Figure 14.11b*).

Rotation of Joints

Rotation is turning around an axis. Medial rotation of the upper arm bone, the humerus, with the elbow flexed brings the palm of the hand toward the body. Lateral rotation moves the palm away from the body (*Figure 14.11c*).

Pronation and Supination

When you lie flat on the ground facedown on your belly with your palms touching the ground, you are **prone**. When you lie flat on your back with your spine on the floor and your palms facing up, you are **supine**.

When you rotate your forearm so that your palm faces the floor, that is **pronation**. When you rotate the forearm so that your palm is facing upward, that is **supination** (*Figure 14.11e*).

WORD	PRONUNCIATION		ELEMENTS	DEFINITION
abduction abduct (verb)	ab-**DUK**-shun ab-**DUKT**	S/ P/ R/	-ion *process, action* ab- *away from* -duct- *lead*	Action of moving away from the midline
adduction adduct (verb)	ah-**DUK**-shun ah-**DUKT**	S/ P/ R/	-ion *process, action* ad- *toward* -duct- *lead*	Action of moving toward the midline
circumduction circumduct (verb)	ser-kum-**DUK**-shun ser-kum-**DUKT**	S/ P/ R/	-ion *process, action* circum- *around* -duct- *lead*	Movement of an extremity in a circular motion
eversion evert (verb)	ee-**VER**-shun ee-**VERT**		Latin *overturn*	A turning outward
extension	eks-**TEN**-shun		Latin *stretch out*	When a joint is straightened to increase its angle
flexion	**FLEK**-shun		Latin *to bend*	When a joint is bent to decrease its angle
inversion invert (verb)	in-**VER**-shun in-**VERT**		Latin *to turn about*	A turning inward
prone pronation pronate (verb)	PRONE proh-**NAY**-shun **PROH**-nate	 S/ R/	Latin *prone, lying down* -ion *process, action* pronat- *bend down*	Lying facedown, flat on your belly Process of lying facedown or of turning a hand or foot with the volar (palm or sole) surface down
supine supinate supination	soo-**PINE** **SOO**-pih-nate soo-pih-**NAY**-shun	 S/ R/	Latin *supine, lying face up* Latin *face up* -ion *process, action* supinat- *bend backward*	Lying face up, flat on your spine Rotate the forearm so that the surface of the palm faces anteriorly in the anatomical position Process of lying face upward or turning an arm or foot so that the palm or sole is facing up

Exercises

A. Some medical terms can act as both a verb (action) and a noun (person, place, or thing). *The following pairs of terms are both verbs and nouns. Write the correct form of each term in the blank.* **LO 14.6, 14.A**

1. circumduct   circumduction

   The baseball pitcher was unable to _____ his arm to wind up his pitch.

2. invert   inversion

   A clubfoot would be an _____ of the foot.

3. abduct   abduction

   Moving away from the midline of the body is called _____.

4. evert   eversion

   The patient was unable to _____ her ankle due to great pain.

5. adduct   adduction

   The patient was asked to _____ his arms from a horizontal plane toward the center of his chest.

B. Translate the following statements that are in layman's terms into medical terminology. *Fill in the blanks.* **LO 14.6, 14.A**

1. Moving your hand so the palm is facing upward: _____

2. Moving your foot so the sole of the foot is facing inward: _____

3. A patient is being prepared for back surgery. What would be his position on the operating room table? _____

By age 65, more than 80% of people have some degree of joint degeneration. Mr. Johnson had always been very physically active, putting a lot of pressure on his weight-bearing joints. At different times in his life, he had been overweight, adding to the pressure.

X-rays of his lower back showed **osteoarthritis** of his lower lumbar intervertebral joints and marked osteoarthritis of his left hip joint *(Figure 14.12a and b)*. He received a left total-hip replacement **(THR)** and physiotherapy **(PT)** for his lower back.

Abbreviations

DJD	degenerative joint disease
MCP	metacarpophalangeal
OA	osteoarthritis
PIP	proximal interphalangeal
PT	physiotherapy (physical therapy)
RA	rheumatoid arthritis
THR	total-hip replacement

LO 14.7 Diseases of Joints

Osteoarthritis (OA) is caused by the breakdown and eventual destruction of cartilage in a joint. It develops as a result of wear and tear and is most common in the weight-bearing joints: the knee, hip, and lower back *(Figure 14.12a)*. Because it is a wear-and-tear disease, it is sometimes called **degenerative joint disease (DJD).** The degenerative process begins in the articular cartilage, which cracks and frays, eventually exposing the underlying bone.

Rheumatoid arthritis (RA) is a chronic, inflammatory disease that can affect many joints, causing deformity and disability. In *Figure 14.12b,* the hand deformities of RA—swelling of the **metacarpophalangeal (MCP)** and **proximal interphalangeal (PIP)** joints with **ulnar deviation** of the fingers—are shown. The disease process initially causes inflammation of the synovial membrane and then spreads to all other parts of the joint. Rheumatoid arthritis is three times as common in women and often begins in the thirties and forties.

Bursitis is inflammation of a **bursa** that can result from overuse of a joint, repeated trauma, or diseases such as RA.

Spinal cord

Compressed vertebrae

Narrowed intervertebral disc space

Degenerative changes

(a) Lumbar vertebrae

(b)

▲ **Figure 14.12** Arthritis. (*a*) Magnetic resonance imaging (MRI) scan of lumbar vertebrae showing degenerative changes due to osteoarthritis. (*b*) Rheumatoid arthritis of the hands. (a) ©Du Cane Medical Imaging Ltd./Photo Researchers, Inc. (b) ©VisualDx

WORD	PRONUNCIATION	ELEMENTS		DEFINITION
bursa bursitis	BURR-sah burr-SIGH-tis	 S/ R/	Latin *purse* -itis *inflammation* burs- *bursa*	A closed sac containing synovial fluid Inflammation of a bursa
degenerative	dee-JEN-er-a-tiv	S/ R/	-ive *quality of* degenerat- *deteriorate*	Relating to the deterioration of a structure
deviation	dee-vee-AY-shun		Latin *turn from straight path*	A turning aside from a normal course
interphalangeal	IN-ter-fah-LAN-jee-al	S/ P/ R/	-eal *pertaining to* inter- *between* -phalang- *phalanx*	Pertaining to the joints between two phalanges
metacarpophalangeal	MET-ah-KAR-poh-fah- LAN-jee-al	S/ P/ R/CF R/	-eal *pertaining to* meta- *after, beyond* -carp/o- *bones of the wrist* -phalang- *phalanx*	Pertaining to the joints between the metacarpal bones and phalanges
osteoarthritis	OS-tee-oh-ar-THRIE-tis	S/ R/CF R/	-itis *inflammation* oste/o- *bone* -arthr- *joint*	Chronic inflammatory disease of the joints with pain and loss of function
rheumatoid arthritis	RHU-mah-toyd ar- THRIE-tis	S/ R/ S/ R/	-oid *resemble* rheumat- *rheumatism* -itis *inflammation* arthr- *joint*	Disease of connective tissue, with arthritis as a major manifestation
ulna ulnar (adj)	UL-nah UL-nar	 S/ R/	Latin *elbow* -ar *pertaining to* uln- *forearm bone*	The medial and larger bone of the forearm Pertaining to the ulna or any of the structures (artery, vein, nerve) named after it

Exercises

A. Use the appropriate abbreviation. *From the given list, choose the abbreviation that best fits the given description. Fill in the blanks.* **LO 14.7, 14.F**

RA   PT   MCP   DJD   THR

1. Due to the wear and tear on the hip joint, the patient needed it to be replaced. She needed a _____.

2. The wear and tear on the joint is also known as _____.

3. The patient demonstrated signs of swelling of the joints where the finger bones meet the hand bones. The area of swelling was at the _____ joints.

4. The physician referred the patient to a specialist to strengthen the muscles in order to relieve pain. This type of therapy is known as _____.

5. The arthritis in the joints was due to an autoimmune disease that caused the body to attack its own tissue. This type of arthritis is termed _____.

B. Deconstruct medical terms. *Deconstruct medical terms into their word elements. Fill in the blanks.* **LO 14.D**

1. osteoarthritis: _____ / _____ / _____ / _____

2. interphalangeal: _____ / _____ / _____

3. degenerative: _____ / _____

Lesson 14.3

Axial Skeleton

Lesson Objectives

The vertebral column is part of the axial skeleton. In this lesson, information about the axial skeleton, with its joints and the muscles that function in an integrated manner, will enable you to use correct medical terminology to:

14.3.1 Define the regions and bones of the vertebral column.

14.3.2 Describe the structure and functions of an intervertebral joint.

14.3.3 Identify the major muscles that hold the vertebral column erect.

14.3.4 Describe the major problems and diseases that affect the vertebral column.

14.3.5 Identify the bones of the skull.

14.3.6 Identify the major muscles of mastication and respiration.

Case Report (CR) 14.3

You are
. . . a physical therapist assistant working in the Physical Therapy Department of Fulwood Medical Center.

Your patient is
. . . Ms. Nancy Cardenas, a 27-year-old jeweler. Ms. Cardenas was waiting in her car at a traffic light 3 days ago when her car was rear-ended.

Ms. Cardenas now has severe neck pain radiating down her left arm, with dizziness and headaches. She is unable to go to work. Dr. Stannard has examined her and diagnosed her condition as a **whiplash** injury. A magnetic resonance image (MRI) shows **herniation** of intervertebral **discs** between C5–C6 and C6–C7. Your role is to implement a regime of physiotherapy, including range-of-motion (ROM) exercises for her neck joints.

LO 14.8 Structure of Axial Skeleton

The axial skeleton comprises the

1. Vertebral column   2. Skull   3. Rib cage

The axial skeleton is the upright axis of the body and protects the brain, **spinal** cord, heart, and lungs—most of the major centers of our physiology.

LO 14.9 Components of the Vertebral Column

The **vertebral column** has 26 bones divided into five regions *(Figure 14.13)*:

1. **Cervical** region, with seven vertebrae, labeled C1 to C7 and curved anteriorly.

2. **Thoracic** region, with 12 vertebrae, labeled T1 to T12 and curved posteriorly.

3. **Lumbar** region, with five vertebrae, labeled L1 to L5 and curved anteriorly.

4. **Sacral** region, with one bone curved posteriorly.

5. **Coccyx** (tailbone), with one bone curved posteriorly.

The spinal cord lies protected in the vertebral canal. Spinal nerves leave the spinal cord through the **intervertebral foramina** to travel to other parts of the body.

Intervertebral discs consist of fibrocartilage and inhabit the intervertebral space between the bodies of adjacent vertebrae. They provide additional support and cushioning for the vertebral column. The center of the disc is a gelatinous nucleus pulposus.

Cervical region (curved anteriorly)

— C1

— C7

— T1

Thoracic region (curved posteriorly)

Intervertebral disc

Twelfth thoracic vertebra (T12)

Intervertebral foramina

First lumbar vertebra (L1)

Lumbar region (curved anteriorly)

Body

Transverse process

Spinous process

Fifth lumbar vertebra (L5)

Sacral promontory

Sacral and coccygeal regions (curved posteriorly)

Sacrum

Coccyx

Lateral view

▲ **Figure 14.13** Vertebral column.

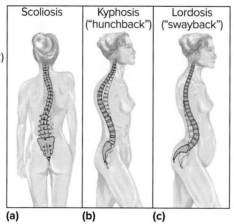

| Scoliosis | Kyphosis ("hunchback") | Lordosis ("swayback") |

(a)   (b)   (c)

▲ **Figure 14.14** Abnormal Spinal Curvatures. (*a*) Scoliosis. (*b*) Kyphosis. (*c*) Lordosis.

LO 14.10 Common Disorders of the Vertebral Column

Abnormal spinal curvatures can result from disease, poor posture, or congenital defects in the vertebrae. The defect that is most common is called **scoliosis**, an abnormal lateral curve in the thoracic region *(Figure 14.14a)*. In older people, particularly those with osteoporosis, an exaggerated thoracic curvature is called **kyphosis** *(Figure 14.14b)*. An exaggerated lumbar curve is called **lordosis** *(Figure 14.14c)*.

WORD	PRONUNCIATION		ELEMENTS	DEFINITION
cervical	**SER**-vih-kal	S/ R/	-al *pertaining to* cervic- *neck*	Pertaining to the neck region
coccyx	**KOK**-siks		Greek *coccyx*	Small tailbone at the lowest end of the vertebral column
disc	DISK		Latin or Greek *disk*	Flattened, round structure. In the skeletal system, a flattened round fibrocartilaginous structure between bones
foramen foramina (pl)	foh-**RAY**-men foh-**RAM**-in-ah		Latin *an aperture*	An opening through a structure
herniation herniate (verb)	**HER**-nee-ay-shun **HER**-nee-ate	S/ R/ S/	-ation *process, being* herni- *rupture* -ate *process*	Protrusion of an anatomical structure from its normal position
intervertebral	**IN**-ter-**VER**-teh-bral	S/ P/ R/	-al *pertaining to* inter- *between* -vertebr- *vertebra*	Located between two vertebrae
kyphosis kyphotic (adj)	kie-**FOH**-sis ki-**FOT**-ik	S/ R/ S/ R/CF	-osis *condition* kyph- *humpback* -tic *pertaining to* kyph/o- *humpback*	A normal posterior curve of the thoracic spine that can be exaggerated in disease Pertaining to kyphosis
lordosis lordotic (adj)	lore-**DOH**-sis lore-**DOT**-ik	S/ R/ S/ R/CF	-osis *condition* lord- *bend backward* -tic *pertaining to* lord/o- *bend backward*	An exaggerated forward curvature of the lumbar spine Pertaining to lordosis
lumbar (adj)	**LUM**-bar		Latin *loin*	Relating to the region in the back and sides between the ribs and pelvis
sacrum sacral (adj)	**SAY**-krum **SAY**-kral	S/ R/	Latin *sacred* -al *pertaining to* sacr- *sacrum*	Segment of the vertebral column that forms part of the pelvis Pertaining to the sacrum
scoliosis scoliotic (adj)	skoh-lee-**OH**-sis **SKOH**-lee-**OT**-ik	S/ R/ S/ R/CF	-osis *condition* scoli- *crooked* -tic *pertaining to* scoli/o- *crooked*	An abnormal lateral curvature of the vertebral column Pertaining to scoliosis
spine spinal (adj)	SPINE **SPY**-nal	S/ R/	Latin *spine* -al *pertaining to* spin- *spine*	Vertebral column, *or a short projection from a bone* Pertaining to the spine
thorax thoracic (adj)	**THOR**-aks thor-**ASS**-ik	S/ R/	Greek *breastplate* -ic *pertaining to* thorac- *chest*	The part of the trunk between the abdomen and neck Pertaining to the chest (thorax)
vertebra vertebrae (pl) vertebral (adj)	**VER**-teh-brah **VER**-teh-bray **VER**-teh-bral	S/ R/	Latin *spinal joint* -al *pertaining to* vertebr- *vertebra*	One of the bones of the spinal column Pertaining to the vertebrae
whiplash	**WHIP**-lash	R/ R/	whip- *to swing* -lash *end of whip*	Symptoms caused by sudden, uncontrolled extension and flexion of the neck, often in an automobile accident

Exercises

A. Deconstruct medical terms associated with the axial skeleton. *Breaking medical terms into their elements will make it easier to decipher their meaning. Fill in the blanks.* **LO 14.D**

1. intervertebral: _____ / _____ / _____

                       P   R/CF   S

2. cervical: _____ / _____

               R   S

3. thoracic: _____ / _____

               R   S

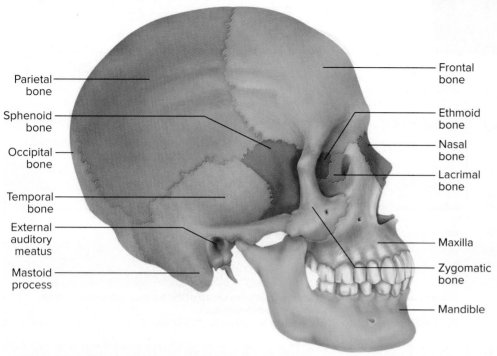

Parietal bone
Sphenoid bone
Occipital bone
Temporal bone
External auditory meatus
Mastoid process

Frontal bone
Ethmoid bone
Nasal bone
Lacrimal bone
Maxilla
Zygomatic bone
Mandible

▲ **Figure 14.15** Skull: Right Lateral View.

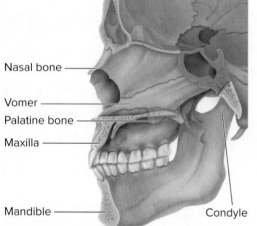

Nasal bone
Vomer
Palatine bone
Maxilla
Mandible
Condyle

▲ **Figure 14.16** Facial Bones.

Abbreviation	
TMJ	temporomandibular joint

LO 14.11 The Skull

The human skull has 22 bones, 8 of which make up the **cranium**, the upper part of the skull that encloses the **cranial cavity** and protects the brain *(Figure 14.15)*. The bones of the cranium are:

1. **Frontal bone**—forms the forehead and the roofs of the orbits and contains a pair of right and left frontal sinuses above the orbits.
2. **Parietal bones** (2)—form the bulging sides and roof of the cranium.
3. **Occipital bone**—forms the back of and part of the base of the cranium.
4. **Temporal bones** (2)—form the sides and part of the base of the cranium.
5. **Sphenoid bone**—forms part of the base of the cranium and the orbits.
6. **Ethmoid bone**—forms parts of the nose and the orbits and is hollow, forming the ethmoid sinuses.

The bones of the cranium are joined together by sutures, joints that appear as seams, covered on the inside and outside by a thin layer of connective tissue.

The lower anterior part of the skull comprises the 14 bones of the facial skeleton *(Figure 14.16; see also Figure 14.15)*:

1. **Maxillary** bones (2)—form the upper jaw, hold the upper teeth, and are hollow, forming the maxillary sinuses.
2. **Palatine** bones (2)—are located behind the maxilla.
3. **Zygomatic** bones (2)—form the prominences of the cheeks below the eyes.
4. **Lacrimal** bones (2)—form the medial wall of each eye orbit.
5. **Nasal** bones (2)—form the sides and bridge of the nose.
6. **Vomer** bone—separates the two nasal cavities *(Figure 14.16)*.
7. Inferior nasal **conchae** (2)—are fragile bones in the lower nasal cavity.
8. **Mandible**—is the lower jawbone, which holds the lower teeth.

The third component of the axial skeleton, the rib cage, is discussed in *Chapter 13*.

Bones and Joints of Mastication

The **temporomandibular joint (TMJ)** connects the condyle of the mandible to a fossa in the temporal bone at the base of the skull. The joint acts like a hinge when you open and close your mouth.

WORD	PRONUNCIATION	ELEMENTS		DEFINITION
concha conchae (pl)	KON-kah KON-kee		Latin *a shell*	Shell-shaped bone on medial wall of nasal cavity
cranium	KRAY-nee-um		Greek *skull*	The upper part of the skull that encloses and protects the brain
cranial (adj)	KRAY-nee-al	S/ R/	-al *pertaining to* crani- *skull*	Pertaining to the skull
ethmoid bone	ETH-moyd BOHN	S/ R/	-oid *resemble* ethm- *sieve* bone Old English *bone*	Bone that forms the back of the nose and part of the orbits and encloses numerous air cells, forming the ethmoid sinuses
lacrimal	LAK-rim-al	S/ R/	-al *pertaining to* lacrim- *tears*	Pertaining to tears
mandible mandibular (adj)	MAN-di-bel man-DIB-you-lar	S/ R/	Latin *jaw* -ar *pertaining to* mandibul- *the jaw*	Lower jawbone Pertaining to the mandible
maxilla maxillary (adj)	mak-SILL-ah MAK-sill-ah-ree	S/ R/	Latin *jawbone* -ary *pertaining to* maxill- *maxilla*	Upper jawbone, containing right and left maxillary sinuses
occiput occipital bone	OK-si-put ok-SIP-it-al BOHN	S/ R/	Latin *occiput* al- *pertaining to* occipit- *back of head* bone Old English *bone*	The back of the skull Bone that forms the back and part of the base of the cranium
palatine	PAL-ah-tine		Latin *palate*	Bone that forms the hard palate and parts of the nose and orbits
parietal bone	pah-RYE-eh-tal BOHN	S/ R/	-al *pertaining to* pariet- *wall* bone Old English *bone*	Bones that form the bulging sides and roof of the cranium
sphenoid bone	SFEE-noyd BOHN	S/ R/	-oid *resemble* sphen- *wedge* bone Old English *bone*	Wedge-shaped bone that forms part of the base of the cranium and the orbits
temporal bones	TEM-por-al BOHNZ	S/ R/	-al *pertaining to* tempor- *temple, side of head* bone Old English *bone*	Bones that form the sides and part of the base of the cranium
temporomandibular joint (TMJ)	TEM-por-oh-man-DIB-you-lar JOYNT	S/ R/CF R/	-ar *pertaining to* temporo- *temple, side of head* -mandibul- *the jaw* joint Middle English *joint*	The joint between the temporal bone and the mandible
vomer	VOH-mer		Latin *ploughshare*	Lower nasal septum
zygoma zygomatic (adj)	zie-GOH-mah zie-goh-MAT-ik	S/ R/	French *yoke* -ic *pertaining to* zygomat- *cheekbone*	Bone that forms the prominence of the cheek

Exercises

A. Construct medical terms related to the bones of the skull. *Given the definition, complete the medical term with the correct word element.* *Fill in the blank.* **LO 14.11, 14.C**

1. Wedge-shaped bone at the base of the skull. _____/oid

2. Bone that forms part of the base and sides of the skull. _____/al

3. Bone that forms the back of the nose and encloses numerous air cells. _____/oid

4. The two bones forming the sidewalls and roof of the cranium. _____/al

B. Not all bones are constructed with word elements. *Some bones are named for their shape. Given the description, enter the name of the bone.* *Fill in the blank.* **LO 14.11**

1. Bone that forms the hard palate and parts of the nose and orbits: _____

2. Shell-shaped bone on medial wall of nasal cavity: _____

3. Bone named because it resembled a *yoke:* _____

4. This bone has the shape of a *plow:* _____

5. The upper jawbone: _____

6. The lower jawbone: _____

Lesson 14.4
SKELETAL SYSTEM

Appendicular Skeleton

Keynotes

• **Shoulder dislocation** occurs when the ball of the humerus slips out of the socket of the scapula, usually anteriorly.

• **Shoulder subluxation** occurs when the ball of the humerus slips partially out of position and then moves back in.

Abbreviation

AC   acromioclavicular

Case Report (CR) 14.4

You are
. . . an emergency technician working in the Emergency Department at Fulwood Medical Center.

Your patient is
. . . Mr. Luke Johnson, a 20-year-old university student.

Mr. Johnson presents with severe pain in his right shoulder area. At rugby practice, Mr. Johnson jumped to catch a pass, was tackled while in the air, and landed on the tip of his left shoulder. He is now complaining of pain in his upper chest near the shoulder, has his left arm held close to his chest, and is supporting it with his right hand. Examination shows swelling and tenderness over the midclavicular region and inability to abduct his left arm.

The emergency physician agrees with your findings and sends Mr. Johnson for an x-ray, which shows a midshaft fracture of his clavicle. He is given analgesia and referred to the orthopedic department, where a surgical procedure of fixation with an 8-hole plate was performed.

LO 14.12. Shoulder Girdle and Upper Arm

The **pectoral** (shoulder) **girdle** connects the axial skeleton to the upper limbs and helps with movements of the upper limb.

The bones of the pectoral girdle are the **scapulae** (shoulder blades) and **clavicles** *(Figure 14.17)*. The scapula extends over the top of the joint to form a roof called the **acromion**. The acromion is attached to the clavicle at the **acromioclavicular (AC)** joint. This also provides a connection between the axial skeleton, pectoral girdle, and upper arm. The clavicle acts as a strut to keep the scapula in place so that the arm hangs freely and can have maximum range of movement. It is commonly fractured by a fall on the shoulder tip *(Case Report 14.4)* or on the outstretched hand.

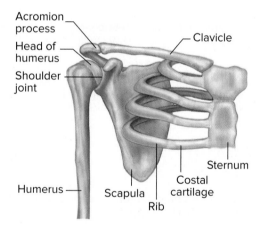

▲ **Figure 14.17** Pectoral Girdle.

The joint that connects the pectoral girdle to the upper limb is the shoulder joint, located between the scapula and the **humerus** bone of the upper arm *(see Figure 14.17)*. This joint is a ball-and-socket joint in which the head of the humerus allows the greatest range of motion of any joint in the body.

Several ligaments hold together the articulating surfaces of the humerus and scapula.

LO 14.13 Common Disorders of the Shoulder

Because of the increased range of motion of this joint, the shoulder joint also is the most unstable joint and is liable to **dislocation**.

Shoulder separation is a dislocation of the acromioclavicular joint, usually due to a fall on the point of the shoulder. The other common injury caused by falling on the point of the shoulder is a fractured clavicle *(Case Report 14.4)*.

WORD	PRONUNCIATION	ELEMENTS		DEFINITION
acromion	ah-**CROH**-mee-on	S/ R/	-ion *action* acrom- *acromion*	Lateral end of the scapula, extending over the shoulder joint
acromioclavicular	ah-**CROH**-mee-oh-klah-**VIK**-you-lar	S/ R/CF R/	-ar *pertaining to* acromi/o *acromion* -clavicul- *clavicle*	Pertaining to the joint between the acromion and the clavicle
clavicle clavicular (adj)	**KLAV**-ih-kul klah-**VIK**-you-lar	S/ R/	Latin *collarbone* -ar *pertaining to* clavicul- *clavicle*	Curved bone that forms the anterior part of the pectoral girdle Pertaining to the clavicle
dislocation	dis-loh-**KAY**-shun	P/ R/	-ion *action* dis- *apart* -locat- *a place*	The state of being completely out of joint
humerus	**HYU**-mer-us		Latin *shoulder*	Single bone of the upper arm
pectoral	**PEK**-tor-al	S/ R/	-al *pertaining to* pector- *chest*	Pertaining to the chest
pectoral girdle	**PEK**-tor-al **GIR**-del		girdle Old English *encircle*	Incomplete bony ring that attaches the upper limb to the axial skeleton
scapula scapulae (pl) scapular (adj)	**SKAP**-you-lah **SKAP**-you-lee **SKAP**-you-lar	S/ R/	Latin *shoulder blade* -ar *pertaining to* scapul- *scapula*	Shoulder blade Pertaining to the shoulder blade
separation	sep-ah-**RAY**-shun	S/ R/	-ion *action* separat *move apart*	A shoulder separation is a dislocation of the acromioclavicular joint
subluxation	sub-luk-**SAY**-shun	S/ P/ R/	-ion *action* sub- *under, slightly* -luxat- *dislocate*	An incomplete dislocation in which some contact between the joint surfaces remains

Exercises

A. Use your knowledge of the *language of orthopedics* to complete the following medical terms. *Each blank represents a word element. If the term has a combining vowel, there is a blank for that as well. The first one has been done for you.* **LO 14.12, 14.13, 14.D**

1. Lateral end of the scapula   _____ acrom _____ / _____ ion _____

2. Incomplete dislocation   _____ / _____ / _____

3. Joint between acromion and clavicle   _____ / _____ / _____

4. Completely out of joint   _____ / _____ / _____

5. Pertaining to the shoulder blade   _____ / _____

B. Implement the *language of orthopedics* to answer the following questions. *Write medical terms for the following layman's terms.* *Fill in the blanks.* **LO 14.12, 14.A**

1. the shoulder girdle (2 words) _____

2. shoulder blades _____

3. collarbones _____

LO 14.14 Upper Arm and Elbow Joint

The **humerus** is the long bone of the upper arm *(Figure 14.18)*. It extends from the scapula to the elbow joint. Muscles connect it to the pectoral girdle, vertebral column, and ribs. These muscles enable the arm to be freely movable at the shoulder joint. The inferior end of the humerus has two **condyles** that articulate with the ulna to form the elbow joint. A lateral projection on each condyle, the **epicondyle**, serves as an attachment for ligaments and tendons to allow for stabilization as well as movement of the joint.

The elbow joint has two **articulations**:

1. A hinge joint between the humerus and **ulna** bone of the forearm, which allows flexion and extension of the elbow.

2. A gliding joint between the humerus and **radius** bone of the forearm, which allows pronation and supination of the forearm and hand.

A joint capsule and ligaments hold the two articulations together.

LO 14.15 Common Disorders of the Elbow

Tennis elbow is caused by overuse of the elbow joint or poor techniques in playing tennis or golf. Tendons of upper-arm and forearm muscles are inserted into the medial and lateral **epicondyles** of the humerus just above the elbow joint *(Figure 14.19)*. Small tears in the tendons at their attachments occur with overuse, and eventually enough tears accumulate to cause pain and restrict elbow movement. The pain occurs when straightening the elbow or opening and closing the fingers.

Ligament strains and **bone fractures** due to a heavy fall or a blow to the elbow are also common injuries.

Anterior surface

▲ **Figure 14.18** Humerus.

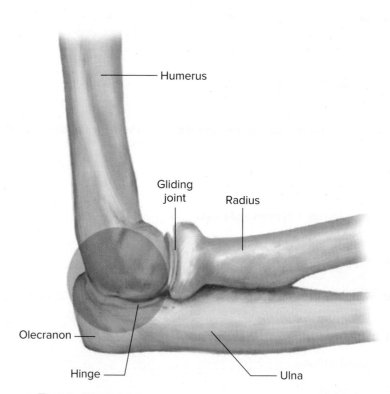

▲ **Figure 14.19** Elbow Joint.

WORD	PRONUNCIATION	ELEMENTS		DEFINITION
condyle epicondyle	KON-dile ep-ih-KON-dile	P/ R/	Greek *knuckle* epi- *above* -condyle *knuckle*	Rounded bone surface that articluates with another bone Projection above the condyle for attachment of a ligament or tendon
radius	RAY-dee-us		Latin *spoke of a wheel*	The forearm bone on the thumb side
ulna ulnar (adj)	UL-nah UL-nar	S/ R/	Latin *elbow* -ar *pertaining to* uln- *forearm bone*	The medial and larger bone of the forearm Pertaining to the ulna or any of the structures (artery, vein, nerve) named after it

Exercises

A. Identify the bone structures of the upper arm. *From the provided definition, provide the term it is describing.* **LO 14.14, 14.A**

1. The forearm bone that is on the thumb side: _____

2. The structure of the humerus that articulates with the ulna: _____

3. The forearm bone that is on the medial side of the forearm: _____

4. The structure of the humerus that serves as an attachment for ligaments and tendons: _____

B. Read the following scenario. *Answer the following questions related to disorders of the upper arm. Select the correct answer that correctly answers the question or completes each statement.* **LO 14.15**

You are working as a physical therapist in an outpatient rehabilitation clinic. You are assess a 53 year-old man who has worked a house painter for 30 years. He is complaining of intense pain in his elbow, especially when he opens and closes his fingers.

1. What condition do you think the patient has?

   a. tennis elbow

   b. closed fracture

   c. osteoarthritis

   d. degenerative bone disease

2. The pain is due to an injury in the

   a. fingers

   b. hand

   c. wrist

   d. elbow

3. The tissue that is injured is a

   a. bone

   b. tendon

   c. ligament

   d. cartilage

LO 14.16 Forearm and Wrist

The forearm has two bones, the **radius** on the thumb side and the **ulna** on the little-finger side. They articulate at the wrist joint with the small **carpal** bones. The muscles of the forearm **supinate** and **pronate** the forearm, flex and extend the wrist joint and hand, and move the hand medially and laterally.

As the tendons pass over the wrist, they are surrounded by sheaths of synovial membrane and held in place on the wrist by a transverse, thick fibrous band called a **retinaculum** *(Figure 14.20)*.

 Case Report (CR) 14.5

You are

. . . an orthopedic technologist working with Kenneth Stannard, MD, at Fulwood Medical Center.

Your patient is

. . . James Fox, a 17-year-old male who complains of severe pain in his right wrist. While playing soccer a few hours earlier, he fell. James pushed his hand out to break his fall and heard his wrist snap. The wrist is now swollen and deformed.

VS are T 98.2, P 92, R 15, BP 110/76. On examination, his right wrist is swollen and tender and has a dinner-fork deformity. An IV has been started, and he has been give 3 mg of morphine IV. An x-ray of the wrist has been ordered.

LO 14.17 Common Disorders of the Wrist

Ganglion cysts are fluid-filled cysts arising when the synovial tendon sheaths that run over the back of the wrist are irritated or inflamed. They often disappear spontaneously.

Colles fracture is a common fracture of the radius just above the wrist joint. It occurs when a person tries to break a fall with an outstretched hand. The distal radius just proximal to the wrist is broken. In some cases, the distal ulna is also fractured and the wrist joint dislocated. The fracture is diagnosed with an x-ray *(Figure 14.21)*.

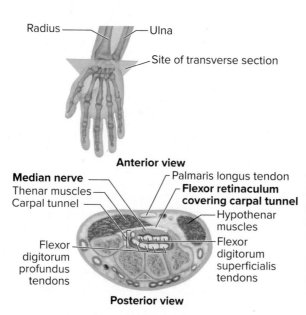

▲ **Figure 14.20** Carpal Tunnel: Transverse Section.

▲ **Figure 14.21** X-ray of Colles fracture with radius and ulna involved. ©Zephyr/ Photo Researchers, Inc.

Word Analysis and Definition

WORD	PRONUNCIATION		ELEMENTS	DEFINITION
carpus carpal (adj)	**KAR**-pus **KAR**-pal	S/ R/	Greek *wrist* **-al** *pertaining to* **carp-** *bones of the wrist*	Collective term for the eight carpal bones of the wrist Pertaining to the wrist
Colles fracture	**KOL**-ez **FRAK**-chur		Abraham Colles, 1773–1843, Irish surgeon	Fracture of the distal radius at the wrist
cyst	SIST		Greek *bladder*	An abnormal, fluid-containing sac
retinaculum	ret-ih-**NAK**-you-lum	S/ R/	**-um** *structure* **retinacul-** *hold back*	Fibrous ligament that keeps the tendons in place on the wrist so that they do not "bowstring" when the forearm muscles contract

Exercises

A. Terms related to the anatomy of the wrist. *Correctly identify the structures of the wrist.* **LO 14.16**

1. The ligament of the wrist that keeps the tendons in place:

   a. ganglion

   b. radius

   c. retinaculum

   d. fascia

2. The medical term that means *wrist:*

   a. carpal

   b. retinaculum

   c. radius

   d. ulna

B. Terms related to disorders of the wrist. *Correctly identify disorders of the wrist.* **LO 14.17, 14. B**

1. A Colles fracture occurs at the:

   a. proximal radius

   b. distal radius

   c. proximal carpals

   d. distals carpals

2. The proper pronunciation for Colles is:

   a. cool ease

   b. cool ess

   c. call ease

   d. call ess

3. In a Colles fracture, the radius is displaced:

   a. medially

   b. laterally

   c. anteriorly

   d. posteriorly

4. The typical treatment for a ganglion cyst is:

   a. lance and drain

   b. observe

   c. splint

LO 14.18 The Hand

Disorders of and injuries to the hand are among the most common reasons for office and Emergency Department visits and for ambulatory surgical procedures.

The complex structure of the hand *(Figure 14.22)* has evolved in response to the complicated and often very fine movements that modern-day activities require the hand to perform. Examples are making jewelry, repairing a watch, and sewing an artery or nerve back together.

The five fingers of one hand together have 14 bones called **phalanges**. The thumb has two phalanges. The remaining four fingers have three each *(Figure 14.22a)*.

In the **palm** of the hand, the five bones proximal to the fingers are **metacarpals**, which connect at the wrist to eight small **carpal** bones. These in turn connect the hand to the bones of the forearm *(Figure 14.22)*.

All these bones require numerous joints with ligaments to connect and stabilize them.

▲ **Figure 14.22** **The Bones of the Hand.** ©McGraw-Hill Education/Christine Eckel, photographer.

WORD	PRONUNCIATION	ELEMENTS		DEFINITION
metacarpal	**MET**-ah-**KAR**-pal	S/ P/ R/	-al *pertaining to* meta- *after* -carp- *bones of the wrist*	The five bones between the carpus and the fingers
phalanx phalanges (pl)	**FAY**-lanks **FAY**-lan-jeez		Greek *line of soldiers*	A bone of a finger or toe

Exercises

A. Because the body has 206 bones, there is an extensive amount of orthopedic vocabulary. *Build your knowledge of hand terminology with this exercise. Select the answer that correctly completes each statement.* **LO 14.18**

1. The suffix -*al* means:

   a. pertaining to

   b. one who does

   c. study of

   d. condition

2. The prefix *meta-* means:

   a. before

   b. during

   c. after

   d. middle

3. The term **metacarpal** refers to the:

   a. arm

   b. elbow

   c. forearm

   d. hand

4. The bone of a finger *or* toe is called a(n):

   a. carpus

   b. fascia

   c. eminence

   d. phalanx

5. The palm of the hand is the _____ surface of the hand.

   a. inferior

   b. posterior

   c. dorsum

   d. anterior

▲ **Figure 14.23** Hand with **Osteoarthritis.** Osteoarthritis of hands showing Heberden nodes. ©Dr. P. Marazzi/ SPL/Photo Researchers, Inc.

Heberden node

▲ **Figure 14.24** Hands with Rheumatoid **Arthritis.** ©John Watney/Science Source

Abbreviations	
JRA	juvenile rheumatoid arthritis
OA	osteoarthritis
RA	rheumatoid arthritis

LO 14.19 Disorders of the Hand

Osteoarthritis (OA) in the hand joints occurs from wear and tear, particularly in the joint at the base of the thumb. It occurs mostly in the elderly. As a finger joint deteriorates, small bony spurs called **Heberden nodes** form over it *(Figure 14.23)*. William Heberden (1710–1801), a surgeon in Cambridge, England, first described these nodes.

Rheumatoid arthritis (RA), with destruction of joint surfaces, joint capsule, and ligaments, leads to marked **deformity** and joint **instability** *(Figure 14.24)*. It occurs mostly in women, with onset between ages 20 and 50.

The great majority of patients have involvement of the hands, where the disease affects the synovial membrane that lines joints and tendons. The abnormal synovial membrane can invade the smooth, gliding joint surfaces and destroy them, or it can invade the surrounding joint capsule and ligaments and cause deformity and joint instability. Lumps known as **rheumatic nodules** form over the small joints of the hand and wrist. The metacarpophalangeal joints can be affected, and this leads to drift of the fingers away from the thumb, called **ulnar deviation**.

Juvenile rheumatoid arthritis (JRA) affects children under the age of 17 with inflammation and stiffness of joints. Many children grow out of it.

Dupuytren contracture is a progressive thickening and **contracture** of the skin and connective tissues of the palm of the hand.

Injuries of the Hand

Flexor tendon injuries occur as a result of lacerations. Because the flexor tendons lie just beneath the skin on the palmar surfaces of the fingers, they are very **susceptible** to injury even with a shallow laceration. Even after repair, there can be **residual** stiffness and limited motion of the fingers.

Open fractures of hand bones, when the skin is broken and the broken bone penetrates through the break in the skin, can lead to infection of hand tissues.

Partial amputation of a fingertip is a common type of injury, particularly in people who work with sharp tools *(Figure 14.25)*. This type of wound also produces an open phalangeal fracture.

▲ **Figure 14.25** Healed Partial **Amputation of Two Fingers.** ©Dr. P. Marazzi/ SPL/Photo Researchers, Inc.

WORD	PRONUNCIATION	ELEMENTS		DEFINITION
amputation	am-pyu-**TAY**-shun	S/ R/	-ation *process* **amput-** *to prune, lop off*	Process of removing a limb, a part of a limb, a breast, or some other projecting part
amputate (verb) amputee (noun)	**AM**-pyu-tate **AM**-pyu-tee	S/ S/	-ate *pertaining to* -ee *one associated with*	The act of amputation A person with an amputation
contracture	kon-**TRAK**-chur	S/ R/	-ure *process* **contract-** *draw together*	Muscle shortening due to spasm or fibrosis
deformity	dee-**FOR**-mih-tee	S/ P/ R/	-ity *condition* **de-** *take away* **-form-** *form, appearance*	A permanent structural deviation from the normal
Dupuytren contracture	du-pweh-**TRAHN** kon-**TRAK**-chur	 S/ R/	Guillaume Dupuytren, 1777–1835, French surgeon -ure *process* **contract-** *draw together*	A thickening and shortening of fibrous bands in the palm of the hand
flexor flex (verb)	**FLEK**-sor FLEKS		Latin *to bend*	Muscle or tendon that flexes a joint To bend a joint so that the two parts come together
Heberden node	**HEH**-ber-den NOHD		William Heberden, 1710–1801, English physician **node** Latin *a knot*	Bony lump on the terminal phalanx of the fingers in osteoarthritis
instability	in-stah-**BIL**-ih-tee	S/ P/ R/	-ity *condition* **in-** *not* **-stabil-** *stand firm*	Abnormal tendency of a joint to partially or fully dislocate
juvenile	**JU**-ven-ile		Latin *youthful*	Between the ages of 2 and 17 years
nodule	**NOD**-yule	S/ R/	-ule *little, small* **nod-** *node*	Small node or knotlike swelling
residue (noun) residual	**REZ**-ih-dyu ree-**ZID**-you-al	S/ R/CF	Latin *left over* -al *pertaining to* **resid/u-** *what is left over*	That which remains or is left over Pertaining to anything left over
rheumatism	**RHU**-mat-izm	S/ R/	-ism *condition* **rheumat-** *a flow*	Pain in various parts of the musculoskeletal system
rheumatic (adj) rheumatoid arthritis	rhu-**MAT**-ik **RHU**-mah-toyd ar-**THRIE**-tis	S/ S/ S/ R/	-ic *pertaining to* -oid *resembling* -itis *inflammation* **arthr-** *joint*	Relating to or characterized by rheumatism Disease of connective tissue, with arthritis as a major manifestation
susceptible	suh-**SEP**-tih-bull		Latin *to take up*	Capable of being affected by

Exercises

A. Demonstrate your knowledge of the difference between these similar terms. *Use the correct form of the term in the appropriate place. Fill in the blanks.* **LO 14.6, 14.18, 14.19**

1. **amputation**   **amputate**   **amputee**

   The surgeon has decided to _____ the patient's left leg below the knee. The _____ will be performed as soon as possible. Following the surgery, the _____ will be fitted for a new leg prosthesis.

2. **flex**   **flexor**

   The _____ tendons _____ a joint so that the two parts of the joint can come together.

3. **residual**   **residue**

   The _____ in the bottom of the test beaker can be referred to as the _____ matter.

4. **rheumatic**   **rheumatoid arthritis**   **rheumatism**

   _____ is a generic term for _____ pain in various parts of the musculoskeletal system. However, _____ is a specific systemic disease affecting many joints.

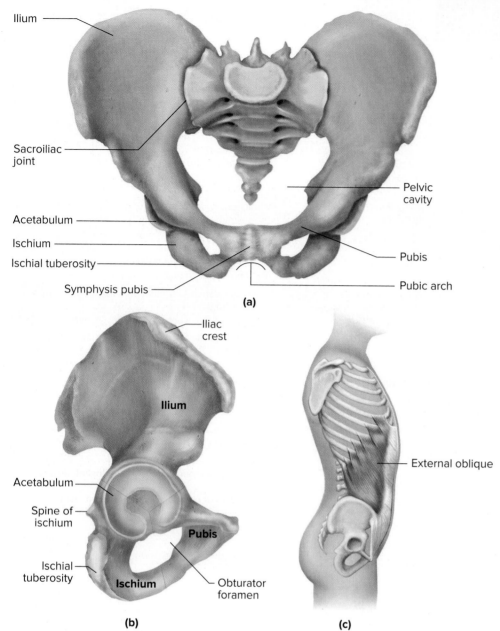

Ilium

Sacroiliac joint

Acetabulum

Ischium

Ischial tuberosity

Symphysis pubis

Pelvic cavity

Pubis

Pubic arch

(a)

Iliac crest

Ilium

Acetabulum

Spine of ischium

Ischial tuberosity

Ischium

Pubis

Obturator foramen

(b)

External oblique

(c)

▲ **Figure 14.26** Pelvic Girdle. (a) Front view. (b) Side view. (c) Abdominal muscles supporting the pelvic girdle.

LO 14.20 Pelvic Girdle

The pelvic girdle (Figure 14.26) is the two hip bones that articulate anteriorly with each other at the **symphysis pubis** and posteriorly with the **sacrum** to form the bowl-shaped **pelvis**. The two joints between the hip bones and the sacrum are the **sacroiliac (SI) joints**.

The pelvic girdle has the following functions:

1. Supports the axial skeleton.
2. Transmits the body's weight through to the lower limbs.
3. Provides attachments for the lower limbs.
4. Protects the internal reproductive organs, urinary bladder, and distal end of the large intestine.

Each hip bone is a fusion of three bones: the **ilium**, **ischium**, and **pubis** (Figure 14.26a). The fusion takes place in the region of the **acetabulum**, a cup-shaped cavity on the lateral surface of each hip bone that receives the **head** of the **femur** (thigh bone, Figure 14.26b).

The lower part of the pelvis is formed by the lower ilium, ischium, and **pubic** bones that surround a short canal-like cavity. This opening is larger in females than males to allow the infant to pass through during childbirth. The outlet from the cavity is spanned by strong muscular layers through which the rectum, vagina, and urethra pass.

Muscles anchor the pelvic girdle to the vertebrae and ribs of the axial skeleton (Figure 14.26c).

LO 14.21 Disorders of the Pelvic Girdle

SI joint strain is a common cause of lower-back pain. Unlike most joints, the sacroiliac joint is only designed to move ¼ inch (approximately 6 mm) during weight bearing and forward flexion. Its main function is to provide shock absorption for the spine.

During pregnancy, hormones enable connective tissue to relax so that the pelvis can expand enough to allow birth. The stretching in the sacroiliac joint ligaments makes it excessively mobile and susceptible to wear-and-tear painful arthritis.

Another cause of pain in the sacroiliac joint is trauma, with tearing of the joint ligaments generating too much motion and pain. The pain is felt in the low back, in the buttock, and sometimes in the back and front of the thigh.

Low back pain can be caused by a variety of problems with the interconnected network of bones, muscles, nerves, and discs in the lumbar spine. In adults 30 to 60 years old, the pain often can arise from disc degeneration or herniation in the lumbar spine or from muscle or other tissue strain. Adults over 60 years can suffer from lumbar joint degeneration and spinal stenosis. In February 2017, the American College of Physicians issued guidelines for the initial treatment of low back pain, recommending nondrug therapies such as superficial heat, massage, acupuncture, or spinal manipulation. If drugs are necessary, nonsteroidal anti-inflammatory drugs (NSAIDs) or skeletal muscle relaxants are recommended.

Diastasis symphysis pubis is another result of the stretching of pelvic ligaments during pregnancy. The softening and stretching of the ligaments of the symphysis pubis stretch the joint between the two pubic bones and lead to pain over the joint and difficulty in walking, climbing stairs, and turning over in bed.

Abbreviations	
NSAIDs	nonsteroidal anti-inflammatory drugs
SI	sacroiliac

WORD	PRONUNCIATION		ELEMENTS	DEFINITION
acetabulum	ass-eh-**TAB**-you-lum		Latin *vinegar cup*	The cup-shaped cavity of the hip bone that receives the head of the femur to form the hip joint
diastasis	die-**ASS**-tah-sis		Greek *separation*	Separation of normally joined parts
femur	**FEE**-mur		Latin *thigh*	The thigh bone
femoral (adj)	**FEM**-oh-ral	S/ R/	-al *pertaining to* femor- *femur*	Pertaining to the femur
ilium (*Note:* The ileum is a section of the small intestine [*Chapter 6*].)	**ILL**-ee-um		Latin *to twist*	Large wing-shaped bone at the upper and posterior part of the pelvis
ilia (pl)	**ILL**-ee-ah			
ischium	**ISS**-kee-um		Greek *hip*	Lower and posterior part of the hip bone
ischia (pl)	**ISS**-kee-ah	S/	-al *pertaining to*	Pertaining to the ischium
ischial (adj)	**ISS**-kee-al	R/CF	isch/i- *ischium*	
pelvis	**PEL**-vis		Latin *basin*	A cup-shaped ring of bone; also a cup-shaped cavity, as in the pelvis of the kidney
pelvic (adj)	**PEL**-vic	S/ R/	-ic *pertaining to* pelv- *pelvis*	Pertaining to the pelvis
pubis	**PYU**-bis	S/	Latin *pubis*	Bony front arch of the pelvis of the hip; also called *pubic bone*
pubic (adj)	**PYU**-bik	R/	-ic *pertaining to* pub- *pubis*	Pertaining to the pubis
sacrum	**SAY**-crum		Latin *sacred*	Segment of the vertebral column that forms part of the pelvis
sacral (adj)	**SAY**-kral	S/ R/	-al sacr- *sacrum*	In the neighborhood of the sacrum
sacroiliac joint	say-kroh-**ILL**-ih-ak JOYNT	S/ R/CF R/	-ac sacr/o- *sacrum* ili- *ilium* **joint** Middle English *joint*	The joint between the sacrum and ilium

Exercises

A. Match the language of the pelvic girdle to the correct definitions. *Match the definition in the first column with its correct term in the second column.* **LO 14.20**

_____ **1.** receives head of femur

_____ **2.** cup-shaped ring of bones

_____ **3.** posterior part of hip bone

_____ **4.** bony anterior arch of the pelvis

_____ **5.** wing-shaped bone, upper part of pelvis

_____ **6.** segment of vertebral column

_____ **7.** thigh bone

a. sacrum

b. ilium

c. pubis

d. femur

e. pelvis

f. ischium

g. acetabulum

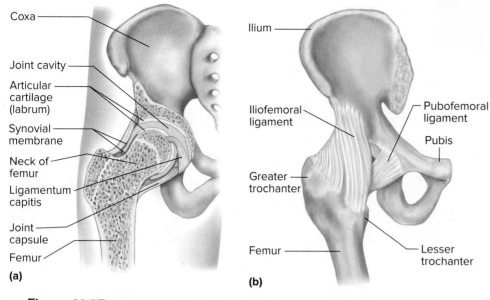

Coxa

Joint cavity

Articular
cartilage
(labrum)

Synovial
membrane

Neck of
femur

Ligamentum
capitis

Joint
capsule

Femur

(a)

Ilium

Iliofemoral
ligament

Greater
trochanter

Femur

(b)

Pubofemoral
ligament

Pubis

Lesser
trochanter

▲ **Figure 14.27** Hip Joint. (*a*) Right frontal view of a section of hip joint. (*b*) Ligaments of hip joint.

LO 14.22 Bones and Joints of the Hip and Thigh

The hip joint is a ball-and-socket synovial joint between the head of the femur and the cup-shaped **acetabulum** of the hip bone (*Figure 14.27a*). A ligament (ligamentum capitis) attached to the head of the femur from the lining of the acetabulum carries blood vessels to the head of the femur to nourish it.

The joint is held in place by a thick joint **capsule** reinforced by strong ligaments that connect the neck of the femur to the rim of the acetabulum (*Figure 14.27*).

The **labrum** is the cartilage that forms a rim around the socket of the joint; it cushions the joint and helps keep the head of the femur in place in the socket.

LO 14.23 Disorders and Injuries of the Hip Joint

Hip pointer, usually a football-related injury, is a blow to the rim of the pelvis that leads to bruising of the bone and surrounding tissues.

Osteoarthritis is common in the hip as a result of aging, weight bearing, and repetitive use of the joint. The cartilage on both the acetabulum and the head of the femur degenerates, and eventually there is total loss of the cartilage cushion. The resulting friction between the bones of the head of the femur and the acetabulum leads to pain and loss of mobility.

Rheumatoid arthritis (RA) also can affect the hip, beginning in the synovial membrane and progressing to destroy cartilage and bone.

Avascular necrosis of the femoral head is the necrosis (death) of bone tissue when the blood supply becomes avascular (is cut off), usually as a result of trauma.

Fractures of the neck of the femur occur as a result of falls, most commonly in elderly women with osteoporosis.

WORD	PRONUNCIATION	ELEMENTS		DEFINITION
arthritis	ar-**THRIE**-tis	S/ R/	-itis *inflammation* arthr- *joint*	Inflammation of a joint or joints
avascular	ay-**VAS**-cue-lar	S/ P/ R/	-ar *pertaining to* a- *without* vascul- *blood vessel*	Without a blood supply
labrum	**LAY**-brum		Latin *lip-shaped*	Cartilage that forms a rim around the socket of the hip joint
necrosis	neh-**KROH**-sis	S/ R/	-osis *condition* necr- *death*	Pathologic death of cells or tissue
necrotic (adj)	neh-**KROT**-ik	S/ R/CF	-tic *pertaining to* necr/o- *death*	Affected by necrosis

Exercises

A. Continue working with the *language of orthopedics.* *Demonstrate your knowledge of the terms by selecting the best answer to each of the following statements* **LO 14.22, 14.23**

1. The head of the femur fits into the _____ of the pelvis.
   a. sacrum
   b. acetabulum
   c. labrum
   d. foramen

2. Inflammation of the bone and joints:
   a. arthritis
   b. osteoarthritis
   c. necrosis
   d. avascular

3. Hip pointer injury results from a blow to the:
   a. femur
   b. sacrum
   c. pelvis
   d. pubic symphysis

4. *Avascular* means no
   a. living tissue
   b. tendon support
   c. movement
   d. blood supply
   e. inflammation

5. The cartilage that forms a ring around the hip joint:
   a. labrum
   b. pubis
   c. acetabulum
   d. symphysis

Case Report (CR) 14.6

Operative Report

Gail Griffith, age 17.

Preoperative Diagnosis: Traumatic ACL tear and tear of medial meniscus right knee.

Postoperative Diagnosis: Same.

Procedure Performed: Repair of medial collateral ligament, ACL reconstruction, repair of torn medial meniscus, right knee.

Operative Findings: An avulsed anterior cruciate ligament off the femoral condyle, with a tear of the posterior horn of the medial meniscus and a tear of the medial collateral ligament.

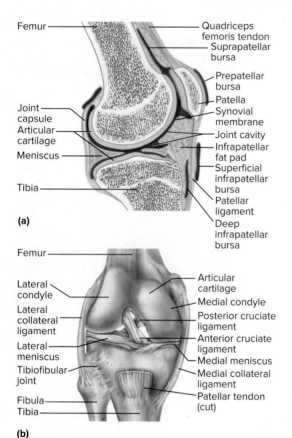

(a)

(b)

▲ **Figure 14.28** **Knee Joint.** (*a*) Section of knee joint. (*b*) Right knee joint: anterior view.

Abbreviations

ACL	anterior cruciate ligament
LCL	lateral collateral ligament
MCL	medial collateral ligament
PCL	posterior cruciate ligament

LO 14.24 Bones and Joints of the Knee and Thigh

Knee Joint

The knee is a hinged joint formed with four bones:

1. The lower end of the **femur**, shaped like a horseshoe. The two ends of the horseshoe are the medial and lateral femoral **condyles** (*Figure 14.28b*).

2. The flat upper end of the **tibia**.

3. The **patella** (kneecap), a flat triangular bone embedded in the **patellar tendon.** The patella articulates with the femur between its two **condyles** (*Figure 14.28a*).

4. The **fibula**, which forms a separate joint by articulating with the tibia. This is called the **tibiofibular joint** (*see Figure 14.28b*).

Mechanically, the role of the patella is to provide an increase of about 30% in the strength of extension of the knee joint.

Within the knee joint, two crescent-shaped pads of cartilage lie on top of the tibia to articulate with the femoral condyles. They are the **medial** and **lateral menisci**. Their function is to distribute weight more evenly across the joint surface to minimize wear and tear. They play a crucial role in joint stability, lubrication, and transmission of force.

The knee joint has a **fibrous capsule** lined with **synovial membrane** to secrete **synovial fluid,** which provides lubrication for the joint. The joint is held together by **ligaments.** The two ligaments outside the joint are the **medial collateral ligament (MCL)** and the **lateral collateral ligament (LCL).** Two other ligaments are located inside the joint cavity and are called the **anterior cruciate ligament (ACL)** and the **posterior cruciate ligament (PCL).** They cross over each other to form an "X" (*Figure 14.28b*). There are numerous bursae associated with the knee joint (*Figure 14.28a*). Their function is to aid the movement of the patella and the patellar tendon over the bones of the joint.

WORD	PRONUNCIATION	ELEMENTS		DEFINITION
collateral	koh-**LAT**-er-al	S/ P/ R/	-al *pertaining to* col- *before* -later- *side*	Situated at the side, often to bypass an obstruction
condyle	**KON**-dile		Greek *knuckle*	Large, smooth, rounded expansion of the end of a bone that forms a joint with another bone
cruciate	**KRU**-shee-ate		Latin *cross*	Shaped like a cross
fibula fibular (adj)	**FIB**-you-lah **FIB**-you-lar	S/ R/	Latin *clasp or buckle* -ar *pertaining to* fibul- *fibula*	The smaller of the two bones of the lower leg Pertaining to the fibula
lateral (opposite of medial)	**LAT**-er-al	S/ R/	-al *pertaining to* later- *side*	Situated at the side of a structure
medial (opposite of lateral)	**ME**-dee-al	S/ R/	-al *pertaining to* medi- *middle*	Nearer to the middle of the body
tibia tibial (adj)	**TIB**-ee-ah **TIB**-ee-al	S/ R/	Latin *large shinbone* -al *pertaining to* tibi- *tibia*	The larger bone of the lower leg Pertaining to the tibia

Exercises

A. Identify the structures that make up the knee joint. *Given the description, identify the structure that makes up the knee joint. Fill in the blanks.* **LO 14.24, 14.A**

1. This cartilage is tough and functions to cushion and add stability to the joint._____

2. This bone protects the anterior portion of the knee joint. It is embedded in a tendon. _____

3. The femur articulates with this leg bone. _____

4. This lower leg bone is on the lateral side of the leg. _____

5. Ligaments that form a "cross" are termed _____ ligaments.

6. Ligaments that stabilize the knee joints on the lateral and medial sides are termed _____ ligaments.

Gail Griffith, a 17-year-old, landed awkwardly after jumping for a ball during a basketball game. "My knee kinda popped as I landed." She had to be assisted off the court. In the Emergency Room, the knee was swollen and unstable. An MRI showed a complete tear of the medial collateral ligament, a complete tear of the anterior cruciate ligament (ACL), and a partial tear (avulsion) of the medial meniscus *(Figure 14.29)*. Gail decided to have surgery, even though full recovery would take 6 months to 1 year of rehabilitation.

LO 14.25 Common Disorders of the Knee

The anterior cruciate ligament (ACL) is the most commonly injured ligament in the knee *(Figure 14.29)*, particularly in female athletes. The injury is often caused by a sudden **hyperextension** of the knee joint when landing awkwardly on flat ground, as in Gail's injury. Because of its poor vascular supply, once torn the ligament does not heal. The knee becomes unstable, risking further joint damage and arthritis.

Other major ligaments that are commonly injured are the medial and lateral collateral ligaments and the posterior cruciate ligament.

Meniscus injuries result from a twist to the knee. Pain and locking are the result of the torn meniscus flipping in and out of the joint as it moves. Because loss of a meniscus leads to arthritic changes, repair of the meniscus, as in Gail's case, rather than removal is preferred. Removal of a meniscus is a **meniscectomy**.

Patellar problems produce pain that is noticed particularly when descending stairs. The force on the patella when descending stairs is about seven times body weight, compared to about two times body weight when ascending stairs.

Chondromalacia patellae (runner's knee) is caused by irritation of the undersurface of the patella.

Patellar subluxation or **dislocation** produces an unstable, painful kneecap.

Prepatellar bursitis (housemaid's knee) produces painful swelling over the bursa at the front of the knee and is seen in people who kneel for extended periods of time, such as carpet layers.

Anterior cruciate ligament (torn)

Medial collateral ligament (torn)

Medial meniscus (torn)

Patellar ligament (cut)

▲ **Figure 14.29** Gail Griffith's Knee.

WORD	PRONUNCIATION	ELEMENTS		DEFINITION
chondromalacia	**KON**-droh-mah-**LAY**-shee-ah	S/ R/CF	-malacia *abnormal softness* chondr/o- *cartilage*	Softening and degeneration of cartilage
hyperflexion	high-per-**FLEK**-shun	S/ P/ R/	-ion *action, condition* hyper- *excess* -flex- *bend*	Flexion of a limb or part beyond the normal limits
meniscus menisci (pl)	meh-**NISS**-kuss meh-**NISS**-kee		Greek *crescent*	Disc of connective tissue cartilage between the bones of a joint; for example, in the knee joint
patella (kneecap (syn)) patellae (pl) patellar (adj)	pah-**TELL**-ah pah-**TELL**-ee pah-**TELL**-ar	 S/ R/	 -ar *pertaining to* patell- *patella*	Thin, circular bone in front of the knee joint and embedded in the patellar tendon Pertaining to the patella (kneecap)
prepatellar	pree-pah-**TELL**-ar	P/	pre- *before, in front of*	In front of the patella

Exercises

A. Use medical terminology in written documentation. *June has come to the emergency department complaining of sudden knee pain. After reading the description, insert the medical term that correctly replaces the description in the reading that appears in italics.* **LO 14.25, 14.A**

June has just recently taken up the sport of running. She ran too many miles her first week, causing a sharp pain to develop *in front of her kneecap* 1.(_____). The physician believes that the pain is due to a *softening of the cartilage* 2.(_____) of the kneecap. June thought it best to not run long distances, and instead practice sprinting with sudden stopping and starting. This resulted in an *over extension of her knee* 3.(_____), which caused a sudden tearing of her ACL.

B. Proper use of singular and plural forms of medical terms. *Using the proper form of the term is critical for communication in healthcare. Select the correct term that completes each statement.* **LO 14.25, 14.A**

1. Datu turned awkwardly and tore a _____ in his right knee.

    a. menisci   **b.** meniscuses   **c.** meniscus

2. The car accident left her with bilateral fractures of the _____.

    a. patella   **b.** patellas   **c.** patellae

C. Disorders of the knee. *Select the correct answer that completes each statement.* **LO 14.25**

1. People with occupations that frequently kneel on the floor may suffer from a condition referred to as:

    a. prepatellar bursitis   **b.** chondromalacia patellae   **c.** patellar subluxation   **d.** a tears of the menisci

2. The medical term for the condition informally known as runner's knee is:

    a. prepatellar bursitis   **b.** chondromalacia patellae   **c.** patellar subluxation   **d.** a tear of the meniscus

Phalanges
Distal phalanx
Middle phalanx
Proximal phalanx

Metatarsals
First metatarsal

Fifth metatarsal

Tarsals
Medial cuneiform
Intermediate cuneiform
Lateral cuneiform
Navicular
Cuboid

Talus

Articular surface
for tibia

Calcaneus

Tuberosity of calcaneus

▲ **Figure 14.30** Twenty-Six Bones and 33 Joints of Right Foot.

LO 14.26 Bones and Joints of the Lower Leg, Ankle, and Foot

The two bones of the lower leg are the larger and medial **tibia** and the thinner and lateral **fibula**. The lower end of the tibia on its medial border forms a prominent process called the medial malleolus. The lower end of the fibula forms the lateral malleolus. You can **palpate** both these prominences at your own ankle.

The ankle has two joints:

1. One between the lateral malleolus of the fibula and the talus.
2. One between the medial malleolus of the tibia and the talus.

The **calcaneus** is the heelbone. The **talus** is the most superior of the seven **tarsal** bones of the ankle and proximal foot *(Figure 14.30)*, and its surface articulates with the tibia. The tarsal bones help the ankle bear the body's weight. Strong ligaments on both sides of the ankle joint hold it together.

Attached to the tarsal bones are the five parallel **metatarsal** bones that form the instep and then fan out to form the ball of the foot, where they bear weight. Each of the toes has three phalanges, except for the big toe, which has only two. This is identical to the thumb and its relation to the hand. The tendons of the leg muscles are inserted into the phalanges.

LO 14.27 Disorders of the Ankle and Foot

Podiatry is a health care specialty concerned with the diagnosis and treatment of disorders and injuries of the foot.

Bunions occur usually at the base of the big toe and are swellings of the bones that cause the metatarsophalangeal joint to be misaligned and stick out medially. This deformity is called **hallux valgus**.

Strains and sprains are more common in the ankle than in any other joint in the body. A strain is an acute injury resulting from overstretching or overcontraction of a muscle or tendon. A sprain is the result of an abnormal stretch or tear of a ligament. Some severe sprains with tearing of the ligament may require surgical repair.

Pott fracture is a term applied to a variety of fractures in which there is a fracture of the fibula near the ankle, often accompanied by a fracture of the medial malleolus of the tibia.

Plantar fasciitis is the overstretching or tearing of the dense sheet of fascia that supports the arch of the foot. If the plantar fascia is weak, **pes planus** (flatfoot) can be present.

Ingrown toenails are nails that grow into the skin folds on either side of the toe. They are often infected and painful and may need surgical repair.

Gout is an extremely painful arthritis of the big toe and other joints caused by a buildup of uric acid in the blood, which forms needlelike crystals that accumulate in the joints.

Talipes equinovarus is a congenital deformity of the foot. The foot is turned inwardly at the ankle and is commonly referred to as "clubfoot."

WORD	PRONUNCIATION		ELEMENTS	DEFINITION
bunion	**BUN**-yun		French *bump*	A swelling at the base of the big toe
calcaneus calcaneal (adj)	kal-**KAY**-nee-us kal-**KAY**-nee-al	 S/ R/	Latin *the heel* **-eal** *pertaining to* **calcan-** *calcaneus*	Bone of the tarsus that forms the heel Pertaining to the calcaneus
fasci̲itis (note spelling)	fash-ee-**IE**-tis	S/ R/	**-itis** *inflammation* **fasci-** *fascia*	Inflammation of the fascia
gout	GOWT		Latin *drop*	Painful arthritis of the big toe and other joints
hallux valgus	**HAL**-uks **VAL**-gus		**hallux** Latin *big toe* **valgus** Latin *turn out*	Deviation of the big toe toward the lateral side of the foot
metatarsus	**MET**-ah-**TAR**-sus	S/ P/ R/	**-us** *structure* **meta-** *behind* **-tars-** *ankle*	A collective term referring to the five parallel bones of the foot between the tarsus and the phalanges
metatarsal (adj)	**MET**-ah-**TAR**-sal	S/	**-al** *pertaining to*	Pertaining to the metatarsus
pes planus	PES **PLAY**-nuss		**pes** Latin *foot* **planus** Latin *flat surface*	A flat foot with no plantar arch
podiatry	poh-**DIE**-ah-tree	S/ R/	**-iatry** *treatment* **pod-** *foot*	Specialty concerned with the diagnosis and treatment of disorders and injuries of the foot
podiatrist	poh-**DIE**-ah-trist	S/	**-iatrist** *practitioner*	Practitioner of podiatry
Pott fracture	POT **FRAK**-chur	 S/ R/	Percival Pott, 1714–1788, London surgeon **-ure** *result of* **fract-** *break*	Fracture of lower end of fibula, often with fracture of tibial malleolus
talipes equinovarus	**TAL**-ip-eez ee-kwie-noh-**VAY**-rus	R/ R/ R/CF S/	**-pes** *foot* **tali-** *ankle bone* **equin/o-** *horse* **-varus** *bent inward, bow-legged*	Deformity of the foot involving the talus
talus	**TAY**-luss		Latin *heel bone*	The tarsal bone that articulates with the tibia to form the ankle joint
tarsus tarsal (adj)	**TAR**-sus **TAR**-sal	 S/ R/	Latin *flat surface* **-al** *pertaining to* **tars-** *tarsus*	The collection of seven bones in the foot that form the ankle and instep Pertaining to the tarsus

Exercises

A. Complete your knowledge of the skeleton by matching the statement in the left column to the appropriate term in the right column. LO 14.26, 14.27

_____ **1.** forms ankle joint

_____ **2.** flatfoot

_____ **3.** forms ankle and instep

_____ **4.** heel bone

_____ **5.** arthritis of big toe

_____ **6.** deviation of big toe

_____ **7.** swelling at base of big toe

_____ **8.** five parallel bones in the foot

_____ **9.** foot deformity involving talus

a. hallux valgus

b. gout

c. tarsus

d. talipes

e. pes planus

f. metatarsus

g. talus

h. calcaneus

i. bunion

Lesson 14.5

Procedures and Pharmacology

LO 14.28 Diagnostic Procedures for Skeletal Disorders

Because the bones are readily visible using x-rays, radiology is a common method to evaluate bone disorders. Radiography, CT scans, and MRI are frequently used to determine the presence of fractures or growths, such as tumors.

Arthrography is an x-ray of a joint taken after the injection of a contrast medium into the joint. A contrast medium makes the inside details of the joint visible.

Diagnostic arthroscopy is an exploratory procedure performed using an **arthroscope** to examine the internal compartments of a joint.

Osteoporosis

Women at risk for osteoporosis should have **bone mineral density (BMD)** screening using a **dual-energy x-ray absorptiometry (DEXA)** scan.

LO 14.29 Therapeutic Procedures for the Skeletal System

Arthroplasty, a total replacement of the hip joint with a metal **prosthesis**, is the most common hip surgery today; 150,000 total hip replacements **(THP)** are performed each year in the United States, mostly for osteoarthritis of the hip joint. The diseased parts of the joint are removed and replaced with artificial parts made of titanium, other metals, and ceramics *(Figure 14.31)*.

Arthrocentesis, the aspiration of fluid from the hip joint and replacement of the fluid with a steroid solution, is also performed frequently for osteoarthritis.

▲ **Figure 14.31** **Total Hip Replacement.** Colored x-ray of prosthetic hip. ©AJPhoto/Photo Researchers, Inc.

Treatment for SI Joint Pain

Fluoroscopic injection of local anesthetic into the joint can relieve the pain temporarily. Treatment is usually **stabilization** of the joint with a **brace** and physical therapy to strengthen the low-back muscles. Occasionally, **arthrodesis** of the joint is necessary.

Surgical Procedures of the Knee Joint

Arthrocentesis, aspiration of fluid from the knee joint, is used to establish a diagnosis by laboratory examination of the fluid and to drain off infected fluid.

Surgical arthroscopy, performed through an arthroscope, can be a **debridement** or removal of torn tissue such as a meniscus **(meniscectomy)** or a ligament. It also can be repair of a torn ligament by suturing, tendon autograft, or repair of a torn meniscus.

Arthroplasty involves a total replacement of the knee joint *(Figure 14.32)*, usually because of osteoarthritis of the joint. The lower end of the femur is replaced with a metal shell. The upper end of the tibia is replaced with a metal trough lined with plastic, and the back of the patella can be replaced with a plastic button.

Surgical Procedures of the Hand

Fasciectomy is the surgical removal of the hypertrophied connective tissue to release a contracture.

The retinaculum may need to be incised and released **(fasciotomy)**.

Arthrodesis is the surgical fixation of a joint to prevent motion. Bone graft, wires, screws, or a plate can be used to stabilize the joint.

Arthroplasty in this setting is the complete replacement of a damaged finger joint with an artificial joint made of silicone rubber.

Reattachment of amputated fingers is performed frequently. The bones are rejoined with plates, wires, or screws. The tendons are reconstructed. Nerves and blood vessels are joined back together by using microsurgical instruments.

▲ **Figure 14.32** **Total Knee Replacement.** Colored x-ray of total knee replacement of left knee. ©ChooChin/Shutterstock.com RF

S = Suffix   P = Prefix   R = Root   R/CF = Combining Form

WORD	PRONUNCIATION		ELEMENTS	DEFINITION
arthrocentesis	AR-throh-sen-TEE-sis	S/ R/CF	-centesis *to puncture* arthr/o *-joint*	Withdrawal of fluid from a joint with a needle
arthrodesis	AR-throh-DEE-sis	S/	-desis *bind together*	Fixation or stiffening of a joint by surgery
arthrography	ar-THROG-rah-fee	S/	-graphy *process of recording*	X-ray of a joint taken after injection of a contrast medium in the joint
arthroplasty	AR-throh-plas-tee	S/	-plasty *surgical repair*	Surgery to restore as far as possible the function of a joint
arthroscope	AR-throh-skope	S/	-scope *instrument for viewing*	Endoscope used to view the interior of a joint
arthroscopy	ar-THROS-koh-pee	S/	-scopy *to view*	Visual examination of the interior of a joint
debridement	day-BREED-mon	S/ P/ R/	-ment *action* de- *take away* -bride- *rubble*	The removal of injured or necrotic tissue
fasciectomy	fash-ee-EK-toh-mee	S/ R/	-ectomy *excision* fasci- *fascia*	Surgical removal of fascia
fasciotomy	fash-ee-OT-oh-mee	S/ R/	-tomy *incision* fasci/o- *fascia*	An incision through a band of fascia, usually to relieve pressure on underlying structures
meniscectomy	men-ih-SEK-toh-me	S/ R/	-ectomy *excision* menisc- *crescent, meniscus*	Excision (cutting out) of all or part of a meniscus
prosthesis	pros-THEE-sis		Greek *addition*	Manufactured substitute for a missing part of the body

Exercises

A. There are several procedures that are specific to the joint. *Use the medical terms below to correctly complete each sentence. Not all terms will be used. Fill in the blanks.* **14.28, 14.29, 14.A**

arthrocentesis   arthrodesis   arthroplasty   arthroscope   arthroscopy

Mr. Johansen is a 54-year-old-man complaining of chronic, intense wrist pain and swelling. Dr. Lee believes that the pain is due to overuse and joint instability as a consequence of Mr. Johansen's years of college cheerleading due to repeated lifting of female cheerleaders.

In order to relieve the swelling, (**1**) _____ of the wrist was performed. In order to visualize the joint, an (**2**) _____ was ordered. During the surgery, Dr. Lee utilized the (**3**) _____ to determine that the best course of action was to fuse the bones of the wrist. Therefore, an (**4**) _____ was performed.

B. Construct medical terms related to therapeutic procedures. *You are given definitions of medical terms along with a few word elements. Fill in the blanks with the missing word elements to create the medical term.* **LO 14.29, 14.C**

1. Surgicial removal of fascia: fasci /_____

2. Excision of a part of a mensicus: menisc /_____

3. Removal of necrotic tissue: _____ /_____/ment

4. An incision through facsci: fasci /_____ /_____

5. Surgical fixation of a joint: _____ /o/_____

LO 14.30 Pharmacology

For osteoporosis, calcium (1200 mg daily) and vitamin D (800 IU daily) are both the accepted baseline prevention and treatment.

For patients at risk of fractures, several medications approved by the U.S. **Food and Drug Administration (FDA)** are available for the treatment of osteoporosis. Most inhibit osteoclast activity to reduce the rate of loss of bone **(resorption)**, but some produce a direct increase in bone mass. As the turnover of bone is very slow, the time needed for assessing the effects of medications takes several years. Drugs that reduce the rate of bone resorption include estrogen, bisphosphonates, and calcitonin. **Bisphosphonates** *(Alendronate, Risedronate,* and others) are poorly absorbed from the gastrointestinal tract and can be given intravenously. **Calcitonin** also decreases osteoclast activity and is available as a subcutaneous injection or nasal spray. Several other drugs are available in other countries and/or are undergoing clinical trials in the United States.

Medications for osteoarthritis are numerous. **Acetaminophen** reduces mild pain but does not affect inflammation or swelling. It is used in combination with aspirin and/or caffeine *(Excedrin)* as an **OTC** medicine, and with codeine, propoxyphene *(Darvon),* or the narcotics hydrocodone *(Vicodin)* or oxycodone *(Percocet)* as prescription medications. Nonsteroidal anti-inflammatory drugs **(NSAIDs)** such as ibubrofen *(Advil)* and naproxen *(Aleve)* work well for pain but cause gastrointestinal problems and an increased risk of heart attacks and strokes.

Corticosteroids such as cortisone, prednisone, triamcinalone, and betamethsone, are used to reduce the pain and inflammation of severe osteoarthritis and are given orally or injected directly into the joint **(intra-articular).** Corticosteroids are also used to reduce inflammation in rheumatoid arthritis **(RA)** but do not slow the progression of the disease. **Disease modifying anti-rheumatic drugs (DMARDs)** such as methotrexate *(Trexall)* are effective in reducing the signs and symptoms of RA, and other DMARDs such as hydrochloroquine *(Plaquenil)* and sulfasalazine *(Azulfidine)* can be added to methotrexate to enhance its effects. **Tumor necrosis factor (TNF)** is produced in RA joints by synovial macrophages and lymphocytes to attack the joint tissues and TNF **inhibitors** such as abatacept *(Orencia)* and rituximab *(Rituxan)* slow or halt the destruction.

WORD	PRONUNCIATION	ELEMENTS		DEFINITION
acetaminophen	ah-seat-ah-**MIN**-oh-fen		Generic drug name	Medication that modifies or relieves pain
bisphosphonate	bis-**FOSS**-foh-nate	S/ P/ R/ R/	-ate *composed of* **bi-** *two* **-phos-** *light* **-phon-** *sound*	Drug that delays the rate of bone resorption
calcitonin	kal-sih-**TONE**-in	S/ R/CF R/	**-in** *chemical compound* **calci-** *calcium* **-ton-** *tension, pressure*	Hormone that moves calcium from blood to bones
corticosteroid	**KOR**-tih-koh-**STEHR**-oyd	S/ R/CF R/	**-oid** *resembling* **cortic/o-** *cortisone* **-ster-** *steroid*	A hormone produced by the adrenal cortex
inhibit (verb) inhibitor (noun)	in-**HIB**-it in-**HIB**-it-or		Latin *to keep back*	To curb or restrain Agent that curbs or restrains
intra-articular	**IN**-trah-ar-**TIK**-you-lar	S/ P/ R/	**-ar** *pertaining to* **intra-** *inside* **-articul-** *joint*	Pertaining to the inside of a joint

Exercises

A. Use terms related to pharmacology. *Use terms and abbreviations to complete the following paragraph. Use the terms provided. Not all terms will be used. Fill in the blanks.* **LO 14.30, 14.A, 14.E, 14.F**

DNARD   podiatrist   **RA**   **OTC**   chiropractor   acetaminophen   calcitonin   corticosteroid

Ms. Walker made an appointment with a _____ for pain in her shoulder. She participates in high-intensity weightlifting and fitness training. She has been taking _____ medication to treat the pain; specifically, the medication _____. She denies a personal or family history of _____.

B. Construct medical terms related to the pharmacology of the skeletal system. *Insert the correct word element that completes each term. Fill in the blanks.* **LO 14.30, 14.C**

1. Hormone that moves calcium from the blood to the bone: calc/i/_____/in

2. Hormone produced by the adrenal cortex: _____/_____/ster/oid

3. Pertaining to the inside of a joint: intra-_____/ar

Chapter 14 Review

©2014 Nucleus Medical Media

Bones and Joints of the Skeletal System

Challenge Your Knowledge

A. **Knowing the exact number of certain body parts, and their relative positions, will ensure precision in your medical documentation.** Match the correct number to the correct term. Use one answer twice. **(LO 14.9)**

_____ 1. Number of lumbar vertebrae: _____   **a.** 7

_____ 2. Number of bones in the vertebral column: _____   **b.** 5

_____ 3. Number of cervical vertebrae: _____   **c.** 4

_____ 4. Number of components in the skeletal system: _____   **d.** 12

_____ 5. Number of regions in the vertebral column: _____   **e.** 26

_____ 6. Number of thoracic vertebrae: _____

B. **Match the health professional in the second column with his or her job description in the first column.** **(LO 14.E)**

_____ 1. Practitioner in the diagnosis and treatment of disorders and injuries of the foot   **a.** orthotist

_____ 2. Practitioner who evaluates and treats pain, disease, or injury by measures   **b.** physiatrist

other than medical or surgical

_____ 3. Practitioner who makes and fits orthopedic appliances   **c.** podiatrist

_____ 4. Physician who specializes in physical medicine and rehabilitation   **d.** chiropractor

_____ 5. Practitioner who focuses on manual adjustment of joints to maintain and restore health   **e.** physical therapist

C. **Correct spelling and formation of plurals are important in medical documentation.** Improve your skill with this exercise. Fill in the blanks the correct spelling of the singular term, and then form the plural. The plural form is not provided for you. **(LO 14.A)**

1. epiphysis   epipisis   ephysis   epyisis

Correct spelling of the term: _____

Plural form of the term: _____

2. laccuna   lacuna   lecuna   lacunna

Correct spelling of the term: _____

Plural form of the term: _____

3. thoraax   torax   thorax   thoraxx

Correct spelling of the term: _____

Plural form of the term: _____

4. palanx   phalanx   phalynx   palanyx

Correct spelling of the term: _____

Plural form of the term: _____

D. The following prefixes have all appeared in this chapter. The meaning of the prefix is given to you—identify the prefix. Fill in the chart. **(LO 14.A)**

Prefix	Meaning of Prefix
1.	*from, out of*
2.	*beyond, making change*
3.	*many*
4.	*without*
5.	*between*
6.	*inside*
7.	*together*
8.	*away from*
9.	*toward*
10.	*around*

E. Demonstrate your knowledge of the upper-body bones and joints by selecting the correct answer to these questions. (LO 14.5, 14.13, 14.14, 14.17, 14.29)

1. What is the long bone of the upper arm called?

a. radius

b. ulna

c. humerus

d. carpal

e. scapula

2. What is a likely shoulder injury?

a. separation

b. anterior cruciate ligament tear

c. Colles fracture

d. Carpal tunnel syndrome

3. What structures hold an articulation together?

a. ligaments

b. tendons

c. joint capsule

d. all of these

4. Incision through a band of fascia is called

a. arthrotomy

b. fasciectomy

c. arthrodesis

d. arthroplasty

e. fasciotomy

5. Where does a Colles fracture occur?

a. shoulder

b. hip

c. shoulder

d. elbow

e. wrist

©2014 Nucleus Medical Media

Bones and Joints of the Skeletal System

F. **Many medical terms come directly from Greek or Latin.** Match the term on the left with its correct Greek or Latin meaning on the right. **(LO 14.A)**

Medical Term

_____ 1. bursa

_____ 2. callus

_____ 3. cartilage

_____ 4. condyle

_____ 5. cortex

_____ 6. lacuna

_____ 7. ligament

_____ 8. matrix

Greek or Latin Meaning

a. mother, womb

b. bark

c. purse

d. hard skin

e. band, sheet

f. knuckle

g. pit, lake

h. gristle

G. **Read the description and then enter the abnormal spinal curvature that it is describing.** Some conditions are used more than once. **(LO 14.10)**

1. An abnormal lateral curvature of the spine: _____

2. An abnormal posterior curvature of the thoracic vertebrae: _____

3. An abnormal anterior curvature of the lumbar vertebrae: _____

4. Osteoporosis can lead to this abnormal spinal curvature: _____

5. Of the three types of abnormal curvatures, this one occurs most frequently: _____

H. **Physical therapists instruct patients in range-of-motion (ROM) exercises to improve mobility.** The exercises are described for you—determine the correct medical term. Use the provided word bank to fill in the blanks with the correct action being described. **(LO 14.6)**

abduction	lateral rotation	rotation	pronation	supination
inversion	circumduction	medial rotation	adduction	eversion

1. Rotating the humerus with the elbow flexed while bringing the palm of the hand toward the body: _____

2. Elbow flexed at 90 degrees, rotating forearm so that palm is facing the floor: _____

3. Sole of the foot facing toward the opposite foot: _____. This is also called _____.

4. Action of moving toward the midline: _____

5. Turning a joint on its axis: _____

6. Sole of the foot facing laterally away from the other foot: _____ or _____

7. Moving the shoulder so that it forms a cone with the shoulder joint as the apex of the cone: _____

8. Spreading fingers apart, away from the middle finger: _____

9. Moving the palm away from the body: _____

10. Lying flat on your back, palms facing up: _____

I. **Choose the correct medical term(s) from the list to complete the sentence.** You will not use all the terms. Use the provided word bank to fill in the blanks with the correct action being described. **(LO 14.1, 14.4, 14.27, 14.29)**

arthrodesis	symphysis	detoxification	intervertebral discs
prosthesis	cancellous	circumduction	pelvis
retinaculum	shoulder girdle	cortex	acetabulum
Colles	arthrocentesis	Pott	labrum

1. Removal of excess fluid from a joint: _____.

2. A transverse, fibrous band on the wrist is called a _____.

3. _____ support and cushion the vertebral column.

4. A fracture of the fibula near the ankle is called a _____ fracture.

5. Moving the arms in a circular motion is termed _____.

6. Cartilaginous joint between two bones is called _____.

7. A _____ is a cartilage rim along a ball and socket joint.

8. Dr. Stannard performed a(n) _____ to remove the excess fluid from the knee.

9. An artificial limb is an example of a _____.

10. The _____ is the hard outer bone shell.

Bones and Joints of the Skeletal System

J. **Many professional certification exams are given in multiple-choice format.** Decide on the answer by quickly eliminating the answers you know to be incorrect. Then select the remaining answer that correctly completes each statement. **(LO 14.2, 14.3, 14.5, 14.6, 14.27, 14.29)**

1. Bone growth occurs at the

   a. origin   d. epicondyle

   b. epiphyseal plate   e. lacuna

   c. diaphysis

2. An inherited condition in which bone formation is incomplete is

   a. osteoarthritis   d. osteogenesis imperfecta

   b. osteomalacia   e. osteopenia

   c. osteomyelitis

3. Lubricant for joint movement is

   a. mucin   d. synovial

   b. mucus   e. meniscus

   c. mucous

4. The following is where two bones come together at a joint:

   a. articulation   d. striation

   b. reduction   e. herniation

   c. mastication

5. An extension of synovial membrane that forms a cushion to prevent structures from rubbing together is

   a. tendon   d. bursa

   b. periosteum   e. muscle

   c. ligament

6. Pulling a bone from the distal end back into alignment is

   a. subluxation   d. resorption

   b. dislocation   e. external fixation

   c. reduction

7. The process of lying face upward, flat on your spine, is

   a. pronation   d. supination

   b. abduction   e. inversion

   c. adduction

8. Overstretching or tearing of the dense sheet of tissue that supports the arch of the foot is

   a. pes planus   d. Achilles tendinitis

   b. plantar fasciitis   e. exostosis

   c. hallux valgus

9. Joints between the teeth and their sockets are called

   a. symphyses   d. syndesmoses

   b. gomphoses   e. synchondroses

   c. sutures

K. **Build your orthopedic terminology by completing the medical terms defined here.** After you fill in the element on the line, write the type of element (prefix, root, combining form, suffix) you have used below the lines. Fill in the blanks. **(LO 14.1, 14.2, 14.3, 14.C)**

1. Removing poison from tissue   de/ _____ / _____

2. Bone softening   osteo/_____

3. Projection above the condyle   _____ /condyle

4. Membrane surrounding a bone   peri/ _____ / _____

5. Region between diaphysis and epiphysis   _____ /physis

6. Decreased calcification of bone   osteo/ _____

7. Bone cell that lives in a lacuna   osteo/ _____

8. Malignant tumor of connective tissue   _____ /oma

9. Moving toward the midline   _____ / _____ /ion

10. Fixation of a joint with surgery   arthro/ _____

L. **Post the OR schedule for the Orthopedic Department.** Convert the description into a medical term for billing the procedure. Fill in the chart. **(LO 14.28, 14.29, 14.A)**

Description	Medical Term
insertion right-hip prosthesis	1.
removing dead tissue from an open wound of the leg	2.
scope examination of left shoulder	3.
surgical removal of torn meniscus of left knee	4.
withdrawal of fluid from the right knee	5.
removal of gangrenous right leg	6.
surgical removal of hypertrophied connective tissue to release a contracture	7.

©2014 Nucleus Medical Media

Bones and Joints of the Skeletal System

M. Identify the elements in each medical term and unlock the meaning of the word. Fill in the chart. If the word does not have a particular word element, write n/a. (**LO 14.D**)

Medical Term	Meaning of Prefix	Meaning of Root/ Combining Form	Meaning of Suffix	Meaning of the Term
syndesmosis	1.	2.	3.	4.
osteogenesis	5.	6.	7.	8.
subluxation	9.	10.	11.	12.
periosteal	13.	14.	15.	16.
pectoral	17.	18.	19.	20.
hyperflexion	21.	22.	23.	24.

N. Write the correctly spelled terms for each of the following definitions. (**LO 14.2, 14.10, 14.12, 14.20, 14.29, 14.A**)

1. Incision and release of retinaculum _____

2. Tailbone _____

3. Joint formed by ligaments _____

4. Lower/posterior part of the hip bone _____

5. Compact bone grows in and forms this line _____

6. Shoulder blades _____

7. Posterior spinal curve _____

O. **Using your knowledge of the terminology in the following report, choose the correct answers for the following questions.** (LO 14.16, 14.A, 14.E, 14.F)

 Case Report (CR) 14.5

You are

. . . an orthopedic technologist working with Kenneth Stannard, MD, at Fulwood Medical Center.

Your patient is

. . . James Fox, a 17-year-old male who complains of severe pain in his right wrist. While playing soccer a few hours earlier, he fell. James pushed his hand out to break his fall and heard his wrist snap. The wrist is now swollen and deformed.

VS are T 98.2, P 92, R 15, BP 110/76. On examination, his right wrist is swollen and tender and has a dinner-fork deformity. An IV has been started, and he has been given 3 mg of morphine IV. An x-ray of the wrist was ordered and reveals a closed Colles Fx.

1. What type of physician is Dr. Stannard?

   a. podiatrist

   b. orthotist

   c. orthopedist

   d. chiropractor

2. The fracture has been described as *closed:*

   a. bones are out of placement

   b. the skin is unbroken

   c. bones are shifted laterally

   d. it is complex and requires surgery

3. The abbreviation *Fx* means:

   a. fracture

   b. fixation

   c. flexion

   d. febrile

4. Why was James given morphine?

   a. reduce swelling

   b. decrease the respiratory rate

   c. reduce the elevated blood pressure

   d. treat the pain

5. In a Colles Fx, a bone that is likely affected is:

   a. ulna

   b. humerus

   c. radius

   d. phalange

©2014 Nucleus Medical Media

The health professionals involved in the diagnosis and treatment of problems of the musculo-skeletal system include:

- **Physiatrists,** who are physicians specializing in physical medicine and rehabilitation.

- **Physical therapists,** who evaluate and treat pain, disease, or injury by physical therapeutic measures as opposed to medical and surgical measures.

- **Physical therapist assistants,** who work under the direction of a physical therapist to assist patients with their physical therapy.

- **Occupational therapists,** who practice occupational therapy (OT) to help patients improve their activities of daily living (ADLs) and adapt to visual and other perceptual deficits.

- **Occupational therapy assistants** (COTAs), who assist occupational therapists.

- **Orthopedic technologists and technicians,** who assist orthopedic surgeons in treating patients.

- **Orthotists,** who make and fit orthopedic appliances (**orthotics**).

Chapter Learning Outcomes

Bones of the skeleton support the body and joints provide mobility between two or more bones. Neither of these functions can occur without attached muscles and their tendons. Information in this chapter provides correct medical terminology to:

LO 15.1   Identify the three different types of muscle in relation to their functions.

LO 15.2   Describe the functions and structure of skeletal muscle.

LO 15.3   Discuss the common disorders of skeletal muscle.

LO 15.4   Describe the muscles and tendons of the shoulder girdle, trunk, and upper limb and their common disorders.

LO 15.5   Describe the muscles and tendons of the pelvic girdle, thigh, leg, and foot.

LO 15.6   Explain diagnostic procedures used in disorders of skeletal muscle and physical medicine and rehabilitation.

LO 15.7   Describe pharmacologic agents used in the treatment of disorders of skeletal muscle and in physical medicine and rehabilitation.

LO 15.8   Define the different types of physical medicine and rehabilitation.

LO 15.9   Discuss the specific areas of stroke rehabilitation and amputations.

LO 15.A   Use the medical terms of the muscular system and rehabilitation to communicate in writing and document accurately and precisely in any health care setting.

LO 15.B   Use the medical terms of the muscular system and rehabilitation to communicate verbally with accuracy and precision in any health care setting.

LO 15.C   Construct medical terms used in rehabilitation medicine from their word elements (roots, combining forms, prefixes, and suffixes).

LO 15.D   Deconstruct medical terms used in rehabilitation medicine into their word elements (roots, combining forms, prefixes, and suffixes).

LO 15.E   Identify health professionals working in muscle disorders and rehabilitation medicine.

LO 15.F   Use abbreviations of medical terms used in rehabilitation medicine.

 ## Case Report (CR) 15.1

You are

. . . an emergency technician working in the Emergency Department at Fulwood Medical Center

Your patient is

. . . Mr. Bruce Adams, a 55-year-old construction worker.

Mr. Adams presents with severe pain in his right shoulder that has made him leave work and seek relief. The pain began 3 or 4 months ago; it is worse at the end of the workday and when he has to work with his arm above the shoulder. In the past week, the pain has awakened him from sleep.

The company physician has diagnosed shoulder bursitis and treated Mr. Adams with anti-inflammatory medication and a heating pad. Mr. Adams has no previous history of work injuries. Physical examination shows marked limitation by pain of all passive and active movements of the right shoulder and weakness in all lifting movements.

Lesson 15.1

MUSCULAR SYSTEM

Muscles and Tendons

Bones of the skeleton support the body and joints provide mobility. Neither of these functions can occur without muscles and their tendons to provide both posture and movement. Information in this lesson will enable you to use correct medical terminology to:

15.1.1 Differentiate the three types of muscle.

15.1.2 Describe the structure of skeletal muscle and tendons.

15.1.3 Identify the functions of skeletal muscle and tendons.

15.1.4 Describe the major problems and diseases that occur in muscles and tendons.

Keynotes

- The **origin** of a muscle is its attachment to a more fixed part of the skeleton.
- The **insertion** of a muscle is its attachment to a more movable part of the skeleton.

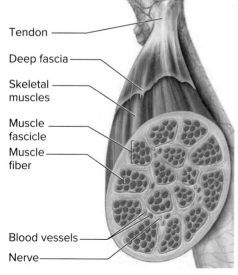

▲ **Figure 15.2** **Structure of Skeletal Muscle.**

Tendon

Deep fascia

Skeletal muscles

Muscle fascicle

Muscle fiber

Blood vessels

Nerve

LO 15.1 Types of Muscle

The three types of muscle are:

- **skeletal**
- **cardiac**
- **smooth**

Skeletal muscle contracts on demand to provide posture and movement.

Cardiac and smooth muscle contract and relax without conscious thought, cardiac muscle to power the heart contractions and smooth muscle to power the movement of food through the gastrointestinal tract (*see Chapter 5*), the process called **peristalsis**.

LO 15.2 Functions and Structure of Skeletal Muscle

Functions of Skeletal Muscle

Skeletal muscle is attached to one or more bones. It is also called **voluntary muscle** because it is under conscious control. Because of their length, muscle cells are usually called muscle **fibers**. Each skeletal muscle consists of bundles of muscle fibers, blood vessels, and nerves, with connective tissue sheets that hold the fibers together and connect the muscle to bone.

Skeletal muscle has the following functions:

1. **Movement.** All skeletal muscles are attached to bones, and when a muscle **contracts**, it causes movement of the bones to which it is attached (*Figure 15.1*). This enables you to walk, run, and work with your hands.

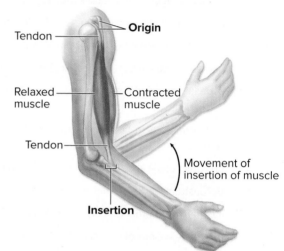

▲ **Figure 15.1** **Muscle Contraction.**

Tendon

Origin

Relaxed muscle

Contracted muscle

Tendon

Movement of insertion of muscle

Insertion

2. **Posture.** The **tone** of skeletal muscles holds you straight when sitting, standing, or moving.

3. **Body heat.** When skeletal muscles contract, heat is produced as a by-product of the energy reaction. This heat is essential to maintain your body temperature.

4. **Respiration.** Skeletal muscles move the chest wall as you breathe.

5. **Communication.** Skeletal muscles enable you to speak, write, type, gesture, and grimace.

Structure of Skeletal Muscle

Skeletal muscle **fibers** (*Figure 5.2*) are narrow and long, up to 1½ inches (approximately 3.7 cm) in length. Each muscle fiber has a thin layer of connective tissue around it. Bundles of muscle fibers are grouped together into **fascicles** that are also surrounded by a layer of connective tissue. Skeletal muscle fibers contain alternating dark and light bands (**striations**) created by the pattern of protein filaments responsible for muscle contraction. Skeletal muscle can be referred to as **striated muscle**.

Bundles of fascicles form a muscle that is separated from adjacent muscles and kept in position by a dense layer of connective tissue called **fascia**. Fascia extends beyond the muscle to form a tendon. The tendon attaches to the **periosteum** of a bone at the origin and insertion of the muscle.

As an adult, you have the same number of muscle fibers as you had in late childhood. When you exercise and/or lift weights and your muscles enlarge or **hypertrophy**, you have increased the thickness of each muscle fiber. If you do not use your muscles, the reverse happens, and the muscles **atrophy**.

WORD	PRONUNCIATION	ELEMENTS		DEFINITION
atrophy	**AT**-roh-fee	P/ R/	**a-** *without* **-trophy** *nourishment*	The wasting away or diminished volume of tissue, an organ, or a body part
contract	kon-**TRAKT**	P/ R/	**con-** *with, together* **-tract** *draw*	Draw together or shorten
fascia	**FASH**-ee-ah		Latin *a band*	Sheet of fibrous connective tissue
fascicle	**FAS**-ih-kull		Latin *small bundle*	Bundle of muscle fibers
fiber	**FIE**-ber		Latin *fiber*	A strand or filament
hypertrophy	high-**PER**-troh-fee	P/ R/	**hyper-** *excessive* **-trophy** *nourishment*	Increase in size, but not in number, of an individual tissue element
insert (verb) insertion	in-**SIRT** in-**SIR**-shun	S/ R/	Latin *to join* **-ion** *action, condition* **insert-** *put together*	The insertion of a muscle is the attachment of a muscle to a more movable part of the skeleton, as distinct from the origin
origin	**OR**-ih-gin		Latin *source of*	Fixed source of a muscle at its attachment to bone
orthotic	or-**THOT**-ik	S/ R/	**-ic** *pertaining to* **orthot-** *correct*	Orthopedic appliance to correct an abnormality
orthotist	or-**THOT**-ist	S/	**-ist** *specialist*	Specialist who makes and fits orthopedic appliances
peristalsis	per-ih-**STAL**-sis	P/ R/	**peri-** *around* **-stalsis** *constrict*	Waves of alternate contraction and relaxation of the alimentary canal wall to move food along the digestive tract
striated muscle	**STRIE**-ay-ted **MUSS**-el		**striated** Latin *stripe* **muscle** Latin *muscle*	Another term for skeletal muscle
striation	strie-**AY**-shun	S/ R/	**-ion** *action, condition* **striat-** *stripe*	Stripes
tone	TONE		Greek *tone*	Tension present in resting muscles
voluntary muscle	**VOL**-un-tare-ee **MUSS**-el	S/ R/	**-ary** *pertaining to* **volunt-** *free will* **muscle** Latin *muscle*	Another term for skeletal muscle. It is under the control of the will

Exercises

A. Deconstruct the following medical terms related to muscles into their basic elements. *Fill in the chart. If the word does not have a particular word element, write n/a.* **LO 15.1, 15.2, 15.D**

Medical Term	Prefix	Meaning of Prefix	Root/ Combining Form	Meaning of Root/ Combining Form	Suffix	Meaning of Suffix
hypertrophy	1.	2.	3.	4.	5.	6.
contract	7.	8.	9.	10.	11.	12.
atrophy	13.	14.	15.	16.	17.	18.

B. Use terms related to skeletal muscle to answer the following questions. *Fill in the blank to complete each statement correctly.* **LO 15.2**

1. Skeletal muscle also can be referred to as _____ muscle.

2. Skeletal muscle attaches to _____.

3. Skeletal muscle is under conscious control; therefore, it is considered a _____ muscle.

4. Skeletal muscle must be used, or _____ (condition) occurs.

LO 15.3 Disorders of Skeletal Muscles

Muscle soreness may be a result of vigorous exercise, particularly if your muscles are not used to it. Exercise causes buildup of lactic acid in muscle fibers, and the resulting inflammation of them and their surrounding connective tissue produces soreness.

Muscle cramps are sudden, painful contractions of a muscle or group of muscles. They are usually of short duration. The etiology of cramps is unknown, but low blood potassium, calcium, and magnesium levels; use of caffeine and tobacco; and diminished blood supply are possible causes. There are no effective medications available. The cramp is usually self-limiting.

Muscle strains range from a simple stretch in the muscle or **tendon** to a partial or complete tear in the muscle or muscle-tendon combination. A **sprain** is a stretching or tearing of a ligament.

Fibromyalgia affects muscles and tendons all over the body, causing chronic pain associated with fatigue and depression. Its etiology is unknown. There are no laboratory tests for it and no specific treatment except pain management, physiotherapy, and stress reduction.

Polymyalgia rheumatica is an inflammatory disease of muscles that causes pain and stiffness on both sides of the body, particularly in the shoulders, neck, upper arms, buttocks, and thighs with a general feeling of not being well. Most people who develop this disorder are older than 65.

Myasthenia gravis is a chronic autoimmune disease *(see Chapter 12)* characterized by varying degrees of weakness of the skeletal muscles. The weakness increases with activity and decreases with rest. Facial muscles are often involved, causing problems with eye and eyelid movements, chewing, and talking. Antibodies produced by the body's own immune system block the passage of **neurotransmitters** from motor nerves to muscles.

Muscular dystrophy is a general term for a group of hereditary, progressive disorders affecting skeletal muscles. **Duchenne muscular dystrophy (DMD)** is the most common, occurring in boys, who begin to have difficulty walking around the age of 3. Generalized muscle weakness and atrophy progress, and few live beyond 20 years. There is no effective treatment.

Rhabdomyolysis is the breakdown of muscle fibers. This releases a protein pigment called **myoglobin** into the bloodstream. Myoglobin breaks down into toxic compounds that cause kidney failure. Rhabdomyolysis can be caused by muscle trauma; severe exertion (marathon running); alcoholism; and use of cocaine, heroin, amphetamines, or phencyclidine (**PCP**).

Tenosynovitis is inflammation of the sheath that surrounds a **tendon**. It is usually related to repetitive use, occurs commonly in the wrist and hands in computer users, and is beginning to be seen in the thumbs of frequent texters. It produces pain, tenderness in the tendon, and difficulty in movement of a joint. Treatment is rest, immobilization, nonsteroidal anti-inflammatory drugs (**NSAIDs**), local corticosteroid injections, and, occasionally, surgery.

Achilles tendinitis results from a small stretch injury that causes the tendon to become swollen and painful. A larger partial or complete tear leads to loss of function with difficulty in walking and no ability to "push off."

Abbreviations

DMD	Duchenne muscular dystrophy
NSAID	nonsteroidal anti-inflammatory drug
PCP	phencyclidine

WORD	PRONUNCIATION		ELEMENTS	DEFINITION
Duchenne muscular dystrophy	DOO-shen MUSS-kyu-lar DISS-troh-fee	S/ R/ P/ R/	Guillaume Benjamin Duchenne, 1806–1875, French neurologist -ar *pertaining to* muscul- *muscle* dys- *bad, difficult* -trophy *nourishment*	A condition with symmetrical weakness and wasting of pelvic, shoulder, and proximal limb muscles
fibromyalgia	fie-broh-my-AL-jee-ah	S/ R/CF R/	-algia *pain* fibr/o- *fiber* -my- *muscle*	Pain in the muscle fibers
myoglobin	MY-oh-GLOH-bin	S/ R/CF R/	-in *substance* my/o- *muscle* -glob- *globe*	Protein of muscle that stores and transports oxygen
neurotransmitter (*Note:* Transmitter is a word in itself and begins with a prefix.)	NYUR-oh-trans-MIT-er	S/ R/CF P/ R/	-er *agent* neur/o- *nerve* -trans- *across* -mitt- *to send*	Chemical agent that relays messages from one nerve cell to the next
rhabdomyolysis	RAB-doh-my-oh-LIE-sis	S/ R/CF R/CF	-lysis *destruction* rhabd/o- *rod shaped* -my/o- *muscle*	Destruction of muscle to produce myoglobin
strain	STRAIN		Latin *to bind*	Overstretch or tear in a muscle or tendon
sprain	SPRAIN		Old English *tear*	A stretching or tearing of ligaments
tendon tendinitis (also spelled tendonitis)	TEN-dun ten-dih-NIE-tis	S/ R/	Latin *sinew* -itis *inflammation* tendin- *tendon*	Fibrous band that connects muscle to bone Inflammation of a tendon
tenosynovitis	TEN-oh-sine-oh-VIE-tis	S/ R/CF R/	-itis *inflammation* ten/o- *tendon* -synov- *synovial membrane*	Inflammation of a tendon and its surrounding synovial sheath

Exercises

A. The following elements are all contained in the above WAD. *Choose the best answer.* **LO 15.3, 15.D**

1. *Dys* is a

   a. suffix   b. prefix   c. root

2. *Fibro* is a

   a. combining form   b. root   c. suffix

B. Interpret definitions of medical terms. *Read the following sentences and determine the condition the patient is likely suffering from. Use the terms from the WAD above. Fill in each blank.* **LO 15.3, 15.A**

1. The patient made an appointment with the nurse practioner. She was complaining of chronic pain and fatigue, and had symptoms of depression. The probable diagnosis is _____.

2. Jon just completed his second marathon. He is now feeling quite ill and visits the emergency department. The note states that he is in acute kidney failure. The physician determines that the patient likely has the muscular condition _____.

3. After five years of no routine exercise, Analisa has decided to begin an aggressive weight-lifting program. The next day she is very sore and it is painful to move from a sitting to a standing position. After consulting a physician assistant, she is diagnosed with severe muscle _____.

4. Over the weekend, Marcus painted his mother's kitchen and living room. On Monday, his hands were achy and painful. He is likely suffering from _____ of the hands.

Muscles and Tendons of the Shoulder Girdle, Trunk, and Upper Limb

The muscles and tendons of your shoulders, arms, and hands are nearly always in motion. You shake hands, point your finger, use a computer, turn doorknobs, and lift various objects throughout the course of any given day. The information in this lesson will enable you to use correct medical terminology to:

15.2.1 Describe the structures and functions of the muscles and tendons of the shoulder girdle.

15.2.2 Identify the common disorders of the muscles and tendons of the shoulder girdle.

15.2.3 Specify the major muscles that join the arm to the trunk.

15.2.4 Explain the structures and functions of the muscles of the arm, elbow, forearm, wrist, and hand.

15.2.5 Name common disorders of the joints, muscles, and tendons of the elbow.

15.2.6 Define common disorders of the joints and muscles of the hand.

Case Report (CR) 15.1 *(continued)*

When Dr. Stannard evaluated Mr. Adams, an MRI revealed a full-thickness tear of his **rotator cuff**. Mr. Adams has been scheduled for **ambulatory** surgery to repair the tear.

LO 15.4 Shoulder Girdle

Your **pectoral girdle (shoulder girdle)** connects your axial skeleton to your upper limbs and helps you to move these limbs. Without your shoulder girdle, you wouldn't be able to throw a ball, drive a car, or reach that top shelf of your closet or kitchen cabinet. In fact, you wouldn't be able to move your upper limbs.

The muscles and tendons in your shoulder girdle get plenty of use. Four muscles originate on your scapula, wrap around the shoulder joint, and fuse together. This fusion forms one large tendon (the **rotator cuff**), which is inserted into the humerus (*Figure 5.3*). Your rotator cuff keeps the ball of the humerus tightly in the scapula's socket and provides stability of the shoulder joint and the kind of strength needed by baseball pitchers.

The rotator cuff muscles are

1. Subscapularis
2. Supraspinatus
3. Infraspinatus
4. Teres minor

LO 15.4 Common Disorders of the Shoulder Girdle

Rotator cuff tears (a frequent injury to the shoulder girdle) are caused by wear and tear from overuse in work situations or in certain sports, such as baseball, football, and golf. These tears can be partial or complete (*Figure 15.3*).

Tendinitis of the shoulder joint is caused when the rotator cuff and/or biceps tendon becomes inflamed from overuse.

Bursitis, inflammation of the lubricating sac of the rotator cuff, also can be produced by overuse.

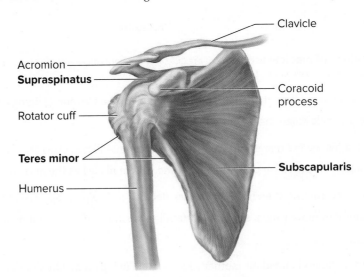

▲ **Figure 15.3** Rotator Cuff Muscles (Anterior view).

WORD	PRONUNCIATION		ELEMENTS	DEFINITION
ambulatory	**AM**-byu-lah-**TOR**-ee	S/ R/	**-ory** *having the function of* **ambulat-** *walking*	Surgery or any other care provided without an overnight stay in a medical facility
infraspinatus	**IN**-frah-spy-**NAY**-tuss	S/ P/ R/	**-us** *pertaining to* **infra-** *below, beneath* **-spinat-** *having spines*	Pertaining to beneath the spine (of the scapula)
rotator cuff	roh-**TAY**-tor CUFF	S/ R/	**-or** *one who does* **rotat-** *rotate* **cuff** Old English *band*	Part of the capsule of the shoulder joint
subscapularis	**SUB**-skap-you-**LA**-ris	S/ P/ R/	**-is** *pertaining to* **sub-** *below* **-scapular-** *scapula*	Pertaining to below the scapula
supraspinatus	sue-prah-spy-**NAY**-tuss	S/ P/ R/	**-us** *pertaining to* **supra-** *above* **-spinat-** *having spines*	Pertaining to above the spine (of the scapula)
teres major	**TER**-eze **MAY**-jor		**teres** Latin *long and round* **major** Latin *large*	One of the muscles that make up the rotator cuff

Exercises

A. Deconstruct the names of the muscles that make up the rotator cuff. *The prefix and root elements explain the location of each muscle. Select the answer that correctly completes each statement.* **LO 15.4**

1. The muscle that is located *above the spine of the scapula*:

   a. supraspinatus

   b. subscapularis

   c. infraspinatus

   d. teres major

2. The muscle that is described as *large, long, and round*:

   a. supraspinatus

   b. subscapularis

   c. infraspinatus

   d. teres major

3. This muscle has a root element that means the *shoulder blade*:

   a. supraspinatus

   b. subscapularis

   c. infraspinatus

   d. teres major

▲ **Figure 15.5** Muscles of Elbow Joint.

Abbreviation	
CTS	Carpal tunnel syndrome

▲ **Figure 15.6** Carpal Tunnel: Transverse Section.

▲ **Figure 15.7** Palmar Surface of the Hand. ©McGraw-Hill Education/Eric Wise, photographer

▲ **Figure 15.4** Muscles Join Arm to Body. (a) Anterior view. (b) Posterior view.

LO 15.4 Upper Arm and Elbow Joint

Muscles connect the humerus (upper arm bone) to the shoulder girdle, vertebral column, and ribs. These muscles enable the arm to move freely at the shoulder joint. The major anterior muscles (those at the front of the body) are the **deltoid** (shoulder muscle) and **pectoralis major** (chest muscle) (*Figure 15.4a*). Among the major posterior muscles is the **latissimus dorsi**, found in the back (*Figure 15.4b*).

Muscles that move the elbow joint and forearm have their **origins** on the humerus or pectoral girdle and are **inserted** into the bones of the forearm. On the front of the arm, a group of three muscles (the **biceps brachii**, **brachialis**, and **brachioradialis**) flexes the forearm at the elbow joint and rotates the forearm and hand laterally (supination) (*Figure 15.5*). On the back of the arm, a single muscle, the **triceps brachii**, extends the elbow joint and forearm.

Common Disorder of the Elbow

Tennis elbow is a common injury. Upper arm and forearm muscle tendons are inserted into the upper arm bone just above the elbow joint. Small tears in these tendons at their attachments can be caused by trauma or overuse of the elbow joint.

LO 15.4 Forearm, Wrist, and Hand

The muscles of the forearm are responsible for various movements. These muscles supinate and pronate the forearm (turning it upward and downward), flex and extend the wrist joint and hand, and move the hand medially and laterally (back and forth cross ways). These terms of movement are detailed in Chapter 3.

Common Disorders of the Wrist

Because you use your hands and wrists almost constantly, your wrists can be prone to disorders and injuries.

Ganglion cysts are fluid-filled cysts on the back of the wrist that result from irritation or inflammation of the synovial tendon sheaths in this area. These cysts usually disappear on their own.

Stenosing tenosynovitis is a painful inflammation of the synovial sheaths on the back of the wrist.

Carpal tunnel syndrome (CTS) develops on the front of the wrist and results from inflammation and swelling of overused tendon sheaths (*Figure 15.6*). Repetitive movements, like typing on a computer keyboard, can lead to CTS. A feeling of "pins and needles" or pain and loss of muscle power in the thumb side of the hand are common.

The Hand

When you look at the palm of your hand, you'll see a prominent pad of muscles (the **thenar eminence**) at the base of your thumb (*Figure 15.7*). A smaller pad of muscles (the **hypothenar eminence**) is located at the base of your little finger. The back of your hand is called the **dorsum**.

WORD	PRONUNCIATION	ELEMENTS		DEFINITION
biceps brachii	**BIE**-sepz **BRAY**-kee-eye	R/ P/ R/CF	-ceps *head* bi- *two* brachi/i *of the arm*	A muscle of the arm that has two heads or points of origin on the scapula
brachialis	**BRAY**-kee-al-is	S/ R/	-alis *pertaining to* brachi- *arm*	Muscle that lies underneath the biceps and is the strongest flexor of the forearm
brachioradialis	**BRAY**-kee-oh-**RAY**-dee-al-is	S/ R/CF R/	-alis *pertaining to* brachi/o- *arm* -radi- *radius*	Muscle that helps flex the forearm
cyst	SIST		Greek *fluid-filled sac*	An abnormal, fluid-containing sac
deltoid	**DEL**-toyd	S/ R/	-oid *resembling* delt- *triangle*	Large, fan-shaped muscle connecting the scapula and clavicle to the humerus
dorsum dorsal (adj)	**DOR**-sum **DOR**-sal	S/ R/	Latin *back* -al *pertaining to* dors- *back*	The back of any part of the body, including the hand Pertaining to the back of any part of the body
ganglion	**GANG**-lee-on		Greek *swelling*	Fluid-containing swelling attached to the synovial sheath of a tendon
latissimus dorsi	lah-**TISS**-ih-muss **DOR**-sigh	S/ R/ R/	-imus *most* latiss- *wide* dorsi *of the back*	The widest (broadest) muscle in the back
stenosis	steh-**NOH**-sis	S/ R/CF	-sis *abnormal condition* sten/o- *narrow*	Narrowing of a passage
thenar eminence	**THAY**-nar **EM**-in-ens	R/	thenar *palm* eminence Latin *stand out*	The fleshy mass at the base of the thumb
hypothenar eminence	high-poh-**THAY**-nar **EM**-in-ens	P/	hypo- *below, smaller*	The fleshy mass at the base of the little finger
triceps brachii	**TRY**-sepz **BRAY**-kee-eye	R/ P/ R/CF	-ceps *head* tri- *three* brachi/i *of the arm*	Muscle of the arm that has three heads or points of origin

Exercises

A. Name the muscles of the upper arm and elbow joint. *Match the name of the muscle in the first column with its correct description listed in the second column.* **LO 15.4**

_____ **1.** biceps brachii

_____ **2.** deltoid

_____ **3.** latissimus dorsi

_____ **4.** triceps brachii

_____ **5.** pectoralis major

a. the largest back muscle

b. located on the chest; moves the arm at the shoulder joint

c. flexes the forearm at the elbow joint

d. moves the arm at the shoulder joint

e. extends the forearm at the elbow joint

B. Identify disorders of the elbow and wrist joints. *Given the description, identify the condition. Fill in the blank to correctly complete each statement.* **LO 15.4, 15.F**

1. A painful wrist condition caused by repetitive movements. Write the abbreviation for this condition: _____

2. Fluid-filled sacs located on the back of the wrist: _____ cysts

3. Painful inflammation of the synovial sheaths on the back of the wrist: stenosing _____

> ### Study Hint
> To help remember the difference between the *thenar* eminence and the *hypothenar*, focus on the prefix *hypo-*, which can mean below or smaller. If you hold the hand open, palm facing you, with the thumb straight up, the *hypothenar* eminence is the fleshy mass at the base of the little finger, which is much smaller than the one below the thumb.

Lesson 15.3

MUSCULAR SYSTEM

Muscles and Tendons of the Pelvic Girdle and Lower Limb

Lesson Objectives

The muscles and tendons of the legs and feet are used so routinely that sometimes these "separate pieces" are forgotten to exist until one of them begins to ache or is injured. The information in this lesson will enable you to use correct medical terminology to:

15.3.1 Discuss the muscles of the hip and thigh.

15.3.2 Describe the muscle tendons of the lower leg, ankle, and foot.

LO 15.5 Muscles of Pelvic Girdle and Lower Limb

Powerful muscles that support the hip joint and move the thigh have their **origins** on the pelvic girdle and their **insertions** into the femur. Prominent among them are the three **gluteus** muscles—**maximus, medius,** and **minimus** (*Figure 15.8*)—and the **adductor** muscles that run down the inner thigh.

Thigh Muscles

The thigh muscles move the knee joint and lower leg. The anterior thigh (the front of the thigh) contains the large **quadriceps femoris** muscle. This muscle has four heads: the rectus femoris, vastus lateralis, vastus medialis, and the vastus intermedius (which lies beneath the rectus femoris). These four muscle heads join into the **quadriceps tendon** (which contains the patella) and continue as the patellar tendon to be inserted into the tibia (*Figure 15.9*). The quadriceps muscle **extends** (straightens) the knee joint and, because of the lower leg's weight, it has to be a very strong muscle.

The posterior (rear) thigh is composed mostly of the three **hamstring muscles:** the **biceps femoris, semimembranosus,** and **semitendinosus** (*Figure 15.10*). These muscles flex (bend) the knee joint and rotate the lower leg. The hollow area at the back of the knee joint between the hamstring tendons is the **popliteal fossa**.

Muscles of the Lower Leg

The muscles of the lower leg move the ankle, foot, and toes. Those on the front of the leg are in a compartment between the tibia and fibula. They dorsiflex the foot at the ankle and extend the toes. Those on the lateral side of the leg evert the foot.

Those on the back of the leg plantar flex the foot at the ankle, flex the toes, and invert the foot (*Figure 15.11*). The **gastrocnemius** muscle forms a large part of the calf. The distal end of it joins with the tendon of the **soleus** muscle to form the **calcaneal (Achilles) tendon,** which is attached to the **calcaneus** (heel bone). The gastrocnemius muscle and the calcaneal tendon enable you to "push off" and start running or jumping.

Gluteus medius

Gluteus maximus

Biceps femoris

Tensor fasciae latae

Sartorius

Rectus femoris

Vastus lateralis

Iliotibial band (fascia)

▲ **Figure 15.8** Muscles of the Hip and Thigh [lateral view].

Rectus femoris

Vastus lateralis

Vastus medialis

Quadriceps femoris tendon

Patella

Patellar tendon

▲ **Figure 15.9** Anterior Muscles of the Thigh.

Hamstring group

Biceps femoris long head

Biceps femoris short head

Semitendinosus

Semimembranosus

Popliteal fossa

▲ **Figure 15.10** Posterior Thigh Muscles.

Gastrocnemius

Medial head

Lateral head

Tendon of gastrocnemius

Achilles (calcaneal) tendon

Calcaneus

▲ **Figure 15.11** Muscles of the Right Lower Leg [posterior view].

WORD	PRONUNCIATION	ELEMENTS		DEFINITION
adductor	ah-**DUK**-tor	S/ P/ R/	**-or** *that which does something* **ad-** *toward* **-duct-** *lead*	Muscle that moves the thigh toward the midline
adduction	ah-**DUK**-shun	S/	**-ion** *action, condition*	Action of moving toward the midline
calcaneus calcaneal tendon (*same as* **Achilles** tendon) Achilles	cal-**KAY**-nee-us kal-**KAY**-knee-al **TEN**-dun ah-**KIL**-eez	S/ R/	Latin *the heel* **-al** *pertaining to* **calcane-** *calcaneus* **tendon** Latin *sinew* **Achilles** mythical Greek warrior	The heel bone The tendon of the heel formed from gastrocne- mius and soleus muscles and inserted into the calcaneus
gastrocnemius	gas-trok-**NEE**-mee-us	S/ R/	**-ius** *pertaining to* **gastrocnem-** *calf of leg*	Major muscle in back of the lower leg (the calf)
gluteus gluteal maximus medius minimus	**GLUE**-tee-us **GLUE**-tee-al **MAKS**-ih-mus **MEE**-dee-us **MIN**-ih-mus	S/ R/	Greek *buttocks* **-eal** *pertaining to* **glut-** *buttocks* Latin *the biggest* Latin *middle* Latin *smallest*	Refers to one of three muscles in the buttocks Pertaining to the buttocks The gluteus maximus muscle is the largest muscle in the body, covering a large part of each buttock The gluteus medius muscle is partly covered by the gluteus maximus The gluteus minimus is the smallest of the gluteal muscles and lies under the gluteus medius
popliteal fossa	pop-**LIT**-ee-al **FOSS**-ah	S/ R/CF	**-al** *pertaining to* **poplit/e-** *ham, back of knee* **fossa** Latin *trench, ditch*	The hollow at the back of the knee
quadriceps femoris	**KWAD**-rih-seps **FEM**-or-is	S/ P/ S/ R/	**-ceps** *head* **quadri-** *four* **-is** *belonging to, pertaining to* **femor-** *femur*	An anterior thigh muscle with four heads (origins)

Exercises

A. Deconstruct the term to decipher its meaning. *Defining the word element provides a clue to its meaning. Choose the correct answer for each statement.* **LO 15.D**

1. The prefix that means *four*:

   a. *ad-*   **b.** *quadri-*   **c.** *ab-*

2. The root that means *lead*:

   a. *calcan-*   **b.** *femor-*   **c.** *glut-*   **d.** *duct-*

3. The suffix that means *that which does something*:

   a. *-is*   **b.** *-ion*   **c.** *-al*   **d.** *-or*

4. The suffix *-ceps* means:

   a. trench, ditch   **b.** muscle   **c.** head   **d.** belong to

B. Identify medical terms that come from Latin. *Given the Latin meaning, write the medical term that it is defining. Fill in the blanks.* **LO 15.5**

1. buttocks: _____

2. smallest: _____

3. the heel: _____

4. middle: _____

5. biggest: _____

Lesson 15.4

Procedures and Pharmacology

Lesson Objectives

Many different health professionals are involved in the diagnosis and treatment of disorders of muscles and tendons in their acute phase, primary care and rehabilitation. It is essential to have a common language and understanding to ensure a high quality of patient care. The information in this lesson will enable you to:

15.4.1 Explain the diagnostic procedures used for disorders of muscles and tendons.

15.4.2 Discuss the treatment procedures used for disorders of the wrist.

15.4.3 Describe the medications used for disorders of muscles and tendons.

Abbreviations

Bx	biopsy
CK	creatine kinase
CT	computed tomography
EMG	electromyography
ESR	erythrocyte sedimentation rate
MRI	magnetic resonance imaging
MSA	myositis specific antibodies

LO 15.6 Diagnostic Procedures for Disorders of Muscles and Tendons

A medical history and physical examination are essential components of a diagnostic examination. Additional diagnostic tests include:

- **Blood tests.** Damaged muscles release **enzymes** such as **creatine kinase** (**CK**) and aldolase into the blood, and their levels can be measured. An **erythrocyte sedimentation rate** (**ESR**) is not specific for any disease process, but it indicates the presence of **inflammation,** and serial readings can be used to measure changes in an inflammatory process.

- **Electromyography** (**EMG**), in which an **electrode** needle is inserted into the muscle to be tested to measure and record the electrical activity in that muscle as the muscle is contracted and relaxed.

- **Nerve conduction studies** are used to measure the speed at which motor or sensory nerves conduct impulses and also can show problems at the neuromuscular junction; for example, in myasthenia gravis.

- **Magnetic resonance imaging** (**MRI**) and **computed tomography scan** (**CT scan**) show detailed images of damage or disease in muscles.

- **Ultrasonography** can identify tears and inflammation of tendons and involves no exposure to radiation, unlike MRI and CT scan.

- **Muscle biopsy** (**Bx**) is performed by removing a small piece of the abnormal muscle through a hollow needle or a small incision to be sent to the laboratory for examination and analysis.

- **Genetic testing** of blood or tissues can show the mutations in some of the genes that cause the different types of muscular dystrophy.

- **Myositis specific antibodies** (**MSA**) can confirm a diagnosis of **dermatomyositis** or polymyositis. Dozens of these antibodies have been identified and research is ongoing to define their significance.

WORD	PRONUNCIATION	ELEMENTS		DEFINITION
antibody	**AN**-tih-body	P/ R/	anti- *against* -body *substance*	Protein produced in response to an antigen
biopsy	**BIE**-op-see	S/ R/	-opsy *to view* bi- *life*	Removal of a tissue from a living person for laboratory examination
electromyography	ee-**LEK**-troh-my-**OG**-rah-fee	S/ R/CF R/CF	-graphy *process of recording* electr/o- *electricity* -my/o- *muscle*	Recording of electrical activity in a muscle
enzyme	**EN**-zime	P/ R	en- *in* -zyme *fermenting*	Protein that induces change in other substances
inflammation	in-flah-**MAY**-shun	S/ P/ R/	-ation *process* in- *in* -flamm- *flame*	A basic complex of reactions in blood vessels and adjacent tissues in response to injury or abnormal stimulation
ultrasonography	**UL**-trah-soh-**NOG**-rah-fee	S/ P/ R/CF	-graphy *process of recording* ultra- *beyond* -son/o- *sound*	Delineation of deep structures using sound waves

Exercises

A. Determine the appropriate diagnostic test. *Read each scenario and determine which diagnostic test is indicated to support the diagnosis. Fill in the blanks. Not all answers will be used.* **LO 15.6, 15.F**

ESR   **EMG**   **CK**   **Bx**   **MSA**

1. The physician ordered a(n) _____ to determine the strength of muscular contraction in the patient with polio.

2. In order to support the diagnosis of myositis, a(n) _____ of the muscle tissue was ordered.

3. Dr. Novak sent a blood sample to the lab to have the medical technologist measure the _____ to determine if the patient had rhabdomyolysis.

4. The patient's blood was sent to the lab with an order for the medical technologist to measure the _____ in order to determine if the patient had a chronic inflammatory condition.

LO 15.7 Musculoskeletal Drugs

NSAIDs inhibit the two cyclooxygenase (**COX**) enzymes that are involved in producing the inflammatory process. They have **analgesic** and **antipyretic** effects and are used for treatment of tissue injury, pyrexia, rheumatoid arthritis, osteoarthritis, gout, and nonspecific joint and tissue pains. The three major NSAIDs, each of which is available OTC, are:

1. **Acetylsalicylic acid** (aspirin), which, in addition to the above effects and uses, also has an antiplatelet effect due to its inhibition of one of the COX enzymes; thus, it is often used in the prevention of heart attacks.

2. **Ibuprofen** (*Advil, Motrin,* and several other trade names), which acts by inhibiting both the COX enzymes, essential elements in the enzyme pathways involved in pain, inflammation, and fever. It is taken orally, but in 2009 an injectable form of ibuprofen (*Caldolor*) was approved for use. In some studies, ibuprofen has been associated with the prevention of Alzheimer and Parkinson diseases, but further studies are needed.

3. **Naproxen** (*Aleve* and many other trade names), which is taken orally once a day and also inhibits both the COX enzymes.

Indomethacin, an NSAID that inhibits both COX enzymes, is a potent drug with many serious side effects. It is not used as an analgesic for minor aches and pains or for fever.

Paracetamol (acetaminophen), an active **metabolite** of phenacetin (not an NSAID), is a widely used OTC analgesic and antipyretic. It is used for the relief of minor aches and pains and is an **ingredient** in many cold and flu remedies.

Skeletal muscle relaxants are FDA-approved for spasticity (baclofen, dantrolene, tizanidine) or for muscular conditions like multiple sclerosis (carisoprodol, chlorzoxazone, cyclobenzaprine, metaxalone, methocarbamol, orphenadrine). The only drug with available evidence of efficacy in spasticity is tizanidine (*Zanaflex, Sirdalud*), but cyclobenzaprine (*Amrix*) appears to be somewhat effective.

Anabolic steroids are related to testosterone but have been altered so that their main effect is to cause skeletal muscle to hypertrophy. They are used illegally in many sports to increase muscle strength. They have marked, often irreversible, side effects, including stunting the height of growing adolescents, shrinking testes and sperm counts, masculinizing women, and causing delusions and paranoid jealousy. In the long term, there are increased risks of heart attacks and strokes, kidney failure, and liver tumors.

Keynote

Spasticity is a state of increased muscular tone with exaggeration of the tendon reflexes.

Abbreviations

COX   cyclooxygenase enzymes
NSAID   nonsteroidal anti-inflammatory drug

WORD	PRONUNCIATION	ELEMENTS		DEFINITION
anabolic steroid	an-ah-**BOL**-ik **STER**-oyd	S/ R/ S/ R/	-ic *pertaining to* **anabol-** *to raise up* -oid *resembling* **ster-** *solid*	Prescription drug used by some athletes to increase muscle mass
analgesia analgesic	an-al-**JEE**-zee-ah	S/ P/ R/ S/	-ia *condition* **an-** *without* **-alges-** *sensation of pain* -ic *pertaining to*	State in which pain is reduced Agent that produces analgesia
antipyretic	**AN**-tee-pie-**RET**-ik	S/ P/ R/	-ic *pertaining to* **anti-** *against* **-pyret-** *fever*	Agent that reduces fever
ingredient	in-**GREE**-dee-ent	S/ P/ R/	**-ent** *end result, pertaining to* **in-** *in, into* **-gredi-** *to go*	An element in a mixture
metabolism metabolite	meh-**TAB**-oh-lizm meh-**TAB**-oh-lite	S/ R/ S/	-ism *condition* **metabol-** *change* -ite *associated with*	The constantly changing physical and chemical processes in the cell Any product of metabolism

Exercises

A. Select the correct medical term to complete the following questions. *Choose the correct answer.* **LO 15.7, 15.F**

1. NSAIDS inhibit enzymes that are involved in the
   _____ process.

   a. respiratory

   b. digestive

   c. urinary

   d. pulmonary

   e. inflammatory

2. The class of medication that treats muscle spasticity:

   a. COX inhibitor

   b. analgesic

   c. muscle relaxant

   d. antipyretic

3. The analgesic listed that is NOT an NSAID:

   a. naproxen

   b. ibuprofen

   c. aspirin

   d. paracetamol

4. An NSAID that is described as a potent pain reliever but is not used for minor aches and pains due to its serious side effects:

   a. orphenadrine

   b. naproxen

   c. indomethacin

   d. cyclobenzaprine

5. A medication that lowers a fever is termed a(n):

   a. metabolite

   b. antipyretic

   c. ingredient

   d. anti-inflammatory

Physical Medicine and Rehabilitation (PM&R)

As a health professional, you may be directly involved in helping a patient through the rehabilitation and recovery process after an illness, surgery, or medical procedure. The information in this lesson will enable you to use correct medical terminology to:

15.5.1 Identify the members of the rehabilitation team.

15.5.2 Discuss the purposes of rehabilitation medicine.

15.5.3 Define the goals for a restorative rehabilitation program for specific common problems.

15.5.4 Define the different types of rehabilitation.

15.5.5 Use the activities of daily living as a measure to assess therapy needs and effectiveness.

Abbreviations

ADLs activities of daily living
COTA certified occupational therapist assistant
PM&R physical medicine and rehabilitation

▲ **Figure 15.12** Assistive Device for Reaching. ©Realistic Reflections

---

Case Report (CR) 15.2

You are

. . . **a certified occupational therapist assistant (COTA)** working in the Rehabilitation Unit at Fulwood Medical Center.

Your patient is

. . . Mr. Hank Johnson, a 65-year-old print shop owner.

One year ago, Mr. Johnson had an elective left total-hip replacement for osteoarthritis. Four months later, he had a myocardial infarction. Two weeks ago, while on his exercise bike, he had a stroke. His right arm and leg were paralyzed, he lost his speech, and he had difficulty swallowing. He arrived in the Emergency Department within 3 hours of the stroke and received thrombolytic **therapy** (see Chapter 9). Mr. Johnson is now receiving **physical therapy**, **occupational therapy**, and speech therapy in the inpatient Rehabilitation Unit. He is able to say some simple words and has begun to have voluntary movements in the arm and leg. Your roles are to help him regain function in his arm and leg and to monitor and record his progress.

LO 15.8 Physical Medicine and Rehabilitation

Physical medicine and rehabilitation (PM&R) health professionals are listed and defined at the beginning of this chapter.

Physical medicine and rehabilitation is also called **physiatry**. Its goal is to develop a comprehensive program to put together the different pieces of a person's life—medical, social, emotional, and **vocational**—after injury or disease. PM&R programs cover a wide spectrum, from prevention of injury in athletes to treating sports-related injuries in sports medicine to coping with complicated multiple trauma.

Mr. Hank Johnson (*see Case Report 15.2*) will need a program designed specifically to get him back on his feet literally and in so many other ways.

LO 15.9 Stroke Rehabilitation

The goals of Mr. Johnson's rehabilitation program are to enable him to:

• Walk safely using an assistive device.

• Use his hands with accuracy.

• Restore his speech abilities.

• Prevent a second stroke.

Because he received thrombolytic therapy (*see Chapter 9*) within 3 hours of his stroke's onset, he has a 50% chance of being left with little or no residual difficulty, compared to a 35% chance had he not received the therapy.

Social workers are helping Mr. Johnson's wife to make their home safe for his return, including obtaining **adaptive equipment**. Raised toilet seats, handrails in the bath and shower, eating devices, and other **assistive devices** (*Figure 15.12*) will help Mr. Johnson perform **activities of daily living (ADLs)** during his recovery. Social workers also will help Mrs. Johnson to work with Medicare to obtain the maximum allowable benefits. Anyone who has had one stroke is at high risk for having a second stroke. Therefore, during this rehabilitative period, Mr. Johnson will be evaluated for such risk factors as narrowing of the carotid arteries with plaque, thrombosis (*see Chapter 6*), and the presence of atrial fibrillation (*see Chapter 6*).

WORD	PRONUNCIATION	ELEMENTS		DEFINITION
assistive device	ah-**SIS**-tiv dee-**VICE**	S/ R/ R/	-ive *nature of* **assist-** *aid, help* **device** *an appliance*	Tool, software, or hardware to assist in performing daily activities
occupational therapy	**OK**-you-**PAY**-shun-al **THAIR**-ah-pee	S/ R/	-al *pertaining to* **occupation-** *work* **therapy** Greek *medical treatment*	Use of work and recreational activities to increase independent function
physiatry (**Note:** The "i" in the root is dropped because "iatry" also begins with "i")	fih-**ZIE**-ah-tree	S/ R/	-iatry *treatment, field of medicine* **phys** *body*	Physical medicine
physiatrist	fih-**ZIE**-ah-trist	S/ R/	-ist *specialist* **iatr-** *treatment*	Specialist in physical medicine
physical medicine	**FIZ**-ih-cal **MED**-ih-sin	S/ R/ S/ R/	-al *pertaining to* **physic-** *body* -ine *pertaining to, substance* **medic-** *medicine*	Diagnosis and treatment by means of remedial agents, such as exercises, manipulation, heat, etc.
physical therapy (also known as physiotherapy)	**FIZ**-ih-cal **THAIR**-ah-pee	S/ R/	-al *pertaining to* **physic-** *body* **therapy** Greek *medical treatment*	Use of remedial processes to overcome a physical defect
physiotherapy (syn)	**FIZ**-ee-oh-**THAIR**-ah-pee	S/ R/CF	-therapy *treatment* **physi/o-** *body*	Another term for physical therapy
rehabilitation	**REE**-hah-bil-ih-**TAY**-shun	S/ P/ R/	-ion *action, condition* **re-** *again* **-habilitat-** *restore*	Therapeutic restoration of an ability to function as before
therapy	**THAIR**-ah-pee		Greek *medical treatment*	Systematic treatment of a disease, dysfunction, or disorder
therapist	**THAIR**-ah-pist	S/ R/	-ist *specialist* **therap-** *treatment*	Professional trained in the practice of a particular therapy
therapeutic (adj)	**THAIR**-ah-**PYU**-tik	S/ R/	-ic *pertaining to* **therapeut-** *treatment*	Relating to the treatment of a disease or disorder

Exercises

A. Use the correct term to complete each sentence. *Use the terms provided to complete each sentence.* **LO 15.8, 15.9, 15.F**

| therapist | therapy | therapeutic | orthotic | orthotist |

1. The physician prescribes two shoe inserts as _____ devices to relieve the patient's foot pain.

2. After breaking her fingers, the patient was prescribed occupational _____ to regain strength and function in her hand.

3. The physiatrist used warm, moist heat as a _____ measure to relieve the muscle strain.

4. The _____ created an ankle brace for the child.

5. After having surgery to repair a rotator cuff tear, the physical _____ created a strengthening plan for the patient.

LO 15.8 Rehabilitation Definitions

Definitions

The following definitions of terms or phrases specific to rehabilitation will help you to understand more precisely the different kinds of rehabilitation in which you may be involved as a health professional.

Rehabilitation medicine focuses on function. Being able to function is essential to an individual's independence and ability to have a good quality of life.

Restorative rehabilitation restores a function that has been lost, such as after a hip fracture, hip replacement, or stroke. This process can be intense, but it's also usually short term.

Maintenance rehabilitation strengthens and maintains a function that is gradually being lost. It is less intense than restorative rehabilitation but often long term. Problems of senescence (old age), like difficulty with balance or flexibility, require this long-term approach.

Rehabilitation medicine is also involved with the **prevention** of function loss and the prevention of injury. In sports medicine, an example is the prevention of shoulder and elbow injuries often experienced by baseball pitchers.

Activities of daily living (ADLs) are the routine activities of personal care. The six basic ADLs are eating, bathing, dressing, grooming, toileting, and transferring. Assistive devices are designed to make ADLs easier to perform and help maintain the patient's independence. Examples of these devices include reachers and grabbers, easy-pull sock aids, long shoehorns, jar openers, and eating aids (*Figure 15.12*). ADLs are also a measurement to assess therapy needs and monitor its effectiveness.

Instrumental activities of daily living (IADLs) relate to independent living. These activities include managing money, using a telephone, cooking, driving, shopping for groceries and personal items, and doing housework.

LO 15.9 Amputations

Seventy-five percent of all **amputations** are performed on people over 65 years of age with **peripheral vascular disease (PVD)**. This includes complications from arteriosclerosis and diabetes. Most of these cases involve **below-the-knee amputations (BKAs).**

Recently, the wars in Iraq and Afghanistan have led to soldiers losing their arms or legs due to the detonation of explosive devices. In some of these cases, amputations are also required, depending on the level of damage an explosion has caused to the soldier's body.

Rehabilitation after amputation (*Figure 5.12*) is an increasingly important component in rehabilitation programs. Immediately after surgery, the objectives of the rehabilitation team are to:

- Promote healing of the stump;
- Strengthen the muscles above the site of the amputation;
- Strengthen arm muscles to assist in ambulation or help with walking using a cane, crutches, or other assistive devices;
- Prevent **contractures** or tightening of the joints above the amputation (knee and hip for BKAs);
- Shrink the post-amputation stump with elastic cuffs or bandages to fit the socket of a temporary **prosthesis** (*Figure 5.13*); and
- Provide emotional, psychological, and family support.

▲ **Figure 15.13** Teenager Doing ADL after Amputation ©Arnd Wiegmann/ Reuters/Alamy Stock Photo

▲ **Figure 15.14** Young man Being Fitted with a Prosthesis ©Johnny Greig/Getty Images RF

WORD	PRONUNCIATION	ELEMENTS		DEFINITION
amputation	am-pyu-**TAY**-shun	S/ R/	**-ation** *process* **amput-** *prune*	Removal of a limb, part of a limb, or other projecting body part
contracture	kon-**TRAK**-chur	S/ R/	**-ure** *result of* **contract-** *pull together*	Muscle shortening due to spasm or fibrosis
prevention	pree-**VEN**-shun	S/ R/	**-ion** *action, condition* **prevent-** *prevent*	Process to prevent occurrence of a disease or health problem
prosthesis	**PROS**-thee-sis		Greek *an addition*	An artificial part to remedy a defect in the body
restorative rehabilitation	ree-**STOR**-ah-tiv **REE**-hah-bil-ih-**TAY**-shun	S/ R/ S/ P/ R/	**-ative** *quality of* **restor-** *renew* **-ion** *action, process* **re-** *begin again* **-habilitat-** *restore*	Therapy that promotes renewal of health and strength

Exercises

A. Describe the treatment of amputations. *Choose the correct answer for each statement.* **LO 15.9**

1. When employing the use of physical therapy for strengthening muscles, the area for strengthening the muscles is
_____ the amputation site.

   a. above   **b.** below   **c.** lateral to   **d.** medial to

2. In order to prepare patients for walking with crutches, which muscles should be strengthened?

   a. back   **b.** chest   **c.** arm   **d.** leg

3. Family support is an important part of rehabilitation therapy for patients with amputation.

   a. True   **b.** False

B. Define terms associated with rehabilitation. *Match the term in the first column with its correct definition in the second column.* **LO 15.8, 15.9**

_____ **1.** maintenance rehabilitation   **a.** activities specific to independent living

_____ **2.** restorative rehabilitation   **b.** short-term therapy, aimed at returning the patient to prior function

_____ **3.** rehabilitation medicine   **c.** routine activities of personal care

_____ **4.** instrumental activities of daily living   **d.** long-term therapy; helps to prevent loss of current strength

_____ **5.** activities of daily living   **e.** focuses on the patient's functional abilities

Muscular System

Challenge Your Knowledge

A. **Match the health professional in the second column with his or her job description in the first column.** (LO 15.E)

_____ 1. Practitioner who evaluates and treats pain, disease, or injury by measures other than medical or surgical

_____ 2. Practitioner who makes and fits orthopedic appliances

_____ 3. Physician who specializes in physical medicine and rehabilitation

_____ 4. Practitioner who focuses on helping patients with activities of daily living

a. orthotist

b. physiatrist

c. occupational therapist

d. physical therapist

B. **Describe the function of skeletal muscle.** From the given example, identify the function being described. Use the provided terms to fill in the blank. (LO 15.2)

movement   posture   heat   respiration   communication

1. The function of skeletal muscles that Mr. Schwartz uses when he greets patients when they arrive to the clinic:

   _____

2. The children were cold, so they ran around the house to warm up. The function of warming up: _____

3. The occupational therapy assistant helped his patient to bring the spoon to her mouth. Bringing the spoon to the mouth is an example of: _____

4. Skeletal muscles contract to keep the back straight: _____

5. Breathing to bring oxygen into the body and move carbon dioxide out: _____

C. Demonstrate your knowledge of the muscular system anatomy and disorders by choosing the correct answer to complete each statement. (LO 15.1, 15.2, 15.3, 15.4)

1. The type of muscle only found in the heart:

   a. smooth

   b. skeletal

   c. cardiac

2. Due to their long size, skeletal muscle cells are also known as muscle:

   a. strings

   b. fascicles

   c. fibers

   d. junction

3. The stripes seen in a microscopic view of skeletal muscle are called:

   a. striations

   b. fascia

   c. interneurons

   d. osteoclasts

4. Muscle that has decreased in size is said to have the condition of:

   a. edema

   b. hypertrophy

   c. atrophy

   d. paralysis

5. Lifting heavy objects over a long period of time can result in muscle:

   a. polymyalgia

   b. tenosynovitis

   c. atrophy

   d. hypertrophy

6. The location where a skeletal muscle attaches to the bone that is moved with muscle contraction is termed the:

   a. origin

   b. insertion

   c. fascicle

   d. fascia

7. The broadest muscle in the back is the:

   a. biceps

   b. triceps

   c. brachii

   d. latissimus dorsi

   e. deltoid

8. Ganglion cysts are fluid-filled cysts arising from the:

   a. muscles

   b. joints

   c. synovial tendon sheaths

   d. articulations

   e. bursa

9. Four muscles that originate on the scapula, wrap around the joint, and fuse to form one large tendon are called the:

   a. articulation

   b. rotator cuff

   c. brachialis

   d. scapulae

   e. pectoral

10. An overstretch or tear in a muscle is termed a:

    a. strain

    b. fasciotomy

    c. sprain

    d. tenosynovitis

    e. cyst

Muscular System

D. Common disorders of skeletal muscle. Match the skeletal muscle disorder in the first column with its correct description in the second column. (**LO 15.3**)

_____ **1.** rhabdomyolysis   **a.** symmetrical weakness and wasting of pelvic, shoulder, and proximal limb muscles

_____ **2.** tenosynovitis   **b.** overstretch of a muscle or tendon

_____ **3.** Duchenne muscular dystrophy   **c.** inflammation of tendon and its surrounding synovial sheath

_____ **4.** tendonitis   **d.** destruction of muscle to produce myoglobin

_____ **5.** fibromyalgia   **e.** inflammation of a tendon

_____ **6.** strain   **f.** pain in the muscle fibers

E. Skeletal muscles that move the arms, legs, and feet. Select the answer that correctly completes each statement. (**LO 15.4, 15.5**)

1. The smallest gluteal muscle is the gluteus:

  a. maximus

  b. medius

  c. minimus

2. The group of muscles located on the anterior side of the femur:

  a. hamstrings

  b. quadriceps

  c. rotator cuff

  d. gluteals

3. A muscle located directly below the spine of the scapula:

  a. vastus lateralis

  b. subscapularis

  c. brachioradialis

  d. infraspinatus

4. The pad of muscle located on the thumb side of your hand:

  a. dorsum

  b. bursa

  c. thenar eminence

  d. hypothenar eminence

5. The origin of all muscles that make up the rotator cuff:

  a. scapula

  b. humerus

  c. clavicle

  d. radius

6. The meaning of the muscle _teres major_:

  a. above the acromion

  b. wide and broad

  c. pertaining to the earth

  d. big, long, and round

7. The muscle that extends the arm at the elbow joint:

  a. triceps brachii

  b. biceps brachii

  c. deltoid

  d. subscapularis

8. The largest muscle that makes up the buttocks is the:

  a. gluteus minimus

  b. gluteus medius

  c. gluteus maximus

  d. vastus lateralis

  e. vastus medialis

F. **Disorders of the muscles of the arm, thigh, leg, and foot.** Given the description, identify the likely disorder related to the muscular system. Match the description in the first column with its matching term in the second column. **(LO 15.3, 15.4)**

_____ 1. Pain and tingling in the hand due to repetitive wrist movements

_____ 2. Injury due to overuse of the shoulder joint

_____ 3. Painful condition caused by overuse of the elbow joint

_____ 4. Inflammation of the lubricating sac found near a joint

a. bursitis

b. tennis elbow

c. rotator cuff tear

d. carpal tunnel syndrome

G. **Deconstructing words related to physical medicine and rehabilitation. Identify the meaning of the element in each medical term.** Select the answer that correctly completes each statement. **(LO 15.4, 15.8, 15.D, 15.E)**

1. The suffix in the term **physiatry** means:

   a. pertaining to

   b. nature

   c. treatment

   d. specialist

2. The root in the term **therapeutic** means:

   a. specialist

   b. treatment

   c. body

   d. pertaining to

3. The word element in the term **rehabilitation** that means *again*:

   a. prefix

   b. root

   c. suffix

4. The root in the term **occupational** means:

   a. work

   b. aid, help

   c. body

   d. treatment

5. The suffix in **assistive** means:

   a. restore

   b. help

   c. nature of

   d. pertaining to

Muscular System

H. **Use medical terms to complete professional documentation.** Read the following case study and replace the words in italics with the medical term it is describing. (**LO 15.3, 15.4, 15.A, 15.C, 15.E**)

Mr. Vernon has arrived to the clinic today to see Dr. Cho, **(1)** *a specialist in the treatment of bone and muscle disorders.* He states that he experienced a constant pain in his shoulder that he thinks may be due to an **(2)** *inflamed tendon.* He was an avid tennis player for over 15 years, which may be related to his condition.

Dr. Cho examines Mr. Vernon and notes that he is limited in his ability to move his arm away from his body. Dr. Cho diagnoses the patient with a tear in the **(3)** *muscles that support the shoulder joint.* He recommends that Mr. Vernon see a **(4)** *specialist in the strengthening of muscles* for five weeks followed by surgery to repair the tear.

1. _____

2. _____

3. _____ _____

4. _____

I. **Prefixes: Match the correct medical term in the first column with the meaning of its prefix in the second column.** (**LO 15.D**)

Medical Term	Meaning of the Prefix
_____ 1. hypothenar	a. two
_____ 2. triceps	b. together
_____ 3. adductor	c. toward
_____ 4. quadriceps	d. above
_____ 5. contract	e. three
_____ 6. supra	f. four
_____ 7. biceps	g. below, deficient

J. **Identify abbreviations that describe medical terms.** Match the abbreviation in the first column to its correct description in the second column. (**LO 15.3, 15.4, 15.7, 15.8, 15.9, 15.E, 15.F**)

_____ 1. COTA	a. examples include toileting, brushing one's hair, brushing one's teeth
_____ 2. NSAID	b. removal of the lower leg and foot
_____ 3. CTS	c. a professional that assists people in improving their activities of daily living
_____ 4. BKA	d. hereditary muscular condition with general muscle weakness and atropy
_____ 5. ADLs	e. repetitive movements that cause a feeling of "pins and needles" in the hand
_____ 6. DMD	f. a type of medication used to treat muscle pain

K. **Read the Case Report presented below. Choose the correct answer to each question.** (LO 15.5, 15.A, 15.E, 15.F)

 Case Report (CR) 15.2

You are

. . . a certified occupational therapist assistant working in the Rehabilitation Unit at Fulwood Medical Center.

Your patient is

. . . Mr. Hank Johnson, a 65-year-old print shop owner.

One year ago, Mr. Johnson had an elective left total-hip replacement for osteoarthritis. Four months later, he had a myocardial infarction. Two weeks ago, while on his exercise bike, he had a stroke. His right arm and leg were paralyzed, he lost his speech, and he had difficulty swallowing. He arrived in the Emergency Department within 3 hours of the stroke and received thrombolytic therapy (see Chapter 9). Mr. Johnson is now receiving physical therapy, occupational therapy, and speech therapy in the inpatient Rehabilitation Unit. He is able to say some simple words and has begun to have voluntary movements in the arm and leg. Your roles are to help him regain function in his arm and leg and to monitor and record his progress.

1. When completing required patient documentation, you would likely abbreviate your job title. Which abbreviation would you use?

   a. PTA   **b.** COTA   **c.** OT   **d.** PT

2. The fact that his movements in his arm and leg are **voluntary** means that:

   a. his arm and leg muscles have atrophied   **c.** his arm and leg are weak

   b. he has no control over the movement of his arm and leg   **d.** he can choose to move his arm and leg

3. Which of the following may be an occupational therapy goal in regards to his arm?

   a. use a cane for walking   **c.** chew and swallow solid food

   b. ride a bicycle   **d.** brush his hair and teeth

L. **Identify the elements in each medical term and unlock the meaning of the word.** *Fill in the chart. If the word does not have a particular word element, write n/a. The first one has been done for you.* (LO 10.D)

Medical Term	Prefix	Meaning of Prefix	Root/ Combining Form	Meaning of Root/ Combining Form	Suffix	Meaning of Suffix	Meaning of Term
dorsal	1. n/a	2. n/a	3. *dors-*	4. back	5. *-al*	6. pertaining to	7. pertaining to the back
analgesia	8.	9.	10.	11.	12.	13.	14.
deltoid	15.	16.	17.	18.	19.	20.	21.
hypertrophy	22.	23.	24.	25.	26.	27.	28.
infraspinatus	29.	30.	31.	32.	33.	34.	35.

©2014 Nucleus Medical Media

In your future career, you may work directly and/or indirectly with the following health professionals in the area of ophthalmology:

- **Ophthalmologists,** who are medical specialists (MDs) in the diagnosis and treatment of diseases of the eye.
- **Optometrists** (ODs), who are doctors of optometry and are skilled in the measurement of vision. They are not medical doctors and cannot prescribe medication.
- **Opticians,** who are licensed to make corrective lenses, adjust and repair spectacles, and fit contact lenses.

The health professionals in the following list perform specific assigned procedures and support ophthalmologists according to the depth of their training:

- Certified ophthalmic medical technicians
- Certified ophthalmic assistants
- Certified ophthalmic technicians
- Certified ophthalmic technologists
- Registered ophthalmic ultrasound biometrists
- Diagnostic ophthalmic sonographers

In the area of otology, you may work directly and/or indirectly with the following health professionals:

- **Otologists,** who are medical specialists in diseases of the ear.
- **Otorhinolaryngologists,** who are medical specialists (MDs) in diseases of the ear, nose, and throat (ENT).
- **Audiologists,** who evaluate hearing function.

Chapter Learning Outcomes

In order to make correct decisions when you see patients with eye or ear problems, to communicate with other health professionals about the patient, to participate in patient education, and to document the patient's care, you need to be able to:

LO 16.1 Relate the structures of the accessory glands of the eye to their functions.

LO 16.2 Describe disorders of the accessory structures of the eye.

LO 16.3 Identify common disorders due to imbalance of the extrinsic muscles of the eye.

LO 16.4 Relate the structure of the different components of the eyeball to their functions.

LO 16.5 Map the visual pathway from the lens to the visual cortex of the brain.

LO 16.6 Describe disorders of the anterior eyeball.

LO 16.7 Explain disorders of the retina.

LO 16.8 Describe diagnostic procedures used for disorders of the eye.

LO 16.9 Explain the therapeutic procedures used for disorders of the eye.

LO 16.10 Discuss medications used in the treatment of disorders of the eye.

LO 16.11 Relate the structure of the external ear to its functions.

LO 16.12 Describe disorders of the external ear.

LO 16.13 Relate the structures of the middle ear to their hearing functions.

LO 16.14 Describe disorders of the middle ear.

LO 16.15 Identify the structures of the inner ear involved in hearing and their disorders.

LO 16.16 Explain the structures of the inner ear involved in balance and their disorders.

LO 16.17 Describe diagnostic procedures used for disorders of the ear.

LO 16.18 Explain therapeutic procedures used for disorders of the ear.

LO 16.19 Discuss medications used for disorders of the ear.

LO 16.A Use the medical terms of ophthalmology and otology to communicate in writing and to document accurately and precisely in any health care setting.

LO 16.B Use the medical terms of ophthalmology and otology to communicate verbally with accuracy and precision in any health care settting.

LO 16.C Construct word elements into the medical terms of ophthalmology and otology.

LO 16.D Deconstruct the medical terms of ophthalmology and otology into their word elements.

LO 16 E Identify the health professionals involved in treating patients with disorders of the eye and ear.

LO 16 F Correctly use approved abbreviations of medical terms in ophthalmology and otology correctly.

Note: The sense of smell is discussed as an integral part of the respiratory system *(Chapter 13),* the sense of taste as an integral part of the digestive system *(Chapter 5),* and the sense of touch as an integral part of the nervous system *(Chapter 9).*

 Case Report (CR) 16.1

You are

. . . an **ophthalmic** technician **(OT)** working in the office of **ophthalmologist** Angela Chun, MD, a member of the Fulwood Medical Group.

Your patient is

. . . Mrs. Jenny Hughes, a 30-year-old computer software consultant, who walked into the office with painful, red, swollen eyelids and a sticky, **purulent** discharge from both eyes. The administrative medical assistant did not hold her in the reception area but brought her directly in to you.

Mrs. Hughes complains of headache and **photophobia**, and her eyelids were stuck together when she woke up this morning. She tells you that, a couple of days earlier, she had gone into a small business office to install software at 10 workstations. One of the employees was absent with "**pink eye**." She wants to know if she could have contracted the disease from that employee's keyboard and how to prevent her husband and two children from getting it.

You have in your hand a clipboard, pen attached, with the office Notice of Privacy Practices and sign-in sheet for her to sign. How do you proceed?

Accessory Structures of the Eye

Lesson Objectives

An understanding of the terminology, anatomy, and physiology of the eye's accessory structures is an essential step to acquire an understanding of how they function to maintain the integrity of the eye.

The information in this lesson will enable you to:

16.1.1 Link the structure of the accessory structures of the eye to their appropriate functions.

16.1.2 Explain the roles of the accessory structures in protecting the eye.

16.1.3 Describe some common abnormalities and disorders of the accessory structures.

16.1.4 Apply the correct medical terminology to the anatomy, physiology, and disorders of the accessory structures.

LO 16.1 Accessory Structures and Their Functions

Mrs. Jenny Hughes's "**pink eye**" involved her **conjunctiva** and **eyelids**, two of the **periorbital** accessory structures of the eye, located around the **orbit** and in front of the **eyeball**. The other accessory structures are the **eyebrows** and **eyelashes** and the **lacrimal (tear) apparatus**. All these structures support and protect the exposed front surface of the eye.

Eyebrows keep sweat from running into the eye and function in nonverbal communication.

Eyelids protect the eye from foreign objects. They blink to move tears across the surface of the eye and sweep debris away. They close in sleep to keep out visual stimuli. They are covered in the body's thinnest layer of skin. They consist mostly of muscle that fans out from each eyelid onto the forehead and cheek to open and close the eyelids.

In the eyelids, a flat, fibrous connective tissue layer (**tarsus**) holds 20 to 25 **tarsal glands**, whose ducts open along the edge of the eyelid. These glands secrete an oily fluid that keeps the eyelids from sticking together. The two corners where the upper and lower eyelids meet are called **canthi** (singular, **canthus**).

Eyelashes are strong hairs that help keep debris out of the eyes. They arise on the edge of the lids from hair follicles (*see Chapter 4*).

The **conjunctiva** is a transparent mucous membrane that lines the inside of both eyelids and covers all of the front of the eye except the central portion, the cornea. In the conjunctiva, numerous goblet cells secrete a thin film of mucin that prevents the surface of the eyeball from dehydrating.

The conjunctiva is freely movable over the eyeball. It has numerous small blood vessels and is richly supplied with nerve endings that make it very sensitive to pain.

The **lacrimal apparatus** (*Figure 16.1*) consists of four structures. The **lacrimal (tear) gland**, located in the upper, lateral corner of the orbit, secretes tears. Short **lacrimal ducts** carry the tears to the surface of the conjunctiva. After washing across the conjunctiva, the tears leave the eye at the medial corner of the eye by draining into the **lacrimal sac**. They then flow through the **nasolacrimal duct** into the nose, from where they are swallowed.

The functions of tears are to:

- *Clean and lubricate* the surface of the eye.
- *Deliver nutrients and oxygen* to the conjunctiva.
- *Prevent infection* through a bactericidal enzyme called **lysozyme**.

Lacrimal gland

Ducts of lacrimal gland

Lacrimal sac

Canthus

Lacrimal canal

Nasolacrimal duct

Inferior meatus of nasal cavity

Nostril

▲ **Figure 16.1** Lacrimal Apparatus and Accessory Structures.

Abbreviations

OD	doctor of optometry
OT	ophthalmic technician

Word Analysis and Definition

WORD	PRONUNCIATION		ELEMENTS	DEFINITION
canthus canthi (pl)	**KAN**-thus **KAN**-thee		Greek *corner of the eye*	Corner of the eye where upper and lower lids meet
conjunctiva conjunctival (adj)	kon-junk-**TIE**-vah kon-junk-**TIE**-val	S/ R/	-al *pertaining to* **conjunctiv-** *conjunctiva*	Inner lining of the eyelids Pertaining to the conjunctiva
lacrimal	**LAK**-rim-al	S/ R/	-al *pertaining to* **lacrim-** *tears*	Pertaining to tears
lacrimal duct lacrimal sac nasolacrimal duct	**LAK**-rim-al DUKT **LAK**-rim-al SAK **NAY**-zoh-**LAK**-rim-al DUKT	R/ R/CF	duct *to lead* sac Latin *bag, pocket* **nas/o-** *nose*	Carries tears to the conjunctiva Where tears leave the eye at the medial corner Passage from the lacrimal sac to the nose
lysozyme	**LIE**-soh-zime	S/ R/CF	-zyme *enzyme* **lys/o-** *decomposition*	Enzyme that dissolves the cell walls of bacteria
ophthalmology ophthalmologist ophthalmic (adj)	off-thal-**MALL**-oh-jee off-thal-**MALL**-oh-jist off-**THAL**-mik	S/ R/CF S/ S/ R/	-logy *study of* **ophthalm/o-** *eye* -logist *one who studies, specialist* -ic *pertaining to* **ophthalm-** *eye*	Medical specialty that diagnoses and treats diseases of the eye Medical specialist in ophthalmology Pertaining to the eye
optician optometrist	op-**TIH**-shun op-**TOM**-eh-trist	S/ R/CF S/ R/CF	-cian *having a skill or art* **opt/i-** *vision* -metrist *skilled in measurement* **opt/o-** *vision*	Someone who is licensed to make corrective lenses, adjust and repair spectacles, and fit contact lenses Someone who is skilled in the measurement of vision but cannot treat eye diseases or prescribe medication
orbit orbital (adj)	**OR**-bit **OR**-bit-al	S/ R/	-al *pertaining to* **orbit-** *orbit*	The bony socket that holds the eyeball Pertaining to the orbit
periorbital	per-ee-**OR**-bit-al	S/ P/ R/	-al *pertaining to* **peri-** *around* **-orbit-** *orbit*	Pertaining to tissues around the orbit
photophobia photophobic (adj)	foh-toh-**FOH**-bee-ah foh-toh-**FOH**-bik	S/ R/CF S/ R/	ia *condition* **phot/o-** *light* -ic *pertaining to* **-phob-** *fear*	Fear of the light because it hurts the eyes Relating to or suffering from photophobia
tarsus (*Note:* Tarsus also is used to refer to the seven bones in the instep of the foot.) tarsal (adj)	**TAR**-sus **TAR**-sal	 S/ R/	Greek *flat* -al *pertaining to* **tars-** *tarsus*	The flat fibrous plate that gives shape to the outer edges of the eyelids Pertaining to the tarsus

Exercises

A. Define the accessory structures of the eye. *Match the accessory structure of the eye with its correct definition.* **LO 16.1, 16.A**

_____ 1. lysozyme

_____ 2. canthus

_____ 3. tarsus

_____ 4. eyelash

_____ 5. eyebrow

_____ 6. lacrimal gland

_____ 7. conjunctiva

_____ 8. tarsal gland

a. corner of the eye where eyelids meet

b. strong hairs that keep debris out of the eye

c. secretes tears

d. secretes an oily substance to keep eyelids from sticking together

e. enzyme that destroys bacteria

f. hair that keeps sweat out of the eyes

g. transparent mucous membrane that lines the eyelids and the front of the eye (except for the cornea)

h. fibrous connective tissue that gives structure to the eyelids

▲ **Figure 16.2** **Conjunctivitis.** ©Bob
Tapper/Diomedia/Medical Images RM

Stye

▲ **Figure 16.3** **Stye Showing Pus-Filled
Cyst.** ©Western Opthamolic Hospital/Photo
Researchers, Inc.

▲ **Figure 16.4** Chalazion in Upper Eyelid.
©SPL/Photo Researchers, Inc.

▲ **Figure 16.5** Ptosis of Right Eyelid.
©ISM/Barraquer, Barcelona/Diomedia/Medical
Images

Case Report (CR) 16.1 *(continued)*

Mrs. Jenny Hughes's "pink eye" is called acute **contagious** conjunctivitis *(see Figure 16.2)*. It responds well to **antibiotic** eyedrops. Her hands were **contaminated** from the keyboard of the employee who had left work and gone home with "pink eye." Mrs. Hughes transmitted the infection from her fingers to her eyes by touching or rubbing.

Your documentation of Mrs. Hughes's office visit could read:

Progress Note 04/10/13

Mrs. Jenny Hughes was brought directly into the clinical area at 1030 hrs with what appeared to be conjunctivitis, "pink eye." Both eyelids were red and swollen with a purulent discharge. She complained of headache and photophobia. Dr. Chun prescribed Neosporin eyedrops, 1–2 drops every four hours (**q.4.h**) for 7 days. A swab was sent to the laboratory. I instructed and watched Mrs. Hughes wash her hands and use an alcohol-based hand gel. I then had her sign in and sign our Notice of Privacy Practices. I instructed her in the use of the drops and emphasized home care and hand care measures to prevent the infection from spreading to her family. She was given a return appointment in 1 week and told to call the office if the drops did not help. Daphne Butras, OT. 1055 hrs.

LO 16.2 Disorders of the Accessory Glands

Conjunctivitis *(Figure 16.2)*, inflammation of the conjunctiva, is more commonly viral than bacterial and also can be caused by irritants such as chlorine, soaps, fumes, and smoke.

Eyelid edema, generalized swelling of the eyelids, is often produced by an allergic reaction due to cosmetics, pollen in the air, or stings and bites from insects.

A **stye**, or **hordeolum**, is an infection of an eyelash follicle producing an abscess *(Figure 16.3)*, with localized pain, swelling, redness, and pus formation at the edge of the eyelid.

A **chalazion** is a small, painless, localized, whitish swelling inside the lid when a tarsal gland becomes blocked *(Figure 16.4)*. It can disappear spontaneously or require surgical removal.

Blepharitis occurs when multiple eyelash follicles and tarsal glands become infected. The margin of the eyelid shows persistent redness and crusting and may become ulcerated. The infection is usually staphylococcal. It is treated with antibiotic ointments.

Dacryostenosis is blockage of the drainage of tears, usually due to narrowing of the nasolacrimal ducts. Approximately 6% of newborns have this condition, but it may not be noticeable at birth because infants do not produce tears until they are several weeks old. Fortunately, nearly all blocked ducts open by the age of one year and do not require surgical opening.

Dacryocystitis is an infection of the lacrimal sac, with swelling and pus at the medial corner of the eye.

Ptosis occurs when the upper eyelid is constantly drooped over the eye due to **paresis** (partial paralysis) of the muscle that raises the upper lid *(Figure 16.5)*. It can be associated with diabetes, myasthenia gravis, brain tumor, and muscular dystrophy, all of which are described in subsequent chapters. The term **blepharoptosis** is used for sagging of the eyelids due to excess skin.

WORD	PRONUNCIATION	ELEMENTS		DEFINITION
blepharitis blepharoptosis	blef-ah-**RIE**-tis **BLEF**-ah-rop-**TOH**-sis	S/ R/ S/ R/CF	-itis *inflammation* **blephar-** *eyelid* **-ptosis** *drooping* **blephar/o-** *eyelid*	Inflammation of the eyelid Drooping of the upper eyelid
chalazion	kah-**LAY**-zee-on		Greek *lump*	Cyst on the outer edge of an eyelid caused by a blocked tarsal gland
conjunctivitis	kon-junk-tih-**VIE**-tis	S/ R/	-itis *inflammation* **conjunctiv-** *conjunctiva*	Inflammation of the conjunctiva
contagious	kon-**TAY**-jus	S/ R/	-ous *pertaining to* **contagi-** *transmissible by contact*	Able to be transmitted, as infections transmitted from person to person, from person to air, or from surface to person
dacryocystitis	**DAK**-ree-oh-sis-**TIE**-tis	S/ R/CF R/	-itis *inflammation* **dacry/o-** *tears* **-cyst-** *sac*	Inflammation of the lacrimal sac
dacryostenosis	**DAK**-ree-oh-steh-**NOH**-sis	S/ R/CF	-sis *abnormal condition* **-sten/o-** *narrowing*	Narrowing of the nasolacrimal duct
hordeolum stye (syn)	hor-**DEE**-oh-lum STY		Latin *stye in the eye*	Abscess in an eyelash follicle
paresis	par-**EE**-sis		Greek *paralysis*	Partial paralysis
ptosis (*Note:* The first consonant is silent.)	**TOH**-sis		Greek *drooping*	Sinking down of an eyelid or an organ

Exercises

A. Disorders: The accessory structures of the eye have their own disorders. *The patient conditions are described in the left column; match the condition with the correct medical term (right column) from this lesson.* **LO 16.2**

_____ 1. allergic reaction to pollen

_____ 2. drooping of upper eyelid over eye

_____ 3. infection of the lacrimal sac

_____ 4. produced by a blocked tarsal gland

_____ 5. blockage of the drainage of tears

_____ 6. red, crusted, and ulcerated eyelid

_____ 7. pus at the edge of the eyelid

a. chalazion

b. hordeolum

c. dacryostenosis

d. blepharitis

e. eyelid edema

f. dacryocystitis

g. ptosis

You are

. . . an ophthalmic technician working with Angela Chun, MD, an ophthalmologist at Fulwood Medical Center.

Your patient is

. . . Sam Hughes, a 2-year-old boy, who has been referred by his pediatrician to Dr. Chun.

His mother, Mrs. Jenny Hughes, states that she has noticed for the past couple of months that his right eye has turned in. The only visual difficulty she has noticed is that he sometimes misses a Cheerio when he tries to grab it. Otherwise, he is healthy.

You are responsible for documenting Sam's diagnostic and therapeutic procedures and explaining the significance of these to his mother.

LO 16.3 Extrinsic Muscles of the Eye

Humans, with their two eyes working closely together, have developed very good three-dimensional perception (**stereopsis**) and hand-eye coordination. Stereopsis depends on an accurate alignment of the two eyes.

This alignment is held in place by the coordination of six **extrinsic eye muscles** in each eye that are attached to the inner wall of the orbit and to the outer surface of the eyeball *(Figure 16.6)*. These muscles move the eye in all directions.

When there is muscle imbalance in one eye, as in Sam's case, the alignment breaks down, and the resulting condition is called **strabismus**, also known in lay terms as "squinting" or "cross-eyed."

Esotropia is the eye turned in toward the nose. In congenital or infantile esotropia, both eyes look in toward the nose—the right eye looks to the left and the left eye looks to the right. These children require surgical intervention.

Accommodative esotropia is an inward eye turn, usually noticed around 2 years of age in 1% to 2% of children *(Figure 16.7)*. In Sam's case, he had an accommodative esotropia in one eye. He will probably respond to treatment using glasses and perhaps a patch over the stronger eye to encourage use of the weaker eye.

Exotropia, an outward turning of one eye, is noticed around 2 to 4 years of age. It will often respond to vision therapy, which includes eye exercises and glasses from an optometrist.

Strabismus is not the same as **amblyopia**, or "lazy eye," which occurs in children when vision in one eye has not developed as well as in the other. It occurs because the eye and the brain are not cooperating for the one eye.

Keynote

Amblyopia is the failure or incomplete development of the pathways of vision to the brain.

▲ **Figure 16.7** **Strabismus with Right Eye Turned Inward.** ©BioPhoto Associates/ Photo Researchers, Inc.

▲ **Figure 16.6** Extrinsic Muscles of the Right Eye (Lateral View).

Word Analysis and Definition

S = Suffix   P = Prefix   R = Root   R/CF = Combining Form

WORD	PRONUNCIATION	ELEMENTS		DEFINITION
accommodate (verb)	ah-**KOM**-oh-date	P/ R/CF	**ac-** *toward* **-commodat/e** *adjust*	To adjust something to make it fit the needs
accommodation	ah-kom-oh-**DAY**-shun	S/ R/	**-ion** *action* **-commodat-** *adjust*	The act of adjusting something to make it fit the needs; in the case of the eye, the lens adjusts itself
amblyopia	am-blee-**OH**-pee-ah	P/ R/	**ambly-** *dull* **-opia** *sight*	Failure or incomplete development of the pathways of vision to the brain
esotropia	es-oh-**TROH**-pee-ah	S/ P/ R/	**-ia** *condition* **eso-** *inward* **-trop-** *turn*	A turning of the eye inward toward the nose
exotropia	ek-soh-**TROH**-pee-ah	S/ P/ R/	**-ia** *condition* **exo-** *outward* **-trop-** *turn*	A turning of the eye outward away from the nose
extrinsic intrinsic	eks-**TRIN**-sik in-**TRIN**-sik		Latin *on the outer side* Latin *on the inner side*	Muscles that are located on the outside of the eye Muscles that are located inside the eye
stereopsis	ster-ee-**OP**-sis	S/ R/	**-opsis** *vision* **stere-** *three-dimensional*	Three-dimensional vision
strabismus	strah-**BIZ**-mus	S/ R/	**-ismus** *take action* **strab-** *squint*	A turning of an eye away from its normal position

Exercises

A. Notice in this exercise that not every medical term needs a prefix and/or a suffix. *However, every medical term does contain one or more roots and/or combining forms.* **Deconstruct** *the following medical terms into their elements. Fill in the chart.* **LO 16.3, 16.D**

Medical Term	Prefix	Root(s)/Combining Form	Suffix
strabismus		1.	2.
exotropia	3.	4.	5.
accommodation	6.	7.	8.
esotropia	9.	10.	11.
amblyopia	12.	13.	
stereopsis		14.	15.

B. Recognize the definitions of disorders of the extrinsic muscles of the eye. *Insert the disorder of the eye that is being described. Fill in the blanks.* **LO 16.3, 16.A**

1. a turning of the eye outward away from the nose _____

2. failure or incomplete development of the pathways of vision to the brain _____

3. turning of the eye inward toward the nose _____

4. a turning of an eye away from its normal position _____

5. three-dimensional vision _____

6. the adjustment of the lens by itself _____

Lesson 16.2

SPECIAL SENSES OF THE EYE AND EAR

The Eyeball and Seeing

Lesson Objectives

The eyeball is a fluid-filled globe about 1 inch in diameter. Knowledge of its terminology, structure, and function enables you to understand how we see and what major problems and disorders of the eyeball can arise.

In this lesson, the information will enable you to:

16.2.1 Identify the principal components of the eyeball.

16.2.2 Explain the role of the cornea and the problems that can occur in that structure.

16.2.3 Describe the structure and functions of the lens and its associated structures.

16.2.4 Link the different components of the retina to their functions.

16.2.5 Discuss common disorders of the eyeball and its components.

16.2.6 Apply correct medical terminology to the anatomy, physiology, and disorders of the eyeball.

Keynotes

- The cornea protects the eye and, by changing shape, provides about 60% of the eye's focusing power.
- The pupil controls the amount of light entering the eye.
- The lens changes its shape to focus rays of light onto the retina.
- Both the cornea and the lens refract light rays. Neither has a blood supply, which compromises healing from injury or disease.

LO 16.4 The Eyeball

The functions of the eyeball are to:

- *Adjust* continuously the amount of light it lets in to reach the retina.
- *Focus* continually on near or distant objects.
- *Produce images* of those objects and instantly transmit them to the brain.

The front of the eyeball (except for the cornea) is covered by the conjunctiva, a thin layer of tissue that covers the inside of the eyelids and curves over the eyeball to meet the **sclera**, the tough, white outer layer of the eye.

The center of the front of the eye is a transparent, dome-shaped membrane called the **cornea**. The cornea has no blood supply and obtains its nutrients from tears and from fluid in the **anterior chamber** behind it.

When light rays strike the eye, they pass through the cornea. Because of its domed curvature, those rays striking the edge of the cornea are bent toward its center. The light rays then go through the **pupil**, the black opening in the center of the colored area (the **iris**) in the front of the eye.

The pupil controls the amount of light entering the eye. The **sphincter pupillae muscle** *(Figure 16.8)* opens and closes the pupil. When you are in a dark place, the sphincter pupillae muscle opens (dilates) to allow more light to enter. When you are in bright light, the sphincter pupillae muscle closes (constricts) to admit less light.

After passing through the pupil, the light rays pass through the transparent **lens**. The ciliary muscle of the **ciliary body** makes the lens thicker and thinner, enabling it to bend the light rays and focus them on the **retina** at the back of the eye. This process of changing focus is called accommodation. The process of bending the light rays by the cornea and lens is called **refraction**.

The lens has no supply of blood vessels or nerves. With increasing age, the lens loses its elasticity.

▲ **Figure 16.8** Anatomy of the Eyeball.

WORD	PRONUNCIATION		ELEMENTS	DEFINITION
ciliary body	**SILL**-ee-air-ee**BOD**-ee	S/ R/ R/	**-ary** *pertaining to* **cili-** *eyelid* **body** *mass*	Muscles that make the lens of the eye thicker and thinner
cornea	**KOR**-nee-ah		Latin *web, tunic*	The central, transparent part of the outer coat of the eye covering the iris and pupil
iris	**EYE**-ris		Greek *diaphragm of the eye*	Colored portion of the eye with the pupil in its center
lens	LENZ		Latin *lentil shape*	Transparent refractive structure behind the iris
pupil pupillae (pl) pupillary (adj)	**PYU**-pill pyu-**PILL**-ee **PYU**-pill-**AH**-ree	 S/ R/	Latin *pupil* **-ary** *pertaining to* **pupill-** *pupil*	The opening in the center of the iris that allows light to reach the lens Pertaining to the pupil
refract (verb) refraction (noun)	ree-**FRAKT** ree-**FRAK**-shun	 S/ R/	Latin *break up* **-ion** *action, condition, process* **refract-** *break up*	Make a change in direction of, or bend, a ray of light The change in direction of a ray of light when it passes from one optic medium to another
retina retinal (adj)	**RET**-ih-nah **RET**-ih-nal	 S/ R/	Latin *net* **-al** *pertaining to* **retin-** *retina*	Light-sensitive innermost layer of eyeball Pertaining to the retina
sclera scleral (adj)	**SKLAIR**-ah **SKLAIR**-al	 S/ R/	Greek *hard* **-al** *pertaining to* **scler-** *hard, white of eye*	Fibrous outer covering of the eyeball and the white of the eye Pertaining to the sclera
sphincter	**SFINK**-ter		Greek *band*	Band of muscle that encircles an opening; when it contracts, the opening squeezes closed

Exercises

A. Components of the eyeball: Enhance your knowledge of the components of the eyeball and their functions. *This will help you to understand the vision process. Match the phrase in the left column with the appropriate medical term in the right column.* **LO 16.4**

_____ 1. Colored portion of the eye

_____ 2. Change direction of a ray of light

_____ 3. Opening in the iris

_____ 4. Band of muscle that encircles an opening

_____ 5. Transparent, refractive structure

_____ 6. Innermost layer of eyeball

_____ 7. White of the eye

_____ 8. Operates the lens

a. lens

b. retina

c. sphincter

d. pupil

e. ciliary body

f. refract

g. iris

h. sclera

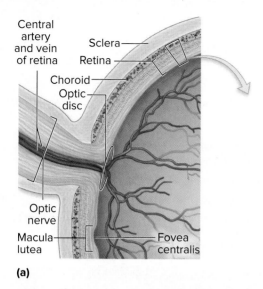

Central artery and vein of retina
Sclera
Retina
Choroid
Optic disc
Optic nerve
Macula lutea
Fovea centralis

(a)

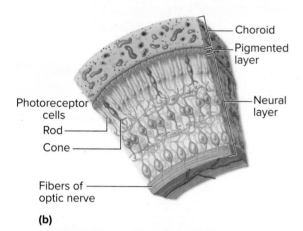

Choroid
Pigmented layer
Neural layer
Photoreceptor cells
Rod
Cone
Fibers of optic nerve

(b)

▲ **Figure 16.9** Structure of the Retina.

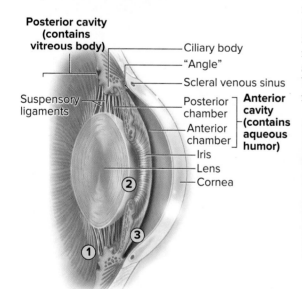

Posterior cavity (contains vitreous body)
Ciliary body
"Angle"
Scleral venous sinus
Suspensory ligaments
Posterior chamber
Anterior chamber
Anterior cavity (contains aqueous humor)
Iris
Lens
Cornea
② ③ ①

▲ **Figure 16.10** Circulation of Aqueous Humor.

LO 16.4 The Eyeball (continued)

The Retina

The final destination of the light rays is the **retina**, the thin lining at the back of your eye *(Figure 16.9a)*. It's an area the size of a small postage stamp that has 10 layers of cells. The retina has 130 million **rods** *(Figure 16.9b)*, which perceive only light, not color, and function mostly when the light is dim. There are 6.5 million **cones** *(see Figure 16.9b)*, which are activated by light and color and have precise **visual acuity**. Different cones respond to red, blue, and green light. The perception of color is based on the intensity of different mixtures of colors from the three types of cones.

Rods and cones are called **photoreceptor** cells. The rods and cones convert the energy of the light rays into electrical impulses, and the **optic nerve**, a bundle of more than a million nerve fibers, transmits these impulses to the **visual cortex** at the back of the brain. The area where the optic nerve leaves the retina is called the **optic disc**. Because it has no rods and cones, the optic disc cannot form images and is called the **blind spot**.

Just lateral to the optic disc at the back of the retina is a circular, yellowish region called the **macula lutea** *(see Figure 16.9a)*. In the center of the macula is a small pit called the **fovea centralis**, which has 4,000 tiny cones and no rods. Each cone has its own nerve fiber, and this makes the fovea the area of sharpest vision. As you read this text, the words are precisely focused on your fovea centralis.

Behind the photoreceptor layer of the retina is a very **vascular** layer called the **choroid**. This layer, together with the iris and **ciliary body**, is called the **uvea**.

Segments of the Eye

The eyeball is divided into two fluid-filled segments separated by the lens and the ciliary muscle. The fluids maintain the shape of the eyeball. In the back, the **posterior cavity** extends from the back of the lens to the retina and contains a transparent jelly called the **vitreous humor**, which helps maintain the shape of the eyeball.

In front, the **anterior cavity** extends from the cornea to the lens and is divided into two chambers. The **anterior chamber** extends from the cornea to the iris, and the **posterior chamber** extends from the iris to the lens *(Figure 16.10)*. **Aqueous humor** is produced in the posterior chamber as a filtrate from plasma (Step 1). It passes through the pupil into the anterior chamber (Step 2) where it is continually reabsorbed into a vascular space called the **scleral venous sinus** (Step 3) and taken into the venous bloodstream. The aqueous humor also removes waste products and helps maintain the internal chemical environment of the eye.

Keynotes

- Rods of the retina perceive only dim light and not color.
- Cones of the retina perceive bright light and color.
- Rods and cones are called photoreceptor cells.

Word Analysis and Definition

WORD	PRONUNCIATION	ELEMENTS		DEFINITION
aqueous humor	**AYK**-wee-us **HEW**-mor	S/ R/CF	**-ous** *pertaining to* **aqu/e-** *watery* **humor** Greek *liquid*	Watery liquid in the anterior and posterior chambers of the eye
choroid	**KOR**-oid		Greek *membrane*	Region of the retina and uvea
fovea centralis	**FOH**-vee-ah sen-**TRAH**-lis		**fovea** Latin *a pit* **centralis** Latin *central, in the center*	Small pit in the center of the macula that has the highest visual acuity
macula lutea	**MAK**-you-lah **LOO**-tee-ah		**macula** Latin *small spot* **lutea** Latin *yellow*	Yellowish spot on the back of the retina; contains the fovea centralis
optic	**OP**-tik	S/ R/	**-ic** *pertaining to* **opt-** *vision, eye*	Pertaining to vision or the eye
optical (adj)	**OP**-tih-kal	S/	**-ical** *pertaining to*	Pertaining to vision or the eye
photoreceptor	foh-toh-ree-**SEP**-tor	S/ R/CF R/	**-or** *that which does something* **phot/o-** *light* **-recept-** *receive*	A photoreceptor cell receives light and converts it into electrical impulses
uvea	**YOU**-vee-ah		Greek *layer of eyeball*	Middle coat of eyeball; includes iris, ciliary body, and choroid
visual acuity	**VIH**-zhoo-wal ah-**KYU**-ih-tee	S/ R/	**-al** *pertaining to* **visu-** *sight* **acuity** Latin *sharpen*	Sharpness and clearness of vision
vitreous humor	**VIT**-ree-us **HEW**-mor	S/ R/	**-ous** *pertaining to* **vitre-** *glassy* **humor** Greek *liquid*	A gelatinous liquid in the posterior cavity of the eyeball with the appearance of glass

Exercises

A. Identify the structures of the eyeball. *Select the best answer.* **LO 16.4, 16.A**

1. Sharpness and clearness of vision is called
   a. optical
   b. acuity
   c. vascular
   d. aqueous
   e. choroid

2. The term **photoreceptor** has
   a. two combining forms and a suffix
   b. a prefix, root, and suffix
   c. a root, a combining form, and a suffix
   d. two roots and a suffix
   e. a suffix and a root

3. The choroid, iris, and ciliary body make up the
   a. optic disc
   b. blind spot
   c. uvea
   d. visual cortex
   e. optic nerve

4. The gel contained in the posterior cavity is called
   a. vitreous humor
   b. ciliary body
   c. visual cortex
   d. aqueous humor
   e. macula lutea

5. This helps maintain the shape of the eyeball:
   a. vitreous humor
   b. rods
   c. fovea centralis
   d. cones
   e. macula lutea

6. The area of sharpest vision is the
   a. cornea
   b. rods
   c. macula lutea
   d. fovea centralis
   e. choroid

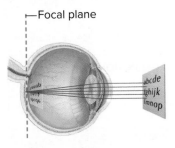

▲ **Figure 16.12** Emmetropia (Normal Vision).

Focal plane

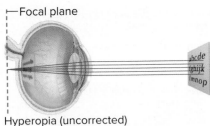

Hyperopia (uncorrected)

Corrected focal plane | Convex corrective lens

▲ **Figure 16.13** Hyperopia (Farsightedness).

Focal plane

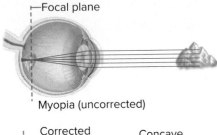

Myopia (uncorrected)

Corrected focal plane | Concave corrective lens

▲ **Figure 16.14** Myopia (Nearsightedness).

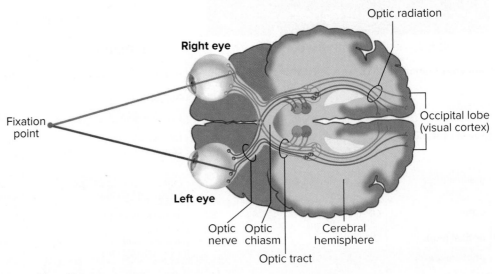

▲ **Figure 16.11** Visual Pathway.

LO 16.5 Visual Pathway

After the optic nerves leave the back of the retina and eyeball, they leave each orbit through the **optic foramen**. They converge into an "X" called the **optic chiasm** *(Figure 16.11)*. Here, the fibers from the medial half of each retina cross to the opposite side of the brain.

After leaving the chiasm, the fibers form the **optic tract** and then the **optic radiation** to take the nerve impulses to the **visual cortex** in the **occipital lobes** at the back of the brain. Here the incoming visual stimuli are interpreted.

Refraction

Light is traveling at a speed of 186,000 miles per second when it hits the eye. Light rays that hit the center of the cornea pass straight through, but because of the curvature of the cornea, rays that hit away from center are bent toward the center. The light rays then hit the lens, are bent again, and, in normal vision, the image is focused sharply on the retina *(Figure 16.12)*. This normal vision is called **emmetropia**.

Disorders of Refraction

Farsighted people are said to have **hyperopia** *(Figure 16.13)* in which only distant objects can be seen clearly. Because the eyeball is shortened, objects close to the eye are focused behind the retina and vision is blurred. Convex lenses are needed to correct the problem.

Nearsighted people are said to have **myopia** *(Figure 16.14)*, in which only close objects can be clearly seen. Because the eyeball is elongated, faraway objects are focused in front of the retina. Vision is blurred. Concave lenses are needed to correct the problem.

In **presbyopia**, the lens loses its flexibility, so there is difficulty focusing for near vision. This happens when you reach your forties. Convex bifocal or progressive lenses are needed for this problem.

In **astigmatism**, unequal curvatures of the cornea cause unequal focusing and blurred images. Cylindrical lenses, which refract light more in one plane than another, are needed to correct this problem.

LO 16.5, 16.A
Word Analysis and Definition

S = Suffix   P = Prefix   R = Root   R/CF = Combining Form

WORD	PRONUNCIATION	ELEMENTS		DEFINITION
astigmatism	ah-**STIG**-mah-tism	S/ P/ R/	-ism *action* a- *without* -stigmat- *focus*	Inability to focus light rays that enter the eye in different planes
chiasm chiasma (alternative term)	**KIE**-asm kie-**AZ**-mah		Greek *cross*	X-shaped crossing of the two optic nerves at the base of the brain
emmetropia	em-eh-**TROH**-pee-ah	P/ R/	emmetr- *measure* -opia *sight*	Normal refractive condition of the eye
hyperopia	high-per-**OH**-pee-ah	P/ R/	hyper- *beyond* -opia *sight*	Able to see distant objects but unable to see close objects
myopia (*Note:* An "o" is removed from the elements.)	my-**OH**-pee-ah	P/ R/	myo- *to blink* -opia *sight*	Able to see close objects but unable to see distant objects
presbyopia	prez-bee-**OH**-pee-ah	R/ R/	presby- *old person* -opia *sight*	Difficulty in nearsighted vision occurring in middle and old age in both sexes
tract	TRAKT		Latin *path*	Bundle of nerve fibers with a common origin and destination

Exercises

A. Create new medical terms by applying different prefixes to the root -*opia*. *The definition of each term is provided; you construct the medical term. Fill in the blanks.* **LO 16.5, 16.A, 16.C**

1. Meaning of -*opia*: _____.

2. Difficulty in nearsighted vision occurring in middle and old age: _____/opia

3. Normal refractive condition of the eye: _____/opia

4. Able to see close objects but unable to see distant ones: _____/opia

5. Able to see distant objects but unable to see close objects: _____/opia

6. *Challenge question:* If *dipl/o* means *double* and *two,* what then is **diplopia**? _____

B. Choose the correct answer, using the *language of ophthalmology*. **LO 16.5, 16.A**

1. Which of the following medical terms does not apply to the visual pathway?

   a. visual cortex

   b. occipital lobes

   c. optic foramen

   d. labyrinth

   e. optic tract

2. Which eye condition requires cylindrical lenses for correction?

   a. astigmatism

   b. myopia

   c. hyperopia

   d. emmetropia

   e. presbyopia

Ulcer

▲ **Figure 16.15** **Fluorescein-Stained Corneal Ulcer.** ©Barbara Galati/Diomedaa/ Medical Images

▲ **Figure 16.16** **Vision with Glaucoma.** Source: National Eye Institute, National Institutes of Health

Cataract

▲ **Figure 16.17** **Cataract.** ©Dr. P. Marazzi/ SPL/Photo Researchers, Inc.

Vision with

▲ **Figure 16.18** **Vision with Cataract.** Source: National Eye Institute, National Institutes of Health

LO 16.6 Disorders of the Anterior Eyeball

Conjunctivitis is the **infectious**, contagious condition that Mrs. Jenny Hughes had in the Case Report 16.1. It can be caused by viruses, many different bacteria, and organisms that cause sexually transmitted diseases (STDs, see *Chapter 8*). It is a cause of "blood-shot" eyes.

Allergic conjunctivitis can be part of seasonal hay fever or be produced by year-round **allergens** such as animal dander and dust mites (*see Chapter 12*). **Irritant conjunctivitis** can be caused by air pollutants (smoke and fumes) and by chemicals such as chlorine and those found in soaps and cosmetics.

Neonatal conjunctivitis (ophthalmia neonatorum) can be caused by a blocked tear duct in the baby, by the antibiotic eyedrops given routinely at birth, or by sexually trans-mitted bacteria in an infected mother's birth canal.

Dry eyes are a common and chronic condition which over 75 million Americans suf-fer from. It is due to the tears losing water and becoming too salty so that the eyes sting and burn and vision becomes blurry.

Corneal abrasions can be caused by foreign bodies, direct trauma (such as being poked by a fingernail), or badly fitting contact lenses. The abrasion can grow into an ulcer (*see Figure 16.15*).

Scleritis, inflammation of the sclera (the white outer covering of the eyeball), can affect one or both eyes. It causes dull pain and intense redness, and is often associated with rheumatoid arthritis (*see Chapter 14*) and the digestive disorder Crohn's disease (*see Chapter 5*).

Uveitis, inflammation of the iris, ciliary body, and choroid, produces pain, intense **photophobia**, blurred vision, and constriction of the pupil. There is usually an underly-ing disease, such as rheumatoid arthritis.

Glaucoma

The circulation of aqueous humor was described earlier in this chapter. If the aqueous humor cannot escape from the eye into the bloodstream, the fluid continues to be pro-duced and pressure builds up inside the eye. The increased **intraocular** pressure inter-feres with the blood supply to the retina, causing death of retinal cells. Eventually the optic nerve fibers are damaged. This condition is called **glaucoma** and is a major cause of blindness (*Figure 16.16*).

Cataracts

A **cataract** is a cloudy or opaque area in the lens (*Figure 16.17*). It is typically caused by deterioration of the lens due to aging and may be associated with diabetes and with cigarette smoke. It presents with blurring of vision and **photosensitivity** or may be dis-covered on routine eye examination. It is another major cause of blindness.

The majority of cataracts occur in the center of the lens, but those associated with diabetes can be cortical (around the outside of the lens). Cortical cataracts can cause diminished **peripheral vision** and photosensitivity. The blurred vision obtained when a cataract is present is shown in *Figure 16.18*.

WORD	PRONUNCIATION	ELEMENTS		DEFINITION
abrasion	ah-**BRAY**-shun	S/ R/	-ion *action, condition, process* **abras-** *scrape off*	Area of skin or mucous membrane that has been scraped off
cataract	**KAT**-ah-rakt		Greek *waterfall*	Complete or partial opacity of the lens
glaucoma	glaw-**KOH**-mah	S/ R/	-oma *mass, tumor* **glauc-** *lens opacity*	Increased intraocular pressure
infectious	in-**FEK**-shus	S/ R/CF	-ous *pertaining to* **infect/i-** *internal invasion*	Capable of being transmitted, or caused by infection by a microorganism
intraocular	in-trah-**OK**-you-lar	S/ P/ R/	-ar *pertaining to* **intra-** *inside* -ocul- *eye*	Pertaining to the inside of the eye
ophthalmia neonatorum	off-**THAL**-mee-ah nee-oh-nay-**TOR**-um	S/ R/ S/ P/ R/	-ia *condition* **ophthalm-** *eye* -orum *function of* **neo-** *new* -nat- *born*	Conjunctivitis of the newborn
peripheral vision	peh-**RIF**-er-al **VIZH**-un	S/ R/	-al *pertaining to* **peripher-** *external boundary* **vision** Latin *to see*	Ability to see objects as they come into the outer edges of the visual field
photophobia	foh-toh-**FOH**-bee-ah	S/ R/CF	-phobia *fear* **phot/o-** *light*	Fear of the light because it hurts the eyes
photophobic (adj)	foh-toh-**FOH**-bik	S/ R/	-ic *pertaining to* -phob- *light*	Relating to or suffering from photophobia
photosensitive (adj)	foh-toh-**SEN**-sih-tiv	R/CF R/CF	**phot/o-** *light* -sensitiv/e *sensitive*	An eye in which light induces pain
photosensitivity	foh-toh-sen-sih-**TIV**-ih-tee	S/ R/	-ity *condition* -sensitiv- *sensitive*	Condition in which light produces pain in the eye

Exercises

A. Review the medical terms in the above WAD. *Use the language of ophthalmology to complete the sentences. Use each term only once. Fill in the blanks.* **LO 16.6, 16.A**

1. _____ is a result of increased intraocular pressure.

2. Sensitivity to light that produces eye pain is _____.

3. Another name for neonatal conjunctivitis is _____ _____ (2 words).

4. Inflammation of the iris, ciliary body, and choroid is termed _____.

B. Deconstruct medical terms into their word elements. **LO 16.6, 16.D**

1. abrasion: _____ / _____
                   R   **S**

2. glaucoma: _____ / _____
                   R   **S**

3. intraocular: _____ / _____ / _____
               P   **R**   **S**

Macular degeneration

▲ **Figure 16.19** Ophthalmoscopic View of Macular Degeneration. ©Paul Parker/ Photo Researchers, Inc.

▲ **Figure 16.20** Vision with Macular Degeneration. ©Spencer Grant/Science Source

Hemorrhage

▲ **Figure 16.21** Ophthalmoscopic View of Diabetic Retinopathy. ©memorisz/Getty Images RF

▲ **Figure 16.22** Vision with Diabetic Retinopathy. Source: National Eye Institute, National Institutes of Health

LO 16.7 Diseases of the Retina

Macular Degeneration

Degeneration of the central macula results in loss of visual acuity, with a dark blurry area of vision loss in the center of the visual field (*Figures 16.19 and 16.20*).

There is photoreceptor cell loss and bleeding, with capillary proliferation and scar formation. The condition can progress to blindness. Most cases occur in people over age 55.

Retinal Detachment

Separation of the retina from its underlying choroid layer may be partial or complete and produces a retinal tear or hole. The detachment can happen suddenly, without pain. The patient sees a dark shadow invading his or her peripheral vision. The detachment can be seen on **ophthalmoscopic** examination.

Diabetic Retinopathy

This disease occurs most frequently in diabetics whose blood sugar levels are not controlled. Some 50% of diabetics have **retinopathy**.

In the early stages, **microaneurysms** of the small retinal blood vessels form. There are usually no symptoms. Later, hemorrhages can occur, leading to destruction of the photoreceptor cells (rods and cones) and visual difficulties (*Figure 16.21*).

Laser photocoagulation is usually effective in controlling the lesions; but once vision is lost from an area of the retina, it usually does not return (*Figure 16.22*).

Papilledema

Papilledema is swelling of the optic disc due to increased **intracranial** pressure. It is not a diagnosis; it is a sign of some underlying pathology. It is seen on ophthalmoscopic examination.

Cancer of the Eye

Tumors of the skin of the eyelids include the **squamous cell** and **basal cell carcinomas** and **melanoma**, described in *Chapter 4*.

Retinoblastoma is the most common cancer in children and is diagnosed most commonly around 18 months of age. Twenty percent have the cancer in both eyes. The condition can be hereditary.

The first symptom is a white appearance of the pupil (**leukocoria**). With early detection and aggressive treatment based on chemotherapy and laser surgery, 90% of cases are cured.

In adults, the most common cancers are **metastases** to the eye from cancer of the lung in men and the breast in women.

Some people have a hereditary lack of response by one or more of the three types of cones and show **color blindness**. The most common form is red-green color blindness, in which these colors and related shades cannot be distinguished from each other.

Night blindness is the inability to see in poor light. It is a symptom of an underlying problem that can be

- Uncorrected nearsightedness.
- Cataracts.
- Retinitis pigmentosa.
- Vitamin A deficiency.
- Glaucoma medications (such as pilocarpine) that constrict the pupil.

WORD	PRONUNCIATION		ELEMENTS	DEFINITION
leukocoria	loo-koh-**KOH**-ree-ah	S/ R/CF R/	**-ia** *condition* **leuk/o-** *white* **-cor-** *pupil*	Reflection in pupil of white mass in the eye
metastasis metastases (pl)	meh-**TAS**-tah-sis meh-**TAS**-tah-sees	P/ R/	**meta-** *beyond* **-stasis** *stay in one place*	Spread of disease from one part of the body to another
microaneurysm	my-kroh-**AN**-yu-rizm	P/ R/	**micro-** *small* **-aneurysm** *dilation*	Focal dilation of retinal capillaries
papilledema	pah-pill-eh-**DEE**-mah	R/ R/	**papill-** *pimple* **-edema** *swelling*	Swelling of the optic disc in the retina
retinoblastoma	**RET**-in-oh-blas-**TOH**-mah	S/ S/ R/CF	**-oma** *tumor, mass* **-blast-** *germ cell* **retin/o-** *retina*	Malignant neoplasm of primitive retinal cells
retinopathy	ret-ih-**NOP**-ah-thee	S/	**-pathy** *disease*	Degenerative disease of the retina

Exercises

A. Identify the disorders of the eye. *Given the description, identify the disease being described. Fill in the blanks.* **LO 16.7, 16.A**

1. This is a cancer of the eye. It is the most common cancer occurring in children: _____.

2. Increased intracranial pressure can lead to swelling of the optic disc, correctly termed as _____.

3. This condition can occur in diabetics and can lead to blindness. This condition is diabetic _____.

4. A loss of central vision due to the degeneration of the retina lateral to the optic disc: _____ degeneration.

B. Define the word elements to decipher the meaning of medical terms. *Word elements provide clues to the meanings of medical terms. Choose the correct answer to complete the following statements.* **LO 16.7, 16.D**

1. In the term **leukocoria,** the root element *cor-* means:
   a. cornea
   b. vessel
   c. white
   d. pupil
   e. condition

2. In the term **retinopathy,** the suffix means:
   a. choroid
   b. disease
   c. uvea
   d. retina
   e. cancer

3. In the term **retinoblastoma,** the word element that means *germ cell* is:
   a. *retin/o*
   b. *-blast*
   c. *-oma*

4. In the term **papilledema,** the root *papill-* means:
   a. pimple
   b. cancer
   c. pupil
   d. swelling

Lesson 16.3

SPECIAL SENSES OF THE EYE AND EAR

Procedures and Pharmacology for the Eye

Lesson Objectives

Diagnostic and therapeutic procedures and the application of medications to the external eye are performed by many different health professionals. The information in this lesson will enable you to:

16.3.1 Explain the diagnostic procedures used for disorders of the eye.

16.3.2 Discuss therapeutic procedures used for disorders of the eye.

16.3.3 Describe medications used for disorders of the eye.

Abbreviation

PERRLA pupils equal, round, reactive to light and accommodation

(a)

(b)

V = .50 D.

The fourteenth of August was the day fixed upon for the sailing of the brig Pilgrim, on her voyage from Boston round Cape Horn, to the western coast of North America. As she was to get under way early in the afternoon, I made my appearance on board at twelve o'clock in full sea-rig, and with my chest, containing an outfit for a two or three years voyage, which I had undertaken from a determination to cure, if possible, by an entire change of life, and by a long absence from books and study, a weakness of the eyes which had obliged me to give up my pursuits, and which no medical aid seemed likely to cure. The change from the tight dress coat, silk cap and kid gloves of an undergraduate at Cambridge, to the

V = .75 D.

loose duck trousers, checked shirt and tarpaulin hat of a sailor, though somewhat of a transformation, was soon made, and I supposed that I should pass very well for a Jack tar. But it is impossible to deceive the practiced eye in these matters; and while I supposed myself to be looking as salt as Neptune himself, I was, no doubt, known for a landsman by every one on board, as soon as I hove in sight. A sailor has a peculiar cut to his clothes, and a way of wear-

V = 1.   D.

ing them which a green hand can never get. The trousers, tight around the hips, and thence hanging long and loose around the feet, a superabundance of checked shirt, a low-crowned, well-varnished black hat, worn on the back of the head, with half a fathom of black ribbon hanging over the left eye, and a peculiar tie to the black silk neckerchief, with sundry other *details*, are signs the want of which betray the beginner at once.

V = 1.25 D.

Beside the points in my dress which were out of the way, doubtless my complexion and hands would distinguish me from the regular *salt*, who, with a sun-browned cheek, wide step and rolling gait, swings his bronzed and toughened hands athwartships half open, as though just to ready to grasp a rope. "With all my imperfections

V = 1.50 D.

on my head," I joined the crew, and we hauled out into the stream and came to anchor for the night. The next day we were employed in preparation for sea, reeving and studding-sail gear, crossing royal yards, putting on chafing gear, and taking on board our powder. On the

▲ **Figure 16.23** **Visual Acuity Tests.** (*a*) Snellen letter chart for distance vision. (*b*) Jaeger reading card. Fig 16.23a: ©McGraw-Hill Education/Rick Brady, photographer. Fig 16.23b: Courtesy Good-Lite Company

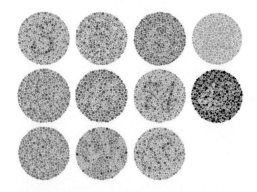

Complete **Ishihara** color test plates

▲ **Figure 16.24** **Test for Color Blindness.** Reproduced with permission from *Ishihara's Tests for Color Deficiency*, published by Kanehara Trading Inc., Tokyo, Japan. Tests for color deficiency cannot be conducted with this figure. For accurate testing, the original plates should be used. ©Alexander Kaludov/Alamy Stock Photo RF

LO 16.8 Ophthalmic Diagnostic Procedures

Examination of the eye includes evaluation of pupillary reaction. Medical shorthand for this quick normal eye examination can be **PERRLA,** which means *p*upils *e*qual, *r*ound, *r*eactive to *l*ight and *a*ccommodation.

Visual acuity, the sharpness and clearness of vision, is tested for each eye with the opposite eye covered with a solid object. For **distance vision**, patients look at a **Snellen letter chart** (*Figure 16.23a*) 20 feet away and vision is recorded as the smallest line in which the patient can read half of the letters. For **near vision**, the patient reads a standard **Jaeger reading card** (*Figure 16.23b*) at a distance of 14 inches.

Color vision is tested using the **Ishihara color system**. In the example shown in *Figure 16.24,* people with red-green color blindness would not be able to detect the number 74 among the colored dots.

Refractive error, the nature and degree to which light is bent by the eye, is measured with a **refractometer**.

Visual fields can be impaired by lesions anywhere in the neural visual pathway and in glaucoma, and can be assessed grossly by **direct confrontation**. The patient maintains a fixed gaze at the examiner's nose and a small object or finger is brought into the patient's visual periphery (**peripheral vision**) in each of the four visual quadrants. The patient indicates when the object is first seen. Each eye is tested separately.

Corneal examination uses **fluorescein** staining to reveal abrasions and ulcers.

Pupillary reaction to light is tested in each eye with a penlight as the patient looks into the distance.

Extrinsic muscles of the eyeball are tested by guiding the patient to look in 8 directions (up, up and right, right, down and right, down, down and left, left, left and up) with a moving finger or penlight.

WORD	PRONUNCIATION	ELEMENTS		DEFINITION
fluorescein	flor-**ESS**-ee-in	P/ R/	**fluo-** *fluorine* **-rescein** *resin*	Dye that produces a vivid green color under a blue light to diagnose corneal abrasions and foreign bodies in the eye
Jaeger reading cards	**YAY**-ger **REED**-ing CARDS	S/ R/	Edward Jaeger, 1818–1884, Austrian ophthalmologist **-ing** *quality of, doing* **read-** *advise, interpret, read* **card** Latin *leaf of papyrus*	Printed in different sizes of print for testing near vision
peripheral vision	peh-**RIF**-er-al **VIZH**-un	S/ R/	**-al** *pertaining to* **peripher-** *external boundary* **vision** Latin *to see*	Ability to see objects as they come into the outer edges of the visual field
refractometer	ree-frak-**TAH**-meh-tur	S/ R/CF	**-meter** *measure, instrument to measure* **refract/o-** *to bend (light)*	Device that measures refractive errors of the cornea
Snellen letter chart	**SNEL**-en **LET**-er CHART		Hermann Snellen, 1834–1908, Dutch ophthalmologist **letter** Latin *letter of the alphabet* **chart** Latin *piece of papyrus, document*	Test for acuity of distance vision

Exercises

A. The ophthalmic technician in Dr. Chun's office needs to be familiar with all these terms in order to communicate with Dr. Chun and her patients. *Show your understanding of the terms by choosing the correct answers.* **LO 16.8**

1. The test used to measure color blindness is
   - **a.** Snellen
   - **b.** Jaeger
   - **c.** Ishihara
   - **d.** visual fields
   - **e.** otoscope

2. Peripheral vision measures the outer edge of the
   - **a.** anterior segment
   - **b.** vitreous body
   - **c.** aqueous humor
   - **d.** posterior segment
   - **e.** visual field

3. A test for near vision is the
   - **a.** Snellen chart
   - **b.** ophthalmoscope
   - **c.** Jaeger card
   - **d.** Ishihara
   - **e.** visual fields

4. This is used to detect corneal abrasions or ulcers
   - **a.** ophthalmoscope
   - **b.** refractometer
   - **c.** tonometer
   - **d.** fluorescein

Optic disc

▲ **Figure 16.25** Ophthalmoscopic **Examination of the Eye.** ©Lisa R. Klancher

LO 16.8 Ophthalmic Diagnostic Procedures (continued)

Fundoscopy using an **ophthalmoscope** *(Figure 16.25)* can detect lens opacities, retinal changes, and retinal vascular changes. The vascular changes can be areas of hemorrhage or changes in the retinal arteries indicating hypertension or arteriosclerosis. The retinal changes can show age-related macular degeneration, retinoblastoma, retinal detachment, signs of diabetes, signs of glaucoma, or signs of raised intracranial pressure (**papilledema**).

Slit-lamp examination focuses the height and width of a beam of light to give a **stereoscopic** view of the interior structures of the eyeball. It is used for identifying corneal foreign bodies and abrasions, and identifying retinal diseases.

Intraocular pressure is measured with a **tonometer,** which determines the eyeball's resistance to tension or indentation. There are several methods of **tonometry,** which include pneumatonometry and Goldmann tonometry.

LO 16.9 Therapeutic Procedures for Diseases of the Eye

Photocoagulation therapy is used to reattach a torn or detached portion of the retina and to prevent further growth of abnormal blood vessels that can cause a detachment. A high-intensity, narrowly focused beam of light from the **argon laser** is absorbed by pigment in the retinal cells and converted into heat, which welds the edge of the retinal detachment against the underlying choroid. **Retinal cryopexy (cryotherapy)** uses intense cold to have the same effects as the heat of photocoagulation.

Photocoagulation therapy is also used to heal bleeding **microaneurysms** of small blood vessels in the early stages of **diabetic retinopathy,** and is used with **chemotherapy** in the treatment of **retinoblastoma**. It also can be used for wet age-related macular degeneration to destroy or seal off new blood vessels to prevent leakage, but the many small retinal scars it creates cause blind spots in the patient's visual field.

When a **cataract** is interfering with vision, the opaque lens is removed by **phacoemulsification** in which ultrasonic waves fragment the cataract to make its removal much easier. The lens is then replaced with an artificial **intraocular** lens, which becomes a permanent part of the eye.

Laser corneal surgery is a procedure that uses a laser to reshape the surface of the eye to change the curvature of the cornea. The surgical procedure **radial keratotomy** is used to treat myopia. Radial cuts, like the spokes of a wheel, flatten the cornea and enable it to refract the light rays to focus on the retina. In flattening the cornea, it can correct myopia (nearsightedness) and astigmatism (uneven curvature of the cornea) and alter the outer edges of the cornea to correct hypermetropia (farsightedness). These procedures are also called **refractive surgery** and **laser-assisted in situ keratomileusis (LASIK)**. An alternative to LASIK is **photorefractive keratectomy (PRK)**, in which spoke-like incisions are cut into the cornea to flatten its surface and correct nearsightedness.

Glaucoma is treated with a combination of eye drops *(see next section on ocular pharmacology)*, pills, laser surgery, and traditional surgery with the goal of preventing loss of vision. The most commonly used laser procedure is **trabeculoplasty**, in which the eye's drainage system is changed by the laser beam to enable the aqueous humor fluid to drain out more easily into the blood stream. **Trabeculectomy** is the most common traditional surgical procedure, in which a passage is created in the sclera to allow excess fluid to drain out of the eye. More recently, a small silicone tube has been placed from the surface of the eye into the anterior chamber to allow drainage of the excess fluid.

y

WORD	PRONUNCIATION	ELEMENTS		DEFINITION
argon laser	**AR**-gon **LAY**-zer		**argon** Greek *lazy* **laser** *acronym for* **L**ight **A**mplification by **S**timulated **E**mission of **R**adiation	Laser used for ophthalmic procedures consisting of photons in the blue and/or green spectrum
cryotherapy	**CRY**-oh-**THAIR**-ah-pee	S/ R/CF	**-therapy** *treatment* **cry/o-** *cold*	The use of cold in the treatment of disease
cryopexy	**CRY**-oh-**PEK**-see	S/	**-pexy** *fixation*	Repair of a detached retina by freezing it to surrounding tissue
fundus	**FUN**-dus		Latin *bottom*	Part farthest from the opening of a hollow organ
fundoscopy	fun-**DOS**-koh-pee	S/ R/CF	**-scopy** *to examine* **fund/o-** *fundus*	Examination of the fundus (retina) of the eye
fundoscopic (adj) Ishihara color system	fun-doh-**SKOP**-ik ish-ee-**HAR**-ah **KUH**-ler **SIS**-tem	S/	**-ic** *pertaining to* Shinobu Ishihara, 1879–1963, Japanese ophthalmologist **color** Latin *color* **system** Greek *to combine*	As a result of fundoscopy Test for color vision defects
in situ	IN **SIGH**-tyu		Latin *in its original place*	In the correct place
keratectomy	**KER**-ah-**TEK**-toh-mee	S/ R/	**-ectomy** *excision* **kerat-** *cornea*	Surgery to remove corneal tissue
keratomileusis	**KER**-ah-toh-mie-**LOO**-sis	R/CF R/	**kerat/o-** *cornea* **-mileusis** *lathe*	A surgical procedure that involves cutting and shaping the cornea
keratotomy	**KER**-ah-**TOT**-oh-mee	S/	**-tomy** *surgical incision*	Incision in the cornea
ophthalmoscope	off-**THAL**-moh-skope	S/ R/CF	**-scope** *instrument for viewing* **ophthalam/o-** *eye*	Instrument for viewing the retina
ophthalmoscopy ophthalmoscopic	**OFF**-thal-**MOS**-koh-pee **OFF**-thal-moh-**SKOP**-ik	S/ S/	**-scopy** *to examine, to view* **-ic** *pertaining to*	The process of viewing the retina Pertaining to the use of an ophthalmoscope
phacoemulsification	**FAK**-oh-ee-mul-sih-fih-**KAY**-shun	S/ R/CF R/	**-ation** *process* **phac/o-** *lens* **-emulsific-** *to milk out*	Technique used to fragment the center of the lens into very tiny pieces and suck them out of the eye
photocoagulation	foh-toh-koh-ah-you-**LAY**-shun	S/ R/CF R/	**-ation** *process* **phot/o-** *light* **-coagul-** *clot*	The use of light (laser beam) to form a clot
photoreactive	foh-toh-ree-**AK**-tiv	P/ R/	**-re-** *again* **-active** *movement*	Initiation by light of a process previously inactive
tonometer	toh-**NOM**-eh-ter	S/	**-meter** *measure, instrument to measure*	Instrument for determining intraocular pressure
		R/CF	**ton/o-** *pressure, tension*	The measurement of intraocular pressure
tonometry	toh-**NOM**-eh-tree	S/	**-metry** *process of measuring*	
trabeculectomy	trah-**BEK**-you-**LEK**-toh-mee	S/ R/	**-ectomy** *excision* **trabecul-** *eye's fluid drainage system*	Surgical creation of passage in sclera to allow fluid to drain out of the eye
trabeculoplasty	trah-**BEK**-you-loh-plas-tee	S/ R/CF	**-plasty** *surgical repair* **trabecul/o-** *eye's fluid drainage system*	Laser repair of eye's fluid drainage system

Exercises

A. Identify the meaning of the word elements related to ophthalmology. *Match the element in the first column with its correct meaning in the second column.* **LO 16.9, 16.C**

Word Element	Meaning
_____ **1.** *kerat-*	**a.** cold
_____ **2.** *cry/o-*	**b.** light
_____ **3.** *-ectomy*	**c.** surgical repair
_____ **4.** *-plasty*	**d.** eye's fluid drainage system
_____ **5.** *phot/o-*	**e.** cornea
_____ **6.** *trabecul-*	**f.** excision

LO 16.10 Ocular Pharmacology

There are a wide variety and number of medications placed directly into the conjunctival sac to treat different eye disorders or to help the clinician examine the eye more thoroughly and more easily.

- **Mydriatics** are drugs that cause the pupil to dilate and are mainly used to examine the eye fundus. **Mydriacil** *(Tropicamide)* takes 15 minutes for the eye to fully dilate and can last for 3 to 6 hours with blurred vision. Other dilating drops, for example, **atropine** and **homatropine,** are long acting, lasting 7 to 10 days.

- **Miotics** are drugs that constrict the pupil (**miosis**); for example **pilocarpine,** which can be part of a regimen for treating glaucoma.

- **Ocular topical anesthetics** temporarily block nerve conduction in the conjunctiva and cornea. They have a quick onset of 10 to 20 seconds and last for 10 to 20 minutes. They are used to assist with eye examinations and visual **acuity** testing and to help treat chemical burns, welding flash, and foreign bodies. Examples are **amethocaine,** 0.5% and 1%, and **oxybupricaine,** 0.4%.

- **Ocular diagnostic drops** stain conjunctival cells to improve diagnostic capabilities; for example, the presence of a foreign body or a corneal abrasion. Examples are **fluorescein** and **Lissamine Green.** The drops do not interfere with vision but are taken up by soft contact lenses, which should be removed prior to instillation of the drops.

- **Ocular lubricant drops** are used to replace tears, treat dry eyes, moisten hard contact lenses, protect the eye during eye surgical procedures, and help treat keratitis. Examples are *Visine, Refresh Optive,* and *Retaine.*

- **Anti-infective eye medications,** both drops and ointments, can be **antibacterial,** for example, **glatifloxacin** *(Zymaxid)* and **sulfacetamide** *(Klaron, Ovace)*; **antifungal,** such as **natamycin** *(Natacyn)*; and **antiviral,** for example, **idoxuridine** *(Herplex)* and **trifluridine** *(Viroptic).*

- **Anti-inflammatory eye medications** are used in allergic disorders, to prevent scarring and visual loss in inflammation of the eye, and to decrease postoperative eye inflammation and scarring. Examples are **corticosteroids** such as **dexamethasone** *(Decadron)* and **nonsteroidal anti-inflammatory agents** such as **flurbiprofen** *(Ocufen)* and **suprofen** *(Profenal).*

- In **glaucoma,** numerous eye medications are available and are used individually, in combinations, and/or with surgery *(see previous section on eye therapeutic procedures).* **Miotics** decrease the size of the pupil and widen the trabecular network to enable fluid to escape more easily. **Beta-adrenergic blockers** decrease production of aqueous humor; examples are **timolol maleate** *(Timoptic)* and **betaxolol** *(Betoptic).* **Carbonic anhydrase inhibitors** reduce production of aqueous humor; examples are **acetazolamide sodium** *(Diamox)* and **dichlorphenamide** *(Daranide)*; **alpha-adrenergic agents** increase the outflow of aqueous humor by unknown mechanisms; examples are **epinephrine** *(Epifrin)* and **phenylephrine** *(Neo-synephrine).*

WORD	PRONUNCIATION	ELEMENTS		DEFINITION
antibacterial	**AN**-teh-bak-**TEER**-ee-al	S/ P/ R/CF	-al *pertaining to* anti- *against* -bacter/i- *bacteria*	Destructive of or preventing the growth of bacteria
antifungal anti-infective	**AN**-teh-**FUN**-gal **AN**-teh-in-**FEK**-tiv	R/ S/ R/	-fung- *fungus* -ive *nature of* -infect- *taint*	Destructive of or preventing the growth of fungi Made incapable of transmitting an infection
anti-inflammatory	**AN**-teh-in-**FLAM**-ah-toh-ree	S/ P/ R/	-ory *having the function of* -in- *in* -flammat- *inflammation*	Reducing, removing, or preventing inflammation
antiviral	an-teh-**VIE**-ral	R/	-vir- *virus*	To weaken or abolish the action or replication of a virus
atropine	**AT**-roh-peen		Greek *belladonna*	Pharmacologic agent used to dilate pupils
inhibitor	in-**HIB**-ih-tor	S/ P/ R/	-or *one who does* in- *in* -hibit- *keep back*	An agent that restrains or retards physiologic, chemical, or enzymatic action
miosis miotic	my-**OH**-sis my-**OT**-ik	S/ R/CF	Greek *lessening* -tic *pertaining to* mi/o- *less*	Contraction of the pupil An agent that causes the pupil to contract
mydriasis mydriatic	mih-**DRY**-ah-sis mid-ree-**AT**-ik	S/ R/	Greek *dilation of the pupil* -atic *pertaining to* mydri- *dilation of the pupil*	Dilation of the pupil Pertaining to or an agent that causes dilation of the pupil

Exercises

A. Identify the medication that would treat each condition. *Match the medication on the left with its correct indicated use.* **LO 16.10**

_____ 1. antibacterial

_____ 2. mydriatic

_____ 3. anti-inflammatory

_____ 4. miotic

_____ 5. ocular topical anesthetic

_____ 6. lubricant

a. a treatment for glaucoma

b. dry eyes

c. bacterial infection of the eye

d. allergic disorder of the eye

e. dilate the pupil in order to view the eye fundus

f. chemical burn to the eyes

Lesson 16.4

The Ear and Hearing

Lesson Objectives

In order to understand what is going on with Eddie in Case Report (CR) 16.3, to communicate with Dr. Lee about him, to respond to the mother's concerns, and to document the office visit, you need to be able to:

16.4.1 Describe the structures and functions of the three regions of the ear.

16.4.2 Explain how sound waves progress through the ear and are transferred to the brain and recognized as sounds.

16.4.3 Identify how common diseases of the ear interfere with the process of hearing.

16.4.4 Apply the correct medical terminology to the anatomy, physiology, and disorders of the ear.

 Case Report (CR) 16.3

You are

. . . a medical assistant working with **primary care** physician Susan Lee, MD, of the Fulwood Medical Group on March 16, 2017.

Your patients are

. . . 3-year-old Eddie Cardenas and his mother, Mrs. Carmen Cardenas.

Mrs. Cardenas has brought in her son, Eddie. She tells you that he has had a cold for a couple of days. Early this morning he woke up screaming, felt hot, and was tugging his ears. She gave him **acetaminophen** with some orange juice, and he threw up. This is the third similar episode in the past year. Since the last time, she is concerned that he is not hearing normally. You see a worried mother and a very unhappy, restless toddler with a green nasal discharge. His oral temperature taken with an electronic digital thermometer is 102.4°F, pulse 100. Dr. Lee examines Eddie and finds that he has an **upper respiratory infection (URI)** with a **bilateral otitis media (BOM)**. She prescribes amoxicillin 250 mg four times a day (q.i.d.) for 10 days, and acetaminophen 160 mg when necessary (p.r.n.) for pain, after which she will see Eddie again. After the acute infection subsides, if there remains an **effusion** in the middle ear, she will refer Eddie to an **otologist**. She explained this to Mrs. Cardenas.—Luisa Guittierez, CMA. 1115 hrs. 3/16/17.

Abbreviations	
BOM	bilateral otitis media
mg	milligram
p.r.n.	when necessary
q.i.d.	four times each day
URI	upper respiratory infection

Figure 16.26 **Anatomical Regions of the Ear.** ▶

You ear has three major sections *(Figure 16.26)*: the external ear, the middle ear, and the inner ear.

Helix
Auricle
Tympanic membrane
External auditory canal
External auditory meatus
Earlobe

Ossicles
Stapes
Incus
Malleus

Semicircular ducts
Vestibular nerve
Cochlear nerve
Cochlea
Round window
Tympanic cavity
Tensor tympani muscle
Eustachian tube

External ear   Middle ear   Inner ear

WORD	PRONUNCIATION	ELEMENTS		DEFINITION
bilateral	by-**LAT**-er-al	S/ P/ R/	-al *pertaining to* bi- *two, twice* -later- *side*	On two sides; for example, in both ears
effusion	eh-**FYU**-shun		Latin *pouring out*	Collection of fluid that has escaped from blood vessels into a cavity or tissues
otitis media	oh-**TIE**-tis **MEE**-dee-ah	S/ R/ R/	-itis *inflammation* ot- *ear* media *middle*	Inflammation of the middle ear
otologist	oh-**TOL**-oh-jist	S/ R/CF	-logist *one who studies, specialist* ot/o- *ear*	Medical specialist in diseases of the ear
otology otorhinolaryngologist	oh-**TOL**-oh-jee oh-toh-**RIE**-noh-**LAH**-rin-**GOL**-oh-jist	S/ R/CF R/CF	-logy *study of* -rhin/o- *nose* -laryng/o- *larynx*	Study of the function and diseases of the ear Ear, nose, and throat medical specialist
primary care	**PRY**-mah-ree KAIR		**primary** Latin *first* **care** Greek *concern*	Comprehensive and preventive health care services that are the first point of care for a patient

Exercises

A. Create medical terms. *Given the definition, insert the missing word element that correctly completes the medical term being described. Fill in the blanks.* **LO 16.13, 16.14, 16.A, 16.C, 16.E**

1. One who specializes in the study of the ear: _____/logist

2. Pertaining to both sides: _____/later/al

3. Medical specialist in the treatment of the ear, nose, and throat: ot/o/rhin/o/_____/logist

4. Infection of the middle ear: otitis _____

5. Collection of fluid _____

6. Initial care of a patient _____

LO 16.11 External Ear

The **auricle**, or **pinna**, is a wing-shaped structure that directs sound waves coming through the air into the **external auditory meatus** and **external auditory canal**. This in turn ends at the **tympanic membrane** (*Figure 16.27*). The external auditory canal not only protects the middle and inner ears but also acts as a resonator to augment the transmission of sound to the middle and inner ears.

The external auditory canal is the only skin-lined cul-de-sac in the body. Its interior is dark, warm, and prone to become moist. These are ideal conditions for bacterial and fungal growth.

The meatus and canal are lined with skin that contains many modified sweat glands called ceruminous glands, which secrete **cerumen**. The cerumen and hairs growing in the meatus help to keep out foreign objects. Cerumen combines with dead skin cells to form **earwax**.

LO 16.12 Disorders of External Ear

Otitis externa (*Figure 16.28*) is an infection of the lining of the external auditory canal. It produces a painful, red, swollen ear canal, sometimes with purulent drainage. The infection can be bacterial or fungal. Fungal infections are responsible for 10% of otitis externa cases and are called **otomycoses.**

Conditions helping to cause otitis externa include trauma to the canal during attempts to self-clean it; use of unclean earplugs, earphones, or hearing aids; and the presence of other skin diseases, such as seborrhea and psoriasis (*see Chapter 4*).

Treatment entails thorough cleansing of the canal, acidification with a topical solution of 2% acetic acid in a hydrocortisone solution, and the use of antibiotic drops. Occasionally, a wick is needed to enable the topical medications to penetrate down the canal.

Swimmer's ear is a form of otitis externa that comes after swimming, particularly if the water is polluted.

Overproduction of cerumen can completely block the external canal (**cerumen impaction**), causing hearing loss and preventing examination of the tympanic membrane with an **otoscope.**

Excessive earwax can be removed in your physician's office by ear **irrigation** or ear syringing. Manual removal with a **curette**, a small metal ring at the end of a handle, or suction is performed for those with narrow ear canals.

If a foreign body, such as a small bead, does get into the canal, or if cerumen becomes **impacted** in the canal, then hearing loss can result.

Helix

Auricle

Tympanic membrane

External auditory canal

External auditory meatus

Earlobe

▲ **Figure 16.27** External Ear.

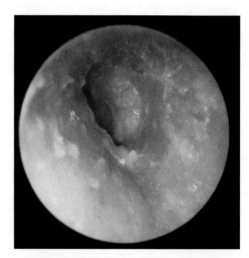

▲ **Figure 16.28** Anatomical Regions of the Ear. Otoscopic view of otitis externa with purulent exudate (shown in yellow). ©Dr. Michael Hawke

Word Analysis and Definition

WORD	PRONUNCIATION		ELEMENTS	DEFINITION
auditory	AW-dih-tor-ee		Latin *hearing*	Pertaining to the sense or organs of hearing
auricle	AW-ri-kul		Latin *ear*	The shell-like external ear
cerumen	seh-ROO-men		Latin *wax*	Waxy secretion of ceruminous glands of external ear canal
curette	kyu-RET	S/ R/	-ette *little* cur- *cleanse, cure*	Scoop-shaped instrument for scraping the interior of a cavity or removing new growths
impacted	im-PAK-ted		Latin *driven in*	Immovably wedged, as with earwax blocking the external ear canal
irrigation	ih-rih-GAY-shun	S/ R/	-ion *process* irrigat- *to water*	Use of water to wash out a canal or wound.
meatus	mee-AY-tus		Latin *passage*	Passage or channel; also used to denote the external opening of a passage
meatal (adj)	mee-AY-tal	S/ R/	-al *pertaining to* meat- *passage or channel*	Pertaining to a meatus
otomycosis	OH-toh-my-KOH-sis	S/ R/CF R/CF	-sis *abnormal condition* ot/o- *ear* -myc/o- *fungus*	Fungal infection of the external ear canal
otoscope	OH-toh-skope	S/ R/CF	-scope *instrument for viewing* ot/o- *ear*	Instrument for examining the ear
pinna pinnae (pl)	PIN-ah PIN-ee		Latin *wing*	Another name for auricle
tympanic	tim-PAN-ik	S/ R/	-ic *pertaining to* tympan- *eardrum, tympanic membrane*	Pertaining to the tympanic membrane or tympanic cavity

Exercises

A. Every part of the body has its own specialized vocabulary. *Test your knowledge of the language of otology by matching correct answers. Match the phrase in the left column with the appropriate medical term in the right column.* **LO 16.11, 16.12, 16.A**

_____ 1. External ear fungal infection

_____ 2. External opening of a passage

_____ 3. Instrument for viewing the ear

_____ 4. Shell-like external ear

_____ 5. "Driven in"

_____ 6. Another name for auricle

_____ 7. Pertaining to the sense or organs of hearing

_____ 8. Earwax

_____ 9. Pertaining to the eardrum

a. pinna

b. auditory

c. auricle

d. tympanic

e. otomycosis

f. meatus

g. otoscope

h. impacted

i. cerumen

Temporal bone

Malleus

Incus

Tendon of stapedius muscle

External auditory canal

Stapes

Tympanic membrane

Tympanic cavity

Tendon of tensor tympani muscle

Tensor tympani muscle

Oval window

Round window

Eustachian tube

▲ **Figure 16.29** Middle Ear.

▲ **Figure 16.30** Otoscopic View of Normal Tympanic Membrane. ©ISM/ Clinica Claros/Diomedia/Medical Images

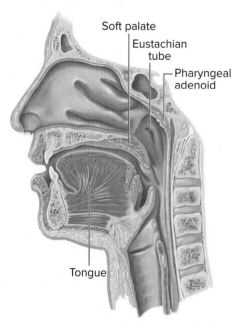

Soft palate

Eustachian tube

Pharyngeal adenoid

Tongue

▲ **Figure 16.31** Nasopharynx (Throat).

LO 16.13 Middle Ear

The middle ear has four components: the tympanic membrane, the tympanic cavity, the **eustachian tube (auditory) tube**, and the ossicles *(Figure 16.29)*.

1. The **tympanic membrane (eardrum)** is located at the inner end of the external auditory canal. It is suspended in a bony groove, is concave on its outer surface, and vibrates freely as sound waves hit it. It has a good nerve supply and is very sensitive to pain. When examined through the **otoscope**, it is transparent and reflects light *(Figure 16.30)*.

2. The **tympanic cavity** is immediately behind the tympanic membrane. It is filled with air that enters through the eustachian (auditory) tube, and the cavity is continuous with the **mastoid** air cells in the bone behind it. The presence of air in the cavity maintains equal air pressure on both sides of the tympanic membrane, which is essential for normal hearing. The cavity contains the **ossicles**.

3. The eustachian (auditory) tube *(Figure 16.29)* connects the middle ear with the **nasopharynx** (throat), into which it opens close to the pharyngeal **tonsil (adenoid)** *(Figure 16.31)*. In children under 5 years, the tube is not fully developed. It is short and horizontal, and the valvelike flaps in the throat that protect it are not developed. When you are landing in an airplane and moving from a high altitude to a lower one, the air pressure in the external auditory canal increases and pushes the tympanic membrane inward. If your eustachian (auditory) tube is blocked, no air can get into the middle ear to equalize the pressure, and your eardrum is painful. If you can force some air up the eustachian (auditory) tube by chewing or swallowing, then your ear "pops" as the tympanic membrane moves back to its normal position.

4. The three **ossicles**—the **malleus**, **incus**, and **stapes** *(Figure 16.29)*—are attached to the wall of the tympanic cavity by tiny ligaments that are covered by a mucous membrane. The malleus is attached to the tympanic membrane and vibrates with the membrane when sound waves hit it. The malleus is also attached to the incus, which also vibrates and passes the vibrations onto the stapes. The stapes is attached to the oval window, an opening that transmits the vibrations to the inner ear. The stapes is the smallest bone in the body.

WORD	PRONUNCIATION		ELEMENTS	DEFINITION
eustachian tube auditory tube (syn)	you-STAY-shun TYUB		Bartolommeo Eustachio, 1524–1574, Italian anatomist **tube** Latin *trumpet*	Tube that connects the middle ear to the nasopharynx
incus	IN-cuss		Latin *anvil*	Middle one of the three ossicles in the middle ear; shaped like an anvil
malleus	MAL-ee-us		Latin *hammer*	Outer (lateral) one of the three ossicles in the middle ear; shaped like a hammer
mastoid	MASS-toyd	S/ R/	**-oid** *resembling* **mast-** *breast*	Small bony protrusion immediately behind the ear
nasopharynx	NAY-zoh-FAIR-inks	R/CF R/	**nas/o-** *nose* **-pharynx** *throat*	Region of the pharynx at the back of the nose and above the soft palate
ossicle	OS-ih-kel	S/ R/CF	**-cle** *small* **oss/i-** *bone*	A small bone, particularly relating to the three bones in the middle ear
stapes	STAY-pees		Latin *stirrup*	Inner (medial) one of the three ossicles of the middle ear; shaped like a stirrup
tonsil	TON-sill		Latin *tonsil*	Mass of lymphoid tissue on either side of the throat at the back of the tongue
tonsillar (adj)	TON-sih-lar	S/ R/	**-ar** *pertaining to* **tonsill-** *tonsil*	Pertaining to the tonsils

Exercises

A. Answers to the following questions can all be found in the above WAD. *Review the terms before you start this exercise. Pay special attention to the spelling. Select the best choice.* **LO 16.13**

1. In the term **mastoid,** the suffix means

   a. condition   **b.** resembling   **c.** inflammation

2. The element *mast-* means

   a. throat   **b.** breast   **c.** ear

3. The **stapes** is a(n)

   a. gland   **b.** ossicle   **c.** mastoid

4. The element *pharynx-* means

   a. throat   **b.** nose   **c.** gland

5. The term *nasopharynx* is composed of

   a. prefix + suffix   **b.** root + root   **c.** combining form + root

6. The _____ is shaped like a hammer.

   a. malleus   **b.** malleolus   **c.** maleus

7. One of the names for the tube that connects the middle ear to the nasopharynx is the _____ tube.

   a. eusstachian   **b.** eustashian   **c.** eustachian

8. The _____ is shaped like an anvil.

   a. incus   **b.** stapes   **c.** adenoid

B. This exercise pertains to the ossicles. *Use the language of otology for your answers.* **LO 16.13**

1. How many bones make up the ossicles? _____

2. Which of the ossicles is the smallest bone in the body? _____

3. Which bone is attached to the tympanic membrane and the incus? _____

4. Are the ossicles in the external ear, the middle ear, or the inner ear? _____

Inflamed membrane

▲ **Figure 16.32 Otoscopic View of Otitis Media (Acute), Showing Inflamed Tympanic Membrane.** ©Lester V. Bergman/Getty Images

Perforation

▲ **Figure 16.33** Otoscopic View of Otitis Media (Chronic) with Perforated Tympanic Membrane. ©ISM/Clinica Claros/Diomedia/Medical Images

Perforation

▲ **Figure 16.34** Perforated Tympanic Membrane. ©ISM/Clinica Claros/Diomedia/Medical Images

Abbreviations

AOM	acute otitis media
COM	chronic otitis media
OME	otitis media with effusion
URI	upper respiratory infection

Case Report (CR) 16.3 *(continued)*

Eddie Cardenas's ear problems began with his eustachian (auditory) tube. His cold (**URI**, or **coryza**) inflamed the mucous membranes of his throat and auditory tube. Because a young child's auditory tube is short and horizontal, the inflammation spread easily into the middle ear, causing Eddie's acute otitis media (**AOM**). The inflammatory process produced fluid (**effusion**) in the middle ear. His tympanic membrane became painful and inflamed, which you could see through an otoscope *(Figure 16.32)*.

LO 16.14 Disorders of Middle Ear

Acute otitis media (AOM) is the presence of pus in the middle ear with pain in the ear, fever, and redness of the tympanic membrane. This occurs most often in the first 2 to 4 years of age because:

- Eustachian tubes in children are shorter and more horizontal than in adults, making it easier for bacteria and viruses to find their way into the middle ear from the nasopharynx.
- Adenoids at the back of the nasopharynx near the eustachian tubes can block the opening of the eustachian tubes.
- Children's immune systems are not fully developed until 7 years of age, and they have difficulty fighting infections.

If the infections are viral, they will go away on their own. If bacterial, oral antibiotics may be necessary.

Chronic otitis media (COM) occurs when the acute infection subsides but the eustachian tube is still blocked. The **effusion** (fluid) in the middle ear cannot drain out and gradually becomes stickier. This is called **chronic otitis media with effusion (OME)** and produces hearing loss because the sticky fluid prevents the ossicles from vibrating. You can see the fluid through the otoscope *(Figure 16.33)*. Dr. Lee was concerned that this had happened to Eddie in his previous ear infection.

A **perforated tympanic membrane** can occur in acute otitis media when pus in the middle ear cannot escape down the eustachian tube. It builds up pressure and perforates the eardrum *(Figures 16.33 and 16.34)*. Other causes of perforation include a puncture by a cotton swab, an open-handed slap to the ear, or large pressure changes (as may be induced in scuba diving). Most perforations will heal spontaneously in a month, leaving a small scar.

Cholesteatoma is a complication of chronic otitis media with effusion or of poor eustachian tube function. Chronically inflamed cells in the middle ear multiply and collect into a tumor. They damage the ossicles and can spread to the inner ear. Surgical removal is required.

Otosclerosis is a middle-ear disease that usually affects people between 18 and 35 years of age. It can affect one ear or both and produces a gradual hearing loss for low and soft sounds. Its etiology is unknown. Spongy bone forms around the junction of the oval window and stapes, preventing the stapes from conducting the sound vibrations to the inner ear. The only treatment is to replace the stapes with a metal or plastic **prosthesis**.

WORD	PRONUNCIATION	ELEMENTS		DEFINITION
cholesteatoma	koh-less-tee-ah-**TOH**-mah	S/ R/CF R/	**-oma** *tumor, mass* **chol/e-** *bile* **-steat-** *fat*	Yellow, waxy tumor arising in the middle ear
effusion	eh-**FYU**-shun		Latin *pouring out*	Collection of fluid that has escaped from blood vessels into a cavity or tissues
otosclerosis	oh-toh-skler-**OH**-sis	S/ R/CF R/CF	**-sis** *abnormal condition* **ot/o-** *ear* **-scler/o-** *hardening*	Hardening at the junction of the stapes and oval window that causes loss of hearing
perforated	**PER**-foh-ray-ted		Latin *to bore through*	Punctured with one or more holes
tympanic	tim-**PAN**-ik	S/ R/	**-ic** *pertaining to* **tympan-** *eardrum, tympanic membrane*	Pertaining to the tympanic membrane or tympanic cavity

Exercises

A. Build medical terms. *Fill in the blanks with the correct element to complete the terms.* **LO 16.14, 16.C**

1. Pertaining to the eardrum: _____ /ic

2. Hardening at the junction of the stapes and oval window:

   ot/o/_____ /sis

3. Yellow, waxy tumor in the middle ear:

   _____ / _____ / _____ /oma

B. Choose the correct answer to each statement. **LO 16.14**

1. The term **effusion** implies

   a. tumor

   b. mass

   c. liquid

   d. tear

   e. blockage

2. In the term **cholesteatoma,** the word element that means *fat* is:

   a. *choles-*

   b. *-steat-*

   c. *-oma*

3. In the term **otosclerosis,** the word element *oto-* means:

   a. pertaining to

   b. hardening

   c. condition of

   d. ear

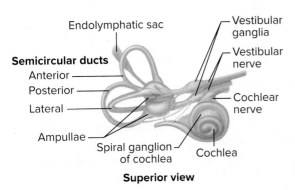

Endolymphatic sac

Semicircular ducts
Anterior
Posterior
Lateral

Ampullae

Spiral ganglion of cochlea

Vestibular ganglia

Vestibular nerve

Cochlear nerve

Cochlea

Superior view

▲ **Figure 16.35** Inner Ear.

LO 16.15 Inner Ear for Hearing

The inner ear is a **labyrinth** (*Figure 16.35*) of complex, intricate systems of passages. The passages in the **cochlea**, a part of the labyrinth, contain receptors to translate vibrations into nerve impulses so that the brain can interpret them as different sounds.

The membrane of the oval window separates the middle ear from the **vestibule** of the inner ear. From the tympanic membrane (① *in Figure 16.36*), the stapes ② moves the oval membrane to generate pressure waves in the fluid inside the cochlea ③. The pressure waves cause **vestibular** and **basilar membranes** inside the cochlea to vibrate ④ and sway fine hair cells attached to the basilar membrane ⑤. The hair cells convert this motion into nerve impulses, which travel via the **cochlear nerve** to the brain. The excess pressure waves in the cochlea escape the inner ear via the round window ⑥.

Hearing Disorders of the Inner Ear

Today, the most common cause of hearing loss is damage to the fine hairs in the cochlea by exposure to repeated loud noise, related either to work (for example, jackhammers, leaf blowers) or to leisure activities (such as amplified music at concerts, personal listening devices, and motorcycles). This is a **sensorineural hearing loss**.

Hearing aids are becoming more sophisticated and smaller, but they do not help people with cochlear damage. **Cochlear implants** are used to bypass the damaged hair cells and directly stimulate cochlear nerve endings.

Keynotes

- Repeated exposure to loud noise causes hearing loss in young people as well as in older people.

- A **conductive hearing loss** occurs when sound is not conducted efficiently through the external auditory canal to the tympanic membrane and the ossicles. Causes include

  – Middle ear pathology, such as acute otitis media, otitis media with effusion, or a perforated eardrum.

  – Impacted cerumen.

  – An infected external auditory canal.

  – A foreign body in the external canal.

Auditory ossicles

Malleus   Stapes
    Incus

Cochlear nerve

Oval window membrane

Scala vestibuli

External auditory canal ①

Vestibular membrane

Basilar membrane

Tympanic membrane

Round window

Auditory (eustachian) tube

▲ **Figure 16.36** Hearing Process in the Inner Ear.

WORD	PRONUNCIATION	ELEMENTS		DEFINITION
basilar	**BAS**-ih-lar	S/ R/	**-ar** *pertaining to* **basil-** *base, support*	Pertaining to the base of a structure
cochlea	**KOK**-lee-ah		Latin *snail shell*	An intricate combination of passages; used to describe the part of the inner ear used in hearing
cochlear (adj)	**KOK**-lee-ar	S/ R/	**-ar** *pertaining to* **cochle-** *cochlea*	Pertaining to the cochlea
conductive hearing loss	kon-**DUK**-tiv **HEER**-ing LOSS	S/ R/	**conductive** Latin *to lead* **-ing** *quality of* **hear-** *to perceive sounds* **loss** Middle English *to lose*	Hearing loss caused by lesions in the outer ear or middle ear
labyrinth labyrinthitis	**LAB**-ih-rinth **LAB**-ih-rin-**THIE**-tis	S/ R/	Greek *labyrinth* **-itis** *inflammation* **labyrinth-** *inner ear*	The inner ear Inflammation of the inner ear
sensorineural hearing loss	**SEN**-sor-ih-**NYUR**-al **HEER**-ing LOSS	S/ R/CF R/ S/ R/	**-al** *pertaining to* **sensor/i-** *sensory* **-neur-** *nerve* **-ing** *quality of* **hear-** *to perceive sounds* **loss** Middle English *to lose*	Hearing loss caused by lesions of the inner ear or the auditory nerve
vestibule vestibular (adj)	**VES**-tih-byul ves-**TIB**-you-lar	S/ R/	Latin *entrance* **-ar** *pertaining to* **vestibul-** *vestibule of the inner ear*	Space at the entrance to a canal Pertaining to the vestibule of the inner ear

Exercises

A. Increase your knowledge of the language of otology by correctly answering the following questions. *Review the material regarding the middle ear structures and their disorders; then choose the best answer.* **LO 16.15**

1. In the term **basilar,** *basil-* is a
   a. prefix   **b.** root   **c.** combining form

2. The **entrance to the inner ear** is the
   a. vestibule   **b.** labyrinth   **c.** cochlea   **d.** aqueous   **e.** choroid

3. **Labyrinthitis** is a(n)
   a. procedure   **b.** symptom   **c.** inflammation

4. The element *neur-* means
   a. never   **b.** nerve   **c.** nose

5. **Hearing loss** caused by lesions of the outer ear is
   a. auditory   **b.** basilar   **c.** sensorineural   **d.** aqueous

6. An **intricate combination of passages** in the ear is the
   a. cochlea   **b.** vestibule   **c.** labyrinth

7. The root meaning *inflammation* can be found in the word
   a. vestibule   **b.** labyrinthitis   **c.** otology

8. **Hearing loss** caused by lesions of the inner ear is called _____ hearing loss.
   a. auditory   **b.** basilar   **c.** sensorineural

9. The suffix meaning *pertaining to* is found in the term
   a. vestibular   **b.** labyrinthitis   **c.** audiometer

Maculae
(in vestibule)

Gelatinous
material — Otoliths

Vestibular nerve
Hair cell
Supporting cell

▲ **Figure 16.37** **Vestibule and Maculae.**

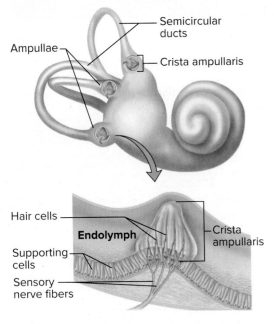

Semicircular
ducts

Ampullae

Crista ampullaris

Hair cells

Endolymph

Crista
ampullaris

Supporting
cells

Sensory
nerve fibers

▲ **Figure 16.38** **Semicircular Ducts.**

Case Report (CR) 16.4

You are

. . . Sonia Ramos, a medical assistant working with Sylvia Thompson, MD, an otolaryngologist at Fulwood Medical Center.

Your patient is

. . . Mr. Ernesto Santiago, a 44-year-old man who was referred to Dr. Thompson by his primary care physician.

Mr. Santiago complains of **recurrent** attacks of nausea and vomiting, a sense of spinning or whirling, and ringing in his ears. The attacks last about 24 hours and are getting more frequent. He has been having trouble hearing quiet speech on his left side.

Your role is to document his investigation, diagnosis, and care and to act as translator between Mr. Santiago and Dr. Thompson.

LO 16.16 Inner Ear for Equilibrium and Balance

The **vestibule** and the three **semicircular canals** *(Figure 16.37)* are the organs of balance.

Inside the fluid-filled vestibule are two raised, flat areas (**maculae**) covered with hair cells and a gelatinous material. This gelatinous material contains crystals of calcium and protein called **otoliths**. The position of the head alters the pressure applied to the hair cells by the gelatinous mass. The hair cells respond to horizontal and vertical changes and send impulses to the brain indicating the position to which the head has tilted.

Each of the three fluid-filled semicircular canals has a dilated end called an **ampulla** that contains a mound of hair cells embedded in a gelatinous material that together are called a **crista ampullaris** *(Figure 16.38)*. They detect rotational movements of the head that distort the hair cells and lead to stimulation of connected nerve cells. The nerve impulses travel via the vestibular nerve and go to the brain. From the brain, nerve impulses travel to the muscles to maintain **equilibrium** and balance.

Disorders of the Inner Ear for Balance

The sensation of spinning or whirling that Mr. Santiago experiences is called **vertigo**, often described by patients as dizziness. The ringing in his ears is called **tinnitus**. Both sensations arise in the inner ear.

Acute labyrinthitis is an acute viral infection of the labyrinth, producing extreme vertigo, nausea, and vomiting. It usually lasts 1 to 2 weeks.

Benign paroxysmal positional vertigo (BPPV) presents with short (less than 60 sec) episodes of vertigo occurring with certain head positions due to displacement of otoliths. It is diagnosed clinically and treated with otolith repositioning maneuvers.

Case Report (CR) 16.4 *(continued)*

The recurrent attacks that Mr. Santiago suffered are called **Ménière disease**. The disease involves the destruction of inner-ear hair cells, but the etiology is unknown and there is no cure. Dr. Thompson prescribed medication to control his nausea and vomiting.

WORD	PRONUNCIATION		ELEMENTS	DEFINITION
ampulla crista ampullaris	am-**PULL**-ah **KRIS**-tah am-pull-**AIR**-is	R/ S/ R/	Latin *two-handled bottle* **crista** *crest* **-aris** *pertaining to* **ampull-** *bottle-shaped*	Dilated portion of canal or duct Mound of hair cells and gelatinous material in the ampulla of a semicircular canal
equilibrium	ee-kwih-**LIB**-ree-um	P/ R/	**equi-** *equal* **-librium** *balance*	Being evenly balanced
macula maculae (pl)	**MAK**-you-lah **MAK**-you-lee		Latin *small spot*	Small area of special function; in the ear, a sensory receptor
Ménière disease	men-**YEAR** diz-**EEZ**	P/ R/	Prosper Ménière, 1799–1862, French physician **dis-** *apart* **-ease** *normal function*	Disorder of inner ear with cluster of symptoms of acute attacks of tinnitus, vertigo, and hearing loss
otolith	**OH**-toh-lith	R/ R/CF	**ot/o-** *ear* **-lith** *stone*	A calcium particle in the vestibule of the inner ear
paroxysmal	par-ok-**SIZ**-mal	S/ R/	**-al** *pertaining to* **paroxysm-** *irritation*	Occurring in sharp, spasmodic episodes
recurrent	ree-**KUR**-ent	S/ P/ R/	**-ent** *pertaining to* **re-** *back* **-curr-** *to run*	Symptoms or lesions returning after an intermission
tinnitus	**TIN**-ih-tus		Latin *jingle*	Persistent ringing, whistling, clicking, or booming noise in the ears
vertigo	**VER**-tih-go		Latin *dizziness*	Sensation of spinning or whirling

Exercises

A. Challenge your knowledge of the ear by filling in the correct terms for the following definitions. *Fill in the blanks.* **LO 16.16**

Definition   Medical Term

1. Persistent ringing in the ears   _____

2. Sensation of spinning or whirling   _____

3. Occurring in sharp, spasmodic episodes _____

4. Evenly balanced   _____

5. Dilated portion of a canal or duct   _____

6. Small area of special function   _____

7. Calcium particle in the vestibule   _____

8. Mound of hair cells found in ampulla   _____

Lesson 16.5

SPECIAL SENSES OF THE EYE AND EAR

Procedures and Pharmacology for the Ear

LO 16.17 Diagnostic Procedures for Diseases of the Ear

Basic hearing test procedures that can be performed in an office include:

- **Whispered speech testing**, which is a simple screening method in which one ear of the patient is covered and the patient is asked to identify whispered sounds.
- **Tuning fork screening tests**, which can identify on which side a hearing loss is located (**Weber test**) and whether the hearing loss is due to loss of bone or air conduction (**Rinne test**).

An **audiometer** is an electronic device that generates sounds in different frequencies and intensities and prints out a graph (**audiogram**) of the patient's responses (*Figure 16.39*). **Audiometry** measures hearing function and is often performed by an **audiologist**. An audiologist is a specialist in **audiology**. **Tympanometry** helps detect problems between the tympanic membrane and the inner ear by using a small earpiece that generates pressure and sound in the ear canal to gather information (**tympanography**) about changes of pressure inside the ear.

When recording the results of hearing testing, **A.D.** is shorthand for the right ear, **A.S.** for the left ear, and **A.U.** for both ears.

Lesson Objectives

Many of the diagnostic tests for hearing function and to determine diseases of the ear can be performed by technicians with physician overview. To communicate clearly and accurately, the terminology of these diagnostic procedures must be clearly understood by everyone involved. The information in this lesson will enable you to:

16.5.1 Describe the different tests that can be performed in a medical office.

16.5.2 Explain the uses of an otoscope.

16.5.3 Discuss the value of specialized tests for inner ear function.

16.5.4 Identify tests to measure the response of the nervous system to sound.

Abbreviations

ABR	auditory brainstem response
AD	right ear
AS	left ear
AU	both ears
CAT	computed axial tomography

▲ **Figure 16.39** Examples of audiometry results.

WORD	PRONUNCIATION	ELEMENTS		DEFINITION
audiology	aw-dee-**OL**-oh-jee	S/ R/CF	**-logy** *study of* **audi/o-** *hearing*	Study of hearing disorders
audiologist	aw-dee-**OL**-oh-jist	S/	**-logist** *specialist*	Specialist in evaluation of hearing function
audiometer	aw-dee-**OM**-eh-ter	R/CF R/	**audi/o-** *hearing* **-meter** *measure*	Instrument to measure hearing
audiometric (adj)	**AW**-dee-oh-**MET**-rik	S/ R/	**-ic** *pertaining to* **-metr-** *measure*	Pertaining to the measurement of hearing
audiometry	aw-dee-**OM**-eh-tree	S/	**-metry** *process of measuring*	The measurement of hearing
auditory	**AW**-dih-tor-ee	S/ R/	**-ory** *having the function of* **audit-** *hearing*	Pertaining to the sense of hearing or to the organs of hearing
Rinne test	**RIN**-eh TEST		Friedrich Rinne, 1819–1868, German otologist **test** Latin *earthen vessel*	Test for conductive hearing loss
tympanocentesis	**TIM**-pah-noh-sen-**TEE**-sis	S/ R/CF	**-centesis** *to puncture* **tympan/o-** *eardrum, tympanic membrane*	Puncture of the tympanic membrane with a needle
tympanography	**TIM**-pan-**OG**-rah-fee	S/	**-graphy** *process of recording*	Recording pressure changes inside the ear
tympanometry	**TIM**-pan-**OM**-eh-tree	S/	**-metry** *process of measuring*	Measurement of pressure changes between the middle and inner ears
Weber test	**VAY**-ber TEST		Ernst Weber, 1794–1878, German physiologist **test** Latin *earthen vessel*	Test for sensorineural hearing loss

Exercises

A. Define the different auditory diagnostic tests. *The different auditory tests are indicated for different disorders of the ear. Knowing what they test for gives clues to the patient's condition. Match the test on the left with its correct description on the right.* **LO 16.17**

_____ 1. tympanometry

_____ 2. Rinne test

_____ 3. otoscopy

_____ 4. Weber test

a. used to view the external ear and tympanic membrane

b. test for conductive hearing loss

c. test for sensorineural hearing loss

d. measures pressure changes between the middle and inner ears

B. Deconstruct medical terms relating to the diagnostic tests of the ear. *Deconstruct the terms in order to decipher their meanings.* **LO 16.17, 16.D**

1. tympanometry: _____ / _____ / _____
            CF   S

2. tympanocentesis: _____ / _____ / _____
            CF   S

3. audiologist: _____ / _____ / _____
            CF   S

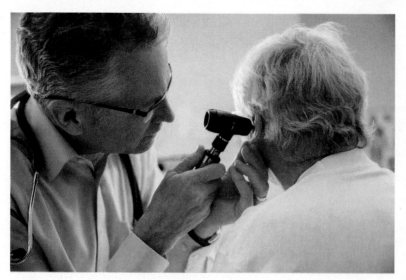

▲ **Figure 16.40** Physician Using an Otoscope to Examine Patient's Ear. ©Hero Images Inc./Alamy Stock Photo RF

LO 16.17 Diagnostic Procedures for Diseases of the Ear (continued)

The pinna (auricle) is examined visually and by touch. The external ear and the middle ear are examined via **otoscopy** with an **otoscope** (*Figure 16.40*). The pinna (auricle) of the ear is gently manipulated in order for a health care provider to obtain an **otoscopic** view of the external and middle ear. The otoscopic view enables the tympanic membrane and the ossicles behind it to be visualized.

A **pneumatic otoscope** pushes air into the ear and enables the examiner to see if the eardrum moves freely. **Tympanocentesis** is puncture of the tympanic membrane with a needle to aspirate fluid from the middle ear that has remained behind after a middle ear infection (chronic otitis media with effusion).

Electrocochleography (ECOG) measures the response to sound by the nervous system. A soft electrode is placed deeply in the external ear canal and other electrodes are placed on the forehead to measure responses to sound.

Auditory brainstem response test (ABR) also measures the nervous system response to sound with a setup and procedure similar to ECOG.

Magnetic resonance imaging (MRI) of structures in the inner ear can be helpful in the diagnosis of some vestibular disorders. **Computerized axial tomography (CAT scan)** can help diagnose problems in and around the inner ear.

Balance

Electronystagmography (ENG) and **videonystagmography (VNG)** evaluate the movement of the eyes as they follow different visual targets to evaluate vestibular dysfunction, ENG uses small electrodes placed on the skin around the eyes and VNG uses goggles with video cameras to monitor the eye movements.

Rotation tests, such as head rotation or a computerized rotary chair, also measure associated eye movements using electrodes or goggles to determine how well the balance organs are functioning.

Abbreviations	
ECOG	electrocochleography
ENG	electronystagmography
MRI	magnetic resonance imaging
VNG	videonystagmography

WORD	PRONUNCIATION		ELEMENTS	DEFINITION
electrocochleography	ee-**LEK**-troh-kok-lee-**OG**-rah-fee	S/ R/CF R/CF	**-graphy** *process of recording* **electr/o-** *electric* **-cochle/o-** *cochlea*	Measurement of the electric potentials generated in the inner ear by sounds
electronystagmography	ee-**LEK**-troh-nys-tag-**MOG**-rah-fee	S/ R/CF R/CF R/CF	**-graphy** *process of recording* **electr/o-** *electric* **-nystagm/o-** *nystagmus* **video-** *visual*	Test using electrodes to measure eye movements to evaluate vestibular dysfunction
videonystagmography	**VID**-ee-oh-nys-tag-**MOG**-rah-fee			Test using goggles with video cameras to measure eye movements to evaluate vestibular dysfunction
otoscope	**OH**-toh-scope	S/ R/CF	**-scope** *instrument for viewing* **ot/o-** *ear*	Instrument for examining the external and middle ears
otoscopic (adj) otoscopy	oh-toh-**SKOP**-ik oh-**TOS**-koh-pee	S/ S/	**-ic** *pertaining to* **-scopy** *to examine*	Pertaining to examination with an otoscope Examination of the ear
pneumatic	new-**MAT**-ik	S/ R/	**-ic** *pertaining to* **pneumat-** *structure filled with air*	Pertaining to a structure filled with air

Exercises

A. Use the following table *to list all the combining forms in the terms given and give their meaning:* **LO 16.17 D**

Terms	Combining Forms	Meaning of Combining Forms
otoscope		
electrocochleography		
electronystagmography		
videonystagmography		

PE tube

▲ **Figure 16.41** Pressure Equalization (PE) Tube in Tympanic Membrane. ©Yoav Levy/Diomedia/Medical Images

Abbreviation	
PE	pressure equalization (tubes)

LO 16.18 Therapeutic Procedures for the Ear

Hearing

Ear clearing to equalize the pressure in the middle ear with the outside air pressure by making the ear(s) "pop" can be performed by yawning, swallowing, or using a method like a **Valsalva maneuver**, in which the nose is pinched, the mouth is closed, and attempts are made to breathe out through the nose.

Ear wax blockage is removed by loosening it with oil, and then flushing, **curetting**, or suctioning out the softened wax.

Debridement is the removal of **necrotic** tissue and debris from the external ear canal in **otitis externa** using dry cotton wipes and/or suction. Mild otitis externa can then be treated with 2% acetic acid and hydrocortisone drops. Moderate infections require the addition of a **topical antibacterial suspension**, and severe infections require the insertion of an ear wick into the canal, wetted four times a day with a topical antibiotic or 5% aluminum acetate solution. Very severe infections may need systemic antibiotics. **Swimmer's ear** is a form of otitis externa and can be prevented by applying a few drops of a 1:1 mixture of rubbing alcohol and vinegar immediately after swimming.

Acute otitis media responds to an antibiotic such as amoxicillin, though some infections may subside spontaneously.

In **chronic otitis media with effusion**, when the sticky fluid persists in the middle ear, a **myringotomy** can be performed and a small, hollow plastic tube inserted through the tympanic membrane to allow the effusion to drain out. These tubes are called **tympanostomy tubes**, or **pressure equalization tubes** (**PE tubes**) (*Figure 16.41*). Surgical removal is required for a **cholesteatoma**.

Hearing aids can help a sensorineural hearing loss and an **audiologist** will recommend the type of device for each patient.

Cochlear implants can be used for a severe hearing loss. Unlike a hearing aid that amplifies sound and directs it through the ear canal, a cochlear implant compensates for damaged or nonworking elements in the cochlea. The devices pick up sound and **digitize** it, convert the digitized sound into electrical signals, and transmit those signals to electrodes embedded in the cochlea. The electrodes stimulate the cochlear nerve, sending signals to the brain.

Balance

Otolith repositioning procedures, performed by physical therapists with specialized training, are employed to return the tiny otolith granules to their correct resting place to resolve positional vertigo.

Exercises taught in a physical therapy setting can help with dizziness and vertigo to improve balance in different positions and activities.

LO 16.19 Medications for the Ear

In the external ear canal, buildup of wax can be loosened with oil or with carbamide peroxide solution *(Debrox)*. Otitis externa can be treated with acetic acid drops to change the pH of the external canal or with drops containing an antibiotic or an antibiotic and steroid such as ciprofloxacin and dexamethazone *(Ciprodex)* or neomycin, polymycin, and hydrocortisone *(Corticosporin)*.

For infections of the middle ear, antibiotics such as penicillin, amoxicillin, and erythromycin are used.

For inner ear disorders, the antihistamine meclizine and the anti-anxiety medication diazepam *(Valium)* are used to diminish the vertigo of BPPV. The treatment of Ménière's disease has been revolutionized with the use of a single transtympanic injection of a low dose of gentamycin.

WORD	PRONUNCIATION	ELEMENTS		DEFINITION
curette **curettage** (Note: the final "e" of curette is dropped because the suffix "–age" begins with a vowel)	kyu-**RET** kyu-reh-**TAHZH**	S/ R/ S/	**-ette** *little* **cur-** *cleanse* **-age** *related to*	Scoop-shaped instrument for scraping the interior of a cavity or removing new growths Scraping the interior of a cavity or removing a new growth
debridement	day-**BREED**-mon	S/ P/ R/	**-ment** *resulting state* **de-** *take away* **-bride-** *rubbish*	The removal of necrotic or injured tissue
digitize	**DIJ**-ih-tize	S/ R/	**-ize** *affect in a specific way* **digit-** *finger, toe, number*	To change analog information into a numerical format to facilitate computer processing
maneuver	mah-**NYU**-ver		French *to work by hand*	A planned movement or procedure
myringotomy	mir-in-**GOT**-oh-mee	S/ R/CF	**-tomy** *surgical incision* **myring/o-** *tympanic membrane*	Incision in the tympanic membrane
necrosis	neh-**KROH**-sis	S/ R/	**-osis** *condition* **necr-** *death*	Pathologic death of one or more cells
necrotic (adj)	neh-**KROT**-ik	S/ R/CF	**-tic** *pertaining to* **necr/o-** *death*	Affected by necrosis
topical	**TOP**-ih-kal	S/ R/	**-al** *pertaining to* **topic-** *local*	Medication applied directly to obtain a local effect
tympanostomy	tim-pan-**OS**-toh-mee	S/ R/CF	**-stomy** *new opening* **tympan/o-** *eardrum, tympanic membrane*	Surgically created new opening in the tympanic membrane to allow fluid to drain from the middle ear
Valsalva	val-**SAL**-vah		Antonio Valsalva, 1666–1723, Italian physician	Any forced expiratory effort against a closed airway

Exercises

A. Identify the therapeutic procedure indicated for each disorder. *Select the correct answer for each question.* **LO 16.18**

1. Chronic otitis media is treated with:

   a. Valsalva maneuver **b.** tympanostomy tubes **c.** rubbing alcohol drops **d.** physical therapy

2. An acute otitis media is treated with:

   a. myringotomy **b.** tympanostomy tubes **c.** oral antibiotics **d.** antihistamines

3. Positional vertigo can be treated with:

   a. physical therapy **b.** anti-anxiety medications **c.** cochlear implants **d.** myringotomy

4. Excessive cerumen in the auditory canal is treated with:

   a. alcohol and vinegar drops **b.** antibiotic drops **c.** myringotomy **d.** curettage

5. Cholesteatoma is treated with:

   a. debridement **b.** excision **c.** acetic acid drops **d.** oral antibiotics

©2014 Nucleus Medical Media

Special Senses of the Eye and Ear
Challenge Your Knowledge

A. **Apply your knowledge of medical terminology to interpret Case Study** (LO 16.17, 16.19, 16.A)

You are

...a medical assistant working with primary care physician Susan Lee, MD, of the Fulwood Medical Group on March 16, 2017. Your patients are Mrs. Cardenas and her 3-year-old son, Eddie.

You see a worried mother and a very unhappy, restless toddler with a green nasal discharge. His oral temperature taken with an electronic digital thermometer is 102.4°F, pulse 100. Dr. Lee examines Eddie and finds that he has an upper respiratory infection (URI) with a bilateral otitis media (BOM). She prescribes amoxicillin 250 mg four times a day (q.i.d.) for 10 days, and acetaminophen 160 mg when necessary (p.r.n.) for pain, after which she will see Eddie again. After the acute infection subsides, if there remains an effusion in the middle ear, she will refer Eddie to an otologist. She explained this to Mrs. Cardenas.
—Luisa Guittierez, CMA. 1115 hrs. 3/16/17.

1. Dr. Lee has recommended the use of acetaminophen as an:
   a. analgesic   b. antibiotic   c. antihistamine

2. What type of medication is the amoxicillin?
   a. antipyretic   b. analgesic   c. antibiotic

3. Which diagnostic tool will Dr. Lee use to determine if there is an effusion in the middle ear?
   a. tonometer   b. otoscope   c. ophthalmoscope   d. curette

B. **Suffixes.** The following terms all have a suffix with a common meaning. Write the suffix for each term. Write it with the hyphen, for example, -itis. Fill in the blanks. (LO 16.A, 16.D)

1. periorbital _____
2. lacrimal _____
3. bactericidal _____
4. intraocular _____
5. neural _____
6. optic _____
7. tarsal _____
8. macular _____
9. retinal _____
10. corneal _____

These suffixes all mean _____.

C. **Prefixes.** Use your knowledge of prefixes to deconstruct the following terms; write the prefix for each term. **(LO 16A, 16.D)**

Term	Prefix
periorbital	1.
esotropia	2.
astigmatism	3.
emmetropia	4.
accommodation	5.
exotropia	6.
bilateral	7.
equilateral	8.
intraocular	9.

D. **Diagnosis.** You are preparing to code the claim forms for various patients seen in the clinic today. The doctor has given each diagnosis in general terms on the charge slip. Write the correct medical term for each general term. **(LO 16.2, 16.6, 16.A)**

1. Pink eye _____

2. Sensitivity to light _____

3. Nearsighted _____

4. Scratched cornea (2 words) _____

5. Inflammation of the iris _____

6. "Lazy eye" _____

7. Farsighted _____

8. Inflamed eyelash and tarsal gland _____

9. Droopy eyelid _____

10. Cross-eyed _____

E. **Match the Latin and Greek terms in the left column to their meanings in the right column. (LO 16.1, 16.2, 16.3, 16.4, 16.8, 16.A)**

_____ 1. orbit

_____ 2. extrinsic

_____ 3. chalazion

_____ 4. cornea

_____ 5. cortex

_____ 6. ptosis

_____ 7. canthus

_____ 8. contagious

_____ 9. tarsus

_____ 10. paresis

a. flat

b. drooping

c. on the outer side

d. paralysis

e. lump

f. corner of the eye

g. web

h. circle

i. outer shell

j. touch closely

©2014 Nucleus Medical Media

Special Senses of the Eye and Ear

F. Refer to Case Report (CR) 16.2. Correctly answer the questions as they relate to the Case Report. **LO 16.3, 16.E**

 Case Report (CR) 16.2

You are

. . . an ophthalmic technician working with Angela Chun, MD, an ophthalmologist at Fulwood Medical Center.

Your patient is

. . . Sam Hughes, a 2-year-old boy, who has been referred by his pediatrician to Dr. Chun.

His mother, Mrs. Jenny Hughes, states that she has noticed for the past couple of months that his right eye has turned in. The only visual difficulty she has noticed is that he sometimes misses a Cheerio when he tries to grab it. Otherwise, he is healthy.

You are responsible for documenting Sam's diagnostic and therapeutic procedures and explaining the significance of these to his mother.

---

1. What is the medical term for *eye turned in toward the nose:*

   a. strabismus

   b. glaucoma

   c. esotropia

   d. ambylopia

2. Can Dr. Chun prescribe medication?

   a. yes

   b. no

3. According to the Case Report, how did Mrs. Hughes decide to seek Dr. Chun's medical opinion?

   a. performed an Internet search

   b. a friend suggested she see Dr. Chun

   c. she was referred by her son's doctor

   d. Dr. Chun was called to see Sam in the ER.

G. Master your documentation—it is a legal record. Select the most appropriate choice, and insert the correct abbreviation where indicated on the line. (LO 16.2, 16. 5, 16.8, 16.9, 16.A, 16.E, 16.F)

1. Patient complains of sticky eyelids with (purulent/perulent) discharge, prescription eye drops prescribed to be given every four

   hours (_____ [abbreviation]). Diagnosis: (scleritis/conjunctivitis)

2. The optometrist (_____ [abbreviation]) determined with the patient's vision now 20/40 in the right eye,

   with correction.

3. The (diagnosis/prognosis) for Mr. Baker is continued decreasing vision in his right eye if his diabetes remains uncontrolled and

   his (retinopathy/retinoblastoma) worsens.

4. (Opthalmoscopic/Ophthalmoscopic) examination of the left eye reveals (microaneurisms/microaneurysms) forming. The (Fluoreseen/Fluorescein) angiography is ordered for more details.

5. The (ophthalmologist/ophthalamologist) determined that the patient's pupils are equal, round, and reactive to light and accommodation (_____ [abbreviation]).

H. Terminology challenge. The following medical terms are associated with either an eye specialist or an ear specialist. Check (√) the appropriate specialist for the term. (LO 16.1, 16.2, 16.6, 16.7, 16.14, 16.15, 16.16, 16.E, 16.F)

Term	Otologist	Ophthalmologist
1. uveitis		
2. otolith		
3. vertigo		
4. cholesteatoma		
5. conjunctivitis		
6. glaucoma		
7. labyrinthitis		
8. papilledema		
9. canthus		
10. audiologist		
11. hordeolum		
12. dacryostenosis		
13. LASIK		
14. ptosis		

Special Senses of the Eye and Ear

I. **Word elements.** Learning word elements is your most valuable tool for increasing your medical vocabulary. Use your knowledge of word elements to answer the following questions. Select the correct answer. **(LO 16.1, 16.2, 16.9, 16.A, 16.C, 16.D)**

1. The root for *tear* is

   a. blephar

   b. tamin

   c. commodat

   d. strab

   e. lacrim

2. The root of this word means *letting go* and is used to indicate partial paralysis:

   a. parietal

   b. periorbital

   c. paresis

   d. ptosis

   e. presbyopia

3. On the basis of its suffix, you can tell that a **keratotomy** is a

   a. body part

   b. procedure

   c. diagnosis

   d. medication

   e. infection

4. The prefix in **microaneurysm** tells you that this aneurysm is

   a. large

   b. black

   c. small

   d. painful

   e. red

5. In the term **amblyopia,** *-opia* means

   a. sound

   b. light

   c. sight

   d. movement

   e. pain

6. **In situ** is a Latin phrase that means *(Be precise!)*

   a. in this place

   b. in another place

   c. in its original place

   d. in the place

   e. in place of

7. In the terms **retinoblastoma** and **retinopathy**, the combining form tells you that both these terms concern the

   a. cornea

   b. iris

   c. lens

   d. vitreous body

   e. retina

8. **Tonometry** is a diagnostic test of a(n)

   a. organ

   b. bone

   c. blood vessel

   d. muscle

   e. gland

9. In the term **periorbital,** *peri-* is a prefix that means

   a. within

   b. outside

   c. on top of

   d. against

   e. around

J. Abbreviations. The following abbreviations are all part of the *language of otology*. Match the abbreviation in the left column with its meaning in the right column. **(LO 16.F)**

_____ 1. PE

_____ 2. BPPV

_____ 3. A.S.

_____ 4. p.r.n.

_____ 5. q.i.d.

_____ 6. OME

_____ 7. A.U.

_____ 8. COM

_____ 9. URI

_____ 10. A.D.

a. ear infection with fluid collection

b. both ears

c. four times each day

d. right ear

e. common cold

f. sensation of spinning or whirling

g. chronic otitis media

h. pressure equalization tubes

i. left ear

j. when necessary

K. Identify the elements in each medical term and unlock the meaning of the word. *Fill in the chart. If the word does not have a particular word element, write n/a. The first one has been done for you.* **(LO 16.10, 16.11, 16.17, 16.18, 16.D)**

Medical Term	Prefix	Meaning of Prefix	Root/Combining Form	Meaning of Root/Combing Form	Suffix	Meaning of Suffix	Meaning of the Term
mydriatic	1. n/a	2. n/a	3. *mydri-*	4. dilation of the pupil	5. *-atic*	6. pertaining to	7. Pertaining to the dilation of the pupil
tympanic	8.	9.	10.	11.	12.	13.	14.
irrigation	15.	16.	17.	18.	19.	20.	21.
myringotomy	22.	23.	24.	25.	26.	27.	28.
otoscope	29.	30.	31.	32.	33.	34.	35.

©2014 Nucleus Medical Media

Special Senses of the Eye and Ear

L. Match the term in the left column with its meaning in the right column. (LO 16.11, 16.12, 16.14, 16.A)

_____	1. chronic	a.	pouring out
_____	2. impacted	b.	wing
_____	3. auricle	c.	sharp
_____	4. vertigo	d.	stirrup
_____	5. meatus	e.	driven in
_____	6. effusion	f.	time
_____	7. cerumen	g.	dizziness
_____	8. pinna	h.	ear
_____	9. stapes	i.	wax
_____	10. acute	j.	go through

M. **Schedule your patients.** The following doctors and ancillary personnel are seeing patients in the clinic today. Based on the patient's needs, schedule the patient for the correct physician or technician. (LO 16.5, 16.9, 16.10, 16.14, 16.18, 16.E, 16.F)

ophthalmologist   ophthalmic technician

otologist   otorhinolaryngologist

Patient Needs/Has	Schedule with
refraction	1.
PE tubes	2.
phacoemulsification	3.
instruction in using eyedrops	4.
cholesteatoma	5.
patient hit in eye with tree branch	6.
removal of tonsils and adenoids	7.
LASIK surgery	8.
child has bubblegum in nose	9.
runny nose, stopped-up ears, sore throat	10.
broken eyeglasses	11.

N. **Apply what you know about the middle ear to choose the answer.** Select the best choice. (LO 16.13, 16.14)

1. Which of these is NOT a component of the middle ear?

    a. tympanic membrane

    b. eustachian (auditory) tube

    c. malleus, incus, stapes

    d. nasopharynx

    e. tympanic cavity

2. The eustachian (auditory) tube connects the

    a. tonsils and nasopharynx

    b. middle ear and nasopharynx

    c. nasopharynx and ossicles

    d. nasopharynx and tympanic membrane

    e. tympanic cavity and tympanic membrane

3. Identify the three ossicles:

    a. pinna, auricle, stapes

    b. eustachian (auditory) tube, mastoid cells, tonsils

    c. nasopharynx, tonsils, middle ear

    d. malleus, incus, stapes

    e. tonsils, stapes, incus

4. What is a complication of chronic otitis media with effusion?

    a. vertigo

    b. acute infection

    c. cholesteatoma

    d. dizziness

    e. nausea

5. Which of these would NOT cause a perforated eardrum?

    a. puncture by a cotton swab

    b. open-handed slap to the ear

    c. scuba diving

    d. pus from acute otitis media

    e. sinusitis

©2014 Nucleus Medical Media

Health professionals involved in the treatment of patients with **endocrinological** problems include:

- **Endocrinologists,** who are medical specialists concerned with the endocrine glands that produce hormonal secretions.

- **Pediatric endocrinologists,** who are medical specialists concerned with the diagnosis and management of children with endocrine disorders and diabetes.

- **Diabetologists,** who are physicians and endocrinologists whose practice and research are concentrated in diabetes care. **Diabetology** is not a recognized medical specialty.

- **Endocrine physician assistants,** who work as a team with endocrinologists to provide care and education to endocrine and diabetes patients.

- **Endocrine nurse practitioners,** who also work as a team with endocrinologists to provide care and education to endocrine and diabetes patients.

- **Certified diabetic educators,** licensed health care professionals including registered nurses, registered dietitians, and pharmacists, who are certified to possess distinct and specialized knowledge in diabetes self-management education and monitoring.

Chapter Learning Outcomes

The **endocrine system** is a communication system. **Hormones** are bloodborne messengers secreted by the endocrine glands. These hormones circulate in the blood stream giving them access to all other cells of the body. They are distributed anywhere blood goes but affect only the target cells that have receptors for each individual hormone and are then able to affect the metabolism of the target cell.
The information in this chapter enables you to:

LO 17.1 Identify the glands of the endocrine system and the hormones each gland secretes.

LO 17.2 Describe the pituitary gland and its hormones.

LO 17.3 Discuss disorders of the pituitary gland.

LO 17.4 Understand the diagnostic procedures for disorders of the pituitary gland.

LO 17.5 Explain the therapeutic procedures for disorders of the pituitary gland.

LO 17.6 Summarize the pharmacologic agents used in the treatment of disorders of the pituitary gland.

LO 17.7 Describe the thyroid gland and its hormones.

LO 17.8 Explain disorders of the thyroid gland.

LO 17.9 Understand the diagnostic procedures for disorders of the thyroid gland.

LO 17.10 Explain the therapeutic procedures for disorders of the thyroid gland.

LO 17.11 Summarize the pharmacologic agents used in the treatment of disorders of the thyroid gland.

LO 17.12 Identify the parathyroid gland and its disorders.

LO 17.13 Recognize the thymus gland and its disorders.

LO 17.14 Describe the adrenal glands and their hormones.

LO 17.15 Define disorders of the adrenal glands.

LO 17.16 Discuss the stress syndrome.

LO 17.17 Understand the diagnostic procedures for disorders of the adrenal glands.

LO 17.18 Explain the therapeutic procedures for disorders of the adrenal glands.

LO 17.19 Summarize the pharmacologic agents used in the treatment of disorders of the adrenal glands.

LO 17.20 Identify the hormones used in hormone replacement therapy.

LO 17.21 Describe the endocrine cells of the pancreas.

LO 17.22 Explain the different types of diabetes mellitus.

LO 17.23 Discuss the diagnostic procedures used in the treatment of diabetes mellitus.

LO 17.24 Explain the therapeutic procedures used in the treatment of diabetes mellitus.

LO 17.25 Describe the pharmacologic agents used in the treatment of diabetes mellitus.

LO 17.A Use the medical terms of endocrinology to communicate and document in writing accurately and precisely in any health care setting.

LO 17.B Use the medical terms of endocrinology to communicate verbally with accuracy and precision in any health care setting.

LO 17.C Construct medical terms associated with the endocrine system from their word roots.

LO 17.D Deconstruct medical terms into their word elements (roots, combining forms, prefixes, and suffixes).

LO 17.E Identify health professionals involved in the care of patients with endocrine disorders.

LO 17.F Correctly use approved abbreviations of medical terms used in endocrinology.

Case Report (CR) 17.1

You are

. . . a registered nurse (**RN**) working with endocrinologist Sabina Khalid, MD, in the Endocrinology Clinic at Fulwood Medical Center.

Your patient is

. . . Mrs. Gina Tacher, a 33-year-old schoolteacher. She complains of coarsening of her facial features and enlargement of the bones of her hands. Over the past 10 years, her nose and jaw have increased in size, and her voice has become husky. She brought photos of herself at ages 9 and 16. She has no other health problems.

Lesson 17.1

Endocrine System Overview: Hypothalamus, Pituitary, and Pineal Glands

LO 17.1 Endocrine System

The endocrine system is composed of 14 major glands *(Figure 14.1)*

- **Pituitary** gland and the nearby hypothalamus
- **Pineal** gland
- Thyroid gland
- **Parathyroid** glands (4)
- Thymus gland
- Adrenal glands (2)
- Pancreas
- Gonads: testes (2) in the male; ovaries (2) in the female

In addition, endocrine cells found in tissues all over the body secrete hormones. Examples are:

- **Cells in the upper GI tract** that secrete the hormone **gastrin**, which stimulates gastric secretions, and the hormone **cholecystokinin**, which contracts the gallbladder *(see Chapter 5).*
- **Cells in the kidney** that secrete **erythropoietin**, which stimulates erythrocyte production *(see Chapter 6).*
- **Fat cells** that secrete **leptin**, which helps suppress appetite. Lack of it can lead to overeating and obesity.

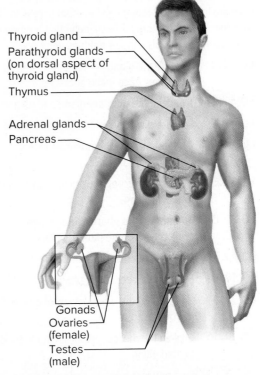

▲ **Figure 17.1** Major Endocrine Glands.

- **Cells in tissues throughout the body** that secrete **prostaglandins**, which act locally to dilate blood vessels, relax airways, stimulate uterine contractions in menstrual cramps or labor, and lower acid secretion in the stomach. When tissues are injured, prostaglandins promote an inflammatory response.

Hypothalamus

The hypothalamus *(Figure 17.2)* forms the floor and walls of the brain's third ventricle *(see Chapter 9)* and produces eight hormones. Six of them are local hormones that regulate the production of hormones by the anterior pituitary gland *(see page 592)*. Two of them, **oxytocin** and **antidiuretic hormone (ADH)**, are transported to the posterior pituitary, where they are stored until they are needed elsewhere in the body.

Pineal Gland

The pineal gland is located on the roof of the third ventricle of the brain, posterior to the hypothalamus *(Figure 17.2)*. It secretes **serotonin** by day and converts it to **melatonin** at night. The gland reaches its maximum size in childhood and may regulate the timing of puberty. It also may play a role in **seasonal affective disorder (SAD)**, in which people are depressed in the dark days of winter.

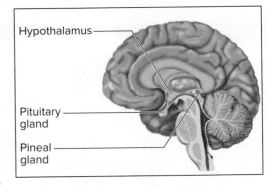

▲ **Figure 17.2** Hypothalamus, Pituitary Gland, and Pineal Gland.

WORD	PRONUNCIATION	ELEMENTS		DEFINITION
antidiuretic (*Note:* This term has two prefixes.)	**AN**-tih-die-you-**RET**-ik	S/ P/ P/ R/	**-ic** *pertaining to* **anti-** *against* **-di-** *complete* **-uret-** *urination*	An agent that decreases urine production
antidiuretic hormone	**AN**-tih-die-you-**RET**-ik **HOR**-mohn		**hormone** Greek *to set in motion*	Posterior pituitary hormone that decreases urine output by acting on the kidney; also called *vasopressin*
endocrine	**EN**-doh-krin	S/ P/	**-crine** *secrete* **endo-** *within*	Pertaining to a gland that produces an internal or hormonal secretion
endocrinology (*Note:* The "e" in -*crine* changes to "o" for easier pronunciation.)	**EN**-doh-krih-**NOL**-oh-jee	S/ R/CF	**-logy** *study of* **-crin/o** *secrete*	Medical specialty concerned with the production and effects of hormones
endocrinologist	**EN**-doh-krih-**NOL**-oh-jist	S/	**-logist** *one who studies, specialist*	A medical specialist in endocrinology
gland	GLAND		Latin *glans, acorn*	A collection of cells functioning as a secretory or excretory organ
hormone	**HOR**-mohn		Greek *to set in motion*	Chemical formed in one tissue or organ and carried by the blood to stimulate or inhibit a function of another tissue or organ
hormonal (adj)	hor-**MOHN**-al	S/ R/	**-al** *pertaining to* **hormon-** *chemical messenger*	Pertaining to a hormone(s) or the endocrine system
leptin	**LEP**-tin	S/ R/	**-in** *chemical compound* **lept-** *thin, small*	Hormone secreted by adipose tissue
melatonin	mel-ah-**TONE**-in	S/ R/ R/	**-in** *chemical compound* **mela-** *black* **-ton-** *tension, pressure*	Hormone formed by the pineal gland
oxytocin	**OK**-see-**TOH**-sin	S/ P/ R/	**-in** *chemical compound* **oxy-** *quick* **-toc-** *labor, birth*	Hypothalamic hormone, stored in the posterior pituitary, that stimulates the uterus to contract
parathyroid	pair-ah-**THIGH**-royd	P/ S/ R/	**para-** *beside* **-oid** *resembling* **-thyr-** *an oblong shield*	Endocrine glands embedded in the back of the thyroid gland
pineal	**PIN**-ee-al		Latin *like a pine cone*	Pertaining to the pineal gland
pituitary	pih-**TOO**-ih-tair-ee	S/ R/	**-ary** *pertaining to* **pituit-** *pituitary*	Pertaining to the pituitary gland
prostaglandin	**PROS**-tah-**GLAN**-din	S/ R/CF R/	**-in** *chemical compound* **prost/a-** *prostate* **-gland-** *gland*	Hormone present in many tissues, but first isolated from prostate gland
seasonal affective disorder (*Note:* The abbreviation for this is SAD, which is how you feel with this disorder.)	**SEE**-zon-al af-**FEK**-tiv dis-**OR**-der	S/ R/ S/ R/ P/ R/	**-al** *pertaining to* **season-** *period of the year* **-ive** *pertaining to* **affect-** *mood* **dis-** *apart, away from* **-order** *arrange*	Depression that occurs at the same time every year, often in winter
serotonin	ser-oh-**TOH**-nin	S/ R/CF R/	**-in** *substance* **ser/o-** *serum* **-ton-** *tension, pressure*	A neurotransmitter in the central and peripheral nervous systems

Exercises

A. Elements are listed in the left column. *In the first blank, write P for prefix, R/CF for root/combining form, or S for suffix. Finish the exercise by writing the meaning of the element in the right column.* **LO 17.1, 17.A, 17.C**

Element	P, R/CF, or S	Meaning of Element
1. *di*	_____	_____
2. *anti*	_____	_____
3. *endo*	_____	_____
4. *mela*	_____	_____

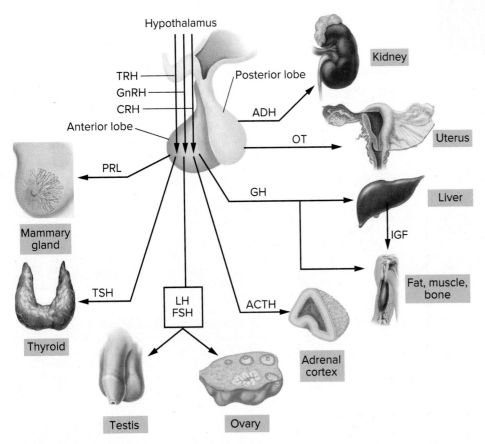

▲ Figure 17.3 Hormones of the Pituitary Gland and Their Target Organs.

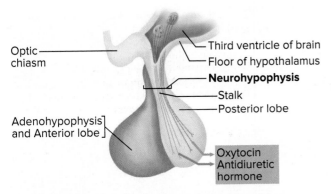

▲ Figure 17.4 Hormones of the Posterior Lobe of the Pituitary Gland.

Abbreviations

ACTH	adrenocorticotropic hormone
ADH	antidiuretic hormone
FSH	follicle-stimulating hormone
GH	growth hormone
GnRH	gonadotropin-releasing hormone
LH	luteinizing hormone
OT	oxytocin
PRL	prolactin
TSH	thyroid-stimulating hormone

LO 17.2 Pituitary Gland

While there is no single conductor of the endocrine orchestra in which each hormone plays its part in maintaining **homeostasis**, the pituitary gland and the hypothalamus work together and often influence the production of hormones in the other endocrine glands.

The pituitary gland (**hypophysis**) is suspended from the hypothalamus. The gland has two components:

1. A large anterior lobe called the **adenohypophysis**.
2. A smaller posterior lobe called the **neurohypophysis**.

Anterior lobe hormones are six in number *(Figure 17.3)*:

- **Follicle-stimulating hormone (FSH)** stimulates target cells in the ovaries to develop eggs and stimulates sperm production in the testes.
- **Luteinizing hormone (LH)** stimulates ovulation and the formation of a corpus luteum in the ovary *(see Chapter 8)* to secrete estrogen and progesterone. In the male, LH stimulates production of testosterone *(see Chapter 7)*.

(FSH and LH are gonadotropins and are released under the control of gonadotropin-releasing hormone [**GnRH**] of the hypothalamus.)

- **Thyroid-stimulating hormone (TSH)**, or **thyrotropin**, stimulates the growth of the thyroid gland and the production of **thyroxine**.
- **Adrenocorticotropic hormone (ACTH)**, or **corticotropin**, stimulates the **adrenal glands** to produce hormones called **corticosteroids**.
- **Prolactin (PRL)** stimulates the mammary glands after pregnancy to produce milk.
- **Growth hormone (GH)**, or **somatotropin**, is produced in quantities at least a thousand times as great as any other pituitary hormone. It stimulates cells to enlarge and divide to produce growth, particularly in childhood and adolescence.

Tropic (also spelled **trophic**) **hormones** are hormones that stimulate other endocrine glands to produce their hormones. All of the anterior lobe hormones except PRL and GH are tropic hormones.

Posterior lobe hormones, which are produced by nuclei in the hypothalamus and then stored in and released by the pituitary posterior lobe, are of two types *(Figure 17.4)*:

- **Oxytocin (OT)** in childbirth stimulates uterine contractions and in lactation forces milk to flow down ducts to the nipple. In both sexes, its production increases during sexual intercourse to help give the feelings of satisfaction and emotional bonding.
- **Antidiuretic hormone (ADH)** reduces the volume of urine produced by the kidneys. It is also called **vasopressin**.

WORD	PRONUNCIATION	ELEMENTS		DEFINITION
adenohypophysis (*Note:* The prefix *hypo-* is part of **hypophysis**, which is a term in itself.)	**AD**-en-oh-high-**POF**-ih-sis	P/ R/CF R/	**-hypo-** *below* **aden/o-** *gland* **-physis** *growth*	Anterior lobe of the pituitary gland
adrenal gland	ah-**DREE**-nal GLAND	S/ P/ R/	**-al** *pertaining to* **ad-** *near, toward* **-ren-** *kidney* **gland** Latin *glans, acorn*	The suprarenal, or adrenal, gland on the upper pole of each kidney
adrenocorticotropic hormone	ah-**DREE**-noh-**KOR**-tih-koh-**TROH**-pik **HOR**-mohn	S/ R/CF R/CF	**-tropic** *stimulator* **adren/o-** *adrenal gland* **-cortic/o-** *cortisone, cortex* **hormone** Greek *to set in motion*	Hormone of the anterior pituitary that stimulates the cortex of the adrenal gland to produce its own hormones
antidiuretic hormone (ADH) (also called **vasopressin**)	**AN**-tih-die-you-**RET**-ik **HOR**-mohn	S/ P/ P/ R/CF	**-ic** *pertaining to* **anti-** *against* **-di-** *complete* **-uret-** *urinary system* **hormone** Greek *to set in motion*	Posterior pituitary hormone that decreases urine output by acting on the kidney
corticosteroid	**KOR**-tih-koh-**STEHR**-oyd	S/ R/CF	**-steroid** *steroid* **cortic/o-** *cortisone, cortex*	A hormone produced by the adrenal cortex
corticotropin	**KOR**-tih-koh-**TROH**-pin	S/ R/CF	**-tropin** *stimulation* **cortic/o-** *cortisone, cortex*	Pituitary hormone that stimulates the cortex of the adrenal gland to secrete cortisone
hypophysis	high-**POF**-ih-sis	P/ R/	**hypo-** *below* **-physis** *growth*	Another name for the pituitary gland
neurohypophysis	**NYUR**-oh-high-**POF**-ih-sis	P/ R/CF R/	**-hypo-** *below* **neur/o-** *nervous tissue* **-physis** *growth*	Posterior lobe of the pituitary gland
prolactin	proh-**LAK**-tin	S/ P/ R/	**-in** *chemical compound* **pro-** *before* **-lact-** *milk*	Pituitary hormone that stimulates the production of milk
somatotropin (also called growth hormone)	**SOH**-mah-toh-**TROH**-pin	S/ R/CF	**-tropin** *stimulation* **somat/o-** *the body*	Hormone of the anterior pituitary that stimulates growth of body tissues
thyroid	**THIGH**-royd	S/ R/	**-oid** *resembling* **thyr-** *an oblong shield*	Endocrine gland in the neck, or a cartilage of the larynx
thyrotropin	thigh-roh-**TROH**-pin	S/ R/CF	**-tropin** *stimulation* **thyr/o-** *thyroid*	Hormone from the anterior pituitary gland that stimulates function of the thyroid gland
thyroxine	thigh-**ROK**-seen	S/ R/ R/	**-ine** *pertaining to* **thyr-** *an oblong shield* **-ox-** *oxygen*	Thyroid hormone T$_4$, tetraiodothyronine
tropin (noun) trophin (alt) tropic (adj) trophic (alt)	**TROH**-pin **TROH**-fin **TROH**-pik **TROH**-fic	S/ R/ R/	Greek *a turning* Greek *nourishment* **-ic** *pertaining to* **trop-** *turning* **troph-** *nourishment*	Hormone Hormone Tropic hormones stimulate other endocrine glands to produce hormones
vasopressin (also called antidiuretic hormone ADH)	vay-soh-**PRESS**-in	S/ R/CF R/	**-in** *chemical compound* **vas/o-** *blood vessel* **-press-** *press, close*	Pituitary hormone that constricts blood vessels and decreases urine output

Exercises

A. Many hormones are known by their abbreviation. *Match the description in the left column to the correct abbreviation in the right column.*
 LO 17.2, 17.F

_____ **1.** Stimulates formation of corpus luteum   **a.** OT

_____ **2.** Stimulates production of corticosteroids   **b.** LH

_____ **3.** Stimulates uterine contractions   **c.** FSH

_____ **4.** Stimulates ovaries to develop eggs   **d.** ACTH

▲ **Figure 17.5** **Pituitary Gigantism.** ©Marcelo Sayao/EPA/Newscom

▲ **Figure 17.6** **Man with Acromegaly, Age 52.** ©Clinical Photography, Central Manchester University Hospitals NHS Foundation Trust, UK/Science Source

 Case Report (CR) 17.1 *(continued)*

Dr. Khalid's examination of Mrs. Gina Tacher showed a protruding mandible (**prognathism**) and an enlarged, deeply grooved tongue. Her feet and hands were enlarged. She had noticed an increase in her shoe size and an inability to remove her wedding band. Her ribs were thickened, her heart was enlarged, and her blood pressure (**BP**) was 140/90. Her body hair was dark and coarse, and she was sweating freely.

X-rays showed a thickened skull with enlarged nasal sinuses and thickened terminal phalanges of her hands. A diagnosis of **acromegaly** was made.

Computed tomography (**CT**) and magnetic resonance imaging (**MRI**) scans showed a tumor in the pituitary that occupies most of the sella turcica *(see Chapter 5)*.

Blood tests showed high levels of growth hormone and **insulin-like growth factor (IGF)**.

LO 17.3 Disorders of Pituitary Hormones

Overproduction of Pituitary Hormones

Overproduction of growth hormone stimulates excessive growth of bones and muscles. It is almost always caused by a benign pituitary adenoma.

In children, the excessive production starts before the growth plates of the long bones have closed. The long bones grow enormously, producing **gigantism** *(Figure 17.5)*. Puberty can be delayed, genitalia may not develop fully, and diabetes can be a problem.

In adults, excessive growth hormone produces **acromegaly** *(Figure 17.6)*. This is the condition Mrs. Gina Tacher has.

Treatment of acromegaly is difficult. In Mrs. Tacher's case, surgery was able to remove much of the pituitary adenoma and was followed by radiation therapy.

A **prolactinoma** is a benign prolactin-secreting tumor of the pituitary gland in both men and women. It can lead to breast milk production in women who are not breast-feeding and produce scanty menstrual periods. In men it leads to breast milk production and impotence. The abnormal production of breast milk is called **galactorrhea** *(see Chapter 13)*.

Underproduction of Pituitary Hormones

Underproduction of growth hormone can be present at birth and leads to **pituitary dwarfism** *(Figure 17.7)*. The short stature becomes evident at around 1 year of age and is associated with episodes of hypoglycemia.

Hypopituitarism is uncommon. It can be caused by a pituitary tumor and cause a decline in the production of several hormones at the same time, a condition called **panhypopituitarism**.

Diabetes insipidus (DI) results from a decreased production of ADH, which helps regulate the amount of water in the body. (Diabetes mellitus is an entirely different disorder; *see Lesson 17.4*.) Antidiuretic hormone is produced in the hypothalamus and stored in the posterior pituitary lobe. Diabetes insipidus can result from insufficient production of ADH in the hypothalamus or failure of the pituitary gland to release it.

Symptoms begin with excessive urine production (polyuria) by day and by night. This leads to thirst and the need to drink up to 40 quarts of fluid per day.

In contrast to diabetes mellitus, urine in diabetes insipidus is dilute and does not contain sugar.

Treatment of diabetes insipidus is with vasopressin or desmopressin, synthetic modified forms of ADH. They are taken as a nasal spray several times daily, the dose being adjusted to maintain a normal urine output.

▲ **Figure 17.7** **Pituitary Dwarfism.** ©Frank Trapper/Getty Images

WORD	PRONUNCIATION	ELEMENTS		DEFINITION
acromegaly	ak-roh-**MEG**-ah-lee	P/ R/	acro- *highest point, extremity* -megaly *enlargement*	Enlargement of the head, face, hands, and feet due to excess growth hormone in an adult
diabetes insipidus	die-ah-**BEE**-teez in-**SIP**-ih-dus	 S/ P/ R/	diabetes Greek *siphon* -us *pertaining to* in- *not, without* -sipid- *flavor*	Excretion of large amounts of dilute urine as a result of inadequate ADH production
dwarfism	**DWORF**-izm	S/ R/	-ism *condition* dwarf- *miniature*	Short stature due to underproduction of growth hormone
gigantism	jie-**GAN**-tizm	S/ R/	-ism *condition* gigant- *giant*	Abnormal height and size of entire body
hypopituitarism	**HIGH**-poh-pih-**TYU**-ih-tah-rizm	S/ P/ R/	-ism *condition* hypo- *deficient* -pituitar- *pituitary*	Condition of one or more deficient pituitary hormones
panhypopituitarism	pan-**HIGH**-poh-pih-**TYU**-ih-tah-rizm	S/ P/ P/ R/	-ism *condition* pan- *all* -hypo- *deficient* -pituitar- *pituitary*	Deficiency of all the pituitary hormones
prognathism	**PROG**-nah-thizm	S/ P/ R/	-ism *condition* pro- *before, in front* -gnath- *jaw*	Condition of a forward-projecting jaw
prolactinoma	proh-lak-tih-**NOH**-mah	S/ S/ P/ R/	-oma *tumor* -in- *chemical compound* pro- *before, in front* -lact- *milk*	Prolactin-producing tumor

Exercises

A. After reading Case Report (CR) 17.1, answer the following questions. *Fill in the blanks with the correct answer or choose the correct letter(s) for the multiple choice questions.* **LO 17.3, 17.A**

1. What is the medical term for *protruding mandible?* _____

2. Which of the following are the signs (observable on the outside) that Mrs. Tacher is exhibiting? (Choose all that apply.)

   a. protruding mandible   **b.** observed sweating   **c.** increase in shoe size

   d. enlarged heart   **e.** change in voice

3. Which of the following are the symptoms (felt by the patient)? (Choose all that apply.)

   a. protruding mandible   **b.** observed sweating   **c.** increase in shoe size

   d. enlarged heart   **e.** change in voice

4. Was her blood pressure elevated?

   a. Yes   **b.** No

5. Which of the following are the diagnostic tests used by her physician to determine a disorder? (Choose all that apply.)

   a. change in shoe size   **b.** CT scan   **c.** tongue appearance

   d. blood tests   **e.** MRI

6. In the diagnosis **acromegaly,** which element means *enlargement?*

   _____

7. Why wasn't her condition considered to be gigantism?

   a. Gigantism is caused by another hormone.   **b.** People with gigantism do not have enlarged feet.

   c. Her disorder occurred after puberty.   **d.** Acromegaly only occurs in females.

8. Mrs. Tacher's acromegaly was caused by:

   a. cancer of her hypothalamus   **b.** inappropriate diet

   c. decreased production of ADH   **d.** tumor of her anterior pituitary gland

Abbreviations

ACTH	adrenocorticotropic hormone, corticotropin
ADH	antidiuretic hormone
IGF-1	insulinlike growth factor-1
MRI	magnetic resonance imaging
TSH	thyroid-stimulating hormone, thyrotropin

Keynote

Pituitary tumors present with symptoms that lead to a complete medical history and physical examination, blood and urine tests, and x-rays.

LO 17.4 Pituitary Diagnostic Procedures

Visual field tests can show the presence of a **pituitary tumor** as the tumor presses on the **optic chiasma** *(see Figure 16.11),* causing loss of vision in the peripheral visual fields.

Levels of pituitary hormones in the blood and/or urine can be measured directly to show the presence of a hormone-producing pituitary **adenoma**.

Examples are the levels of **growth hormone** and **insulinlike growth factor-1** (IGF-1). When growth hormone levels are high, they cause the liver to produce more IGF-1. When both levels are very high, a pituitary tumor is the diagnosis. If the levels are only slightly increased, a **glucose suppression test** is performed. Ingestion of a large amount of sugar normally leads to a drop in growth hormone levels. If growth hormones remain high, a pituitary adenoma is the cause. High levels of growth hormone are found in gigantism, beginning in children, and acromegaly, beginning in adults.

Blood **prolactin** levels can be measured to check for a prolactinoma; **ACTH (corticotropin)** levels help distinguish ACTH-secreting pituitary tumors from adrenal gland tumors: **TSH (thyrotropin)** levels usually identify thyrotropin-secreting adenomas.

Diabetes insipidus, caused by failure in production of **ADH (antidiuretic hormone)** by the hypothalamus or by failure of the posterior pituitary to release it due to an adenoma, is diagnosed primarily by measurement of the amount of urine and its **osmolality**.

Magnetic resonance imaging (MRI) can show pituitary tumors greater than 3 mm across.

Biopsy of the tumor is sometimes needed to make a firm diagnosis. When pituitary tumors are removed surgically, they are always examined under a microscope to confirm the exact diagnosis.

WORD	PRONUNCIATION	ELEMENTS		DEFINITION
adenoma	AD-eh-NOH-mah	S/ R/	-oma *tumor* aden- *gland*	A benign neoplasm of epithelial tissue
biopsy (*Note:* the extra "o" is dropped)	BIE-op-see	S/ R/	-opsy *to view* bio- *life*	Process of removing tissue from living patients for microscopic examination
chiasm chiasma (alt)	KIE-asm kie-AZ-mah		Greek *cross*	X-shaped crossing of the two optic nerves at the base of the brain
optic	OP-tik	S/ R/	-ic *pertaining to* opt- *vision*	Pertaining to the eye
osmolality	OZ-moh-LAL-ih-tee	S/ S/ R/	-ity *state* -al- *pertaining to* osmol- *concentration*	The concentration of a solution
tumor	TOO-mer		Latin *swelling*	Any abnormal swelling

Exercises

A. Use abbreviations to describe the condition. *Health care professionals often use abbreviations in documentation; therefore, it is important to know the meanings of abbreviations. Given the description, write the abbreviation for the hormone. Fill in the blank.* **LO 17.3, 17.4, 17.A, 17.F**

1. Lack of this hormone would increase urine production. _____

2. This hormone will be increased with thyrotropin-secreting adenomas. _____

3. Helps distinguish corticotropin pituitary tumors from adrenal gland tumors. _____

B. Define the word elements to quickly decipher the meaning of the medical term. *Knowing the meaning of the word elements makes short work of defining medical terms. Identify the meaning of the element on the left with its correct meaning on the right.* **LO 17.D**

_____	1. *osmol-*	**a.**	tumor
_____	2. *-oma*	**b.**	gland
_____	3. *bio-*	**c.**	to view
_____	4. *-opsy*	**d.**	concentration
_____	5. *aden-*	**e.**	life

LO 17.5 Pituitary Therapeutic Procedures

Surgical removal of a pituitary tumor is necessary if the tumor is pressing on the optic nerves or if it is overproducing hormones. In 99% of cases, this is performed by an **endoscopic transnasal transsphenoidal approach** in which the surgery is performed through the nose and sphenoid sinus using an **endoscope**. **Craniotomy**, in which a very large tumor is removed through the upper part of the skull, is occasionally necessary. The surgery can be made more efficient by using **image-guided stereotactic surgery** in which advanced computers create a three-dimensional image of the tumor to guide the surgeon.

Radiation therapy can be used alone, after surgery, or if the tumor persists or returns after surgery. Methods of radiation therapy include:

- **Gamma knife stereotactic radiosurgery**, which delivers a single high-dose radiation beam the size and shape of the tumor using special brain-imaging techniques.

- **Proton beam therapy**, which delivers positively charged ions (protons) rather than x-rays in beams that are finely controlled with minimal risk to surrounding healthy tissues.

- **External beam radiation**, which delivers x-rays in small increments, usually five times a week over a four- to six-week period. It may damage surrounding healthy pituitary and brain tissues.

LO 17.6 Pituitary Medications and Hormone Replacement Therapy

Medications can help to block excessive hormone secretion and sometimes reduce pituitary tumor size:

- **Growth hormone-secreting tumors** have two types of drugs used if surgery has been unsuccessful in normalizing growth hormone production. **Somatostatin analogs** *(Sandostatin, Somatuline Depot)* cause a decrease in growth hormone production and are given by injection every four weeks. The second type, **pegvisomant** *(Somavert)*, blocks the effect of excess growth hormone, is given by daily injection, and may cause liver damage.

- **Prolactin-secreting tumors (prolactinomas)** are treated with two drugs, **cabergoline** *(Dostinex)* and **bromocriptine** *(Parlodel)*, that decrease prolactin secretion, but they can have serious side effects, including developing compulsive behaviors.

Pituitary hormone replacement therapy is needed after surgery or radiation therapy to maintain normal hormone levels. The medication taken depends on the hormones that need to be replaced, which include adrenocorticotropic hormone (ACTH), thyroxine, estrogen and progesterone, testosterone, antidiuretic hormone (ADH), and synthetic growth hormones.

WORD	PRONUNCIATION		ELEMENTS	DEFINITION
analog	**AN**-ah-log		Greek *proportionate*	A compound that resembles another in structure but not in function; analog is a means of the transmission of continuous information to our senses, in contrast with the digital transmission of only zeros and ones.
craniotomy	kray-nee-**OT**-oh-mee	S/ R/	**-tomy** *incision* **crani/o** *cranium*	Incision of the skull
endoscope	**EN**-doh-skope	P/ R/	**endo-** *inside* **-scope** *instrument for viewing*	Instrument for viewing the inside of a tubular or hollow organ
endoscopic	**EN**-doh-**SKOP**-ik	S/	**-ic** *pertaining to*	Pertaining to an endoscope.
gamma knife	**GAM**-ah NIFE		**gamma** *third letter in Greek alphabet* **knife** *Old English knife*	A minimally invasive radiosurgical system
proton	**PROH**-ton		Greek *first*	The positively charged unit of the nuclear mass
stereotactic	**STER**-ee-oh-**TAK**-tik	S/ R/CF R/	**-ic** *pertaining to* **stere/o** *three- dimensional* **-tact-** *orderly arrangement*	Pertaining to a precise three-dimensional method to locate a lesion or a tumor
transnasal	trans-**NAY**-zal	S/ P/ R/	**-al** *pertaining to* **trans-** *across, through* **-nas-** *nose*	Through the nose
transsphenoid	trans-**SFEE**-noyd	S/ P/ R/CF	**-oid** *resembling* **trans-** *through* **sphen/o** *wedge*	Through the sphenoid sinus

Exercises

A. Explain the therapeutic procedures for disorders of the pituitary gland. *Choose the correct answer to complete the sentence or answer the question.* **LO 17.5**

1. Treatment of pituitary tumors is aimed at:

   a. shrinking or removing the tumor

   b. removing the entire pituitary gland

   c. increasing pituitary hormone levels

   d. suppressing adrenal gland secretion

2. Large pituitary tumors may require a:

   a. MRI   **b.** craniotomy   **c.** lithotripsy   **d.** lobectomy

3. After treatment of pituitary tumors, what type of therapy is often begun?

   a. physical   **b.** occupational   **c.** radiation   **d.** hormone-replacement

B. Deconstruct the terms relating to therapeutic procedures to treat disorders of the pituitary gland. *Identifying the word elements will help you understand the purpose of the procedure. Choose the correct answer.* **LO 17.5, 17.D**

1. The suffix of the term **endoscopic** means

   a. process of viewing   **b.** use of a microscope   **c.** across   **d.** pertaining to

2. The suffix in the term **transsphenoid** means:

   a. pertaining to   **b.** bony projection   **c.** resembling   **d.** across   **e.** butterfly

3. The suffix in the term **craniotomy** means:

   a. incision into   **b.** removal of   **c.** skull   **d.** treatment of   **e.** covering

Lesson 17.2

ENDOCRINE SYSTEM

Thyroid, Parathyroid, and Thymus Glands

Case Report (CR) 17.2

You are

... an emergency medical technician (**EMT**) working in the Emergency Room at Fulwood Medical Center at 0200 hours.

Your patient is

... Ms. Norma Leary, a 22-year-old college student living with her parents for the summer.

Ms. Leary is **emaciated**, extremely agitated, restless, and at times disoriented and confused. Her parents tell you that, in the past 3 or 4 days, she has been coughing and not feeling well. In the past 12 hours, she has become feverish and been complaining of a left-sided chest pain. With questioning, the parents reveal that prior to this acute illness, she had lost about 20 pounds in weight, although she was eating voraciously. Her vital signs (VS) are T 105.2°F, P 180 and irregular, R 24, BP 160/85.

You call for Dr. Hilinski **STAT** (immediately). On his initial examination, he believes that the patient is in **thyroid storm**. This is a medical emergency. There are no immediate laboratory tests that can confirm this diagnosis.

LO 17.7 Thyroid Gland

The thyroid gland lies just beneath the skin of the neck and below the thyroid cartilage (Adam's apple). It is about 2 inches (5 cm) across and shaped like a bow tie. Two lobes extend up on either side of the trachea and are joined by an isthmus *(Figure 17.8).*

The thyroid is a soft, very vascular organ composed mostly of small follicles lined with epithelial cells. These cells secrete the two thyroid hormones: **triiodothyronine (T_3)** and **thyroxine (T_4)**. The term **thyroid hormone** refers to T_3 and T_4 collectively.

Superior thyroid artery and vein

Thyroid cartilage

Thyroid gland

Thyroid gland

Isthmus

Inferior thyroid vein

Trachea

▲ **Figure 17.8** **Anatomy of the Thyroid Gland.**

Thyroid hormone acts in three interrelated ways:

- **Stimulates** almost every tissue in the body to produce proteins.
- **Increases** the amount of oxygen that cells use.
- **Controls** the speed at which the body's chemical functions proceed (**metabolic rate**).

The thyroid gland extracts **iodine** from the blood to produce T_3 and T_4. The hormones are produced in response to **thyroid-stimulating hormone (TSH)** from the anterior pituitary gland. The pituitary gland, in turn, increases or slows the release of TSH in response to the level of thyroid hormone in the blood.

The thyroid also produces the hormone **calcitonin** from the **C cells** found between the follicles. Calcitonin stimulates osteoblastic activity *(see Chapter 14)* to promote calcium deposition and bone formation. It is secreted in response to **hypercalcemia**.

WORD	PRONUNCIATION	ELEMENTS		DEFINITION
calcitonin	kal-sih-**TONE**-in	S/ R/CF R/	**-in** chemical compound **calc/i-** calcium **-ton-** pressure, tension	Thyroid hormone that moves calcium from blood to bones
emaciation	ee-**MAY**-see-**AY**-shun	S/ R/CF	**-ation** process **emac/i-** make thin	Abnormal thinness
emaciated (adv)	ee-**MAY**-see-**ATE**-ed	S/	**-ated** composed of	Abnormally thin and wasted
hypercalcemia	**HIGH**-per-kal-**SEE**-mee-ah	S/ P/ R/	**-emia** condition of the blood **hyper-** above, excessive **-calc-** calcium	Excessive level of calcium in the blood
iodine	**EYE**-oh-dine or **EYE**-oh-deen	S/ R/	**-ine** pertaining to **iod-** violet, iodine	Chemical element, the lack of which causes thyroid disease
thyroid hormone	**THIGH**-royd **HOR**-mohn	S/ R/	**-oid** resembling **thyr-** an oblong shield **hormone** Greek to set in motion	Collective term for the two thyroid hormones, T_3 and T_4
thyroid storm	**THIGH**-royd STORM	S/ R/	**-oid** resembling **thyr-** an oblong shield **storm** Old High German storm, crisis	Medical crisis and emergency due to excess thyroid hormones
thyroxine	thigh-**ROK**-seen	S/ R/ R/	**-ine** pertaining to **thyr-** an oblong shield **-ox-** oxygen	Thyroid hormone T_4, tetraiodothyronine
triiodothyronine	trie-**EYE**-oh-doh-**THIE**-roh-neen	S/ P/ R/CF R/CF R/	**-ine** pertaining to **tri-** three **-iod/o-** violet, iodine **-thyr-** an oblong shield **-on** chemical substance	Thyroid hormone T_3

Exercises

A. After reading Case Report (CR) 17.2, answer the following questions. LO 17.7, 17.A, 17.F

1. Someone who appears **emaciated** is:

   a. obese   **b.** sleepy   **c.** rude   **d.** thin

2. Which of the following are *signs* that a disorder is present? (choose all that apply)

   a. agitation   **b.** not feeling well   **c.** pain

   d. increased body temperature   **e.** rapid respirations

3. Which of the following are *symptoms* felt by Ms. Leary?

   a. agitation   **b.** not feeling well   **c.** pain

   d. increased body temperature   **e.** rapid respirations

4. What is her diagnosed condition? (choose all that apply)

   a. diabetes insipidus   **b.** thyroid storm   **c.** dyspnea

   d. bradycardia   **e.** osteoporosis

5. Which of the following terms in the Case Report means *immediately:*

   a. feverish   **b.** voraciously   **c.** disoriented   **d.** irregular   **e.** STAT

6. *Thyroid storm* is due to:

   a. excessive thyroid hormones   **b.** increased somatostatin

   c. shrinking isthmus   **d.** decreased blood iodine

Thyroid storm is the condition Ms. Norma Leary presented with in the Emergency Department. It shows severely exaggerated effects of the thyroid hormones. This explains her hyperpyrexia, tachycardia, agitation, and delirium. The weight loss before her illness became acute was part of her undiagnosed Graves disease. Ms. Leary's immediate treatment included supplemental oxygen, intravenous (IV) fluids with dextrose solutions, ice packs and cooling blanket, propranolol, **antithyroid** medications, and oral iodine compounds.

▲ **Figure 17.9** **Hyperthyroidism May Cause the Eyes to Protrude (Exophthalmos).**
©Biophoto Associates/Photo Researchers, Inc.

LO 17.8 Disorders of the Thyroid Gland

Hyperthyroidism (Thyrotoxicosis)

Whatever the cause of **hyperthyroidism(thyrotoxicosis)**, the symptoms are those of increased body metabolism. These include tachycardia, hypertension, sweating, shakiness, anxiety, weight loss despite increased appetite, and diarrhea.

Graves disease is an autoimmune disorder *(see Chapter 12)* in which an antibody stimulates the thyroid to produce and secrete excessive quantities of thyroid hormones into the blood. It is associated with one or more symptoms of **goiter** (enlarged thyroid gland), **exophthalmos**, and pretibial **myxedema**.

Exophthalmos, in which the eyes bulge outward *(Figure 17.9)*, is caused by a substance that builds up behind the eyes. The same substance is occasionally deposited in the skin over the shins and called *pretibial myxedema*.

Thyroiditis is an inflammation of the thyroid gland. It presents in three forms:

- **Silent lymphocytic thyroiditis** is characterized by some thyroid enlargement and a **self-limiting** hyperthyroid phase of a few weeks, followed by recovery to the normal **euthyroid** state.

- **Subacute thyroiditis** has a history of an antecedent viral upper respiratory infection (URI) followed by signs of hyperthyroidism with a diffusely enlarged thyroid gland. It is self-limiting.

- **Hashimoto disease** is an autoimmune disease with lymphocytic infiltration of the thyroid gland. Hypothyroidism results, necessitating lifelong synthetic thyroid hormone replacement therapy.

Toxic thyroid adenoma is a nodule in the gland that produces thyroid hormones without stimulation by the pituitary's TSH. The nodule can be removed surgically.

Goiter *(Figure 17.10)* is an enlargement of the thyroid gland that, as it enlarges, can cause difficulty in swallowing and breathing. It can occur in any of the disorders listed previously and also in pregnancy.

▲ **Figure 17.10** **Woman with Goiter.**
©Lester V. Bergman/Getty Images

LO 17.8, 17.A
Word Analysis and Definition

S = Suffix   P = Prefix   R = Root   R/CF = Combining Form

WORD	PRONUNCIATION		ELEMENTS	DEFINITION
antithyroid	an-tee-**THIGH**-royd	S/ P/ R/	**-oid** *resembling* **anti-** *against* **-thyr-** *an oblong shield*	A substance that inhibits production of thyroid hormones
euthyroid	you-**THIGH**-royd	S/ P/ R/	**-oid-** *resembling* **eu-** *good, normal* **-thyr-** *an oblong shield*	Normal thyroid function
exophthalmos	ek-sof-**THAL**-mos	P/ R/	**ex-** *out, out of* **-ophthalmos** *eye*	Protrusion of the eyeball
goiter	**GOY**-ter		Latin *throat*	Enlargement of the thyroid gland
Graves disease	GRAYVZ diz-**EEZ**	P/ R/	Robert Graves, 1796–1853, Irish physician **dis-** *apart* **-ease** *normal function*	Hyperthyroidism with toxic goiter
Hashimoto disease Hashimoto thyroiditis (syn)	hah-shee-**MOH**-toh diz-**EEZ**	P/ R/	Hakaru Hashimoto, 1881–1934, Japanese surgeon **dis-** *apart* **-ease** *normal function*	Autoimmune disease of the thyroid gland
hyperthyroidism	high-per-**THIGH**-royd-ism	S/ S/ P/ R/	**-ism** *condition, process* **-oid-** *resembling* **hyper-** *excessive* **-thyr-** *an oblong shield*	Excessive production of thyroid hormones
myxedema	mik-seh-**DEE**-mah	P/ R/	**myx-** *mucus* **-edema** *swelling*	Waxy, nonpitting edema of the skin
thyroiditis	thigh-roy-**DIE**-tis	S/ S/ R/	**-itis** *inflammation* **-oid-** *resembling* **thyr-** *an oblong shield*	Inflammation of the thyroid gland
thyrotoxicosis	**THIGH**-roh-tok-sih-**KOH**-sis	S/ R/CF R/CF	**-sis** *abnormal condition* **thyr/o-** *an oblong shield* **-toxic/o-** *poison*	Disorder caused by excessive thyroid hormone production

Exercises

A. Elements: One word or phrase in each of the descriptions in the following questions is in bold. *This is your clue to finding the correct medical term in the word bank. Fill in the blanks with the language of endocrinology.* **LO 17.8**

thyroiditis   euthyroid   antithyroid   exophthalmos

thyrotoxicosis   hyperthyroidism   myxedema

1. **Excessive production** of thyroid hormones: _____

2. **Swelling** with a waxy substance: _____

3. **Inhibition** of production of thyroid hormone: _____

4. **Normal** thyroid function: _____

5. **Inflammation** of the thyroid gland: _____

6. **Protrusion** of the eyeball: _____

LO 17.8 Disorders of the Thyroid Gland (continued)
Hypothyroidism

Hypothyroidism results from an inadequate production of thyroid hormone, leading to a slowing of the body's metabolism. Primary hypothyroidism, in which no specific cause is found, affects 10% of older women. Severe hypothyroidism is called *myxedema*. In developing countries, a common cause is lack of iodine in the diet. In the United States, iodine is added to table salt to prevent hypothyroidism, and iodine is also found in dairy products and seafood.

Hypothyroidism causes the body to function slowly. Symptoms develop gradually. They include loss of hair; dry, scaly skin; puffy face and eyes; slow, hoarse speech; weight gain; constipation; and inability to tolerate cold (*Figure 17.11*).

Diagnosis of primary hypothyroidism is confirmed with a TSH blood level that is high. Treatment is to replace the thyroid hormone with synthetic T_4 (L-thyroxine), which is started in small doses.

Cretinism (*Figure 17.12*) is a congenital form of thyroid deficiency that severely retards mental and physical growth. If it is diagnosed and treated early with thyroid hormones, significant improvement can be achieved.

Thyroid cancer usually presents as a symptomless **nodule** in the thyroid gland.

▲ **Figure 17.11** **Elderly Woman with Hypothyroidism.** ©Dr. P. Marazzi/SPL/Photo Researchers, Inc.

LO 17.9 Diagnostic Procedures for Disorders of the Thyroid Gland

Thyroid-stimulating hormone (TSH) levels in the blood are low if the gland is overactive.

Thyroid hormone levels in the blood detail the activity of the gland; the levels are high if the gland is overactive.

Antithyroid antibodies are associated with autoimmune inflammatory diseases of the thyroid.

Isotopic thyroid scans detail the nature of the thyroid enlargement and the function of the gland.

Serum calcitonin level is elevated in medullary carcinoma.

Fine needle aspiration biopsy distinguishes benign from malignant nodules.

Ultrasonography reveals the size of the gland and the presence of nodules.

LO 17.10 Therapeutic Procedures for Disorders of the Thyroid Gland

Radioactive iodine (I-131) therapy uses the **isotope** of iodine that emits radiation to treat hyperthyroidism and thyroid cancer. When a small dose of the isotope is swallowed, it is absorbed into the bloodstream, taken up from the blood, and concentrated by the cells of the thyroid gland, where it begins destroying the gland's cells.

Hypothyroidism, in most cases, can be treated adequately with a constant daily dose of **levothyroxine (LT4)**. For hypothyroidism due to destruction of thyroid cells, **TSH** levels are monitored. For central (pituitary or hypothalamic) hypothyroidism, T_4 levels are used for monitoring.

Thyroid surgery is indicated for a variety of conditions including **cancerous** and **benign nodules**, **goiters**, and **overactive thyroid glands**. The types of surgery that can be performed include:

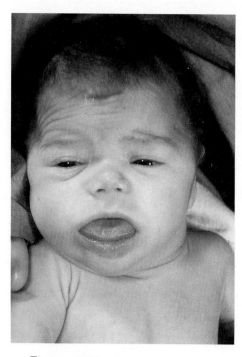

▲ **Figure 17.12** **Infant with Cretinism.** ©Alamy Stock Photo

- **Excisional biopsy**: removal of a small part of the gland.
- **Lobectomy**: removal of half of the thyroid gland (**hemilobectomy**).
- **Total thyroidectomy**: removal of all thyroid tissue.
- **Near-total thyroidectomy**: removal of all but a very small part of the gland.
- **Endoscopic thyroidectomy**: performed through a single small incision using a flexible lighted tube and video monitor to guide the surgical procedure.
- **Laser ablation**: a minimally invasive procedure used to remove benign thyroid nodules using ultrasound guidance without affecting the surrounding organ.

LO 17.11 Thyroid Pharmacology

Antithyroid medications prevent formation of thyroid hormones in the gland's cells.

Propylthiouracil and **methimazole** both decrease the amount of thyroid hormone produced by the gland's cells and can be used to treat hyperthyroidism. Unfortunately, they both have the major and frequent side effects of agranulocytosis and aplastic anemia, and are no longer recognized as a front-line medication.

Thyroid replacements are:

- L-thyroxine. This synthetic T_4 is a preferred replacement.
- Liothyronine sodium. This synthetic T_3 has a rapid turnover and has to be monitored frequently.

S = Suffix   P = Prefix   R = Root   R/CF = Combining Form

WORD	PRONUNCIATION	ELEMENTS		DEFINITION
ablation	ab-**LAY**-shun	S/ R/	-ion *process* ablat- *take away*	Removal of tissue to destroy its function
aspiration	**AS**-pih-**RAY**-shun	S/ R/	-ion *process* aspirat- *breathe in*	Removal by suction of fluid or gas from a body cavity
cretin cretinism	**KREH**-tin **KREH**-tin-ism	S/ R/	French *cretin* -ism *condition, process* cretin- *cretin*	A person with severe congenital hypothyroidism Condition of severe congenital hypothyroidism
hypothyroidism	high-poh-**THIGH**-royd-ism	S/ S/ P/ R/	-ism *condition, process* -oid- *resmbling* hypo- *deficient* -thyr- *an oblong shield*	Deficient production of thyroid hormones
isotope isotopic (adj)	**EYE**-so-tope	P/ R/ S/ R/	iso- *equal* -tope *part* -ic *pertaining to* -top- *part*	Radioactive element; some of these elements are used in diagnostic procedures Of identical chemical composition
lobectomy	loh-**BEK**-toh-mee	S/ R/	-ectomy *surgical excision* lob- *lobe*	Surgical removal of a lobe of the lungs or the thyroid gland
lymphadenectomy	lim-**FAD**-eh-**NEK**-toh-mee	S/ R/	-ectomy *surgical excision* lymphaden- *lymph node*	Surgical excision of a lymph node
nodule	**NOD**-yule		Latin *small knot*	Small node or knotlike swelling
radioactive iodine	**RAY**-dee-oh-**AK**-tiv **EYE**-oh-dine	S/ R/CF R/	-ive *pertaining to* radi/o- *radiation* -act- *performance* iodine *nonmetallic element*	Any of the various tracers that emit alpha, beta, or gamma rays
ultrasonography	**UL**-trah-soh-**NOG**-rah-fee	S/ P/ R/CF	-graphy *recording* ultra- *beyond* son/o- *sound*	Delineation of deep structures using sound waves

Exercises

A. Certain kinds of tests are performed for the purpose of arriving at the correct diagnosis for treatment. *Select the correct diagnostic test for each described condition.* **LO 17.7, 17.8, 17.9, 17.10**

1. Is associated with autoimmune inflammatory disease of the thyroid:

   a. serum calcitonin levels

   c. antithyroid hormone levels

   b. thyroid-stimulating hormone levels

   d. fine needle aspiration biopsy

2. Blood test to measure activity of the thyroid gland:

   a. serum calcitonin levels

   c. antithyroid hormone levels

   b. thyroid hormone levels

   d. fine needle aspiration biopsy

3. Level becomes elevated in medullary carcinoma:

   a. serum calcitonin levels

   c. antithyroid hormone levels

   b. thyroid-stimulating hormone levels

   d. fine needle aspiration biopsy

4. Reveals the size of the gland and the presence of nodules:

   a. radioactive iodine therapy

   c. ultrasonography

   b. fine needle aspiration biopsy

   d. serum calcitonin levels

5. Distinguishes benign from malignant nodules:

   a. radioactive iodine therapy

   b. fine needle aspiration biopsy

   c. ultrasonography

   d. isotopic thyroid scans

6. Details the nature of the thyroid enlargement and the function of the gland:

   a. isotopic thyroid scans

   c. ultrasonography

   b. fine needle aspiration biopsy

   d. serum calcitonin levels

LO 17.12, 17.13 Other Endocrine Glands

Parathyroid Glands

The **parathyroid glands** are usually four in number and are partially embedded in the posterior surface of the thyroid gland *(Figure 17.13)*. They secrete **parathyroid hormone (PTH)** in response to hypocalcemia. Calcitonin and PTH are **antagonistic**: PTH stimulates osteoclasts to reabsorb bone and bring calcium back into the blood while calcitonin takes calcium from the blood and stimulates osteoblasts to lay down bone *(see Chapter 14)*.

Disorders of Parathyroid Glands

Hypoparathyroidism is a deficiency of parathyroid hormone that lowers levels of blood calcium (hypocalcemia). Most symptoms are neuromuscular, ranging from tingling in the fingers to muscle cramps and the painful muscle spasms of **tetany** (*not* **tetanus**). A genetically engineered recombinant form of parathyroid hormone is now available, but classic treatment for hypoparathyroidism still involves high-dose calcium and vitamin D supplements.

Hyperparathyroidism is an excess of parathyroid hormone. It is seen more often than hypoparathyroidism and is usually caused by one of the four glands enlarging and secreting excess parathyroid hormone in an unregulated manner. It leads to four major abnormalities:

1. Bones are depleted of calcium (osteopenia) and become brittle.
2. High blood calcium levels (hypercalcemia) lead to decreased bowel motility and constipation and to increased gastric acidity and heartburn.
3. Extra excretion of calcium in the urine leads to kidney stones (nephrolithiasis).
4. High blood calcium leads to mental symptoms such as depression and fatigue and can lead to coma.

Surgical removal of the enlarged gland is **curative**.

Thymus Gland

The thymus **gland** is located in the mediastinum behind the sternum between the lungs and above the heart *(Figure 17.14)*. It is large in children and decreases in size until, in the elderly, it is mostly fibrous tissue. It secretes a group of hormones that stimulate the production of T lymphocytes *(see Chapter 12)*.

Disorders of Thymus Gland

DiGeorge syndrome is a genetic immunodeficiency disorder *(see Chapter 12)* in which the thymus is underdeveloped or absent at birth. Abnormalities of the thymus and parathyroid glands, heart, and facial structure are present, with few or no T lymphocytes. Transplantation of stem cells or thymus tissue can cure the immunodeficiency.

Thymomas, benign tumors, and **thymic carcinomas** are rare tumors that can be associated with myasthenia gravis *(see Chapter 9)* and other autoimmune syndromes, such as lupus erythematosus and rheumatoid arthritis. Treatment is usually surgical removal of the tumor or the gland (**thymectomy**), followed by **adjuvant** radiotherapy.

Pharynx (posterior view)

Thyroid gland

Parathyroid glands

Esophagus

Trachea

▲ **Figure 17.13** Site of Parathyroid Glands: Posterior View.

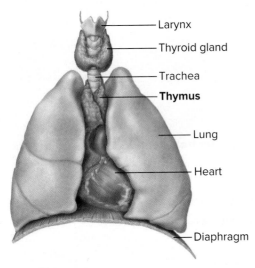

Larynx

Thyroid gland

Trachea

Thymus

Lung

Heart

Diaphragm

▲ **Figure 17.14** Position of Thymus Gland in the Mediastinum.

Abbreviation	
PTH	parathyroid hormone

WORD	PRONUNCIATION	ELEMENTS		DEFINITION
adjuvant	**AD**-joo-vant	S/ R/	-ant *pertaining to* adjuv- *give help*	Additional treatment after a primary treatment has been used
antagonist	an-**TAG**-oh-nist	S/ P/ R/	-ist *agent* ant- *against* -agon- *to fight*	An opposing structure, agent, disease, or process
antagonistic (adj) (*Note:* Two suffixes.)	an-**TAG**-oh-nis-tik	S/	-ic *pertaining to*	Having an opposite function
curative	**KYUR**-ah-tiv	S/ R/	-ive *quality of* curat- *to care for*	That which heals or cures
DiGeorge syndrome	dee-**JORJ SIN**-drome	P/ R/	Angelo M. DiGeorge, 1921–2009, U.S. pediatrician, described syndrome in 1921 syn- *together* -drome *course*	Congenital absence of the thymus gland
parathyroid	pair-ah-**THIGH**-royd	S/ P/ R/	-oid *resembling* para- *adjacent* -thyr- *an oblong shield*	Endocrine glands embedded in the back of the thyroid gland
hyperparathyroidism	**HIGH**-per-pair-ah-**THIGH**-royd-ism	S/ P/	-ism *condition, process* hyper- *excessive*	Excessive levels of parathyroid hormone
hypoparathyroidism	**HIGH**-poh-pair-ah-**THIGH**-royd-ism	P/	hypo- *deficient*	Deficient levels of parathyroid hormone
tetany tetanic (adj)	**TET**-ah-nee teh-**TAN**-ik	S/ R/	Greek *convulsive tension* -ic *pertaining to* tetan- *tetany, tetanus*	Severe muscle twitches, cramps, and spasms Pertaining to tetany or tetanus
thymectomy	thigh-**MEK**-toh-mee	S/ R/	-ectomy *surgical excision* thym- *thymus gland*	Surgical removal of the thymus gland
thymoma	thigh-**MOH**-mah	S/ R/	-oma *tumor, mass* thym- *thymus gland*	Benign tumor of the thymus gland
thymus	**THIGH**-mus		Greek *sweetbread*	Endocrine gland located in the mediastinum

Exercises

A. Describe the location and function of the parathyroid glands and the thymus gland. *Choose the correct answer for each of the following statements.* **LO 17.12, 17.13**

1. There are normally _____ parathyroid glands.

   a. two   **b.** three   **c.** four   **d.** five

2. The parathyroid glands are located on the _____ surface of the thyroid gland.

   a. lateral   **b.** medial   **c.** anterior   **d.** posterior

3. The thymus gland is located _____ to the heart.

   a. anterior   **b.** posterior   **c.** inferior   **d.** superior

4. This hormone is released when blood calcium levels are low.

   a. parathyroid hormone   **b.** calcitonin   **c.** thyroxine   **d.** somatostatin

5. The function of the thymus gland is to:

   a. increase calcium levels in the blood.   **b.** decrease the body's metabolic rate.

   c. stimulate the production of T lymphocytes.   **d.** secrete testosterone.

Lesson 17.3

Adrenal Glands and Hormones

Lesson Objectives

The information in this lesson will enable you to use correct medical terminology to:

17.3.1 Locate the adrenal glands.

17.3.2 Identify the functions of the hormones produced by the cortex and medulla.

17.3.3 Describe how the body adapts to stress.

17.3.4 Explain common disorders of the adrenal glands.

Case Report (CR) 17.3

John Fitzgerald Kennedy (1917–1963) was elected president of the United States of America in 1960 at the age of 43, the youngest person ever elected to that office *(Figure 17.15)*. Since the age of 13, when he was diagnosed as having colitis, he had health problems. At age 27, he had low-back pain necessitating lower-back surgery, and he was then diagnosed as having adrenal gland insufficiency (**Addison disease**) with osteoporosis of his lumbar spine. This required lower-back surgery on three more occasions. Kennedy received adrenal hormone replacement therapy for the rest of his life, together with pain medication for his low-back pain, until his assassination in Dallas, Texas, in 1963.

In medical retrospect, instead of colitis, he probably had celiac disease *(see Chapter 5)*, which has strong associations with Addison disease.

▲ **Figure 17.15 John F. Kennedy.**
©Corbis/Getty Images

LO 17.14 Adrenal Glands and Hormones

An **adrenal (suprarenal) gland** is anchored like a cap on the upper pole of each kidney *(Figure 17.16)*.

The outer layer of the gland, the **adrenal cortex**, synthesizes more than 25 steroid hormones known collectively as **adrenocortical hormones**, **corticosteroids**, or **corticoids**. There are three groups of corticosteroids:

1. **Glucocorticoids**—particularly **hydrocortisone (cortisol)**. These hormones stimulate fat and protein catabolism and help regulate blood glucose levels, particularly as the body resists stress *(see Lesson 17.4)*. Hydrocortisone also has an anti-inflammatory effect and is used in ointments to relieve inflammation.

2. **Mineralocorticoids**—the principal one of which is called **aldosterone**. This hormone promotes sodium retention and potassium excretion by the kidneys.

3. **Sex steroids:**

   a. **Androgens**—principally **dehydroepiandrosterone (DHEA)**, which is a weak androgen but is converted by other tissues into testosterone *(see Chapter 7)*.

   b. **Estrogens**—principally estradiol, which is produced in much smaller quantities than in the ovaries *(see Chapter 8)*.

The inner layer of the adrenal gland, the **adrenal medulla**, secretes hormones called **catecholamines**, principally **epinephrine (adrenaline)** and **norepinephrine**. These hormones prepare the body for physical activity. They raise blood pressure, increase circulation to muscles, increase pulmonary blood flow, and stimulate gluconeogenesis.

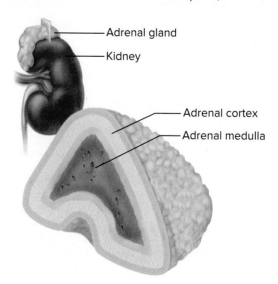

Adrenal gland

Kidney

Adrenal cortex

Adrenal medulla

▲ **Figure 17.16** Adrenal Gland.

WORD	PRONUNCIATION	ELEMENTS		DEFINITION
Addison disease	ADD-ih-son diz-EEZ	P/ R/	Thomas Addison, 1793–1860, English physician dis- apart -ease normal function	An autoimmune disease leading to decreased production of adrenocortical steroids
adrenal gland	ah-DREE-nal GLAND	S/ R/	-al pertaining to adren- adrenal gland gland Latin glans, acorn	The suprarenal, or adrenal, gland on the upper pole of each kidney
adrenaline epinephrine (syn)	ah-DREN-ah-lin ep-ih-NEF-rin	S/	-ine pertaining to	One of the catecholamines
adrenocortical	ah-DREE-noh-KOR-tih-kal	S/ R/CF R/	-al pertaining to adren/o- adrenal gland -cortic- cortex, cortisone	Pertaining to the cortex of the adrenal gland
aldosterone	al-DOS-ter-ohn	S/ R/CF R/	-one hormone ald/o- organic compound -ster- steroid	Mineralocorticoid hormone of the adrenal cortex
catecholamine	kat-eh-KOHL-ah-meen	S/ R/	-amine nitrogen-containing catechol- benzene derivative	Any major hormones in stress response; includes epinephrine and norepinephrine
corticoid corticosteroid (syn)	KOR-tih-koyd KOR-tih-koh-STEHR-oyd	S/ R/ R/CF R/	-oid resemble cortic- cortex, cortisone cortic/o- cortex, cortisone -ster- steroid	One of the steroid hormones produced by the adrenal cortex A hormone produced by the adrenal cortex
cortisol hydrocortisone (syn)	KOR-tih-sol	S/ R/	-ol chemical substance cortis- cortisone	One of the glucocorticoids produced by the adrenal cortex; has anti-inflammatory effects
dehydroepian- drosterone (DHEA)	dee-HIGH-droh-eh-pee-an-DROS-ter-ohn	S/ P/ R/CF P/ R/CF R/	-one hormone de- without, change of -hydr/o- water -epi- above -andr/o- male, masculine -ster- steroid	Precursor to testosterone; produced in the adrenal cortex
epinephrine adrenaline (syn)	ep-ih-NEF-rin	S/ P/ R/	-ine pertaining to epi- above -nephr- kidney	Main catecholamine produced by the adrenal medulla
glucocorticoid	glue-koh-KOR-tih-koyd	S/ R/CF R/	-oid resemble gluc/o- glucose -cortic- cortex, cortisone	Hormone of the adrenal cortex that helps regulate glucose metabolism
hydrocortisone cortisol (syn)	high-droh-KOR-tih-sohn	S/ R/CF R/	-one hormone hydr/o- water -cortis- cortisone	Potent glucocorticoid with anti-inflammatory properties
mineralocorticoid	MIN-er-al-oh-KOR-tih-koyd	S/ R/CF R/	-oid resemble mineral/o- inorganic materials -cortic- cortex, cortisone	Hormone of the adrenal cortex that influences sodium and potassium metabolism
norepinephrine noradrenaline (syn)	NOR-ep-ih-NEF-rin	S/ P/ P/ R/	-ine pertaining to nor- normal -epi- above -nephr- kidney	Parasympathetic neurotransmitter that is a catecholamine hormone of the adrenal gland

Exercises

A. Word elements are the building blocks that enable you to define the meaning of unknown words. *Match the elements in 1–10 to their correct meanings in a-j.* **LO 17.14, 17.D**

_____ **1.** *hydro*   **a.** normal   _____ **6.** *andr/o*   **f.** steroid

_____ **2.** *adren/o*   **b.** resemble   _____ **7.** *gluc/o*   **g.** kidney

_____ **3.** *oid*   **c.** hormone   _____ **8.** *nor*   **h.** adrenal

_____ **4.** *epi*   **d.** glucose   _____ **9.** *one*   **i.** above

_____ **5.** *ster*   **e.** water   _____ **10.** *nephr*   **j.** male

Keynotes

- Prolonged or repeated stress can cause physical illness.
- Stress reduction techniques are an important part of modern life.

LO 17.15 Disorders of Adrenal Glands

Adrenal cortical hypofunction can be primary when the disorder is in the adrenal cortex (Addison disease) or secondary when there is a lack of ACTH from the pituitary gland.

Addison disease is caused mostly by idiopathic atrophy of the adrenal cortex. Production of the three groups of adrenocortical steroids is diminished or absent:

- **Decreased cortisol production** leads to weakness, fatigue, diminished resistance to stress, increased susceptibility to infection, and weight loss.
- **Decreased aldosterone production** leads to dehydration, decreased circulatory volume, hypotension, and circulatory collapse.

Replacement therapy in Addison disease is daily hydrocortisone **by mouth (PO)**. Additionally, fluorocortisone is given PO to replace aldosterone. **Intercurrent** infections require that the hydrocortisone dose be doubled. John F. Kennedy received replacement therapy from his late twenties until he died.

Acute adrenocortical insufficiency in patients with Addison disease is called an **adrenal crisis**. It can be precipitated by an infection or trauma and leads to peripheral vascular collapse and kidney failure. Treatment is with IV fluids and IV hydrocortisone.

Adrenal cortical hyperfunction is due to excessive production of the groups of the corticosteroids.

Hypersecretion of glucocorticoids produces **Cushing syndrome** (*Figure 17.17*). Clinical manifestations include "moon" **facies**, obesity of the trunk, muscle wasting and weakness, osteoporosis, kidney stones, and reduced resistance to infection. Most cases of Cushing syndrome are due to a pituitary tumor secreting too much ACTH, thereby causing the normal adrenal glands to produce too much cortisol.

Often, the symptoms of Cushing syndrome can result from therapeutic administration of excess cortisol medications.

Hypersecretion of aldosterone (**aldosteronism**, or **Conn syndrome**) leads to sodium retention and potassium loss with increased blood volume, hypertension, excessive thirst, and excessive urination. A benign adenoma (**aldosteronoma**) is the most common cause and can be removed by laparoscopic **adrenalectomy**.

Hypersecretion of androgens is called **adrenal virilism** or **adrenogenital syndrome**. In adult women, manifestations include **hirsutism**, baldness, acne, deepened voice, decreased breast size, and other signs of masculinization. If a tumor is found by CT or MRI scan, it can be removed surgically.

Pheochromocytoma is a tumor of the adrenal medulla that overproduces the catecholamines epinephrine and norepinephrine. It produces marked hypertension that is difficult to control, with severe headaches, tachycardia, palpitations, and feelings of impending death.

(a)   **(b)**

▲ **Figure 17.17** Cushing Syndrome.
(a) Patient before onset of the syndrome. (b) The same person, only 4 months later, showing the "moon face" characteristic of Cushing syndrome. ©Mikkel Juul Jensen/ Science Source

LO 17.16 Stress Syndrome

Is there an exam at the end of the week? Is the babysitter sick? You know what stress is and how it affects your physical and emotional well-being.

Your body reacts to stress in a consistent way called *the stress response* or *general adaptation syndrome.*

The initial stage of the stress response is an **alarm reaction** ("fight or flight") initiated by catecholamines that raise blood pressure and increase glucose production from stored glycogen. This source of glucose is soon exhausted, and the feelings of anxiety, irritability, and insecurity are replaced by headache and back and neck pain. If the stress is allowed to persist, the physical priority is to provide alternative fuels to provide energy. In the second stage of the stress reaction, the adrenal gland increases its output of cortisol to stimulate glucose synthesis. Fatigue, indigestion, and diminished sex drive become dominant.

The third stage of a prolonged stress response is exhaustion when glycogen and fat stores have gone. The immune system cannot find the energy to continue functioning. This is when deep physical illness takes over. Body muscle wastes away, and heart and kidney failure or overwhelming infection are the end result.

WORD	PRONUNCIATION	ELEMENTS		DEFINITION
adrenalectomy	ah-**DREE**-nal-**EK**-toh-mee	S/ S/ R/	**-ectomy** *surgical excision* **-al-** *pertaining to* **adren-** *adrenal gland*	Removal of part or all of an adrenal gland
adrenogenital syndrome	ah-**DREE**-noh-**JEN**-it-al **SIN**-drome	S/ R/CF R/ P/ R/	**-al** *pertaining to* **adren/o-** *adrenal gland* **-genit-** *primary male or female sex organs* **syn-** *together* **-drome** *course*	Hypersecretion of androgens from the adrenal gland
aldosteronism	al-**DOS**-ter-ohn-izm	S/ R/CF R/	**-ism** *condition, process* **ald/o-** *organic compound* **-steron-** *steroid*	Condition caused by excessive secretion of aldosterone
aldosteronoma Conn syndrome (syn)	al-**DOS**-ter-oh-**NOH**-mah KON **SIN**-drome	S/ P/ R/	**-oma** *tumor, mass* Jerome W. Conn, 1907–1981, American endocrinologist **syn-** *together* **-drome** *course*	Benign adenoma of the adrenal cortex
Cushing syndrome	**KUSH**-ing **SIN**-drome	 P/ R/	Harvey Cushing, 1869–1939, American neurosurgeon **syn-** *together* **-drome** *course*	Hypersecretion of cortisol (hydrocortisone) by the adrenal cortex
facies	**FASH**-eez		Latin *appearance*	Facial expression and features characteristic of a specific disease
hirsutism	**HER**-sue-tizm		Latin *shaggy*	Excessive body and facial hair
intercurrent	**IN**-ter-**KUR**-ent	S/ P/ R/	**-ent** *end result, pertaining to* **inter-** *among, between* **-curr-** *to run*	A disease attacking a person who already has another disease
pheochromocytoma	fee-oh-**KROH**-moh-sigh-**TOH**-mah	S/ P/ R/CF R/	**-oma** *tumor* **pheo-** *gray* **-chrom/o-** *color* **-cyt-** *cell*	Adenoma of the adrenal medulla secreting excessive catecholamines
virilism	**VIR**-ih-lizm	S/ R/	**-ism** *condition, process* **viril-** *masculine*	Development of masculine characteristics by a woman or girl

Exercises

A. Language of endocrinology: The meaning of a word element never changes, regardless of the term that contains it. *Demonstrate your knowledge of word elements by making the correct choice in the following multiple-choice questions.* **LO 17.15, 17.D**

1. On the basis of its suffix, an **aldosteronoma** is a

   a. condition   **b.** facial hair   **c.** tumor   **d.** facial expression   **e.** gland

2. In the term **pheochromocytoma,** the prefix is one of

   a. size   **b.** shape   **c.** direction   **d.** color   **e.** gender

3. Select the term with a root that means *masculine:*

   a. hirsutism   **b.** aldosteronism   **c.** facies   **d.** virilism   **e.** aldosteronoma

4. The suffix in this term means *surgical excision:*

   a. adrenalectomy   **b.** virilism   **c.** aldosteronoma   **d.** facies   **e.** pheochromocytoma

B. Discuss the stress response. *Place the events of the stress response in the correct order starting with A for the first stage and C for the last stage.* **LO 17.16**

_____   **1.** body uses alternative metabolic pathways to produce glucose

_____   **2.** fight or flight response is initiated and glucose is released

_____   **3.** glycogen and fat stores are depleted

LO 17.17 Diagnostic Procedures for Disorders of the Adrenal Glands

Congenital adrenal hyperplasia can be diagnosed in the fetus using amniocentesis and chorionic villus sampling (*see Chapter 8*) and in the newborn through a heel stick to obtain a blood sample. The test detects elevated levels of 17-hydroxy-progesterone (17-HP) and, as with all screening tests, a confirmatory test(s) has to be performed. Treatment can then be started in the womb or immediately after birth.

Cushing syndrome can be confirmed with three tests: elevated cortisol levels in saliva, elevated cortisol levels in 24-hour urine, and suppression of cortisol production by the synthetic steroid dexamethasone.

Addison disease can be diagnosed based on routine blood tests showing hypercalcemia, hypoglycemia, hyponatremia, and hyperkalemia; the diagnosis is confirmed by the ACTH stimulation test, in which the synthetic pituitary ACTH hormone **tetracosactide** fails to stimulate the production of cortisol.

Pheochromocytoma is diagnosed by measuring **catecholamines** and **metanephrines** in plasma or by 24-hour urinary collection. CT scan or MRI can localize the tumor.

Hyperaldosteronism (Conn syndrome) is diagnosed by high levels of aldosterone and low levels of potassium in blood or urine tests. CT scan or MRI can locate the tumor in the adrenal gland.

LO 17.18 Therapeutic Procedures for Disorders of the Adrenal Glands

Congenital adrenal hyperplasia, when diagnosed in a female fetus, can require the pregnant mother to take a **corticosteroid** drug such as **dexamethasone** during pregnancy. This drug crosses the placenta to reduce the secretion of the fetal male hormones and allow the female genitals to develop normally. When diagnosed in childhood, dexamethasone or hydrocortisone are needed daily, and in some infant girls who have **ambiguous external genitalia**, reconstructive surgery to correct the appearance and function of the **genitals** is performed.

Addison disease requires lifelong replacement of the absent hormones by taking oral corticosteroids such as hydrocortisone and fludrocortisone.

Pheochromocytoma is treated with surgery to remove the adrenal tumor, usually by **laparoscopic** surgery.

Adrenal cortical carcinomas or benign adenomas are usually treated with surgery.

LO 17.19 Adrenal Pharmacology

The **adrenal medulla** secretes **epinephrine (adrenaline)**. The **adrenal cortex** synthesizes **steroids** from cholesterol. The outer zona glomerulosa secretes **mineralocorticoids**, which regulate salt and water metabolism (aldosterone) by affecting excretory organs such as the kidney, colon, salivary glands, sweat glands, and brain. The middle zona fasciculate synthesizes **glucocorticoids**, which regulate normal metabolism and resistance to stress (cortisol) by affecting every organ in the body including the brain. The inner zona reticularis secretes adrenal **androgens** that control the development and activity of the male sex organs and male secondary sex characteristics. Androgens are the precursor of all **estrogens**. The primary androgen is testosterone, present in males and females.

WORD	PRONUNCIATION		ELEMENTS	DEFINITION
ambiguous	am-**BIG**-you-us		Latin *to wander*	Uncertain
androgen	**AN**-droh-jen	S/ R/CF	-gen *to produce* andr/o- *male*	Hormone that produces masculine characteristics
cortex	**KOR**-teks		Latin *outer covering*	Outer portion of an organ
genital	**JEN**-ih-tal	S/ R/	-al *pertaining to* genit- *primary male or female sex organs*	Relating to the primary male or female sex organs
hyperplasia	high-per-**PLAY**-zee-ah	S/ P/ R/	-ia *condition* hyper- *excessive* -plas- *formation*	Increase in the number of cells in a tissue or organ
medulla	meh-**DULL**-ah		Latin *marrow*	Central part of a structure surrounded by cortex
steroid	**STER**-oyd	S/ R/	-oid *resemble* ster- *solid*	Large family of chemical substances found in hormones, body components, and drugs

Exercises

A. Deconstruct medical terms into their component parts. *Using the terms in the WAD above, place the correct element on each blank.*
LO 17.17, 17.18, 17.19, 17.D

1. Increase in the number of cells in a tissue: _____ / _____ / _____

2. Hormone that produces masculine characteristics: _____ / _____ / _____

3. Large family of chemical substances found in hormones: _____ / _____

B. Explain the therapeutic procedures for disorders of the adrenal glands. *Choose the correct answer for each statement.* **LO 17.18**

1. Treatment for this condition requires lifelong hormone replacement with hydrocortisone:

   a. pheochromocytoma

   b. Addison disease

   c. Cushing syndrome

   d. adrenal cortex carcinoma

2. In this condition, it is the mother who takes medication to treat the fetal condition:

   a. congenital adrenal hyperplasia

   b. pheochromocytoma

   c. Addison disease

   d. Cushing syndrome

3. A condition that is often treated with laparoscopic surgery and removal of the adrenal tumor:

   a. Cushing syndrome

   b. Addison disease

   c. pheochromocytoma

   d. congenital adrenal hyperplasia

Hormone replacement therapy (HRT) (also called **hormone therapy** or **HT**) uses estrogen and progestin to treat symptoms of menopause *(see Chapter 8)*. HRT comes as a tablet, patch, injection, vaginal cream, or vaginal ring; protects against osteoporosis *(see Chapter 14)*; and reduces the risk for uterine cancer, but it may increase the risk for blood clots, breast cancer, heart disease, stroke, and gallstones. At this time, short-term (up to 5 years) use of HRT given in the lowest possible dose to treat the symptoms of menopause appears to be safe for many women.

Estrogen makes hormone-receptor-positive breast cancers *(see Chapter 8)* grow. HRT medications treat hormone-receptor-positive breast cancers by lowering the amount of estrogen in the body and/or blocking the action of estrogen on breast cancer cells. They are used after surgery to help slow the growth of advanced-stage or metastatic hormone-receptor-positive breast cancers. There are three main types of HRT agents:

- **Aromatase inhibitors (AIs)**, which stop the production of estrogen from androgen in post-menopausal women. These medications are anastrozole *(Arimidex)*, exemestane *(Aromasin)*, and letrozole *(Femara)*. Each is given in a pill form taken once a day. Anastrozole and letrozole are available in generic form.

- **Selective estrogen receptor modulators (SERMs)**, which block estrogen in the estrogen receptors of breast cells so that the cells can't grow and multiply. The SERMs are tamoxifen *(Nolvadex)*, raloxifene *(Evista)*, and toremifene *(Fareston)*.

- **Estrogen-receptor downregulators (ERDs)** act just like SERMs, sitting in the receptors of breast cells to block estrogen. Fulvestrant *(Faslodex)* is the only approved ERD at this time.

LO 17.20 Word Analysis and Definition

S = Suffix   P = Prefix   R = Root   R/CF = Combining Form

WORD	PRONUNCIATION	ELEMENTS		DEFINITION
aromatase	ah-**ROH**-mah-taze	S/ R/	-ase enzyme aromat- *spice*	An enzyme responsible for a key step in the production of estrogens from androgens
aromatase inhibitor	ah-**ROH**-mah-taze in-**HIB**-ih-tor	S/ R/	-or *a doer* inhibit- *repress*	An agent that stops the production of estrogen in post-menopausal women
estrogen	**ES**-troh-jen	S/ R/CF	-gen *produce, create* estr/o *woman*	Generic term for hormones that stimulate female secondary sex characteristics
hormone	**HOR**-mohn		Greek *set in motion*	Chemical formed in one tissue or organ that is then carried by the blood to stimulate or inhibit a function of another tissue or organ
modulator	mod-you-**LAY**-tor		Latin *to measure off properly*	An agent that regulates or adjusts
therapy therapeutic	**THAIR**-ah-pee **THAIR**-ah-PYU-tik	S/ R/	Greek *medical treatment* -ic *pertaining to* therapeut- *treatment*	Systematic treatment of a disease, dysfunction, or disorder Relating to the treatment of a disease, dysfunction, or disorder

Exercises

A. Answer the questions employing the medical language of pharmacology. *Match the abbreviation to its correct description.* **LO 17.20, 17.F**

Description

_____ 1. block estrogen receptor cells; tamoxifen

_____ 2. stop production of estrogen from androgen

_____ 3. used to relieve symptoms of menopause

_____ 4. block estrogen receptors; fulvestrant

Abbreviation

a. ERD

b. SERMs

c. AI

d. HRT

Lesson 17.4

ENDOCRINE SYSTEM

Pancreas

Lesson Objectives

The information provided in this lesson will enable you to:

17.4.1 Distinguish between the different cells of the pancreas and their secretions.

17.4.2 Identify the functions of the hormones produced by the pancreas.

17.4.3 Explain common disorders of the pancreatic hormones.

Case Report (CR) 17.4

You are

. . . a medical assistant working with Susan Lee, MD, in her primary care clinic at Fulwood Medical Center.

Your patient is

. . . Mrs. Martha Jones, who is here for her monthly checkup.

Mrs. Martha Jones is a 53-year-old type 2 diabetic on insulin, with diabetic retinopathy and diabetic neuropathy of her feet. Bariatric surgery has enabled her to reduce her weight from 275 to 156 pounds. The time is 0930 hrs. She is complaining of having a cold and cough for the past few days. Now she is feeling drowsy and nauseous and has a dry mouth. As you talk with her, you notice that her speech is slurred. She cannot remember if she gave herself her morning insulin. Examination of her lungs reveals rales at her right base. Her vital signs are T 97.8°F, P 120, R 20, BP 100/50. You perform her blood glucose measurement. The reading is 525 mg/dL (a recommended value 2 hours after breakfast is < 145 mg/dL).

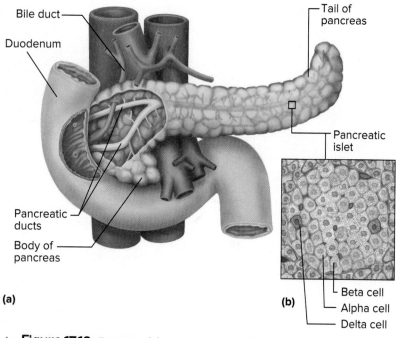

▲ **Figure 17.18** Pancreas. (*a*) General anatomy. (*b*) Alpha, beta, and delta cells.

Keynotes

Glucagon is not the only hormone that raises blood glucose; epinephrine, cortisol, and growth hormone also have that effect. Insulin is the only hormone that lowers blood glucose.

LO 17.21 Pancreas

The location and structure of the **pancreas** are detailed in *Chapter 5*. Most of the pancreas is an exocrine gland that secretes digestive juices into the duodenum through a duct (*Figure 17.18*). Scattered throughout the pancreas are clusters of endocrine cells grouped around blood vessels. These clusters are called **pancreatic islets (islets of Langerhans)**. Within the islets are three distinct cell types:

1. **Alpha cells**, which secrete the hormone **glucagon** in response to a low blood glucose. Glucagon's actions are:

   a. In the liver, to stimulate **gluconeogenesis**, **glycogenolysis**, and the release of glucose into the bloodstream.

   b. In adipose tissue, to stimulate fat catabolism and the release of free fatty acids.

2. **Beta cells**, which secrete **insulin** in response to a high blood glucose. Insulin has the opposite effects of glucagon:

   a. In muscle and fat cells, to encourage absorption of glucose and to store glycogen and fat.

   b. In the liver, to stimulate the conversion of glucose to glycogen and to inhibit the conversion of noncarbohydrates to glucose.

3. **Delta cells**, which secrete **somatostatin**, which acts within the pancreas to inhibit the secretion of glucagon and insulin.

   These three types of cell secrete their hormones directly into the bloodstream.

WORD	PRONUNCIATION	ELEMENTS		DEFINITION
glucagon	**GLUE**-kah-gon	S/ R/	-agon *contest* gluc- *glucose*	Pancreatic hormone that supports blood glucose levels
gluconeogenesis	**GLUE**-koh-nee-oh-**JEN**-eh-sis	S/ P/ R/CF	-genesis *creation* -neo- *new* gluc/o- *glucose*	Formation of glucose from noncarbohydrate sources
glycogenolysis	**GLIE**-koh-jeh-**NOL**-ih-sis	S/ R/CF R/CF	-lysis *break down* glyc/o- *glycogen* -gen/o- *to create*	Conversion of glycogen to glucose
insulin	**IN**-syu-lin	S/ R/	-in *chemical compound* insul- *island*	A hormone secreted by the islet cells of the pancreas
pancreas	**PAN**-kree-ass		Greek *sweetbread*	Lobulated gland, the head of which is tucked into the curve of the duodenum
pancreatic (adj)	pan-kree-**AT**-ik	S/ R/	-ic *pertaining to* pancreat- *pancreas*	Pertaining to the pancreas
pancreatic islets	pan-kree-**AT**-ik **EYE**-lets	S/ R/ S/ R/	-ic *pertaining to* pancreat- *pancreas* -et *little* isl- *island*	Areas of pancreatic cells that produce insulin and glucagon
islets of Langerhans (syn)	**EYE**-lets of **LAHNG**-er-hahnz		Paul Langerhans, 1847–1888, German anatomist	
somatostatin	**SOH**-mah-toh-**STAT**-in	S/ R/CF	-statin *inhibit* somat/o- *body*	Hormone that inhibits release of growth hormone and insulin

Exercises

A. Describe the functions of the pancreas. *Choose the correct answer for each of the following statements.* **LO 17.21**

1. The effect of glucagon is:

   a. decrease blood sugar levels   **b.** increase blood sugar levels

2. Glucagon is secreted by the _____ cells.

   a. alpha   **b.** beta   **c.** delta

3. Clusters of alpha, beta, and delta cells in the pancreas are called:

   a. pancreatic clusters   **b.** pancreatic islets   **c.** pancreatitis   **d.** gluconeogenesis

4. The process of gluconeogenesis will cause blood sugar levels to:

   a. increase   **b.** decrease   **c.** stay the same

5. Storage of glycogen is stimulated by the hormone:

   a. somatostatin   **b.** glucagon   **c.** insulin

B. Identify the meaning of word elements. *Recognizing the meaning of the word elements makes short work of knowing the meaning of the entire medical term. Choose the correct answer.* **LO 17.21, 17.D**

1. The suffix in the term **glycogenolysis** means:

   a. creation   **b.** contest   **c.** break down   **d.** store

2. The root in the term **glucagon** means:

   a. chemical compound   **b.** create   **c.** sugar   **d.** contest

3. The suffix in the term **somatostatin** means:

   a. inhibit   **b.** pertaining to   **c.** creation   **d.** body

4. The prefix in the term **gluconeogenesis** means:

   a. sugar   **b.** new   **c.** creation   **d.** pertaining to

Abbreviations

DM	diabetes mellitus
IDDM	insulin-dependent diabetes mellitus
MODY	mature-onset diabetes of youth
NIDDM	non-insulin-dependent diabetes mellitus

Keynotes

- Type 2 diabetes used to occur primarily after the age of 45 but is now seen also in children, adolescents, and young adults.

- Stress can raise blood glucose levels in type 2 diabetes by having a direct effect on insulin response and effectiveness but also by disturbing the patient's pattern of disease management.

- The brain is the first organ affected by hypoglycemia.

- **Diabetics** should always carry candy or glucose tablets and an identification card, bracelet, or neck chain indicating they are diabetic.

LO 17.22 Disorders of Pancreatic Hormones: Diabetes Mellitus

Diabetes mellitus (DM) is a syndrome characterized by hyperglycemia resulting from an absolute or relative impairment of insulin secretion and/or insulin action. This leads to a disruption of carbohydrate, fat, and protein metabolism. It is the world's most prevalent metabolic disease and the leading cause of blindness, renal failure, and gangrene. There are four categories of diabetes mellitus:

1. **Type 1 diabetes**, also called **insulin-dependent diabetes mellitus (IDDM)**, accounts for 10% to 15% of all cases of DM but is the predominant type of DM under the age of 30. When symptoms become apparent, 90% of the pancreatic insulin-producing cells have been destroyed by **autoantibodies**. The incidence of type 1 diabetes is increased in patients with Graves disease, Hashimoto disease, and Addison disease.

2. **Type 2 diabetes**, also called **non-insulin-dependent diabetes mellitus (NIDDM)**, accounts for 85% to 90% of all cases of DM. Almost 7% of U.S. residents are diagnosed with type 2 diabetes, and the incidence is increasing rapidly. Not only is there some impairment of insulin response, but there is decreased insulin effectiveness in stimulating glucose uptake by tissues and in restraining hepatic glucose production. This is called **insulin resistance**. In addition to type 2 diabetes, insulin resistance leads to other common disorders such as obesity, hypertension, hyperlipidemia, and coronary artery disease. Type 2 diabetes can be secondary to Cushing syndrome, acromegaly, pheochromocytoma, and aldosteronism.

3. **Gestational diabetes** is seen in the latter half of 5% of pregnancies. While most cases of gestational diabetes resolve after the pregnancy, a woman who has this complication of pregnancy has a 30% chance of developing type 2 diabetes within 10 years.

4. **Mature-onset diabetes of youth (MODY)** is genetically inherited, occurs in thin individuals who are in their teens and twenties, and is comparable to type 2 diabetes in its severity.

Hypoglycemia is present when blood glucose is below 70 mg/dL. Hormonal defense mechanisms (glucagon and adrenaline) are activated as the blood glucose drops below 55 mg/dL. Because brain metabolism depends primarily on glucose, the brain is the first organ affected by hypoglycemia. Impaired mental efficiency starts to be seen when the blood glucose falls below 65 mg/dL. It becomes very obvious (shakiness, anxiety, confusion, tremor) around 40 mg/dL, and below that figure seizures can occur. If the blood glucose falls below 10 mg/dL, the neurons become electrically silent, resulting in diabetic **coma**. Symptomatic hypoglycemia is sometimes called **insulin shock**.

Low blood glucose can be raised to normal in minutes by taking 3 to 4 ounces of orange, apple, or grape juice. Symptoms should begin to improve in 5 minutes, with full recovery in 10 to 15 minutes. In an emergency, if the patient is not able to take oral sugar, treatment is begun with a rapid IV **bolus** of 25 mL of 50% glucose solution, followed by an intravenous infusion of glucose.

WORD	PRONUNCIATION	ELEMENTS		DEFINITION
autoantibody	aw-toh-**AN**-tee-bod-ee	P/ P/ R/	**auto-** self, same **-anti-** against **-body** body	Antibody produced in response to an antigen from the host's own tissue
bolus	**BOH**-lus		Greek *a lump*	Single mass of a substance
coma	**KOH**-mah		Greek *deep sleep*	State of deep unconsciousness
diabetes mellitus	die-ah-**BEE**-teez **MEL**-ih-tus		**diabetes** Greek *a siphon* **mellitus** Latin *sweetened with honey*	Metabolic syndrome caused by absolute or relative insulin deficiency and/or insulin ineffectiveness
diabetic (adj)	die-ah-**BET**-ik	S/ R/	**-ic** *pertaining to* **diabet-** *diabetes*	Pertaining to or suffering from diabetes
hypoglycemia	**HIGH**-poh-glie-**SEE**-mee-ah	S/ P/ R/	**-emia** *blood condition* **hypo-** *below, deficient* **-glyc-** *glucose*	Low level of glucose (sugar) in the blood
hypoglycemic (adj)	**HIGH**-poh-glie-**SEE**-mik	S/	**-emic** *in the blood*	Pertaining to or suffering from hypoglycemia

Exercises

A. Diabetes is the world's most prevalent metabolic disease. *Many patients have diabetes as a concurrent condition with other health problems—which always makes it a consideration in treatment and prescribing medications. Test your knowledge of this disease by answering the following questions. Choose the correct answer.* **LO 17.22, 17.F**

1. Diabetes mellitus is the leading cause of
   a. blindness   **b.** hypotension   **c.** hemorrhage   **d.** kidney stones   **e.** reflux disease

2. The first organ affected by hypoglycemia is the
   a. kidney   **b.** heart   **c.** pancreas   **d.** brain   **e.** liver

3. The predominant type of diabetes mellitus in patients under the age of 30 is
   a. type 1   **b.** type 2   **c.** non-insulin-dependent DM   **d.** gestational diabetes type 3

4. Impairment of insulin response and decreased insulin effectiveness are termed insulin
   a. production   **b.** resistance   **c.** autoantibodies   **d.** control   **e.** conversion

5. Most cases of gestational diabetes resolve after
   a. medication   **b.** treatment   **c.** testing   **d.** delivery   **e.** surgery

6. Symptomatic hypoglycemia is sometimes called
   a. insulin resistance   **b.** coma   **c.** insulin shock   **d.** glucolysis   **e.** bolus

7. Type 1 diabetes is also known as
   a. IDDM   **b.** NIDDM   **c.** hypoglycemia   **d.** hyperglycemia   **e.** coma

8. Insulin resistance can lead to
   a. obesity   **b.** aldosteronoma   **c.** hirsutism   **d.** myxedema   **e.** virilism

9. Low blood glucose can be raised to normal with a
   a. vitamin   **b.** hormone   **c.** enzyme   **d.** carbohydrate   **e.** electrolyte

10. What can raise blood glucose levels in type 2 diabetes?
    a. stress   **b.** dehydration   **c.** nausea   **d.** coughing   **e.** vomiting

LO 17.22 Disorders of Pancreatic Hormones: Diabetes Mellitus (continued)

Hyperglycemia

The classic symptoms of hyperglycemia are **polyuria** (excessive urination), **polydipsia** (excessive thirst), and **polyphagia** (excessive hunger), with unexplained weight loss.

Symptomatic hyperglycemia is how type 1 diabetes usually presents. Type 2 diabetes can be symptomatic or asymptomatic and is often found during a routine health examination.

Because of high glucose levels, hyperglycemia damages capillary endothelial cells in the retina and renal glomerulus and neurons and neurolemmocytes in peripheral nerves. Of all diabetics, 85% develop some degree of diabetic retinopathy, while 30% develop diabetic nephropathy, which can progress to end-stage renal disease *(see Chapter 6)*. Diabetic neuropathy causes sensory defects with numbness, tingling, and **paresthesias** in the stocking-glove (feet-hands) distribution.

In larger blood vessels, the hyperglycemia contributes to endothelial cell lining damage and atherosclerosis. Coronary artery disease and peripheral vascular disease with claudication *(see Chapter 10)* are complications. Hyperglycemia is the most common cause of foot ulcers followed by gangrene of the lower extremity, sometimes necessitating amputation. The risk of infection is increased by the cellular hyperglycemia and the circulatory deficits.

The complications of hyperglycemia can be kept at bay by strict control of blood glucose levels.

Diabetic ketoacidosis (DKA) is a state of marked hyperglycemia with dehydration, **metabolic acidosis**, and **ketone formation**. It is seen mostly in type 1 diabetes and is usually the result of a lapse in insulin treatment, acute infection, or trauma that renders the usual insulin treatment inadequate.

DKA presents with polyuria, vomiting, and lethargy and can progress to coma. **Acetone** (a ketone) can be smelled on the breath. Diabetic ketoacidosis is a medical emergency and requires rapid fluid volume expansion, correction of hyperglycemia, prevention of hypokalemia, and treatment of any infection. There is a 2% to 5% mortality from circulatory collapse.

Diabetic coma, a severe medical emergency, has three causes, which have been described earlier:

- **Diabetic ketoacidosis (DKA).**

- **Hyperglycemia** with dehydration, but not the ketosis and acidosis of DKA. This condition is called **hyperosmolar coma**. This is the condition that Mrs. Jones presented with. She was on the verge of going into a coma.

- **Hypoglycemic coma.** A blood glucose test will differentiate hypoglycemia from the other two causes.

 ### Case Report (CR) 17.4 *(continued)*

Mrs. Martha Jones is in the early stages of a **hyperglycemic**, nonketotic (hyperosmolar) coma, probably initiated by a right-lower-lobe pneumonia. A urine specimen is obtained. Dr. Lee is notified. Blood is taken for a full chemistry panel, and arterial blood gases are drawn. An IV infusion **bolus** of 550 mL of isotonic sodium chloride is given, followed by 1.5 L of isotonic **saline** over the next 2 hours. Mrs. Jones is given 10 units of regular insulin IV and admitted to the hospital.

WORD	PRONUNCIATION	ELEMENTS		DEFINITION
acetone	**ASS**-eh-tone		Latin *vinegar*	Ketone that is found in blood, urine, and breath when diabetes mellitus is out of control
bolus	**BOW**-luss		Greek *lump*	A single, relatively large quantity of a substance; for example a bolus dose of an intravenously injected drug.
hyperglycemia	**HIGH**-per-glie-**SEE**-mee-ah	S/ P/ R/	-emia *blood condition* hyper- *above* -glyc- *glucose*	High level of glucose (sugar) in blood
hyperglycemic (adj)	**HIGH**-per-glie-**SEE**-mik	S/	-emic *in the blood*	Pertaining to high blood sugar
hyperosmolar	**HIGH**-per-os-**MOH**-lar	S/ P/ R/	-ar *pertaining to* hyper- *above* -osmol- *concentration*	Marked hyperglycemia without ketoacidosis
ketoacidosis	**KEY**-toh-ass-ih-**DOH**-sis	S/ R/CF R/	-osis *condition* ket/o- *ketone* -acid- *acid*	Excessive production of ketones, making the blood acid
ketone	**KEY**-tone		Greek *acetone*	Chemical formed in uncontrolled diabetes or in starvation
ketosis (*Note:* With the "o" in ket/o- preceding the "o" in -osis, one "o" drops out for simpler pronunciation.)	key-**TOH**-sis	S/ R/	-osis *condition* ket- *ketone*	Excessive production of ketones
metabolic acidosis	met-ah-**BOL**-ik ass-ih-**DOH**-sis	S/ R/ S/ R/	-ic *pertaining to* metabol- *change* -osis *condition* acid- *acid*	Decreased pH in blood and body tissues as a result of an upset in metabolism
paresthesia paresthesias (pl)	par-es-**THEE**-zee-ah par-es-**THEE**-zee-as	S/ P/ R/	-ia *condition* par- *abnormal* -esthes- *sensation*	An abnormal sensation; for example, tingling, burning, pricking
polydipsia	pol-ee-**DIP**-see-ah	S/ P/ R/	-ia *condition* poly- *many, much* -dips- *thirst*	Excessive thirst
polyphagia	pol-ee-**FAY**-jee-ah	S/ P/ R/	-ia *condition* poly- *many, much* -phag- *to eat*	Excessive eating
polyuria	pol-ee-**YOU**-ree-ah	S/ P/ R/	-ia *condition* poly- *many, much* -ur- *urine*	Excessive production of urine
saline	**SAY**-leen		Latin *salt*	Salt solution, usually sodium chloride

Exercises

A. After reading Case Report (CR) 17.4, answer the following questions. *Fill in the blanks.* **LO 17.22, 17.A**

1. **Hyperglycemic** means that the level of _____ is too high in the patient's blood.

2. **Hyperosmolar coma** is the same thing as _____.

B. Translate the explanation of a condition into the medical term it is describing. *As a health care provider, you will need to be able to correctly interpret conditions into a medical term. You will need to be able to correctly spell the term. Fill in the blanks.* **LO 17.22, 17.A, 17.F**

1. The abbreviation for the condition that has the signs of ketone formation, metabolic acidosis, and marked hyperglycemia: _____

2. Excessive thirst: _____

3. Excessive urination: _____

4. Pertaining to high sugar in the blood: _____

5. Condition of excess ketones: _____

6. Excessive eating: _____

7. Condition of excess ketones causing the blood to be acidic: _____

- Maintaining normal plasma glucose levels is the basis for good management of DM.

- Many insulin-dependent diabetics need multiple subcutaneous insulin injections each day.

- An **oral glucose tolerance test (OGTT)** is used occasionally in diagnosing type 2 diabetes.

Abbreviations

BUN	blood urea nitrogen
ECG	electrocardiogram
Hb A1c	glycosylated hemoglobin (hemoglobin A one-C)
OGTT	oral glucose tolerance test
SGLT2	sodium-glucose cotransporter-2
U	unit

LO 17.23, 17.24 Diagnosis and Treatment of Diabetes Mellitus

Criteria for the Diagnosis of Diabetes Mellitus

The accepted **criteria** for the diagnosis of diabetes mellitus (DM) include either a fasting (8 hours) plasma glucose of 126 mg/dL or greater; or symptoms (polyuria, polydipsia, polyphagia, unexplained weight loss) and a random plasma glucose of 200 mg/dL or higher.

Treatment of Diabetes Mellitus

The basic principle of diabetes treatment is to avoid hyperglycemia and hypoglycemia. The following are the areas of treatment:

- **Diet and exercise.** To achieve weight reduction of 2 pounds per week in overweight type 2 patients is essential. For insulin-treated diabetics, detailed diet management restricts variations in timing, size, and content of meals.

- **Patient education.** Patients are taught to understand the disease process, to recognize the indications for seeking immediate medical care, and to follow a regimen of foot care.

- **Plasma glucose monitoring.** This is an essential skill that all diabetics must learn. Patients on insulin must learn to adjust their insulin doses. Home glucose analyzers use a drop of blood obtained by a spring-powered lancet from the fingertip or forearm. The frequency of testing is varied individually. As a rule, insulin-treated patients should test their plasma glucose before meals, 2 hours after meals, and at bedtime.

- **Routine physician visits.** The patient is assessed for symptoms or signs of complications. Skin condition, pulses, and sensation in feet are tested. Urine is tested for **microalbuminuria** by using **immunoassays**. This detects smaller increases in urinary albumin than does conventional urine testing.

- **Periodic laboratory evaluation.** This includes **blood urea nitrogen (BUN)** and serum creatinine (kidney function), lipid profile, electrocardiogram (**ECG**), and an annual complete ophthalmologic evaluation.

    Glycosylated hemoglobin (Hb A1c) is used to monitor plasma glucose control during the preceding 1 to 3 months. It is formed at rates that increase with plasma glucose levels. Normal Hb A1c is less than 6%. In poor control, the value is 9% to 12%. It is also part of a periodic laboratory evaluation.

    Fructosamine is formed by glucose combining with plasma protein and reflects plasma glucose control over the preceding 1 to 3 weeks. A standard reference range for this test is not available.

    Insulin preparations routinely contain 100 units (U/mL) (**U-100 insulin**). The insulin is injected subcutaneously by using disposable syringes that hold 0.5 mL. In addition, already prepared mixtures of intermediate and regular insulins in different ratios are available. An **insulin pen** is an injection device that holds several days' dosage.

    Continuous subcutaneous insulin infusion is given by a battery-powered, programmable pump that provides continuous insulin through a small needle in the abdominal wall.

LO 17.25 Classes of Insulin

Insulin Type	Onset of Action*	Peak of Action*	Duration of Action*	Examples
Rapid acting	15 min	30–60 min	3–5 hr	Humalog, NovoLog
Regular acting	30–60 min	100–120 min	5–8 hr	Humulin R, Novolin R
Intermediate acting (NPH)	1–3 hr	7–8 hr	18–24 hr	Humulin N, Novolin N
Long acting	4–8 hr	minimal peak effects	16–24 hr	Lantus, Levemir

*min = minutes; hr = hours.

LO 17.25 Pharmacology of Diabetes Mellitus

Oral antidiabetic drugs are used for type 2 but not type 1 diabetes. These drugs include:

- **Metformin,** which acts by decreasing hepatic glucose production. It also promotes weight loss and decreases lipid levels. It is **synergistic** in combination with sulfonylureas.

- **Sulfonylureas,** which act by stimulating the beta cells to secrete insulin.

WORD	PRONUNCIATION	ELEMENTS		DEFINITION
criterion criteria (pl)	kri-**TEER**-ee-on kri-**TEER**-ee-ah		Greek *a standard*	Standard or rule for judging
fructosamine	**FRUK**-toh-sah-meen	S/ R/	**-amine** *nitrogen-containing* **fructos-** *fruit sugar*	Organic compound with fructose as its base
glycosylated hemoglobin (Hb A1c)	**GLIE**-koh-sih-lay-ted **HEE**-moh-**GLOH**-bin	S/ R/CF R/CF R/	**-sylated** *linked* **glyc/o-** *glucose* **hem/o-** *blood* **-globin** *protein*	Hemoglobin A fraction linked to glucose; used as index of glucose control
immunoassay	**IM**-you-noh-**ASS**-ay	R/CF R	**immun/o-** *immune response* **-assay** *evaluate*	Biochemical test that uses the reaction of an antibody to its antigen to measure the amount of a substance in a liquid
microalbuminuria	**MY**-kroh-al-byu-min-**YOU**-ree-ah	S/ P/ R/ R/	**-ia** *condition* **micro-** *small* **-albumin-** *albumin* **-ur-** *urine*	Presence of very small quantities of albumin in urine that cannot be detected by conventional urine testing
synergist	**SIN**-er-jist	S/ P/ R/	**-ist** *specialist* **syn-** *together* **-erg-** *work*	Agent or process that aids the action of another
synergistic (adj)		S/	**-ic** *pertaining to*	Working together

Exercises

A. Medications: Diabetics will deal with medications for the rest of their lives. *Choose the correct medication that is being described. Select the one drug that is the correct answer for each statement.* **LO 17.25**

1. Act(s) by stimulating the beta cells to secrete insulin

    a. metformin   **b.** sulfonylureas   **c.** thiazolidinedione

2. Suppress(es) hepatic glucose production

    a. metformin   **b.** sulfonylureas   **c.** thiazolidinedione

3. Improve(s) insulin sensitivity in skeletal muscle

    a. metformin   **b.** sulfonylureas   **c.** thiazolidinedione

B. Treatment of diabetes mellitus. *Health care providers involved with the care of patients with diabetes mellitus must constantly educate them regarding the proper treatment and self care. Test your knowledge of the treatment of patients with diabetes mellitus by identifying statements as T for true and F for false.* **LO 17.23, 17.24**

1. All patients with diabetes mellitus follow the same plasma glucose monitoring schedule.   **T**   **F**

2. An important part of the daily routine is foot care.   **T**   **F**

3. The standard reference for fructosamine levels is 0.5U/dl   **T**   **F**

4. The HbA1c is a record of blood sugar control over the preceding 1 to 3 months.   **T**   **F**

5. An option for some patients is a continuous infusion of insulin via a programmable pump.   **T**   **F**

Endocrine System

Challenge Your Knowledge

A. Diseases and disorders. Identify the diseases and disorders of the endocrine system as described in the following statements. Special attention to the prefixes will aid you in matching your correct choice. **(LO 17.8)**

_____ 1. Autoimmune disease with lymphocytic infiltration manifesting with hypothyroidism

_____ 2. Congenital form of thyroid deficiency

_____ 3. Excess of parathyroid hormone

_____ 4. Severe hypothyroidism

_____ 5. Presents as symptomless thyroid nodule

_____ 6. Inflammation of the thyroid gland

_____ 7. Hyperthyroidism associated with a goiter

_____ 8. Deficiency of parathyroid hormone

_____ 9. Enlargement of the thyroid gland

_____ 10. Eyes bulging outward

a. Graves disease

b. thyroid cancer

c. hypoparathyroidism

d. thyroiditis

e. Hashimoto disease

f. goiter

g. exophthalmos

h. hyperparathyroidism

i. myxedema

j. cretinism

B. Latin and Greek terms. Latin and Greek terms cannot be further deconstructed into prefix, root, or suffix. You must know them for what they are. Test your knowledge of these terms with the following exercise. Match the meaning in the left column with the correct medical term in the right column. **(LO 17.A)**

_____ 1. Outer covering

_____ 2. Cross

_____ 3. Deep sleep

_____ 4. Stimulation, change

_____ 5. Sweet bread

_____ 6. A lump

_____ 7. Convulsive tension

_____ 8. Appearance

_____ 9. Shaggy or hairy

_____ 10. To set in motion

a. tetany

b. coma

c. tropin

d. cortex

e. chiasm

f. facies

g. hirsutism

h. bolus

i. hormone

j. thymus

C. Language of endocrinology. Knowing the endocrine system will aid you in understanding the overall body process of *homeostasis*. Apply the *language of endocrinology* to the following questions about the anatomy and physiology of the endocrine system; choose the correct answer. **(LO 17.1, 17.3, 17.7)**

1. Which of the following is *not* a part of the endocrine system?

    a. pancreas

    b. pituitary

    c. pineal

    d. parathyroid

    e. palatine

2. The abnormal production of breast milk is called

    a. dysmenorrhea

    b. polydipsia

    c. galactorrhea

    d. dysphagia

    e. menorrhagia

3. The speed at which the body's chemical functions proceed is called

    a. cardiac rate

    b. vasoconstriction

    c. metabolic rate

    d. blood pressure

    e. homeostasis

4. The only hormone that lowers blood glucose is

    a. glucagon

    b. cortisol

    c. aldosterone

    d. corticosterone

    e. insulin

D. Language of endocrinology. Apply the *language of endocrinology* to the following questions about the anatomy and physiology of the endocrine system; choose the correct answer. **(LO 17.1, 17.3, 17.8, 17.14)**

1. A congenital form of thyroid deficiency that severely retards mental and physical growth is

    a. goiter

    b. thyroid adenoma

    c. cretinism

    d. pretibial myxedema

    e. hyperthyroidism

2. **Tetany** is

    a. lockjaw

    b. painful muscle spasm

    c. protrusion of the eyeball

    d. enlargement of the thyroid gland

    e. excessive production of thyroid hormones

3. A condition produced by a pituitary tumor that causes a decline in the production of several hormones at the same time is called

    a. hypopituitarism

    b. hyperpituitarism

    c. panhypopituitarism

    d. prolactinoma

    e. diabetes mellitus

4. Another name for **epinephrine** is

    a. corticosteroid

    b. corticosterone

    c. adrenalin

    d. hydrocortisone

    e. cortisol

5. The pineal gland secretes **serotonin** by day and converts it to _____ at night.

    a. melatonin

    b. a vasodilator

    c. vasopressin

    d. prolactin

    e. an enzyme

Endocrine System

E. **Hormones.** Hormones are bloodborne messengers secreted by endocrine glands. Each has a specific purpose. Correctly use the following terms or abbreviations to fill in the blanks after each definition. (**LO 17.1, 17.2**)

ACTH	FSH	somatotropin	PRL	tropic
insulin	glucocorticoid	melatonin	LH	thyrotropin

1. Hormone that stimulates the growth of the thyroid gland: _____

2. Hormones that stimulate other endocrine glands to produce hormones: _____

3. Hormone that stimulates ovulation and testosterone production: _____

4. Hormone of the adrenal cortex that helps regulate glucose metabolism: _____

5. Hormone that stimulates cells to enlarge and divide: _____

6. Hormone that regulates blood sugar: _____

7. Hormone of the anterior pituitary that stimulates cortex of adrenal gland to produce its own hormones: _____

8. Hormone that stimulates target cells in the ovaries and testes: _____

9. Hormone that replaces serotonin at night: _____

10. Hormone that stimulates the mammary glands after pregnancy to produce milk: _____

F. **Plurals.** Enhance your command of plurals in medical terminology by completing this exercise. Select the best choice for the correct form of the plural in the sentence. Fill in the blank. (**LO 17.A**)

1. Patient complains of multiple _____ (paresthesiae/paresthesias) on her left side.

2. There are several _____ (criterion/criteria) by which to judge this patient's recovery.

3. _____ (Catecholamines/Catecholamina) are major elements in stress response.

G. After rereading Case Report (CR) 17.2, answer the following questions. (LO 17.7, 17.8, 17.A, 17.B, 17.E)

Case Report (CR) 17.2

You are

. . . an emergency medical technician (**EMT**) working in the Emergency Room at Fulwood Medical Center at 0200 hours.

Your patient is

. . . Ms. Norma Leary, a 22-year-old college student living with her parents for the summer.

Ms. Leary is **emaciated,** extremely agitated, restless, and at times disoriented and confused. Her parents tell you that, in the past 3 or 4 days, she has been coughing and not feeling well. In the past 12 hours she has become feverish and been complaining of a left-sided chest pain. With questioning, the parents reveal that prior to this acute illness she had lost about 20 pounds in weight, although she was eating voraciously. Her vital signs (VS) are T 105.2°F, P 180 and irregular, R 24, BP 160/85.

You call for Dr. Hilinski **STAT** (immediately). On his initial examination, he believes that the patient is in **thyroid storm.** This is a medical emergency. There are no immediate laboratory tests that can confirm this diagnosis.

---

1. What does the term **emaciated** mean?

    a. exhausted

    b. anxious

    c. irritated

    d. thin

2. After reviewing her vital signs, what term describes her heart rate?

    a. hypotensive

    b. febrile

    c. tachycardic

    d. bradypneic

3. Ms. Leary's signs and symptoms are due to:

    a. decreased thyroid hormones

    b. increased thyroid hormones

    c. dehydration

    d. overhydration

4. The thyroid storm:

    a. came about suddenly

    b. has been occurring for a long period of time

    c. is diagnosed with a measure of serum electrolytes

    d. requires an MRI to confirm Dr. Hilinski's diagnosis

H. Terminology construction. Construct the *language of endocrinology*. Build the term for the definition provided. Fill in the blanks. (LO 17.1, 17.3, 17.8, 17.14, 17.18, 17.C)

    1. Hormone formed by the pineal gland   _____ /tonin

    2. Protrusion of the eyeball   ex/ _____

    3. Hormone produced by the adrenal cortex   _____ /o/steroid

    4. Deficiency of all the pituitary hormones   _____ /hypo/pituitar/ism

    5. Another name for the pituitary gland   _____ /physis

    6. Hormone that stimulates the uterus to contract   oxy/ _____ /in

    7. Removal of part or all of the adrenal gland   adrenal/_____

    8. Prolactin-producing tumor   prolactin/ _____

    9. Waxy, nonpitting edema of skin   _____ /edema

    10. Excess of growth hormone that produces enlarged hands and feet   _____ /megaly

Endocrine System

I. Elements. Use your knowledge of word elements to answer the following questions about hormones in other body systems. Fill in the blanks. **(LO 17.D)**

1. Based on its root, the hormone gastrin would have a connection with which body organ? _____

2. Based on its root, the hormone cholecystokinin has an effect on which body organ? _____

3. Both of the above organs are part of which body system that you have already studied? _____ (answer is one word)

4. Based on its root, the hormone erythropoietin stimulates production of _____.

J. Deconstruction. Deconstruct these medical terms into the meanings of their basic elements. Fill in the chart. If the term does not have an element, write n/a. **(LO 17.2, 17.3, 17.12, 17.22, 17.D)**

Medical Term	Meaning of Prefix	Meaning of Root/ Combining Form	Meaning of Suffix	Meaning of Medical Term
polyuria	1.	2.	3.	4.
parathyroid	5.	6.	7.	8.
thyrotropin	9.	10.	11.	12.
oxytocin	13.	14.	15.	16.
prognathism	17.	18.	19.	20.

K. Abbreviations. This exercise contains all the letters you need to form the correct abbreviations for the terms described. Fill in the blanks. **(LO 17.1, 17.2, 17.12, 17.21, 17.22, 17.A, 17.F)**

A   D   G   H   I   K   M   N   O   P   S   T

1. Stored in the posterior pituitary: _____

2. Type 2 diabetes: _____

3. Thyrotropin: _____

4. Somatotropin: _____

5. Secreted in response to hypocalcemia: _____

6. Type 1 diabetes: _____

7. Winter depression: _____

8. Marked hyperglycemia with dehydration: _____

9. Used occasionally to diagnose type 2 diabetes: _____

10. Disorder caused by insulin deficiency: _____

L. **Terminology challenge.** An element may have more than one meaning. For example, *hypo-* can mean either *below* (location) or *deficient* (less in quantity or number). The following five terms all start with *hypo-*. Choose the meaning of the prefix in the following section. **(LO 17.A, 17.D)**

1. hypoglycemia

   a. below

   b. deficient

2. hypodermic

   a. below

   b. deficient

3. hypothalamus

   a. below

   b. deficient

4. hypopituitarism

   a. below

   b. deficient

5. hypophysis

   a. below

   b. deficient

Now match the term to its correct definition. **(LO 17.8)**

_____ 6. hypoglycemia

_____ 7. hypodermic

_____ 8. hypothalamus

_____ 9. hypopituitarism

_____10. hypophysis

a. another name for the pituitary gland

b. produces eight hormones

c. pertaining to below the skin

d. condition of one or more deficient pituitary hormones

e. pertaining to low blood sugar

You are ultimately responsible for everything you communicate regarding patient care!

©2014 Nucleus Medical Media

The health professionals involved in the diagnosis and treatment of patients with mental health disorders include:

- **Psychiatrists**, who are medical doctors licensed in the diagnosis and treatment of mental disorders.

- **Clinical psychologists**, who are professionals licensed in the science concerned with the behavior of the human mind.

- **Psychiatric and mental health nurses or nurse practitioners**, who evaluate and provide care for patients with psychiatric disorders, medical mental conditions, and substance abuse problems.

- **Psychiatric social workers**, who assess, develop treatment plans, and provide case management and rights advocacy to patients with mental health problems.

- **Psychiatric technicians**, who provide front-line care to patients with mental illnesses and/or developmental disabilities and who carry out doctors' orders and serve as the eyes and ears of the diagnosing professional.

Chapter Learning Outcomes

To be an effective member of the mental health team that will be responsible for Mr. Diment's care *(see Case Report (CR) 18.1)*, you will need to be able to:

LO 18.1 Define key medical terms unique to psychiatry and psychology to relate to a uniform system for classifying and describing mental disorders.

LO 18.2 Describe the major types of affective disorders.

LO 18.3 Discuss anxiety disorders.

LO 18.4 Explain psychosomatic and somatoform disorders.

LO 18.5 Discuss schizophrenia.

LO 18.6 Identify the main personality disorders.

LO 18.7 Discuss diagnostic methods used for mental health disorders.

LO 18.8 Explain therapeutic methods used for mental health disorders.

LO 18.9 Describe pharmacologic agents used for mental health disorders.

LO 18.A Use the medical terms of mental health to communicate in writing and document accurately and precisely in any health care setting.

LO 18.B Use the medical terms of mental health to communicate verbally with accuracy and precision in any health care setting.

LO 18.C Construct medical terms used in mental health from their word elements (roots, combining forms, prefixes, and suffixes).

LO 18.D Deconstruct medical terms used in mental health into their word elements (roots, combining forms, prefixes, and suffixes).

LO 18.E Identify health professionals involved in the care of patients with mental disorders.

LO 18.F Identify correct abbreviations for medical terms used in mental health.

Case Report (CR) 18.1

You are

. . . a **psychiatric technician** employed in the Psychiatric Department of Fulwood Medical Center. Your patient has been referred from the Emergency Department, where he was seen earlier this morning.

Your patient is

. . . Mr. Harlan Diment, a 40-year-old construction worker. He was brought to the Emergency Department by his roommate, who says that Mr. Diment has slept only a couple of hours each night for the past 3 weeks. He stays up most of the night, cleaning their apartment and drinking beer. He has bought a new home entertainment set, including a big-screen plasma TV, that he cannot afford. He is very irritable and explosive when challenged about his behavior. His roommate has seen no signs of drugs and is not aware of any medical problems. Mr. Diment is usually very quiet, thoughtful, and introverted.

A mental status examination shows Mr. Diment to be alternately irritable and excited. He is wearing a bright orange top and camouflage slacks and is carrying a soft green cap. His speech is rapid and loud, and it is difficult to interrupt him. He paces the room, claims to feel "great," and is angry with his roommate for insisting that he come to the hospital. His thought processes and verbalization go off on different **tangents (tangentiality)**. He says he has no suicidal thoughts, **hallucinations**, or **delusions**.

Lesson 18.1

Mental Health and Affective Disorders

In this lesson, you will be given information about mental health disorders including affective disorders, mood disorders, schizophrenia, anxiety disorders, and psychosomatic and somatoform disorders.

This lesson and the introduction will enable you to use correct medical terminology to:

18.1.1 Distinguish between psychology and psychiatry.

18.1.2 Define mental disorder and insanity.

18.1.3 Discuss affective disorders.

18.1.4 Describe the differences between the two main types of mood disorder.

Keynotes

- Psychologists are not licensed to prescribe medications.
- As physicians, psychiatrists are licensed to prescribe medications.
- The *Diagnostic and Statistical Manual of Mental Disorders*, fifth edition (DSM-5) classifies and describes psychiatric disorders.
- The DSM-5 contains over 200 diagnoses grouped into 17 major categories.

Abbreviations

PhD	doctorate in philosophy
PsyD	doctorate in psychology

LO 18.1 Definitions in Mental Health

Mental health is defined as emotional, behavioral, and social well-being such that an individual can cope with internal and external events.

Psychology is defined as the scientific study of behavior and mental processes. **Behavior** is anything you do—talking, sleeping, reading, interacting with others. **Mental processes** are your private, internal experiences—thinking, feeling, remembering, dreaming.

A licensed specialist in psychology is called a **psychologist**. Psychologists can have a master's degree or a doctorate in philosophy **(PhD)** or a doctorate in psychology **(PsyD)**. They can practice in many different career specialties, including being a **psychotherapist** or a **psychoanalyst**.

Psychiatry is the medical specialty concerned with the origin, diagnosis, prevention, and treatment of mental, emotional, and behavioral disorders. **Psychiatrists** have an MD or DO degree and a minimum of 4 years of residency training in the specialty.

Many psychiatrists and psychologists work together in a team approach to therapy. Other health professionals in the mental health team include **clinical social workers**, **psychiatric nurses**, and **psychiatric technicians**.

Mental disorder can be defined as any behavior or emotional state that:

- Causes a person to suffer emotional distress (e.g., depression, anxiety).

- Is harmful to the individual sufferer (impairs the individual's ability to work, take care of personal needs, or get along with others).

- Is self-destructive (e.g., substance abuse, gambling and other addictions, self-injury).

- Endangers others or the community (antisocial behaviors, **homicidal** intent, **pyromania** [setting fires]).

Insanity is a *legal* term for a severe mental illness, present at the time a crime was committed, that impaired the defendant's capacity to understand the moral wrong of the act. *It is not a medical diagnosis.*

S = Suffix   P = Prefix   R = Root   R/CF = Combining Form

WORD	PRONUNCIATION	ELEMENTS		DEFINITION
hallucination	hah-loo-sih-**NAY**-shun	S/ R/	-ation *process* hallucin- *imagination*	Perception of an object or event when there is no such thing present
homicide	**HOM**-ih-side	S/ R/CF	-cide *to kill* hom/i- *man*	Killing of one human by another
homicidal (adj)	hom-ih-**SIDE**-al	S/	-cidal *pertaining to killing*	Having a tendency to commit homicide
insanity	in-**SAN**-ih-tee	S/ P/ R/	-ity *condition* in- *not* -san- *sound, healthy*	Nonmedical term for person unable to be responsible for actions
psychiatry	sigh-**KIE**-ah-tree	S/ R/	-iatry *treatment* psych- *mind*	Diagnosis and treatment of mental disorders
psychiatric (adj) psychiatrist	sigh-kee-**AH**-trik sigh-**KIE**-ah-trist	S/ S/	-ic *pertaining to* -iatrist *one who treats, practitioner*	Pertaining to psychiatry Licensed medical specialist in psychiatry
psychology	sigh-**KOL**-oh-jee	S/ R/CF	-logy *study of* psych/o- *mind*	Scientific study of the human mind and behavior
psychological psychologist psychoanalysis psychoanalyst psychotherapy psychotherapist	sigh-koh-**LOJ**-ik-al sigh-**KOL**-oh-jist sigh-koh-ah-**NAL**-ih-sis sigh-koh-**AN**-ah-list sigh-koh-**THAIR**-ah-pee sigh-koh-**THAIR**-ah-pist	S/ S/ R/ R/ S/ S/	-ical *pertaining to* -logist *specialist* -analysis *process to define* -analyst *one who defines* -therapy *treatment* -therapist *one who treats*	Pertaining to psychology Licensed specialist in psychology Method of psychotherapy Practitioner of psychoanalysis Treatment of mental disorders through communication Practitioner of psychotherapy
pyromania	pie-roh-**MAY**-nee-ah	S/ R/CF	-mania *frenzy* pyr/o- *fire*	Morbid impulse to set fires

Exercises

A. Reinforce your learning of the *languages of psychology and psychiatry* by providing the term that is being defined.
Fill in the blank. **LO 18.1, 18.E**

1. A medical doctor who specializes in the origin, diagnosis, prevention, and treatment of mental, emotional, and behavioral

   disorders: _____

2. A front-line worker who directly cares for those with mental illnesses and/or developmental disabilities: _____

   technician.

3. The general term for a licensed specialist in psychology: _____

B. Choose the correct answer for the question. LO 18.1

1. Which of the following choices cannot be classified under the term *behavior*?

   a. talking

   b. sleeping

   c. reading

   d. depression

   e. interacting with others

2. Which of the following statements *best* describes a mental process?

   a. your private, internal experiences

   b. thinking

   c. feeling

   d. remembering

   e. dreaming

3. Which of the following terms contains a prefix, root, and suffix?

   a. psychology

   b. hallucination

   c. insanity

   d. homicidal

   e. psychiatry

LO 18.2 Affective Disorders

Affective disorders are not a clearly delineated group of disorders. Included are the **mood disorders** of **unipolar** and **bipolar depression**.

Mood Disorders

▲ **Figure 18.1** Depressed Woman at Window. ©Bojan Kontrec/Getty Images RF

You will feel sad and blue and down in the dumps from time to time and occasionally feel the grief of the death of a loved one and the tragedy of injury or severe emotional hurt. Everyone does. But people with **major depression** are so deeply sad for at least 2 weeks that they feel despairing and hopeless, see nothing but sorrow in the future, and may not want to live anymore *(Figure 18.1)*. They see themselves as worthless and unlovable. They have difficulty getting up and going to school or work. One person's depression can hurt everyone in the entire family.

    Physical symptoms occur. These may include difficulty concentrating, difficulty falling asleep, feeling tired all the time, and losing weight. Violent behavior or substance abuse occurs more often in depressed men than in women, though depression is more common in women.

    Some people rebound to the opposite extreme of depression called **mania**, an excessive state of overexcitement and impulsive behavior. This alternation of episodes of depression with mania is called **bipolar disorder**. It used to be called **manic-depressive disorder**. Approximately 6 million Americans suffer from bipolar disorder. A study published in 2017 from the University of Texas at Houston linked a volume decrease in specific parts of the brain's hippocampus *(see Chapter 9)*.

    In the **manic** phase, the person is hyperactive and distractible and may not sleep for days, yet shows no fatigue. Thinking and speech are rapid and disjointed and cannot be interrupted. The person may give away possessions or go on a spending spree. Untreated pure manic episodes usually last 6 weeks. Untreated mixed (manic and depressive) episodes usually last 17 weeks.

    Dysphoric mania, a form of bipolar disorder, combines the frenetic energy of mania with dark thoughts and paranoid delusions. It may be the cause of some mass shootings.

    Seasonal affective disorder (SAD) is a mood disorder associated with episodes of depression during the fall and winter months, subsiding during spring and summer. It appears to be related to a lack of sunshine causing increased melatonin production by the pineal gland *(see Chapter 14)*. It can be helped by phototherapy with bright white fluorescent lights. Antidepressant drugs also can be helpful.

Abbreviation	
SAD	seasonal affective disorder

Case Report (CR) 18.1 *(continued)*

Mr. Harlan Diment is clearly in a manic phase. When Dr. Robert Nguyen, a psychiatrist, examined him in the Emergency Department, he believed the most likely diagnosis to be bipolar disorder. He has asked you to obtain a urine specimen to test for drugs of abuse and to do a blood test for his alcohol level, to exclude those as causes. Dr. Nguyen has ordered that Mr. Diment be admitted to the Psychiatric Unit. He will need treatment with a mood stabilizer such as lithium. If he resists admission, he can be placed on a 72-hour hold because he is a danger to himself and to others.

Word Analysis and Definition

S = Suffix   P = Prefix   R = Root   R/CF = Combining Form

WORD	PRONUNCIATION	ELEMENTS		DEFINITION
affect	**AF**-fekt		Latin *state of mind*	External display of feelings, thoughts, and emotions
affective	af-**FEK**-tiv	S/	-ive *pertaining to*	Expressing emotion
		R/	affect- *mood*	
bipolar disorder	bi-**POH**-lar dis-**OR**-der	S/	-ar *pertaining to*	A mood disorder with alternating episodes of depression and mania, the two poles of the disorder
		P/	bi- *two*	
		R/	-pol- *pole*	
		P/	dis- *apart, away from*	
		R/	-order *arrange*	
depression	de-**PRESH**-un	S/	-ion *condition, process*	Mental disorder with feelings of deep sadness and despair
		R/	depress- *press down*	
dysphoria	dis-**FOR**-ee-ah	S/	-ia *condition*	A condition of severe depression, agitation, and paranoid delusions
		P/	dys- *bad, difficult*	
		R/	-phor- *carry, bear*	
dysphoric (adj)		S/	-ic *pertaining to*	Pertaining to dysphoria
mania	**MAY**-nee-ah		Greek *frenzy*	Mood disorder with hyperactivity, irritability, and rapid speech
manic (adj)	**MAN**-ik	S/	-ic *pertaining to*	Pertaining to or characterized by mania
		R/	man- *affected by frenzy*	
manic-depressive disorder	**MAN**-ik dee-**PRESS**-iv dis-**OR**-der	S/	-ive *quality of*	An outdated name for bipolar disorder
		R/	depress- *press down*	
		P/	dis- *apart, away from*	
		R/	-order *arrange*	
unipolar disorder	you-nih-**POLE**-ar dis-**OR**-der	S/	-ar *pertaining to*	Depression
		P/	uni- *one*	
		R/	-pol- *pole (at the pole of depression)*	
		P/	dis- *apart, away from*	
		R/	-order *arrange*	

Exercises

A. Differentiate between the conditions and signs of bipolar and unipolar disorders. *Use the words below to fill in the blanks in the following sentences.* **LO 18.2**

bipolar   unipolar   mania   manic   depression

1. A patient who experiences episodes of mania with episodes of depression is diagnosed with _____ disorder.

2. While experiencing the periods of hyperactivity, irritability, and paranoid delusions, the patient is said to be

   in a _____ state.

3. A patient whose symptoms are limited to deep sadness suffers from _____.

4. Clinical depression is the same as _____ disorder.

5. A person with bipolar disorder is experiencing _____ when he speaks very rapidly, is irritable, and is

   hyperactive.

Lesson 18.2

Anxiety Disorders

To work effectively with patients with anxiety disorders, you will need to be able to use correct medical terminology to:

18.2.1 Define the five major categories of anxiety disorders.

18.2.2 Discuss the symptoms of the five major types of anxiety disorders.

18.2.3 Specify the diagnostic criteria for posttraumatic stress disorder (PTSD).

18.2.4 Identify some of the drugs used to treat anxiety disorders.

18.2.5 Differentiate between psychosomatic and somatoform disorders.

 Case Report (CR) 18.2

You are

. . . a readjustment counseling technician in a Veterans Administration Counseling Center attached to Fulwood Medical Center.

Your patient is

. . . Sergeant Mike West, an Army reservist who has recently returned from his second tour of duty in Afghanistan.

As you interview Sergeant West, you learn that he is having difficulty coping with what he experienced during wartime. The vehicle he was driving ran over an improvised explosive device (*Figure 18.2*). Two of his comrades died, and Sergeant West received shrapnel wounds in his leg and hand. He plays the tape of the incident in his mind over and over again. Loud noises, like thunderstorms, trigger paralysis. The smell of diesel brings back the memory of the vehicle on fire. Chicken on the barbecue smells like searing flesh. He can't sleep more than 3 or 4 hours a night, and then he wakes up in cold sweats. Sergeant West has become quick-tempered and doesn't like the way he is treating his wife. He is frightened to have children because of his outbursts of anger at seemingly minor upsets.

▲ **Figure 18.2** The remains of an American Humvee, one of four that were disabled by massive IEDs, lies on a dirt road on August 4, 2007, in Hawr Rajab, Iraq. ©Benjamin Lowy/Getty Images

Abbreviations

GAD generalized anxiety disorder

PTSD posttraumatic stress disorder

LO 18.3 Anxiety Disorders

Anxiety disorders are the most common category of mental disorders found in the United States. They are characterized by an **unreasonable anxiety** or **fear** that is inappropriate to the circumstances and so intense and chronic that it disrupts the person's life.

There are five major categories of anxiety disorder:

1. **Generalized anxiety disorder (GAD)** consists of persistent, excessive worrying and uncontrollable anxiety that is not focused on one particular situation and has lasted for at least 6 months. People with this disorder are frightened of something but are unable to articulate a specific fear. They develop physical fear reactions including palpitations, **insomnia**, difficulty concentrating, and irritability.

2. **Posttraumatic** stress disorder (PTSD) occurs when a person who has gone through a significant trauma shows stress symptoms that last for longer than a month and impair the person's ability to function. The trauma can be a life-threatening accident, a natural disaster, loss of a loved one, torture or abuse, or combat and its related incidents. Posttraumatic stress disorder is the diagnosis for Sergeant West.

636 CHAPTER 18 Mental Health The Languages of Psychology and Psychiatry

WORD	PRONUNCIATION		ELEMENTS	DEFINITION
anxiety	ang-**ZIE**-eh-tee		Greek *distress, anxiety*	Distress caused by fear
insomnia	in-**SOM**-nee-ah	S/ P/ R/	**-ia** *condition* **in-** *not* **-somn-** *sleep*	Inability to sleep
posttraumatic	post-traw-**MAT**-ik	S/ P/ R/	**-ic** *pertaining to* **post-** *after* **-traumat-** *wound*	Occurring after and caused by trauma

Exercises

A. Identify the word elements in each medical term. *Choose the correct answer for each question below.* **LO 18.2, 18.D**

1. Which of the following terms has a word element that means *not*?

    a. insomnia

    b. posttraumatic

    c. anxiety

2. Which of the following terms has a word element that means *wound*?

    a. insomnia

    b. posttraumatic

    c. anxiety

3. Which of the following terms has a word element that means *condition*?

    a. insomnia

    b. posttraumatic

    c. anxiety

LO 18.3 Anxiety Disorders (continued)

3. **Panic disorder** is characterized by sudden, brief attacks of **intense fear** that cause physical symptoms. The fear rises abruptly, often for no reason, and peaks in 10 minutes or less. The frequency of the attacks varies widely over many years. The disorder runs in families, but whether it is due to genetics or a shared environment is not clear.

4. **Phobias** differ from generalized anxiety and panic attacks in that a specific situation or object brings on the strong fear response. The danger is small, and the person realizes the fear is irrational, but there is still overwhelming anxiety. There are two categories of phobia:

   - **Situational phobias** involve a fear of specific situations. Examples include **agoraphobia** (fear of crowded places, buses, and elevators), **acrophobia** (fear of heights), fear of flying or driving in tunnels, and fear of specific animals (snakes, mice). The basic fear of being trapped in a confined space is called **claustrophobia**.

   - **Social phobias** involve fear of being embarrassed in social situations. The most common are fear of public speaking (stage fright) and of eating in public. In many, the fear is so strong that it makes normal life impossible.

5. In **obsessive-compulsive disorder (OCD)**, a majority of patients have both **obsessions** and **compulsions**. The obsessions are recurrent thoughts, fears, doubts, images, or impulses. The compulsions are recurrent, irresistible impulses to perform actions such as counting, hand washing, checking, and systematically arranging things. The recurrent thoughts can be violent or sexual.

Most patients recognize the senselessness of their behaviors; but if they resist doing them, the fear and anxiety become intolerable.

LO 18.4 Psychosomatic and Somatoform Disorders

Psychosomatic disorder is a real, physical disorder that, at least in part, has a psychologic cause. Tension headaches have real pain caused by muscle spasm, but stress and anxiety play a role in causing the symptoms.

Somatoform disorder occurs when there is no identifiable physical cause to explain physical symptoms. The symptoms are real to the patient and are not under voluntary control.

In **conversion disorder**, symptoms progress to involve loss of feeling, paralysis, deafness, or blindness.

Somatic symptom disorder (SSD) is a condition in which the patient has distressing physical (somatic) symptoms together with abnormal thoughts, feelings, and behaviors in response to these symptoms.

Keynote

- The DSM-5 has replaced the disorder **hypochondriasis** with the diagnosis of **somatic symptom disorder** and **illness anxiety disorder.**

Abbreviations

OCD obsessive-compulsive disorder
SSD somatic symptom disorder

WORD	PRONUNCIATION	ELEMENTS		DEFINITION
acrophobia	ak-roh-**FOH**-bee-ah	S/ R/CF	-phobia *fear* acr/o- *peak, highest point*	Pathologic fear of heights
agoraphobia	ah-gor-ah-**FOH**-bee-ah	S/ R/CF	-phobia *fear* agor/a- *marketplace*	Pathologic fear of being trapped in a public place
claustrophobia	klaw-stroh-**FOH**-bee-ah	S/ R/CF	-phobia *fear* claustr/o- *confined space*	Pathologic fear of being trapped in a confined space
compulsion	kom-**PUL**-shun	S/ R/	-ion *action, condition* compuls- *drive, compel*	Uncontrollable impulses to perform an act repetitively
compulsive (adj)	kom-**PUL**-siv	S/	-ive *nature of, quality of*	Possessing uncontrollable impulses to perform an act repetitively
conversion disorder	kon-**VER**-shun dis-**OR**-der	S/ P/ R/ P/ R/	-ion *action, condition* con- *with, together* -vers- *turned* dis- *apart, away from* -order *arrange*	An unconscious emotional conflict is expressed as physical symptoms with no organic basis
hypochondriasis	**HIGH**-poh-kon-**DRIE**-ah-sis	S/ P/ R/	-iasis *condition, state of* hypo- *below* -chondr- *rib, cartilage*	Belief that a minor symptom indicates a severe disease
obsession	ob-**SESH**-un	S/ R/	-ion *action, condition* obsess- *besieged by thoughts*	Persistent, recurrent, uncontrollable thoughts or impulses
obsessive (adj)	ob-**SES**-iv	S/	-ive *nature of, quality of*	Possessing persistent, recurrent, uncontrollable thoughts or impulses
phobia	**FOH**-bee-ah		Greek *fear*	Pathologic fear or dread
psychosomatic	sigh-koh-soh-**MAT**-ik	S/ R/CF R/	-ic *pertaining to* psych/o- *mind* -somat- *body*	Pertaining to disorders of the body usually resulting from disturbances of the mind
somatic symptom disorder	soh-**MAT**-ik **SIMP**-tum dis-**OR**-der	S/ R/ P/ R/	-ic *pertaining to* somat- *body* symptom Greek *sign* dis- *apart, away from* -order *arrange*	Distressing physical symptoms occur, causing abnormal thoughts, feelings, and behaviors
somatoform	soh-**MAT**-oh-form	S/ R/CF	-form *appearance of* somat/o- *body*	Physical symptoms occurring without identifiable physical cause

Exercises

A. Match the term to its correct definition. *Pay close attention to the word elements to assist you in choosing the correct definition for each term.*
LO 18.3, 18.4

_____ 1. psychosomatic

_____ 2. acrophobia

_____ 3. obsessive

_____ 4. hypochondriasis

_____ 5. somatoform

_____ 6. agoraphobia

_____ 7. compulsion

a. Fear of being trapped in a public space

b. Fear of heights

c. Physical symptoms occurring without a physical cause

d. Disorder of body due to disturbance of the mind

e. Belief that a minor symptom indicates a severe disease

f. Uncontrollable impulses to perform act repetitively

g. Persistent, recurrent, uncontrollable thoughts

Schizophrenia and Personality Disorders

The information in this lesson will enable you to use correct medical terminology to:

18.3.1 Detail the symptoms and treatment of schizophrenia.

18.3.2 Describe the different types of personality disorders.

18.3.3 Discuss the classes of psychoactive drugs.

▲ **Figure 18.3** **Artwork by Schizophrenic Patient.**
©Wellcome Images/Photo Researchers, Inc.

▲ **Figure 18.4** **Homeless Schizophrenic Man on the Street.** ©George Rose/Getty Images

Case Report (CR) 18.3

You are

. . . an emergency medical technician (EMT) working in the Emergency Department at Fulwood Medical Center.

Your patient is

. . . Mr. Dante Costello, a 21-year-old homeless man brought in by the police after he was found sitting in the middle of a main street.

Mr. Costello's explanation is "the voices told me to do it." He has heard voices telling him to do things for the past year. The voices often comment on his behavior. He has isolated himself from other people because "they are not who they say they are, and they are trying to get me." He is taking no drugs or medications and denies any **suicidal** or homicidal intent. Mr. Costello is dirty and disheveled, with poor hygiene. He can give no home or family address. His **affect** is **congruent**, though expressionless. His speech is slow, and his thoughts are disorganized and confused. The most probable diagnosis is **schizophrenia**. He needs to be admitted to the hospital because he is a danger to himself and other people.

LO 18.5 Schizophrenia

Schizophrenia is a form of **psychosis** in which there is a loss of contact with reality. People with schizophrenia do *not* have a split personality, but their words are separated from the meaning, their perceptions are separated from reality, and their behaviors are separated from their thought processes *(Figure 18.3)*.

People with schizophrenia have their sensory perceptions jumbled and distorted, have difficulty concentrating, and perceive things without a stimulation—**hallucinations**. Hallucinations can occur in any of the senses but are most often auditory. These people also suffer from **delusions**, mistaken beliefs that are contrary to facts. The delusions can be **paranoid**, with pervasive distrust and suspicion of others. People with schizophrenia can withdraw from society, become homeless, and refuse to communicate *(Figure 18.4)*.

Their speech is disorganized and can be incoherent. Their behaviors are often totally inappropriate. Their blunted emotions and withdrawal can progress to **catatonia**, motor immobility that can last for hours. **Mutism** is the inability or refusal to speak.

Symptoms of schizophrenia typically come on in the late teens and twenties. Although there is no cure, it can be effectively treated with medications and programs of psychological rehabilitation *(see Lesson 18.4)*.

Case Report (CR) 18.3 *(continued)*

Mr. Costello stated he was hearing voices of people who were not there speaking to him (hallucination). Mr. Costello was also paranoid, believing that people were "out to get him." He withdrew from society and became homeless. His behavior of sitting immobile in the middle of the street for long periods is inappropriate and is **catatonic**.

WORD	PRONUNCIATION	ELEMENTS		DEFINITION
affect (noun)	**AF**-fekt		Latin *state of mind*	External display of feelings, thoughts, and emotions
catatonia	kat-ah-**TOH**-nee-ah	S/ P/ R/	-ia *condition* cata- *down* -ton- *pressure, tension*	Syndrome characterized by physical immobility and mental stupor
catatonic (adj)	kat-ah-**TON**-ik	S/	-ic *pertaining to*	Pertaining to or characterized by catatonia
congruent	**KON**-gru-ent	S/ P/ R/	-ent *end result* con- *with* -gru- *to move*	Coinciding or agreeing with
delusion	dee-**LOO**-shun	S/ R/	-ion *condition, process* delus- *deceive*	Fixed, unyielding, false belief or judgment held despite strong evidence to the contrary
delusional (adj)	dee-**LOO**-shun-al	S/	-al *pertaining to*	Pertaining to having delusions
hallucination	hah-loo-sih-**NAY**-shun	S/ R/	-ation *process* hallucin- *imagination*	Perception of an object or event when there is no such thing present
mute mutism	MYUT **MYU**-tizm	 S/ R/	Latin *silent* -ism *condition, process* mut- *silent*	Unable or unwilling to speak Absence of speech
paranoia	pair-ah-**NOY**-ah	P/ R/	para- *abnormal, beside* -noia *to think*	Mental disorder with persecutory delusions
paranoid (adj)	**PAIR**-ah-noyd	R/	-noid *abnormal thinking*	Having delusions of persecution
psychosis	sigh-**KOH**-sis	S/ R/	-osis *condition* psych- *mind*	Disorder causing mental disruption and loss of contact with reality
schizophrenia	skitz-oh-**FREE**-nee-ah	S/ R/CF R/	-ia *condition* schiz/o- *to split, cleave* -phren- *mind*	Disorder of perception, thought, emotion, and behavior
schizophrenic (adj)	skitz-oh-**FREN**-ik	S/	-ic *pertaining to*	Relating to, or suffering from, schizophrenia
suicide	**SOO**-ih-side	S/ R/CF	-cide *to kill* su/i- *self*	The act of killing oneself
suicidal (adj)	**SOO**-ih-**SIGH**-dal	S/	-cidal *pertaining to killing*	Wanting to kill oneself

Exercises

A. After reading Case Report (CR) 18.3, *choose the correct answer to complete each statement.* **LO 18.5**

1. The term that means *wanting to kill oneself:*

   a. homicidal

   b. schizophrenic

   c. suicidal

   d. psychotic

2. Mr. Costello's inappropriate behavior is due to:

   a. homicidal thoughts

   b. poor hygiene

   c. hearing voices

   d. homelessness

3. In the statement "His affect is congruent, though expressionless," the term **congruent** means:

   a. the behavior matches his appearance

   b. he is not speaking

   c. he believes people are out to get him

   d. his behavior points to hurting other people

4. His behavior of sitting in the street for long periods of time describes which condition?

   a. paranoia

   b. mutism

   c. homicidal

   d. catatonia

LO 18.6 Personality Disorders

Personality is defined as an individual's unique and stable patterns of thoughts, feelings, and behaviors. When these patterns become rigid and inflexible in response to different situations, they can cause impairment of the individual's ability to deal with other people (i.e., to function socially).

Borderline personality disorder (BPD) is a frequent diagnosis in people who are impulsive, unstable in mood, and manipulative. They can be exciting, charming, and friendly one moment and angry, irritable, and sarcastic the next. Their identity is fragile and insecure, their self-worth low. They can be promiscuous and self-destructive; for example, committing **self-mutilation (self-injury)** *(Figure 18.5)* or suicide. People with **narcissistic personality disorder** have an exaggerated sense of self-importance and seek constant attention.

Antisocial personality disorder, used interchangeably with the terms **sociopath** and **psychopath**, describes people who lie, cheat, steal, make trouble for others, and have no sense of responsibility and no anxiety or guilt about their behavior. The psychopaths have these characteristics but tend to be more violent and anger more easily than sociopaths.

Schizoid and **paranoid personality disorders** describe people who are absorbed with themselves, untrusting, and fearful of closeness with others.

Treatment for personality disorders is not successful.

Dissociative Disorders

Dissociative disorders involve a disassociation (splitting apart) of past experiences from present memory or consciousness. Being unable to recall identity is called **dissociative amnesia**. The development of distinctly separate personalities is called **dissociative identity disorder (DID)**. It was formerly called **multiple personality disorder (MPD)**.

The basic origin of all these disorders is the need to escape, usually from extreme trauma, and most often from sexual, emotional, or physical abuse in childhood.

The most severe of this group of disorders is DID. Two or more distinct personalities, each with their own memories and behaviors, inhabit the same person at the same time *(Figure 18.6)*. Treatment is with psychotherapy.

Impulse Control Disorders

Impulse control disorders are an inability to resist an impulse to perform an action that is harmful to the individual or to others. These disorders include:

- **Intermittent explosive disorder**, which is characterized by recurrent episodes of unrestrained aggression toward people, furniture, or property, with violent resistance to attempts to restrain. The etiology is thought to be epileptic-like activity in the brain.
- **Kleptomania**, which is characterized by stealing—not for gain, but to satisfy an irresistible urge to steal.
- **Trichotillomania (TTM)**, which is characterized by the repeated urge to pull out scalp, beard, pubic, and other body hair.
- **Substance abuse** and **chemical dependence**, which involve a person's continued use of drugs or alcohol despite having had significant problems or distress related to their use. This **addiction** affects the brain and behavior, and develops an increased need for the substance and an inability to stop using it.
- **Pyromania**, which is repeated fire setting with no motive other than a fascination with fire and fire engines. Some pyromaniacs end up as volunteer firefighters. Treatment with behavioral therapy is sometimes successful.

▲ **Figure 18.5** Self-Mutilated Arm.
©Dr. P. Marazzi/SPL/Photo Researchers, Inc.

▲ **Figure 18.6** Dissociative Identity Disorder (Multiple Personality Disorder).
©John Lund/Getty Images

Abbreviations

BPD	borderline personality disorder
DID	dissociative identity disorder
MPD	multiple personality disorder
TTM	trichotillomania

WORD	PRONUNCIATION	ELEMENTS		DEFINITION
addict addiction	**AD**-ikt ah-**DIK**-shun	P/ R/ S/	**ad-** *toward* **-dict** *surrender* **-ion** *condition, action*	Person with a psychologic or physical dependence on a substance or practice Habitual psychologic and physiologic dependence on a substance or practice
amnesia	am-**NEE**-zee-ah		Greek *forgetfulness*	Total or partial inability to remember past experiences
antisocial personality disorder	**AN**-tee-**SOH**-shal person-**AL**-ih-tee dis-**OR**-der	S/ P/ R/ S/ S/ R/ P/ R/	**-al** *pertaining to* **anti-** *against* **-soci-** *partner, ally, community* **-ity** *condition, state* **-al-** *pertaining to* **person-** *person* **dis-** *apart, away from* **-order** *arrange*	Disorder of people who lie, cheat, steal, and have no guilt about their behavior
dissociative identity disorder	di-**SO**-see-ah-tiv eye-**DEN**-tih-tee dis-**OR**-der	S/ P/ R/ R/	**-ative** *quality of* **dis-** *apart, away from* **-soci-** *partner, ally, community* **identity** Latin *repeatedly, again and again* **-order** *arrange*	Mental disorder in which part of an individual's personality is separated from the rest, leading to multiple personalities
kleptomania	klep-toh-**MAY**-nee-ah	S/ R/CF	**-mania** *frenzy* **klept/o-** *to steal*	Uncontrollable need to steal
narcissism narcissistic (adj)	**NAR**-sih-sizm **NAR**-sih-**SIS**-tik	 S/ R/ S/	**Narcissus**, Greek mythical character who was in love with his own reflection in water **-ism** *a process* **narciss-** *self-love* **-istic** *pertaining to*	Self-love; person interprets everything purely in relation to himself or herself Relating everything to oneself; pertaining to, or suffering from, narcissism
psychopath	**SIGH**-koh-path	S/ R/CF	**-path** *disease* **psych/o-** *mind*	Person with antisocial personality disorder who is prone to anger and violence
pyromania	pie-roh-**MAY**-nee-ah	S/ R/CF	**-mania** *frenzy* **pyr/o-** *fire*	Morbid impulse to set fires
schizoid	**SKITZ**-oyd	S/ R/	**-oid** *resemble* **schiz-** *split*	Withdrawn, socially isolated
self-mutilation	self-myu-tih-**LAY**-shun	S/ R/ R/	**-ation** *process* **self-** *own individual* **-mutil-** *to maim*	Injury or disfigurement made to one's own body
sociopath	**SOH**-see-oh-path	S/ R/CF	**-path** *disease* **soci/o-** *partner, ally, community*	Person with antisocial personality disorder

Exercises

A. Use the correct abbreviation for personality disorders. *Read the description of the personality disorder and give the correct abbreviation for which it is describing.* **LO 18.6, 18.A, 18.F**

1. A person who pulls the hairs from the eyebrows and eyelids: _____

2. The current title for a condition in which a person states that he or she has two separate and distinct personalities: _____

3. The older abbreviation for a person with two separate and distinct personalities: _____

4. This person is known to be manipulative, yet charming. His or her moods are unstable and behavior is impulsive:_____

Lesson 18.4

Procedures and Pharmacology for Mental Disorders

Abbreviations

CBT	cognitive behavioral therapy
CPT	cognitive processing therapy
DSM-5	*Diagnostic and Statistical Manual of Mental Disorders*, fifth edition

LO 18.7 Diagnostic Methods for Mental Disorders

At this time, there are no tests (examination of blood or body fluids) for mental illnesses as is the case with a physical health condition, though research to identify markers for schizophrenia and depression is ongoing. To define a mental health diagnosis, the following steps can be taken:

- A **physical examination** by a primary care physician to rule out physical problems that could be causing the symptoms.

- **Lab tests** to rule out physical causes of the symptoms; for example, tests of thyroid function and screening for alcohol and drugs.

- A **psychological evaluation** by a psychiatrist or psychologist to determine the patient's symptoms, thoughts, feelings, and behavior patterns by talking to the patient and using questionnaires. The defining symptoms of each mental illness are detailed in the *Diagnostic and Statistical Manual of Mental Disorders*, **fifth edition (DSM-5)**, compiled by the American Psychiatric Association, which is used by mental health providers to make the diagnosis of mental health disorders and by insurance companies to set reimbursements for treatment.

Brain imaging scans (neuroimaging scans) are being used to help detect and diagnose medical disorders, but their use for mental disorders is in research to try to learn more about the mental disorders.

The diagnosis of mental disorders is even more challenging in children, where the U.S. Surgeon General estimates that one in five children has a diagnosable mental illness. Children are developing mentally as well as physically and actions such as anger, anxiety, or shyness can be a temporary condition as part of developmental growth rather than an illness. When troubling behaviors occur over a period of time or in a way that disrupts daily life, they can then be considered symptoms of a disorder.

LO 18.8 Therapeutic Methods for Mental Disorders

Mental disorders are characterized by changes in mood, thought, and/or behavior that interfere with the daily activities of living and impair the ability to work and interact with family and the community. The National Survey on Drug Use and Health Data for 2014 shows that 43.6 million adults aged 18 and older experienced some form of mental illness in that year, about 18.1% of the population.

Psychotherapy, also called talk therapy, explores with a trained mental health professional thoughts, feelings, and behaviors on the assumption that the cure for a person's suffering lies within that person. The therapist's roles are to generate emotional awareness and insight to help the person identify the source of the problems and consider alternatives for dealing with them. There are six types of psychotherapy:

1. **Supportive psychotherapy**, in which the expression of feelings is encouraged and the therapist provides help with problem solving.

2. **Psychoanalysis**, which is the oldest form of psychotherapy, developed by Sigmund Freud in the early 20th century. It encourages the person to say whatever comes to mind and helps the person develop an understanding of how the past affects the present, enabling the person to develop new and more adaptive ways of functioning.

3. **Psychodynamic psychotherapy**, which is similar to psychoanalysis and focuses on identifying unconscious patterns in current thoughts, feelings, and behaviors.

4. **Cognitive therapy**, which helps people identify distortions in interpreting experiences and learn to think in different ways about the experiences, which leads to an improvement in behavior and feelings.

5. **Behavioral therapy**, which is similar to cognitive therapy. A combination of the two—**cognitive behavioral therapy (CBT)**—is often used. Behavioral therapy believes that abnormal behaviors are due to faulty learning, and these maladaptive behaviors can be unlearned and corrected.

6. **Interpersonal therapy** involves treatment for depression and focuses on unresolved grief and conflicts that arise when people have to fill roles that differ from their expectations both at work and in the family.

WORD	PRONUNCIATION	ELEMENTS		DEFINITION
behavioral	be-**HAYV**-yur-al	S/ S/ R/	-al *pertaining to* -ior- *pertaining to* behav- *mental activity*	Pertaining to any mental or motor activity
multimodal	mul-tee-**MOH**-dal	S/ P/ R/	-al *pertaining to* multi- *many* -mod- *method*	Using many methods
psychoanalysis	sigh-koh-ah-**NAL**-ih-sis	R/CF R/	psych/o- *mind* -analysis *process to define*	Method of psychotherapy
psychodynamic	sigh-koh-die-**NAM**-ik	S/ R/CF R/	-ic *pertaining to* psych/o- *mind* -dynam- *power*	The interplay between motivation and emotion
psychological	sigh-koh-**LOJ**-ih-kal	S/ R/ R/CF	-ical *pertaining to* -logy *study of* psych/o- *mind*	Pertaining to psychology—the study of the mind
psychotherapy	sigh-koh-**THAIR**-ah-pee	R/CF R/	psych/o- *mind* -therapy *treatment*	Treatment of mental disorders through talking
transcranial	trans-**KRAY**-nee-al	S/ P/ R/CF	-al *pertaining to* trans- *through* -crani- *skull*	Through the skull

Exercises

A. Identify the meaning of the word element to help you determine the meaning of the medical term. *One word element can change the entire meaning of the word. Match the term on the left with its correct definition on the right.* **LO 18.8, 18.D**

1. _____ psychotherapy

2. _____ psychoanalysis

3. _____ psychological

4. _____ psychodynamic

a. method of psychotherapy

b. pertaining to the study of the mind

c. interplay between motivation and emotion

d. treatment of mental disorders through talking

▲ **Figure 18.7** Patient Receiving Biofeedback Therapy. ©Will & Deni McInytre/ Photo Researchers, Inc.

LO 18.8 Therapeutic Methods for Mental Disorders (continued)

Psychotherapy is often combined with medications (*see below*). Group psychotherapy, couples therapy, and family therapy also are used frequently.

Eye movement desensitization and reprocessing (**EMDR**) is an eight-phase treatment found to be as effective as CBT for patients suffering from PTSD and for patients who have experienced traumatic situations. The process involves the patient recalling painful memories while the clinician provides sensory input for the patient, such as side-to-side eye movements.

Biofeedback (*Figure 18.7*) and relaxation techniques can be helpful in reducing the tension and spasm associated with psychosomatic disorders.

Brain stimulation treatment, in the form of **electroconvulsive therapy (ECT)**, is an effective treatment for severe depression that is unresponsive to other treatments. Electrodes are attached to the head and a series of electrical shocks are delivered to the brain to induce a brief seizure. The effect of this on the brain cells is not fully understood. Other brain stimulation therapies such as **repetitive transcranial magnetic stimulation** and **deep brain stimulation** are experimental.

The treatment of **posttraumatic stress disorder** is **multimodal**, involving **psychotherapy**, social interventions, and family and patient education. Forms of psychotherapy are **cognitive behavioral therapy (CBT)** and **cognitive processing therapy (CPT)**, in which thoughts and beliefs generated by the trauma are reframed.

Care in a **psychiatric hospital** may be necessary for severe mental illness and can take the form of 24-hour inpatient care, partial or day hospitalization, or residential treatment to provide a temporary supportive place to live.

Abbreviations

ECT	electroconvulsive therapy
EMDR	eye movement desensitization and reprocessing

WORD	PRONUNCIATION	ELEMENTS		DEFINITION
biofeedback (**Note:** This term has no prefix or suffix.)	bye-oh-**FEED**-back	S/ R/ R/	**-back** *back, return* **bio-** *life* **-feed-** *to nourish*	Training techniques to achieve voluntary control of responses to stimuli
cognitive behavioral therapy (**Note:** Behavioral has two suffixes.)	KOG-nih-tiv be-**HAYV**-yur-al **THAIR**-ah-pee	S/ R/ S/ S/ R/	**-ive** *quality of* **cognit-** *thinking* **-al** *pertaining to* **-ior-** *pertaining to* **behav-** *mental activity*	Psychotherapy that emphasizes thoughts and attitudes in one's behavior
cognitive processing therapy	KOG-nih-tiv PROSS-es-ing THAIR-ah-pee	S/ R/ S/ P/ R/	**-ive** *quality of* **cognit-** *thinking* **-ing** *doing* **pro-** *before* **cess-** *going forward* **therapy** Greek *medical treatment*	Psychotherapy to build skills to deal with the effects of trauma in other areas of life
electroconvulsive	ee-**LEK**-troh-kon-**VUL**-siv	S/ R/CF P/ R/	**-ive** *quality of* **electr/o-** *electricity* **-con-** *with* **-vuls-** *tear, pull*	Use of electrical current to produce convulsions

Exercises

A. Elements remain your best clue to the meaning of a medical term. *Match the element in the left column with its correct meaning in the right column.* **LO 18.8**

_____ 1. *electr/o*

_____ 2. *cognit*

_____ 3. *bio*

_____ 4. *pro*

_____ 5. *vuls*

_____ 6. *behav*

_____ 7. *con*

_____ 8. *ior*

_____ 9. *ive*

_____ 10. *feed*

a. mental activity

b. before

c. nourish

d. pertaining to

e. tear

f. life

g. quality of

h. electricity

i. with

j. thinking

B. Apply the elements of the language of medical terminology to answer the following questions. *Fill in the blanks.* **LO 18.8**

1. What are the differences between *behavioral, processing,* and *feedback* therapies?

a. Behavioral therapy _____

_____

b. Processing therapy _____

_____

c. Biofeedback therapy _____

_____

LO 18.9 Pharmacologic Agents Used for Mental Disorders

Psychiatric medications do not cure mental disorders, but they can significantly improve symptoms and help to make other treatments such as psychotherapy more effective. Commonly used classes of prescription medications are discussed below.

Antidepressants work by affecting **neurotransmitters**, especially **serotonin** and **norepinephrine**, and classes of these medications include:

- **Selective serotonin reuptake inhibitors (SSRIs)**, with generic and brand names fluoxetine *(Prozac)*, fluoxamine *(Luvox)*, paroxeline *(Paxil)*, and sertraline *(Zoloft)*.
- **Serotonin and norepinephrine reuptake inhibitors (SNRIs)**, with generic and brand names veriafaxine *(Effexor)*, milnacipran *(Dalcipran)*, and duloxetine *(Cymbalta)*.
- **Tricyclic antidepressants (TCAs)**, with generic names amitriptyline, protryptyline, clomipramine, imipramine, and trimipramine.
- **Monoamine oxidase inhibitors (MAOIs)**, with generic and brand names isocarboxazid *(Marplan)*, phenelzine *(Nardil)*, selegiline *(Ensam)*, and tranylcypromine *(Parnate)*.

Several different classes of medications are used to treat **bipolar disorder:**

- **Mood stabilizers** to control manic or hypomanic episodes are lithium *(Lithobid)*, valproic acid *(Depakene)*, divalproex *(Depakote)*, carbamazepine *(Tegretol)*, and iamotrigine *(Lamictal)*.
- **Antipsychotics** to help persistent symptoms of depression or mania are the newer, second-generation antipsychotics olanzapine *(Zyprexa)*, risperidone *(Risperdal)*, quetiapine *(Seroquel)*, and anipiprazole *(Abilify)*. These medications are also used to treat **schizophrenia**, often in combination with a **benzodiazepine** *(see below)*.
- **Antidepressants** to help manage persistent depression.
- **Antidepressant-psychotic**—the medication *Symbyax* is a combination of the antidepressant fluoxetine and the antipsychotic olanzapine and is approved for the treatment of depressive disorders in bipolar disorder.

Anti-anxiety medications include **benzodiazepines** such as diazepam *(Valium)*, alazolam *(Xanax)*, clonazepam *(Klonopin)*, and lorazepam *(Ativan)* and the **SSRIs** named above *(also see Table 18.1)*.

Stimulants such as dextroamphetamine *(Adderal, Dexedrene)* and methylphenidate *(Ritalin, Metylin)* are used to treat **attention-deficit/hyperactivity disorder (ADHD)** and are also available in long-acting formats.

Sedatives such as **barbiturates** and **benzodiazepines** quiet nervous excitement and newer sedative **hypnotics** such as zolpidem *(Ambien)*, zaleplon *(Sonata)*, and eszopiclone *(Lunesta)* also are used to treat insomnia.

Tranquilizers such as chlorpromazine *(Thorazine)*, haloperidol *(Aloperidin)*, and the benzodiazepines calm like sedatives but without a sleep-inducing effect.

Abbreviations

ADHD	attention-deficit/hyperactivity disorder
MAOI	monoamine oxidase inhibitor
SNRI	serotonin and norepinephrine reuptake inhibitor
SSRI	selective serotonin reuptake inhibitor
TCA	tricyclic antidepressant

Table 18.1 Pharmacotherapy of Panic Disorder

Type of Drug	Effect
Benzodiazepines:	Effective prophylaxis
alprazolam *(Xanax)*	Reduce anticipatory anxiety
clonazepam *(Klonopin)*	Rapid onset of action
lorazepam *(Ativan)*	
diazepam *(Valium)*	
Selective Serotonin Reuptake Inhibitors (SSRIs):	Reduce frequency of attacks
sertraline *(Zoloft)*	Reduce intensity of panic
paroxetine *(Paxil)*	Take 2 weeks to produce effect
fluvoxamine *(Luvox)*	

WORD	PRONUNCIATION	ELEMENTS		DEFINITION
antidepressant	**AN**-tih-dee-**PRESS**-ant	S/ P/ R/	-ant *agent* anti- *against* -depress- *press down*	An agent to suppress the symptoms of depression
antipsychotic	**AN**-tih-sigh-**KOT**-ik	S/ P/ R/CF	-tic *pertaining to* anti- *against* -psych/o *mind*	An agent helpful in the treatment of psychosis
barbiturate	bar-**BIT**-chu-rat	S/ R/	-urate *salt of uric acid* barbit- *barbituric acid*	Central nervous system depressant used as a hyp- notic, anxiolytic, or anticonvulsant
benzodiazepine	ben-zoh-die-**AZ**-ah-peen	S/ P/ R/CF	-pine *pine* -diaze- *organic compound* benz/o- *benzene*	Central nervous system depressant used as a hypnotic, anxiolytic, or anticonvulsant, or to produce amnesia
hypnotic	hip-**NOT**-ik	S/ R/CF	-tic *pertaining to* hypn/o- *sleep*	An agent that promotes sleep
sedative	**SED**-ah-tiv	S/ R/	-tive *quality of* sedat- *to calm*	Agent that calms nervous excitement
stabilizer	**STAY**-bill-ize-er	S/ S/ R/	-er *agent* -ize- *action* stabil- *fixed, steady*	Agent that helps create a steady state
stimulant	**STIM**-you-lant	S/ R/	-ant *forming* stimul- *excite*	Agent that excites functional activity
tranquilizer	**TRANG**-kwih-lie-zer	S/ R/	-izer *affects in a* *particular way* tranquil- *calm, serene*	Agent that calms without sedating or depressing

Exercises

A. Define the types of medications used to treat mental disorders. *Choose the correct definition for the given medication.* **LO 18.9**

1. The action of a **sedative** is to:
   a. suppress the symptoms of depression
   c. promote wakefulness
   b. calm without depressing
   d. calm nervous excitement

2. The action of a **stabilizer** is to:
   a. create a steady state in mood
   c. treat psychosis
   b. excite functional activity
   d. promote sleep

3. The difference between a **tranquilizer** and a **sedative** is:
   a. tranquilizers treat psychosis and sedatives treat mania
   c. tranquilizers are used for inducing sleep and a sedative does not
   b. sedatives treat depression and tranquilizers treat mania
   d. sedatives induce sleep and tranquilizers do not

4. A patient may be prescribed a **hypnotic** to:
   a. promote sleep   b. reduce anxiety   c. prevent hallucinations   d. improve psychotherapy

5. A reason why a physician would prescribe a **benzodiazepine** would be due to its ability to induce:
   a. seizures   b. muscle spasms   c. memory loss   d. insomnia

B. Identify the action of medications and provide the abbreviation. *Read the description of the medications and treatments for mental disorders. Write the correct abbreviation for what is being described.* **LO 18.9, 18.F**

1. This medication affects the neurotransmitters serotonin and norepinephrine: _____

2. This medication is old and works by inhibiting an enzyme that breaks down neurotransmitters: _____

3. This medication prevents the reuptake of only serotonin: _____

Abbreviations

LSD	lysergic acid diethylamide
MDMA	methylenedioxy-methamphetamine
PCP	phencyclidine
THC	tetrahydrocannabinol

LO 18.9 Psychoactive Drugs

Psychoactive drugs are chemicals that change consciousness, awareness, or perception *(Table 18.2)*. The most commonly used drugs are caffeine, tobacco, and alcohol.

Drug abuse refers to the use of drugs that cause emotional or physical harm to an individual as consumption becomes frequent and compulsive.

Addiction occurs when a person feels compelled to use a drug or perform a certain activity and cannot control the use.

Psychological dependence is the mental desire or **craving** for the effects produced by a drug.

Physical dependence is the changes in the body processes that make the drug necessary for daily functioning. If the drug is stopped, the withdrawal symptoms include physical pain as well as intense cravings.

Tolerance occurs when the body adjusts to the effects of the drug, and higher and higher doses produce less and less effect. The brain, liver, heart, and other organs can be damaged.

Comorbidity is the presence of a combination of disorders. It is very common. Alcohol dependence and abuse overlap with almost all other mental disorders, including anxiety disorders, mood disorders, and personality disorders. In such cases, stopping drinking alcohol is only the first step in solving the problem.

Table 18.2 Psychoactive Drugs

Type/Mode of Action	Name	Common Effects	Effects of Abuse
Stimulants ("uppers")	caffeine	Wakefulness, shorter reaction time, alertness	Restlessness, insomnia, heartbeat irregularities
Speed up activity in the central nervous system (CNS)	nicotine	Varies from alertness to calmness, appetite for carbohydrates decreases	Heart disease; high blood pressure; vasoconstriction; bronchitis; emphysema; lung, throat, mouth cancer
	amphetamines	Wakefulness, alertness, increased metabolism, decreased appetite	Nervousness, high blood pressure, delusions, psychosis, convulsions, death
	cocaine	**Euphoria**, high energy, illusions of power	Excitability, paranoia, anxiety, panic, depression, heart failure, death
Depressants ("downers")	alcohol	**1–2 drinks**—reduced inhibitions and anxiety	Blackouts, mental and neurologic impairment, psychosis, cirrhosis of liver, death
Slow down activity in the CNS		**Many drinks**—slow reaction time, poor coordination and memory	Impaired motor and sensory functions, amnesia, loss of consciousness, death
	barbiturates and tranquilizers	Reduced anxiety and tension, sedation	
Narcotics	codeine, opium, morphine, heroin	Euphoria, pleasure, relief of pain	High tolerance of pain, nausea, vomiting, constipation, convulsions, coma, death
Mimic the actions of natural **endorphins**			
Psychedelics	marijuana **(THC)**	Relaxation, euphoria, increased appetite, pain relief	Sensory distortion, hallucinations, paranoia, throat and lung damage
Disrupt normal thought processes	**LSD**, mescaline, **MDMA** (ecstasy), **PCP** (angel dust)	Exhilaration, euphoria, hallucinations, insightful experiences	Panic, extreme delusions, bad trips, paranoia, psychosis

WORD	PRONUNCIATION	ELEMENTS		DEFINITION
comorbidity	koh-mor-**BID**-ih-tee	S/ P/ R/	-ity *condition, state* co- *with, together* -morbid- *disease*	Presence of two or more diseases at the same time
craving	**KRAY**-ving		Latin *desire*	Deep longing or desire
dependence	dee-**PEN**-dense	S/ R/	-ence *forming, quality of* depend- *relying on*	State of needing someone or something
depressant	dee-**PRESS**-ant	S/ P/ R/	-ant *agent* de- *away from* -press- *press down*	Substance that diminishes activity, sensation, or tone
endorphin	en-**DOR**-fin	P/ R/	end- *within* -orphin *morphine*	Natural substance in the brain that has same effect as opium
euphoria	yoo-**FOR**-ee-ah	S/ P/ R/	-ia *condition* eu- *normal* -phor- *bear, carry*	Exaggerated feeling of well-being
narcotic	nar-**KOT**-ik	S/ R/CF	-tic *pertaining to* narc/o- *sleep, stupor*	Drug derived from opium or a synthetic drug with similar effects
psychedelic	sigh-keh-**DEL**-ik	S/ R/CF R/	-ic *pertaining to* psych/e- *mind, soul* -del- *manifest, visible*	Agent that intensifies sensory perception
psychoactive	sigh-koh-**AK**-tiv	S/ R/CF R/	-ive *quality of, nature of* psych/o- *mind, soul* -act- *performance*	Able to alter mood, behavior, and/or cognition
stimulant	**STIM**-you-lant	S/ R/	-ant *agent* stimul- *excite*	Agent that excites or strengthens functional activity
tolerance	**TOL**-er-ants	S/ R/	-ance *condition, state of* toler- *endure*	The capacity to become accustomed to a stimulus or drug

Exercises

A. Review all the new terms you have learned in Table 18.2 and in the above WAD. *From the provided terms below, choose the correct medical term to insert into each of the following sentences. Fill in the blanks.* **LO 18.9, 18.A**

craving   endorphins   narcotic   psychoactive   psychedelic   stimulant   tolerance

1. After repeated use of a drug, a person can build up a _____, which would cause the person to need a higher dose of the drug to get the same effect.

2. Marathon runners can experience the natural stimulatory effect from _____.

3. A(n) _____ mimics the effect of the naturally occurring substance endorphin.

4. A broad category of drugs that can alter mood, behavior, and/or cognition is _____.

5. A(n) _____ is an agent that can create feelings of euphoria along with pain relief and increased appetite.

6. Deep longing or desire is a(n) _____.

7. Nicotine is classified as a(n) _____.

Mental Health

Challenge Your Knowledge

A. Abbreviations. Apply your knowledge of abbreviations to complete the following patient documentation. Choose from the following abbreviations to correctly fill in the blanks. You will have more answers than questions. **(LO 18.1, 18.A, 18.F)**

ECT	CNS	PTSD	BPD	DID	CBT	SSRI	STAT

1. Patient now has developed three distinct, separate personalities. Her _____ is rapidly progressing.

2. Patient is suffering from unipolar depression, and a(n) _____ medication will be prescribed.

3. Patient's nightmares are increasing and are always the same replay of his automobile accident. I am sending him

for _____ in the hopes this can alleviate some of his _____ and help him sleep better. Sleep medication is also prescribed.

4. Patient exhibits frequent mood changes and has become manipulative in her relationship with her parents.

Her _____ is escalating her insecurity.

5. _____ will be prescribed for this patient as a last resort for treatment of his mania.

B. Prefixes. Test your recall of word element meanings by answering the following questions about prefixes. The medical term is given; fill in the blank with the word element that is the prefix, then select the best answer. **(LO 18.2, 18.4, 18.6, 18.D)**

1. *bipolar:* Prefix is _____ and means

  a. one

  b. two

  c. three

  d. four

  e. five

2. *hypochondriasis:* Prefix is _____ and means

  a. after

  b. around

  c. deficient

  d. next to

  e. excessive

3. *depressant:* Prefix is _____ and means

  a. toward

  b. forming

  c. within

  d. away from

  e. around

4. *catatonia:* Prefix is _____ and means

  a. up

  b. around

  c. through

  d. down

  e. beside

5. *addiction:* Prefix is _____ and means

  a. toward

  b. from

  c. for

  d. with

  e. up

6. *euphoria:* Prefix is _____ and means

  a. marketplace

  b. mind

  c. normal

  d. madness

  e. wound

7. *paranoia:* Prefix is _____ and means

    a. above

    b. excessive

    c. abnormal

    d. condition

    e. study of

8. *unipolar:* Prefix is _____ and means

    a. one

    b. four

    c. many

    d. few

    e. none

9. *dissociative:* Prefix is _____ and means

    a. painful

    b. apart

    c. abnormal

    d. irregular

    e. together

10. *convulsive:* Prefix is _____ and means

    a. in front of

    b. with

    c. next to

    d. yellow

    e. small

C. **Language of psychology and psychiatry.** Employ your knowledge of the *language of mental health* to match the statement in the left column with the correct medical vocabulary in the right column. **(LO 18.2, 18.4, 18.6, 18.A)**

_____ **1.** lack of contact with reality	**a.** delusion
_____ **2.** symptoms with no physical cause	**b.** mutism
_____ **3.** refusal or inability to speak	**c.** dissociative amnesia
_____ **4.** legal term, not a diagnosis	**d.** personality
_____ **5.** motor immobility for hours	**e.** mental disorder
_____ **6.** deep sadness and despair	**f.** catatonia
_____ **7.** mistaken belief, contrary to fact	**g.** somatoform
_____ **8.** individual's unique pattern of thought	**h.** psychosis
_____ **9.** unable to recall identity	**i.** depression
_____ **10.** emotional state that is self-destructive	**j.** insanity

Mental Health

D. Define terms that are unique to psychiatry and psychology. Match the terms on the left with their correct description on the right. (LO 18.1, 18.A, 18.E)

_____ 1. psychologist

_____ 2. psychiatrist

_____ 3. psychotherapist

_____ 4. insanity

_____ 5. homicidal

_____ 6. delusion

_____ 7. suicidal

_____ 8. mental disorder

a. wanting to kill oneself

b. fixed false belief held despite strong evidence to the contrary

c. condition in which person is unable to be responsible for his actions

d. licensed specialist in treatment of human mind and behavior

e. wanting to kill another human being

f. medical doctor who diagnoses and treats mental disorders

g. behavior that causes a person to suffer emotional distress

h. practitioner who uses communication to treat mental disorders

Using the terms above in the left column, write the term that best defines the following sentences.

Mr. Robinson has a **(9.)** _____ that he and a female celebrity have a romantic relationship. The celebrity does not know Mr. Robinson. His family recommends that he talk to a professional to talk about this belief. He would benefit from speaking with a **(10.)** _____.

A patient comes to a hospital's emergency department because she feels like taking her life. She is **(11.)** _____. The emergency department contacts a **(12.)** _____, who can effectively diagnose and treat her current condition.

The police have been called to a residence because the adult male in the home has been threatening to kill the other people in the home. He is being suspected of having **(13.)** _____ thoughts. His family has reported that he talks to people that are not in the room and behaves oddly, leading them to think he may be suffering from **(14.)** _____.

E. Latin and Greek terms cannot be further deconstructed into prefix, root, or suffix. You must know them for what they are. Test your knowledge of these terms with this exercise. Match the meaning in the first column with the correct medical term in the second column. (LO 18.1, 18.A)

_____ 1. silent

_____ 2. medical treatment

_____ 3. knowledge

_____ 4. frenzy

_____ 5. desire

_____ 6. forgetfulness

_____ 7. fear

_____ 8. distress

_____ 9. state of mind

a. mania

b. affect

c. mute

d. phobia

e. craving

f. anxiety

g. amnesia

h. cognitive

i. therapy

F. Deconstruction. Deconstruct these medical terms into the meanings of their basic elements. Fill in the chart. If the term does not have an element, write n/a. **(LO 18.D)**

Medical Term	Prefix	Meaning of Prefix	Root/ Combining Form	Meaning of Root/ Combining Form	Suffix	Meaning of Suffix	Meaning of Term
antipsychotic	1.	2.	3.	4.	5.	6.	7.
pyromania	8.	9.	10.	11.	12.	13.	14.
insomnia	15.	16.	17.	18.	19.	20.	21.
comorbidity	22.	23.	24.	25.	26.	27.	28.
endorphin	29.	30.	31.	32.	33.	34.	35.

G. Use your knowledge of the language of psychology and psychiatry. Choose the correct answer to the following questions. *Remember*: There is only one *best* answer. **(LO 18.2, 18.3, 18.6, 18.9, 18.F)**

1. A personality disorder in which a person pulls out his or her body hairs:

   a. PTSD

   b. SAD

   c. TTM

   d. OCD

   e. MPD

2. Manic-depressive disorder is now known as

   a. borderline personality

   b. unipolar disorder

   c. generalized anxiety disorder

   d. mania

   e. bipolar disorder

3. A TCA used to treat depression is

   a. *Prozac*

   b. *Paxil*

   c. amitriptyline

   d. *Zoloft*

   e. duloxetine

4. Significant trauma can lead to

   a. OCD

   b. TTM

   c. SAD

   d. DID

   e. PTSD

5. Select the drug NOT prescribed for a panic disorder:

   a. *Tegretol*

   b. *Paxil*

   c. *Xanax*

   d. *Zoloft*

   e. *Klonopin*

Mental Health

H. Apply your knowledge of the language of psychology and psychiatry. Choose the correct answer to the following questions. *Remember*: There is only one *best* answer. **(LO 18.3, 18.4, 18.5, 18.9, 18.F)**

1. A combination of CBT and EMDR would be treatment for

   a. MPD

   b. DID

   c. OCD

   d. PTSD

   e. TTM

2. No identifiable physical cause to explain physical symptoms characterizes

   a. hypochondriasis

   b. acrophobia

   c. conversion disorder

   d. agoraphobia

   e. somatoform disorder

3. Perceiving things without a stimulation is a(n)

   a. compulsion

   b. delusion

   c. hallucination

   d. obsession

   e. tangent

4. Higher doses of a drug produce less effect:

   a. psychological dependence

   b. addiction

   c. tolerance

   d. physical dependence

   e. comorbidity

5. Schizophrenia is a form of

   a. delusion

   b. phobia

   c. psychosis

   d. mood disorder

   e. obsession

I. Suffixes. Mental health practitioners can be either *psych*ologists or *psych*iatrists. The root/combining form *psych/o-* is present in all the following terms. The suffix is what makes the difference. Challenge your knowledge of the language of mental health by applying the correct term to the following statements. Fill in the blanks, using the choices below. **(LO 18.1, 18.2, 18.D)**

psychopath	psychiatry	psychiatric	psychotherapy
psychotic	psychopharmacotherapy	psychoanalysis	psychology
psychiatrist	psychoanalyst	psychologist	psychological
psychosomatic	psychotherapist	psychosis	psychoactive

1. An agent able to alter mood, behavior, or cognition is _____.

2. Treatment of mental disorders through communication is called _____.

3. _____ is the science concerned with the behavior of humans.

4. A licensed specialist in psychology is known as a _____.

5. The patient's _____ state was starting to affect his physical well-being.

6. A method of psychotherapy is _____.

7. What type of technician is the health care worker in the first CR at the beginning of this chapter?

_____ *technician*

8. Drug treatment of mental disorders is known as _____.

9. A medical specialist in psychiatry is a _____.

10. A practitioner of psychoanalysis is called a _____.

11. Disorder causing mental disruption and loss of contact with reality is _____.

12. _____ is the medical specialty dealing with the diagnosis and treatment of mental disorders.

13. A practitioner of psychotherapy is a _____.

14. A real, physical disorder that, at least in part, has a psychological cause is _____.

15. Pertaining to or affected by psychosis is _____.

16. A serial killer can be termed a _____.

J. **Review Case Study (CR) 18.3 presented below.** Answer the questions as they relate to the Case Study. **(LO 18.5, 18.A)**

Case Report (CR) 18.3

You are

. . . an emergency medical technician (EMT) working in the Emergency Department at Fulwood Medical Center.

Your patient is

. . . Mr. Dante Costello, a 21-year-old homeless man, brought in by the police after he was found sitting in the middle of a main street.

Mr. Costello's explanation is "the voices told me to do it." He has heard voices telling him to do things for the past year. The voices often comment on his behavior. He has isolated himself from other people because "they are not who they say they are, and they are trying to get me." He is taking no drugs or medications and denies any **suicidal** or homicidal intent. Mr. Costello is dirty and disheveled, with poor hygiene. He can give no home or family address. His **affect** is **congruent**, though expressionless. His speech is slow, and his thoughts are disorganized and confused. The most probable diagnosis is **schizophrenia**. He needs to be admitted to the hospital because he is a danger to himself and other people.

---

1. The medical term that defines Mr. Costello's feelings that *"they are trying to get me"* is

   a. paranoia   **b.** catatonia   **c.** mania   **d.** psychotic

2. Which of the following statements best describes the observation that Mr. Costello's *affect is congruent*?

   a. Mr. Costello's thoughts of people trying to get me is unreasonable.

   b. His poor hygiene is due to his homelessness.

   c. The way Mr. Costello describes the way he feels matches what he is experiencing.

   d. Mr. Costello acts upset, but he should not be feeling this way.

3. What signs and symptoms lead to the probable diagnosis of schizophrenia?

   a. thoughts that tell him to harm himself   **b.** slow, disorganized speech

   c. expressionless affect that is opposite of his situation   **d.** he hears voices telling him to do things

©2014 Nucleus Medical Media

In many situations, a team of health professionals can work together to meet the different needs of older patients. The team can include:

- **Geriatricians**, who are physicians who specialize in the care of elderly people.

- **Gerontologists**, who are professionals who study the aging process.

- **Geriatric nurse practitioners (NP)**, who are nurses with special training in the care of the elderly.

- **Social workers, nutritionists, and physical and occupational therapists**, who are also members of the geriatric care team as needs for their services arise.

Chapter Learning Outcomes

To understand the physical and mental changes occurring in the elderly and to communicate these to other health professionals, the patients, and their families, you need to be able to:

LO 19.1 Compare and contrast geriatrics and gerontology.

LO 19.2 Define aging.

LO 19.3 Describe the most up-to-date profile of older Americans.

LO 19.4 Identify disorders of aging.

LO 19.5 Discuss dementia.

LO 19.6 Explain the effects of senescence on the major organ systems.

LO 19.7 Describe the theories of the process of senescence.

LO 19.8 Explain the complex effects of aging.

LO 19.9 Discuss dying and death.

LO 19.10 Recognize important legal issues surrounding dying and death.

LO 19.11 Define death and conditions similar to death.

LO 19.12 Explain the diagnostic and therapeutic procedures and medications used in geriatrics.

LO 19.A Use the medical terms of geriatrics to communicate in writing and document accurately and precisely in any health care setting.

LO 19.B Use the medical terms of geriatrics to communicate verbally with accuracy and precision in any health care setting.

LO 19.C Construct geriatric terms from their word elements (roots, combining forms, prefixes, and suffixes).

LO 19.D Deconstruct geriatric terms into their word elements (roots, combining forms, prefixes, and suffixes).

LO 19.E Identify health professionals involved in the care of geriatric patients.

LO 19.F Identify correct abbreviations for medical terms used in geriatrics.

 ## Case Report (CR) 19.1

You are

. . . a medical assistant working in the Geriatric Clinic at Fulwood Medical Center.

Your patient is

. . . 85-year-old Mr. Mathew Hickman, who has an early dementia and a slow-growing prostate cancer for which he has opted to have no treatment.

With the help of his two daughters and day care providers, he is struggling to stay at home. His daughter, Mrs. Anna Hotteling, is with him.

Mr. Hickman:

"I'm still here, you know, somewhere inside this frail old body. I can remember yesteryear, though I'm a bit hazy about today. I can't hear you like I used to. I have difficulty starting to pee. But I can still put my socks on and tie my shoelaces. I'm not frightened of death, but the process of getting there scares the heck out of me. I've lived my life with dignity. I want to live my death the same way, you know . . . and leave with dry pants."

Lesson 19.1
GERIATRICS

Aging and Senescence

Lesson Objectives

The information in this lesson will enable you to:

19.1.1 Describe the links between geriatrics and gerontology.

19.1.2 Discuss the profile of the elderly population in America.

19.1.3 Discuss aging and senescence.

19.1.4 Describe changes that occur with senescence in major organ systems.

19.1.5 Outline major theories of senescence.

19.1.6 Define death and the key issues in preparing for death.

Keynotes

• **Life span** is the age to which individual humans aspire to live and the process of getting there.

• **Life expectancy** is the average length of life for any given population.

• **Longevity** is living beyond the normal life expectancy.

• **Senescence** is the loss over time of the ability of cells to divide, grow, and function, a process that terminates in death. It is sometimes used interchangeably with the term *aging*.

LO 19.1, 19.2 Aging

Aging is the gradual, spontaneous changes resulting in maturation through childhood, adolescence, and young adulthood and causing a decline in function (rather than maturation) through late adulthood and old age.

Senile is a term used to refer to the characteristics of old age, and **senility** is the general term used in referring to a person who demonstrates a variety of conditions of mental disorders occurring in old age.

Gerontology is the study of the social, mental, and physical aspects of aging. Professionals from diverse fields call themselves **gerontologists**. The medical field that involves the study, care, and treatment of the elderly *(Figure 19.1)* is called **geriatrics**, and a medical specialist in geriatrics is called a **geriatrician**.

LO 19.3 Profile of Older Americans

According to the latest statistics published by the Administration on Aging (AoA) of the U.S. Department of Health and Human Services in 2016:

• The population aged 65 and older numbered 47.8 million in 2015, compared to 40.4 million in 2010, and is projected to more than double to 98 million in 2060.

• About one in every seven, or 14.9% of the population, is 65 or older.

• Persons reaching age 65 have an average life expectancy of an additional 19.4 years (20.6 years for females and 18 years for males).

• Older women outnumber older men at 26.7 million older women to 21.1 million older men.

• In 2015, 22% of persons 65+ were members of racial or ethnic minority populations: 9% were African American, 4% were Asian, and 8% were Hispanic.

• About 29% (13.3 million) of noninstitutionalized older persons live alone (9.3 million women, 4.3 million men).

• The 85+ population is projected to increase from 6.2 million to 14.6 million in 2040.

• Over 4.5 million adults (10%) were below the poverty level in 2015.

• Most older people have at least one chronic medical condition, and the average is six conditions.

• The most frequently occurring conditions among the elderly are:

  • Arthritis (50%)

  • Hypertension (38%)

  • All types of heart disease (32%)

  • Any cancer (22%)

  • Diabetes (18%)

  • **Alzheimer disease** (13%). It accounts for 70% of all **dementias**.

▲ **Figure 19.1** **Elderly Couple.**
©Darren Greenwood/Design Pics RF

WORD	PRONUNCIATION	ELEMENTS		DEFINITION
aging aged	AY-jing AY-jid		Latin *aging* Latin *being old*	The process of human maturation and decline Having lived to an advanced age
Alzheimer disease	AWLZ-high-mer diz-EEZ	P/ R/	Alois Alzheimer, 1864–1915, German neurologist dis- *apart* -ease *normal function*	Common form of dementia
dementia	dee-MEN-shee-ah	S/ P/ R/	-ia *condition* de- *without* -ment- *mind*	Chronic, progressive, irreversible loss of the mind's cognitive and intellectual functions
geriatrics (**Note:** This term contains two roots.) geriatrician	jer-ee-AT-riks jer-ee-ah-TRISH-an	S/ R/ R/ S/	-ics *knowledge of* ger- *old age* -iatr- *medical treatment* -ician *expert*	Medical specialty that deals with the problems of old age Medical specialist in geriatrics
gerontology	jer-on-TOL-oh-jee	S/ R/CF	-logy *study of* geront/o- *process* *of aging*	Study of the process and problems of aging
life expectancy life span	LIFE ek-SPEK-tan-see LIFE SPAN	S/ R/	-ancy *state of* expect- *await* **life** Old English *life* **span** Old English *reach* or *stretch*	Statistical determination of the number of years an individual is expected to live The age that a person reaches
longevity	lon-JEV-ih-tee	S/ R/	-ity *condition, state* longev- *long life*	Duration of life beyond the normal expectation
senescence	seh-NES-ens	S/ R/	-ence *state of, quality of* senesc- *growing old*	The state of being old
senile senility	SEE-nile seh-NIL-ih-tee	S/ R/ S/ R/	-ile *capability* sen- *old age* -ity *condition, state* senil- *characteristic of* *old age*	Characteristic of old age Mental disorders occurring in old age

Exercise

A. Choose the correct definition for each of the following medical terms from the *languages of geriatrics and gerontology*.
Match the medical term in the first column with its correct meaning in the second column. **LO 19.1, 19.2, 19.3**

_____ **1.** senile

_____ **2.** longevity

_____ **3.** senility

_____ **4.** geriatrics

_____ **5.** Alzheimer disease

_____ **6.** gerontology

_____ **7.** life expectancy

_____ **8.** life span

a. mental disorders that occur in old age

b. new field that involves study, care, and treatment of the elderly

c. common form of dementia

d. characteristic of old age

e. duration of life beyond the normal expected time

f. the age a person reaches

g. study of the process and problems of aging

h. the number of years a person is expected to live

▲ **Figure 19.2** Elderly Woman Injured in a Fall. ©Cristina Pedrazzini/Photo Researchers, Inc.

LO 19.4 Specific Disorders of Aging

The major categories of impairment in elderly people as they begin to fail (the so-called **Geriatric Giants**) include:

• immobility

• instability

• incontinence

• impaired intellect/memory

    Immobility is a common pathway produced by many diseases and problems, particularly those that involve prolonged bed rest, immobilization, or inactivity. It can also occur when it is self-imposed—when elderly patients do not exercise to keep limbs flexible, promote circulation, and improve well-being. Many factors influencing the elderly's state of immobility are **iatrogenic**, or arising from medical regimens, institutional policies, and resident and staff characteristics in nursing homes. The negative consequences of immobility often can be avoided with careful and vigilant medical and nursing management.

    Instability, or difficulty in balance *(Figure 19.2)*, is often the first problem that the elderly person encounters. The instability and associated falls can result from a single disease process or the accumulated effects of multiple diseases. It is essential to take a careful, detailed history and examination to define all the factors contributing to the instability and to develop the appropriate interventions to prevent future falls. Instability and falling are not inevitable in aging but are problems that arise from identifiable disabilities that are often treatable.

    Incontinence is the inability to prevent the discharge of urine or feces. It is a common, but never normal, part of aging. In the nursing home population, some 50% of residents have urinary incontinence. There are five main types of urinary incontinence:

• **Urge incontinence,** the loss of urine before one can get to the toilet, is the most common form in the elderly. It can be caused by strokes, multiple sclerosis, dementia, and pelvic floor atrophy in women or prostate enlargement in men.

• **Stress incontinence** is caused by weak bladder muscles. It occurs when the abdominal pressure when you cough, sneeze, laugh, or climb stairs overcomes the closing pressure of the bladder.

• **Overflow incontinence** is rare. It occurs when the bladder never completely empties and leaks small amounts of urine.

• **Functional incontinence** is an inability to reach the toilet in time; for example, due to arthritis, stroke, or dementia.

• **Mixed incontinence** is usually a combination of stress and urge incontinence.

    Fecal incontinence occurs in about one-third of the elderly in institutional care, and is the second most common reason for committing the elderly to a nursing home. It can be produced by local causes such as chronic laxative abuse or muscle damage to the sphincter muscles in surgery or childbirth. It also is seen in dementia, multiple sclerosis, and diabetes.

    Impaired intellect/memory that is present for at least six months is called **dementia**. The **cognitive** functions that are affected include decision making, judgment, memory, thinking, reasoning, and verbal communication. Dementia is not a normal part of aging, but advancing age is the greatest risk factor. More than 5 million people aged 65 and older have dementia and more than 500,000 people under 65 have early-onset dementia.

    Alzheimer disease accounts for 70% of all dementias; it is progressive and there is no cure. Other types of dementia are vascular dementia, frontotemporal dementia, and dementia with **Lewy bodies**.

    Delirium is a set of symptoms including an inability to focus attention; mental confusion; impairments in awareness, time, and space; and perhaps **hallucinations**. It often has a fluctuating course, and it can follow head trauma, stroke, drug withdrawal, hypoxia, hypoglycemia, physical illness of almost every type, and the use of opiates and benzodiazepines. Delirium is probably the single most common disorder affecting adults in hospitals and occurs in 30–40% of elderly hospitalized patients and in up to 80% of intensive care unit (ICU) patients. Treatment is targeted on the underlying disease causing the delirium.

WORD	PRONUNCIATION	ELEMENTS		DEFINITION
cognition	kog-**NIH**-shun	S/	-ion *process*	Process of acquiring knowledge through thinking and learning
		R/	**cognit-** *thinking*	
cognitive (adj)	**KOG**-nih-tiv	S/	-ive *quality of*	Pertaining to the mental activities of thinking and learning
dementia	dee-**MEN**-she-ah	S/	-ia *condition*	Chronic, progressive, and irreversible loss of the mind's cognitive and intellectual functions
		P/	**de-** *without*	
		R/	**-ment-** *mind*	
hallucination	hah-loo-sih-**NAY**-shun	S/	-ation *process*	Perception of an object or event when there is no such thing present
		R/	**hallucin-** *imagination*	
iatrogenic	eye-at-roh-**JEN**-ik	S/	-ic *pertaining to*	An unfavorable response to medical or surgical treatment, caused by the treatment itself
		P/	**iatro-** *medical treatment*	
		R/	**-gen-** *producing*	

Exercises

A. Medical terms related to geriatrics. *Select the correct answer as it relates to terms and elements related to geriatrics.* **LO 19.4, 19.D**

1. The patient does not have the strength to walk because he is confined to a bed. The inability to walk has a(n) _____ cause.

   a. cognitive   **b.** iatrogenic   **c.** dementia   **d.** skeletal

2. The general term that relates to a progressive, irreversible loss of cognitive and intellectual functions:

   a. senility   **b.** incontinence   **c.** dementia   **d.** Alzheimer disease

3. The medical term that contains the root meaning **thinking:**

   a. iatrogenic   **b.** dementia   **c.** hallucination   **d.** cognition

4. The root in the term **hallucination** means:

   a. recognition   **b.** mind   **c.** imagination   **d.** physician

5. The suffix *-ia* means:

   a. condition   **b.** pertaining to   **c.** producing   **d.** without

B. Use the new medical terminology you have learned in this chapter to select the correct answer for each question. **LO 19.4**

1. What is incontinence? (Read carefully and choose the BEST answer.)

   a. inability to prevent the discharge of urine

   b. inability to prevent the discharge of feces

   c. inability to prevent the discharge of flatus

   d. inability to prevent the discharge of urine or feces

   e. inability to prevent diarrhea

2. Coughing can cause a specific type of urinary incontinence. What is the medical term for this condition?

   a. stress incontinence

   b. urge incontinence

   c. overflow incontinence

   d. functional incontinence

   e. mixed incontinence

(a)

(b)

▲ **Figure 19.3** MRI Scans. (a) Normal brain; (b) brain scan of individual with Alzheimer disease showing cerebral atrophy (yellow). ©Howard J. Radzyner/Diomedia/Medical Images RM

Abbreviations

AD	Alzheimer disease
ADLs	activities of daily living
DLB	dementia with Lewy bodies
FTLD	frontotemporal lobar degeneration
PD	Parkinson disease
PDA	personal digital assistant
PET	positron emission tomography
RT	reminiscence therapy
SPECT	single photon emission computerized tomography

LO 19.5 Dementia

Dementia is an overall term for diseases characterized by a decline in memory and **cognitive** (thinking) skills. In mild dementia, there is evidence of cognitive decline and recent memory loss that do not interfere with **activities of daily living (ADLs)**. Then dementia progresses to cause significant cognitive decline in memory, language, and learning, sufficient to interfere with independence in ADLs. Ultimately confusion; disorientation; and difficulty speaking, swallowing, and walking take away independent living. All dementias are caused by damage inside and around the brain's neurons with different pathological changes. There is no cure.

Alzheimer disease (AD) accounts for 60% to 80% of dementias and is a slowly progressive dementia that begins well before clinical symptoms arise. **Vascular dementia** arises from infarcts (strokes) or bleeding into the brain and accounts for about 10% of dementia cases. In older individuals, pathologic changes of both Alzheimer and vascular dementia are found; this is called **mixed dementia**.

Dementia with Lewy bodies (DLB), frontotemporal lobar degeneration (FTLD), and **Parkinson disease (PD)** are other causes of dementia.

Diagnosis of dementia is often difficult in the early stages, particularly as there is no one simple test for it. Initial assessment involves a detailed history from the patient and a close family member; physical examination and blood tests to identify other conditions present; and tests of mental abilities using both pen-and-paper tests and questions. These will test memory, language, and **visuospatial** skills, and can provide a baseline to measure future changes. Computerized tomography (CT) and magnetic resonance imaging (MRI) scans can show structural brain changes (*Figure 19.3*). If the diagnosis of the type of dementia is still unclear, single photon emission computerized tomography **(SPECT)** and positron emission tomography **(PET)** scans showing changes in brain activity may help clarify the diagnosis.

Treatment options, as there is no cure, aim to maximize the patient's quality of life and ability to communicate. **Environmental modifications** such as reducing visual and auditory clutter, providing cues (simple signs), and displaying personal items can improve memory, awareness, and orientation. External memory aids such as personal digital assistants **(PDAs)**, message boards, and pictures can help with memory difficulties.

Reminiscence therapy (RT) uses photographs, familiar items, past activities and experiences to improve the patient's memory to reinforce understanding and awareness of the environment. Other similar programs attempt to achieve similar goals.

Medications cannot stop dementia from progressing, but they may lessen symptoms of memory loss and confusion for a limited time. For treating Alzheimer disease, the FDA has approved two types of medications: **cholinesterase inhibitors** donepezil *(Ancept)*, rivastigmine *(Exelon)*, and galantamine *(Razadyne)*, as well as **memantine** *(Namenda)*, which has benefits similar to those induced by cholinesterase inhibitors.

WORD	PRONUNCIATION		ELEMENTS	DEFINITION
Alzheimer disease	**AWLZ**-high-mer diz-**EEZ**	P/ R/	Alois Alzheimer, 1894-1915, German neurologist **dis-** *apart* **-ease** *normal function*	Most common form of dementia
Lewy body	**LOO**-ee **BOD**-ee		Frederic Lewy, 1895–1950, German neurologist **body** Old English *body*	Abnormal cell found in brain in this form of dementia
visuospatial	**VIZ**-you-oh-**SPAY**-shall	S/ R/CF R/	**-ial** *pertaining to* **visu/o-** *vision* **-spat-** *space*	Denoting the ability to conceptualize visual representations and spatial relationships in learning

Exercises

A. Use abbreviations within medical documentation. *Read the descriptions of the conditions and diagnosis related to dementia. Use the appropriate abbreviation to complete the sentence. Fill in the blanks.* **LO 19.5, 19.F**

1. Cholinesterase inhibitors can be used to treat _____.

2. People with dementia may not be able to perform _____, such as brushing their hair, cooking meals, and routine cleaning tasks.

3. If all other diagnostic methods are unable to confirm the diagnosis of dementia, a(n) _____ scan may show changes in brain activity to clarify the diagnosis.

B. Diagnosis and treatment for dementia. *Choose the correct answer for each statement.* **LO 19.5**

1. Use of past activities and experiences to help patient with dementia with understanding of current environment:

   a. Namenda medication

   b. physical therapy

   c. environmental modifications

   d. reminiscence therapy

2. There is no definitive diagnosis for dementia.

   a. True

   b. False

3. Medications such as rivastigmine *(Exelon)* will cure Alzheimer disease.

   a. True

   b. False

▲ **Figure 19.4** Senescence of the Skin. Elderly Tibetan woman with her granddaughter. ©Jane Sweeney/Art Directors & TRIP/Alamy Stock Photo

Keynotes

- Visual acuity starts to decline very early in life. Eye exercises can help prevent this normal occurrence.

- Exercise and good nutrition help prevent osteopenia.

- Exercise and good nutrition help prevent muscle degeneration.

- Exercising your brain enhances your quality of life in old age.

- Exercise and good nutrition extend **longevity** and enhance the quality of life.

- Bronchitis and emphysema, the **chronic obstructive pulmonary diseases (COPDs),** are the cumulative effects of cigarette smoking and are a leading cause of death in old age.

- The kidneys of an 80-year-old receive only half as much blood as those of a 30-year-old because of atherosclerosis.

- Because they have lowered immunity, the elderly are advised to receive vaccinations against influenza and other infections.

LO 19.6 Senescence of Organ Systems

Organ systems begin to show signs of senescence at very different ages and do not degenerate at the same speed. Most physiologic studies show general peak physical performance occurs during a person's twenties, but surprisingly, **autopsies (postmortems)** in children will often reveal atherosclerosis in the arteries supplying the heart. Autopsies are usually performed by a **pathologist** or a medical examiner.

Integumentary system *(see Chapter 4)* changes begin in a person's forties. Melanocytes die, and hair becomes gray and thinner. The skin becomes paper thin, loses elasticity, and hangs loose, and wrinkles appear *(Figure 19.4)*. Flat brown-black spots called **senile lentigines** (age spots) appear on the back of the hands and areas exposed to sunlight.

Special senses start to decline in the twenties. Visual acuity declines at that time. In the forties, presbyopia *(see Chapter 16)* begins, and many people develop cataracts later, in old age. Hearing loss occurs as the ossicles become stiffer and the number of cochlear hair cells *(see Chapter 16)* declines—the cause of Mr. Hickman's hearing loss in Case Report 19.1. Taste and smell also are blunted late in life, as taste cells and olfactory buds decline in number.

Skeletal system *(see Chapter 14)* changes appear during a person's thirties, as osteoblasts become less active than osteoclasts. The result is osteopenia, which later develops into osteoporosis—particularly in postmenopausal women. The joints of people in their later years have less synovial fluid and thinner articular cartilage, and often, osteoarthritis results.

Muscular system *(see Chapter 15)* changes occur with age as muscle mass is lost (**sarcopenia**) and replaced with fat. As muscle **atrophies**, there are fewer muscle fibers to do the work; as a result, the available blood supply decreases. Tasks that used to be easy become difficult, such as buttoning shirts and tying shoelaces—one of the daily triumphs Mr. Hickman mentioned in Case Report 19.1.

Nervous system *(see Chapter 9)* changes begin around age 30, when the brain weighs twice as much as it does at age 75. Motor coordination, intellectual function, and short-term memory decline more quickly than long-term memory and language skills.

Cardiovascular systems *(see Chapter 10)* always have coronary artery atherosclerosis, even at a very early age. As a result, when aging myocardial cells die, the heart wall gets thinner and weaker, and cardiac output declines. This causes the decline in physical capabilities with aging. Atherosclerotic plaques narrow arteries and trigger thrombosis, leading to strokes and heart attacks. In veins, valves become weaker, and blood flows back and pools in the legs, leading to poor venous return to the heart and heart failure.

Respiratory system *(see Chapter 13)* changes are noticeable in the thirties, as pulmonary ventilation declines. This decline is a factor in the gradual loss of stamina that occurs as people age. The rib cage becomes less flexible, and the lungs become less elastic and have fewer alveoli. Respiratory function declines. As respiratory health declines, hypoxic degenerative changes occur in all the other organ systems.

Urinary system *(see Chapter 6)* changes begin in a person's twenties, when the number of nephrons starts to decline. Later in life, many of the remaining glomeruli become atherosclerotic. The body's glomerular filtration rate (GFR) decreases, and the kidneys become less efficient. For example, drug doses in the elderly are generally lower than those for younger people because drugs cannot be cleared from the elderly's blood as rapidly.

Immune system *(see Chapter 12)* function declines in the elderly, as the amounts of lymphatic tissue and red bone marrow in their bodies decrease with age. This leads to a reduction in both cellular and humoral (antibody) immunity. As a result, the elderly have lower levels of protection against infectious diseases and cancer.

Specific **disorders of senescence** and their terminology are described in each of the body system chapters in this book.

WORD	PRONUNCIATION		ELEMENTS	DEFINITION
atrophy atrophies (verb)	**AT**-roh-fee **AT**-roh-feez	P/ R/	a- *without* -trophy *development, nourishment*	Wasting or diminished volume of a tissue or organ
autopsy postmortem (syn)	**AWE**-top-see post-**MOR**-tem	S/ P/ P/	-opsy *to view* aut- *self, same* post- *after* mortem Latin *death*	Examination of the body and organs of a dead person to determine the cause of death
lentigo lentigines (pl)	len-**TIE**-go len-**TIHJ**-ih-neez		Greek *lentil*	Age spot; small, flat, brown-black spot in the skin of older people
pathologist	pa-**THOL**-oh-jist	S/ R/CF	-logist *one who studies, specialist* path/o- *disease*	A specialist in pathology (study of disease or characteristics of a particular disease)
sarcopenia	sar-koh-**PEE**-nee-ah	S/ R/CF	-penia *deficiency* sarc/o- *flesh*	Progressive loss of muscle mass and strength in aging

Exercises

A. Proper pronunciation of medical terms. *Identify the proper pronunciation of the bolded area of each medical term.* **LO 19.B, 19.D**

1. sarco**pe**nia

    a. pie   **b.** pay   **c.** pee   **d.** peh

2. len**ti**go

    a. tie   **b.** tay   **c.** tee   **d.** the

3. lentig**i**nes

    a. nighs   **b.** nays   **c.** knees   **d.** nose

B. Choose the correct answer for the following questions. **LO 19.6**

1. What does the medical term **lentigo** identify?

    a. skin lesion   **b.** skin tumor   **c.** skin type   **d.** skin spots   **e.** skin wrinkles

2. What is the correct plural of **lentigo**?

    a. lentigos   **b.** lentigoes   **c.** lentigones   **d.** lentigines   **e.** lentigons

3. Another medical term used for **autopsy** is

    a. senescence   **b.** senility   **c.** geriatrics   **d.** atrophy   **e.** postmortem

4. What is the correct element that means *after*?

    a. *post*   **b.** *em*   **c.** *mort*   **d.** *auto*   **e.** *patho*

5. What is the purpose of a *postmortem*?

    a. to discover the patient's blood type

    c. to discover the weight of the body organs

    b. to discover the cause of death

    d. to discover the body's final blood volume

    e. to discover the presence of foreign bodies

▲ **Figure 19.5** Elderly Woman Confused about Her Medications.

©Dennis MacDonald/PhotoEdit Inc.

LO 19.7 Theories of Senescence

The causes of **senescence** are unknown. **Heredity** plays a role because longevity or early death tends to run in families. Theories of senescence include:

- **Protein abnormalities.** One-quarter of the body's protein is collagen. With age, collagen and other proteins show abnormal structures in their cells and tissues, and become less soluble and more rigid. The cells accumulate more of these dysfunctional proteins as they age, and their functions are impaired, leading to **senescent** changes.

- **Free radicals.** These are chemical particles with an extra electron. For example, the stable oxygen molecule (O_2) has two atoms with many electrons. If it picks up an extra electron through some metabolic reaction, by radiation, or by chemical action, it becomes a free radical. The free radical's life is short because it combines quickly with other molecules that, in turn, become free radicals with the addition of the extra electron. A chain reaction occurs as more and more molecules become free radicals. Among the damage they cause are cancer, myocardial infarction, and perhaps senescence. They can be neutralized by **antioxidants.**

- **Autoimmune-altered molecules** (*see Chapter 12*). These molecules may be recognized as foreign antigens, and an immune response may be generated against the body's own tissues. This theory is helped by the fact that autoimmune diseases such as rheumatoid arthritis are more common in old age.

LO 19.8 Complex Effects of Aging

The appearance of symptoms of aging depends on the remaining healthy reserves of organs as they decline with age. For example, renal **impairment** can be part of aging, but renal **failure** is not. This decline in physiological reserve can produce complications from mild problems. For example, dehydration in mild gastroenteritis can cause confusion in the elderly, which in turn can lead to a fall and a fractured femur.

Many diseases in elderly persons may present with very vague and nonspecific symptoms. For example, pneumonia can present with low-grade fever, confusion, or falls rather than with the high fever and cough seen in younger adults. **Delirium** in the elderly can be caused by something as simple as constipation. Some elderly people may have difficulty describing their symptoms, particularly if they have cognitive impairment. Therefore, time and care have to be taken to discover the root cause.

Many elderly patients take multiple **medications**, sometimes prescribed by different specialists without reference to other medications prescribed by other specialists. This **polypharmacy** can result in **adverse** drug interactions (*Figure 19.5*). In addition, most drugs are excreted by the liver or kidneys, either of which can be impaired in the elderly. As a result, the dosage of medications may need to be adjusted to avoid excessive levels in the blood and undesirable side effects.

Aging has some benefits and advantages for many people. These include:

- Increased knowledge of life (wisdom).
- Freedom from many of the day-to-day responsibilities that working adults face.
- Freedom to be gentle and grow with oneself.
- Time to enjoy family.
- Freedom to choose to participate in childrearing for grandchildren or other relatives.
- Increased participation in volunteer organizations.

Keynotes

- People older than 65 make up 13% of the population and use about 30% of all prescriptions written.
- A study of 27,600 Medicare patients documented more than 1,500 adverse drug effects (**ADEs**) in a single year.
- When a physician or nurse practitioner or a pharmacist oversees an elderly patient's medication regimen, drug-related problems are less likely to occur.
- The elderly patient should bring all of his/her medications to every hospital or office visit, including prescription, over-the-counter (**OTC**) drugs, and all supplements.

Abbreviations

ADE	adverse drug effect
OTC	over the counter

WORD	PRONUNCIATION	ELEMENTS		DEFINITION
antioxidant	an-tee-**OKS**-ih-dant	S/ P/ R/	-ant *forming* **anti-** *against* **-oxid-** *oxidize*	Substance that can prevent cell damage by neutralizing free radicals
delirium	deh-**LIR**-ee-um	S/ R/	-um *structure* **deliri-** *confusion, disorientation*	Acute altered state of consciousness with agitation and disorientation
free radical	FREE **RAD**-ih-kal	 S/ R/	**free** Old English *free* -al *pertaining to* **radic-** *root*	Short-lived product of oxidation in a cell that can be damaging to the cell
heredity	heh-**RED**-ih-tee	S/ R/	-ity *condition, state* **hered-** *inherited through genes*	Transmission of characteristics from parents to offspring through genes
polypharmacy	pol-ee-**FAR**-mah-see	P/ R/	**poly-** *many* **-pharmacy** *drug*	The administration of many drugs at the same time
senescence senescent (adj)	seh-**NES**-ens	S/ R/ S/	-ence *state of, quality of* **senesc-** *growing old* -ent *end result, state of*	The state of being old Growing old

Exercises

A. Complete the sentences with the correct medical term. *Fill in the blanks.* **LO 19.8, 19.A**

1. Elderly persons often need care from several health care providers. Often, the specialists prescribe medications without knowing all of the other medications a patient may be taking. It is possible for patients to suffer from the interaction *multiple medications* (1) _____.

2. A person's life span can be affected by *inherited traits* (2) _____. The effect of *products that can damage cells* (3) _____ can also play a role. A healthy diet rich in *substances that neutralize free radicals* (4) _____ can be helpful.

B. Use the appropriate abbreviation to complete the sentence. *Fill in the blanks.* **LO 19.F**

1. Medications that do not require a prescription: _____

2. Unintended effects of medications: _____

Lesson 19.2
GERIATRICS

Dying and Death

Lesson Objectives

In the past century in the United States, life expectancy has risen from age 47 to 84 and individuals over 90 are now the most rapidly growing portion of the population. While death can occur without warning in assaults and trauma, and sudden death can occur in certain illnesses, death usually comes at the end of a chronic illness or the frailty of old age. As a result, more and more health professionals of different disciplines are becoming involved in the care of dying elderly patients. The information in this lesson will enable you to:

19.2.1 Describe the components of an advance medical directive.

19.2.2 Recognize the value of a Physician's Order for Life-Sustaining Treatment (POLST) document.

19.2.3 Define palliative care.

19.2.4 Differentiate between brain death, persistent vegetative state, and minimally conscious state.

Keynote

- Both PVS and MCS differ from **coma,** in which the individual is unresponsive and keeps his/her eyes closed.

Abbreviations

DNR	do not resuscitate
HIPAA	Health Insurance Portability and Accountability Act
MCS	minimally conscious state
POLST	Physician's Orders for Life-Sustaining Treatment

📁 Case Report (CR) 19.2

You are
. . . a social worker in the Breast Care Clinic at Fulwood Medical Center.

Your patient is
. . . Mrs. Faye Hampson, a 42-year-old woman who has breast cancer that has metastasized to the bones in her arms and spine, generating pain for which she takes morphine orally five or six times each day. She also has metastases in her brain. She has two daughters, aged 10 and 6.

Mrs. Hampson has mutation of the genes BRCA1 and BRCA2. She has requested that the two girls not be genetically tested until they are old enough to request the tests themselves.

Mrs. Hampson is having difficulty sitting, standing, walking, and sleeping because of bone pain. She remarks, "I want to be as comfortable as possible, even if it shortens my life."

After conducting the interview with Mrs. Hampson, you decide to recommend to her and to the team caring for her that she be admitted to hospice care.

LO 19.9 Death

Dying is inevitable. Just as fetal life in the womb is a preparation for birth, living and aging are a preparation for **death**. Death is a deeply personal, yet highly subjective experience. You can prepare for death in different ways, most of which are done with your family's involvement and many of which require legal assistance.

LO 19.10 Legal Issues in Dying and Death

Medical issues are clearly significant in the process of dying. Your views on the types and extent of medical treatment you wish to have during the process of dying should be clearly stated. This is done through an **advance medical directive**, which consists of two documents:

1. **Medical (durable) power of attorney**, in which you appoint someone you know and trust as your agent and authorize that person to make medical decisions for you when you cannot.

2. **Living will**, in which you provide a set of instructions detailing what treatment you do and do not want in a terminal illness, including **hospice** treatment. If there are special instructions, such as **do not resuscitate (DNR),** these must be stated clearly. It should also include a Health Insurance Portability and Accountability Act **(HIPAA) authorization** that enables your agent to receive the medical information about you that is necessary for making decisions about treatment. This is needed because HIPAA imposes tough privacy-of-medical-information rules on doctors and hospitals.

Your primary care doctor should have a copy of your advance medical directive and read the document with you. This document should be part of your medical record. In some states, a document known as **Physician's Orders for Life-Sustaining Treatment (POLST)** is now available. This formal document is effectively a physician's order statement that is based on the patient's current medical condition and wishes. It has specific sections that list the patient's wishes for cardiopulmonary resuscitation (CPR), medical interventions, and artificially administered nutrition. It becomes a valid, durable component of the patient's medical record that health professionals must obey.

WORD	PRONUNCIATION	ELEMENTS		DEFINITION
advance medical directive	ad-**VANTS** **MED**-ih-kal die-**REK**-tiv	S/ R/ S/ R/	**advance** Latin *in front* **-al** *pertaining to* **medic-** *medicine* **-ive** *nature of, pertaining to* **direct-** *straight*	Legal document signed by the patient dealing with issues of prolonging or ending life in the event of life-threatening illness
death	DETH		Old English *to die*	Total and permanent cessation of all vital functions

Exercises

A. Use abbreviations that are commonly part of verbal and written communication. *Choose the correct abbreviation for the described medical term.* **LO 19.10, 19.F**

1. Document that allows the release of a patient's private medical information.

   a. DNR   **b.** POLST   **c.** ADL   **d.** HIPAA

2. This document provides instructions for a patient's care in a specific condition, such as which medical interventions should be administered:

   a. POLST   **b.** HIPAA   **c.** DNR   **d.** BD

B. List the documents that form a complete Advance Medical Directive. **LO 19.10**

_____

_____

_____

C. What is the single critical difference between an Advance Medical Directive and a POLST document? **LO 19.10, 19.F**

_____

_____

▲ **Figure 19.6** Flat Line on Electroencephalogram Shows Brain Death. ©Pasieka/SPL/Photo Researchers, Inc.

LO 19.10 Legal Issues in Dying and Death (continued)

The process of dying, rather than death itself, is of concern to most elderly people. Dying should be free from physical and emotional pain and dignified, and occurring in the place most acceptable, usually the home. Death with Dignity state laws allow terminally ill adults to voluntarily request and receive a prescription medication from their physician to enable them to die in a peaceful, humane, and dignified manner. As of December 2016, these laws have been passed in Oregon, Vermont, Washington, Colorado, Montana, and California. In January 2017, bills to pass similar laws were introduced in New York, Maryland, Massachusetts, and Pennsylvania.

A **hospice** provides **palliative care** and provides for the emotional and spiritual needs of terminally ill patients and their loved ones at an inpatient facility or in the patient's home. Palliative care is designed to provide pain and symptom management to maintain the highest quality of life for as long as life remains.

LO 19.11 Legal Definition of Death

Just as the moment life begins is controversial, there is no universally accepted moment of biological death.

In most states in the United States, death is now defined in terms of **brain death (BD),** when there is no cerebral or brainstem activity and the electroencephalogram (EEG) is flat for a specific length of time *(Figure 19.6)*. Two other conditions involving brain damage and loss of brain function cause medical difficulty and should be addressed in your living will:

1. **Persistent vegetative state (PVS)** occurs in people who suffer enough brain damage that they are unaware of themselves or their surroundings, even though their eyes are open. Yet they still have certain reflexes and can breathe and pump blood because the brainstem still functions. Even reflex events like crying and smiling and the sleep–wake cycle can be seen. With medical care and artificial feeding, patients can survive for decades.

2. **Minimally conscious state (MCS)** is a condition of severely altered consciousness in which minimal evidence of awareness of self or surroundings is demonstrated. There is inconsistent communication or command following. However, positron emission tomography (PET) scans of MCS patients show cortical function when their loved ones speak to them. They are more likely to improve than are PVS patients.

LO 19.12 Diagnostic and Therapeutic Procedures and Medications

Abbreviations	
BD	brain death
PVS	persistent vegetative state

The procedures used in geriatrics are identical to the procedures used for other patients and have been described in previous chapters on body systems. However, history taking and observing the elderly patient to determine his or her ability to live independently are of great importance. A Katz Activities of Daily Living Scale uses history taking to score patients in the areas of eating, dressing, bathing, transferring (e.g., moving in and out of bed), toileting, and continence.

WORD	PRONUNCIATION		ELEMENTS	DEFINITION
hospice	**HOS**-pis		Latin *lodging*	Facility or program that provides care to the dying and their families
palliative care	**PAL**-ee-ah-tiv KAIR	S/ R/ R/	**-ive** *nature of, pertaining to* **palliat-** *reduce suffering* **care** *be responsible for*	Care that relieves symptoms and pain without curing
vegetative	**VEJ**-eh-tay-tiv	S/ R/	**-ive** *nature of, pertaining to* **vegetat-** *growth*	Functioning unconsciously as plant life is assumed to do

Exercises

A. Differentiate between medical terms associated with death and dying. *Match the term on the left with its correct definition on the right.*
LO 19.10, 19.11

_____ 1. hospice

_____ 2. minimally conscious state

_____ 3. palliative care

_____ 4. vegetative state

_____ 5. death

a. cessation of life

b. patient is completely unaware of surroundings

c. facility to provide care for dying patients and their families

d. patient that does not demonstrate awareness of self or surroundings

e. care that treats but does not cure

Geriatrics

Challenge Your Knowledge

A. **Abbreviations.** Regardless of whether you are an administrative or clinical health care worker, you will be reading patient documentation with abbreviations, which can mean a diagnosis, procedure, disease, and so on. To interpret this documentation correctly and safely, you must know the meanings of the abbreviations. Challenge yourself to *define* each of the following abbreviations correctly. Fill in the chart. **(LO 19.F)**

Abbreviation	Meaning of Abbreviation
BD	1.
MCS	2.
PVS	3.

B. **Elements.** Even though these elements do not appear here in the context of a medical term, you should be able to recognize their meaning out of context. Match the correct element in the left column with its meaning in the right column. Fill in the blanks. **(LO 19.D)**

_____ **1.** *ician*   **a.** after

_____ **2.** *ity*   **b.** old age

_____ **3.** *trophy*   **c.** against

_____ **4.** *sarc/o*   **d.** without

_____ **5.** *ile*   **e.** confusion

_____ **6.** *post*   **f.** expert

_____ **7.** *anti*   **g.** capability

_____ **8.** *a or an*   **h.** condition, state

_____ **9.** *deliri*   **i.** many

_____ **10.** *poly*   **j.** muscle

_____ **11.** *geront/o*   **k.** development

C. Read the following Case Report 19.3. Choose the correct answer as it pertains to the Case Report. **(LO 19.5, 19.A)**

 Case Report (CR) 19.3

You are

. . . a family physician in a small group practice.

Your patient is

. . . Mrs. Virtanen, who is an 85-year-old female who is seeing you today for her annual well visit. Mrs. Virtanen is accompanied by her two daughters. They communicate to you that their mother is beginning to forget routine facts and she also has a decreased appetite. Two months ago, Mrs. Virtanen was involved in a minor traffic accident. She entered traffic in front of a car and misjudged the distance and speed of the oncoming car. The daughters are concerned that their mother should perhaps not drive. Mrs. Virtanen becomes very upset, as she does not want to lose her ability to come and go as she wants.

You perform a checkup and note the following: VS P 82, RR 18, BP 115/72, T 98.4 F. Her weight is down 15 pounds from last year's visit.

1. How would you classify Mrs. Virtanen's blood pressure?

  a. hypotensive   **b.** hypertensive   **c.** within normal limits

2. What is the likely explanation for her decreased appetite?

  a. dementia   **b.** decreased sensation of taste

  c. probable malignancy   **d.** abnormally low body temperature

3. Her inability to judge the speed and distance of the car may represent:

  a. early onset Alzheimer disease   **b.** a decline in her visuospatial skills

  c. low oxygen delivery to the brain   **d.** presence of lentigines

D. Latin and Greek terms cannot be further deconstructed into prefix, root, or suffix. You must know them for what they are. Test your knowledge of these terms with this exercise. Match the meaning in the left column with the correct medical term in the right column. **(LO 19.3, 19.4)**

_____ **1.** death	**a.** hospice
_____ **2.** age spots	**b.** mortem
_____ **3.** lodging	**c.** lentigo

E. Medical language. Employ the _languages of geriatrics and gerontology_ to answer the following multiple-choice questions. Select the correct answer. **(LO 19.3, 19.8, 19.9, 19.10)**

1. Impaired intellect or memory that is present for at least six months is called

  a. dementia

  b. delirium

  c. hallucinations

  d. senescence

  e. cognition

2. In most U.S. states, _death_ is described in terms of

  a. lack of breathing

  b. lack of blood flow to the body

  c. brain death

  d. lack of muscle response

  e. lack of speech and hearing

Geriatrics

3. It is highly likely that senescence has more than one

   a. result

   b. free radical

   c. cause

   d. antioxidant

   e. autoimmune reaction

4. This condition is not a normal part of aging:

   a. renal failure

   b. renal impairment

   c. cataracts

   d. arthritis

   e. osteoporosis

5. A document that appoints someone you trust to make medical decisions for you is called a

   a. living will

   b. medical power of attorney

   c. DNR order

   d. consent form

   e. HIPAA authorization

6. The term meaning an unfavorable response to medical or surgical treatment, caused by the treatment itself, is

   a. polypharmacy

   b. iatrogenic

   c. senescence

   d. heredity

   e. dementia

7. The condition sarcopenia affects the _____ system.

   a. skeletal

   b. integumentary

   c. nervous

   d. muscular

   e. urinary

8. Free radicals can be neutralized by

   a. T lymphocytes (T cells)

   b. organ systems

   c. antioxidants

   d. enzymes

   e. hormones

9. What medical term describes an acute, altered state of consciousness with agitation and disorientation?

   a. delirium

   b. dementia

   c. hallucination

   d. persistent vegetative state

   e. migraine

10. Which of the following is NOT one of the so-called geriatric giants?

    a. immobility

    b. impaired intellect/memory

    c. instability

    d. incontinence

    e. loss of hearing

11. Which type of incontinence is caused by weak bladder muscles?

    a. overflow incontinence

    b. urge incontinence

    c. stress incontinence

    d. mixed incontinence

    e. functional incontinence

12. What disease accounts for 70% of all dementias?

    a. delirium

    b. Alzheimer disease

    c. fecal incontinence

    d. Lewy bodies

    e. impaired memory

13. Exercise and good nutrition are helpful in preventing

   a. wrinkles

   b. hair loss

   c. freckles

   d. osteopenia

   e. COPD

14. Which of the following statements is NOT true about hospice and the palliative care it provides?

   a. Hospice care can be provided in a hospital or in your home.

   b. Palliative care cannot cure anything.

   c. The main purpose of hospice is to alleviate pain and make you comfortable until you die.

   d. Hospice care does not charge the patient any fees.

   e. Hospice provides emotional support to the patient's family as well.

15. Which of the following statements applies to brain death?

   a. You have no cerebral or brainstem activity, and your EEG is flat for a specific length of time.

   b. You lose your sense of smell.

   c. You cannot hear anything around you.

   d. You cannot speak.

   e. You cannot walk.

F. Use one of the following words to fill in the appropriate spaces with the *language of gerontology*. Use each term only once; some terms will not be used. (LO 19.1, 19.3, 19.8, 19.9, 19.E)

sarcopenia	pathologist	postmortem	hospice
polypharmacy	adverse	incontinence	cognitive
dementia	iatrogenic	gerontologist	

1. Because she of her _____, the patient needs to wear diapers.

2. The _____ will perform the autopsy tomorrow morning.

3. The patient is suffering from _____ and needs physical therapy to strengthen his weakened muscles.

4. A(n) _____ drug reaction is not beneficial to the patient.

5. The family decided that _____ would be appropriate for their dying father.

G. Prefixes and suffixes are good clues to the meaning of a medical term. Analyze each medical term for the meaning of its prefix and suffix. Then give the complete meaning of the medical term in the last column. Every term may not have both a prefix and a suffix. If it does not have a particular word element, write n/a. Fill in the blanks. (LO 19.4, 19.5, 19.6, 19.10, 19.A, 19.D)

Medical Term	Meaning of Prefix	Meaning of Root/ Combining Form	Meaning of Suffix	Meaning of Term
palliative	1.	2.	3.	4.
iatrogenic	5.	6.	7.	8.
dementia	9.	10.	11.	12.
atrophy	13.	14.	15.	16.

©2014 Nucleus Medical Media

Health professionals involved in the diagnosis and treatment of cancer include:

- **Oncologists**, who are physicians who specialize in the diagnosis and treatment of patients with cancer. There are many subspecialties of oncologists, including medical oncologists, surgical oncologists, pediatric oncologists, and radiation oncologists; their titles are self-explanatory.

- **Oncology clinical nurse specialists**, who are registered nurses with advanced clinical practice in the care of cancer patients.

- **Oncology social workers**, who have master's degrees in medical social work and provide for the social and emotional needs of cancer patients and their families.

Chapter Learning Outcomes

To understand the possible etiologies of cancer, its pathology and staging, and its treatment and prognosis, and to communicate among the health care team as you care for Mrs. Sacco, you will need to be able to:

LO 20.1 Discuss the different types of cancer.

LO 20.2 Explain carcinogenesis.

LO 20.3 Describe the roles of environmental pollution in causing cancer.

LO 20.4 Specify ways in which cancer can be prevented.

LO 20.5 Describe methods of screening for and detecting cancer.

LO 20.6 Define methods of treating cancer.

LO 20.7 Discuss the chemical and biologic agents used to treat cancer.

LO 20.A Use the medical terms of oncology to communicate in writing and document accurately and precisely in any health care setting.

LO 20.B Use the medical terms of oncology to communicate verbally with accuracy and precision in any health care setting.

LO 20.C Construct terms used in oncology from their word elements (roots, combining forms, prefixes, and suffixes).

LO 20.D Deconstruct oncology terms into their word elements (roots, combining forms, prefixes, and suffixes).

LO 20.E Identify health professionals involved in the care of cancer patients.

LO 20.F Identify correct abbreviations for medical terms used in oncology.

Note: In previous chapters on individual body systems, the terminology of cancers specific to each body system has been detailed. In this chapter, the terminology that relates to cancer in general will be explored by using lung cancer as an example.

Case Report (CR) 20.1

You are

. . . an advanced-level respiratory therapist employed by Fulwood Medical Center, working with Tavis Senko, MD, a pulmonologist.

Your patient is

. . . Mrs. Raquel Sacco, a 44-year-old mother of two teenage boys, who is the owner of a quilting fabrics store. She is 2 days postop from lung surgery for non–small cell lung cancer. From her records, you see that she has two secondary (2°) metastases in her brain. She has been a nonsmoker all her life. Her 70-year-old father is a two-pack-a-day smoker, as is her husband. They both show no evidence of cancer on chest x-rays. Before Mrs. Sacco is discharged, as part of her postoperative respiratory care plan, you are using incentive spirometry to increase her inspiratory volume and improve her inspiratory muscle performance. You also will be taking an arterial blood sample to check her arterial oxygen pressure (PaO_2).

Lesson 20.1
CANCER

Types of Cancer

Normal tissue development is a balance between cell growth and cell death. If cells multiply more quickly than cells die, tumors (neoplasms) are formed. The study of tumors is called oncology, and medical specialists in this field are called oncologists.

Neoplasms whose cells proliferate rapidly and spread to distant sites (metastasize) are called malignant. Neoplasms that grow slowly, stay localized, do not invade surrounding tissues, and do not metastasize are called benign.

The information in this lesson will enable you to use correct medical terminology to:

20.1.1 Distinguish between benign and malignant neoplasms.

20.1.2 Classify the types of cancer by the type of cell from which it originates.

20.1.3 Explain the process of carcinogenesis.

20.1.4 Discuss the roles of environmental factors in carcinogenesis.

Abbreviations

CA	cancer
2°	secondary

LO 20.1 Types of Cancer

Cancer (CA) is a class of malignant diseases characterized by uncontrolled cell division. The basic cause of this uncontrolled growth is damage to the cells' DNA. This damage produces **mutations** to the genes that control cell division. These mutations, which can be inherited or acquired, lead to the uncontrolled cell division and malignant tumor formation. Thus, all cancer is genetic; that is, it develops because something in a cell's genes has changed (mutated).

Less than 10% of all cancers are inherited; that is, the genetic change is passed from parent to child. Almost 90% of cancers are acquired—something has caused the gene mutation in specific cells in a particular individual. A few genes mutated within a cell nucleus are enough to cause cancer. These gene mutations give the cells a superpower to proliferate in an uncontrolled way.

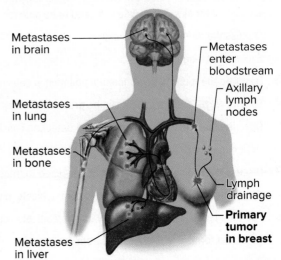

Metastases in brain
Metastases enter bloodstream
Metastases in lung
Axillary lymph nodes
Metastases in bone
Lymph drainage
Primary tumor in breast
Metastases in liver

▲ **Figure 20.1** **Metastases from Primary Breast Cancer.** Metastases may be via lymph drainage to the axillary lymph nodes or via the bloodstream to the brain, lung, liver, and bone.

The Cells of Malignant Tumors

- Have unlimited, unregulated growth potential.
- Grow directly into adjacent tissues (invasion or **infiltration**).
- Invade the lymphatic system and are carried to local and distant lymph nodes *(Figure 20.1)*.
- Invade the bloodstream and are carried to other distant organs and tissues (**metastasis**; *Figure 20.1*).

In contrast, **benign** tumors do not show such unregulated, invasive growth.

The Cells of Benign Tumors

- Grow slowly.
- Are surrounded by a connective tissue capsule.
- Do not invade or infiltrate adjacent tissues.
- Do not spread to other organs (metastasize) or to lymph nodes.
- Can compress surrounding tissues, causing functional problems.

Causes of Death

In the United States, the three most common causes of death are:

1. Cardiovascular disease (28.5% of all deaths).
2. Cancer (22.8% of all deaths).
3. Cerebrovascular disease, primarily stroke (6.7% of all deaths).

Environmental factors, particularly cigarette smoke, are associated with many forms of cancer. In this chapter, we will use a case of lung cancer to illustrate the characteristics of an acquired cancer and to discuss methods of detection and treatment.

Keynotes

- The American Cancer Society estimates 1,688,780 new cases of cancer in 2017 with 600,92 cancer deaths.

- In females, 30% of new cancers are in the breast, 12% in the lungs, and 8% in the colon and rectum.

- In males, 19% are in the prostate, 14% in the lungs, and 9% in the colon and rectum.

- Between 2004 and 2013, the most recent years for which data are available, overall death rates for cancer decreased by 13% in the United States.

- The decline in cancer death rates is due to better prevention efforts, new screening methods, and more effective treatments.

WORD	PRONUNCIATION		ELEMENTS	DEFINITION
benign (adj)	bee-**NINE**		Latin *kind*	Denoting the nonmalignant character of a neoplasm or illness
cancer cancerous (adj)	**KAN**-ser **KAN**-ser-us	S/ R/	Latin *crab* -ous *pertaining to* **cancer-** *cancer*	General term for a malignant neoplasm Pertaining to a malignant neoplasm
infiltrate infiltration	**IN**-fil-trate in-fil-**TRAY**-shun	S/ P/ R/ S/	-ate *composed of, pertaining to* in- *in* -filtr- *strain through* -ation *process*	To penetrate and invade a tissue or cell The invasion into a tissue or cell
malignant (adj) malignancy (noun)	mah-**LIG**-nant mah-**LIG**-nan-see	 S/ R/	Latin *hurtful* -ancy *state of* **malign-** *cancer*	Capable of invading surrounding tissues and metastasizing to distant organs Tumor that invades surrounding tissues and metastasizes to distant organs
metastasis (noun) metastases (pl) metastatic (adj)	meh-**TAS**-tah-sis meh-**TAS**-tah-seez meh-tah-**STAT**-ik	P/ R/ S/ R/	meta- *after, beyond* -stasis *stay in one place* -ic *pertaining to* -stat- *stand still*	Spread of disease from one part of the body to another Able to metastasize
mutation mutagen	myu-**TAY**-shun **MYU**-tah-jen	S/ R/ S/	-tion *process* **muta-** *genetic change* -gen *produce*	A change in the chemistry of a gene that is continued in subsequent divisions of the cell Agent that produces a mutation in a gene
neoplasm (noun) neoplastic (adj) (**Note:** The "m" in *-plasm* is removed to allow the elements to flow.) neoplasia	**NEE**-oh-plazm **NEE**-oh-**PLAS**-tic **NEE**-oh-**PLAY**-zee-ah	P/ R/ S/ S/	neo- *new* -plasm *to form* -tic *pertaining to* -plasia *formation, growth*	A new growth, either a benign or malignant tumor Pertaining to a neoplasm Process that results in formation of a tumor
oncology oncologist	on-**KOL**-oh-jee on-**KOL**-oh-jist	S/ R/CF S/	-logy *study of* onc/o- *tumor* -logist *one who studies, specialist*	The science dealing with cancer Medical specialist in oncology
proliferate	proh-**LIF**-eh-rate	S/ R/CF R/	-ate *composed of, pertaining to* prol/i- *bear offspring* -fer- *to bear*	To increase in number through reproduction
tumor	**TOO**-mor		Latin *swelling*	Any abnormal swelling

Exercises

A. Demonstrate that you can use various forms of the same term correctly. *Insert the appropriate medical term in the following blanks.* **LO 20.1, 20.A**

neoplasm   **neoplastic**   **neoplasia**

1. The process of _____ results in the formation of a tumor, which can be either malignant or benign.

2. Another name for a tumor is a _____.

3. The tumor exhibited _____ behavior and was immediately biopsied.

metastases   **metastatic**   **metastasis**

4. A _____ carcinoma is cancer that has spread to a different site than the primary tumor.

5. The patient has _____ in his brain and kidneys.

6. Finding a primary tumor before _____ has occurred increases the chances for a cure.

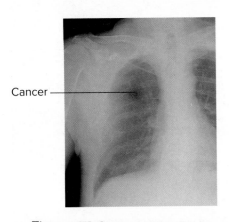

Cancer ──────

▲ **Figure 20.2** X-ray of Small Cell Cancer of Right Upper Lung. ©Steve Gschmeissner/Science Photo Library/Photo Researchers, Inc.

LO 20.1 Types of Cancer (continued)

Within the broad classes of cancer *(Table 20.1)* are many subgroups, depending on the type of cells in the cancer.

Lung Cancer

Lung cancer has three main subgroups:

1. **Non–small cell lung cancer** accounts for 85% of cases, and 80% of patients die within 5 years of diagnosis. Included in this type are:

   a. **Squamous cell carcinoma**, arising from *round cells* that have replaced damaged cells in the epithelial lining cells of a major bronchus. It accounts for 25% to 40% of lung cancers.

   b. **Adenocarcinoma**, arising from the *mucus-producing cells* in the bronchi. It accounts for between 30% and 50% of lung cancers. It is the most common lung cancer in women, and its incidence is increasing.

   c. **Large cell carcinoma**, which includes cancers that cannot be identified under the microscope as squamous cell or adenocarcinoma. It accounts for 10% to 20% of lung cancers.

Abbreviations

CIS	carcinoma in situ
1°	primary

 Case Report (CR) 20.1 *(Continued)*

Adenocarcinoma was found in Raquel Sacco. It was diagnosed because she had a seizure, and neurologic tests revealed the presence of two metastases in her brain. This led to a search for the primary (1°) tumor, which was found in her lung *(Figure 20.2)*.

Keynotes

The term **carcinoma in situ (CIS)** describes an early form of carcinoma in which there is no invasion of surrounding tissues. In many instances, it is a precursor that will transform into an invasive or malignant cancer.

- The three most common cancers in men and the three leading causes of cancer death are prostate cancer, lung cancer, and colorectal cancer.

- The three most common cancers in women are breast cancer, lung cancer, and colorectal cancer.

2. **Small cell lung cancer,** like squamous cell carcinoma, is derived from the epithelial cells of the bronchi but replicates at a faster rate, producing smaller cells. It accounts for 14% of all lung cancers; most patients die within 18 months of diagnosis.

3. **Mesothelioma** is a rare tumor arising from the cells lining the pleura and is associated with asbestosis.

Table 20.1 Types of Cancer

Class of Cancer	Cells of Origin	Examples
carcinoma	Epithelial	Cervical cancer, stomach cancer, squamous cell skin cancer, lung cancer
sarcoma	Connective tissue, bone cartilage, muscle	**Osteosarcoma, chondrosarcoma, rhabdomyosarcoma**
leukemia	Blood-forming tissues	Acute lymphocytic leukemia, chronic myelogenous leukemia
lymphoma	Lymph nodes	Hodgkin disease, non-Hodgkin lymphoma
melanoma	Melanocytes (pigment-producing skin cells)	Malignant melanoma

WORD	PRONUNCIATION		ELEMENTS	DEFINITION
adenocarcinoma	AD-eh-noh-kar-sih-NOH-mah	S/ R/CF R/	-oma *tumor* aden/o- *gland* -carcin- *cancer*	A cancer arising from glandular epithelial cells
carcinoma	kar-sih-NOH-mah	S/ R/	-oma *tumor* carcin- *cancer*	A malignant and invasive epithelial tumor
carcinoma in situ (CIS)	kar-sih-NOH-mah IN SIGH-tyu		in situ Latin *in its place*	Carcinoma that has not invaded surrounding tissues
chondrosarcoma	KON-droh-sar-KOH-mah	S/ R/CF R/	-oma *tumor* chondr/o- *cartilage* -sarc- *flesh*	Cancer arising from cartilage cells
leukemia	loo-KEE-mee-ah	S/ R/	-emia *blood condition* leuk- *white*	Disease in which the blood is taken over by white blood cells and their precursors
lymphoma	lim-FOH-mah	S/ R/	-oma *tumor* lymph- *lymph*	Any neoplasm of lymphatic tissue
melanoma	MEL-ah-NOH-mah	S/ R/	-oma *tumor, mass* melan- *black*	Malignant neoplasm formed from cells that produce melanin
mesothelioma	MEEZ-oh-thee-lee-OH-mah	S/ P/ R/	-oma *tumor* meso- *middle* -theli- *lining*	Cancer arising from the cells lining the pleura or peritoneum
osteosarcoma	OS-tee-oh-sar-KOH-mah	S/ R/CF R/	-oma *tumor* oste/o- *bone* -sarc- *flesh*	Cancer arising in bone-forming cells
rhabdomyosarcoma	RAB-doh-MY-oh-sar-KOH-mah	S/ R/CF R/CF R/	-oma *tumor* rhabd/o- *rod-shaped, striated* -my/o- *muscle* -sarc- *flesh*	Cancer derived from skeletal muscle
sarcoma	sar-KOH-mah	S/ R/	-oma *tumor* sarc- *flesh*	A malignant tumor originating in connective tissue

Exercises

A. Deconstruct the following language of oncology into elements. *These elements will form the basis for many additional oncologic terms. Give the one-word definition for the following word elements. Fill in the blank.* **LO 20.1, 20.D**

1. *sarc/o* _____

2. *oste/o* _____

3. *-oma* _____

4. *my/o* _____

5. *chondr/o* _____

6. *aden/o* _____

7. *carcin-* _____

8. *mes/o* _____

9. *leuk-* _____

10. *melan-* _____

▲ **Figure 20.3** **End Stage of Mitosis.** For simplicity, the schematic drawing of the cell *(bottom)* is shown with only two chromosome pairs. ©Ed Reschke/ Getty Images

Abbreviations

ETS	environmental tobacco smoke
PCD	programmed cell death
TS	tumor suppressor

Keynotes

- A pack-year equals the number of packs of cigarettes smoked per day multiplied by the number of years the person has smoked.
- Cigarette smoke contains over 60 known carcinogens.
- Several countries and states in the United States ban cigarette smoking in a car with minors to protect them from ETS

LO 20.2 Carcinogenesis

Carcinogenesis, literally the creation of cancer, is the abnormal rate of cell division as a result of damaged DNA causing gene mutation. Normally, the balance between cell division and proliferation and cell death **(apoptosis, or programmed cell death [PCD])** is tightly controlled to maintain the integrity of organs and tissues. Gene mutations that cause cancer disrupt this orderly process. Mutation in a single gene is usually not enough to cause cancer, and carcinogenesis requires multiple mutations in many genes.

Most normal cells cannot divide unless a **growth factor** binds to a receptor on the cell's surface. This growth factor then stimulates the cell to undergo mitosis *(see Chapter 3)* and **differentiate** into mature, functional cells *(Figure 20.3)*.

Two types of genes have been identified that play a part in the abnormal cell division and proliferation of cancer cells:

1. **Protooncogenes** are healthy genes that promote normal cell growth. Mutated **oncogenes** cause malfunctions in the normal growth mechanisms. For example, an oncogene called *SIS* stimulates blood vessels to grow into a tumor and provide the rich blood supply it needs to proliferate rapidly. An oncogene called *RAS* generates abnormal growth-factor receptors that switch on constant cell division signals. An oncogene called *HER-2* causes many cases of breast and ovarian cancer. The drug *Herceptin* is an antibody that targets the *HER-2* receptors on the cancer cells. This cuts off the chemical signals that the cell needs to keep proliferating. It also marks the abnormal cells for destruction by the immune system.

2. **Tumor suppressor (TS) genes** normally suppress mitosis and are activated by DNA damage. Their function is to stop cell division so that the abnormal genetic structure cannot be passed on to daughter cells. **Mutated TS genes** cannot do this, so the abnormal cells can divide and proliferate. A mutated TS gene called *p53* is present in half of all cancers and is associated with a poor prognosis and resistance to chemotherapy.

Mutations in both types of genes are usually required for cancer to develop. The oncogenes turn on the abnormal cell growth, and the mutated TS genes cannot stop it.

Cancer is due to the accumulation of genetic injury and mutations. Agents that cause these mutations are called **mutagens**, and mutagens that cause cancer are called **carcinogens**. Particular carcinogens are linked to specific types of cancer. Examples are inhalation of asbestos fibers with mesothelioma, prolonged exposure to radiation and ultraviolet radiation with melanoma and other skin malignancies, and tobacco smoking with lung cancer. Although the link between cigarette smoking and lung cancer is well established, only 15% to 20% of smokers develop lung cancer. In addition, about 10% of the population carries a gene that protects against lung cancer.

Studies in 2004 and 2005 of the epithelial cells in the large bronchi found a large number of genes altered by cigarette smoking. The studies defined genes whose alteration correlated with cumulative pack-years of smoking, and they identified 13 genes whose alterations do not return to normal after smoking is stopped. This could explain the persistent risk of lung cancer in former smokers. In addition, a subset of smokers was identified whose gene alterations have a different profile from that of other smokers. It is possible that this subset is the group who develop lung cancer.

Secondhand smoke, called **environmental tobacco smoke (ETS),** contains the same chemicals and carcinogens as those inhaled by smokers. It is responsible for 3,000 lung cancer cases each year in America. The genetic mutations caused by the carcinogens are probably similar to those in the subset of smokers discussed earlier, even though exposure to the carcinogens is much less than that for smokers.

 Case Report (CR) 20.1 *(Continued)*

Raquel Sacco probably developed her lung cancer as a result of inhaling secondhand smoke all her life (from her father and husband).

WORD	PRONUNCIATION	ELEMENTS		DEFINITION
apoptosis	AP-op-TOH-sis	R/ P/	-ptosis *drooping* apo- *separation from*	Programmed normal cell death
carcinogen	kar-SIN-oh-jen	S/ R/CF	-gen *produce* carcin/o *cancer*	Cancer-producing agent
carcinogenic (adj) carcinogenesis	KAR-sin-oh-JEN-ik KAR-sin-oh-JEN-eh-sis	S/ S/	-ic *pertaining to* -genesis *creation*	Causing cancer Origin and development of cancer
oncogene	ONG-koh-jeen	S/ R/CF	-gene *producer, give birth* onc/o- **tumor**	One of a family of genes involved in cell growth that work in concert to cause cancer
oncogenic (adj)	ONG-koh-JEN-ik	S/	-genic *creation, producing*	Capable of producing a neoplasm
protooncogene	pro-toh-ONG-koh-jeen	S/ P/ R/CF	-gene *producer, give birth* proto- *first* -onc/o- *tumor*	A normal gene involved in normal cell growth

Exercises

A. Use the language of oncology to answer questions. *The following questions can be either true or false. Choose T if the statement is true. Choose F if the answer is false.* **LO 20.2**

1. Carcinogenesis is the creation of cancer. T F

2. Damaged blood cells cause gene mutation. T F

3. Programmed cell death is another term for apoptosis. T F

4. Mutagens that cause cancer are called carcinogens. T F

5. It is not possible to get cancer from secondhand smoke. T F

B. Many medical terms can be deconstructed into their word elements. *Choose the correct meaning of the word elements.* **LO 20.2, 20.D**

1. In the medical term **protooncogene,** the root means:

   a. produce   **b.** pertaining to   **c.** first   **d.** tumor

2. The prefix in the medical term **apoptosis** means:

   a. separation from   **b.** source   **c.** without   **d.** tumor

3. The root in the medical term **carcinogenic** means:

   a. produce   **b.** cancer   **c.** genetic change   **d.** tumor

4. The suffix in the medical term **oncogene** means:

   a. tumor   **b.** cancer   **c.** producer   **d.** first

> 💡 **Study Hint**
>
> **Ptosis** is a medical term in its own right. Another example is the term **hemolysis,** in which **lysis** is also a medical term in and of itself.

▲ **Figure 20.4** Woman Smoking.
©McGraw-Hill Education/Gary He, photographer.

▲ **Figure 20.5** Air Pollution over a
Large City. ©Patrick Clark/Getty Images RF

▲ **Figure 20.6** Pesticide Spraying of
Field of Vegetables. ©Garry D. McMichael/
Photo Researchers, Inc.

▲ **Figure 20.7** No Smoking Sign.
©Medical Elements PhotoDisc/Getty Images RF

LO 20.3 Environmental Pollution

Pollution is a trigger of many cancers. For example, cigarette smoke *(Figure 20.4)* causes 87% of all lung cancers and acts in the following way: In the smoke are approximately 4,000 chemicals, some 60 of which are known to be carcinogenic and trigger genetic mutations that lead to cancer. Among the inhaled chemicals are cyanide, benzene, formaldehyde, acetylene, tar, arsenic, and ammonia, all of which can increase the risk for cancer.

Radon, a radioactive gas that you cannot see or smell, is the second leading cause of lung cancer (after smoking). It is produced by decaying **uranium** and is found in nearly all soils. In underground miners, it increases the risk of cancer to 40%. It gets into homes through cracks in the foundations or construction joints and is a problem in 1 out of 15 homes. Cigarette smoking on top of radon significantly increases the risk of lung cancer. Testing for radon is cheap and easy.

Air pollution may be the cause of the 10% to 40% increase in lung cancer mortality between urban and rural areas *(Figure 20.5)*. **Particulate matter,** especially very small **particles,** includes soot; organic material such as hydrocarbons; and metals such as arsenic, chromium, and nickel—all of which are known mutagens and carcinogens. A new analysis shows that premature death from cardiovascular ailments is increased by 24% among people exposed to tiny soot particles.

Chemical toxins are estimated to cause more than 75% of all cancers. Some 77,000 chemicals are used in this country. Over 3,000 are added to our food, and most Americans have between 400 and 800 chemicals stored in their bodies, mostly in fat cells. The toxins known to cause cancer include:

- **Chlorine.** Used in drinking water, chlorine produces carcinogenic compounds. Cancer risk among people drinking chlorinated water is 93% higher than that of people not drinking chlorinated water.

- **Lead.** Found in lead-based paint and contaminated air, water, and soil, lead poisoning can severely affect mental and physical development, particularly in children younger than 6. In 2014, over 100,000 residents of Flint, Michigan, including 12,000 children, were exposed to high levels of lead in their drinking water. The lead came from the polluted river source of water and from lead pipes used to supply the water.

- **Polychlorinated biphenyls (PCBs).** These were banned years ago but still persist in the environment, and are found in farmed salmon.

- **Pesticides.** According to the **Environmental Protection Agency (EPA),** 60% of herbicides, 90% of fungicides, and 30% of insecticides are known to be carcinogenic *(Figure 20.6)*. Farmers using pesticides have a 14% greater risk for developing prostate cancer than do organic farmers.

- **Dioxins.** These are chemical compounds produced by combustion processes from waste incineration and from burning fuels like wood, coal, and oil.

- **Asbestos.** This insulating material was used in the 1950s to 1970s on floors, ceilings, water pipes, and heating ducts. When the material becomes old and crumbly, it releases fibers into the air. Inhalation of the fibers is the cause of mesothelioma.

- **Arsenic.** This is used by insecticide and herbicide sprayers and oil refinery workers.

Occupational Safety and Health Administration **(OSHA)** regulations are designed to protect workers from these environmental hazards.

LO 20.4 Prevention of Cancer

More than 50% of cancers could be prevented by **changes in lifestyle and environment.** The same carcinogens that affect the lining of the respiratory tract cause cancer of the oral cavity, pharynx, larynx, and esophagus. They also are absorbed into the bloodstream and disseminated, thereby becoming factors that can cause cancer in the pancreas, stomach, kidney, bladder, prostate, and cervix. **Stopping smoking** alone would reduce most of the 30% of all deaths due to lung cancer and reduce the incidence of many of the other cancers related to smoking *(Figure 20.7)*.

Clean air measures that are being implemented to reduce the more than 2 billion pounds of toxic air pollutants emitted into the atmosphere annually in this country can reduce the incidence of cancer.

Obesity is said to be linked to about 10% of breast and colorectal cancers and up to 40% of kidney, esophageal, and endometrial cancers. The mechanisms of obesity linked to these cancers are not understood.

Abbreviations	
EPA	Environmental Protection Agency
OSHA	Occupational Safety and Health Administration
PCBs	polychlorinated biphenyls

WORD	PRONUNCIATION		ELEMENTS	DEFINITION
chlorine	**KLOR**-een		Greek *greenish-yellow*	A toxic agent used as a disinfectant and bleaching agent
dioxin	die-**OK**-sin	S/ P/ R/	**-in** *chemical compound* **di-** *two* **-ox-** *oxygen*	Carcinogenic contaminant in pesticides
environment	en-**VIE**-ron-ment	S/ R/	**-ment** *resulting state* **environ-** *surroundings*	All the external conditions affecting the life of an organism
environmental (adj)	en-**VIE**-ron-**MEN**-tal	S/	**-al** *pertaining to*	Pertaining to the environment
particle particulate (adj)	**PAR**-tih-kul par-**TIK**-you-let	S/ R/	Latin *little piece* **-ate** *composed of, pertaining to* **particul-** *little piece*	A small piece of matter Relating to a fine particle
pesticide	**PES**-tih-side	S/ R/CF	**-cide** *to kill* **pest/i-** *pest*	Agent for destroying flies, mosquitoes, and other pests
pollution	poh-**LOO**-shun		Latin *dirty*	Condition that is unclean, impure, and a danger to health
radon	**RAY**-don		German *radium*	Colorless, tasteless, and odorless gas that can cause lung cancer
uranium	you-**RAY**-nee-um		Greek mythological character, Uranus	Radioactive metallic element

Exercises

A. Demonstrate your knowledge of the following terminology by deconstructing the terms into their elements. *Fill in the blanks. If the term does not a particular word element, leave the blank empty.* **LO 20.3, 20.D**

1. particulate _____/_____/_____
  P   R/CF   S

2. environment _____/_____/_____
  P   R/CF   S

3. pesticide _____/_____/_____
  P   R/CF   S

4. dioxin _____/_____/_____
  P   R/CF   S

B. Use the medical terms in context. *Use terms related to Environment Pollution to complete the following sentences. Fill in the blanks.* **LO 20.3, 20.A**

1. Decaying _____ causes the release of radon, which can lead to lung cancer.

2. Consumption of water treated with _____ can increase the incidence of cancer.

3. Burning fuels such as coal releases the toxin _____, which can cause cancer.

4. Small bits of material are called _____.

5. A farmer may spray a chemical _____ on his produce to prevent insects from destroying the crops.

Lesson 20.2

CANCER

Detecting Cancer

Lesson Objectives

One genetic mutation in one cell, the mother or progenitor cell, can produce cancer, and the daughter cells can reproduce rapidly. But clinical detection is rare for a tumor mass less than 1 cm in diameter, which can include 1 billion cancer cells. The earlier and the more localized the tumor is detected, the better the chance of a cure.

The information in this lesson will enable you to use correct medical terminology to:

20.2.1 Explain the roles of different screening tests for different cancers.

20.2.2 Discuss the value of self-examination methods for detecting cancer.

20.2.3 Describe the factors that increase the risk of developing different cancers.

20.2.4 List methods of preventing cancer.

Abbreviations

AMAS	anti-malignin antibody screen
BAL	bronchoalveolar lavage
BSE	breast self-examination
CEA	carcinoembryonic antigen
CT	computed tomography
DRE	digital rectal examination
FOBT	fecal occult blood test
MRI	magnetic resonance imaging
Pap	Papanicolaou cervical smear test
PCA3	prostate cancer antigen 3
PET	positron emission tomography
PSA	prostate-specific antigen

LO 20.5 Screening for and Detecting Cancers

For the four major types of cancer (lung, breast, prostate, colorectal) combined, the National Cancer Institute estimates that in 2017 there will be 772,000 new cases and 133,470 deaths in the United States alone. The ability to find cancers before they cause symptoms (like a lump that can be felt) and have spread would greatly improve the **prognosis** for people with this disease. The goal of **screening** tests is to achieve this outcome.

Breast Cancer Screening

The medical procedures used in screening for breast cancer include:

Examination and **palpation.**

Self-examination of the breast following a period.

Mammograms to record images of the breast on x-ray film.

Digital mammography to record images in computer code.

Computer-aided mammography using a laser beam to produce a digital signal that can be processed by a computer to highlight suspicious areas.

Ultrasound using sound waves to make a computer image of the inside of the breast, particularly to see changes in women with dense breast tissue and to tell the difference between benign fluid-filled cysts and a possibly malignant solid mass.

Magnetic resonance imaging (MRI) creating detailed images of the breast in different planes.

Ductal lavage using saline solution introducd through a fine catheter inserted into a milk duct through its opening on the surface of the nipple. The solution is **aspirated** out and examined microscopically to check for abnormal cells.

Biopsy of a suspicious lesion can detect the type of lung cancer (*see Chapter 13*). X-rays or ultrasound are used to guide accurate insertion of a needle into the suspicious lesion.

Several national organizations have developed guidelines for the age when screening for breast cancer should be started and how often procedures should be performed. Unfortunately, they are all slightly different, making it confusing for patients.

▲ **Figure 20.8** **Mammography.** ©Keith Brofsky/Vol. 40 PhotoDisc/GettyImages RF

WORD	PRONUNCIATION		ELEMENTS	DEFINITION
biopsy	**BI**-op-see	S/	-opsy *to view* bi- *life*	Removal of tissue from a living person for laboratory examination
duct	DUKT		Latin *to lead*	A tubular structure allowing any fluid to flow through it
ductal	**DUCK**-tal	S/ R/	-al *pertaining to* duct- *to lead*	Pertaining to a duct
lavage	lah-**VAHZH**		Latin *to wash*	Washing out of a hollow tube, cavity, or organ
mammogram	**MAM**-oh-gram	S/ R/	-gram *a record* mammo- *breast*	The record produced by x-ray imaging of the breast
mammography	mah-**MOG**-rah-fee	S/	graphy *process of recording*	Process of x-ray examination of the breast
palpate (verb)	**PAL**-pate		Latin *to touch*	Examination with the fingers and hand
palpation (noun)	pal-**PAY**-shun	S/ R/	-ion *action* palpat- *touch, stroke*	To examine using the fingers and hands
progenitor	pro-**JEN**-ih-tor	P/ R/	pro- *before* -genitor *offspring*	Founder; beginning of an ancestry
prognosis	prog-**NO**-sis	P/ R/	pro- *before* -gnosis *knowledge*	Forecasting of the probable course of a disease
screen (verb) screening (noun)	SKREEN **SKREEN**-ing		French *examine*	To evaluate a group The evaluation of a group
self-examination	**SELF**-ek-zam-ih-**NAY**-shun	S/ R/ R/	-ation *process* examin- *test* self- *me*	To examine part of one's own body

Exercises

A. Learning word elements are the key to quickly knowing the medical term. *Match the element in the left column with its correct meaning in the right column.* **LO 20.1, 20.5**

_____ **1.** *ion*

_____ **2.** *opsy*

_____ **3.** *gram*

_____ **4.** *ation*

_____ **5.** *pro*

_____ **6.** *bi*

_____ **7.** *duct*

a. before

b. to lead

c. process

d. life

e. action

f. to view

g. a record

LO 20.5 Screening for and Detecting Cancers (continued)

The medical terms used in screening for and detecting lung cancer are:

Chest x-rays are thought of as **the** screening method for lung cancer. Frequently when lung cancer is detectable on chest x-ray it has spread beyond the lungs.

Computed tomography (CT) scans are more effective at identifying early lung cancers than are chest x-rays.

Magnetic resonance imaging (MRI) is being used to screen for lung cancer in high risk patients.

Sputum analysis of coughed up sputum can be a useful and cost-effective method of identifying cancer cells arising from the lining of the airways.

Biomarkers are substances released by specific cancers and can be found in blood, sputum, and tissue samples. The blood test **anti-malignin antibody screen** can detect the presence of any kind of cancer and is non-specific.

More specific tests for detecting the presence of lung cancer cells include:

Positron emission tomography (PET) scans are expensive and not widely available. They are the most accurate non-invasive test for identifying if the cancer has spread outside lung tissue.

Scintigraphy uses low-level **radioactive** agents that bind to cancer cells and can be tracked by special cameras to reveal the exact locations of cancer cells.

Bronchoscopy can locate cancers in the linings of the major airways. Biopsy specimens are obtained by cutting tissue, by brushings, or by a washing process called **bronchoalveolar lavage (BAL)**.

Mediastinoscopy uses a fiber-optic tube with a camera and is inserted into the mediastinum via the suprasternal notch to locate affected mediastinal lymph nodes for biopsy.

Needle biopsy of tumors in the periphery of the lungs is performed by inserting a needle between the ribs and guiding it to the tumor with **fluoroscopy** or CT scan.

Brain metastases are identified by MRI and bone metastases by technetium-99m radionuclide bone scans.

Staging Lung Cancer

The **tumor-node-metastasis (TNM) system** is used to stage cancer:

- **T** stands for *tumor* and describes its size and its spread within the lung and to nearby tissues such as the pleura, diaphragm, and pericardium.

- **N** stands for spread to lymph *nodes* around the affected lung.

- **M** stands for *metastasis* to distant sites such as brain liver and bones.

- **O**nce the TNM categories have been assigned, the information is combined and given an overall stage of O, I, II, III, or IV.

LO 20.5 Word Analysis and Definition

WORD	PRONUNCIATION	ELEMENTS		DEFINITION
biomarker	BI-oh-MARK-er	P/ R/	bio- *life* -marker *sign*	A biological marker or product by which a cell can be identified
bronchoalveolar	BRONG-koh-al-VEE-oh-lar	S/ R/CF R/	-ar *pertaining to* bronch/o- *bronchus* -alveol- *alveolus*	Pertaining to the bronchi and alveoli
bronchoscope bronchoscopy	BRONG-koh-scope brong-KOS-koh-pee	S/ R/CF S/	-scope *instrument for viewing* bronch/o- *bronchus* -scopy *to examine*	Endoscope used for bronchoscopy Examination of the interior of the tracheobronchial tree with an endoscope
fluoroscopy	flor-OS-koh-pee	S/ R/CF	-scopy *to examine* fluor/o- *x-ray beam*	Examination of the structure of the body by x-rays
mediastinoscopy	ME-dee-ass-tih-NOS-koh-pee	S/ R/CF	-scopy *to examine* mediastin/o- *mediastinum*	Examination of the mediastinum using an endoscope
scintigraphy	sin-TIG-rah-fee	S/ R/	-graphy *process of recording* scinti- *spark*	Recording of radioactivity using a special camera
stage staging	STAYJ STAY-jing		Latin *to stand*	Definition of extent and dissemination of a malignant neoplasm Process of determination of the extent of the distribution of a neoplasm

Exercises

A. Language of Oncology: Test your knowledge of the language of oncology with this exercise. *Select the best answer(s).*
LO 20.1, 20.5

1. Which of the following terms contains a prefix?

   a. biomarker

   b. bronchoscopy

   c. pathologist

   d. scintigraphy

2. Which term contains the suffix meaning *to examine*?

   a. bronchoscope

   b. fluoroscopy

   c. scintigraphy

   d. staging

3. Which term would mean a recording with a special camera?

   a. biomarker

   b. fluoroscopy

   c. scintigraphy

   d. bronchoscope

4. Which of the following terms is a procedure on the chest?

   a. mediastinoscopy

   b. scintigraphy

   c. bronchoalveolar

   d. biomarker

LO 20.6 Treating Cancer

Treatment of any cancer depends on its location, its size, its localization or spread to surrounding tissues and lymph nodes, the presence of metastases, and the cancer's aggressiveness (as determined by pathologic findings on biopsy or surgical removal).

If the cancer is still localized, it can be removed and cure is possible. Unfortunately, few patients are diagnosed at such an early stage, particularly with lung cancer. Even if the original tumor is removed, cancer recurrence rates are high. Additional treatments with **radiation** and **chemotherapy** are used and can produce unpleasant side effects. A patient will have to balance a diminished quality of life against a chance for a modestly prolonged survival.

In the elderly, studies have shown that survival rates are the same for therapies aimed at relieving pain as they are for aggressive, unpleasant treatment **regimens** with their diminished quality of life.

Surgical Procedures

Surgical procedures for specific body system cancers are discussed in the relevant chapters. For example, surgery for breast cancer is covered in *Chapter 8* and for prostate cancer in *Chapter 7.*

The type of surgery for lung cancer depends on the amount of lung tissue that has to be removed.

Wedge resection (segmentectomy) removes only a small part of the lung. It is used for carcinoma in situ, small tumors, frailer patients who cannot tolerate lobectomy, or patients with lung disease.

Lobectomy is removal of one lobe of the lung and is used if the cancer has not spread beyond the lobe or into lymph nodes.

Pneumonectomy removes an entire lung and has a mortality of 5% to 8%.

▲ **Figure 20.9** Radioactive Seeds Implanted in a Tumor. Courtesy of Varian Medical Systems

 Case Report (CR) 20.1 *(Continued)*

Lobectomy was the procedure performed on Mrs. Raquel Sacco. The respiratory therapy she is having is designed to enhance the function of her residual lung tissue.

Radiation Procedures (Radiotherapy)

Radiotherapy does not remove the lesion but distorts the DNA of the cancer cells so that they lose their ability to reproduce and to retain fluids; the cells shrink over time. Side effects of radiotherapy depend on the type of therapy used, and occur when healthy cells are damaged during the treatment. Tiredness, nausea, loss of appetite, and sore skin in the treatment area can be short-term effects.

External-beam radiation focuses a beam of radiation directly on the tumor. It is generally used for metastasized cancer.

Brachytherapy implants radioactive seeds through thin tubes directly into the tumor to give high doses of radiation to the tumor while reducing radiation exposure to the surrounding tissues *(Figure 20.9)*. It can be used for inoperable cancers.

Continuous hyperfractionated accelerated radiotherapy (CHART) administers standard doses of radiation multiple times per day. It allows the total dose of radiation to be administered in a shorter period of time than the standard 6 weeks.

Stereotactic radiosurgery (SRS) uses three-dimensional computer programming to deliver a precise, single high dose of radiation in a 1-day session. The most common form of SRS used in the United States is a cobalt-60–based machine called the gamma knife. Though this technique is labeled and implied as "surgery," there is no actual surgery involved.

Abbreviations

CHART	continuous hyperfractionated accelerated radiotherapy
SRS	stereotactic radiosurgery

S = Suffix   P = Prefix   R = Root   R/CF = Combining Form

WORD	PRONUNCIATION	ELEMENTS		DEFINITION
brachytherapy	brah-kee-**THAIR**-ah-pee	P/ R/	**brachy-** *short* **-therapy** *medical treatment*	Radiation therapy in which the source of irradiation is implanted in the tissue to be treated
chemotherapy	**KEE**-moh-**THAIR**-ah-pee	R/CF R/	**chem/o-** *chemical* **-therapy** *medical treatment*	Treatment using chemical agents
hyperfractionated (adj)	high-per-**FRAK**-shun-ay-ted	S/ P/ R/	**-ated** *process* **hyper-** *excessive* **-fraction-** *small amount*	Given in smaller amounts and more frequently
lobectomy	loh-**BEK**-toh-mee	S/ R/	**-ectomy** *surgical excision* **lob-** *lobe*	Surgical removal of a lobe of the lungs
pneumonectomy	**NEW**-moh-**NEK**-toh-mee	S/ R/	**-ectomy** *surgical excision* **pneumon-** *lung*	Surgical removal of a whole lung
radiation	ray-dee-**AY**-shun	S/ R/	**-ation** *process* **radi-** *x-ray, radiation*	Treatment with x-rays
radiotherapy	**RAY**-dee-oh-**THAIR**-ah-pee	R/CF R/	**radi/o-** *x-ray, radiation* **-therapy** *medical treatment*	Treatment using radiation
regimen	**REJ**-ih-men		Latin *direction*	Program of treatment
segmentectomy	seg-men-**TEK**-toh-mee	S/ R/	**-ectomy** *surgical excision* **segment-** *section*	Surgical excision of a segment of a tissue or organ

Exercises

A. Match the word element in the first column with its correct meaning found in the second column. *Some of these elements have appeared in earlier chapters as well.* **LO 20.6**

_____ **1.** *chemo*

_____ **2.** *pneumon*

_____ **3.** *brachy*

_____ **4.** *hyper*

_____ **5.** *ectomy*

_____ **6.** *lob*

_____ **7.** *therapy*

_____ **8.** *fraction*

a. small amount

b. lobe

c. excessive

d. treatment

e. lung

f. short

g. chemical

h. surgical excision

LO 20.6 Treating Cancer (continued)

Medications

Chemotherapy (chemo) is the use of any drug to treat any disease, but the term is mostly used for drugs that treat cancer. Chemotherapy drugs target cells at different phases of the process of forming new cells. Cancer cells form new cells more quickly than normal cells and this makes them a better target for chemotherapy. But chemotherapy drugs cannot tell the difference between healthy cells and cancer cells. This means that normal cells are damaged along with cancer cells, and this causes **side effects.** Fatigue, nausea, vomiting, and hair loss are common side effects. Anemia and blood-clotting problems can arise from side effects on the bone marrow.

Sometimes cancer can be treated solely with chemotherapy, either as a single drug or with several drugs commonly given at regular intervals, called cycles. A cycle can be a dose of chemotherapy followed by several days or weeks without therapy. This gives normal cells time to recover from the effects of the chemotherapy.

More often, chemotherapy is used with surgery or radiation therapy, or both:

- Chemotherapy can be used to shrink a tumor before surgery or radiation therapy.

- Chemotherapy can be used after surgery or radiation therapy to help kill any remaining cancer cells.

In many cases, with treatment the cancer does not go away but can be controlled and managed as a chronic disease. In other cases, the cancer may seem to have gone away but returns. Chemotherapy can then be given again.

When the cancer is at an advanced stage, is not under control, and has metastasized to other parts of the body, chemotherapy can help shrink a tumor that is causing pain or pressure to improve the quality of life for the patient. This is called **palliation.**

There are more than 100 chemotherapy drugs of a dozen different types.

Biologic Therapies (Immunotherapy)

Biologic therapies use the body's immune system, directly or indirectly, to attack cancer cells or to lessen the side effects that can be caused by radiation and chemotherapy. **Biologic response modifiers** alter the immune system's response to cancer cells and include interferons, interleukins, monoclonal antibodies, vaccines, and gene therapy.

Monoclonal antibodies (MOABs) are antibodies produced by a single type of cell and are specific for a single antigen. Examples of MOABs are rituximab (*Rituxan*), used for non-Hodgkin lymphoma, and trastuzumab (*Herceptin*), used in breast cancer for tumors that produce a protein called *HER-2*.

Cytostatics inhibit cell division. Examples include cyclophosphamide (*Cytoxan*) which is a potent agent; methotrexate (*Amethopterin*); cyclosporine (*Cyclosporin A*); mechlorethamine (*Nitrogen mustard*).

Antiangiogenesis therapy interferes with the genetic mechanisms that increase blood supply for the active growth of cancer cells. The drug *Avastin* has led to a great increase in the survival of patients with colon cancer and also is being used in lung and breast cancer.

Gene therapy is now a focus of cancer therapy. In 2005, the **National Cancer Institute (NCI)** and the **National Human Genome Research Institute (NHGRI)** announced a 3-year pilot project to map the genetic alterations in cancer cells. New technologies called **microarrays** or **gene chips** (small slivers of glass or nylon that can be coated with genes) enable every gene that is active in a cancer cell to be identified.

Gene therapy involves introducing a normal gene into a person's cells to replace an abnormal disease-producing gene *(see Chapter 21)*. Numerous trials are under way to define gene therapy's applications in the biologic treatment of cancer.

Immune therapy is a recent focus of cancer therapy research. **Vaccines** against lymphoma, prostate cancer, breast cancer, and pancreatic cancer have shown promise in stimulating the immune system to attack cancer cells and extend survival rates. In 2010, the **FDA** approved the first-ever tumor vaccine, called *Provenge,* to treat prostate cancer. Another FDA-approved immunotherapy, *Yervoy,* is used in metastatic melanoma, but it only extends average survival by a few months.

Targeted immune modulators are new drugs used for diseases such as rheumatoid arthritis and psoriatic arthritis.Evidence of their effectiveness is evolving.

Many types of biological therapy are still in clinical trials, and biological therapy for cancer is a very active area of cancer research. In 2016, the FDA approved the immunotherapy drug pembrolizumab (*Keytruda*) as a first-line treatment for non–small cell lung cancer prior to chemotherapy and also to treat people who had already received chemotherapy.

WORD	PRONUNCIATION	ELEMENTS		DEFINITION
angiogenesis	AN-jee-oh-JEN-eh-sis	S/	-genesis origin, creation, formation	Creation of new blood vessels
		R/CF	angi/o- blood vessel	
antiangiogenesis	An-tee-AN-jee-oh-JEN-eh-sis	P/	anti- against	The prevention of growth of new blood vessels
biology	bie-OL-oh-jee	S/	-logy study of	Science concerned with life and living organisms
		R/CF	bio- life	
biologic (adj)	BI-oh-LOJ-ik	S/	-ic pertaining to	Pertaining to life and living organisms
clone	KLOHN		Greek cutting used for propagation	A colony of organisms or cells all having identical genetic constitutions
monoclonal (adj)	MON-oh-KLOH-nal	S/	-al pertaining to	Derived from a protein from a single clone of cells, all molecules of which are the same
		P/	mono- one	
		R/	-clon- cutting used for propagation	
microarray (also called gene chips)	MY-kroh-ah-RAY	P/	micro- small	Technique for studying one gene in one experiment
		R/	-array place in order	

Exercises

A. Review the content related to the pharmacologic treatment of cancer to find the answers to the following questions. *Choose the best answer.* **LO 20.6, 20.7**

1. The term containing a combining form that means *blood vessel* is

   a. hemolysis   **b.** angiogenesis   **c.** environmental

2. The prefix in this term means *one:*

   a. biologic   **b.** dioxin   **c.** monoclonal

3. The suffix in this term means *study of:*

   a. microarray   **b.** biology   **c.** brachytherapy

4. The suffix in this term means *origin:*

   a. biologic   **b.** antiangiogenesis   **c.** microarray

5. The term containing a word element that means *small* is

   a. lobectomy   **b.** stereotactic   **c.** microarray

6. The term that does NOT contain a prefix is

   a. biology   **b.** monoclonal   **c.** microarray

B. Medications used to treat cancer. *From the provided terms, complete the statements regarding medications that are used to treat cancer. Fill in the blank.* **LO 20.7**

   palliation   chemotherapy   tumor   nausea   cycles

1. The use of drugs to treat cancer is termed _____.

2. Medication can shrink a _____ prior to its surgical removal.

3. Doses of medication are given at scheduled _____ to allow the patient to recover from its side effects.

4. Side effects of chemotherapy include fatigue, hair loss, and _____.

5. Chemotherapy that relieves symptoms but does not cure would be _____ therapy.

Cancer

Challenge Your Knowledge

A. Prefixes. Not every medical term will have a prefix, but when they do, it is an extra clue for you in determining the meaning of the term. Given the definition, identify the correct prefix it is describing. Fill in the blank. **(LO 20.C)**

1. Programmed normal cell death: _____ ptosis

2. Carcinogenic released from burning wood: _____ oxin

3. Given in smaller amounts, more often: _____ fractionated

4. Cancer arising from the cells lining the pleural cavity or peritoneum: _____ thelioma

5. Spread of disease to another body part: _____ stasis

6. Technique for studying one gene in one experiment: _____ array

7. Derived from a single protein from a single clone of cells: _____ clonal

8. New growth, benign or malignant: _____ plasm

9. Founder, beginning of an ancestry: _____ genitor

10. A normal gene, in normal cell growth: _____ oncogene

B. Roots. Identify the meaning of the root/combining form in each term below. **(LO 20.1, 20.5, 20.6, 20.7, 20.D)**

_____ 1. mediastinoscopy   **a.** to form

_____ 2. neoplastic   **b.** offspring

_____ 3. antiangiogenesis   **c.** cutting used for propagation

_____ 4. palpation   **d.** mediastinum

_____ 5. monoclonal   **e.** touch

_____ 6. apoptosis   **f.** lobe

_____ 7. lobectomy   **g.** blood vessel

_____ 8. progenitor   **h.** falling

C. Complete the sentence with the correct term. From the words provided, complete the sentences with the best answer. Fill in the blanks. (**LO 20.1, 20.2, 20.5, 20.6, 20.F**)

lavage   neoplasm   infiltrate   carcinogen   metastasis

pneumonectomy   digital   fluoroscopy   oncologist   chemotherapy

1. The family practice physician referred the patient to a(n) _____ for the proper treatment of her cancer.

2. The annual mammogram revealed a _____ in the right breast.

3. The physician ordered a ductal _____ to determine the presence of abnormal breast cells.

4. Because the tumor invaded the entire lung, a _____ was performed.

5. The tumor in the breast began to _____ healthy tissue.

6. The osteosarcoma is a result of the _____ of the liver cancer.

7. Modern radiography utilizes _____ imaging.

8. The radiologist utilized _____ to guide the needle to the tumor.

9. After removing the small cancerous growth, the oncologist recommended five weeks of _____.

10. Radon gas is a known _____.

D. Suffixes can provide additional information about a medical term. Analyze the suffix in each of the following terms, and use it to provide a clue about the term. Fill in the blanks. The first one has been done for you. (**LO 20.D**)

Medical Term	Suffix	Meaning of Suffix	Meaning of Term
angiogenesis	1. -genesis	2. origin, creation, production	3. Creation of new blood vessels
neoplasia	4.	5.	6.
oncology	7.	8.	9.
oncologist	10.	11.	12.
pneumonectomy	13.	14.	15.
chondrosarcoma	16.	17.	18.
proliferate	19.	20.	21.
scintigraphy	22.	23.	24.
malignancy	25.	26.	27.
mammogram	28.	29.	30.

©2014 Nucleus Medical Media

Cancer

E. Compare and contrast benign and malignant tumors to meet a lesson objective. You are given a statement about a tumor. Indicate whether it refers to a benign or malignant tumor by writing B for benign and M for malignant. **(LO 20.2)**

1. Grows slowly: _____

2. Invades the lymph system: _____

3. Does not metastasize to other organs: _____

4. Invades the bloodstream and travels to other organs: _____

5. Lipoma: _____

6. Surrounded by connective tissue capsule: _____

7. Can compress surrounding tissues and cause functional problems: _____

8. Does not invade or infiltrate adjacent tissues: _____

9. Unlimited, unregulated growth potential: _____

10. Invades or infiltrates adjacent tissues: _____

11. Does not spread to lymph nodes: _____

12. Mesothelioma: _____

F. Correct usage. Demonstrate your knowledge of the *language of oncology*. These are similar medical terms, but each has only one correct use in the paragraph. Fill in the blanks. **(LO 20.2)**

carcinogen   carcinoma   carcinogenic   carcinogenesis

1. Raquel Sacco was unknowingly exposed to a _____ in the form of secondhand smoke. This _____

substance brought about the _____ of her tumors. Her primary _____ has already metastasized;

her prognosis is poor.

metastasis   metastasized   metastases   metastatic

2. The _____ of Raquel's primary cancer to a secondary site was discovered after diagnostic study.

The _____ in her brain were not the site of her current surgery. Her _____ lesions may require radiation

therapy if they are inoperable. Because her cancer has already _____ , her chances of survival are poor.

G. **Cancer quiz.** Assess your knowledge of this chapter by correctly answering the following questions on cancer. The *language of oncology* will aid your understanding of the questions and possible answers. Choose the correct choice, and remember there is only one *best* answer. **(LO 20.3, 20.4, 20.5, 20.F)**

1. Second-leading cause of lung cancer (after smoking):

   a. air pollution

   b. radon

   c. chemical toxins

   d. polychlorinated biphenyls

   e. particulate matter

2. Used to vacuum out suspicious breast tissue through a needle:

   a. gamma knife

   b. lavage

   c. bronchoscopy

   d. mammatome

   e. mammogram

3. In the TNM staging system for cancer, the "N" stands for

   a. nothing

   b. normal

   c. neoplasm

   d. node

   e. noninvasive

4. A medication that halts cell division:

   a. oncogene

   b. cytostatic

   c. antineoplastic

   d. protooncogene

5. A tumor that has invaded or infiltrated has

   a. grown into adjacent tissue

   b. died

   c. become weaker

   d. mutated

   e. necrotized

6. Healthy genes that promote normal cell growth are called

   a. tumor suppressor genes

   b. mutated tumor suppressor genes

   c. protooncogenes

   d. mutated genes

   e. receptor genes

7. A benign tumor is

   a. surrounded by a capsule

   b. cytostatic

   c. metastatic

   d. necrotic

   e. invasive

8. An early form of carcinoma in which there is no invasion of surrounding tissues is

   a. large cell carcinoma

   b. small cell carcinoma

   c. adenocarcinoma

   d. carcinoma in situ

   e. squamous cell carcinoma

9. The abbreviation PCD means the same as

   a. protooncogene

   b. apoptosis

   c. oncogene

   d. polychlorinated biphenyls

   e. progenitor

10. Detecting an abnormal growth by touch is defined as:

    a. palpation

    b. lavage

    c. curettage

    d. aspiration

    e. ultrasound

©2014 Nucleus Medical Media

Cancer

H. Abbreviations. Use with care to ensure you are conveying precise information. Demonstrate your knowledge of this chapter's abbreviations by correctly matching the definition in the first column to the abbreviation in the second column. **(LO 20.F)**

_____ 1. genes normally suppress mitosis   **a.** PCD

_____ 2. chemical toxin banned years ago   **b.** FOBT

_____ 3. general test for detecting cancer   **c.** AMAS

_____ 4. tests for blood in stool   **d.** MRI

_____ 5. washing process with a scope   **e.** TS

_____ 6. apoptosis   **f.** PCB

_____ 7. detailed images in planes   **g.** BAL

I. Procedures. There are many different procedures associated with cancer diagnosis and treatment. Can you correctly identify these procedures used for cancer patients? Choose the best answer. **(LO 20.5, 20.6, 20.F)**

1. Removal of the entire lung:

   a. pneumonectomy   **b.** bronchoscopy   **c.** lobectomy

2. The most accurate non-invasive test for identifying if the cancer has metastasized:

   a. thoracoscopy   **b.** cytoscopy   **c.** positron emission tomography

3. Treatment aimed at decreasing pain or discomfort; not curative

   a. brachytherapy   **b.** chemotherapy   **c.** palliation

4. Fiber-optic tube with a camera is inserted into the space between the lungs:

   a. computed tomography   **b.** mediastinoscopy   **c.** fluoroscopy

5. Implants radioactive seeds into the tumor for direct radiation:

   a. brachytherapy   **b.** stereotactic radiosurgery   **c.** scintigraphy

6. Removal of only a small part of the lung; used for carcinoma in situ:

   a. SRS   **b.** segmentectomy   **c.** pneumonectomy

7. Creates three-dimensional images of a lesion for accurate insertion of a needle:

   a. positron emission tomography   **b.** stereotactic-guided biopsy   **c.** ductal lavage

8. A program of therapy:

   a. aspiration   **b.** prognosis   **c.** regimen

9. Employed for cutting tissue, collecting brushings, and performing washings in the lung:

   a. bronchoscopy   **b.** scintigraphy   **c.** chest x-ray

10. More effective than chest x-rays at identifying early tumors:

   a. CT   **b.** PET   **c.** MRI

J. Build your knowledge of elements with this exercise in the language of oncology. The element is given to you in the left column; fill in the meaning of the element in the middle column and identify the type of element (prefix, root, combining form, or suffix) in the right column. Fill in the blanks. **(LO 20.1, 20.2, 20.D)**

Element	Meaning of Element	Type of Element (P, R, CF, S)
proto	1. _____	2. _____
apo	3. _____	4. _____
muta	5. _____	6. _____
genesis	7. _____	8. _____
gen	9. _____	10. _____
onco	11. _____	12. _____
carcino	13. _____	14. _____
ptosis	15. _____	16. _____
gene	17. _____	18. _____

K. Elements. You are given the meaning of the element. Choose the term in which it appears. **(LO 20.D)**

1. The root meaning *surroundings* is in the term

    a. environment   **b.** dioxin   **c.** pollution

2. The suffix meaning *produce* is in the term

    a. carcinogen   **b.** pesticide   **c.** particle

3. The prefix meaning *new* is in the term

    a. proliferate   **b.** neoplastic   **c.** dioxin

4. The suffix meaning *to kill* is in the term

    a. cytostatic   **b.** pesticide   **c.** pollution

5. The suffix meaning *pertaining to* is in the term

    a. pollution   **b.** environmental   **c.** prognosis

6. The prefix meaning *two* is in the term

    a. pesticide   **b.** dioxin   **c.** monoclonal

7. The combining form meaning *spark* is in the term

    a. fluoroscopy   **b.** osteosarcoma   **c.** scintigraphy

8. The root meaning *flesh* is in the term

    a. sarcoma   **b.** leukemia   **c.** carcinoma

©2014 Nucleus Medical Media

Cancer

L. Elements can provide a clue to the origin of a tumor. Analyze the medical terms in the left column and match them to the cancer source in the right column. (**LO 20.1, 20.D**)

Medical Term

_____ 1. mesothelioma

_____ 2. sarcoma

_____ 3. adenocarcinoma

_____ 4. osteosarcoma

_____ 5. melanoma

_____ 6. chondrosarcoma

_____ 7. carcinoma

_____ 8. lymphoma

_____ 9. rhabdomyosarcoma

Cancer Arises from

a. epithelial cells

b. lymph nodes

c. cells lining pleural cavity

d. connective tissue cells

e. glandular epithelial cells

f. skeletal muscle

g. bone-forming cells

h. pigment-producing skin cells

i. cartilage cells

M. Commonalities. Analyze the following medical terms and discover what they all have in common. Choose the correct answer. (**LO 20.1, 20.6, 20.C**)

1. Lobectomy, segmentectomy, and mastectomy are all

    a. diagnoses   b. procedures   c. diagnostic tests

2. Chondrosarcoma, adenocarcinoma, and osteosarcoma are all

    a. neoplasms   b. genes   c. flavonoids

3. PET, MRI, and CT are all

    a. blood tests   b. diagnostic tests   c. surgeries

4. Bronchoscopy, and mediastinoscopy are

    a. chest procedures   b. pelvic procedures   c. abdominal procedures

5. Pathologist, oncologist, and histologist are all

    a. diseases   b. specialists   c. conditions

N. Procedures. An important distinction to learn about procedures is understanding which ones are diagnostic (used to determine a diagnosis) and which ones are therapeutic (carry out treatment). Analyze the following list of medical terms and abbreviations to determine whether they are diagnostic or therapeutic procedures. Write the letter D if it is a diagnostic term and the letter T if it is therapeutic. (**LO 20.5, 20.6, 20.F**)

1. segmentectomy: _____

2. BAL: _____

3. brachytherapy: _____

4. DRE: _____

5. stereotactic biopsy: _____

6. pneumonectomy: _____

7. ductal lavage: _____

8. mediastinoscopy: _____

9. CHART: _____

O. Case Report. The following exercise is based entirely on the Case Report of Raquel Sacco, which was presented in this chapter. **(LO 20.B)**

    1. Reread this entire Case Report out loud to yourself for pronunciation practice. The medical terms you should pay particular attention to have been underlined.

    2. Utilize your knowledge of the *language of oncology* (and previous chapters) to answer the following questions based on the Case Report. Fill in the blanks.

 ## Case Report (CR) 20.1

You are

. . . an advanced-level <u>respiratory therapist</u> employed by Fulwood Medical Center working with Tavis Senko, MD, a <u>pulmonologist</u>.

Your patient is

. . . Raquel Sacco, a 44-year-old mother of two teenage boys, who is the owner of a quilting fabrics store. She is 2 days postop from a lung surgery for non–small cell lung cancer. From her records, you see that she has two <u>secondary metastases</u> in her brain. She has been a nonsmoker all her life. Her 70-year-old father is a two-pack-a-day smoker, as is her husband. They both show no evidence of cancer on chest x-rays. Before Raquel is discharged, as part of her <u>postoperative</u> respiratory care plan, you are using <u>incentive spirometry</u>—also called <u>sustained maximal inspiration (SMI)</u>—to increase her <u>inspiratory</u> volume and improve her inspiratory muscle performance. You also will be taking an arterial blood sample to check her <u>arterial</u> oxygen pressure (PaO_2).

<u>Adenocarcinoma</u> was found in Raquel Sacco. It was <u>diagnosed</u> because she had a <u>seizure</u>, and <u>neurologic</u> tests revealed the presence of two metastases in her brain, leading to a search for the <u>primary</u> tumor, which was found in her lung. Raquel Sacco probably developed her lung cancer as a result of inhaling <u>secondhand</u> smoke all her life (from her father and husband). Because Raquel Sacco's cancer has <u>metastasized</u> to her brain, she is placed in stage IV. The outlook for Mrs. Sacco is bleak.

Non–Small Cell Lung Cancer Survival

Stage	5-Year Relative Survival Rate
I	47%
II	26%
III	8%
IV	2%

    1. Which term means *after surgery*? _____

    2. Does Mrs. Sacco have a personal history of smoking? _____

    3. Is there anyone in her immediate family with a history of cancer? (yes or no) _____

    4. Did her cancer spread? (yes or no) _____

    5. Where did the metastases appear? _____

    6. Are the metastases the 1° or 2° cancer? _____

    7. Where does her 1° cancer originate? _____

    8. What specific type of cancer is the 1° cancer? _____

    9. What problem first brought Mrs. Sacco to the doctor? _____

    10. What stage of cancer has Mrs. Sacco been diagnosed with? _____

RADIOLOGY AND NUCLEAR MEDICINE
The Language of Medical Imaging

©2014 Nucleus Medical Media

The health professionals involved in radiology and nuclear medicine include:

- **Radiologists,** who are physicians with specialized training in obtaining and interpreting medical images.

- **Radiographers, radiologic technologists, radiologic technicians,** and **radiologic assistants,** who provide radiologists with the images they need to diagnose and treat medical conditions.

- **Sonographers,** who operate ultrasound imaging devices to produce diagnostic images.

- **Nuclear medicine specialists,** who are radiologists with specialized training in the use of **radiopharmaceuticals** for the purpose of diagnosis, treatment, and research.

- **Nuclear medicine technologists,** who administer radiopharmaceuticals to patients and operate cameras to detect and map the radioactive drug in the patient's body to create diagnostic images.

- **Radiotherapists,** who are physicians who specialize in the treatment of disease using x-rays and radioactive materials.

Chapter Learning Outcomes

Radiology is a medical specialty that uses imaging techniques to diagnose and treat disease that can be visualized within the human body.
Nuclear medicine is a branch of medical imaging that uses **radioactive** material to pinpoint **molecular** activity within the body in order to diagnose and treat a variety of diseases. The information in this chapter will enable you to:

LO 21.1   Describe the nature and characteristics of x-rays.

LO 21.2   Identify the positions and views of the patient's body used in x-ray examinations.

LO 21.3   Discuss the different techniques for acquiring radiologic diagnostic images.

LO 21.4   Describe the nature and characteristics of radioactive materials used in medical imaging.

LO 21.5   Discuss the nuclear imaging procedures used in the diagnosis of disease.

LO 21.6   Explain the different radiologic techniques used in the treatment of disease.

LO 21.7   Describe the different nuclear medicine therapies and their effectiveness.

LO 21.A   Use the medical terms of medical imaging to communicate in writing and document accurately and precisely in any health care setting.

LO 21.B   Use the medical terms of medical imaging to communicate verbally with accuracy and precision in any health care setting.

LO 21.C   Construct medical terms used in medical imaging from their word elements (roots, combining forms, prefixes, and suffixes).

LO 21.D   Deconstruct medical terms used in medical imaging into their word elements (roots, combining forms, prefixes, and suffixes).

LO 21.E   Identify health professionals involved in medical imaging.

LO 21.F   Identify correct abbreviations for medical terms used in medical imaging.

 ## Case Report (CR) 21.1

You are

. . . Anita Scherraga, a radiologic technologist working in the radiology department at Fulwood Medical Center.

Your patient is

. . . Mrs. Carole Coffrey, a 46-year-old health information technologist with two children who is complaining of pain in her breasts. You are to perform a **mammogram** on Mrs. Coffrey using parallel-plate compression in a **full-field digital mammography** (FFDM) unit. You will be taking two views of Mrs. Coffrey's breasts: a head-to-foot (**craniocaudal [CC]**) and an angled side view (**mediolateral oblique [MLO]**).

Production of X-ray Images

X-rays were first discovered in 1895 by Wilhelm Conrad Röntgen. These x-rays, like light and radio waves, are a form of electromagnetic radiation. The information in this lesson will enable you to:

21.1.1 Discuss the wavelength characteristics of x-rays.

21.1.2 Describe how x-rays interact with and affect matter.

21.1.3 Explain how x-ray images are recorded.

21.1.4 Describe the different alignments of the body in order to produce the most informative x-ray image.

▲ **Figure 21.3** Radiation Monitor. Film badge used to determine a person's exposure to radiation. The badge is worn on a person's clothing and contains a piece of photographic film. Radiation affects the film in a similar way to light.
©Martyn F. Chillmaid/Photo Researchers, Inc.

Abbreviations

CC	craniocaudal
FFDM	full-field digital mammography
MLO	mediolateral oblique

LO 21.1 X-ray Characteristics and Effects

The characteristics of x-rays include:

- **Velocity.** Because they are electromagnetic, x-rays in a vacuum travel at the speed of light, 186,000 miles per second. This velocity is reduced as x-rays penetrate the different substances of the body according to their density.

- **Wavelength.** X-rays have a very short wavelength compared with other electromagnetic waveforms. Only gamma rays from an atomic explosion have a shorter wavelength. This short wavelength is a major factor in enabling x-rays to pass through many materials and tissues to different degrees. Air is the most **radiolucent** and allows the greatest penetration (photographic plates show black, *Figure 21.1*). Fat is denser than air, water is more dense, and bone is the most dense (**radiopaque**) (photographic plates show white, *Figure 21.2*).

- **Invisibility.** X-rays cannot be detected by sight, sound, or touch, so health professionals working in radiology wear a film badge to detect and record radiation to which they are exposed (*Figure 21.3*).

- **Ionization.** An **ion** is an atom or group of atoms carrying an electric charge by having gained or lost one or more electrons. When x-rays **ionize** matter, they can both kill cancerous cells and damage normal cells to produce the side effects of radiation as well as genetic mutations that cause malignant changes. Radiation also can cause damage to a fetus, so the use of x-rays in pregnancy is kept to a minimum.

Recording of X-ray Images

A special type of photographic film is used to record x-ray pictures. The x-rays are converted into light, and the more energy that passes through body tissues to reach the photographic film or plate, the darker that region of film will be. Lungs will be dark; bones that prevent the passage of energy will be white. X-rays can now also be detected electronically using a recorder similar to that used in a digital camera. This means that they can be read immediately and stored more easily.

▲ **Figure 21.1** X-ray Image of a Female Chest. ©UIG/Getty Images

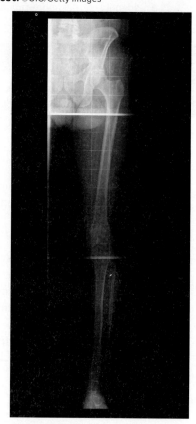

▲ **Figure 21.2** X-ray Image of a Femur. ©Warrick G./Photo Researchers, Inc.

WORD	PRONUNCIATION	ELEMENTS		DEFINITION
craniocaudal	KRAY-nee-oh-KAW-dal	S/ R/CF R/	-al *pertaining to* crani/o- *skull* -caud- *tail*	A view of a structure from head to foot
electromagnetic	ee-LEK-troh-mag-NET-ik	S/ R/CF R/	-ic *pertaining to* electr/o- *electricity* -magnet- *magnet*	Pertaining to energy propagated through matter and space
ion	EYE-on		Greek *going*	An atom or group of atoms having gained or lost one or more electrons
ionization (noun)	EYE-on-ih-ZA-shun	S/ R/	-ization *process of affecting in a specific way* ion- *atom or group of atoms carrying an electric charge*	The process of causing an atom or group of atoms to gain or lose one or more electrons
ionize (verb)		S/	-ize *to affect in a specific way*	To cause the process of ionization
mammography	mah-MOG-rah-fee	S/ R/CF	-graphy *process of recording* mamm/o- *breast*	X-ray imaging of the breast
mammogram	MAM-oh-gram	S/	-gram *a record*	The x-ray record produced by mammography
radioactive	RAY-dee-oh-AK-tiv	R/CF R/CF	radi/o- *radiation* -activ/e *movement*	Spontaneously emitting alpha, beta, or gamma rays
radiograph	RAY-dee-oh-graf	S/ R/CF	-graph *record* radi/o- *radiation*	Image made by exposure to x-rays
radiographer radiographic	ray-dee-OG-rah-fer ray-dee-oh-GRAF-ik	S/ S/	-er *one who records* -ic *pertaining to*	Technologist who performs x-ray procedures Pertaining to x-rays
radiology	ray-dee-OL-oh-jee	S/ R/CF	-logy *study of* radi/o- *radiation*	The study of medical imaging
radiologic radiologist	ray-dee-oh-LOJ-ik ray-dee-OL-oh-jist	S/ S/	-ic *pertaining to* -logist *specialist*	Pertaining to radiology Specialist in radiology
radiolucent	ray-dee-oh-LOO-sent	S/ R/CF	-lucent *open* radi/o- *radiation*	Penetrable by x-rays or other forms of radiation
radiopaque	ray-dee-oh-PAKE	S/	-paque *shady*	Impenetrable to x-rays or other forms of radiation
radiopharmaceutical	RAY-dee-oh-far-mah-SOO-tik-al	S/ S/ R/CF R/CF	-ical *pertaining to* -ceut- *relating to* radi/o- *radiation* -pharm/a- *drug industry*	Relating to a product produced by the drug industry that is radioactive
radiotherapy	RAY-dee-oh-THER-ah-pee	R/CF R/	radi/o- *radiation* -therapy *treatment*	Treatment using radiation
radiotherapist	RAY-dee-oh-THER-ah-pist	S/ R/	-ist *specialist* -therap- *treatment*	Specialist in the use of radiation in the treatment of patients

Exercises

A. Answer the following questions about the characteristics of x-rays. *Select the correct answer.* **LO 21.1**

1. Which of the following is NOT a characteristic of an x-ray?

   a. velocity   **b.** wavelength   **c.** ionization   **d.** invisibility   **e.** weight

2. Which of the following characteristics of x-rays is most damaging to a fetus?

   a. velocity   **b.** radiation   **c.** wavelength   **d.** ionization   **e.** speed

3. X-rays in a vacuum travel at the speed of light. This is called

   a. wavelength   **b.** radiolucent   **c.** velocity   **d.** radiopaque   **e.** invisibility

▲ **Figure 21.4** Radiologist Dictates a Report. ©Spencer Grant/ PhotoEdit Inc.

Duodenum——
Pylorus——
                                    └Stomach

▲ **Figure 21.5** Barium Meal Showing Stomach, **Pylorus, and Duodenum.** ©Biophoto Associates/Photo Researchers, Inc.

Abbreviations	
AP	anteroposterior
DR	digital radiography
EGD	esophagogastroduo-denoscopy
GI	gastrointestinal
PA	posteroanterior

LO 21.2 Patient Alignment

In many situations where x-ray images are taken, the x-ray tube that produces the radiation, the patient, and the photographic film must be aligned to direct the x-ray beam to the lesion being examined in the best possible way. Terms describing the direction of the projection of x-ray beams are of importance in chest x-rays and are:

- **Posteroanterior (PA)**, in which x-rays travel from a posterior source to an anteriorly placed image receiver. This is the most common chest x-ray view.

- **Anteroposterior (AP)**, in which x-rays travel from an anterior source to a posteriorly placed image receiver.

- **Lateral view**. In a left lateral view, x-rays travel from a source located to the right of a patient and travel to an image recorder to the left of the patient. This is reversed in a right lateral view.

- **Mediolateral oblique (MLO)**, which is commonly used in mammography.

- **Oblique**, in which x-rays travel at an angle from the perpendicular plane and pass behind the heart and lung hilum to show structures normally hidden in PA and AP views.

The terms *anterior, posterior,* and other directional terms are described in *Chapter 3.*

LO 21.3 Acquisition of Radiologic Images

Plain (Projectional) Radiography

Plain radiography was the only modality available in the first 50 years of radiology. The x-rays that pass through a patient strike an undeveloped film held in a light-tight cassette. The film is then developed chemically to produce an image on the film. Now, **digital radiography** (**DR**) is replacing film screen radiography; x-rays strike a plate of sensors that convert the signals generated into digital information and an image on a computer screen. Because of its lower cost and availability, plain radiography is the first-line examination of choice in radiologic diagnosis *(Figure 21.4).* Lead aprons can be used to protect patients and technicians from receiving unwanted radiation.

Fluoroscopy

In **fluoroscopy**, a continuous x-ray image is shown on a monitor like an x-ray movie. This allows real-time imaging of structures in motion; for example, blood vessels or the gastrointestinal (**GI**) tract. **Radiocontrast** agents, such as barium sulfate and iodine, are administered orally, rectally, intravenously, or into an artery and enhance the real-time imaging of dynamic processes such as blood flow in arteries and veins (**angiography**) or peristalsis in the GI tract. Iodine contrast also may be concentrated in tumors, cysts, or inflamed areas to make them more **opaque** and conspicuous in imaging. A barium meal *(Figure 21.5),* also known as an upper gastrointestinal series, enables radiographs of the esophagus, stomach, and duodenum to be taken after barium sulfate is ingested. However, the diagnostic use of a barium meal has declined with the increasing use of esophagogastroduodenoscopy (**EGD**), which allows direct visual inspection of suspicious areas in the esophagus, stomach, and duodenum.

WORD	PRONUNCIATION	ELEMENTS		DEFINITION
angiography	an-jee-**OG**-rah-fee	S/ R/CF	**-graphy** *process of recording* **angi/o-** *blood vessel*	Radiography of blood vessels after injection of contrast material
angiogram	**AN**-jee-oh-gram	S/	**-gram** *a record*	The radiograph obtained by angiography
angioplasty	**AN**-jee-oh-**PLAS**-tee	S/	**-plasty** *surgical repair*	Recanalization of a blood vessel by surgery
anteroposterior	**AN**-teh-roh-pos-**TEER**-ee-or	S/ R/CF R/	**-ior** *pertaining to* **anter/o-** *coming before* **-poster-** *coming behind*	The direction the x-ray beam passes through the patient: from front to back (AP)
fluoroscopy	flor-**OS**-koh-pee	S/ R/CF	**-scopy** *to examine* **fluor/o** *x-ray beam*	Examination of the structures of the body by x-rays
oblique	ob-**LEEK**		Latin *slanting*	Slanting; in radiology, a projection that is neither frontal nor lateral
mediolateral oblique	**MEE**-dee-oh-**LAT**-er-al ob-**LEEK**	S/ P/ R/	**-al** *pertaining to* **medio-** *middle* **-later-** *side*	An angled side view of a structure
opaque	oh-**PAKE**		Latin *shady*	Impervious to light; impenetrable by x-rays or other forms of radiation
posteroanterior	**POS**-ter-oh-an-**TEER**-ee-or	S/ R/CF R/	**-ior** *pertaining to* **poster/o-** *coming behind* **-anter-** *coming before*	The direction the x-ray beam passes through the patient: from back to front (PA)
radiocontrast	**RAY**-dee-oh-**CON**-trast	S/ R/CF	**-contrast** *against* **radi/o-** *radiation*	Agents that make structures stand out in x-ray imaging

Exercises

A. Define the views used in radiography. *Match the term in the first column with its correct description in the second column.* **LO 21.2**

_____ 1. posteroanterior

_____ 2. anteroposterior

_____ 3. oblique

_____ 4. mediolateral

a x-ray beam passes through the body at an angle

b. x-ray beam passes through the structure from the middle to the side

c. x-ray beam passes through the patient from back to front

d. x-ray beam passes through the patient from front to back

B. Using the three medical terms below, insert the appropriate medical terms into the paragraph. **LO 21.4, 21.A**

angioplasty   **angiogram**   **angiography**

1. The doctor is using _____ as a diagnostic tool.

2. After seeing the _____, he has decided to schedule the patient for a surgical procedure.

3. He has asked you to schedule the patient's _____ for tomorrow morning.

▲ **Figure 21.6** Brain Hemorrhage, Colored Computed Tomography (CT) Scan. The front of the brain is at top, and a large mass of blood (hematoma, purple) is seen at upper left in the frontal lobe. Bleeding (hemorrhage) in the brain occurs when a blood vessel, such as an artery, ruptures. It may be caused by a head injury, high blood pressure, or vascular disease. In this case, a tree fell on the patient's head. The area of the brain supplied by the ruptured artery may die due to lack of oxygenated blood, leading to a stroke. ©Du Cane Medical Imaging Ltd./Photo Researchers, Inc.

▲ **Figure 21.7** Twins, Ultrasound Biometry. ©VEM/Photo Researchers, Inc.

▲ **Figure 21.8** MRI of Brain Showing Metastases. ©BSIP/Photo Researchers, Inc.

Abbreviations

CT	computed tomography
IR	interventional radiology
MRI	magnetic resonance imaging
US	ultrasound

LO 21.3 Acquisition of Radiologic Images (continued)

Interventional Radiology

Interventional radiology (**IR**) uses minimally invasive procedures both for diagnostic purposes (e.g., angiogram) and for treatment (e.g., **angioplasty**). X-ray images are used for guidance, and the basic instruments used are needles and catheters. The images provide a road map to enable the instruments to be guided to the areas containing disease for diagnosis and for treatment. Benefits from these procedures include short recovery time, shortened hospital stays, reduced infection rates, and reduced costs.

Computed Tomography

The first commercially viable **computed tomography (CT)** scanner was produced at EMI Labs in England in 1972. EMI owned the rights to the Beatles music, and their profits funded the research. CT scans use x-rays in conjunction with computer **algorithms** to produce a computer-generated cross-sectional image (**tomogram**) in the **axial** plane. From these images, the computer can reconstruct **coronal** and **sagittal** images. Radiocontrast agents can be used with CT to enhance the delineation of anatomy. CT scans have become the test of choice in diagnosing some emergency conditions such as cerebral hemorrhage *(Figure 21.6)*, pulmonary embolism *(see Chapter 13)*, aortic dissection *(see Chapter 10)*, and kidney stones *(see Chapter 6)* and in identifying small lung cancers *(see Chapter 13)*. Unfortunately, CT scans expose the patient to much more ionizing radiation than does an x-ray.

Ultrasound

Medical **ultrasonography** uses **ultrasound (US)** (high-frequency sound waves) functioning in real time to visualize soft tissue structures in the body. No ionizing radiation is involved. Because of this, it plays a vital role in obstetrics, enabling early diagnosis of fetal abnormalities and multiple gestations *(Figure 21.7)*. Ultrasound measures the severity of peripheral vascular disease and evaluates the dynamic function of the heart, heart valves, and major blood vessels. In trauma victims, it also can assess the integrity of the major viscera (including liver, spleen, and kidneys) and the presence of bleeding into the peritoneum.

Magnetic Resonance Imaging

Magnetic resonance imaging (MRI) uses strong magnetic fields to align atomic nuclei in tissues, then it uses a radio signal to disrupt the nuclei and observes the radio frequency signal as the nuclei return to their baseline states. MRI can produce images in axial, coronal, sagittal, and oblique planes and also can give the best soft tissue contrast of all imaging modalities. It is an important tool in musculoskeletal radiology and neuroradiology *(Figure 21.8)*. Its disadvantages are that the patient has to lie in a noisy, confined space (tube) for long periods of time, and it cannot be used for patients with pacemakers or any metallic implant such as artificial joints or implanted surgical hardware (plates, rods etc.). For patients with **claustrophobia**, anti-anxiety medication can be prescribed to be taken before entering the scanner.

Teleradiology involves the transmission of radiographic digital images from one location to another for interpretation by a radiologist. It can provide real-time emergency radiology services and expert consultation around the clock.

WORD	PRONUNCIATION		ELEMENTS	DEFINITION
axis axial (adj)	**AK**-sis **AK**-see-al	 S/ R/	Greek *central support* -ial *pertaining to* ax- *central support*	A line of central support Pertaining to an axis
coronal	**KOR**-oh-nal	S/ R/	-al *pertaining to* coron- *crown*	Vertical plane dividing the body into anterior and posterior portions
fibroglandular	fie-broh-**GLAN**-dyu-lar	S/ R/CF R/	-ar *pertaining to* fibr/o- *fiber* -glandul- *little gland*	A mixture of fibrous and glandular tissue
interventional	**IN**-ter-**VEN**-shun-al	S/ S/ R/	-al *pertaining to* -ion- *action, process* intervent- *to come between*	Pertaining to an overt act to change an event or outcome
sagittal	**SAJ**-ih-tal	S/ R/	-al *pertaining to* sagitt- *arrow*	Pertaining to the vertical plane dividing the body into right and left portions
teleradiology	**TEL**-eh-ray-dee-**OL**-oh-jee	S/ P/ R/CF	-logy *study of* tele- *distant* -radi/o- *radiation, x-ray*	The interpretation of digitized diagnostic images transmitted from a distance
tomogram tomography	**TOH**-moh-gram toh-**MOG**-rah-fee	S/ R/CF S/	-gram *a record* tom/o- *section* -graphy *process of recording*	Radiographic image of a selected section or slice of tissue Process of taking a tomogram
ultrasound ultrasonography	**UL**-trah-sownd **UL**-trah-soh-**NOG**-rah-fee	P/ R/ S/ R/CF	ultra- *higher, beyond* -sound *noise* -graphy *process of recording* -son/o- *sound*	Very-high-frequency sound waves Delineation of dynamic structures using sound waves

Exercises

A. Analyze the continuation of the Case Report for Mrs. Coffrey, and then answer the following questions. LO 21.1, 21.3, 21.D

1. The type of image that the radiologist read:

   a. mammography   **b.** mammogram   **c.** angiography   **d.** angiogram

2. Were there any malignancies found in Mrs. Coffrey's report?

   a. yes   **b.** no

3. *Associated mass* would be another term for _____.

4. The medical term in the Case Report that mean *both sides:* _____

B. Improve your knowledge of diagnostic procedures by matching the definition to the appropriate abbreviation. LO 21.3, 21.F

_____ 1. This uses minimally invasive procedures for diagnosis and treatment.   **a.** MRI

_____ 2. This is the test of choice for diagnosing some emergency conditions.   **b.** IR

_____ 3. This uses high-frequency sound waves to visualize soft tissue.   **c.** CT

_____ 4. Patients with pacemakers are unable to use this modality.   **d.** US

Lesson 21.2

RADIOLOGY AND NUCLEAR MEDICINE

Nuclear Medicine

Lesson Objectives

Nuclear medicine imaging uses small amounts of radiopharmaceuticals that are administered to the patient and have an affinity for specific tissues to show their physiological function rather than the anatomical detail of traditional x-ray imaging. The information in this lesson will enable you to:

21.2.1 Describe characteristics and types of radiopharmaceuticals.

21.2.2 Detail imaging devices used in nuclear medicine.

21.2.3 Discuss common diagnostic uses of nuclear medicine imaging procedures.

21.2.4 Describe common nuclear medicine therapies.

Abbreviations

FDG	fludeoxyglucose
PET	positron emission tomography
SPECT	single-photon emission computed tomography

LO 21.4, 21.5 Radiopharmaceuticals

In nuclear medicine, **radionuclides** can be combined with pharmaceutical compounds to form radiopharmaceuticals, which are labeled with a radioactive **tracer**. When administered to a patient orally, injected intravenously, or inhaled as a gas, these compounds can localize to a specific organ or cells. Then, external detectors (gamma cameras) capture and form images from the radiation emitted by the tracers. This two-dimensional imaging is called **scintigraphy**. With computer processing, the information can be displayed as axial, coronal, and sagittal images *(see Chapter 3)*, known as single-**photon** emission computed tomography **(SPECT)** images, to produce an image of a "slice" of a patient in a particular plane. A collection of parallel slices form a slice-stack, a three-dimensional representation of how the radionuclide is distributed in the patient.

The most commonly used tracers include:

· **Technetium-99m,** used in 85% of all nuclear medicine imaging including for bone scans, liver scans, renal function studies, labeling of red blood cells, and use as a gas/aerosol.

· **Iodine-123,** used mainly for thyroid scans.

· **Iodine-131,** used mainly for the destruction of thyroid tissues.

· **Gallium-67,** used in **positron emission tomography (PET)** scans *(see the following)* and for localizing infections.

· **Indium-111,** used to label and identify the movements of white blood cells.

· **Thallium-201,** used for myocardial perfusion scans in stress tests.

· **18F-FDG** (fludeoxyglucose), used in the diagnosis and staging of cancer and most commonly in PET scans.

Positron emission tomography (**PET**) scanning produces two opposite traveling gamma rays to be detected concurrently to improve resolution. 18F-FDG is injected intravenously into the patient, and the radiation emitted is detected to produce multiplanar images of the body. Tissues, such as cancer, that are most metabolically active concentrate the 18F-FDG more than normal tissues. PET images can be fused with an anatomical CT image to improve diagnostic accuracy. In academic and research settings, PET images are now being fused with MRI images.

Radiation Dose

The radiation doses delivered to a patient in a nuclear medicine procedure present a very small risk of inducing cancer. The radiopharmaceuticals are inside the body and emit ionizing radiation that travels a short distance, thus minimizing unwanted side effects and damage to noninvolved nearby structures. The radiopharmaceuticals decay and are excreted from the body through normal bodily functions.

S = Suffix   P = Prefix   R = Root   R/CF = Combining Form

WORD	PRONUNCIATION	ELEMENTS		DEFINITION
photon	**FOH**-ton		Greek *light*	A particle of light or other electromagnetic radiation
positron	**POZ**-ih-tron		Greek *positive element*	A subatomic particle equal in mass to an electron but with the opposite (positive) charge
radionuclide	**RAY**-dee-oh-**NYU**-klide	S/ R/CF R/	**-ide** *having a particular quality* **radi/o-** *radiation* **-nucl-** *nucleus*	Radioactive agent used in nuclear medicine
radiopharmaceutical	**RAY**-dee-oh-far-mah-**SOO**-tik-al	S/ S/ R/CF R/CF	**-ical** *pertaining to* **-ceut-** *relating to* **radi/o-** *radiation* **-pharm/a-** *drug industry*	Radioactive drugs
scintigraphy	sin-**TIG**-rah-fee	S/ R/CF	**-graphy** *process of recording* **scint/i-** *spark*	Recording of radioactivity with gamma cameras
tracer	**TRAY**-ser		Latin *track*	Radioactive agent used to trace metabolic processes

Exercises

A. To improve your knowledge of radiology terms, complete the following exercises by selecting the correct answer.
LO 21.4, 21.5, 21.F

1. Which term best describes two-dimensional imaging?

   a. ultrasound

   b. scintigraphy

   c. PET scan

   d. MRI scan

   e. interventional

2. What is a tracer?

   a. a red line that appears on the scan

   b. a radioactive agent

   c. a plastic object you swallow for the test

   d. a record produced by the test

   e. a tiny camera you swallow for the test

3. A tracer is used in which type of imaging?

   a. ultrasound

   b. MRI

   c. scintigraphy

   d. radiation

4. The type of radioactive positron that is used to detect thyroid disorders:

   a. glucose

   b. iodine

   c. thallium

   d. technetium

5. The production of "slice" views of body structures used with scintigraphy:

   a. SPECT

   b. PET

   c. FDG

   d. IR

LO 21.6 Radiation Therapy

Radiation therapy is defined as treatment with x-rays or radionuclides.

X-ray Therapy

Ionizing radiation works by damaging the DNA of tissues exposed to it. However, the x-rays often have to pass through skin and other organs to reach a target tumor. To spare normal tissues from the harmful side effects of x-rays, narrow radiation beams are aimed from several angles to intersect at the target tumor. This provides a much larger local dose to the tumor than to the surrounding healthy tissues. It is also common to combine x-ray therapy with surgery, chemotherapy, hormone therapy, immunotherapy, or any combination.

There are five types of x-ray therapy:

- **Conventional external-beam radiation therapy** consists of a single beam of radiation delivered to the tumor from several directions. The concern is the effect of the radiation on the healthy tissues close to the tumor being irradiated. For complex reasons, large tumors respond less well to radiation than small tumors. Strategies to overcome this include surgical resection prior to chemotherapy (as in the treatment of breast cancer), chemotherapy to shrink the tumor prior to radiation therapy, and the administration of radiosensitizing drugs during radiation therapy. Examples are cisplatin *(Platinol)* and cetuximab *(Erbitux)*.

- **Stereotactic radiation** is a specialized form of external-beam radiation therapy. It focuses radiation beams by using detailed imaging scans. In **stereotactic radiosurgery (SRS),** radiation is applied to the tumor with multiple (as many as 200), separate narrow beams, so that the tumor receives a very high dose of radiation in one treatment, yet the surrounding tissues are minimally irradiated. In areas of the body where there is motion by breathing or blood flow, a combination of continuous imaging, motion detection, and robotic guidance enable the beams to remain focused on the tumor. **Stereotactic body radiation treatment (SBRT)** refers to the use of these techniques in such areas as the lungs. A technique called **hypofractionation** is the giving of a much higher dose of radiation per session with greater accuracy and the sparing of normal surrounding tissue. Brand names for these stereotactic radiation therapies include Gamma Knife, Cyberknife, Tomotherapy, and Truebeam.

- **3-dimensional conformal radiation therapy (3DCRT)** is the result of being able to delineate tumors and surrounding normal tissues in three dimensions using CT or MRI scanners and planning software. The profile of each radiation beam and the treatment volume conform to the shape of the tumor, allowing a higher dose of radiation to be delivered to the tumor with a reduced toxicity to the surrounding normal tissues.

- **Intensity-modulated radiation therapy (IMRT)** is the next generation of 3DCRT in which, if the tumor is wrapped around a vulnerable structure such as a blood vessel or major organ, the pattern of radiation delivery can avoid the normal structure.

- **Proton beam therapy** has the advantage that the proton only gives up its energy when it hits the tumor and does not continue on through the tumor to hit normal tissue on the far side. Very high doses of radiation can be given without adjacent normal tissue damage. Prostate cancer is the most common cancer to be treated by proton beam therapy.

LO 21.7 Nuclear Medicine Therapy

In **radioactive iodine (I-131) therapy,** the I-131 is taken orally and absorbed into the bloodstream from the GI tract. From the blood, it is concentrated by the thyroid gland, where it destroys cells in that organ and is used to treat thyroid cancer, thyroid nodules, and hyperthyroidism. Common nuclear medicine therapies treat lymphoma, neuroendocrine tumors, and palliative bone pain. Implanted capsules of isotopes **(brachytherapy)** are used for such cancers as prostate and breast cancer.

Radioimmunotherapy (RIT) combines radiation therapy and immunotherapy. In immunotherapy, a laboratory-produced molecule called a **monoclonal antibody** is designed to recognize and bind to the surface of cancer cells; this mimics the body's naturally produced antibodies. In RIT, a monoclonal antibody is fused with a radioactive material and injected into the patient's bloodstream. The antibody travels to and binds to the cancer cells, delivering a high dose of radiation directly to the cells in the cancer.

WORD	PRONUNCIATION	ELEMENTS		DEFINITION
brachytherapy	brah-kee-**THAIR**-ah-pee	P/ R/	**brachy-** *short* **-therapy** *medical treatment*	Internal radiation therapy delivered by placing radiation sources into the tumor
hypofractionation	**HIGH**-poh-frak-shun-**AY**-shun	S/ S/ P/ R/	**-ation** *process* **-ion-** *action, process* **hypo-** *below* **-fract-** *small amount*	Larger measures of a dose of radiation given less frequently
monoclonal	**MON**-oh-**KLOH**-nal	S/ P/ R/	**-al** *pertaining to* **mono-** *one, single* **-clon-** *cutting*	Pertaining to protein from a single clone of cells
proton	**PROH**-ton		Greek *first*	The positively charged unit of the nuclear mass
radioimmunotherapy	**RAY**-dee-oh-**IM**-you-noh-**THAIR**-ah-pee	R/CF R/CF R/	**radi/o-** *radiation* **-immun/o-** *immune response* **-therapy** *medical treatment*	The combination of radiotherapy and the use of antibodies, e.g., monoclonal antibodies
stereotactic	**STER**-ee-oh-**TAK**-tik	S/ R/CF R/	**-ic** *-pertaining to* **stere/o-** *three-dimensional* **-tact-** *orderly arrangement*	Pertaining to a precise three-dimensional method to locate a lesion or a tumor

Exercises

A. Differentiate between the different types of x-ray therapy for malignant tumors. *Choose the best answer for each question.* **LO 21.6, 21.7**

1. A brand name for this type of therapy is Gamma Knife:

   a. proton beam therapy

   b. conventional external-beam radiation therapy

   c. intensity-modulated radiation therapy

   d. stereotactic radiation

2. Of all of the types of x-ray therapy, this one has the greatest incidence of radiation being applied to normal, healthy tissue:

   a. proton beam therapy

   b. conventional external-beam radiation therapy

   c. intensity-modulated radiation therapy

   d. stereotactic radiation

3. The next generation of 3DCRT is:

   a. proton beam therapy

   b. conventional external-beam radiation therapy

   c. intensity-modulated radiation therapy

   d. stereotactic radiation

4. This therapy can treat cancer with high doses of radiation without adjacent normal tissue damage:

   a. proton beam therapy

   b. conventional external-beam radiation therapy

   c. intensity-modulated radiation therapy

   d. stereotactic radiation

B. Identify the following elements that appear in the above WAD and the text on this spread. *Match the word element in the first column to its correct definition in the second column.* **LO 21.6, 21.7, 21.D**

_____ 1. *stereo*

_____ 2. *hypo*

_____ 3. *fract*

_____ 4. *mono*

_____ 5. *clon*

_____ 6. *brachy*

a. short

b. broken

c. below

d. three-dimensional

e. cutting

f. one

Radiology and Nuclear Medicine

Challenge Your Knowledge

A. Review the planes and directional terms because they are very important in diagnostic radiology. Fill in the blanks. **(LO 21.2, 21.A)**

1. front of the body _____

2. divides the body into upper and lower portions _____

3. side of the body _____

4. toward the midline of the body _____

5. head of the body _____

6. back of the body _____

7. divides the body into right and left portions _____

8. only horizontal plane in the body _____

9. head to foot _____

B. Choose the correct answer. **(LO 21.1)**

1. Which x-ray characteristic is electromagnetic?

   a. speed

   b. velocity

   c. wavelength

   d. ionization

C. The most basic element in any medical term is its root or combining form. In each of these terms, identify the root/combining form and define the meaning of the element and the term. **(LO 21.1, 21.5, 21.7, 21.D)**

Term	Identify Root/ Combining Form	Meaning of Element	Meaning of Term
mammogram	1.	2.	3.
fluoroscopy	4.	5.	6.
sagittal	7.	8.	9.
scintigraphy	10.	11.	12.
monoclonal	13.	14.	15.
radiograph	16.	17.	18.

D. **Each of these medical terms has a function in radiology.** Write the correct term with its correct definition. Fill in the blank. (LO 21.6, 21.A)

1. Materials placed into the body to enhance the image of an organ or structure in radiographic procedures. _____

2. Internal radiation therapy delivered by placing radiation sources into the tumor. _____

3. Radioactive agent used in nuclear medicine to visualize metabolic processes of cells and organs. _____

4. The use of high-frequency sound waves to visualize structures. _____

5. A computer-generated cross-sectional image. _____

E. **Choose the best answer.** (LO 21.2, 21.4, 21.A)

1. Which pair of terms could appear in a radiology report?

a. impacted   cerumen

b. oblique   opaque

c. sublingual   subcutaneous

d. tonometer   otolith

e. cannula   catheter

F. **Read the following paragraph and then choose the correct answers.** (LO 21.1, 21.3, 21.4, 21.5, 21.A)

In fluoroscopy and angiography, a fluorescent screen and image intensifier tube are connected to a closed-circuit television system. This allows real-time imaging of structures in motion; for example, blood vessels or the GI tract. Radiocontrast agents, such as barium sulfate and iodine, are administered orally, rectally, intravenously, or into an artery and enhance the real-time imaging of dynamic processes such as blood flow in arteries and veins or peristalsis in the GI tract. Iodine contrast also may be concentrated in tumors, cysts, or inflamed areas to make them more opaque and conspicuous.

1. What is *real-time imaging*?

a. You take pictures during a scan and view them later.

b. You see images on a screen as the scan is actually happening.

c. You take pictures before any tracer is administered.

d. You can only take pictures at night.

e. You can only take pictures in the morning.

2. What does *angiography* look at specifically?

a. organs

b. tissue

c. blood vessels

d. muscle

e. tendons

3. What is the purpose of a radiocontrast agent?

a. to enhance the image being filmed

b. to soften the structure being filmed

c. to block out of the picture any organs not being filmed

d. to administer chemotherapy to a tumor being filmed

e. to add more liquid volume to the body

4. What does radiocontrast specifically identify in the GI tract?

a. outline of organs

b. tumors or masses

c. peristalsis

d. edema

e. clots

Radiology and Nuclear Medicine

G. **Alphabet soup.** Use the correct letters to form the abbreviations necessary to match the definitions. Fill in the blanks with the correct abbreviation. **(LO 21.5, 21.6, 21.F)**

A B C D E F G H I J K L M N O P Q R S T U V W X Y Z

1. This term refers to the stomach and intestines. _____

2. This replaces film screen radiography. _____

3. X-rays travel from an anterior source to a posterior receiver. _____

4. This uses minimally invasive procedures. _____

5. High-frequency sound waves are used to visualize soft tissue structures. _____

6. This test gives the best soft tissue contrast of all the imaging modalities. _____

7. This scan produces a computer-generated cross-sectional image in the axial plane. _____

8. This scan will produce multiplanar images of the body. _____

H. **All the following terms are composed of various combinations of elements.** Answer the questions, using your knowledge of the elements of the language of radiology. Fill in the blank. Not all terms will be used. **(LO 21.2, 21.3, 21.6, 21.A)**

anteroposterior	opaque	fluoroscopy	posteroanterior
claustrophobia	teleradiology	coronal	tomography
ultrasound	radiopharmaceutical	oblique	

1. Which of the above terms means *impervious to light*? _____

2. Which of the above terms means *fear of closed spaces*? _____

3. Which of the above terms has an element meaning *distant*? _____

4. Which of the above terms pertains to a *vertical plane*? _____

5. Which of the above terms has an element meaning *section*? _____

6. Which of the above terms has an element meaning *drugs*? _____

I. **Build the correct medical terms by using elements from the element bank that follows (you will not use all the elements provided) to complete the terms.** **(LO 21.7, 21.C)**

| hypo | immune | mono | stereo | ary |
| brachy | fract | bi | al | mammo |

1. therapy of short duration: _____/therapy

2. larger measures of a dose of radiation given less frequently: _____/ionation

3. protein from a single clone of cells: _____/clon/_____

4. record of the breast: _____/gram

J. Construct medical terms with your knowledge of the language of radiology. **(LO 21.3, 21.A, 21.C)**

1. Combine the R/CF *mamm/o* with various suffixes to complete the sentences below.

graphy   **plasty**   **gram**

The patient underwent _____ at her physician's request. After she read the _____, she

recommended that the patient undergo a _____ to repair her breast.

2. Select the correct terms to complete the sentences below.

radiographer   **radiologist**   **radiographic**   **radiographs**

The chief _____ ordered various _____ studies to help determine the patient's diag-

nosis. The _____ performed the requested studies and after viewing the _____, the

doctor was able to determine a diagnosis for the patient.

K. Which of the following medical terms are diagnostic, and which are therapeutic? Write D is the term is diagnostic. Write T if the term is therapeutic. **(LO 21.2, 21.6, 21.7, 21.D)**

Medical Term	D (Diagnostic) or T (Therapeutic)
brachytherapy	1.
radiotherapy	2.
hypofractionation	3.
Cyberknife	4.
mammogram	5.
angiography	6.
PET scan	7.
fluoroscopy	8.

L. In the following exercise, which statement is incorrect? Choose T if the statement is true. Choose F if the statement is false. **(LO 21.3, 21.5, 21.6, 21.F)**

1. A tracer is a radioactive agent.   T   F

2. MRIs use gamma cameras.   T   F

3. Nuclear medicine uses high doses of radiation.   T   F

4. Ionizing radiation works by damaging the DNA of tissues exposed to it.   T   F

5. *Hypofractionation* refers to the dosage of radiation.   T   F

Radiology and Nuclear Medicine

M. Choose the correct answer. (LO 21.2)

1. Which of the following pairs of terms would *not* appear in a radiology report?

   a. anterior   posterior

   b. medial   lateral

   c. coronal   caudal

   d. platelet   capillary

   e. tarsus   malleolus

N. Assign the correct term from the word bank (you will have more choices than you will need) to complete the statements. Fill in the blank. (LO 21.2, 21.3, 21.5, 21.6, 21.A, 21.F)

Word Bank:

intravenously	back	teleradiology	CT scan
radiocontrast agents	ultrasonography	tomogram	concurrently
sagittal	interventional	scintigraphy	front

1. Barium sulfate and iodine are _____.

2. Delineation of dynamic structures using sound waves is _____.

3. Radiocontrast agents are administered orally, rectally, and _____.

4. A radiographic image of a selected section or slice of tissue is a(n) _____.

5. Anteroposterior x-ray beams pass through the patient from _____ to _____.

6. Digitized diagnostic images transmitted from a distance are called _____.

7. A _____ produces two-dimensional imaging.

8. The term _____ means *happening together* or *at the same time.*

O. **Review Case Report (CR) 21.1 presented below.** Correctly answer the questions that pertain to the Case Report. **(LO 21.A, 21.F)**

 ## Case Report (CR) 21.1

You are

. . . Anita Scherraga, a radiologic technologist working in the radiology department at Fulwood Medical Center.

Your patient is

. . . Mrs. Carole Coffrey, a 46-year-old health information technologist with two children who is complaining of pain in her breasts. You are to obtain a **mammogram** on Mrs. Coffrey using parallel-plate compression in a **full-field digital mammography** (**FFDM**) unit. You will be taking two views of Mrs. Coffrey's breasts, a head-to-foot (**craniocaudal [CC]**) and an angled side view (**mediolateral oblique [MLO]**).

Mrs. Coffrey's mammogram report was sent to her in writing. It reads, "There are scattered fibroglandular densities bilaterally. There is a benign-appearing area of glandular tissue in the right lower inner breast. There are a few faint calcifications in the lower inner and central left breast. There is no associated mass or distortion."

---

1. From the information in the mammogram report, does Mrs. Coffrey have breast cancer?

   a. Yes

   b. No

2. What term in the report led you to this conclusion? (fill in the blank) _____

3. In which breast(s) is/are the fibroglandular densities located?

   a. left only

   b. right only

   c. left and right

4. Which medical professional created the mammogram report?

   a. gerontologist

   b. podiatrist

   c. sonographer

   d. radiologist

PHARMACOLOGY
The Language of Pharmacology

©2014 Nucleus Medical Media

No matter in which health profession you are working, the following medical terms will be used frequently:

- **Pharmacology** is the study of drugs (**medications**) and their sources, preparation, chemistry, actions, and uses.

- A **pharmacologist**, usually a medical professional with an additional PhD, is a specialist who develops and tests drugs for medicinal use.

- A **pharmacist** is licensed to prepare and dispense drugs and compounds when given written orders from a physician. Pharmacists are knowledgeable about drugs' properties and are able to advise patients and practitioners about their effects and interactions.

- A **pharmacy** is a facility licensed to prepare and dispense drugs (medications) to the public.

- A **pharmacy technician** is trained to work under the supervision of a pharmacist to provide medications to patients.

- A **medication aide** is licensed by the state to assist competent individuals, caretakers, and licensed health care professionals to administer medications. They work mostly in nursing homes and assisted living facilities.

Chapter Learning Outcomes

Pharmacology is a branch of medicine concerned with the action of **drugs.** A **drug** is defined as a man-made chemical or natural substance that exerts a physiologic effect on a cell, tissue, organ, and organism. A drug that is manufactured is called a **pharmaceutical.** In patient care, pharmaceuticals are used frequently, and you need to be able to:

LO 22.1 Recognize the differences between the chemical name, generic name, and brand name of a drug.

LO 22.2 Define the methods used for setting and referencing the standards for the effectiveness and purity of drugs used in the United States.

LO 22.3 Define controlled substance schedules.

LO 22.4 Differentiate the different routes of administration of drugs.

LO 22.5 Explain the methods used to ensure safety and accuracy in drug administration by the different persons administering the drugs.

LO 22.A Use the medical terms of pharmacology to communicate in writing and document accurately and precisely in any health care setting.

LO 22.B Use the medical terms of pharmacology to communicate verbally with accuracy and precision in any health care setting.

LO 22.C Construct medical terms used in pharmacology from their word (roots, combining forms, prefixes, and suffixes).

LO 22.D Deconstruct medical terms used in pharmacology into their word elements (roots, combining forms, prefixes, and suffixes).

LO 22.E Identify health professionals involved in the preparation and administration of drugs.

LO 22.F Identify correct abbreviations for medical terms used in pharmacology.

Case Report (CR) 22.1

You are

. . . a pharmacist in the pharmacy at Fulwood Medical Center. Your patient has been sent to you by Susan Lee, MD, a primary care physician at Fulwood Medical Center.

Your patient is

. . . Mrs. Rebecca Borodin, a frail 80-year-old widow living in an assisted living facility. She has recently begun to complain that she has difficulty recognizing and naming her fellow residents and knowing when to go to the facility's dining room for meals. In addition, it has been hard for her to eat because she suffers from dry mouth and difficulty in swallowing. She also has complained of dizziness and problems with balance; recently, she fell as a result of these problems. Her past medical history includes osteoarthritis, osteopenia, hypertension, congestive heart failure, persistent pain following herpes zoster, and stress incontinence.

Mrs. Borodin has brought in a bag containing all her medications, which include cimetidine, acetaminophen with codeine (*Tylenol #2*), oxybutynin, digoxin, atenolol, alprazolam, zolpidem (*Ambien*), and naproxen. In addition, she takes an over-the-counter (OTC) multivitamin and melatonin.

Dr. Lee has asked you to make sure that Mrs. Borodin knows what each of the medications is for and when to take it. She also has asked you to review the drugs themselves to see if any of them could be causing her recent symptoms.

Drug Names, Standards, and References

LO 22.1 Drug Names

There are more than 3,000 drugs that can be **prescribed** by licensed practitioners. Each drug has three different names:

- The drug's **chemical** name (for example, 8-chloro-1-methyl-6-phenyl4H-s-triazolo-benzodiazepine), which specifies the chemical makeup of the drug, is often long and complicated.

- The drug's **generic** name (for example, alprazolam), which identifies the drug legally and scientifically; there is only one generic name for each drug.

- The drug's **brand (trade)** name (for example, *Xanax*), which each manufacturer gives to the drug. These names are the manufacturer's private property. There can be several brand names of a particular drug, depending on how many different companies are manufacturing the drug. The brand names are always capitalized (e.g., *Xanax*).

When a drug manufacturer receives U.S. **Food and Drug Administration (FDA)** approval to sell a particular drug, it is allowed to have 20 years of protected proprietary manufacture of the drug (patent) from the date of invention, which means that no other company can manufacture and sell the same drug during that period of time. After that period of time, however, the generic name of the drug becomes public property, and any drug manufacturer can manufacture and sell the drug under that generic name.

However, if a specific brand name is ordered on a **prescription** by a physician and is designated "dispense as written," no generic or other brand name may be substituted. Generic drugs are usually cheaper than brand-name drugs because several companies are competing with one another to sell them and the generic companies have not had the initial research and development costs.

▲ **Figure 22.1** Shopping in a Pharmacy for Over-the-Counter (OTC) Medicines.
©McGraw-Hill Education/Ken Karp, photographer

LO 22.2 Drug Standards
Over-the-Counter (OTC) Drugs

Over-the-counter (OTC) drugs *(Figure 22.1)*, which also are called nonprescription drugs, are used to treat conditions that do not generally require care or a prescription from a health professional. Examples of these drugs include **analgesics**, such as aspirin or acetaminophen; **antihistamines**, such as *Chlor-Trimeton* and *Dramamine;* and some sleeping aids, such as doxylamine (an antihistamine) and melatonin. In addition, herbal preparations, vitamins, minerals, and food supplements are available without a prescription.

WORD	PRONUNCIATION	ELEMENTS		DEFINITION
antihistamine	an-tee-**HISS**-tah-meen	P/ R/ R/CF	anti- *against* -hist- *derived from histidine* -amin/e *nitrogen compound*	Drug used to treat allergic symptoms because of its action antagonistic to histamine
histamine	**HISS**-tah-meen			Compound liberated in tissues as a result of injury or an allergic response
drug	DRUG		Old English *drug*	A therapeutic agent or an addictive substance
generic	jeh-**NER**-ik	S/ R/	-ic *pertaining to* gener- *birth*	A nonproprietary name for a drug
pharmacist	**FAR**-mah-sist	S/ R/	-ist *specialist* pharmac- *drug*	Person licensed by the state to prepare and dispense drugs
pharmacy	**FAR**-mah-see		Greek *to administer drugs*	Facility licensed to prepare and dispense drugs
pharmacology	far-mah-**KOL**-oh-jee	S/ R/CF	-logy *study* pharmac/o- *drug*	Science of the preparation, uses, and effects of drugs
pharmacologist	far-mah-**KOL**-oh jist	S/	-logist *specialist*	A medical specialist in pharmacology
prescribe	pree-**SKRIBE**	P/ R/	pre- *before* -scribe *write*	To give directions in writing for the preparation and administration of a remedy
prescription	pree-**SKRIP**-shun	S/ R/	-ion *process, action* -script- *writing*	A written direction for the preparation and administration of a remedy

Exercises

A. The differences between the chemical name, generic name, and brand name of a drug. *Match the name in the first column with its correct definition in the second column.* **LO 22.1**

_____ **1.** chemical name

_____ **2.** brand name

_____ **3.** generic name

a. identifies the drug legally and scientifically

b. specifies the chemical makeup of the drug

c. name of the drug given by the manufacturer

B. Identify the different names given to the one drug. *All of the following names are applied to the same drug. Identify its name type by choosing the correct answer.* **LO 22.1**

1. diphenhydramine

   a. chemical name

   b. brand name

   c. generic name

2. 2-(diphenylmethoxy)-N,N-dimethylethanamine

   a. chemical name

   b. brand name

   c. generic name

3. *Benadryl*

   a. chemical name

   b. brand name

   c. generic name

▲ **Figure 22.2** Paper
Prescription Pad. ©Siede
Preis/Getty Images RF

Keynotes

- The *Physicians' Desk Reference* (PDR) contains detailed information on individual drugs, including their intended effects, side effects, interactions, dosage, and administration. The information is provided by the manufacturers and is updated yearly.

- A **hospital formulary** provides similar information about the medications the hospital's physicians can prescribe.

- An insurance company's formulary provides similar information about the medications it will pay for.

Abbreviations

LSD	lysergic acid diethylamide
PDR	*Physicians' Desk Reference*
USP	United States Pharmacopeia

LO 22.2 Drug Standards (continued)

Prescription Drugs

A prescription **medication** is legally regulated, which means that a person needs a medical prescription to purchase it *(Figure 22.2)*. Prescriptions can only be written by physicians, licensed medical practitioners, dentists, optometrists, veterinarians, and advanced nurse practitioners. Prescribed drugs must have a package insert detailing the intended effects of the drug and its **side effects**.

Regulating the safety and effectiveness of prescription drugs in the United States is the responsibility of the **FDA.** Another agency, the **United States Pharmacopeia (USP)**, sets the standards for the quality, purity, and safety of the medications to be enforced by the FDA to protect the public health.

22.3 Controlled Substance Schedules

Certain groups of prescription drugs that are considered to have a potential for abuse are called **controlled drugs.** Regulation of these drugs is the responsibility of the U.S. Department of Justice **Drug Enforcement Administration (DEA)**. These controlled substances are divided into five schedules, depending on their currently accepted medical use in treatment, their potential for abuse, and their likelihood of causing dependence.

- **Schedule I** controlled substances have a high potential for abuse and have no accepted medical use in treatment in the United States. Examples include heroin, marijuana, and **LSD**. Drugs listed in Schedule I cannot be prescribed, administered, or dispensed, but marijuana is legal for medical use in some states, and now in 2018 is legal in some states for recreational use. However, the current federal government is against recreational use.

- **Schedule II** controlled substances have a high potential for abuse. Abuse of these substances may lead to severe psychological or physical dependence. Examples include some **narcotics**, such as morphine, methadone, meperidine (*Demerol*), and oxycodone (*OxyContin*); **stimulants**, such as amphetamine, methamphetamine, and methylphenidate (*Ritalin*); cocaine; and barbiturates, such as pentobarbital.

- **Schedule III** controlled substances have less potential for abuse than substances in Schedules I and II. Abuse of these substances may lead to moderate or low physical dependence or high psychological dependence. Examples include certain narcotics, including combination products with less than 15 milligrams of hydrocodone per dose (for example, *Vicodin*) and combination products with less than 90 milligrams of codeine per dose (for example, acetaminophen [*Tylenol*] with codeine). Other Schedule III nonnarcotics include **anabolic steroids**, such as oxandrolone.

- **Schedule IV** controlled substances have a lower potential for abuse than Schedule III drugs. Schedule IV substances include benzodiazepines (for example, alprazolam [*Xanax*] and diazepam [*Valium*]).

- **Schedule V** controlled substances have a lower potential for abuse compared to Schedule IV substances and consist primarily of preparations containing limited quantities of certain narcotics. These are generally used for **antitussive**, **antidiarrheal**, and **analgesic** purposes. Examples include *Robitussin AC* and *Phenergan* with codeine.

Drugs listed in Schedules II through V have accepted medical uses and therefore may be prescribed, administered, or dispensed for medical use.

WORD	PRONUNCIATION	ELEMENTS		DEFINITION
anabolic steroid	an-a-**BOL**-ik **STER**-oyd	S/ R/ S/ R/	-ic *pertaining to* anabol- *to raise up* -oid *resemble* ster- *solid*	Prescription drug abused by some athletes to increase muscle mass
analgesic	an-al-**JEE**-zik	S/ P/ R/	-ic *pertaining to* an- *without* -alges- *sensation of pain*	Substance that produces a reduction in the sensation of pain
antitussive	an-tee-**TUS**-iv	S/ P/ R/	-ive *nature of, quality of* anti- *against* -tuss- *cough*	A cough remedy
control	kon-**TROLE**		Latin *to check an account*	To regulate, correct
formulary	**FORM**-you-lair-ee	S/ R/	-ary *pertaining to* formul- *form*	An official list of drugs approved for use by a hospital or group of physicians
medication	med-ih-**KAY**-shun	R/ R/	medic- *physician* -ation *healing*	A substance having curative properties
narcotic	nar-**KOT**-ik	S/ R/CF	-tic *pertaining to* narc/o *sleep, stupor*	Drug derived from opium, or a synthetic drug with similar effects
side effect	SIDE ee-**fekt**		side Old English *side* effect Old English *result*	An undesirable result of drug or other therapy
stimulant	**STIM**-you-lant	S/ R/	-ant *agent* stimul- *excite*	Agent that excites or strengthens functional activity

Exercises

A. Use the words of the language of pharmacology in context. *Use the terms from the provided word bank to complete the sentences. Not all terms will be used. Fill in the blanks.* **LO 22.2, 22.F**

USP   FDA   DEA   narcotic   antitussive   analgesic   I   II   IV   V

Mr. Hatfield arrives to the clinic complaining of a cough that occurs frequently. The physician prescribed a(n) _____ **(1)** to control the coughing episodes. The medication contains a(n) _____ **(2)**. Because of this, the _____ **(3)** regulates the drug. Generally speaking, this type of drug is usually a Schedule _____ **(4)** drug.

B. Create words using the correct root/combining form. *Construct medical terms related to pharmacology using the correct root/combining form. Fill in the blank.* **LO 22.2, 22.C**

1. Agent that excites or strengthens functional activity: _____ /ant

2. A cough remedy: anti/_____ /ive

3. Official list of drugs approved for use in a hospital: _____ /ary

4. Agent that reduces the sensation of pain: an/_____ /ic

5. A medication that treats pain but also induces sleep: _____ /ic

Lesson 22.2

PHARMACOLOGY

The Administration of Drugs

Lesson Objectives

A route of administration in pharmacology and toxicology is the path by which a drug or other substance is taken into the body. Routes of administration are usually classified according to the location on the body to which the drug is applied. The routes of administration distinguish whether a drug's effect is local (as in topical) or systemic (as in enteral or parenteral administration).

The bioavailability of a drug reveals what proportion of the drug reaches the systemic blood circulation and is available to reach the intended site(s) of action. A drug's route of administration (for example, oral or intravenous [IV]) and its formulation (for example, tablet, capsule, or liquid) clearly influence its bioavailability.

The path that a drug takes from the point of its application to reach the tissue where its effect is targeted is part of pharmacokinetics—the absorption, distribution, metabolism, and elimination of drugs. A drug's interaction at its target site(s) of action is called pharmacodynamics. The information in this lesson will enable you to:

22.2.1 Define terms relating to a drug's ability to reach and affect a particular tissue.

22.2.2 Discuss the different routes for administering drugs.

22.2.3 Identify abbreviations used in writing medication orders.

Case Report (CR) 22.1 *(continued)*

All the drugs that Mrs. Borodin has brought in for your inspection are administered orally.

Her medications, and their times of administration, include cimetidine 300 mg four times each day **(q.i.d.)**; *Tylenol #2* when necessary **(p.r.n.)** for pain; oxybutinin 5 mg three times each day **(t.i.d.)**; digoxin 0.25 mg twice each day **(b.i.d.)**; atenolol 100 mg at night **(on)**; alprazolam 0.5 mg b.i.d.; *Ambien* 5 mg **on**; and naproxen 500 mg b.i.d. In addition, she takes an OTC multivitamin **q.d.** and melatonin 1 mg **on**.

LO 22.4 Routes of Administration

Enteral Administration

Enteral administration is through the gastrointestinal **(GI)** tract. **Oral** is the most frequently used, convenient, and economical method of drug administration *(Figure 22.3)*. However, absorption of a drug by this route is affected by the unpredictable nature of the GI tract. For example, by affecting the gastric motility and emptying time, the presence of food influences the rate and extent of drug absorption. Solid-dose forms such as tablets and capsules have a high degree of drug stability and provide accurate dosage. The use of liquids and soluble preparations is less reliable. Modified-release preparations aim to maintain plasma drug concentrations for extended periods. If they are chewed or crushed, the full dose is released immediately, leading to **toxicity**.

▲ **Figure 22.3** Mother Gives Medication. ©Image Source/Alamy Stock Photo RF

The **sublingual** and **buccal** routes provide a rich supply of blood vessels through which drugs can be directly absorbed into the systemic circulation. Wafer-based versions of drugs, such as glyceryl trinitrate in the treatment of acute angina pectoris *(see Chapter 10)*, placed under the tongue give rapid responses to their effects.

Rectal administration in the form of **suppositories** or **enemas** is popular in some European countries but is not easily accepted by patients in America. **Antiemetics** can be administered rectally for nausea and vomiting.

Topical Administration

Topical administration allows a drug to be available directly at the site of action without going through the systemic circulation. For example, topical applications include steroid ointments for treating dermatitis *(Chapter 4)*, beta blocker eye drops for treating glaucoma *(Chapter 16)*, nasal medications instilled via drops or a spray, bronchodilators that are inhaled to treat asthma *(Chapter 13)*, and **pessaries** or creams containing clotrimazole *(Lotrimin, Mycelex)* that are inserted to treat vaginal candidiasis *(Chapter 8)*. Thus, *topical* refers to more than just application on the skin.

Drugs also can be administered into the systemic circulation through the skin. Adhesive **transdermal** patches can contain drugs that migrate across the epidermis into the blood vessel–rich dermis, where they are absorbed into the systemic circulation. Medications for motion sickness, cardiac problems, birth control, and the chemicals testosterone and nicotine are administered by transdermal patches.

Abbreviations Used in Prescribing	
a.c.	before meals
b.i.d.	twice each day
GI	gastrointestinal
IV	intravenous
on	at night
p.c.	after meals
p.o.	by mouth
pr	per rectum
p.r.n.	when necessary
q.d.	every day
q.i.d.	four times each day
Rx	prescribe
STAT	immediately
t.i.d.	three times each day

WORD	PRONUNCIATION		ELEMENTS	DEFINITION
antiemetic	**AN**-tee-eh-**MET**-ik	S/ P/ R/	-tic *pertaining to* anti- *against* -eme- *to vomit*	A medication that helps to control nausea and vomiting
bioavailability	**BIE**-oh-ah-**VALE**-ah-**BIL**-ih-tee	S/ R/ R/	-ity *condition, state* bio- *life* -availabil- *to be worth*	The amount of a drug that reaches the systemic circulation and is available to reach the intended site of action
buccal	**BUK**-al	S/ R/	-al *pertaining to* bucc- *cheek*	Inside the cheek—a site for the administration of certain medications
enema	**EN**-eh-mah		Greek *injection*	An injection of fluid into the rectum
enteral	**EN**-ter-al	S/ R/	-al *pertaining to* enter- *intestine*	Administration of medications by way of the GI tract
formulation	**FORM**-you-**LAY**-shun	S/ R/	-ation *process* formul- *form*	The form in which a drug is presented—tablet, capsule, liquid, etc.
oral	**OR**-al	S/ R/	-al *pertaining to* or- *mouth*	Pertaining to the mouth
pessary	**PES**-ah-ree		Greek *an oval stone*	Appliance inserted into the vagina
pharmacodynamics	**FAR**-mah-coh-die-**NAM**-iks	S/ R/CF R/	-ics *pertaining to* pharmac/o- *drug* -dynam- *force*	The uptake and action of drugs at their tissue site(s) of action
pharmacokinetics	**FAR**-mah-coh-ki-**NET**-iks	S/ R/CF R/	-ics *pertaining to* pharmac/o- *drug* -kinet- *moving*	The movement of drugs within the body affecting absorption, distribution, metabolism, and excretion
rectal	**REK**-tal	S/ R/	-al *pertaining to* rect- *rectum*	Pertaining to the rectum
sublingual	sub-**LING**-wal	S/ P/ R/	-al *pertaining to* sub- *underneath* -lingu- *tongue*	Underneath the tongue
suppository	suh-**PAH**-zih-tor-ee		Latin *placed underneath*	A small solid body containing medication that is placed in a body orifice other than the mouth to release the medication
topical	**TOP**-ih-kal	S/ R/	-al *pertaining to* topic- *local*	Medication applied to a local area
toxin toxicity	**TOK**-sin tok-**SIS**-ih-tee	S/ S/ R/	Greek *poison* -ity *state, condition* -ic- *pertaining to* tox- *poison*	Poisonous substance formed by a cell or organism The state of being poisonous
toxicology	tok-sih-**KOL**-oh-jee	S/ R/CF	-logy *study of* toxic/o- *poison*	The science of poisons, including their source, chemistry, actions, and antidotes
transdermal	trans-**DER**-mal	S/ P/ R/	-al *pertaining to* trans- *across, through* -derm- *skin*	Going across or through the skin

Exercises

A. Differentiate the different routes of administration of drugs. *Match the route of administration in the first column with its correct definition in the second column.* **LO 22.4**

_____ 1. *rectal*

_____ 2. *sublingual*

_____ 3. *oral*

_____ 4. *transdermal*

_____ 5. *buccal*

_____ 6. *topical*

_____ 7. *enteral*

a. applied to a local area

b. inside the cheek

c. medication given via the GI tract

d. under the tongue

e. pertaining to the mouth

f. going across the skin

g. pertaining to the rectum

LO 22.4 Routes of Administration (continued)

Parenteral Administration

Parenteral administration, which literally means *not through the GI tract,* is the injection of a drug directly into the body that bypasses the skin and mucous membranes.

The common routes of parenteral administration are:

- **intramuscular (IM)** *(Figure 22.4a)*
- **intravenous (IV)** *(Figure 22.4b)*
- **subcutaneous (SC)**

Less common routes include:

- **intradermal (ID)**
- **intrathecal** *(Figure 22.4c)*

Intramuscular and **subcutaneous injections** establish a "depot" for a drug that is released gradually, depending on the drug's formulation, into the systemic circulation. For example, oil-based medications are released more slowly than water-based. An IM injection of *Depo-Provera,* a birth control drug, works steadily for a three-month period. An **intradermal** route for medications is rarely used, except in allergy testing.

Intravenous injections enable a drug to reach its sites of action within seconds. An IV **infusion** also can deliver continuous medication—for example, morphine to patients in continuous pain or a saline drip for people needing fluids. The medications also can be given in a small solution through a **port** in intravenous tubing (**bolus**), or attached in smaller infusion containers to a larger infusion (piggyback).

Disadvantages of IV injections or infusions include the fact that patients are not typically able to self-administer them and the fact that, because it bypasses most of the body's natural defenses, IV is the most dangerous route of administration. Also, the preparation and administration of IV drugs require the use of **aseptic** techniques. Careful training is necessary to achieve competence in the administration of IV medications.

Intrathecal injections are given into the subarachnoid space surrounding the spinal cord in the spinal canal *(see Chapter 9).* An epidural block, which is an injection of a local anesthetic agent into the epidural space *(Figure 22.4c),* is used often for pain management during labor *(see Chapter 8)* and occasionally for chemotherapy. An intrathecal injection's primary advantage is that the drug avoids the blood–brain barrier (BBB; *see Chapter 9*).

Methods to ensure accuracy and safety in the administration of drugs are described in the next lesson of this chapter.

(a) (b) (c)

▲ **Figure 22.4** **Routes for Parenteral Administration.** (*a*) Inserting an intravenous (IV) cannula, (*b*) IM injection, (*c*) intrathecal injection.

WORD	PRONUNCIATION	ELEMENTS		DEFINITION
aseptic (adj) (Note: The final "s" of the root is not used to allow the pronunciation to flow)	ay-**SEP**-tik	S/ P/ R/	-tic *pertaining to* a- *without* -seps- *decay*	Pertaining to the absence of living organisms
bolus	**BOH**-lus		Greek *a lump*	Single mass of a substance
infusion	in-**FYU**-zhun	P/ R/	in- *in* -fusion *to pour*	Introduction intravenously of a substance other than blood
injection	in-**JEK**-shun	R/	-jection *to throw*	Introduction of a medical substance parenterally
intradermal	**IN**-trah-**DER**-mal	S/ P/ R/	-al *pertaining to* intra- *within* -derm- *skin*	Within the dermis
intramuscular	**IN**-trah-**MUS**-kew-lar	S/ R/	-ar *pertaining to* -muscul- *muscle*	Within the muscle
intrathecal	**IN**-trah-**THEE**-kal	R/	-thec- *sheath*	Within the subarachnoid or subdural space
intravenous	**IN**-trah-**VEE**-nus	S/ R/	-ous *pertaining to* -ven- *vein*	Inside a vein
parenteral	pah-**REN**-ter-al	S/ P/ R/	-al *pertaining to* par- *abnormal, beside* -enter- *intestine*	Administering medication by any means other than the GI tract
port	PORT		Latin *gate*	A point of entry into an IV system
subcutaneous	sub-kew-**TAY**-nee-us	S/ P/ R/	-ous *pertaining to* sub- *below* -cutane- *skin*	Below the skin
hypodermic (syn)	high-poh-**DER**-mik			

Exercises

A. Use the correct abbreviation for the described procedure. *Abbreviations are commonly used when communicating verbally and in writing. Use the correct abbreviation for the words written in italics.* **LO 22.3, 22.4, 22.A, 22.B**

1. The injection was *given into the muscles* of the buttocks. _____

2. The nurse practitioner ordered that the medication be given *under the subcutaneous tissue.* _____

3. The allergy test involves placing an allergen *within the skin.* _____

4. Give the patient his medication *via his vein.* _____

B. The definitions of the terms are given to you. *Write the correct terms on the lines.* **LO 22.4**

1. absence of living organisms: _____

2. within the dermis: _____

3. point of entry into an IV system: _____

4. same as hypodermic: _____

5. single mass of a substance: _____

Lesson 22.3

Accuracy and Safety in Drug Administration

Lesson Objectives

The Centers for Disease Control and Prevention (CDC) report that in 2016, the latest year for which statistics are available, 64,000 patients in the United States died from improperly prescribed, overprescribed, or unmonitored use of tranquilizers, painkillers, and stimulant drugs. This total exceeds the number of deaths from motor vehicle accidents (33,736) and firearms (33,599). According to the CDC, in 2015 more than 33,000 people died from overdoses involving prescription opioids. *Vicodin,* the most prescribed medicine nationwide, kills the most pain and the most people.

The information in this lesson will enable you to:

22.3.1 Understand that every drug has side effects that can be harmful.

22.3.2 Describe patterns of taking multiple self-administered drugs.

22.3.3 Identify the five "rights" to be addressed by patients and caregivers in administering drugs.

22.3.4 Discuss the importance for accurate documentation of each administration of a drug and of any error in its administration.

Abbreviations

ADR	adverse drug reaction
AE	adverse effect
CDC	Centers for Disease Control and Prevention
CNS	central nervous system
PCP	primary care physician

Case Report (CR) 22.1 *(continued)*

After reviewing Mrs. Borodin's medications with her *(Figure 22.5),* you found that she had a poor grasp of the indications for several of her medications. In addition, you found that side effects and **interactions** of several of her medications could be causing her recent symptoms of confusion, dry mouth, difficulty in swallowing, dizziness, difficulty with her balance, and falling.

For example, the benzodiazepine alprazolam *(Xanax)* has the side effects of fainting and dizziness, and accidental falls are common. In addition, zolpidem *(Ambien),* a sedative and hypnotic, interacts with *Xanax* and **synergistically** increases these central nervous system **(CNS)** side effects of *Xanax.* Mrs. Borodin is also taking over-the-counter melatonin at night. You doubt that it is necessary for her to take both *Ambien* and melatonin. *Ambien* and oxybutynin list confusion, dry mouth, and dizziness among their side effects.

You ask for a conference with Dr. Lee, Mrs. Borodin's primary care physician **(PCP),** to review and possibly change her medications. Following that, you will set up a meeting with Mrs. Borodin and medication aides from the assisted living facility where she lives in order to ensure that her new medication regimen is understood and can be implemented safely and accurately.

▲ **Figure 22.5**
Pharmacist Consults with Elderly Patient. ©Keith Brofsky/ Getty Images RF

LO 22.5 Self-Administration of Medications in the Elderly

The most common route of administration of medications is the self-administered oral route. Seventy-nine percent of adults older than 65 are on medications, with 39% of them taking five or more prescription drugs and 90% of them also taking over-the-counter (OTC) drugs. In a 2002 large study of women older than 65, 12% took 10 or more medications and 35% experienced an **adverse effect (AE)** from a drug. Adverse effects are harmful and undesired effects secondary to the main or therapeutic effect of the medication. Research also has found that **adverse drug reactions (ADR)** caused by intolerance, susceptibility, or interaction with another drug occurred in the hospitalization of some 35% of patients. In addition to hospitalization, severe adverse drug reactions can result in death or permanent **impairment** of physical activities and/or quality of life.

Opioids such as morphine and codeine are naturally derived from opium poppy plants. Hydrocodone *(Vicodin)* and oxycodone *(Percocet)* are manufactured semi-synthetic opioids. Fentanyl is a fully synthetic opioid, 100 times more powerful than morphine. Methadone is another fully synthetic opioid. Heroin is an illegal drug synthesized from morphine and caused 13,219 deaths in 2016.

Naloxone *(Narcan)* blocks the effects of opioids, particularly in overdose. Given IV, it works within 2 minutes, IM within 5 minutes. Sprayed into the nose, the effect is variable.

LO 22.5 Word Analysis and Definition

WORD	PRONUNCIATION	ELEMENTS		DEFINITION
adverse	**AD**-vers	P/ R/	ad- *to, into* -verse *turned*	Noxious, unintended, undesired
impairment	im-**PAIR**-ment	S/ R/	-ment *action, state* impair- *worsen*	Diminishing of normal function
interaction	in-ter-**AK**-shun	P/ R/	inter- *between* -action *to do*	The action between two entities to produce or prevent an effect
opioid	**OH**-pee-oyd		Latin *bringing sleep*	A narcotic substance, either natural or synthetic.
reaction	ree-**AK**-shun	P/ R/	re- *again, backward* -action *to do*	The response of a living tissue or organism to a stimulus
synergist	**SIN**-er-jist	S/ P/ R/	-ist *specialist* syn- *together* -erg- *work*	Agent or process that aids the actions of another
synergism	**SIN**-er-jism	S/	-ism *condition, process*	Coordinated action of two or more agents or processes so that the combined action is greater than that of each acting separately
synergistic (adj)	sin-er-**JIS**-tik	S/	-ic *pertaining to*	Pertaining to synergism
tranquilizer	**TRANG**-kwih-lie-zer	S/ R/	-izer *affects in a particular way* tranquil- *calm, serene*	Agent that calms without sedating or depressing

Exercises

A. WAD search and find. *Review the above WAD before doing this exercise. The elements are given in the first column. Fill in the answers to the element questions in columns 2 and 3.* **LO 22.A**

Name of Element	Identity of Element (Prefix, Root, Combining Form, Suffix)	Meaning of Element
syn	1.	2.
impair	3.	4.
erg	5.	6.
ic	7.	8.
ist	9.	10.

B. Which of the following statements is true? *Choose T if the statement is true. Choose F if the statement is false.* **LO 22.5**

1. A synergist is a medical professional.   T   F

2. A tranquilizer will make you sleep.   T   F

3. A reaction is a response to a stimulus.   T   F

4. An impairment is the inability to sleep.   T   F

5. An interaction involves at least five entities.   T   F

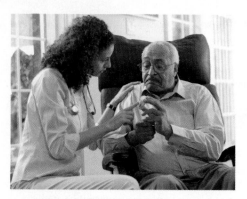

▲ **Figure 22.6** **Patient Is Shown How to Check a Medication Label.** ©Fuse/Getty Images RF

LO 22.5 Caregiver Administration of Medications

Five Rights

Before a caregiver administers a drug (medication) to a patient by any route, five factors should be addressed by the caregiver *(Figure 22.6)*.

- **Right patient**
  - Identify the patient by a bracelet or name badge. Asking the patient's name can lead to confusion, particularly in the assisted living environment.
- **Right drug**
  - Check the medication record for the name of the drug and compare with the drug in hand at three points:
    1. When taking hold of the package that contains the drug.
    2. When opening the package.
    3. When returning the package to storage.
- **Right route**
  - Check the medication record for how to administer the drug and check the labeling of the drug to make sure it matches the prescribed route.
- **Right dose**
  - Check that the medication record orders the same **dose** as that in hand.
- **Right time**
  - Check that the time ordered or the frequency matches the current time.

In addition, the caregiver must actually watch the patient take the medication. Caregivers should not leave medications unattended and should ensure that the medication does not come into contact with any potentially **contaminated** surface or object.

Documentation of having given medication is a vital responsibility of the caregiver. Medication errors must be documented, and should clearly state if it was one or more of the **Five Wrongs**—namely the **wrong patient**, the **wrong drug**, the **wrong route**, the **wrong dose**, or the **wrong time**.

LO 22.5 Self-Administration of Drugs

For a patient at home administering his/her own medications, usually orally, the Five Rights also apply at the time of administration:

- **Right Patient:** The patient should make sure that the container or package holding the medication has his or her name on it.
- **Right Drug:** The patient should check his or her own medication record to ensure that the medication has been prescribed and stored correctly.
- **Right Route:** The patient should check whether the medication should be swallowed whole as a **capsule** or **tablet**, or taken as directed if a liquid.
- **Right Dose:** The patient should check with his or her medication record and the label on the package that the number of tablets or capsules or the amount of liquid is correct.
- **Right Time:** The patient should check his or her medication record and the label on the package to ensure that the medication is being taken at the right time.

Documentation of the administration of all drugs as part of the patient's medical record should be encouraged, particularly among the elderly.

Self-Administration of Insulin

▲ **Figure 22.7** **Injecting Insulin Using a Pen Device.** Insulin pens are pen-like devices that allow diabetics to give themselves insulin injections without using vials and syringes. ©Mark Harmel/Photo Researchers, Inc.

Some 19 million people in the United States have been diagnosed with **diabetes**. Five million of them self-administer insulin into their subcutaneous tissue either by **syringe**, **pen injection**, high-pressure jet injection, or subcutaneous infusion pumps *(Figure 22.7)*. Inhalation of an insulin solution is also available. It is essential that the right dose of the right drug (i.e., the right type of insulin *[see Chapter 17]*) is given in response to the patient's blood sugar level.

The different drugs used in each body system are described in the appropriate chapter.

WORD	PRONUNCIATION	ELEMENTS		DEFINITION
capsule	**KAP**-syul	S/ R/	-ule *little* caps- *box*	A solid dosage form in which a drug is enclosed in a hard or soft shell
document (verb)	**DOK**-you-ment	S/ R/	-ment *resulting state, action* docu- *to teach*	To provide written proof
documentation (noun)	**DOK**-you-men-**TAY**-shun	S/	-ation *process*	The process of providing written proof
dose	DOHS		Greek *a giving*	The quantity of a drug to be taken at one time
syringe	si-**RINJ**		Greek *pipe* or *tube*	An instrument used for injecting or withdrawing fluids
tablet	**TAB**-let		Latin *small table*	A solid, flattish dosage form containing medication

Exercises

A. Match the form of the medication with the route by which it is given. *The form of a drug is specific to the route by which it is to be given. Given the medication, choose the correct route by which it is to be given.* **LO 22.5**

1. tablet
   - **a.** rectal
   - **b.** topical
   - **c.** oral
   - **d.** intravenous

2. ointment
   - **a.** rectal
   - **b.** topical
   - **c.** oral
   - **d.** intravenous

3. capsule
   - **a.** rectal
   - **b.** topical
   - **c.** oral
   - **d.** intravenous

4. syringe with attached needle
   - **a.** rectal
   - **b.** topical
   - **c.** oral
   - **d.** intravenous

5. suppository
   - **a.** rectal
   - **b.** topical
   - **c.** oral
   - **d.** intravenous

Pharmacology

Challenge Your Knowledge

A. Abbreviations are an important part of clinical documentation. Make sure you know what they mean. Insert the correct abbreviation in the appropriate space. **(LO 22.4, 22.A, 22.B, 22.F)**

a.c. b.i.d. t.i.d. q.i.d. on p.o. p.r.n. GI IM p.c.

1. Mr. Baker's doctor has told you to administer his medication _____ (before meals).

2. The medicine prescribed by the doctor will help Mr. Baker's _____ (gastrointestinal) problem.

3. This medication is to be given to the patient _____ (at night).

4. The patient needs the medication _____ (three times each day).

5. Because her coughing is improving, the patient only needs the medication _____ (when necessary).

6. This medicine should be given _____ (after meals); otherwise, it will upset the patient's stomach.

7. Administer this medication for the patient by _____ (intramuscular) injection.

8. The prescription was written to be taken _____ (four times each day) _____ (by mouth).

9. Do not confuse _____ (twice each day) with _____ (three times each day).

B. What is the purpose of a port? Choose the correct answer. **(LO 22.4)**

1. to divert fluids away from the site

2. to provide an entry site for IV fluids

3. to separate veins and arteries

4. to speed the process of blood circulation

5. to help prevent clots

C. Deconstruction. Deconstruction of medical terms is a tool for analyzing the meaning. In the following chart, you are given a medical term. Deconstruct the term into its prefix, root (or combining form), and suffix. Write the element and its meaning in the appropriate column and the meaning of the term in the last column. If the term does not have a word element, write n/a. *The first one is done for you.* **(LO 22.1, 22.2, 22.4, 22.5, 22.D)**

Medical Term	Prefix	Meaning of Prefix	Root/ Combining Form	Meaning of Root/ Combining Form	Suffix	Meaning of Suffix	Meaning of Term
synergism	syn-	together	-erg-	work	-ism	process	Coordinated action of two agents so that the combined action is greater than that of each acting separately
subcutaneous	1.	2.	3.	4.	5.	6.	7.
prescription	8.	9.	10.	11.	12.	13.	14.
interaction	15.	16.	17.	18.	19.	20.	21.
tranquilizer	22.	23.	24.	25.	26.	27.	28.
antitussive	29.	30.	31.	32.	33.	34.	35.

D. **Who are the only health care personnel licensed to write prescriptions?** Choose Yes if the particular health care professional can prescribe medications; choose No if they cannot. **(LO 22.2, 22.E)**

1. dentist

   a. Yes

   b. No

2. pharmacist

   a. Yes

   b. No

3. nurse practitioner

   a. Yes

   b. No

4. optometrist

   a. Yes

   b. No

5. registered nurse

   a. Yes

   b. No

6. physical therapist

   a. Yes

   b. No

7. doctor of osteopathy

   a. Yes

   b. No

8. pediatrician

   a. Yes

   b. No

9. obstetrician

   a. Yes

   b. No

10. physician assistant

   a. Yes

   b. No

E. **One element changes the meaning of medical terms.** *Many medical terms are similar, with one element making the difference between terms. Given the definition, complete each term with the correct element.* **(LO 22.C)**

1. Specialist that is licensed to dispense and prepare medications: pharmac _____

2. The study of the preparation, uses, and effects of drugs: pharmac_____

3. Specialist in the study of the science of the preparation, uses, and effects of drugs: pharmac _____

4. Substance given into the skin: intra_____al

5. Substance given into the subarachnoid space: intra_____al

6. The movement of drugs within the body: pharmaco_____ics

7. The uptake of drugs at the site(s) of action: pharmaco_____ics

F. **Fill in the blanks with the correct abbreviations. (LO 22.2, 22.4, 22.F)**

1. by mouth _____

2. doctors check drugs in this book _____

3. federal government agency that sets standards for drug quality, purity, and safety _____

4. when necessary _____

5. medication that does not need a prescription _____

Pharmacology

G. **Practice the language of pharmacology.** Choose the correct answer that answers each question. **(LO 22.1–22.F)**

1. The path by which a drug or other substance is taken into the body is called:

   a. bioavailability

   b. digestion

   c. absorption

   d. a route of administration

   e. biokinetics

2. The method by which a medication is prepared for administration is called its:

   a. formulation

   b. route

   c. pharmacokinetics

   d. prescription

3. What would an ENT physician prescribe for a patient with a heavy cough?

   a. antiemetic

   b. antihistamine

   c. antitussive

   d. anticoagulant

   e. antidepressant

4. Which of the following does *not* refer to a drug name?

   a. chemical

   b. generic

   c. brand

   d. trade

   e. popular

5. Which U.S. agency sets the standards for the quality, purity, and safety of medications?

   a. USP

   b. USPS

   c. CDC

   d. BATF

   e. AAP

6. The physician wrote for the medication to be placed in the buccal cavity. You would instruct the patient to place it:

   a. under the tongue

   b. in the nose

   c. between the cheek and gum

   d. in the eye

7. You are online researching antibiotics. The following medication is listed as: metronidazole, *Flagyl*, 2-Methyl-5-nitroimidazole-1-ethanol. *Flagyl* is the:

   a. chemical name

   b. brand name

   c. generic name

8. A prescription medication that has a high potential for abuse would be classified as Schedule:

   a. I

   b. II

   c. III

   d. IV

   e. V

9. The federal agency that monitors prescriptions written by physicians:

   a. USP

   b. DEA

   c. FBI

   d. PDR

10. A professional that dispenses medication under the supervision of a pharmacist:

    a. occupational therapist

    b. pharmacologist

    c. medication aide

    d. pharmacy technician

H. Identify the different routes of drug administration. Choose from the following terms the correct route of administration. Fill in the blanks. You will not use all the choices. **LO 22.4**

enteral   oral   rectal   buccal   sublingual   transdermal   intravenous

1. You have placed a patch containing pain medicine on the skin of your patient's back. Which route of administration is that? _____

2. Mr. Matthews has to put his medicine under his tongue. Which route of administration is that? _____

3. Dr. Philips has ordered a suppository for Mrs. Johnson. Which route of administration is that? _____

4. Dr. Mallard prescribed pain pills for Mr. Cosmos. Which route of administration is that? _____

I. Reread the Case Report and use your knowledge of medical language to create answers to the following questions. **(LO 22.1, 22.A)**

Case Report (CR) 22.1

You are

. . . a pharmacist in the pharmacy at Fulwood Medical Center. Your patient has been sent to you by Susan Lee, MD, a primary care physician at Fulwood Medical Center.

Your patient is

. . . Mrs. Rebecca Borodin, a frail 80-year-old widow living in an assisted living facility. She has recently begun to complain that she has difficulty recognizing and naming her fellow residents and knowing when to go to the facility's dining room for meals. In addition, it has been hard for her to eat because she suffers from dry mouth and difficulty in swallowing. She also has complained of dizziness and problems with balance; recently, she fell as a result of these problems. Her past medical history includes osteoarthritis, osteopenia, hypertension, congestive heart failure, persistent pain following herpes zoster, and stress incontinence.

Mrs. Borodin has brought in a bag containing all her medications, which include cimetidine, acetaminophen with codeine (*Tylenol #2*), oxybutynin, digoxin, atenolol, alprazolam, zolpidem (*Ambien*), and naproxen. In addition, she takes an over-the-counter (OTC) multivitamin and melatonin.

Dr. Lee has asked you to make sure that Mrs. Borodin knows what each of the medications is for and when to take it. She also has asked you to review the drugs themselves to see if any of them could be causing her recent symptoms.

---

1. Which of the medications is classified as a Schedule IV drug?

   a. naproxen   **b.** cimetidine   **c.** digoxin   **d.** alprazolam

2. What condition does zolpidem treat?

   a. insomnia   **b.** depression   **c.** stress incontinence   **d.** osteoarthritis

3. List the medications that do not require a prescription: _____

4. List the medications that are scheduled drugs: _____

J. Identify abbreviations used to describe drugs, their routes of administration, and their timing. Match the abbreviation to the correct statement. **(LO 22.F)**

_____ 1. p.r.n.   **a.** intramuscular

_____ 2. t.i.d.   **b.** by mouth

_____ 3. b.i.d.   **c.** when necessary

_____ 4. IM   **d.** twice each day

_____ 5. p.o.   **e.** three times each day

Appendices

Word Parts

Note: For easy identification, the word parts in this appendix appear in the same colors as they do in the Word Analysis and Definition boxes: suffix, prefix, root, root/combining form. Any term that is used in the text in both root and combining form is shown in this appendix only as a combining form. Sometimes the same element (for example, "ac") can function in different parts of the medical term.

WORD PART	DEFINITION
a-	not, without, into
ab-	away from
abdomin/o	abdomen
ability	competence
ablat	take away
-able	capable of
abort	fail at onset
absorpt	to swallow, take in
ac-	toward
-ac	pertaining to
-acea	condition, remedy
acetyl	acetyl
acid/o	acid, low pH
acin	grape
acous	hearing
acr/o	peak, extremity, highest point
acromi/o	acromion
act	to do, perform, performance
activ/e	movement
acu-	sharp
acu	needle, sharp
acumin	to sharpen
ad-	to, toward, near, into
adapt	to adjust
-ade	process
aden/o	gland
adipos/e	fat
adjust	alter
adjuv	give help
adnex	connected parts
adolesc	beginning of adulthood
adren/o	adrenal gland
aer/o	air, gas
ag-	to

WORD PART	DEFINITION
-age	related to
agglutin	sticking together, clumping
-ago	disease
-agon	contest
agon	contest against, fight against
agor/a	marketplace
-agra	rough
-al	pertaining to
alanine	an amino acid, protein synthesized in muscle
albin/o	white
albumin	albumin
ald/o	organic compound
-ale	pertaining to
alges	sensation of pain
-algia	pain, painful condition
aliment	nourishment
-alis	pertaining to
alkal	base
all/o	strange, other, different
aller	allergy
allo-	other, different, strange
alopec	baldness, mange
alpha-	first letter in Greek alphabet
alveol	alveolus, air sac
-aly	condition
ambi-	both double
ambly-	dull
ambulat	to walk, walking
amin/o	nitrogen compound
-amine	nitrogen-containing
ammon	ammonia
amni/o	amnion, fetal membrane
amoeb	amoeba

S = Suffix   P = Prefix   R = Root   R/CF = Combining Form

WORD PART	DEFINITION
amph-	around
ampull	bottle-shaped
amput	to prune, lop off
amyl	starch
-an	pertaining to
an-	not, lack of, without
an/o	anus
ana-	away from, excessive
anabol	build up
analysis	process to define
analyst	one who defines
anastom	join together
-ance	condition, state of
-ancy	state of
andr/o	male, masculine
aneurysm	dilation
angi/o	blood vessel, lymph vessel
angina	sore throat, chest pain radiating to throat
ankyl	stiff
-ant	forming, pertaining to, agent
ante-	before, forward
anter	before, front part
anthrac	coal
anti-	against
aort	aorta
apo-	different from, separation from, off
append	appendix
apse	clasp
aqu/a	watery
-ar	pertaining to
arachn	cobweb, spider
-arche	beginning
aria	air
-arian	one who is
-aris	pertaining to
aroma	smell, sweet herb
array	place in order
arteri/o	artery
arteriosus	like an artery
arthr/o	joint

WORD PART	DEFINITION
articul	joint
-ary	pertaining to
asbest	asbestos
asc	belly
ascit	fluid in the belly
-ase	enzyme
aspartate	an amino acid
aspirat	remove by suction
assay	evaluate
assist	aid, help
astr/o	star
-ata	action, place, use
-ate	composed of, pertaining to, process
-ated	process, composed of
atel	incomplete
ather/o	porridge, gruel, fatty substance
athet	without position, uncontrolled
-atic	pertaining to
-ation	process
-ative	pertaining to, quality of
-ator	agent, instrument, person or thing that does something
atri/o	entrance, atrium
-atric	treatment
attent	awareness
attenu	to weaken
audi/o	to hear
audit	hearing
aur	ear
auscult	listen to
auto-	self, same
avail	useful
axill	armpit
ayur-	life
azot	nitrogen
back	back, return
bacter	bacterium
bacteri/o	bacteria
balan	glans penis
bar	pressure, weight

APPENDIX A

WORD PART	DEFINITION
bas/o	base, opposite of acid
basal/e	deepest part
basil	base, support
be	life
behav	mental activity
beta	second letter of Greek alphabet
bi-	two, twice, double
-bic	life
-bil	able
bil/i	bile
bio	life
biot	life
-blast	embryo, germ cell, immature cell
blast/o	immature cell, germ cell
blephar/o	eyelid
body	body, mass, substance
bov	cattle
brachi/o	arm
brachy-	short
brady-	slow
bride	rubbish, rubble
bronch/o	bronchus
bucc	cheek
buccin	cheek
bulb/o	bulb
burs	bursa
calc/i	calcium
calcan/e	calcaneus
calcul	stone, little stone
callos	thickening
calor	heat
cancer	cancer
candid	*Candida*, a yeast
capill	hairlike structure, capillary
capit	head
capn	carbon dioxide
caps	box, cover, shell
capsul	little box
carb/o	carbon
carboxy	group of organic compounds

WORD PART	DEFINITION
carcin/o	cancerous, cancer
cardi	heart
cardi/o	heart
care	be responsible for
caroten/e	yellow-red pigment
carotid	large neck artery
carp/o	bones of the wrist
cartilag/e	cartilage
cata-	down
catabol	break down
catechol	benzene derivative
cathet	insert, catheter
caud/a	tail
cava	cave
cavern	cave
cec	cecum
-cele	cave, hernia, swelling
celi	abdomen
cellul	small cell
cent-	hundred
cent	hundred
-centesis	to puncture
centr/o	central
cephal/o	head
-cephalus	head
cephalus	head
cephaly	condition of the head
-ceps	head
cept	to receive
cerebell	little brain, cerebellum
cerebr/o	brain
cervic	neck, cervix
cess	going forward
chancr	chancre
chem/o	chemical
chemic	chemical
-chete	hair
-chezia	pass a stool
chir/o	hand
chlor/o	green

WORD PART	DEFINITION
chol/e	bile
cholangi	bile duct
cholecyst	gallbladder
choledoch/o	common bile duct
choline	choline
chondr/o	cartilage, rib
chori/o	chorion, membrane
chorion	chorion
chrom/o	color
chromat	color
chron/o	time
chym/o	chyme
-cidal	pertaining to killing
-cide	to kill
cili	hairlike structure, eyelid
circum-	around
cirrh	yellow
cis	to cut
-clast	break, break down
claudic	limp
claustr/o	confined space
clav	clavicle
clave	lock
clavicul	clavicle
-cle	small
clitor	clitoris
clon	cutting used for propagation
-clonus	violent action
co-	with, together
coagul/o	clotting, clump
coarct	press together, narrow
cobal	cobalt
cocc	spherical bacterium, berry
cochle	cochlea
code	information system
cognit	thinking
coit	sexual intercourse
col-	before
col	colon
coll/a	glue

WORD PART	DEFINITION
colon	colony
colp/o	vagina
com-	with, together
combin	combine
comminut	break into small pieces
commodat	adjust
compat	tolerate
compet	strive together
complete	fill in
complex	woven together
compli	fulfill
compress	press together
compuls	drive, compel
con-	with, together
concav	arched, hollow
concept	become pregnant
concuss	shake violently
condyl	knuckle
confus	bewildered
congest	accumulation of fluid
coni	dust
coniz	cone
conjunctiv	conjunctiva
conscious	aware
constip	press together
constrict	narrow, to narrow
contagi/o	transmissible by contact
contamin	to corrupt, make unclean
contin	hold together
contra-	against
contract	draw together, pull together
contus	bruise
convalesc	recover
cor	heart, pupil
cori	skin
corne/o	cornea
coron	crown, coronary
corpor/a	body
corpus	body
cort	cortex

S = Suffix   P = Prefix   R = Root   R/CF = Combining Form

WORD PART	DEFINITION
cortic/o	cortex, cortisone
cortis	cortisone
cost	rib
crani/o	cranium, skull
cre	separation
crease	groove
creat	flesh
creatin	creatine
cret	to separate
cretin	cretin
crimin	distinguish
crin/o	secrete
-crine	secrete
crista	crest
-crit	to separate
crown	crown
crur	leg
cry/o	icy cold
crypt-	hidden
cub	cube
cubit	elbow
cubitus	lying down
cune/i	wedge
cur	cleanse, cure
curat	to care for
curett	to cleanse
curr	to run
cursor	run
cusp	point
cutane/o	skin
cyan/o	blue
-cyst	cyst, sac, bladder
cyst/o	bladder, sac, cyst
cysteine	an amino acid
cyt/o	cell
-cyte	cell
dacry/o	tears, lacrimal duct
dai	day
de-	from, take away, out of, without
defec	clear out waste

WORD PART	DEFINITION
deferens	carry away
defici	failure, lacking, inadequate
degenerat	deteriorate
deglutit	to swallow
del	visible, manifest
deliri	confusion, disorientation
delt	Greek letter delta
delus	deceive
demi-	half
dendr/o	treelike, branching structure
dent	tooth
depend	relying on
depress	press down
derm/a	skin
dermat/o	skin
dermis	skin
-desis	bind together, fixation of bone or joint
di-	two, complete
dia-	complete, through
diabet	diabetes
diagnost	decision
diaphragm/a	diaphragm
dict	consent, surrender
didym/o	testis
didymis	testis
diet	a way of life
different	not identical
digest	to break down, break up
digit	finger or toe
dilat	open up, expand, open out
dips	thirst
dis-	apart, away from
discipl	understand
disciplin	disciple, instruction
dist	away from the center
-dium	appearance
diverticul	by-road
dorm	sleep
dors/i	back
drome	running

WORD PART	DEFINITION
duce	to lead
ducer	to lead, leader
duct	to lead
ductus	leading
duoden	twelve, duodenum
dur/a	hard, dura mater
dwarf	miniature
dynam	power
-dynia	pain
dys-	bad, difficult, painful
e-	out of, from
-eal	pertaining to
ease	normal function, freedom from pain
ec-	out, outside
ech/o	sound wave
eclamps	shining forth
eco-	environment
-ectasis	dilation
-ectomy	excision, surgical excision
ectop	on the outside, displaced
eczema	eczema
-ed	pertaining to
edema	edema, swelling
efface	wipe out
ejacul	shoot out
electr/o	electric, electricity
elimin	throw away, expel
-elle	small
em-	in, into
-ema	result
emac/i	make thin
embol	plug
embry/o	embryo, fertilized egg
eme	to vomit
-emesis	to vomit, vomiting
-emia	blood, blood condition
-emic	in the blood
emmetr-	measure
emuls	suspend in a liquid
emulsific	to milk out, to drain out

WORD PART	DEFINITION
en-	in
-ence	forming, quality of, state of
encephal/o	brain
encephaly	condition of the brain
-ency	condition, state of, quality, quality of
end-	inside, within
endo-	inner, inside, within
-ent	end result, pertaining to, state of, end, forming
enter/o	intestine
entery	intestine
enur	urinate
environ	surroundings
-eon	one who does
eosin/o	dawn
ependym	lining membrane
epi-	above, upon, over
epilep	seizure
epiphys/e	growth
episi/o	vulva
equi-	equal
equin/a	horse
-er	agent, one who does
erect	straight, to set up
erg/o	work
-ergy	process of working
-ery	condition, process of
erythemat	redness
erythr/o	red
-escent	process
-esis	abnormal condition
eso-	inward
esophag/e	esophagus
esthes	sensation
esthet	sensation, perception
estr/o	woman
ethm	sieve
eti/o	cause
-etic	pertaining to
-etics	pertaining to
-ette	little

APPENDIX A

S = Suffix   P = Prefix   R = Root   R/CF = Combining Form

WORD PART	DEFINITION
eu-	good, normal
ex-	away from, out, out of
exacerb	increase, aggravate
examin	test, examine
excret	separate, discharge
exo-	outside, outward
expect	await
expir	breathe out
extra-	out of, outside
fac/i	face
factor	maker
farct	stuff
fasci/o	fascia
febr	fever
fec	feces
feed	to give food, nourish
femor	femur
fer	to bear, carry
ferrit	iron
fertil	able to conceive
fertiliz	to bear, make fruitful
fet/o	fetus
fibr/o	fiber, fibrous
fibril	small fiber
fibrin/o	fibrin
-fication	remove
fida	split
field	definite area
filtr	strain through
fiss	split
fistul	tube, pipe
flatul	excessive gas
flavon	yellow
flex	bend
fluid/o	to flow
fluo-	fluorine
fluor/o	flux, flow, x-ray beam
flux	flow
foc	center, focus
follicul	follicle

WORD PART	DEFINITION
foramin	opening, foramen
fore-	in front
-form	appearance of, resembling
fract	break
free	free
frequ	repeated, often
front	front, forehead
fruct	fruit
funct	perform
fund/o	fundus
fung/i	fungus
fusion	to pour
galact/o	milk
gall	bile
gastr/o	stomach
gastrin	stomach hormone
gastrocnem	calf of leg
gemin	twin, double
-gen	create, produce, form
-gene	producer, give birth
gener	produce
-genesis	creation, origin, formation, source
genet	origin
-genic	creation, producing
genit	bring forth, birth, primary male or female sex organ
genitor	offspring
ger	old age
geront/o	process of aging
gest	gestation, pregnancy, produce
gestat	gestation, pregnancy, to bear
gigant	giant
gingiv	gums
gland	gland
glauc	lens opacity, gray
gli/o	glue, supportive tissue of nervous system
glia	glue, supportive tissue of nervous system
glob	globe
globin/o	protein
globul	globular, protein

S = Suffix   P = Prefix   R = Root   R/CF = Combining Form

WORD PART	DEFINITION
glomerul/o	glomerulus
gloss/o	tongue
glottis	windpipe
gluc/o	glucose, sugar
glut/e	buttocks
glutin	glue, stick together
glyc/o	glycogen, glucose, sugar
glycer	glycerol, sweet
gnath	jaw
gnose	recognize an abnormal condition
gnosis	knowledge
gomph	bolt, nail
gon/o	seed
gonad/o	gonads, testes or ovaries
-grade	going, level
graft	splice, transplant
graine	head pain
-gram	a record, drawing, recording
grand-	big
granul/o	granule, small grain
-graph	to record, write
-grapher	one who records
-graphy	process of recording
gravid	pregnant
gravida	pregnant woman
gravis	serious
green	green
gru	to move
guan	dung
gurgit	flood
gynec/o	woman, female
habilitat	restore
hale	breathe
halit	breath
hallucin	imagination
hallux	big toe
hem/o	blood
hemangi/o	blood vessel
hemat/o	blood
heme	red iron-containing pigment

WORD PART	DEFINITION
hemi-	half
hepar	liver
hepat/o	liver
hered	inherited through genes
herni/o	hernia, rupture
herp	blister
hetero-	different
hist	derived from histidine
hist/o	tissue
holist	entire, whole
hom/i	man
home/o	the same
homo-	same, alike
humor	fluid
hyal	glass
hydr/o	water
hyp-	below
hyper-	above, beyond, excess, excessive
hypn/o	sleep
hypo-	below, deficient, smaller, low, under
hyster/o	uterus
-ia	condition
-iac	pertaining to
-ial	pertaining to
-ian	one who does, specialist
-ias	condition
-iasis	condition, state of
-iatric	relating to medicine, medical knowledge
-iatrist	practitioner, one who treats
iatro-	medical treatment, treatment
-iatry	treatment, field of medicine
-ible	can do, able to
-ic	pertaining to
-ica	pertaining to
-ical	pertaining to
-ician	expert, specialist
-ics	knowledge of
ict	seizure
icterus	jaundice
-id	having a particular quality, pertaining to

S = Suffix   P = Prefix   R = Root   R/CF = Combining Form

WORD PART	DEFINITION
-ide	having a particular quality
idi/o	personal, distinct, unknown
ifer	to bear, carry
-ify	to become
-il	capability
-ile	capable, capability, pertaining to
ile/o	ileum
-ility	having the quality of, state of
im-	not, in
immun/o	immune, immune response, immunity
impair	worsen
imperfecta	unfinished
-imus	most
-in	chemical, chemical compound, substance
in-	not, into, in, without
incis	cut into
incub	sit on, lie on, hatch
index	to declare
-ine	pertaining to, substance
infect/i	tainted, internal invasion
infer-	below, beneath
infest	invade, attack
inflammat	set on fire
inflat	blow up
infra-	below, beneath
-ing	quality of, doing
ingest	carry in
inguin	groin
inhal	breathe in
inhibit	repress
inject	force in
ino	sinew
insect/i	insect
insert	put together
inspir	breathe in
insul	island
integ/u	covering of the body
integr	whole
intellect/u	perception, discernment
inter-	between

WORD PART	DEFINITION
interstit	spaces within tissues
intestin	gut, intestine
intra-	inside, within
intrins	on the inside
intus-	within
iod/o	violet, iodine
-ion	action, condition, process
-ior	pertaining to, suffix for comparatives
-iosum	pertaining to
-ious	pertaining to
irrigat	to water
-is	belonging to, pertaining to, condition
isch	to keep back
-ism	action, condition, process
-ismus	take action
iso-	equal
-isone	cortisone
-ist	agent, specialist
-istic	pertaining to
-istry	specialty
-isy	inflammation
-ite	resembling
-ites	associated with
-itic	pertaining to
-ition	process
-itis	inflammation, infection
-ity	condition, state
-ium	structure
-ius	pertaining to
-ive	nature of, quality of, pertaining to
-ization	process of creating, process of affecting in a specific way
-ize	action, affect in a specific way, policy
-ized	affected in a specific way
-izer	affects in a particular way, line of action
jejun	jejunum
jugul	throat
junct	joining together
juxta-	beside, near, close to
kal	potassium

WORD PART	DEFINITION
kary/o	nucleus
kel/o	tumor
kerat/o	cornea
keratin/o	keratin
kern	nucleus
ket/o	ketone
keton	ketone
ketone	organic compound, ketone
kin	motion
kinase	enzyme
-kine	movement
kines/i	movement
kinet	motion
-kinin	move in
klept/o	to steal
kyph/o	bent
labi	lip
labyrinth	inner ear
lacer	to tear
lacrim	tears, tear duct
lact/e	milk
lactat	secrete milk
lapar/o	abdomen in general
-lapse	fall together, slide
lapse	clasp, fall together
laryng/o	larynx
laser	acronym for light amplification by stimulated emission of radiation
lash	end of whip
lat	to take
later	side, at the side
latiss	wide
-le	small
lei/o	smooth
-lemma	covering
-lepsy	seizure
lept	thin, small
-let	small
leuk/o	white
lex	word

WORD PART	DEFINITION
librium	balance
ligament	ligament
ligat	tie up, tie off
lign	line
line	a mark
-ling	small
lingu	tongue
lip/o	fat, fatty tissue
lipid	fat
lith/o	stone
liv	life
lob	lobe
locat	a place
log	to study, study of
-logist	one who studies, specialist
logous	relation
-logy	to study, study of
longev	long life
lord	curve, swayback
lubric	make slippery
lucid	bright, clear
lumb	lower back, loin
lump	piece
lun	moon
-lus	small
lute	yellow
luxat	dislocate
-ly	going toward, every
ly	break down, separate
lymph/o	lymph
lymphaden/o	lymph node
lymphangi/o	lymphatic vessels
lys/o	decompose, decomposition, dissolve
-lysis	destroy, destruction, dissolve, separate, break down
lyt	dissolve
-lyte	soluble
-lytic	relating to destruction
lyze	destruct, dissolve, destroy
macro-	large

S = Suffix   P = Prefix   R = Root   R/CF = Combining Form

WORD PART	DEFINITION
macul	spot
-maker	one who makes
mal-	bad, inadequate
mal	bad
-malacia	abnormal softness
malign	harmful, bad, cancer
malleol	small hammer, malleolus
mamm/o	breast
man/o	pressure
mandibul	the jaw
-mania	frenzy, madness
mania	frenzy
manic	affected by frenzy
manipul	handful, use of hands
marker	sign
mast	breast
mastic	chew
mastoid	mastoid process
mater	mother
matern	mother
matur	ripe, ready
mature	ripe, ready, fully developed
medi	middle
media-	middle
medic	medicine
medulla	middle
mega-	enormous
-megaly	enlargement
mei	lessening
mela	black
melan/o	melanin, black pigment, black
mellit	sweetened with honey
membran/o	cover, skin
men/o	menses, monthly, month
mening/o	meninges
meningi/o	membranes
menisc	crescent, meniscus
menstru	menses, occurring monthly
-ment	action, state, resulting state
ment	mind, chin

WORD PART	DEFINITION
mere	part
mero-	partial
mes-	middle
meso-	middle
meta-	after, subsequent to, beyond
metabol	change
metacarp	bones of the hand
metatars	bones of the foot
-meter	measure, instrument to measure
meter	measure
metr/o	uterus
mi-	derived from hemi, half
micro-	small
mictur	make urine, pass urine
mid-	middle
mileusis	lathe
milli-	one-thousandth
miner	mines
mineral/o	inorganic materials
miss	send
mit/o	thread, threadlike structure
mitr-	having two points
mitt	to send
mod	nature, form, method
molec	mass
mollusc	soft
mon	single
mono-	one, single
morbid	disease
morph/o	shape
morphin	morphine
mort	death
mot	move
motiv	move
muc/o	mucous membrane, mucus
mucos/a	lining of a cavity
multi-	many
muscul/o	muscle
mut	silent
muta	genetic change

S = Suffix   P = Prefix   R = Root   R/CF = Combining Form

WORD PART	DEFINITION
mutil	to maim
my/o	muscle
myc/o	fungus
myel/o	spinal cord, bone marrow
myelin	in the spinal cord, myelin
myo-	to blink
myring/o	tympanic membrane, eardrum
myx-	mucus
narc/o	stupor, sleep
narciss	self-love
nas/o	nose
nat/e	birth, born
natr/i	sodium
nebul	cloud
necr/o	death
neo-	new
nephr/o	kidney
nerv	nerve
-ness	quality, state
neur/o	nerve, nervous tissue, nerve tissue
neutr/o	neutral
-nic	pertaining to
nitr/o	nitrogen
noct-	night
noia	to think
nom	law
non-	no
nor-	normal
norm-	normal
nos/o	disease
nucl	nucleus
nucle/o	nucleus
nucleol	small nucleus
nutri	nourish
nutrit	nourishment
o/o	egg
oblong	elongated
obsess	besieged by thoughts
obstetr	midwifery
occipit	back of head

WORD PART	DEFINITION
occult/a	hidden
occupation	work
ocul/o	eye
ode	way, road, path
odont	tooth
-oid	appearance of, resemble, resembling
-ol	alcohol, chemical substance
-ole	small
olfact	smell
oligo-	too little, scanty
-oma	tumor, mass
onc/o	tumor
-one	chemical substance, hormone
onych/o	nail
ophthalm/o	eye
opia	sight
opportun	take advantage of
-opsis	vision
-opsy	to view
opt/o	vision
-or	a doer, one who does, that which does something
or/o	mouth
orbit	orbit
orch/o	testicle
ordin	arrange
orex	appetite
organ	organ, tool, instrument, organic
orth/o	straight
orthot	correct
-orum	function of
-ory	having the function of
os	mouth
-osa	like
-ose	full of, condition
-osis	condition
osmo	push
osmol	concentration
oss/i	bone
oste/o	bone

APPENDIX A

S = Suffix   P = Prefix   R = Root   R/CF = Combining Form

WORD PART	DEFINITION
-osus	condition
ot/o	ear
-otomy	incision
-ous	pertaining to
ov/i	egg
ovari	ovary
ovul	ovum, egg
ox/y	oxygen
-oxia	oxygen condition
oxid	oxidize
oxytoc	swift birth
pace	step, pace
pact	driven in
palat	palate
palliat	reduce suffering
palpat	touch, stroke
palpit	throb
pan-	all
pancreat	pancreas
papill/o	pimple
par-	abnormal, beside
para-	adjacent to, alongside, beside, abnormal
para	to bring forth
parasit	parasite
paresis	weakness
pareun	lying beside, sexual intercourse
pariet	wall
paroxysm	irritation
particul	little piece
partum	childbirth, to bring forth
pat	lie open
patell	patella
patent	lie open
path/o	disease
pathet	suffering
pathic	pertaining to a disease
pathy	emotion, disease
pause	cessation
pector	chest
ped	child, foot

WORD PART	DEFINITION
pedicul	louse
pelv	pelvis
pen	penis
-penia	deficient, deficiency
peps	digestion
pepsin/o	pepsin
pept/i	digest, digestion, amino acid
per-	intense, through
perforat	bore through
perfus/e	to pour
peri-	around
perin/e	perineum
peripher	external boundary, outer part, outer edge
periton/e	stretch over, peritoneum
perium	bringing forth
perm/e	pass through
person	person
pes	foot
pest/i	pest, nuisance
petit-	small
-pexy	fixation, surgical fixation
phac/o	lens
phag/e	to eat
phagia	swallowing, eating
phalang/e	phalanx
pharmac/o	drug
pharyng/e	pharynx
pharynx	throat, pharynx
pheo-	gray
pher-	carrying
-pheresis	removal
phery	outer edge
-phil	attraction
-phile	attraction
-philia	attraction
phim	muzzle
phleb/o	vein
-phobia	fear
phobia	fear
phon/o	sound, voice

S = Suffix   P = Prefix   R = Root   R/CF = Combining Form

WORD PART	DEFINITION	WORD PART	DEFINITION
phor/e	bear, carry	pollut	to defile
phosph	phosphorus	poly-	excessive, many, much
phot/o	light	polyp	polyp
phren	mind	poplit/e	ham, back of knee
phylac	protect	por/o	opening
phylaxis	protection	post-	after
phys	nature	poster	coming behind
physema	blowing	pract	efficient, practical
physi/o	body	prand/i	breakfast
physic	body	pre-	before, in front of
physis	growth	precis	accurate
phyt/o	plant	predn	a derivative of cholesterol
pia	delicate	pregn	with child, pregnant
pituit	pituitary	presby	old person
placed	in an area	press	press close, press down, squeeze
plak	plate, plaque	prevent	prevent
plant	insert, plant	primi-	first
planus	flat surface	pro-	before, in front, projecting forward
plas	molding, formation	proct/o	anus and rectum
-plasia	formation	product	lead forth
-plasm	something formed	prol/i	bear offspring
plasm/o	to form	prolifer	bear offspring
-plasty	formation, repair, surgical repair	pronat	bend down
plate	flat	prost/a	prostate
pleg	paralysis	prot/e	protein
plete	filled	protein	protein
pleur	pleura	proto-	first
plexy	stroke	proton	first
-pnea	to breathe	provis	provide
pneum/o	air, lung	proxim	nearest
pneumat	structure filled with air	prurit	itch
pneumon	air, lung	pseudo-	false
pod	foot	psych/o	mind, soul
-poiesis	to make	pteryg	wing
-poiet	the making	-ptosis	drooping
-poietin	the maker	ptysis	spit
poikilo-	irregular	pub	pubis
point	to pierce	puber	growing up
pol	pole	pubesc	to reach puberty
polio-	gray matter	puer	child

S = Suffix   P = Prefix   R = Root   R/CF = Combining Form

WORD PART	DEFINITION
pulmon/o	lung
puls	to drive
pump	pump
punct	puncture
pur	pus
purg	cleanse, evacuate, throw up
purif	make pure
purul	pus
py/o	pus
pyel/o	renal pelvis
pylor	gate, pylorus
pyr/o	fire, heat, fever
pyret	fever
pyrex	fever, heat
quadr	four
quadri-	four
radi/o	x-ray, radiation, radius
radial	radius
radic	root
re-	again, back, backward
recept	receive
rect/o	rectum
reflex/o	to reflect, bend back
regul	to rule
remiss	send back, give up
ren	kidney
replic	reply
rescein	resin
resect/o	cut off
resid/u	left over, what is left over
resist	to withstand
restor	renew
resuscit	revival from apparent death
reticul	fine net, network
retin/o	retina
retinacul	hold back
retro-	backward
rhabd/o	rod-shaped, striated
-rhaphy	suture, repair
rheumat	a flow, rheumatism

WORD PART	DEFINITION
rhin/o	nose
rhythm	rhythm
rib/o	like a rib
rigid	stiff
rotat	rotate
-rrhage	to flow profusely
-rrhagia	excessive flow, discharge
-rrhaphy	suture
-rrhea	flow, discharge
-rrhoid	flow
rrhythm	rhythm
-rubin	rust colored
rumin	throat
-ry	occupation
sacchar	sugar
sacr/o	sacrum
sagitt	arrow
saliv	saliva
salping/o	fallopian tube, uterine tube
salpinx	trumpet
san	sound, healthy
sarc/o	flesh, sarcoma, muscle
satur	to fill
scapul	scapula
schiz/o	to split, cleave
scinti	spark
scler/o	hard, white of eye, hardness
-scope	instrument for viewing, instrument
scope	instrument for viewing
-scopy	to examine, to view, visual examination
script	writing, thing copied
scrot	scrotum
seb/o	sebum
sebac/e	wax
secret	secrete, produce, separate
sect	cut off
sedat	to calm
sedent	sitting
segment	section
seiz	to grab, convulse

WORD PART	DEFINITION
self	me, own individual
semi-	half
semin	scatter seed
semin/i	semen
sen	old age
senesc	growing old
senil	characteristic of old age
sens	feel
sensitiv	sensitive, feeling, sensitivity
sensor/i	sensation, sensory
separat	move apart
seps	decay, infection
sept/o	septum, partition
septic	infected
ser/o	serum, serous
sib	relative
sigm	Greek letter sigma, "S"
sigmoid/o	sigmoid colon
silic	silicon, glass
simul	imitate
sin/o	sinus
sinus	sinus
sipid	flavor
-sis	abnormal condition, process
sit/u	place
skelet	skeleton
soci/o	partner, ally, community
soma	body
somat/o	body
somn/o	sleep
somy	chromosome
son/o	sound
sorpt	swallow
sound	noise
spad	tear or cut
spasm	spasm, sudden involuntary tightening
spast	tight
specif	species
sperm/i	sperm
spermat/o	sperm

WORD PART	DEFINITION
sphen	wedge
spher/o	sphere
sphygm/o	pulse
spin/o	spine, spinal cord
spir/o	spiral, coil
spirat	breathe
spiro-	spiral, coil
splen/o	spleen
spondyl	vertebra
spong/i	sponge
spongios	sponge
stabil	stand firm
stalsis	to constrict
staphyl/o	bunch of grapes
-stasis	control, stop, stand still
stat	stand still
-static	to make stand, stop
-statin	inhibit
stax	fall in drops
steat	fat
stein	stone
sten/o	narrow, contract
ster	solid, steroid
stere/o	three-dimensional
steril	barren
stern	chest, breastbone
-steroid	steroid
-sterol	steroid
steron	steroid
-sterone	sterol
steth/o	chest
sthen	strength
stick	branch, twig
stigmat	focus
stimul	excite, strengthen
stin	partition
stit/i	space
stoma	mouth
-stomy	new opening
stone	stone, pebble

S = Suffix   P = Prefix   R = Root   R/CF = Combining Form

WORD PART	DEFINITION
storm	crisis
strab	squint
strat	layer
strepto-	curved
su/i	self
sub-	below, under, slightly, underneath
sucr	sucrose, table sugar
suffic/i	enough
sulf	sulfur
super	above
supinat	bend backward
suppress	pressed under, push under
supra-	above, excessive
surf	surface
surg	operate
suscept	to take up
-sylated	linked
sym-	together
symptomat	symptom
syn-	together
syndesm	bind together
synov	synovial membrane
syring/o	tube, pipe
system	body system
systol/e	contraction
tachy-	rapid
tact	orderly arrangement
tali	ankle bone
tamin	touch
tampon	plug
tangent/i	touch
tars/o	ankle
tax	coordination
tect/o	to shelter
tempor/o	time, temple, side of head
ten/o	tendon
tendin	tendon
tens	pressure
-tensin	tense, taut
terat/o	monster, malformed fetus

WORD PART	DEFINITION
term	normal gestation
test/o	testis, testicle
testicul	testicle, testis
tetra-	four
thalam	thalamus
thalass	sea
thec	sheath
thel	breast, nipple
thel/i	lining
thenar	palm
therap/o	healing, treatment
therapeut	healing, treatment
therapy	medical treatment
therm/o	heat
thesis	to arrange, place
thet	place, arrange
thora	chest
thorac/o	chest
-thorax	chest
thromb/o	blood clot, clot
thrombin	clot
thym	thymus gland, the mind
thyr/o	an oblong shield, thyroid
thyroid	an oblong shield, thyroid
-tic	pertaining to
-tion	process, being
-tiz	pertaining to
toc	labor, birth
toler	endure
tom/o	section, incise, cut
-tome	instrument to cut
-tomy	surgical incision
-tory	pertaining to
ton/o	pressure, tension
tonsil	tonsil
tonsill/o	tonsil
tope	part, location
topic	local
-tous	pertaining to
tox/o	poison

WORD PART	DEFINITION
-toxic	able to kill
toxic/o	poison
toxin	poison
trache/o	trachea, windpipe
tract	draw, pull
tranquil	calm
trans-	across, through
trauma	wound, injury
tresia	a hole
tri-	three
trich/o	hair, flagellum
trichin/o	hair
-tripsy	to crush
-tripter	crusher
trochle	pulley
trop	turn, turning
troph	development, nourishment
trophy	development, nourishment
-tropic	stimulator, change
-tropin	nourishing, stimulation
tryps	friction
tub/a	tube
tubercul	swelling, tuberculosis, nodule
tubul	small tube
tuss/i	cough
tussis	cough
-ty	quality, state
tympan/o	eardrum, tympanic membrane
-type	model, particular kind, group
-ula	small thing
ulcer	a sore
-ule	little, small
-ulent	abounding in
uln/a	forearm bone
ultra-	higher, beyond
-um	tissue, structure
umbilic	belly button, navel, umbilicus
un-	not
un	one
uni-	one

WORD PART	DEFINITION
ur/o	urinary system
-ure	process, result of
uresis	to urinate
uret	ureter, urine, urination
ureter/o	ureter
urethr/o	urethra
urin/a	urine
-us	pertaining to
uter/o	uterus
uve	uvea
uvul	uvula
vaccin	vaccine, giving a vaccine
vag	vagus nerve
vagin	sheath, vagina
valgus	turn out
valv	valve
varic/o	varicosity; dilated, tortuous vein
vas/o	blood vessel, duct
vascul	blood vessel
vegetat	growth
ven/o	vein
ventil	wind
ventr	belly
ventricul	ventricle
vers	turned
verse	travel
-version	change
vert	to turn
vertebr/a	vertebra
vesic	sac containing fluid
vestibul/o	vestibule of inner ear
via	the way
violet	bluish purple
vir	virus
viril	masculine
virus	poison
visc/o	sticky
viscer	an internal organ
visu	sight
vit/a	life

S = Suffix   P = Prefix   R = Root   R/CF = Combining Form

WORD PART	DEFINITION
voc	voice
vol	volume
volunt	free will
-volut	rolled up
volut/e	shrink, roll up
vuls	tear, pull
vulv/o	vulva
whip	to swing

WORD PART	DEFINITION
xanth	yellow
xeno-	foreign
-yl	substance
-zoa	animal
zyg	zygote
-zyme	enzyme
zyme	fermenting, enzyme, transform

Abbreviations

ABBREVIATION	DEFINITION
↑	increase/ above
↓	decrease/ below
1°	primary
2°	secondary
99mTc	technetium 99m, a radionuclide
ABG	arterial blood gas
ABI	ankle/brachial index
ABO	a blood group system
AC	acromioclavicular
ACE	angiotensin-converting enzyme
ACEP	American College of Emergency Physicians
ACL	anterior cruciate ligament
ACTH	adrenocorticotropic hormone
AD	right ear
ADD	attention deficit disorder
ADH	antidiuretic hormone
ADHD	attention deficit hyperactivity disorder
ADLs	activities of daily living
AED	automatic external defibrillator
AFP	alpha-fetoprotein
AIDS	acquired immunodeficiency syndrome
ALL	acute lymphoblastic leukemia
ALP	alkaline phosphatase
ALS	amyotrophic lateral sclerosis
ALT	alanine aminotransferase
AMAS	anti-malignin antibody screen
ANS	autonomic nervous system
AOM	acute otitis media
AP	anteroposterior
APP	advanced practice provider
aPTT	activated partial thromboplastin time
ARDS	acute respiratory distress syndrome
ARF	acute respiratory failure
ARF	acute renal failure
AROM	active range of motion
AS	left ear

ABBREVIATION	DEFINITION
ASD	atrial septal defect
ASD	autism spectrum disorder
ASHD	arteriosclerotic heart disease
AST	aspartate aminotransferase
AU	both ears
AV	atrioventricular
AVM	arteriovenous malformation
BAL	bronchoalveolar lavage
BBB	blood-brain barrier
BD	brain death
BKA	below-the-knee amputation
BM	bowel movement
BMD	bone mineral density
BMR	basal metabolic rate
BNP	B-type natriuretic peptide
BOM	bilateral otitis media
BP	blood pressure
BPD	borderline personality disorder
BPH	benign prostatic hyperplasia
BPPV	benign paroxysmal positional vertigo
BRCA1	a gene that, when mutated, increases risk for breast and ovarian cancer (BReast CAncer 1)
BRCA2	a gene that, when mutated, increases risk for breast cancer (BReast CAncer 2)
BSE	bovine spongiform encephalopathy
BSE	breast self-examination
BUN	blood urea nitrogen
C1–C8	cervical spinal nerves
C5	fifth cervical vertebra or nerve
CA	cancer
CABG	coronary artery bypass graft
CAD	coronary artery disease
CAO	chronic airway obstruction
CAPD	continuous ambulatory peritoneal dialysis
CBC	complete blood count
CBT	cognitive behavioral therapy

ABBREVIATION	DEFINITION
CD	cluster of differentiation; coreceptors of cell membranes to recognize specific antigens
CD	conduct disorder
CD8	helper T cell
CDC	Centers for Disease Control and Prevention
CEA	carcinoembryonic antigen
CF	cystic fibrosis
CHART	continuous hyperfractionated accelerated radiotherapy
CHD	congenital heart disease
CHES	Certified Health Education Specialist
CHF	congestive heart failure
CIS	carcinoma in situ
CJD	Creutzfeldt-Jakob disease
CK	creatine kinase
CKD	chronic kidney disease
CMA	Certified Medical Assistant
CMV	cytomegalovirus
CNA	Certified Nurse Assistant
CNS	central nervous system
c/o	complains of
CO2	carbon dioxide
COPD	chronic obstructive pulmonary disease
COT	Certified Occupational Therapist
COTA	Certified Occupational Therapist Assistant
CP	cerebral palsy
CPAP	continuous positive airway pressure
CPR	cardiopulmonary resuscitation
CPT	cognitive processing therapy
CRF	chronic renal failure
CRP	C-reactive protein
C-section	cesarean section
CSF	cerebrospinal fluid
CT	computed tomography
CVA	cerebrovascular accident
CVP	central venous pressure
CVS	cardiovascular system
CVT	cardiovascular technician
CXR	chest x-ray
D&C	dilation and curettage
DEXA	dual-energy x-ray absorptiometry
DHEA	dehydroepiandrosterone
DI	diabetes insipidus

ABBREVIATION	DEFINITION
DIC	disseminated intravascular coagulation
DID	dissociative identity disorder
DIFF	differential white blood cell count
DJD	degenerative joint disease
DKA	diabetic ketoacidosis
dL	deciliter; one-tenth of a liter
DM	diabetes mellitus
DMD	Duchenne muscular dystrophy
DNA	deoxyribonucleic acid
DNR	do not resuscitate
DO	doctor of osteopathy
DRE	digital rectal examination
DSM-IV	*Diagnostic and Statistical Manual of Mental Disorders,* fourth edition
DSM-V	*Diagnostic and Statistical Manual of Mental Disorders*, fifth edition
DUB	dysfunctional uterine bleeding
DVT	deep vein thrombosis
Dx	diagnosis
EBT	electron beam tomography
EBV	Epstein-Barr virus
ECG	electrocardiogram
E. coli	*Escherichia coli*
ECT	electroconvulsive therapy
ED	erectile dysfunction
EEG	electroencephalogram
EKG	electrocardiogram
ELISA	enzyme-linked immunosorbent assay
EMDR	eye movement desensitization and reprocessing
EMG	electromyogram
EMR	emergency medical responder
EMS	emergency medical services
EMT	emergency medical technician
EP	evoked potential
EPA	U.S. Environmental Protection Agency
ER	Emergency Room
ERCP	endoscopic retrograde cholangiopancreatography
ESR	erythrocyte sedimentation rate
ESRD	end-stage renal disease
ESWL	extracorporeal shock wave lithotripsy
ETS	environmental tobacco smoke
FAS	fetal alcohol syndrome
FDA	U.S. Food and Drug Administration

ABBREVIATION	DEFINITION
FEV1	forced expiratory volume in 1 second
fL	femtoliter; one-quadrillionth of a liter
FOBT	fecal occult blood test
FSH	follicle-stimulating hormone
FTT	failure to thrive
FVC	forced vital capacity
Fx	fracture
g	gram
GAD	generalized anxiety disorder
GDM	gestational diabetes mellitus
GERD	gastroesophageal reflux disease
GFR	glomerular filtration rate
GGT	gamma-glutamyl transpeptidase
GH	growth hormone, somatotropin
GI	gastrointestinal
GI	glycemic index
GL	glycemic load
GnRH	gonadotropin-releasing hormone
GSR	galvanic skin response
GTT	glucose tolerance test
GYN	gynecology
H1N1	swine flu virus
H2-blocker	histamine-2 receptor antagonist
H5N1	subtype of avian influenza virus
HAV	hepatitis A virus
Hb	hemoglobin
Hb A1c	glycosylated hemoglobin A1c
HBV	hepatitis B virus
HCG	human chorionic gonadotropin
HCL	hydrochloric acid
Hct	hematocrit
HCV	hepatitis C virus
HDL	high-density lipoprotein
HDN	hemolytic disease of the newborn
Hg	mercury
Hgb	hemoglobin
HIPAA	Health Insurance Portability and Accountability Act
HIV	human immunodeficiency virus
HLA	human leukocyte antigen
HLD	high-level disinfection
HMD	hyaline membrane disease
H/O	history of

ABBREVIATION	DEFINITION
HPI	history of present illness
HPV	human papillomavirus
HRT	hormone replacement therapy
HSV	herpes simplex virus
HSV-1	herpes simplex virus, type 1
HUS	hemolytic uremic syndrome
IADLs	instrumental activities of daily living
IBS	irritable bowel syndrome
ICD	implantable cardioverter/defibrillator
IDDM	insulin-dependent diabetes mellitus
Ig	immunoglobulin
IgA	immunoglobulin A
IgD	immunoglobulin D
IgE	immunoglobulin E
IGF	insulinlike growth factor
IgG	immunoglobulin G
IgM	immunoglobulin M
IM	intramuscular
INR	international normalized ratio
ITP	idiopathic (or immunologic) thrombocytopenic purpura
IU	international unit(s)
IUD	intrauterine device
IV	intravenous
IVC	inferior vena cava
IVF	in vitro fertilization
IVP	intravenous pyelogram
JC	Joint Commission
JRA	juvenile rheumatoid arthritis
KUB	x-ray of abdomen to show kidneys, ureters, and bladder
L	liter
L1–L5	lumbar spinal nerves or vertebrae
LASER	light amplification by stimulated emission of radiation
LCC-ST	Liaison Council on Certification for the Surgical Technologist
LD	learning disability
LDL	low-density lipoprotein
LED	light-emitting diode
LEEP	loop electrosurgical excision procedure
LFT	liver function test
LH	luteinizing hormone
LLQ	left lower quadrant

ABBREVIATION	DEFINITION
LOC	loss of consciousness
LPN	licensed practical nurse
LSD	lysergic acid diethylamide (acid)
LUQ	left upper quadrant
LVN	licensed vocational nurse
MAOI	monoamine oxidase inhibitor
mcg	microgram; one-millionth of a gram
MCH	mean corpuscular hemoglobin (the average amount of hemoglobin in the average red blood cell)
MCHC	mean corpuscular hemoglobin concentration (the average concentration of hemoglobin in a given volume of red blood cells)
MCP	metacarpophalangeal
MCS	minimally conscious state
MCV	mean corpuscular volume (the average volume of a red blood cell)
MD	doctor of medicine
MDMA	methylenedioxymethamphetamine (ecstasy)
mg	milligram
MHC	major histocompatibility complex
MI	myocardial infarction
mL	milliliter
mm3	cubic millimeter
MOAB	monoclonal antibody
MODY	mature-onset diabetes of youth
MPD	multiple personality disorder
MRA	magnetic resonance angiography
MRI	magnetic resonance imaging
mRNA	messenger RNA
MRSA	methicillin-resistant *Staphylococcus aureus*
MS	multiple sclerosis
NCI	National Cancer Institute
NHGRI	National Human Genome Research Institute
NHLBI	National Heart, Lung, and Blood Institute
NIDDM	non-insulin-dependent diabetes mellitus
NIH	National Institutes of Health
NKA	no known allergies
NLM	National Library of Medicine
NMS	neurally mediated syncope
NO	nitric oxide
NPH	neutral protamine Hagedorn insulin
NRDS	neonatal respiratory distress syndrome
NSAID	nonsteroidal anti-inflammatory drug

ABBREVIATION	DEFINITION
O2	oxygen
OA	osteoarthritis
OB	obstetrics
OCD	obsessive-compulsive disorder
OD	doctor of osteopathy
OD	right eye
OGTT	oral glucose tolerance test
OME	otitis media with effusion
omega-3	alpha-linolenic acid
OR	operating room
OS	left eye
OSHA	Occupational Safety and Health Administration
OT	ophthalmic technician
OXT	oxytocin
OT	occupational therapist, occupational therapy
OTC	over-the-counter
OU	both eyes
P	pulse (rate)
PA	posteroanterior
PaO2	partial pressure of arterial oxygen
Pap	Papanicolaou (Pap test, Pap smear)
PAT	paroxysmal atrial tachycardia
PCBs	polychlorinated biphenyls
PCD	programmed cell death
PCL	posterior cruciate ligament
PCOS	polycystic ovarian syndrome
PCP	phencyclidine (angel dust), primary care provider
PDA	patent ductus arteriosus
PDT	postural drainage therapy
PE	pressure equalization (tube)
PEEP	positive end-expiratory pressure
PEFR	peak expiratory flow rate
PET	positron emission tomography
PFT	pulmonary function test
pg	picogram; one-trillionth of a gram
PGY	pregnancy
pH	hydrogen ion concentration
PhD	doctor of philosophy
PID	pelvic inflammatory disease
PIP	proximal interphalangeal (joint)
PKD	polycystic kidney disease
PMDD	premenstrual dysphoric disorder

ABBREVIATION	DEFINITION
PMNL	polymorphonuclear leukocyte
PMS	premenstrual syndrome
PNS	peripheral nervous system
p.o.	by mouth
polio	poliomyelitis
PPH	postpartum hemorrhage
PPI	proton pump inhibitor
PPS	postpolio syndrome
PRL	prolactin
p.r.n.	when necessary
PSA	prostate-specific antigen
PsyD	doctor of psychology
PT	physiotherapy
PT	prothrombin time
PT	physical therapy, physical therapist
PTA	physical therapy assistant
PTCA	percutaneous transluminal coronary angioplasty
PTH	parathyroid hormone
PTSD	posttraumatic stress disorder
PVC	premature ventricular contraction
PVD	peripheral vascular disease
PVS	persistent vegetative state
q.4.h.	every 4 hours
q.i.d.	four times a day
R	respiration (rate)
RA	rheumatoid arthritis
RBC	red blood cell
RDS	respiratory distress syndrome
RF	radiofrequency
Rh	Rhesus
RhoGAM	Rhesus immune globulin
RLQ	right lower quadrant
RN	registered nurse
RNA	ribonucleic acid
ROM	range of motion
RSV	respiratory syncytial virus
RT	radiology technician
RU-486	mifepristone
RUQ	right upper quadrant
S1–S5	sacral nerves or vertebrae
SA	sinoatrial
SAD	seasonal affective disorder

ABBREVIATION	DEFINITION
SBS	shaken baby syndrome
SC	subcutaneous
SCI	spinal cord injury
SET	self-examination of the testes
SG	specific gravity
SGOT	serum glutamic oxaloacetic acid transaminase (AST)
SGPT	serum glutamic-pyruvic transaminase (ALT)
SI	sacroiliac
SLE	systemic lupus erythematosus
SMI	sustained maximal inspiration
SNRI	serotonin and norepinephrine reuptake inhibitor
SOB	short(ness) of breath
SRS	stereotactic radiosurgery
SSA	Sjögren syndrome antibodies A
SSB	Sjögren syndrome antibodies B
SSRI	selective serotonin reuptake inhibitor
STAT	immediately
STD	sexually transmitted disease
SVC	superior vena cava
T	temperature
T1	first thoracic vertebra or nerve
T1–T12	thoracic spinal nerves or vertebrae
T3	triiodothyronine
T4	tetraiodothyronine (thyroxine)
TB	tuberculosis
TBI	traumatic brain injury
TCA	tricyclic antidepressant
TEE	transesophageal echocardiography
TENS	transcutaneous electrical nerve stimulation
THC	tetrahydrocannabinol (marijuana)
THR	total hip replacement
TIA	transient ischemic attack
TIBC	total iron-binding capacity
t.i.d.	(Latin *ter in die*) three times a day
TMJ	temporomandibular joint
TNM	tumor-node-metastasis (staging system for cancer)
TOF	tetralogy of Fallot
tPA	tissue plasminogen activator
TS	tumor suppressor
TSH	thyroid-stimulating hormone

ABBREVIATION	DEFINITION
TTM	trichotillomania
TTP	thrombotic thrombocytopenic purpura
TURP	transurethral resection of the prostate
U	unit
UA	urinalysis
URI	upper respiratory infection
UTI	urinary tract infection
UV	ultraviolet
VCUG	voiding cystourethrogram

ABBREVIATION	DEFINITION
VEP	visual evoked potential
V-fib	ventricular fibrillation
VS	vital signs
VSD	ventricular septal defect
vWD	von Willebrand disease
vWF	von Willebrand factor
WAD	Word Analysis and Definition (box)
WBC	white blood cell; white blood (cell) count
WNL	within normal limits

A

abdomen (AB-doh-men) Part of the trunk between the thorax and the pelvis.

abdominal (ab-DOM-in-al) Pertaining to the abdomen.

abdominopelvic (ab-DOM-ih-noh-PEL-vik) Pertaining to the abdomen and pelvis.

abducens (ab-DYU-senz) Sixth (VI) cranial nerve; responsible for eye movement.

abduction (ab-DUK-shun) Action of moving away from the midline.

ablation (ab-LAY-shun) Removal of tissue to destroy its function.

abortus (ah-BOR-tus) Product of abortion.

abrasion (ah-BRAY-shun) Area of skin or mucous membrane that has been scraped off.

abruptio (ab-RUP-shee-oh) Placenta abruptio is the premature detachment of the placenta.

absorption (ab-SORP-shun) Uptake of nutrients and water by cells in the GI tract.

accessory (ak-SESS-oh-ree) Eleventh (XI) cranial nerve; supplying neck muscles, pharynx, and larynx.

acetabulum (ass-eh-TAB-you-lum) The cup-shaped cavity of the hip bone that receives the head of the femur to form the hip joint.

acetaminophen (ah-seet-ah-MIN-oh-fen) Medication that is an analgesic and an antipyretic.

acetone (ASS-eh-tone) Ketone that is found in blood, urine, and breath when diabetes mellitus is out of control.

acetylcholine (AS-eh-til-KOH-leen) Parasympathetic neurotransmitter.

Achilles tendon (ah-KIL-eez TEN-dun) A tendon formed from the gastrocnemius and soleus muscles and inserted into the calcaneus. Also called *calcaneal tendon.*

achondroplasia (ay-kon-droh-PLAY-zee-ah) Condition with abnormal conversion of cartilage into bone, leading to dwarfism.

acid (ASS-id) Substance with a pH below 7.0.

acinar cells (ASS-in-ar SELLS) Enzyme-secreting cells of the pancreas.

acne (AK-nee) Inflammatory disease of sebaceous glands and hair follicles.

acquired immunodeficiency syndrome (AIDS) (ah-KWIRED IM-you-noh-dee-FISH-en-see SIN-drome) Infection with the HIV virus.

acromegaly (ak-roh-MEG-ah-lee) Enlargement of the head, face, hands, and feet due to excess growth hormone in an adult.

acromioclavicular (AC) (ah-CROH-mee-oh-klah-VIK-you-lar) The joint between the acromion and the clavicle.

acromion (ah-CROH-mee-on) Lateral end of the scapula, extending over the shoulder joint.

acrophobia (ak-roh-FOH-bee-ah) Pathologic fear of heights.

actinic (ak-TIN-ik) Pertaining to the sun.

activities of daily living (ADLs) (ak-TIV-ih-teez of DAY-lee LIV-ing) Daily routines for mobility and personal care: bathing, dressing, eating, and moving.

acuminata (a-KYU-min-AH-ta) Tapering to a point.

addiction (ah-DIK-shun) Habitual psychological and physiologic dependence on a substance or practice.

addictive (ah-DIK-tiv) Pertaining to or causing addiction.

Addison disease (ADD-ih-son diz-EEZ) An autoimmune disease leading to decreased production of adrenocortical steroids.

adduction (ah-DUK-shun) Action of moving toward the midline.

adenocarcinoma (AD-eh-noh-kar-sih-NOH-mah) A cancer arising from glandular epithelial cells.

adenohypophysis (AD-en-oh-high-POF-ih-sis) Anterior lobe of the pituitary gland.

adenoid (ADD-eh-noyd) Single mass of lymphoid tissue in the midline at the back of the throat.

adenoma (AD-eh-NOH-mah) Benign tumor that originates from glandular tissue.

adherence (ad-HEER-ents) The act of sticking to something.

adipose (ADD-i-pose) Containing fat.

adjuvant (AD-joo-vant) Additional treatment after a primary treatment has been used.

adnexa (ad-NEK-sa) Parts accessory to an organ or structure. Singular *adnexum.*

adrenal gland (ah-DREE-nal GLAND) The suprarenal, or adrenal, gland on the upper pole of each kidney.

adrenalectomy (ah-DREE-nal-EK-toh-mee) Removal of part or all of an adrenal gland.

adrenaline (ah-DREN-ah-lin) One of the catecholamines. Also called *epinephrine.*

adrenocortical (ah-DREE-noh-KOR-tih-kal) Pertaining to the cortex of the adrenal gland.

adrenocorticotropic hormone (ah-DREE-noh-KOR-tih-koh-TROH-pik HOR-mohn) Hormone of the anterior pituitary that stimulates the cortex of the adrenal gland to produce its own hormones.

adrenogenital syndrome (ah-DREE-noh-JEN-it-al SIN-drome) Hypersecretion of androgens from the adrenal gland.

advance medical directive (ad-VANTS MED-ih-kal die-REK-tiv) Legal document signed by the patient dealing with issues of prolonging or ending life in the event of life-threatening illness.

adventitia (ad-ven-TISH-ah) Outer layer of connective tissue covering blood vessels or organs.

affect (AF-fekt) External display of feelings, thoughts, and emotions.

afferent (AF-eh-rent) Conducting impulses inward *toward* the spinal cord or brain.

agglutinate (ah-GLUE-tin-ate) Stick together to form clumps.

agglutination (ah-glue-tih-NAY-shun) Process by which cells or other particles adhere to each other to form clumps.

aging (AY-jing) The process of human maturation and decline.

agonist (AG-on-ist) Agent that combines with receptors to initiate drug actions.

agoraphobia (ah-gor-ah-FOH-bee-ah) Pathologic fear of being trapped in a public place.

agranulocyte (ay-GRAN-you-loh-site) A white blood cell without any granules in its cytoplasm.

alanine aminotransferase (ALT) (AL-ah-neen ah-MEE-nh-TRANS-fer-aze) Enzyme that is found in liver cells and leaks out into the bloodstream when the cells are damaged, enabling liver damage to be diagnosed.

albinism (AL-bih-nizm) Genetic disorder with lack of melanin.

albumin (al-BYU-min) Simple, soluble protein.

aldosterone (al-DOS-ter-ohn) Mineralocorticoid hormone of the adrenal cortex.

aldosteronism (al-DOS-ter-ohn-izm) Condition caused by excessive secretion of aldosterone. Also called *Conn syndrome.*

aldosteronoma (al-DOS-ter-oh-NOH-mah) Benign adenoma of the adrenal cortex.

alimentary (al-ih-MEN-tar-ee) Pertaining to the digestive tract.

alkaline (AL-kah-line) Substance with a pH above 7.0. Also called *basic.*

alkaloid (AL-ka-loyd) Alkaline substances with pharmacologic activity synthesized from plants.

allergen (AL-er-jen) Substance producing a hypersensitivity (allergic) reaction.

allergic (ah-LER-jik) Pertaining to being hypersensitive.

allergy (AL-er-jee) Hypersensitivity to an allergen.

allogen (AL-oh-jen) Antigen from someone else in the same species.

allograft (AL-oh-graft) Tissue graft from another person or cadaver.

alloimmune (AL-oh-im-YUNE) Reaction directed against foreign tissue.

alopecia (al-oh-PEE-shah) Partial or complete loss of hair, naturally or from medication.

alpha-fetoprotein (AL-fah-fee-toh-PROH-teen) Protein normally produced only by the fetus.

alveolus (al-VEE-oh-lus) Small empty hollow or sac. It is a terminal element of the respiratory tract. Plural *alveoli.*

Alzheimer disease (AWLZ-high-mer diz-EEZ) Common form of dementia.

amblyopia (am-blee-OH-pee-ah) Failure or incomplete development of the pathways of vision to the brain.

amenorrhea (a-men-oh-REE-ah) Absence or abnormal cessation of menstrual flow.

amino acid (ah-MEE-noh ASS-id) The basic building block of protein.

ammonia (ah-MOHN-ih-ah) Toxic breakdown product of amino acids.

amnesia (am-NEE-zee-ah) Total or partial inability to remember past experiences.

amniocentesis (AM-nee-oh-sen-TEE-sis) Removal of amniotic fluid for diagnostic purposes.

amnion (AM-nee-on) Membrane around the fetus that contains amniotic fluid.

ampulla (am-PULL-ah) Dilated portion of a canal or duct.

amputation (am-pyu-TAY-shun) Process of removing a limb, a part of a limb, a breast, or some other projecting part.

amylase (AM-il-aze) One of a group of enzymes that break down starch.

amyotrophic (a-my-oh-TROH-fik) Pertaining to muscular atrophy.

anabolism (an-AB-oh-lizm) The buildup of complex substances in the cell from simpler ones as a part of metabolism.

analgesic (an-al-JEE-zik) Substance that reduces the response to pain.

anaphylactic (AN-ah-fih-LAK-tik) Pertaining to anaphylaxis.

anaphylaxis (AN-ah-fih-LAK-sis) Immediate severe allergic response.

anastomosis (ah-NAS-to-MOH-sis) A surgically made union between two tubular structures. Plural *anastomoses.*

anatomic (an-ah-TOM-ik) Pertaining to anatomy.

androgen (AN-droh-jen) Hormone that promotes masculine characteristics.

anemia (ah-NEE-mee-ah) Decreased number of red blood cells.

anencephaly (AN-en-SEF-ah-lee) Born without cerebral hemispheres.

anesthesiologist (AN-es-thee-zee-OL-oh-jist) Medical specialist in anesthesia.

anesthetic (an-es-THET-ik) Substance that takes away feeling and pain.

aneurysm (AN-yur-izm) Circumscribed dilation of an artery or cardiac chamber.

angiogram (AN-jee-oh-gram) Radiograph obtained after injection of radiopaque contrast material into blood vessels.

angiography (an-jee-OG-rah-fee) Radiography of vessels after injection of contrast material.

angioplasty (AN-jee-oh-PLAS-tee) Recanalization of a blood vessel by surgery.

anomaly (ah-NOM-ah-lee) A structural abnormality.

anorchism (an-OR-kizm) Absence of testes.

anorexia (an-oh-RECK-see-ah) Severe lack of appetite; *or* an aversion to food.

anoscopy (A-nos-koh-pee) Endoscopic examination of the anus.

anoxia (an-OK-see-ah) Without oxygen.

antacid (ant-ASS-id) Agent that neutralizes acidity.

antagonist (an-TAG-oh-nist) An opposing structure, agent, disease, or process.

antagonistic (an-TAG-oh-nis-tik) Having an opposite function.

anterior (an-TER-ee-or) Front surface of body; situated in front.

anteverted (an-teh-VERT-ed) Tilted forward.

anthracosis (an-thra-KOH-sis) Lung disease caused by the inhalation of coal dust.

anti-inflammatory (AN-tee-in-FLAM-ah-tor-ee) Agent that reduces inflammation by acting on the body's response mechanisms without affecting the causative agent.

antiangiogenesis (AN-tee-AN-jee-oh-JEN-eh-sis) The prevention of growth of new blood vessels.

antibiotic (AN-tih-bye-OT-ik) A substance that has the capacity to destroy bacteria and other microorganisms.

antibody (AN-tih-body) Protein produced in response to an antigen. Plural *antibodies.*

anticoagulant (AN-tee-koh-AG-you-lant) Substance that prevents clotting.

antidiuretic hormone (ADH) (AN-tih-die-you-RET-ik HOR-mohn) Posterior pituitary hormone that decreases urine output by acting on the kidney. Also called *vasopressin.*

antiemetic (AN-tee-eh-MEH-tik) Agent that prevents vomiting.

antiepileptic (AN-tee-eh-pih-LEP-tik) A pharmacologic agent capable of preventing or arresting epilepsy.

antigen (AN-tih-jen) Substance capable of triggering an immune response.

antihistamine (an-tee-HISS-tah-meen) Drug used to treat allergic symptoms because of its action antagonistic to histamine. Some can also be effective against vomiting.

antioxidant (an-tee-OKS-ih-dant) Substance that can prevent cell damage by neutralizing free radicals.

antipruritic (AN-tee-pru-RIT-ik) Medication against itching.

antipsychotic (AN-tih-sigh-KOT-ik) An agent helpful in the treatment of psychosis.

antipyretic (AN-tee-pie-RET-ik) Agent that reduces fever.

antisocial personality disorder (AN-tee-SOH-shal per-son-AL-ih-tee dis-OR-der) Disorder of people who lie, cheat, and steal and have no guilt about their behavior.

antithyroid (an-tee-THIGH-royd) A substance that inhibits production of thyroid hormones.

antrum (AN-trum) A nearly closed cavity or chamber.

anuria (an-YOU-ree-ah) Absence of urine production.

anus (AY-nuss) Terminal opening of the digestive tract through which feces are discharged.

anxiety (ang-ZIE-eh-tee) Distress caused by fear.

aorta (ay-OR-tuh) Main trunk of the systemic arterial system.

apex (AY-peks) Tip or end of cone-shaped structure, such as the heart.

aphonia (ay-FOH-nee-ah) Loss of voice.

aphthous ulcer (AF-thus UL-ser) Painful small oral ulcer (canker sore).

aplastic anemia (ay-PLAS-tik ah-NEE-mee-ah) Condition in which the bone marrow is unable to produce sufficient red cells, white cells, and platelets.

apnea (AP-nee-ah) Absence of spontaneous respiration.

apocrine (AP-oh-krin) Apocrine sweat glands that open into the hair follicle.

apoptosis (AP-op-TOH-sis) Programmed normal cell death.

appendicitis (ah-pen-dih-SIGH-tis) Inflammation of the appendix.

appendix (ah-PEN-dicks) Small blind projection from the pouch of the cecum.

aqueous humor (AYK-wee-us HEW-mor) Watery liquid in the anterior and posterior chambers of the eye.

arachnoid mater (ah-RAK-noyd MAY-ter) Weblike middle layer of the three meninges.

areola (ah-REE-oh-luh) Circular reddish area surrounding the nipple.

arrhythmia (ah-RITH-mee-ah) An abnormal heart rhythm.

arteriography (ar-teer-ee-OG-rah-fee) X-ray visualization of an artery after injection of contrast material.

arteriole (ar-TEER-ee-ole) Small terminal artery leading into the capillary network.

arteriosclerosis (ar-TEER-ee-oh-skler-OH-sis) Hardening of the arteries.

arteriosclerotic (ar-TEER-ee-oh-skler-OT-ik) Pertaining to or suffering from arteriosclerosis.

arteriovenous malformation (ar-TEER-ee-oh-VEE-nus mal-for-MAY-shun) An abnormal communication between an artery and a vein.

artery (AR-ter-ee) Thick-walled blood vessel carrying blood away from the heart.

arthrocentesis (AR-throh-sen-TEE-sis) Withdrawal of fluid from a joint through a needle.

arthrodesis (AR-throh-DEE-sis) Fixation or stiffening of a joint by surgery.

arthrography (ar-THROG-rah-fee) X-ray of a joint taken after the injection of a contrast medium into the joint.

arthroplasty (AR-throh-plas-tee) Surgery to restore as far as possible the function of a joint.

arthroscope (AR-throh-skope) Endoscope used to examine the interior of a joint.

arthroscopy (ar-THROS-koh-pee) Visual examination of the interior of a joint.

articulation (ar-tik-you-LAY-shun) Joint formed to allow movement.

asbestosis (as-bes-TOH-sis) Lung disease caused by the inhalation of asbestos particles.

ascites (ah-SIGH-teez) Accumulation of fluid in the abdominal cavity.

aspartate aminotransferase (AST) (as-PAR-tate ah-MEE-noh-TRANS-fer-aze) Enzyme that is found in liver cells and leaks out into the bloodstream when the cells are damaged, enabling liver damage to be diagnosed.

aspiration (AS-pih-RAY-shun) Removal by suction of fluid or gas from a body cavity.

assistive device (ah-SIS-tiv dee-VICE) Tool, software, or hardware to assist in performing daily activities.

asthma (AZ-mah) Episodes of breathing difficulty due to narrowed or obstructed airways.

astigmatism (ah-STIG-mah-tism) Inability to focus light rays that enter the eye in different planes.

astrocyte (ASS-troh-site) Star-shaped connective tissue cell in the nervous system.

asystole (ay-SIS-toh-lee) Absence of contractions of the heart.

ataxia (a-TAK-see-ah) Inability to coordinate muscle activity, leading to jerky movements.

atelectasis (at-el-EK-tah-sis) Collapse of part of a lung.

atherectomy (ath-er-EK-toh-mee) Surgical removal of the atheroma.

atheroma (ath-er-ROH-mah) Lipid deposit in the lining of an artery.

atherosclerosis (ATH-er-oh-skler-OH-sis) Atheroma in arteries.

athetosis (ath-eh-TOH-sis) Slow, writhing involuntary movements.

atom (AT-om) A small unit of matter.

atopy (AY-toh-pee) State of hypersensitivity to an allergen; allergic.

atrioventricular (AV) (AY-tree-oh-ven-TRIK-you-lar) Pertaining to both the atrium and the ventricle.

atrium (AY-tree-um) Chamber where blood enters the heart on both right and left sides. Plural *atria*.

atrophy (AT-roh-fee) The wasting away or diminished volume of tissue, an organ, or a body part.

atropine (AT-roh-peen) Pharmacologic agent used to dilate pupils.

attenuated (ah-TEN-you-ay-ted) Weakened.

audiologist (aw-dee-OL-oh-jist) Specialist in evaluation of hearing function.

audiology (aw-dee-OL-oh-jee) Study of hearing disorders.

audiometer (aw-dee-OM-eh-ter) Instrument to measure hearing.

auditory (AW-dih-tor-ee) Pertaining to the sense or the organs of hearing.

aura (AWE-rah) Sensory experience preceding an epileptic seizure or a migraine headache.

auricle (AW-ri-kul) The shell-like external ear.

auscultation (aws-kul-TAY-shun) Diagnostic method of listening to body sounds with a stethoscope.

autoantibody (aw-toh-AN-tee-bod-ee) Antibody produced in response to an antigen from the host's own tissue.

autograft (AWE-toh-graft) A graft using tissue taken from the individual who is receiving the graft.

autoimmune (aw-toh-im-YUNE) Immune reaction directed against a person's own tissue.

autologous (awe-TOL-oh-gus) Blood transfusion with the same person as donor and recipient.

autolysis (awe-TOL-ih-sis) Self-destruction of cells by enzymes within the cells.

autonomic (awe-toh-NOM-ik) Not voluntary; pertaining to the self-governing visceral motor division of the peripheral nervous system.

autopsy (AWE-top-see) Examination of the body and organs of a dead person to determine the cause of death.

avascular (ay-VAS-cue-lar) Without a blood supply.

axilla (AK-sill-ah) Medical name for the armpit. Plural *axillae*.

axon (AK-son) Single process of a nerve cell carrying nervous impulses away from the cell body.

azotemia (az-oh-TEE-me-ah) Excess nitrogenous waste products in the blood.

B

bacterium (bak-TEER-ee-um) A unicellular, simple, microscopic organism. Plural *bacteria*.

balanitis (bal-ah-NIE-tis) Inflammation of the glans and prepuce of the penis.

bariatric (bar-ee-AT-rik) Treatment of obesity.

basal metabolic rate (BAY-sal met-ah-BOL-ic RATE) Energy the body requires to function at rest.

basilar (BAS-ih-lar) Pertaining to the base of a structure.

basophil (BAY-so-fill) A basophil's granules attract a basic blue stain in the laboratory.

Bell palsy (BELL PAWL-zee) Paresis or paralysis of one side of the face.

benign (bee-NINE) Denoting the nonmalignant character of a neoplasm or illness.

beta (BAY-tah) Second letter in the Greek alphabet.

biceps brachii (BIE-sepz BRAY-kee-eye) A muscle of the upper arm that has two heads or points of origin on the scapula.

biconcave (BIE-kon-KAVE) Having a hollowed surface on both sides of a structure.

bicuspid (by-KUSS-pid) Having two points; a bicuspid heart valve has two flaps, and a bicuspid (premolar) tooth has two points.

bilateral (by-LAT-er-al) On two sides; for example, in both ears.

bile (BILE) Fluid secreted by the liver into the duodenum.

bile acids (BILE ASS-ids) Steroids synthesized from cholesterol.

biliary (BILL-ee-air-ee) Pertaining to bile or the biliary tract.

bilirubin (bill-ee-RU-bin) Bile pigment formed in the liver from hemoglobin.

biofeedback (bie-oh-FEED-bak) Training techniques to achieve voluntary control of responses to stimuli.

biomarker (BIE-oh-MARK-er) A biological marker or product by which a cell can be identified.

biopsy (BIE-op-see) Removing tissue from a living person for laboratory examination.

biopsy removal (BI-op-see re-MUV-al) Used for small tumors when complete removal provides tissue for a biopsy and cures the lesion. Also called *excisional biopsy*.

bipolar disorder (bi-POH-lar dis-OR-der) A mood disorder with alternating episodes of depression and mania.

bladder (BLAD-er) Hollow sac that holds fluid; for example, urine or bile.

blastocyst (BLAS-toh-sist) The developing embryo during the first 2 weeks.

blepharitis (blef-ah-RIE-tis) Inflammation of the eyelid.

blepharoptosis (BLEF-ah-rop-TOH-sis) Drooping of the upper eyelid.

blood-brain barrier (BBB) (BLUD BRAYN BAIR-ee-er) A selective mechanism that protects the brain from toxins and infections.

bolus (BOH-lus) Single mass of a substance.

botulism (BOT-you-lizm) Food poisoning caused by the neurotoxin produced by *Clostridium botulinum*.

bovine spongiform encephalopathy (BOH-vine SPON-jee-form en-sef-ah-LOP-ah-thee) Disease of cattle (mad cow disease) that can be transmitted to humans, causing Creutzfeldt-Jakob disease.

bowel (BOUGH-el) Another name for intestine.

brace (BRAYS) Appliance to support a part of the body in its correct position.

brachial (BRAY-kee-al) Pertaining to the arm.

brachialis (BRAY-kee-al-is) Muscle that lies underneath the biceps and is the strongest flexor of the forearm.

brachiocephalic (BRAY-kee-oh-seh-FAL-ik) Pertaining to the head and arm, as an artery supplying blood to both.

brachioradialis (BRAY-kee-oh-RAY-dee-al-is) Muscle that helps flex the forearm.

brachytherapy (brah-kee-THAIR-ah-pee) Radiation therapy in which the source of irradiation is implanted in the tissue to be treated.

bradycardia (brad-ee-KAR-dee-ah) Slow heart rate (below 60 beats per minute).

bradypnea (brad-ip-NEE-ah) Slow breathing.

brainstem (BRAYN-stem) Region of the brain that includes the thalamus, pineal gland, pons, fourth ventricle, and medulla oblongata.

breech (BREECH) Buttocks-first presentation of the fetus at delivery.

bronchiectasis (brong-kee-EK-tah-sis) Chronic dilation of the bronchi following inflammatory disease and obstruction.

bronchiole (BRONG-key-ole) Increasingly smaller subdivisions of bronchi.

bronchiolitis (brong-kee-oh-LIE-tis) Inflammation of the small bronchioles.

bronchoalveolar (BRONG-koh-al-VEE-oh-lar) Pertaining to the bronchi and alveoli.

bronchoconstriction (BRONG-koh-kon-STRIK-shun) Reduction in diameter of a bronchus.

bronchodilator (BRONG-koh-die-LAY-tor) Agent that increases the diameter of a bronchus.

bronchogenic (brong-koh-JEN-ik) Arising from a bronchus.

bronchopneumonia (BRONG-koh-new-MOH-nee-ah) Acute inflammation of the walls of smaller bronchioles with spread to lung parenchyma.

bronchoscope (BRONG-koh-skope) Endoscope used for bronchoscopy.

bronchoscopy (brong-KOS-koh-pee) Examination of the interior of the tracheobronchial tree with an endoscope.

bronchus (BRONG-kuss) One of two subdivisions of the trachea. Plural *bronchi.*

buffer (BUFF-er) Substance that resists a change in pH.

bulbourethral (BUL-boh-you-REE-thral) Pertaining to the bulbous penis and urethra.

bulla (BULL-ah) Bubblelike dilated structure. Plural *bullae.*

bundle of Hiss (BUN-del of Hiss) Pathway for electrical signals to be transmitted to the ventricles of the heart.

bunion (BUN-yun) A swelling at the base of the big toe.

bursa (BURR-sah) A closed sac containing synovial fluid.

bursitis (burr-SIGH-tis) Inflammation of a bursa.

C

calcaneus (kal-KAY-nee-us) Bone of the tarsus that forms the heel.

calcitonin (kal-sih-TONE-in) Thyroid hormone that moves calcium from blood to bones.

calculus (KAL-kyu-lus) Small stone. Plural *calculi.*

callus (KAL-us) The mass of fibrous connective tissue that forms at a fracture site and becomes the foundation for the formation of new bone.

calyx (KAY-licks) Funnel-shaped structure. Plural *calyces.*

cancellous (KAN-sell-us) Bone that has a spongy or latticelike structure.

cancer (KAN-ser) General term for a malignant neoplasm.

Candida **(KAN-did-ah)** A yeastlike fungus.

candidiasis (kan-dih-DIE-ah-sis) Infection with the yeastlike fungus *Candida.* Also called *thrush.*

canker; canker sore (KANG-ker SOAR) Nonmedical term for aphthous ulcer. Also called *mouth ulcer.*

canthus (KAN-thus) Corner of the eye where the upper and lower lids meet. Plural *canthi.*

capillary (KAP-ih-lair-ee) Minute blood vessel between the arterial and venous systems.

capsule (KAP-syul) Fibrous tissue layer surrounding a joint or some other structure; or a solid dosage form in which a drug is enclosed in a hard or soft shell.

carbohydrate (kar-boh-HIGH-drate) Group of organic food compounds that includes sugars, starch, glycogen, and cellulose.

carboxypeptidase (kar-box-ee-PEP-tid-ase) Enzyme that breaks down protein.

carbuncle (KAR-bunk-ul) Infection of many furuncles in a small area, often on the back of the neck.

carcinogen (kar-SIN-oh-jen) Cancer-producing agent.

carcinogenesis (KAR-sin-oh-JEN-eh-sis) Origin and development of cancer.

carcinoma (kar-sih-NOH-mah) A cancerous (malignant) and invasive epithelial tumor.

carcinoma in situ (kar-sih-NOH-mah IN SIGH-tyu) Carcinoma that has not invaded surrounding tissues.

cardiac (KAR-dee-ak) Pertaining to the heart.

cardiogenic (KAR-dee-oh-JEN-ik) Of cardiac origin.

cardiologist (kar-dee-OL-oh-jist) A medical specialist in diagnosis and treatment of the heart (cardiology).

cardiology (kar-dee-OL-oh-jee) Medical specialty of diseases of the heart.

cardiomegaly (KAR-dee-oh-MEG-ah-lee) Enlargement of the heart.

cardiomyopathy (KAR-dee-oh-my-OP-ah-thee) Disease of heart muscle, the myocardium.

cardiopulmonary resuscitation (KAR-dee-oh-PUL-moh-nair-ee ree-sus-ih-TAY-shun) The attempt to restore cardiac and pulmonary function.

cardiovascular (KAR-dee-oh-VAS-kyu-lar) Pertaining to the heart and blood vessels.

cardioversion (KAR-dee-oh-VER-shun) Restoration of a normal heart rhythm by electrical shock. Also called *defibrillation.*

cardioverter (KAR-dee-oh-VER-ter) Device used to generate electrical shock for cardioversion.

caries (KARE-eez) Bacterial destruction of teeth.

carotid (kah-ROT-id) Main artery of the neck.

carpal (KAR-pal) Pertaining to the wrist.

cartilage (KAR-tih-lij) Nonvascular, firm connective tissue found mostly in joints.

cast (KAST) A cylindrical mold formed by materials in kidney tubules.

catabolism (kah-TAB-oh-lizm) Breakdown of complex substances into simpler ones as a part of metabolism.

cataplexy (KAT-ah-plek-see) Sudden loss of muscle tone with brief paralysis.

cataract (KAT-ah-rakt) Complete or partial opacity of the lens.

catatonia (kat-ah-TOH-nee-ah) Syndrome characterized by physical immobility and mental stupor.

catecholamine (kat-eh-KOHL-ah-meen) Any major hormones in stress response; includes epinephrine and norepinephrine.

catheter (KATH-eh-ter) Hollow tube that allows passage of fluid into or out of a body cavity, organ, or vessel.

catheterization (KATH-eh-ter-ih-ZAY-shun) Introduction of a catheter.

cauda equina (KAW-dah eh-KWIE-nah) Bundle of spinal nerves in the vertebral canal below the ending of the spinal cord.

caudal (KAW-dal) Pertaining to or nearer to the tail.

cautery (KAW-ter-ee) Agent or device used to burn or scar a tissue.

cavernosa (kav-er-NOH-sah) Resembling a cave.

cavity (KAV-ih-tee) Hollow space or body compartment. Plural *cavities.*

cecum (SEE-kum) Blind pouch that is the first part of the large intestine.

celiac disease (SEE-lee-ak diz-EEZ) Disease caused by sensitivity to gluten.

cell (SELL) The smallest unit capable of independent existence.

cellular (SELL-you-lar) Pertaining to a cell.

cellulitis (sell-you-LIE-tis) Infection of subcutaneous connective tissue.

cephalic (se-FAL-ik) Pertaining to or nearer to the head.

cerebellum (ser-eh-BELL-um) The most posterior area of the brain.

cerebrospinal fluid (CSF) (SER-eh-broh-SPY-nal FLU-id) Fluid formed in the ventricles of the brain; surrounds the brain and spinal cord.

cerebrum (ser-EE-brum) The major portion of the brain divided into two hemispheres (cerebral hemispheres) separated by a fissure.

cerumen (seh-ROO-men) Waxy secretion of the ceruminous glands of the external ear.

cervical (SER-vih-kal) Pertaining to the cervix or to the neck region.

cesarean section (seh-ZAH-ree-an SEK-shun) Extraction of the fetus through an incision in the abdomen and uterine wall. Also called *C-section.*

chalazion (kah-LAY-zee-on) Cyst on the outer edge of an eyelid.

chancre (SHAN-ker) Primary lesion of syphilis.

chancroid (SHAN-kroyd) Infectious, painful, ulcerative STD not related to syphilis.

Charcot joint (SHAR-koh JOYNT) Bone and joint destruction secondary to a neuropathy and loss of sensation.

chemotherapy (KEE-moh-THAIR-ah-pee) Treatment using chemical agents.

chiasm (KIE-asm) X-shaped crossing of the two optic nerves at the base of the brain. Alternative term *chiasma.*

chickenpox (CHICK-en-pocks) Acute, contagious viral disease. Also called *varicella.*

chiropractor (kie-roh-PRAK-tor) Practitioner of chiropractic.

chlamydia (klah-MID-ee-ah) A species of bacteria causing a sexually transmitted disease.

chlorine (KLOR-een) A toxic agent used as a disinfectant and bleaching agent.

cholecystitis (KOH-leh-sis-TIE-tis) Inflammation of the gallbladder.

cholecystokinin (KOH-leh-sis-toh-KIE-nin) Hormone secreted by the lining of the intestine that stimulates secretion of pancreatic enzymes and contraction of the gallbladder.

choledocholithiasis (koh-leh-DOH-koh-lih-THIGH-ah-sis) Presence of a gallstone in the common bile duct.

cholelithiasis (KOH-leh-lih-THIGH-ah-sis) Condition of having bile stones (gallstones).

cholelithotomy (KOH-leh-lih-THOT-oh-mee) Surgical removal of a gallstone(s).

cholesteatoma (koh-less-tee-ah-TOH-mah) Yellow, waxy tumor arising in the middle ear.

cholesterol (koh-LESS-ter-ol) Steroid formed in liver cells; it is the most abundant steroid in tissues and circulates in the plasma attached to proteins of different densities.

chondromalacia (KON-droh-mah-LAY-shee-ah) Softening and degeneration of cartilage.

chondrosarcoma (KON-droh-sar-KOH-mah) Cancer arising from cartilage cells.

chordae tendineae (KOR-dee ten-DIN-ee) Tendinous cords attaching the bicuspid and tricuspid valves to the heart wall.

chorea (kor-EE-ah) Involuntary, irregular spasms of limb and facial muscles.

choriocarcinoma (KOH-ree-oh-kar-sih-NOH-mah) Highly malignant cancer in a testis or ovary.

chorion (KOH-ree-on) The fetal membrane that forms the placenta.

chorionic (koh-ree-ON-ik) Pertaining to the chorion.

chorionic villus (koh-ree-ON-ik VILL-us) Vascular process of the embryonic chorion to form the placenta.

choroid (KOR-oid) Region of the retina and uvea.

chromatin (KROH-ma-tin) Substance composed of DNA that forms chromosomes during cell division.

chromosome (KROH-moh-sohm) Body in the nucleus that contains DNA and genes.

chronic (KRON-ik) Describes a persistent, long-term disease.

chronotropic (KRONE-oh-TROH-pik) Affecting the heart rate.

chyle (KILE) A milky fluid that results from the digestion and absorption of fats in the small intestine.

chyme (KIME) Semifluid, partially digested food passed from the stomach into the duodenum.

chymotrypsin (kie-moh-TRIP-sin) Trypsin found in chyme.

ciliary body (SILL-ee-air-ee BOD-ee) Muscles that make the eye lens thicker and thinner.

cilium (SILL-ee-um) Hairlike motile projection from the surface of a cell. Plural *cilia.*

circulation (SER-kyu-LAY-shun) Continuous movement of blood through the heart and blood vessels.

circumcision (ser-kum-SIZH-un) To remove part or all of the prepuce.

circumduction (ser-kum-DUK-shun) Movement of an extremity in a circular motion.

cirrhosis (sir-ROH-sis) Extensive fibrotic liver disease.

claudication (klaw-dih-KAY-shun) Intermittent leg pain and limping.

claustrophobia (klaw-stroh-FOH-bee-ah) Pathologic fear of being trapped in a confined space.

clavicle (KLAV-ih-kul) Curved bone that forms the anterior part of the pectoral girdle.

clitoris (KLIT-oh-ris) Erectile organ of the vulva.

clonic (KLON-ik) State of rapid successions of muscular contractions and relaxations.

closed fracture (KLOHZD FRAK-chur) A bone is broken, but the skin over it is intact.

Clostridium botulinum **(klos-TRID-ee-um bot-you-LIE-num)** Bacterium that causes food poisoning.

clot (KLOT) The mass of fibrin and cells that is produced in a wound.

coagulation (koh-ag-you-LAY-shun) The process of blood clotting.

coagulopathy (koh-ag-you-LOP-ah-thee) Disorder of blood clotting. Plural *coagulopathies.*

coarctation (koh-ark-TAY-shun) Constriction, stenosis, particularly of the aorta.

coccyx (KOK-siks) Small tailbone at the lower end of the vertebral column.

cochlea (KOK-lee-ah) An intricate combination of passages; used to describe the part of the inner ear used in hearing.

cochlear (KOK-lee-ar) Pertaining to the cochlea.

cognition (kog-NIH-shun) Process of acquiring knowledge through thinking, learning, and memory.

cognitive (KOG-nih-tiv) Pertaining to the mental activities of thinking and learning.

cognitive behavioral therapy (CBT) (KOG-nih-tiv be-HAYV-yur-al THAIR-ah-pee) Psychotherapy that emphasizes thoughts and attitudes in one's behavior.

cognitive processing therapy (KOG-nih-tiv PROS-es-ing THAIR-ah-pee) Psychotherapy to build skills to deal with effects of the trauma in other areas of life.

coitus (KOH-it-us) Sexual intercourse.

colic (KOL-ik) Spasmodic, crampy pains in the abdomen; in young infants, persistent crying and irritability thought to be arising from pain in the intestines.

colitis (koh-LIE-tis) Inflammation of the colon.

collagen (KOL-ah-jen) Major protein of connective tissue, cartilage, and bone.

collateral (koh-LAT-er-al) Situated at the side, often to bypass an obstruction.

Colles fracture (KOL-ez FRAK-chur) Fracture of the distal radius at the wrist.

colloid (COLL-oyd) Liquid containing suspended particles.

colon (KOH-lon) The large intestine, extending from the cecum to the rectum.

colonoscopy (koh-lon-OSS-koh-pee) Examination of the inside of the colon by endoscopy.

color Doppler ultrasonography (DOP-ler UL-trah-soh-NOG-rah-fee) Computer-generated color image to show directions of blood flow.

colostomy (ko-LOS-toh-mee) Artificial opening from the colon to the outside of the body.

colostrum (koh-LOSS-trum) The first breast secretion at the end of pregnancy.

colpopexy (KOL-poh-pek-see) Surgical fixation of the vagina.

coma (KOH-mah) State of deep unconsciousness.

comedo (KOM-ee-doh) A whitehead or blackhead caused by too much sebum and too many keratin cells blocking the hair follicle. Plural *comedones.*

comminuted fracture (KOM-ih-nyu-ted FRAK-chur) A fracture in which the bone is broken into pieces.

comorbidity (koh-mor-BID-ih-tee) Presence of two or more diseases at the same time.

complement (KOM-pleh-ment) Group of proteins in serum destroy bacteria and other cells.

complete fracture (kom-PLEET FRAK-chur) A bone is fractured into at least two separate pieces.

compliance (kom-PLY-ance) Measure of the capacity of a chamber or hollow viscus to expand; for example, compliance of the lungs.

compression (kom-PRESH-un) A squeezing together so as to increase density and/or decrease a dimension of a structure.

compression fracture (kom-PRESH-un FRAK-chur) Fracture of a vertebra causing loss of height of the vertebra.

compulsion (kom-PUL-shun) Uncontrollable impulses to perform an act repetitively.

compulsive (kom-PUL-siv) Possessing uncontrollable impulses to perform an act repetitively.

conception (kon-SEP-shun) Fertilization of the egg by sperm to form a zygote.

concha (KON-kah) Shell-shaped bone on the medial wall of the nasal cavity. Plural *conchae.*

concussion (kon-KUSH-un) Mild head injury.

condom (KON-dom) A sheath or cover for the penis or vagina to prevent conception and infection.

conduction (kon-DUCK-shun) Process of transmitting energy.

conductive hearing loss (kon-DUK-tiv HEER-ing LOSS) Hearing loss caused by lesions in the outer ear or middle ear.

condyle (KON-dile) Large, smooth, rounded expansion of the end of a bone that forms a joint with another bone.

condyloma (kon-dih-LOH-ma) Warty growth on external genitalia. Plural *condylomata.*

confusion (kon-FEW-zhun) Mental state in which environmental stimuli are not processed appropriately.

congenital (kon-JEN-ih-tal) Present at birth, either inherited or due to an event during gestation up to the moment of birth.

congruent (KON-gru-ent) Coinciding or agreeing with.

conization (koh-nih-ZAY-shun) Surgical excision of a cone-shaped piece of tissue.

conjunctiva (kon-junk-TIE-vah) Inner lining of the eyelids.

conjunctivitis (kon-junk-tih-VIE-tis) Inflammation of the conjunctiva.

Conn syndrome (KON SIN-drohm) Condition caused by excessive secretion of aldosterone. Also called *aldosteronism.*

consciousness (KON-shus-ness) The state of being aware of and responsive to the environment.

constipation (kon-stih-PAY-shun) Hard, infrequent bowel movements.

contagious (kon-TAY-jus) Able to be transmitted, as infections transmitted from person to person or from person to air or surface to person.

contaminate (kon-TAM-in-ate) To cause the presence of an infectious agent to be on any surface.

contraception (kon-trah-SEP-shun) Prevention of conception.

contraceptive (kon-trah-SEP-tiv) An agent that prevents conception.

contract (kon-TRAKT) Draw together or shorten.

contracture (kon-TRAK-chur) Muscle shortening due to spasm or fibrosis.

contrecoup (KON-treh-koo) Injury to the brain at a point directly opposite the point of original contact.

contusion (kon-TOO-zhun) Bruising of a tissue, including the brain.

conversion disorder (kon-VER-shun dis-OR-der) An unconscious emotional conflict is expressed as physical symptoms with no organic basis.

cor pulmonale (KOR pul-moh-NAH-lee) Right-sided heart failure arising from chronic lung disease.

coreceptor (koh-ree-SEP-tor) Cell surface protein that enhances the sensitivity of an antigen receptor.

cornea (KOR-nee-ah) The central, transparent part of the outer coat of the eye covering the iris and pupil.

coronal (KOR-oh-nal) Pertaining to the vertical plane dividing the body into anterior and posterior portions.

coronal plane (KOR-oh-nal PLAIN) Vertical plane dividing the body into anterior and posterior portions.

coronary circulation (KOR-oh-nair-ee SER-kyu-LAY-shun) Blood flow through the vessels supplying the heart.

corpus (KOR-pus) Major part of a structure. Plural corpora.

corpus albicans (KOR-pus AL-bih-kanz) An atrophied corpus luteum.

corpus callosum (KOR-pus kah-LOH-sum) Bridge of nerve fibers connecting the two cerebral hemispheres.

corpus luteum (KOR-pus LOO-tee-um) Yellow structure formed at the site of a ruptured ovarian follicle.

cortex (KOR-teks) Outer portion of an organ, such as bone; or gray covering of cerebral hemispheres. Plural cortices.

corticoid (KOR-tih-koyd) One of the steroid hormones produced by the adrenal cortex. Also called corticosteroid.

corticosteroid (KOR-tih-koh-STEHR-oyd) A hormone produced by the adrenal cortex.

corticotropin (KOR-tih-koh-TROH-pin) Pituitary hormone that stimulates the cortex of the adrenal gland to secrete corticosteroids.

cortisol (KOR-tih-sol) One of the glucocorticoids produced by the adrenal cortex; has anti-inflammatory effects. Also called hydrocortisone.

coryza (koh-RIE-zah) Viral inflammation of the mucous membrane of the nose. Also called rhinitis.

cosmetic (koz-MET-ik) A concern for appearance.

coup (KOO) Injury to the brain occurring directly under the skull at the point of impact.

cranial (KRAY-nee-al) Pertaining to the skull.

cranium (KRAY-nee-um) The upper part of the skull that encloses and protects the brain.

craving (KRAY-ving) Deep longing or desire.

creatine kinase (KREE-ah-teen KIE-naze) Enzyme elevated in plasma following heart muscle damage in myocardial infarction.

creatinine (kree-AT-ih-neen) Breakdown product of the skeletal muscle protein creatine.

cretinism (KREH-tin-ism) Condition of severe congenital hypothyroidism.

Creutzfeldt-Jakob disease (KROITS-felt-YAK-op diz-EEZ) Progressive incurable neurologic disease caused by infectious prions.

cricoid (CRY-koyd) Ring-shaped cartilage in the larynx.

crista ampullaris (KRIS-tah am-pull-AIR-is) Mound of hair cells and gelatinous material in the ampulla of a semicircular canal.

criterion (krie-TEER-ee-on) Standard or rule for judging. Plural criteria.

Crohn's disease (KRONES diz-EEZ) Inflammatory bowel disease with narrowing and thickening of the terminal small bowel. Also called regional enteritis.

croup (KROOP) Infection of the upper airways in children; characterized by a barking cough. Also called laryngotracheobronchitis.

crown (KROWN) Part of tooth above the gum.

crowning (KROWN-ing) During childbirth, when the maximum diameter of the baby's head comes through the vulvar ring.

cruciate (KRU-shee-ate) Shaped like a cross.

cryopexy (CRY-oh-PEK-see) Repair of a detached retina by freezing it to surrounding tissue.

cryosurgery (cry-oh-SUR-jer-ee) Use of liquid nitrogen or argon gas in a probe to freeze and kill abnormal tissue.

cryotherapy (CRY-oh-THAIR-ah-pee) The use of cold in the treatment of injury.

cryptorchism (krip-TOR-kizm) Failure of one or both testes to descend into the scrotum.

culture (KUL-chur) The growth of microorganisms on or in media.

curative (KYUR-ah-tiv) That which heals or cures.

curettage (kyu-reh-TAHZH) Scraping of the interior of a cavity.

curette (kyu-RET) Scoop-shaped instrument for scraping the interior of a cavity or removing new growths.

Cushing syndrome (KUSH-ing SIN-drome) Hypersecretion of cortisol (hydrocortisone) by the adrenal cortex.

cuspid (KUSS-pid) Tooth with one point.

cutaneous (kyu-TAY-nee-us) Pertaining to the skin.

cuticle (KEW-tih-cul) Nonliving epidermis at the base of the fingernails and toenails, and the outer layer of hair.

cyanosis (sigh-ah-NOH-sis) Blue discoloration of the skin, lips, and nail beds due to low levels of oxygen in the blood.

cyst (SIST) An abnormal, fluid-containing sac.

cystic (SIS-tik) Relating to a cyst.

cystic fibrosis (CF) (SIS-tik fie-BROH-sis) Genetic disease in which excessive viscid mucus obstructs passages, including in the pancreas and in the bronchi of the lungs.

cystitis (sis-TIE-tis) Inflammation of the urinary bladder.

cystocele (SIS-toh-seal) Hernia of the bladder into the vagina.

cystopexy (SIS-toh-pek-see) Surgical procedure to support the urinary bladder.

cystoscope (SIS-toh-skope) An endoscope inserted to view the inside of the bladder.

cystoscopy (sis-TOS-koh-pee) The process of using a cystoscope.

cystourethrogram (sis-toh-you-REETH-roh-gram) X-ray image during voiding to show the structure and function of the bladder and urethra.

cytogenetics (SIGH-toh-jeh-NET-iks) Study of chromosomal abnormalities in a cell.

cytokine (SIGH-toh-kine) Proteins produced by different cells that communicate with other cells in the immune system.

cytology (SIGH-tol-oh-gee) Study of the cell.

cytoplasm (SIGH-toh-plazm) Clear, gelatinous substance that forms the substance of a cell except for the nucleus.

cytosol (SIGH-toe-sawl) Liquid portion of the cell between the cell membrane and the nucleus.

cytotoxic (sigh-toh-TOK-sik) Destructive to cells.

D

dacryocystitis (DAK-ree-oh-sis-TIE-tis) Inflammation of the lacrimal sac.

dacryostenosis (DAK-ree-oh-steh-NOH-sis) Narrowing of the nasolacrimal duct.

dandruff (DAN-druff) Seborrheic scales from the scalp.

death (DETH) Total and permanent cessation of all vital functions.

debridement (day-BREED-mon) The removal of injured or necrotic tissue.

decongestant (dee-con-JESS-tant) Agent that reduces the swelling and fluid in the nose and sinuses.

decubitus ulcer (de-KYU-bit-us UL-ser) Sore caused by lying down for long periods of time.

decussate (DEE-kuss-ate) Cross over like the arms of an "X."

defecation (def-eh-KAY-shun) Evacuation of feces from the rectum and anus.

defect (DEE-fect) An absence, malformation, or imperfection.

defibrillation (dee-fib-rih-LAY-shun) Restoration of uncontrolled twitching of cardiac muscle fibers to normal rhythm.

defibrillator (dee-FIB-rih-lay-tor) Instrument for defibrillation.

deformity (dee-FOR-mih-tee) A permanent structural deviation from the normal.

degenerative (dee-JEN-er-a-tiv) Relating to the deterioration of a structure.

deglutition (dee-glue-TISH-un) The act of swallowing.

dehydration (dee-high-DRAY-shun) Process of losing body water.

dehydroepiandrosterone (DHEA) (dee-HIGH-droh-eh-pee-an-DROS-ter-ohn) Precursor to testosterone; produced in the adrenal cortex.

delirium (deh-LIR-ee-um) Acute altered state of consciousness with agitation and disorientation; condition is reversible.

deltoid (DEL-toyd) Large, fan-shaped muscle connecting the scapula and clavicle to the humerus.

delusion (dee-LOO-shun) Fixed, unyielding, false belief or judgment held despite strong evidence to the contrary.

dementia (dee-MEN-shee-ah) Chronic, progressive, irreversible loss of the mind's cognitive and intellectual functions.

demyelination (dee-MY-eh-lin-A-shun) Process of losing the myelin sheath of a nerve fiber.

dendrite (DEN-dright) Branched extension of the nerve cell body that receives nervous stimuli.

dental (DEN-tal) Pertaining to the teeth.

dentin (DEN-tin) Dense, ivorylike substance located under the enamel in a tooth.

deoxyribonucleic acid (DNA) (dee-OCK-see-RYE-boh-noo-KLEE-ik ASS-id) Source of hereditary characteristics found in chromosomes.

dependence (dee-PEN-dense) State of needing someone or something.

depressant (dee-PRESS-ant) Substance that diminishes activity, sensation, or tone.

depression (dee-PRESH-un) Mental disorder with feelings of deep sadness and despair.

dermatitis (der-mah-TYE-tis) Inflammation of the skin.

dermatologist (der-mah-TOL-oh-jist) Medical specialist in diseases of the skin.

dermatology (der-mah-TOL-oh-jee) Medical specialty concerned with disorders of the skin.

dermatome (DER-mah-tome) The area of skin supplied by a single spinal nerve; alternatively, an instrument used for cutting thin slices.

dermatomyositis (DER-mah-toh-MY-oh-SIGH-tis) Inflammation of the skin and muscles.

dermis (DER-miss) Connective tissue layer of the skin beneath the epidermis.

detoxification (dee-TOKS-ih-fih-KAY-shun) Removal of poison from a tissue or substance.

deviation (dee-vee-AY-shun) A turning aside from a normal course.

diabetes insipidus (die-ah-BEE-teez in-SIP-ih-dus) Excretion of large amounts of dilute urine as a result of inadequate ADH production.

diabetes mellitus (die-ah-BEE-teez MEL-ih-tus) Metabolic syndrome caused by absolute or relative insulin deficiency and/or insulin ineffectiveness.

diabetic (die-ah-BET-ik) Pertaining to or suffering from diabetes.

diagnosis (die-ag-NO-sis) The determination of the cause of a disease. Plural *diagnoses*.

diagnostic (die-ag-NOS-tik) Pertaining to or establishing a diagnosis.

dialysis (die-AL-ih-sis) An artificial method of filtration to remove excess waste materials and water from the body.

dialyzer (DIE-ah-lie-zer) Machine for dialysis.

diaphoresis (DIE-ah-foh-REE-sis) Abnormal amount of sweat or perspiration.

diaphoretic (DIE-ah-foh-RET-ic) Pertaining to sweat or perspiration.

diaphragm (DIE-ah-fram) A ring and dome-shaped material inserted in the vagina to prevent pregnancy; or the musculomembranous partition separating the abdominal and thoracic cavities.

diaphysis (die-AF-ih-sis) The shaft of a long bone.

diarrhea (die-ah-REE-ah) Abnormally frequent and loose stools.

diascopy (die-AS-koh-pee) Examination of superficial skin lesions with pressure.

diastasis (die-ASS-tah-sis) Separation of normally joined parts.

diastole (die-AS-toh-lee) Dilation of heart cavities, during which they fill with blood.

diffusion (dih-FYU-zhun) The means by which small particles move between tissues.

DiGeorge syndrome (dee-JORJ SIN-drome) Congenital absence of the thymus gland.

digestion (die-JEST-shun) Breakdown of food into elements suitable for cell metabolism.

digestive (die-JEST-iv) Relating to digestion.

digital (DIJ-ih-tal) Pertaining to a finger or toe.

dilation (die-LAY-shun) Stretching or enlarging of an opening.

dioxin (die-OK-sin) Carcinogenic contaminant in pesticides.

diplegia (die-PLEE-jee-ah) Paralysis of all four limbs, with the two legs affected most severely.

disability (dis-ah-BILL-ih-tee) Diminished capacity to perform certain activities or functions.

disaccharide (die-SACK-ah-ride) A combination of two monosaccharides; for example, table sugar.

discrimination (DIS-krim-ih-NAY-shun) Ability to distinguish between different things.

dislocation (dis-loh-KAY-shun) The state of being completely out of joint.

displaced fracture (dis-PLAYSD FRAK-chur) A fracture in which the fragments are separated and are not in alignment.

disseminate (dih-SEM-in-ate) Widely scattered throughout the body or an organ.

dissociative identity disorder (dih-SOH-see-ah-tiv eye-DEN-tih-tee dis-OR-der) Mental disorder in which of an individual's personality is separated from the rest, leading to multiple personalities.

distal (DISS-tal) Situated away from the center of the body.

diuresis (die-you-REE-sis) Excretion of large volumes of urine.

diuretic (die-you-REH-tik) Agent that increases urine output.

diverticulitis (DIE-ver-tick-you-LIE-tis) Inflammation of the diverticula.

diverticulosis (DIE-ver-tick-you-LOH-sis) Presence of a number of small pouches in the wall of the large intestine.

diverticulum (die-ver-TICK-you-lum) A pouchlike opening or sac from a tubular structure (e.g., gut). Plural *diverticula*.

dizygotic (die-zie-GOT-ik) Twins from two separate zygotes.

dopamine (DOH-pah-meen) Neurotransmitter in some specific small areas of the brain.

dormant (DOR-mant) Inactive.

dorsal (DOR-sal) Pertaining to the back or situated behind.

dorsum (DOR-sum) Upper, posterior, or back surface.

Duchenne muscular dystrophy (DOO-shen MUSS-kyu-lar DISS-troh-fee) A condition with symmetrical weakness and wasting of pelvic, shoulder, and proximal limb muscles.

duct (DUKT) A tube to carry gas or fluid.

ductus deferens (DUK-tus DEH-fuh-renz) Tube that receives sperm from the epididymis. Also known as *vas deferens*.

duodenum (du-oh-DEE-num) The first part of the small intestine; approximately 12 finger-breadths (9 to 10 inches) in length.

Dupuytren contracture (du-pweh-TRAHN kon-TRAK-chur) A thickening and shortening of fibrous bands in the palm of the hand.

dura mater (DYU-rah MAY-ter) Hard, fibrous outer layer of the meninges.

dwarfism (DWORF-izm) Short stature due to underproduction of growth hormone.

dysentery (DIS-en-tare-ee) Disease with diarrhea, bowel spasms, fever, and dehydration.

dysfunctional (dis-FUNK-shun-al) Having difficulty in performing.

dysmenorrhea (dis-men-oh-REE-ah) Painful and difficult menstruation.

dysmorphic (dis-MOR-fik) Possessing a developmental structural defect.

dyspareunia (dis-pah-RUE-nee-ah) Pain during sexual intercourse.

dyspepsia (dis-PEP-see-ah) "Upset stomach," epigastric pain, nausea, and gas.

dysphagia (dis-FAY-jee-ah) Difficulty in swallowing.

dysplasia (dis-PLAY-zee-ah) Abnormal tissue formation.

dyspnea (disp-NEE-ah) Difficulty breathing.

dysrhythmia (dis-RITH-mee-ah) An abnormal heart rhythm.

dysuria (dis-YOU-ree-ah) Difficulty or pain with urination.

E

eccrine (EK-rin) Coiled sweat gland that occurs in skin all over the body.

echocardiography (EK-oh-kar-dee-OG-rah-fee) Ultrasound recording of heart function.

echoencephalography (EK-oh-en-sef-ah-LOG-rah-fee) Use of ultrasound in the diagnosis of intracranial lesions.

eclampsia (eh-KLAMP-see-uh) Convulsions in a patient with preeclampsia.

ectopic (ek-TOP-ik) Out of place, not in a normal position.

eczema (EK-zeh-mah) Inflammatory skin disease often with a serous discharge.

edema (ee-DEE-mah) Excessive accumulation of fluid in cells and tissues.

edematous (ee-DEM-ah-tus) Pertaining to or marked by edema.

effacement (ee-FACE-ment) Thinning of the cervix in relation to labor.

efferent (EF-eh-rent) Conducting impulses outward away from the brain or spinal cord.

effusion (eh-FYU-shun) Collection of fluid that has escaped from blood vessels into a cavity or tissues.

ejaculate (ee-JACK-you-late) To expel suddenly; *or* the semen expelled in ejaculation.

ejaculation (ee-JACK-you-LAY-shun) Process of expelling semen suddenly.

electrocardiogram (ECG or EKG) (ee-LEK-troh-KAR-dee-oh-gram) Record of the electrical signals of the heart.

electrocardiograph (ee-LEK-troh-KAR-dee-oh-graf) Machine that makes the electrocardiogram.

electroconvulsive therapy (ee-LEK-troh-kon-VUL-siv THAIR-ah-pee) Passage of electric current through the brain to produce convulsions and treat persistent depression, mania, and other disorders.

electrode (ee-LEK-trode) A device for conducting electricity.

electroencephalogram (EEG) (ee-LEK-troh-en-SEF-ah-loh-gram) Record of the electrical activity of the brain.

electroencephalography (ee-LEK-troh-en-SEF-ah-LOG-rah-fee) The process of recording the electrical activity of the brain.

electrolyte (ee-LEK-troh-lite) Substance that, when dissolved in a suitable medium, forms electrically charged particles.

electromagnetic (ee-LEK-troh-mag-NET-ik) Pertaining to energy propagated through matter and space.

electromyography (ee-LEK-troh-my-OG-rah-fee) Recording of electrical activity in muscle.

electroneurodiagnostic (ee-LEK-troh-NYUR-oh-die-ag-NOS-tik) Pertaining to the use of electricity in the diagnosis of a neurologic disorder.

elimination (e-lim-ih-NAY-shun) Removal of waste material from the digestive tract.

embolus (EM-boh-lus) Detached piece of thrombus, mass of bacteria, quantity of air, or foreign body that blocks a vessel.

embryo (EM-bree-oh) Developing organism from conception until the end of the eighth week.

embryonic (em-bree-ON-ic) Pertaining to the embryo.

emesis (EM-eh-sis) Vomit.

emmetropia (em-eh-TROH-pee-ah) Normal refractive condition of the eye.

empathy (EM-pah-thee) Ability to place yourself into the feelings, emotions, and reactions of another person.

emphysema (em-fih-SEE-mah) Dilation of respiratory bronchioles and alveoli.

empyema (EM-pie-EE-mah) Pus in a body cavity, particularly in the pleural cavity.

emulsify (eh-MUL-sih-fie) Break up into very small droplets to suspend in a solution (emulsion).

enamel (ee-NAM-el) Hard substance covering a tooth.

encephalitis (en-SEF-ah-LIE-tis) Inflammation of brain cells and tissues.

encephalomyelitis (en-SEF-ah-loh-MY-eh-LIE-tis) Inflammation of the brain and spinal cord.

endarterectomy (END-ar-ter-EK-toh-mee) Surgical removal of plaque from an artery.

endocarditis (EN-doh-kar-DIE-tis) Inflammation of the lining of the heart.

endocardium (EN-doh-KAR-dee-um) The inside lining of the heart.

endocrine (EN-doh-krin) Pertaining to a gland that produces an internal or hormonal secretion and secretes it into the bloodstream.

endocrine gland (EN-doh-krin GLAND) A gland that produces an internal or hormonal secretion and secretes it into the bloodstream.

endocrinologist (EN-doh-krih-NOL-oh-jist) A medical specialist in endocrinology.

endocrinology (EN-doh-krih-NOL-oh-jee) Medical specialty concerned with the production and effects of hormones.

endometriosis (EN-doh-mee-tree-OH-sis) Endometrial tissue in the abdomen outside the uterus.

endometrium (en-doh-MEE-tree-um) Inner lining of the uterus.

endoplasmic reticulum (EN-doh-PLAZ-mik reh-TIC-you-lum) Structure inside a cell that synthesizes steroids, detoxifies drugs, and manufactures cell membranes.

endorphin (en-DOR-fin) Natural substance in the brain that has the same effect as opium.

endoscope (EN-doh-skope) Instrument for examining the inside of a tubular or hollow organ.

endoscopy (en-DOSS-koh-pee) The use of an endoscope.

endosteum (en-DOSS-tee-um) A membrane of tissue lining the inner (medullary) cavity of a long bone.

endothelial (en-doh-THEE-lee-al) A type of epithelial cell that lines the inside of blood vessels, lymphatic vessels, and the heart.

endothelium (en-doh-THEE-lee-um) Tissue found lining the inside of blood vessels and lymphatic vessels.

endotracheal (en-doh-TRAY-kee-al) Pertaining to being inside the trachea.

enema (EN-eh-mah) An injection of fluid into the rectum.

enteroscopy (en-ter-OSS-koh-pee) The examination of the lining of the digestive tract.

environment (en-VIE-ron-ment) All the external conditions affecting the life of an organism.

environmental (en-VIE-ron-MEN-tal) Pertaining to the environment.

enzyme (EN-zime) Protein that induces changes in other substances.

eosinophil (ee-oh-SIN-oh-fill) An eosinophil's granules attract a rosy-red color on staining.

ependyma (ep-EN-dih-mah) Membrane lining the central canal of the spinal cord and the ventricles of the brain.

epicardium (EP-ih-KAR-dee-um) The outer layer of the heart wall.

epicondyle (ep-ih-KON-dile) Projection above the condyle for attachment of a ligament or tendon.

epidermis (ep-ih-DER-miss) Top layer of the skin.

epididymis (EP-ih-DID-ih-miss) Coiled tube attached to the testis.

epididymitis (EP-ih-did-ih-MY-tis) Inflammation of the epididymis.

epididymoorchitis (ep-ih-DID-ih-moh-or-KIE-tis) Inflammation of the epididymis and testicle. Also called *orchitis*.

epidural (ep-ih-DYU-ral) Above the dura.

epidural space (ep-ih-DYU-ral SPASE) Space between the dura mater and the wall of the vertebral canal or skull.

epigastric (ep-ih-GAS-trik) Abdominal region above the stomach.

epigenetics (EP-ih-jeh-NET-iks) The study of disorders produced by the effects of chemical compounds (e.g., pollutants) or environmental influences (such as diet) on genes.

epiglottis (ep-ih-GLOT-is) Leaf-shaped plate of cartilage that shuts off the larynx during swallowing.

epiglottitis (ep-ih-glot-TIE-tis) Inflammation of the epiglottis.

epilepsy (EP-ih-LEP-see) Chronic brain disorder due to paroxysmal excessive neuronal discharges.

epinephrine (ep-ih-NEF-rin) Main catecholamine produced by the adrenal medulla. Also called *adrenaline*.

epiphyseal plate (eh-pih-FIZ-ee-al PLATE) Layer of cartilage between the epiphysis and metaphysis where bone growth occurs.

epiphysis (eh-PIF-ih-sis) Expanded area at the proximal and distal ends of a long bone that provides increased surface area for attachment of ligaments and tendons.

episiotomy (eh-peez-ee-OT-oh-mee) Surgical incision of the vulva.

epispadias (ep-ih-SPAY-dee-as) Condition in which the urethral opening is on the dorsum of the penis.

epistaxis (ep-ih-STAK-sis) Nosebleed.

epithelium (ep-ih-THEE-lee-um) Tissue that covers surfaces or lines cavities.

equilibrium (ee-kwih-LIB-ree-um) Being evenly balanced.

erectile (ee-REK-tile) Capable of erection or being distended with blood.

erection (ee-REK-shun) Distended and rigid state of an organ.

erosion (ee-ROH-shun) A shallow ulcer in the lining of a structure.

erythroblast (eh-RITH-roh-blast) Precursor to a red blood cell.

erythroblastosis fetalis (eh-RITH-roh-blas-TOH-sis fee-TAH-lis) Hemolytic disease of the newborn due to Rh incompatibility.

erythrocyte (eh-RITH-roh-site) Another name for a red blood cell.

erythropoiesis (eh-RITH-roh-poy-EE-sis) The formation of red blood cells.

erythropoietin (eh-RITH-roh-POY-ee-tin) Protein secreted by the kidney that stimulates red blood cell production.

eschar (ESS-kar) The burned, dead tissue lying on top of third-degree burns.

esophagitis (ee-SOF-ah-JIE-tis) Inflammation of the lining of the esophagus.

esophagus (ee-SOF-ah-gus) Tube linking the pharynx and the stomach.

esotropia (es-oh-TROH-pee-ah) A turning of the eye inward toward the nose.

estrogen (ES-troh-jen) Generic term for hormones that stimulate female secondary sex characteristics.

ethmoid bone (ETH-moyd BOHN) Bone that forms the back of the nose and part of the orbits and encloses numerous air cells, forming the ethmoid sinuses.

eumelanin (YOU-mel-ah-nin) The dark form of the pigment melanin.

euphoria (yoo-FOR-ee-ah) Exaggerated feeling of well-being.

eupnea (yoop-NEE-ah) Normal breathing.

eustachian tube (you-STAY-shun TYUB) Tube that connects the middle ear to the nasopharynx. Also called *auditory tube*.

euthyroid (you-THIGH-royd) Normal thyroid function.

eversion (ee-VER-shun) A turning outward.

exacerbation (ek-zas-er-BAY-shun) Period in which there is an increase in the severity of a disease.

excoriate (eks-KOR-ee-ate) To scratch.

excrete (eks-KREET) To pass out of the body waste products of metabolism.

excretion (eks-KREE-shun) Removal of waste products of metabolism out of the body.

exhale (EKS-hail) Breathe out.

exocrine gland (EK-soh-krin GLAND) A gland that secretes outwardly through excretory ducts.

exophthalmos (ek-sof-THAL-mos) Protrusion of the eyeball.

exotropia (ek-soh-TROH-pee-ah) A turning of the eye outward away from the nose.

expectorate (ek-SPEC-toh-rate) Cough up and spit out mucus from the respiratory tract.

expiration (EKS-pih-RAY-shun) Breathe out.

extension (eks-TEN-shun) Straighten a joint to increase its angle.

extracorporeal (EKS-trah-kor-POH-ree-al) Outside the body.

extravasate (eks-TRAV-ah-sate) To ooze out from a vessel into the tissues.

extrinsic (eks-TRIN-sik) Extrinsic eye muscles are located on the outside of the eye, as opposed to intrinsic muscles, which are located inside the eye.

F

facet (FAS-et) Small smooth area around a pain-producing nerve.

facial (FAY-shal) Seventh (VII) cranial nerve; supplying the forehead, nose, eyes, mouth, and jaws.

facies (FASH-eez) Facial expression and features characteristic of a specific disease.

fallopian tubes (fah-LOH-pee-an TUBES) Uterine tubes connected to the fundus of the uterus.

fascia (FASH-ee-ah) Sheet of fibrous connective tissue.

fascicle (FAS-ih-kull) Bundle of muscle fibers.

fasciectomy (fash-ee-EK-toh-mee) Surgical removal of fascia.

fasciitis (fash-ee-IE-tis) Inflammation of the fascia.

fasciotomy (fash-ee-OT-oh-mee) An incision through a band of fascia, usually to relieve pressure on underlying structures.

fatty acid (FAT-ee ASS-id) An acid obtained from the hydrolysis of fats.

fecal (FEE-kal) Pertaining to feces.

feces (FEE-sees) Undigested waste material discharged from the bowel.

femoral (FEM-oh-ral) Pertaining to the femur.

femur (FEE-mur) The thigh bone.

ferritin (FER-ih-tin) Iron-protein complex that regulates iron storage and transport.

fertilization (FER-til-eye-ZAY-shun) Union of a male sperm and a female egg.

fertilize (FER-til-ize) To penetrate an oocyte with a sperm so as to impregnate.

festinant (FES-tih-nant) Shuffling, falling-forward gait.

fetal (FEE-tal) Pertaining to the fetus.

fetus (FEE-tus) Human organism from the end of the eighth week after conception to birth.

fiber (FIE-ber) Carbohydrate not digested by intestinal enzymes; *or* a strand or filament.

fibrillation (fih-brih-LAY-shun) Uncontrolled quivering or twitching of the heart muscle.

fibrin (FIE-brin) Stringy protein fiber that is a component of a blood clot.

fibrinogen (fie-BRIN-oh-jen) Precursor of fibrin in blood-clotting process.

fibroadenoma (FIE-broh-ad-en-OH-mah) Benign tumor containing much fibrous tissue.

fibroblast (FIE-broh-blast) Cell that forms collagen fibers.

fibrocartilage (fie-broh-KAR-til-ij) Cartilage containing collagen fibers.

fibrocystic disease (fie-broh-SIS-tik diz-EEZ) Benign breast disease with multiple tiny lumps and cysts.

fibroid (FIE-broyd) Uterine tumor resembling fibrous tissue.

fibromyalgia (fie-broh-my-AL-jee-ah) Pain in the muscle fibers.

fibromyoma (FIE-broh-my-OH-mah) Benign neoplasm derived from smooth muscle containing fibrous tissue.

fibrosis (fie-BROH-sis) Repair of dead tissue cells by formation of fibrous tissue.

fibrous (FIE-brus) Tissue containing fibroblasts and fibers.

fibula (FIB-you-lah) The smaller of the two bones of the lower leg.

filter (FIL-ter) A porous substance through which a liquid or gas is passed to separate out contained particles; or to use a filter.

filtrate (FIL-trate) That which has passed through a filter.

fimbria (FIM-bree-ah) A fringelike structure on the surface of a cell or microorganism. Plural *fimbriae*.

fissure (FISH-ur) Deep furrow or cleft. Plural *fissures*.

fistula (FIS-tyu-lah) Abnormal passage.

flagellum (fla-JELL-um) Tail of a sperm. Plural *flagella*.

flatus (FLAY-tus) Gas or air expelled through the anus.

flexion (FLEK-shun) Bend a joint to decrease its angle.

flexor (FLEK-sor) Muscle or tendon that flexes a joint.

flexure (FLEK-shur) A bend in a structure.

fluoresce (flor-ESS) Emit a bright-colored light when irradiated with ultraviolet or violet-blue rays.

fluorescein (flor-ESS-ee-in) Dye that produces a vivid green color under a blue light to diagnose corneal abrasions and foreign bodies.

fluoroscopy (flor-OS-koh-pee) Examination of the structures of the body by x-rays.

folic acid (FOH-lik ASS-id) Synthetic B_9 vitamin.

follicle (FOLL-ih-kull) Spherical mass of cells containing a cavity or a small cul-de-sac, such as a hair follicle.

follicular (fo-LIK-you-lar) Pertaining to a follicle.

foramen (foh-RAY-men) An opening through a structure. Plural *foramina*.

forceps extraction (FOR-seps ek-STRAK-shun) Assisted delivery of the baby by an instrument that grasps the head of the baby.

fornix (FOR-niks) Arch-shaped, blind-ended part of the vagina behind and around the cervix. Plural *fornices*.

fovea centralis (FOH-vee-ah sen-TRAH-lis) Small pit in the center of the macula that has the highest visual acuity.

free radical (FREE RAD-ih-kal) Short-lived product of oxidation in a cell that can be damaging to the cell.

frenulum (FREN-you-lum) Fold of mucous membrane between the glans and the prepuce.

frequency (FREE-kwen-see) The number of times something happens in a given time (e.g., passing urine).

frontal (FRON-tal) Pertaining to the vertical plane dividing the body into anterior and posterior portions.

frontal bone (FRON-tal BOHN) Bone that forms the forehead and the roofs of the orbits and contains a pair of right and left frontal sinuses above the orbits.

frontal lobe (FRON-tal LOBE) Area of brain behind the frontal bone.

fructosamine (FRUK-toe-sah-meen) Organic compound with fructose as its base.

function (FUNK-shun) The ability of an organ or tissue to perform its special work.

fundoscopy (fun-DOS-koh-pee) Examination of the fundus (retina) of the eye.

fundus (FUN-dus) Part farthest from the opening of a hollow organ.

furuncle (FU-rung-kel) An infected hair follicle that spreads into the tissues around the follicle.

G

galactorrhea (gah-LAK-toh-REE-ah) Abnormal flow of milk from the breasts.

gallbladder (GAWL-blad-er) Receptacle on the inferior surface of the liver for storing bile.

gallstone (GAWL-stone) Hard mass of cholesterol, calcium, and bilirubin that can be formed in the gallbladder and bile duct.

ganglion (GANG-lee-on) Collection of nerve cell bodies outside the CNS; *or* a fluid-containing swelling attached to the synovial sheath of a tendon. Plural *ganglia*.

gastric (GAS-trik) Pertaining to the stomach.

gastrin (GAS-trin) Hormone secreted in the stomach that stimulates secretion of HCl and increases gastric motility.

gastritis (gas-TRY-tis) Inflammation of the lining of the stomach.

gastrocnemius (gas-trok-NEE-mee-us) Major muscle in back of the lower leg (the calf).

gastrocolic reflex (gas-troh-KOL-ik REE-fleks) Taking food into the stomach leads to mass movement of feces in the colon and the desire to defecate.

gastroenteritis (GAS-troh-en-ter-EYE-tis) Inflammation of the stomach and intestines.

gastroenterologist (GAS-troh-en-ter-OL-oh-jist) Medical specialist in gastroenterology.

gastroenterology (GAS-troh-en-ter-OL-oh-gee) Medical specialty of the stomach and intestines.

gastroesophageal (GAS-troh-ee-sof-ah-JEE-al) Pertaining to the stomach and esophagus.

gastrointestinal (GI) (GAS-troh-in-TESS-tin-al) Relating to the stomach and intestines.

gastroscopy (gas-TROS-koh-pee) Endoscopic examination of the stomach.

gene (JEEN) Functional segment of the DNA molecule.

genetic (jeh-NET-ik) Pertaining to a gene.

genetics (jeh-NET-iks) Science of the inheritance of characteristics.

genital (JEN-ih-tal) Relating to reproduction or to the male or female sex organs.

genitalia (JEN-ih-TAY-lee-ah) External and internal organs of reproduction.

genome (JEE-nome) Complete set of genes.

geriatrician (jer-ee-ah-TRISH-an) Medical specialist in geriatrics.

geriatrics (jer-ee-AT-riks) Medical specialty that deals with the problems of old age.

gerontologist (jer-on-TOL-oh-jist) Medical specialist in gerontology.

GLOSSARY

gerontology (jer-on-TOL-oh-jee) Study of the process and problems of aging.

Giardia **(jee-AR-dee-ah)** Parasite in the small intestine.

gigantism (jie-GAN-tizm) Abnormal height and size of the entire body.

gingiva (JIN-jih-vah) Tissue surrounding teeth and covering the jaw.

gingivitis (jin-jih-VIE-tis) Inflammation of the gums.

glans (GLANZ) Head of the penis or clitoris.

glaucoma (glaw-KOH-mah) Increased intraocular pressure.

glia (GLEE-ah) Connective tissue that holds a structure together.

glioblastoma multiforme (GLIE-oh-blas-TOH-mah MULL-tih-FOR-mee) A malignant form of brain cancer.

glioma (glie-OH-mah) Tumor arising in a glial cell.

globulin (GLOB-you-lin) Family of blood proteins.

glomerulonephritis (glo-MER-you-loh-nef-RIE-tis) Infection of the glomeruli of the kidney.

glomerulus (glo-MER-you-lus) Plexus of capillaries; part of a nephron. Plural *glomeruli*.

glossodynia (gloss-oh-DIN-ee-ah) Painful, burning tongue.

glossopharyngeal (GLOSS-oh-fah-RIN-jee-al) Ninth (IX) cranial nerve; supplying the tongue and pharynx.

glottis (GLOT-is) Vocal apparatus of the larynx.

glucagon (GLUE-kah-gon) Pancreatic hormone that supports blood glucose levels.

glucocorticoid (glue-koh-KOR-tih-koyd) Hormone of the adrenal cortex that helps regulate glucose metabolism.

gluconeogenesis (GLUE-koh-nee-oh-JEN-eh-sis) Formation of glucose from noncarbohydrate sources.

glucose (GLU-kose) The final product of carbohydrate digestion and the main sugar in the blood.

gluten (GLU-ten) Insoluble protein found in wheat, rye, and barley.

gluteus (GLUE-tee-us) Term that refers to a muscle in the buttocks.

glycogen (GLIE-koh-jen) The body's principal carbohydrate reserve, stored in the liver and skeletal muscle.

glycogenolysis (GLIE-koh-jeh-NOL-ih-sis) Conversion of glycogen to glucose.

glycosuria (GLIE-koh-SYU-ree-ah) Presence of glucose in urine.

glycosylated hemoglobin (Hb A1c) (GLIE-koh-sih-lay-ted HEE-moh-GLOH-bin) Hemoglobin A fraction linked to glucose; used as an index of glucose control.

goiter (GOY-ter) Enlargement of the thyroid gland.

gomphosis (gom-FOH-sis) Joint formed by a peg and socket. Plural *gomphoses*.

gonad (GOH-nad) Testis or ovary. Plural *gonads*.

gonadotropin (GOH-nad-oh-TROH-pin) Hormone capable of promoting gonad function.

gonorrhea (gon-oh-REE-ah) Specific contagious sexually transmitted infection.

gout (GOWT) Painful arthritis of the big toe and other joints.

grade (GRAYD) In cancer pathology, a classification of the rate of growth of cancer cells.

grand mal (GRAHN MAL) Old name for a generalized tonic-clonic seizure.

granulation (gran-you-LAY-shun) New fibrous tissue formed during wound healing.

granulocyte (GRAN-you-loh-site) A white blood cell that contains multiple small granules in its cytoplasm.

granulosa cell (gran-you-LOH-sah SELL) Cell lining the ovarian follicle.

Graves disease (GRAYVZ diz-EEZ) Hyperthyroidism with toxic goiter.

gravida (GRAV-ih-dah) A pregnant woman.

gravidarum (gra-vih-DAR-um) Relating to pregnant women.

gray matter (GRAY MATT-er) Regions of the brain and spinal cord occupied by cell bodies and dendrites.

greenstick fracture (GREEN-stik FRAK-chur) A fracture in which one side of the bone is partially broken and the other side is bent; occurs mostly in children.

Guillain-Barré syndrome (GEE-yan-bah-RAY SIN-drome) Disorder in which the body makes antibodies against myelin, disrupting nerve conduction.

gynecologist (guy-nih-KOL-oh-jist) Specialist in gynecology.

gynecology (guy-nih-KOL-oh-jee) Medical specialty for the care of the female reproductive system.

gynecomastia (GUY-nih-koh-MAS-tee-ah) Enlargement of the breast.

gyrus (JIE-rus) Rounded elevation on the surface of the cerebral hemispheres. Plural *gyri*.

H

hairline fracture (HAIR-line FRAK-chur) A fracture without separation of the fragments.

halitosis (hal-ih-TOE-sis) Bad odor of the breath.

hallucination (hah-loo-sih-NAY-shun) Perception of an object or event when there is no such thing present.

hallux valgus (HAL-uks VAL-gus) Deviation of the big toe toward the lateral side of the foot.

handicap (HAND-ee-cap) Condition that interferes with a person's ability to function normally.

hapten (HAP-ten) Small molecule that has to bind to a larger molecule to form an antigen.

Hashimoto disease (hah-shee-MOH-toh diz-EEZ) Autoimmune disease of the thyroid gland. Also called *Hashimoto thyroiditis*.

haversian canals (hah-VER-shan ka-NALS) Vascular canals in bone. Also called *central canals*.

head (HED) The rounded extremity of a bone.

Heberden node (HEH-ber-den NOHD) Bony lump on the terminal phalanx of the fingers in osteoarthritis.

helix (HEE-liks) A line in the shape of a coil.

hematemesis (he-mah-TEM-eh-sis) Vomiting of red blood.

hematochezia (he-mat-oh-KEY-zee-ah) The passage of red, bloody stools.

hematocrit (Hct) (hee-MAT-oh-krit) Percentage of red blood cells in blood.

hematology (hee-mah-TOL-oh-jee) Medical specialty of disorders of blood.

hematoma (hee-mah-TOH-mah) Collection of blood that has escaped from the blood vessels into tissue. Also called *bruise*.

hematopoietic (HEE-mah-toh-poy-ET-ik) Pertaining to the making of red blood cells.

hematuria (hee-mah-TYU-ree-ah) Blood in the urine.

heme (HEEM) The iron-based component of hemoglobin that carries oxygen.

hemifacial (hem-ee-FAY-shal) Pertaining to one side of the face.

hemiparesis (HEM-ee-pah-REE-sis) Weakness of one side of the body.

hemiplegia (hem-ee-PLEE-jee-ah) Paralysis of one side of the body.

Hemoccult test (HEEM-oh-kult TEST) Trade name for a fecal occult blood test.

hemochromatosis (HEE-moh-kroh-mah-TOH-sis) Dangerously high levels of iron in the body with deposition of iron pigments in tissues.

hemodialysis (HEE-moh-die-AL-ih-sis) An artificial method of filtration to remove excess waste materials and water directly from the blood.

hemoglobin (HEE-moh-GLOH-bin) Red-pigmented protein that is the main component of red blood cells.

hemoglobinopathy (HEE-moh-GLOH-bih-NOP-ah-thee) Disease caused by the presence of an abnormal hemoglobin in the red blood cells.

hemolysis (hee-MOL-ih-sis) Destruction of red blood cells so that hemoglobin is liberated.

hemolytic (hee-moh-LIT-ik) Pertaining to the process of destruction of red blood cells.

hemophilia (hee-moh-FILL-ee-ah) An inherited disease from a deficiency of clotting factor VIII.

hemoptysis (hee-MOP-tih-sis) Bloody sputum.

hemorrhage (HEM-oh-raj) To bleed profusely.

hemorrhoid (HEM-oh-royd) Dilated rectal vein producing painful anal swelling. Plural *hemorrhoids*.

hemostasis (hee-moh-STAY-sis) Controlling or stopping bleeding.

hemothorax (hee-moh-THOR-aks) Blood in the pleural cavity.

heparin (HEP-ah-rin) An anticoagulant secreted particularly by liver cells.

hepatic (hep-AT-ik) Pertaining to the liver.

hepatitis (hep-ah-TIE-tis) Inflammation of the liver.

hepatocellular (HEP-ah-toh-SELL-you-lar) Pertaining to liver cells.

heredity (heh-RED-ih-tee) Transmission of characteristics from parents to offspring through genes.

hernia (HER-nee-ah) Protrusion of a structure through the tissue that normally contains it.

herniate (HER-nee-ate) To protrude.

herniation (HER-nee-AY-shun) Protrusion of an anatomical structure from its normal location.

herniorrhaphy (HER-nee-OR-ah-fee) Repair of a hernia.

herpes simplex virus (HSV) (HER-peez SIM-pleks VIE-rus) Disease that manifests with painful, watery blisters on the skin and mucous membranes.

herpes zoster (HER-pees ZOS-ter) Painful eruption of vesicles that follows a dermatome or nerve root on one side of the body. Also called *shingles*.

heterograft (HET-er-oh-graft) A graft using tissue taken from another species. Also known as *xenograft*.

hiatus (high-AY-tus) An opening through a structure.

hilum (HIGH-lum) The site where the nerves and blood vessels enter and leave an organ. Plural *hila*.

hirsutism (HER-sue-tizm) Excessive body and facial hair.

histamine (HISS-tah-meen) Compound liberated in tissues as a result of injury or an allergic response.

histology (his-TOL-oh-jee) Structure and function of cells, tissues, and organs.

histone (HIS-tone) A simple protein found in the cell nucleus.

Hodgkin lymphoma (HOJ-kin lim-FOH-muh) Disease marked by chronic enlargement of lymph nodes, spreading to other nodes in an orderly way.

homeostasis (hoh-mee-oh-STAY-sis) Stability or equilibrium of a system or the body's internal environment.

homicidal (hom-ih-SIDE-al) Having a tendency to commit homicide.

homocysteine (hoh-moh-SIS-teen) An amino acid similar to cysteine.

homograft (HOH-moh-graft) Skin graft from another person or a cadaver.

hordeolum (hor-DEE-oh-lum) Abscess in an eyelash follicle. Also called *stye*.

hormone (HOR-mohn) Chemical formed in one tissue or organ and carried by the blood to stimulate or inhibit a function of another tissue or organ.

Horner syndrome (HOR-ner SIN-drome) Disorder of the sympathetic nerves to the face and eye.

hospice (HOS-pis) Facility or program that provides care to the dying and their families.

human immunodeficiency virus (HIV) (HYU-man IM-you-noh-dee-FISH-en-see VIE-rus) Etiologic agent of acquired immunodeficiency syndrome (AIDS).

human papilloma virus (HPV) (HYU-man pap-ih-LOH-mah VIE-rus) Causes warts on the skin and genitalia and can increase the risk for cervical cancer.

humerus (HYU-mer-us) Single bone of the upper arm.

humoral immunity (HYU-mor-al im-YOU-nih-tee) Defense mechanism arising from antibodies in the blood.

Huntington disease (HUN-ting-ton diz-EEZ) Progressive inherited, degenerative, incurable neurologic disease. Also called *Huntington chorea*.

hyaline (HIGH-ah-line) Cartilage that looks like glass and contains fine collagen fibers.

hyaline membrane disease (HIGH-ah-line MEM-brain diz-EEZ) Respiratory distress syndrome of the newborn.

hydrocele (HIGH-droh-seal) Collection of fluid in the space of the tunica vaginalis.

hydrocephalus (HIGH-droh-SEF-ah-lus) Enlarged head due to excess CSF in the cerebral ventricles.

hydrochloric acid (HCl) (high-droh-KLOR-ic ASS-id) The acid of gastric juice.

hydrocortisone (high-droh-KOR-tih-sohn) Potent glucocorticoid with anti-inflammatory properties. Also called *cortisol*.

hydronephrosis (HIGH-droh-neh-FROH-sis) Dilation of the pelvis and calyces of a kidney.

hymen (HIGH-men) Thin membrane partly occluding the vaginal orifice.

hypercalcemia (HIGH-per-kal-SEE-mee-ah) Excessive level of calcium in the blood.

hyperemesis (high-per-EM-eh-sis) Excessive vomiting.

hyperflexion (high-per-FLEK-shun) Flexion of a limb or part beyond the normal limits.

hyperfractionated (high-per-FRAK-shun-ay-ted) Given in smaller amounts and more frequently.

hyperglycemia (HIGH-per-glie-SEE-mee-ah) High level of glucose (sugar) in blood.

hyperglycemic (HIGH-per-glie-SEE-mik) Pertaining to high blood sugar.

hyperinflation (HIGH-per-in-FLAY-shun) Overdistension of pulmonary alveoli with air resulting from airway obstruction.

hyperopia (high-per-OH-pee-ah) Able to see distant objects but unable to see close objects.

hyperosmolar (HIGH-per-os-MOH-lar) Marked hyperglycemia without ketoacidosis.

hyperparathyroidism (HIGH-per-pair-ah-THIGH-royd-ism) Excessive levels of parathyroid hormone.

hyperplasia (high-per-PLAY-zee-ah) Increase in the *number* of the cells in a tissue or organ.

hyperpnea (high-perp-NEE-ah) Deeper and more rapid breathing than normal.

hypersecretion (HIGH-per-seh-KREE-shun) Excessive secretion of mucus (or enzymes or waste products).

hypersensitivity (HIGH-per-sen-sih-TIV-ih-tee) Exaggerated abnormal reaction to an allergen.

hypersplenism (high-per-SPLEN-izm) Condition in which the spleen removes blood components at an excessive rate.

hypertension (HIGH-per-TEN-shun) Persistent high arterial blood pressure.

hyperthyroidism (high-per-THIGH-royd-ism) Excessive production of thyroid hormones.

hypertrophy (high-PER-troh-fee) Increase in size, but not in number, of an individual tissue element.

hypochondriac (high-poh-KON-dree-ack) A person who exaggerates the significance of symptoms; *or* pertaining to below the cartilage below the ribs.

hypochondriasis (HIGH-poh-kon-DRIE-ah-sis) Belief that a minor symptom indicates a severe disease.

hypochromic (high-poh-CROH-mik) Pale in color, as in RBCs when hemoglobin is deficient.

hypodermis (high-poh-DER-miss) Tissue layer below the dermis.

hypogastric (high-poh-GAS-trik) Abdominal region below the stomach.

hypoglossal (high-poh-GLOSS-al) Twelfth (XII) cranial nerve; supplying muscles of the tongue.

hypoglycemia (HIGH-poh-glie-SEE-mee-ah) Low level of glucose (sugar) in the blood.

hypogonadism (HIGH-poh-GOH-nad-izm) Deficient gonad production of sperm or eggs or hormones.

hypokalemia (HIGH-poh-kah-LEE-mee-ah) Low level of potassium in the blood.

hypoparathyroidism (HIGH-poh-pair-ah-THIGH-royd-ism) Deficient levels of parathyroid hormone.

hypophysis (high-POF-ih-sis) Another name for the pituitary gland.

hypopigmentation (HIGH-poh-pig-men-TAY-shun) Below-normal melanin relative to the surrounding skin.

hypopituitarism (HIGH-poh-pih-TYU-ih-tah-rizm) Condition of one or more deficient pituitary hormones.

hypospadias (high-poh-SPAY-dee-as) Urethral opening more proximal than normal on the ventral surface of the penis.

hypotension (HIGH-poh-TEN-shun) Persistent low arterial blood pressure.

hypothalamus (high-poh-THAL-ah-muss) Area of gray matter forming part of the walls and floor of the third ventricle.

hypothenar (high-poh-THAY-nar) Fleshy eminence at the base of the little finger.

hypothyroidism (high-poh-THIGH-royd-ism) Deficient production of thyroid hormones.

hypovolemic (HIGH-poh-voh-LEE-mik) Having decreased blood volume in the body.

hypoxia (high-POK-see-ah) Decrease below normal levels of oxygen in tissues, gases, or blood.

hypoxic (high-POK-sik) Deficient in oxygen.

hysterectomy (his-ter-EK-toh-mee) Surgical removal of the uterus.

hysterosalpingogram (HIS-ter-oh-sal-PING-oh-gram) Radiograph of the uterus and uterine tubes after injection of contrast material.

hysteroscopy (his-ter-OS-koh-pee) Visual inspection of the uterine cavity using an endoscope.

I

ictal (IK-tal) Pertaining to, or condition caused by, a stroke or epilepsy.

icterus (ICK-ter-us) Yellow staining of tissues with bile pigments, including bilirubin.

idiopathic (ID-ih-oh-PATH-ik) Pertaining to a disease of unknown etiology.

ileocecal (ILL-ee-oh-SEE-cal) Pertaining to the junction of the ileum and cecum.

ileocecal sphincter (ILL-ee-oh-SEE-cal SFINK-ter) Band of muscle that encircles the junction of the ileum and cecum.

ileostomy (ill-ee-OS-toh-mee) Artificial opening from the ileum to the outside of the body.

ileum (ILL-ee-um) Third portion of the small intestine.

ilium (ILL-ee-um) Large wing-shaped bone at the upper and posterior part of the pelvis. Plural *ilia*.

immune (im-YUNE) Protected from an infectious disease.

immune serum (im-YUNE SEER-um) Serum taken from another human or animal that has antibodies to a disease. Also called *antiserum*.

immunity (im-YOU-nih-tee) State of being protected.

immunization (im-you-nih-ZAY-shun) Administration of an agent to provide immunity.

immunoassay (IM-you-noh-ASS-ay) Biochemical test to measure the amount of a substance in a liquid, using the reaction of an antibody to its antigen.

immunodeficiency (IM-you-noh-dee-FISH-en-see) Failure of the immune system.

immunoglobulin (IM-you-noh-GLOB-you-lin) Specific protein evoked by an antigen. All antibodies are immunoglobulins.

immunologist (im-you-NOL-oh-jist) Medical specialist in immunology.

immunology (im-you-NOL-oh-jee) The science and practice of immunity and allergy.

immunosuppression (IM-you-noh-suh-PRESH-un) Suppression of the immune response by an outside agent, such as a drug.

impacted (im-PAK-ted) Immovably wedged, as with earwax blocking the external canal.

impacted fracture (im-PAK-ted FRAK-chur) A fracture in which one bone fragment is driven into the other.

impairment (im-PAIR-ment) Diminishing of normal function.

impetigo (im-peh-TIE-go) Infection of the skin producing thick, yellow crusts.

implantable (im-PLAN-tah-bul) Able to be inserted into tissues.

implantation (im-plan-TAY-shun) Attachment of a fertilized egg to the endometrium.

impotence (IM-poh-tence) Inability to achieve an erection.

in situ (IN SIGH-tyu) In the correct place.

in vitro fertilization (IVF) (IN VEE-troh FER-til-eye-ZAY-shun) Process of combining a sperm and egg in a laboratory dish and placing the resulting embryos inside a uterus.

incision (in-SIZH-un) A cut or surgical wound.

incisor (in-SIGH-zor) Chisel-shaped tooth.

incompatible (in-kom-PAT-ih-bul) Substances that interfere with each other physiologically.

incompetence (in-KOM-peh-tense) Failure of valves to close completely.

incomplete fracture (in-kom-PLEET FRAK-chur) A fracture that does not extend across the bone, as in a hairline fracture.

incontinence (in-KON-tin-ens) Inability to prevent discharge of urine or feces.

incubation (in-kyu-BAY-shun) Process of developing an infection.

incus (IN-cuss) Middle one of the three ossicles in the middle ear; shaped like an anvil.

index (IN-deks) A standard indicator of measurement. Plural *indices.*

infarction (in-FARK-shun) Sudden blockage of an artery.

infection (in-FEK-shun) Invasion of the body by disease-producing microorganisms.

infectious (in-FEK-shus) Capable of being transmitted; *or* caused by infection by a microorganism.

inferior (in-FEE-ree-or) Situated below.

infertility (in-fer-TIL-ih-tee) Inability to conceive over a long period of time.

infestation (in-fes-TAY-shun) Act of being invaded on the skin by a troublesome other species, such as a parasite.

infiltration (in-fil-TRAY-shun) The invasion into a tissue or cell.

inflation (in-FLAY-shun) Process of expanding with air.

infundibulum (IN-fun-DIB-you-lum) Funnel-shaped structure. Plural *infundibula.*

infusion (in-FYU-zhun) Introduction intravenously of a substance other than blood.

ingestion (in-JEST-shun) Intake of food, either by mouth or through a nasogastric tube.

inguinal (IN-gwin-al) Pertaining to the groin.

inhale (IN-hail) Breathe in.

inotropic (IN-oh-TROH-pik) Affecting the contractility of cardiac muscle.

insanity (in-SAN-ih-tee) Nonmedical term for a person unable to be responsible for his or her actions.

insecticide (in-SEK-tih-side) Agent for destroying insects.

insemination (in-sem-ih-NAY-shun) Introduction of semen into the vagina.

insertion (in-SIR-shun) The attachment of a muscle to a more movable part of the skeleton, as distinct from the origin.

insomnia (in-SOM-nee-ah) Inability to sleep.

inspiration (in-spih-RAY-shun) Breathe in.

instability (in-stah-BIL-ih-tee) Abnormal tendency of a joint to partially or fully dislocate; *or* difficulty in balance.

insufficiency (in-suh-FISH-en-see) Lack of completeness of function; in the heart, failure of a valve to close properly.

insulin (IN-syu-lin) A hormone secreted by the pancreas.

integumentary (in-TEG-you-MEN-tah-ree) Pertaining to the covering of the body.

interatrial (IN-ter-AY-tree-al) Between the atria of the heart.

intercostal (IN-ter-KOS-tal) The space between two ribs.

intermittent (IN-ter-MIT-ent) Alternately ceasing and beginning again.

interphalangeal (IN-ter-fah-LAN-jee-al) Pertaining to the joints between two phalanges.

interstitial (in-ter-STISH-al) Pertaining to spaces between cells in a tissue or organ.

interventricular (IN-ter-ven-TRIK-you-lar) Between the ventricles of the heart.

intervertebral (IN-ter-VER-teh-bral) The space between two vertebrae.

intestine (in-TES-tin) The digestive tube from stomach to anus.

intima (IN-tih-ma) Inner layer of a structure, particularly a blood vessel.

intolerance (in-TOL-er-ance) Inability of the small intestine to digest and dispose of a particular dietary constituent.

intracellular (in-trah-SELL-you-lar) Within the cell.

intracranial (in-trah-KRAY-nee-al) Within the cranium (skull).

intradermal (IN-trah-DER-mal) Within the dermis.

intramuscular (IN-trah-MUS-kew-lar) Within the muscle.

intraocular (in-trah-OK-you-lar) Pertaining to the inside of the eye.

intrathecal (IN-trah-THEE-kal) Within the subarachnoid or subdural space.

intrauterine (IN-trah-YOU-ter-ine) Inside the uterine cavity.

intravenous (IN-trah-VEE-nus) Inside a vein.

intrinsic (in-TRIN-sik) Any muscle whose origin and insertion are entirely within the structure under consideration; for example, muscles inside the vocal cords or the eye.

intrinsic factor (in-TRIN-sik FAK-tor) Substance that makes the absorption of vitamin B$_{12}$ happen.

intubation (IN-tyu-BAY-shun) Insertion of a tube into the trachea.

intussusception (IN-tuss-sus-SEP-shun) The slipping of one part of the bowel inside another to cause obstruction.

inversion (in-VER-shun) A turning inward.

involute (in-voh-LUTE) To return to a former condition; *or* decline associated with advanced age.

involution (in-voh-LOO-shun) A decrease in size or vigor.

iodine (EYE-oh-dine or EYE-oh-deen) Chemical element, the lack of which causes thyroid disease.

iris (EYE-ris) Colored portion of the eye with the pupil in its center.

irrigation (ih-rih-GAY-shun) Use of water to wash out a canal or wound.

ischemia (is-KEE-mee-ah) Lack of blood supply to a tissue.

ischium (ISS-kee-um) Lower and posterior part of the hip bone. Plural *ischia*.

Ishihara color system (ish-ee-HAR-ah KUH-ler SIS-tem) Test for color vision defects.

islet cells (EYE-let SELLS) Hormone-secreting cells of the pancreas.

islets of Langerhans (EYE-lets ov LAHNG-er-hahnz) Areas of pancreatic cells that produce insulin and glucagon.

isotope (EYE-soh-tope) Radioactive element used in diagnostic procedures.

isthmus (IS-mus) Part connecting two larger parts; for example, the uterus to the uterine tube.

J

Jaeger reading card (YAY-ger REED-ing CARD) Type in different sizes of print for testing near vision.

jaundice (JAWN-dis) Yellow staining of tissues with bile pigments, including bilirubin.

jejunum (je-JEW-num) Segment of small intestine between the duodenum and the ileum where most of the nutrients are absorbed.

jugular (JUG-you-lar) Pertaining to the throat.

juvenile (JU-ven-ile) Between the ages of 2 and 17 years.

K

Kaposi sarcoma (ka-POH-see sar-KOH-mah) A malignancy often seen in AIDS patients.

karyotype (KAIR-ee-oh-type) Map of chromosomes of an individual cell.

Kegel exercises (KEE-gal EKS-er-size-ez) Contraction and relaxation of the pelvic floor muscles to improve urethral and rectal sphincter function.

keloid (KEY-loyd) Raised, irregular, lumpy, shiny scar due to excess collagen fiber production during healing of a wound.

keratin (KER-ah-tin) Protein found in the dead outer layer of skin and in nails and hair.

keratinocyte (ke-RAT-in-oh-site) Cell producing a tough, horny protein (keratin) in the process of differentiating into the dead cells of the stratum corneum.

keratomileusis (KER-ah-toh-mie-LOO-sis) A surgical procedure that involves cutting and shaping the cornea.

keratosis (ker-ah-TOH-sis) Epidermal lesion of circumscribed overgrowth of the horny layer.

keratotomy (KER-ah-TOT-oh-mee) Incision in the cornea.

kernicterus (ker-NIK-ter-us) Bilirubin staining of the basal nuclei of the brain.

ketoacidosis (KEY-toh-ass-ih-DOH-sis) Excessive production of ketones, making the blood acid.

ketone (KEY-tone) Chemical formed in uncontrolled diabetes or in starvation.

ketosis (key-TOH-sis) Excess production of ketones.

kidney (KID-nee) Organ of excretion.

kleptomania (klep-toh-MAY-nee-ah) Uncontrollable need to steal.

kyphosis (kie-FOH-sis) A normal posterior curve of the thoracic spine that can be exaggerated in disease.

L

labium (LAY-bee-um) Fold of the vulva. Plural *labia*.

labor (LAY-bore) Process of expulsion of the fetus.

labrum (LAY-brum) Cartilage that forms a rim around the socket of the hip joint.

labyrinth (LAB-ih-rinth) The inner ear.

laceration (lass-eh-RAY-shun) A tear of the skin.

lacrimal (LAK-rim-al) Pertaining to tears.

lactase (LAK-tase) Enzyme that breaks down lactose to glucose and galactose.

lactation (lak-TAY-shun) Production of milk.

lacteal (LAK-tee-al) A lymphatic vessel carrying chyle away from the intestine.

lactiferous (lak-TIF-er-us) Pertaining to or yielding milk.

lactose (LAK-toes) The disaccharide found in cow's milk.

lacuna (la-KOO-nah) Small space or cavity within the matrix of bone. Plural *lacunae*.

lanugo (la-NYU-go) Fine, soft hair on the fetal body.

laparoscope (LAP-ah-roh-skope) Instrument (endoscope) used for viewing the abdominal contents.

laparoscopic (LAP-ah-rah-SKOP-ik) Pertaining to laparoscopy.

laparoscopy (lap-ah-ROS-koh-pee) Examination of the contents of the abdomen using an endoscope.

laryngitis (lair-in-JIE-tis) Inflammation of the larynx.

laryngopharynx (lah-RING-oh-FAIR-inks) Region of the pharynx below the epiglottis that includes the larynx.

laryngoscope (lah-RING-oh-skope) Hollow tube with a light and camera used to visualize or operate on the larynx.

laryngotracheobronchitis (lah-RING-oh-TRAY-kee-oh-brong-KIE-tis) Inflammation of the larynx, trachea, and bronchi. Also called *croup*.

larynx (LAIR-inks) Organ of voice production.

laser (LAY-zer) Intense, narrow beam of monochromatic light.

laser surgery (LAY-zer SUR-jer-ee) Use of a concentrated, intense narrow beam of electromagnetic radiation for surgery.

lateral (LAT-er-al) Situated at the side of a structure.

latex (LAY-tecks) Manufactured from the milky liquid in rubber plants; used for gloves in patient care.

latissimus dorsi (lah-TISS-ih-muss DOR-sigh) The widest (broadest) muscle in the back.

lavage (lah-VAHZH) Washing out of a hollow cavity, tube, or organ.

leiomyoma (LIE-oh-my-OH-mah) Benign neoplasm derived from smooth muscle.

lens (LENZ) Transparent refractive structure behind the iris.

lentigo (len-TIE-goh) Age spot; small, flat, brown-black spot in the skin of older people. Plural *lentigines.*

leptin (LEP-tin) Hormone secreted by adipose tissue.

lesion (LEE-zhun) Pathologic change or injury in a tissue.

leukemia (loo-KEE-mee-ah) Disease in which the blood is taken over by white blood cells and their precursors.

leukocoria (loo-koh-KOH-ree-ah) Reflection in the pupil of a white mass in the eye.

leukocyte (LOO-koh-site) Another term for *white blood cell.* Alternative spelling *leucocyte.*

leukocytosis (LOO-koh-sigh-TOH-sis) An excessive number of white blood cells.

leukopenia (loo-koh-PEE-nee-ah) A deficient number of white blood cells.

leukoplakia (loo-koh-PLAY-kee-ah) White patch on the oral mucous membrane, often precancerous.

libido (li-BEE-doh) Sexual desire.

life expectancy (LIFE ek-SPEK-tan-see) Statistical determination of the number of years an individual is expected to live.

life span (LIFE SPAN) The age that a person reaches.

ligament (LIG-ah-ment) Band of fibrous tissue connecting two structures.

ligate (LIE-gate) Tie off a structure, such as a bleeding blood vessel.

ligation (lie-GAY-shun) Use of a tie to close a tube.

limbic (LIM-bic) Pertaining to the limbic system, an array of nerve fibers surrounding the thalamus.

linear fracture (LIN-ee-ar FRAK-chur) A fracture running parallel to the length of the bone.

lipase (LIE-paze) Enzyme that breaks down fat.

lipectomy (lip-EK-toh-mee) Surgical removal of adipose tissue.

lipid (LIP-id) General term for all types of fatty compounds; for example, cholesterol, triglycerides, and fatty acids.

lipoprotein (LIE-poh-proh-teen) Molecules made of combinations of fat and protein.

lithotripsy (LITH-oh-trip-see) Crushing stones by sound waves.

lithotripter (LITH-oh-trip-ter) Instrument that generates sound waves.

liver (LIV-er) Body's largest internal organ, located in the right upper quadrant of the abdomen.

lobe (LOBE) Subdivision of an organ or some other part.

lobectomy (loh-BEK-toh-mee) Surgical removal of a lobe of the lungs or the thyroid gland.

lochia (LOH-kee-uh) Vaginal discharge following childbirth.

longevity (lon-JEV-ih-tee) Duration of life beyond the normal expectation.

loop of Henle (LOOP of HEN-lee) Part of the renal tubule where reabsorption occurs.

lordosis (lore-DOH-sis) An exaggerated forward curvature of the lumbar spine.

louse (LOWSE) Parasitic insect. Plural *lice.*

lumbar (LUM-bar) Pertaining to the region in the back and sides between the ribs and pelvis.

lumen (LOO-men) The interior space of a tubelike structure.

lumpectomy (lump-EK-toh-mee) Removal of a lesion with preservation of surrounding tissue.

lutein (LOO-tee-in) Yellow pigment.

Lyme disease (LIME diz-EEZ) Disease transmitted by the bite of an infected deer tick.

lymph (LIMF) A clear fluid collected from tissues and transported by lymph vessels to the venous circulation.

lymphadenectomy (lim-FAD-eh-NEK-toh-mee) Surgical excision of a lymph node.

lymphadenitis (lim-FAD-eh-NIE-tis) Inflammation of a lymph node.

lymphadenopathy (lim-FAD-eh-NOP-ah-thee) Any disease process affecting a lymph node.

lymphangiogram (lim-FAN-jee-oh-gram) Radiographic images of lymph vessels and nodes following injection of contrast material.

lymphatic (lim-FAT-ik) Pertaining to lymph or the lymphatic system.

lymphedema (LIMF-eh-DEE-mah) Tissue swelling due to lymphatic obstruction.

lymphocyte (LIM-foh-site) Small white blood cell with a large nucleus.

lymphoid (LIM-foyd) Resembling lymphatic tissue.

lymphoma (lim-FOH-mah) Any neoplasm of lymphatic tissue.

lysosome (LIE-soh-sohm) Enzyme that digests foreign material and worn-out cell components.

lysozyme (LIE-soh-zime) Enzyme that dissolves the cell walls of bacteria.

M

macrocytic (mak-roh-SIT-ik) Pertaining to macrocytes.

macrophage (MAK-roh-fayj) Large white blood cell that removes bacteria, foreign particles, and dead cells.

macula (MAK-you-lah) Small area of special function; in the ear, a sensory receptor. Plural *maculae.*

macula lutea (MAK-you-lah LOO-tee-ah) Yellowish spot on the back of the retina; contains the fovea centralis.

majus (MAY-jus) Bigger or greater; for example, labia majora. Plural *majora.*

malabsorption (mal-ab-SORP-shun) Inadequate gastrointestinal absorption of nutrients.

malfunction (mal-FUNK-shun) Inadequate or abnormal function.

malignant (mah-LIG-nant) Capable of invading surrounding tissues and metastasizing to distant organs.

malleus (MAL-ee-us) Outer (lateral) one of the three ossicles in the middle ear; shaped like a hammer.

malnutrition (mal-nyu-TRISH-un) Inadequate nutrition from poor diet or inadequate absorption of nutrients.

mammary (MAM-ah-ree) Relating to the lactating breast.

mammogram (MAM-oh-gram) The record produced by x-ray imaging of the breast.

mammography (mah-MOG-rah-fee) Process of x-ray examination of the breast.

mandible (MAN-di-bel) Lower jawbone.

mania (MAY-nee-ah) Mood disorder with hyperactivity, irritability, and rapid speech.

manic-depressive disorder (MAN-ik dee-PRESS-iv dis-OR-der) An outdated name for bipolar disorder.

marijuana (mar-ih-HWAN-ah) Dried, flowering leaves of the plant *Cannabis sativa*.

marrow (MAH-roh) Fatty, blood-forming tissue in the cavities of long bones.

mastalgia (mass-TAL-jee-uh) Pain in the breast.

mastectomy (mass-TEK-toh-mee) Surgical excision of the breast.

masticate (MAS-tih-kate) To chew.

mastitis (mass-TIE-tis) Inflammation of the breast.

mastoid (MASS-toyd) Small bony protrusion immediately behind the ear.

maternal (mah-TER-nal) Pertaining to or derived from the mother.

matrix (MAY-triks) Substance that surrounds cells, is manufactured by the cells, and holds them together.

maximus (MAKS-ih-mus) The gluteus maximus muscle is the largest muscle in the body, covering a large part of each buttock.

McBurney point (mack-BUR-nee POYNT) One-third the distance from the anterior superior iliac spine to the umbilicus.

meatus (mee-AY-tus) Passage or channel; also used to denote the external opening of a passage.

meconium (meh-KOH-nee-um) The first bowel movement of the newborn.

media (MEE-dee-ah) Middle layer of a structure, particularly a blood vessel.

medial (MEE-dee-al) Nearer to the middle of the body.

mediastinoscopy (MEE-dee-ass-tih-NOS-koh-pee) Examination of the mediastinum using an endoscope.

mediastinum (MEE-dee-ah-STIE-num) Area between the lungs containing the heart, aorta, venae cavae, esophagus, and trachea.

medius (MEE-dee-us) The gluteus medius muscle is partly covered by the gluteus maximus; it originates on the ilium and is inserted into the femur.

medulla (meh-DULL-ah) Central portion of a structure surrounded by cortex.

medulla oblongata (meh-DULL-ah ob-lon-GAH-tah) Most posterior subdivision of the brainstem; continuation of the spinal cord.

megakaryocyte (MEG-ah-KAIR-ee-oh-site) Large cell with a large nucleus. Parts of the cytoplasm break off to form platelets.

meiosis (my-OH-sis) Two rapid cell divisions, resulting in half the number of chromosomes.

melanin (MEL-ah-nin) Black pigment found in the skin, hair, and retina.

melanocyte (MEL-an-oh-cyte) Cell that synthesizes (produces) melanin.

melanoma (MEL-ah-NOH-mah) Malignant neoplasm formed from cells that produce melanin.

melasma (meh-LAZ-mah) Patchy pigmentation of the skin.

melatonin (mel-ah-TONE-in) Hormone formed by the pineal gland.

melena (mel-EN-ah) The passage of black, tarry stools.

membrane (MEM-brain) Thin layer of tissue covering a structure or cavity.

Ménière disease (men-YEAR diz-EEZ) Disorder of the inner ear with a cluster of symptoms of acute attacks of tinnitus, vertigo, and hearing loss.

meninges (meh-NIN-jeez) Three-layered covering of the brain and spinal cord.

meningioma (meh-NIN-jee-OH-mah) Tumor arising from the arachnoid layer of the meninges.

meningitis (men-in-JIE-tis) Acute infectious disease of children and young adults.

meningocele (meh-NING-oh-seal) Protrusion of the meninges from the spinal cord or brain through a defect in the vertebral column or cranium.

meningococcal (meh-nin-goh-KOK-al) Pertaining to the *meningococcus* bacterium.

meningomyelocele (meh-NING-oh-MY-el-oh-seal) Protrusion of the spinal cord and meninges through a defect in the vertebral arch of one or more vertebrae.

meniscectomy (men-ih-SEK-toh-mee) Excision (cutting out) of all or part of a meniscus.

meniscus (meh-NISS-kuss) Disc of connective tissue cartilage between the bones of a joint; for example, in the knee joint. Plural *menisci*.

menopause (MEN-oh-paws) Permanent ending of menstrual periods.

menorrhagia (men-oh-RAY-jee-ah) Excessive menstrual bleeding.

menstruation (men-stru-AY-shun) Synonym of *menses*.

merocrine (MARE-oh-krin) Another name for *eccrine*.

mesentery (MESS-en-ter-ree) A double layer of peritoneum enclosing the abdominal viscera.

mesothelioma (MEEZ-oh-thee-lee-OH-mah) Cancer arising from the cells lining the pleura or peritoneum.

metabolic acidosis (met-ah-BOL-ik ass-ih-DOH-sis) Decreased pH in the blood and body tissues as a result of an upset in metabolism.

metabolism (meh-TAB-oh-lizm) The constantly changing physical and chemical processes occurring in the cell.

metacarpal (MET-ah-KAR-pal) The five bones between the carpus and the fingers.

metacarpophalangeal (MET-ah-KAR-poh-fah-LAN-jee-al) Pertaining to the joints between the metacarpal bones and the phalanges.

metaphysis (meh-TAF-ih-sis) Region between the diaphysis and the epiphysis where bone growth occurs.

metastasis (meh-TAS-tah-sis) Spread of a disease from one part of the body to another. Plural *metastases*.

metastasize (meh-TAS-tah-size) To spread to distant parts.

metrorrhagia (MEH-troh-RAY-jee-ah) Irregular uterine bleeding between menses.

microalbuminuria (MY-kroh-al-byu-min-YOU-ree-ah) Presence of very small quantities of albumin in urine that cannot be detected by conventional urine testing.

microaneurysm (my-kroh-AN-yu-rizm) Focal dilation of retinal capillaries.

microangiopathy (MY-kroh-an-jee-OP-ah-thee) Disease of the very small blood vessels (capillaries).

microarray (MY-kroh-ah-RAY) Technique for studying one gene in one experiment. Also called *gene chips.*

microcephaly (MY-kroh-SEF-ah-lee) An abnormally small head.

microcytic (my-kroh-SIT-ik) Pertaining to a small cell.

microglia (my-KROH-glee-ah) Small nervous tissue cells that are phagocytes.

microscope (MY-kroh-skope) Instrument for viewing something small that cannot be seen in detail by the naked eye.

micturition (mik-choo-RISH-un) Act of passing urine.

migraine (MY-grain) Paroxysmal severe headache confined to one side of the head.

mineral (MIN-er-al) Inorganic compound usually found in earth's crust.

mineralocorticoid (MIN-er-al-oh-KOR-tih-koyd) Hormone of the adrenal cortex that influences sodium and potassium metabolism.

minimus (MIN-ih-mus) The gluteus minimus is the smallest of the gluteal muscles and lies under the gluteus medius.

minus (MY-nus) Smaller or lesser; for example, labia minora. Plural *minora.*

mitochondrion (my-toe-KON-dree-on) Organelle that generates, stores, and releases energy for cell activities. Plural *mitochondria.*

mitosis (my-TOH-sis) Cell division to create two identical cells, each with 46 chromosomes.

mitral (MY-tral) Shaped like the headdress of a Catholic bishop.

molar (MOH-lar) One of six teeth in each jaw that grind food.

mole (MOLE) Benign localized area of melanin-producing cells.

molecule (MOLL-eh-kyul) Very small particle consisting of two or more atoms held tightly together.

molluscum contagiosum (moh-LUS-kum kon-TAY-jee-oh-sum) An STD caused by a virus.

monoclonal (MON-oh-KLOH-nal) Derived from a protein from a single clone of cells, all molecules of which are the same.

monocyte (MON-oh-site) Large white blood cell with a single nucleus.

monoglyceride (mon-oh-GLISS-eh-ride) A fatty substance with a single fatty acid.

mononeuropathy (MON-oh-nyu-ROP-ah-thee) Disorder affecting a single nerve.

mononucleosis (MON-oh-nyu-klee-OH-sis) Presence of large numbers of mononuclear leukocytes.

monoplegia (MON-oh-PLEE-jee-ah) Paralysis of one limb.

monosaccharide (MON-oh-SACK-ah-ride) Simplest form of sugar; for example, glucose.

Monospot test (MON-oh-spot TEST) Detects heterophile antibodies in infectious mononucleosis.

monozygotic (MON-oh-zie-GOT-ik) Twins from a single zygote.

mons pubis (MONZ PYU-bis) Fleshy pad with pubic hair, overlying the pubic bone.

morphine (MOR-feen) Derivative of opium used as an analgesic or sedative.

mortality (mor-TAL-ih-tee) Fatal outcome or death rate.

morula (MOR-you-lah) Ball of cells formed from divisions of a zygote.

motile (MOH-til) Capable of spontaneous movement.

motility (moh-TILL-ih-tee) The ability for spontaneous movement.

motor (MOH-tor) Pertaining to nerves that send impulses out to cause muscles to contract or glands to secrete.

mouth (MOWTH) External opening of a cavity or canal.

mucin (MYU-sin) Protein element of mucus.

mucolytic (MYU-koh-LIT-ik) Agent capable of dissolving or liquefying mucus.

mucopurulent (myu-koh-PYUR-you-lent) Mixture of pus and mucus.

mucosa (myu-KOH-sah) Lining of a tubular structure. Another name for *mucous membrane.*

mucus (MYU-kus) Sticky secretion of cells in mucous membranes.

multimodal (mul-tee-MOH-dal) Using many methods.

multipara (mul-TIP-ah-ruh) Woman who has given birth to two or more children.

murmur (MUR-mur) Abnormal sound heard on auscultation of the heart or blood vessels.

Murphy sign (MUR-fee SINE) Tenderness in the right subcostal area on inspiration, associated with acute cholecystitis.

muscle (MUSS-el) Tissue consisting of contractile cells.

muscular (MUSS-kyu-lar) Pertaining to muscle or muscles.

muscularis (muss-kyu-LAR-is) The muscular layer of a hollow organ or tube.

mutagen (MYU-tah-jen) Agent that produces a mutation in a gene.

mutation (myu-TAY-shun) Change in the chemistry of a gene.

mutism (MYU-tizm) Absence of speech.

myasthenia gravis (my-as-THEE-nee-ah GRAH-vis) Disorder of fluctuating muscle weakness.

myelin (MY-eh-lin) Material of the sheath around the axon of a nerve.

myelitis (MY-eh-LIE-tis) Inflammation of the spinal cord.

myelography (my-eh-LOG-rah-fee) Radiography of the spinal cord and nerve roots after injection of a contrast medium into the subarachnoid space.

myeloid (MY-eh-loyd) Resembling cells derived from bone marrow.

myocarditis (MY-oh-kar-DIE-tis) Inflammation of the heart muscle.

myocardium (MY-oh-KAR-dee-um) All the heart muscle.

myoglobin (MY-oh-GLOH-bin) Protein of muscle that stores and transports oxygen.

myoma (my-OH-mah) Benign tumor of muscle.

myomectomy (my-oh-MEK-toh-mee) Surgical removal of a myoma (fibroid).

myometrium (my-oh-MEE-tree-um) Muscle wall of the uterus.

myopia (my-OH-pee-ah) Able to see close objects but unable to see distant objects.

myringotomy (mir-in-GOT-oh-mee) Incision in the tympanic membrane.

myxedema (mik-seh-DEE-mah) Severe hypothyroidism.

N

narcissistic (NAR-sih-SIS-tik) Relating everything to oneself.

narcolepsy (NAR-coh-lep-see) Condition with frequent incidents of sudden, involuntary deep sleep.

narcotic (nar-KOT-ik) Drug derived from opium, or a synthetic drug with similar effects.

naris (NAH-ris) Nostril. Plural *nares.*

nasal (NAY-zal) Pertaining to the nose.

nasolacrimal duct (NAY-zoh-LAK-rim-al DUKT) Passage from the lacrimal sac to the nose.

nasopharynx (NAY-zoh-FAIR-inks) Region of the pharynx at the back of the nose and above the soft palate.

natriuretic peptide (NAH-tree-you-RET-ik PEP-tide) Protein that increases the excretion of sodium.

nebulizer (NEB-you-lize-er) Device used to deliver liquid medicine in a fine mist.

necrosis (neh-KROH-sis) Pathologic death of cells or tissue.

necrotic (neh-KROT-ik) Affected by necrosis.

necrotizing fasciitis (neh-kroh-TIZE-ing fash-eh-EYE-tis) Inflammation of fascia, producing death of the tissue.

neonate (NEE-oh-nate) A newborn infant.

neoplasm (NEE-oh-plazm) A new growth, either a benign or malignant tumor.

nephritis (neh-FRIE-tis) Inflammation of the kidney.

nephroblastoma (NEF-roh-blas-TOH-mah) Cancerous kidney tumor of childhood. Also known as *Wilms tumor.*

nephrolithiasis (NEF-roh-lih-THIGH-ah-sis) Presence of a kidney stone.

nephrolithotomy (NEF-roh-lih-THOT-oh-mee) Incision for removal of a stone.

nephrologist (neh-FROL-oh-jist) Medical specialist in disorders of the kidney.

nephron (NEF-ron) Filtration unit of the kidney; glomerulus + renal tubule.

nephropathy (neh-FROP-ah-thee) Any disease of the kidney.

nephroscope (NEF-roh-skope) Endoscope used to view the inside of the kidney.

nephrotic syndrome (neh-FROT-ik SIN-drome) Glomerular disease with marked loss of protein. Also known as *nephrosis.*

nerve (NERV) A cord of fibers in connective tissue that conduct impulses.

nerve conduction study (NERV kon-DUK-shun STUD-ee) Procedure for measuring the speed at which an electrical impulse travels along a nerve.

nervous (NER-vus) Pertaining to a nerve.

neural tube (NYU-ral TYUB) Embryologic tubelike structure that forms the brain and spinal cord.

neuralgia (nyu-RAL-jee-ah) Pain in the distribution of a nerve.

neurilemma (nyu-ri-LEM-ah) Covering of a nerve around the myelin sheath.

neuroglia (nyu-ROH-glee-ah) Connective tissue holding nervous tissue together.

neurohypophysis (NYUR-oh-high-POF-ih-sis) Posterior lobe of the pituitary gland.

neurologist (nyu-ROL-oh-jist) Medical specialist in disorders of the nervous system.

neurology (nyu-ROL-oh-jee) Medical specialty of disorders of the nervous system.

neuromuscular (NYUR-oh-MUSS-kyu-lar) Pertaining to both nerves and muscles.

neuron (NYUR-on) Technical term for a nerve cell; consists of the cell body with its dendrites and axons.

neuropathy (nyu-ROP-ah-thee) Any disease of the nervous system.

neurosurgeon (NYU-roh-SUR-jun) Specialist in operating on the nervous system.

neurosurgery (NYU-roh-SUR-jer-ee) Medical specialty in surgery of the nervous system.

neurotoxin (NYUR-oh-tock-sin) Agent that poisons the nervous system.

neurotransmitter (NYUR-oh-trans-MIT-er) Chemical agent that relays messages from one nerve cell to the next.

neutropenia (NEW-troh-PEE-nee-ah) A deficiency of neutrophils.

neutrophil (NEW-troh-fill) A neutrophil's granules take up (purple) stain equally, whether the stain is acid or alkaline.

neutrophilia (NEW-troh-FILL-ee-ah) An increase in neutrophils.

nevus (NEE-vus) Congenital or acquired lesion of the skin. Plural *nevi.*

nipple (NIP-el) Projection from the breast into which the lactiferous ducts open.

nitrite (NIE-trite) Chemical formed in urine by *E. coli* and other microorganisms.

nitrogenous (ni-TROJ-en-us) Containing or generating nitrogen.

nocturia (nok-TYU-ree-ah) Excessive urination at night.

node (NOHD) A circumscribed mass of tissue.

nodule (NOD-yule) Small node or knotlike swelling.

norepinephrine (NOR-ep-ih-NEF-rin) Parasympathetic neurotransmitter that is a catecholamine hormone of the adrenal gland. Also called *noradrenaline.*

nuchal cord (NYU-kul KORD) Loop of umbilical cord around the fetal neck.

nucleolus (nyu-KLEE-oh-lus) Small mass within the nucleus.

nucleotide (NYU-klee-oh-tide) Combination of a DNA base, a sugar molecule, and a phosphate molecule.

nucleus (NYU-klee-us) Functional center of a cell or structure.

null cells (NULL SELLS) Lymphocytes with no surface markers, unlike T cells or B cells.

nutrient (NYU-tree-ent) A substance in food required for normal physiologic function.

nutrition (nyu-TRISH-un) The study of food and liquid requirements for normal function of the human body.

O

obesity (oh-BEE-sih-tee) Excessive amount of fat in the body.

oblique fracture (ob-LEEK FRAK-chur) A diagonal fracture across the long axis of the bone.

obsession (ob-SESH-un) Persistent, recurrent, uncontrollable thoughts or impulses.

obsessive (ob-SES-iv) Possessing persistent, recurrent, uncontrollable thoughts or impulses.

obstetrician (ob-steh-TRISH-un) Medical specialist in obstetrics.

obstetrics (OB) (ob-STET-riks) Medical specialty for the care of women during pregnancy and the postpartum period.

occipital bone (ok-SIP-it-al BOHN) Bone that forms the back and part of the base of the cranium.

occipital lobe (ok-SIP-it-al LOBE) Posterior area of the cerebral hemispheres.

occlude (ok-KLUDE) To close, plug, or completely obstruct.

occult (oh-KULT) Not visible on the surface.

occupational therapy (OK-you-PAY-shun-al THAIR-ah-pee) Use of work and recreational activities to increase independent function.

oculomotor (OK-you-loh-MOH-tor) Third (III) cranial nerve; moves the eye.

olfaction (ol-FAK-shun) Sense of smell.

olfactory (ol-FAK-toh-ree) First (I) cranial nerve; carries information related to the sense of smell.

oligodendrocyte (OL-ih-goh-DEN-droh-site) Connective tissue cell of the central nervous system that forms a myelin sheath.

oligohydramnios (OL-ih-goh-high-DRAM-nee-os) Too little amniotic fluid.

oliguria (ol-ih-GYUR-ee-ah) Scanty production of urine.

omentum (oh-MEN-tum) Membrane that encloses the bowels.

oncogene (ONG-koh-jeen) One of a family of genes involved in cell growth that work in concert to cause cancer.

oncologist (on-KOL-oh-jist) Medical specialist in oncology.

oncology (on-KOL-oh-jee) The science dealing with cancer.

onychomycosis (oh-ni-koh-my-KOH-sis) Condition of a fungus infection in a nail.

oocyte (OH-oh-site) Female egg cell.

oogenesis (oh-oh-JEN-eh-sis) Development of a female egg cell.

open fracture (OH-pen FRAK-chur) The skin over the fracture is broken.

ophthalmia neonatorum (off-THAL-mee-ah nee-oh-nay-TOR-um) Conjunctivitis of the newborn.

ophthalmologist (off-thal-MALL-oh-jist) Medical specialist in ophthalmology.

ophthalmoscope (off-THAL-moh-skope) Instrument for viewing the retina.

ophthalmoscopic (OFF-thal-moh-SKOP-ik) Pertaining to the use of an ophthalmoscope.

opiate (OH-pee-ate) A drug derived from opium.

opportunistic (OP-or-tyu-NIS-tik) An organism or a disease in a host with lowered resistance.

opportunistic infection (OP-or-tyu-NIS-tik in-FEK-shun) An infection that causes disease when the immune system is compromised for other reasons.

optic (OP-tik) Pertaining to the eye; *or* second (II) cranial nerve, which carries visual information.

optometrist (op-TOM-eh-trist) Someone who is skilled in the measurement of vision but cannot treat eye diseases or prescribe medication.

oral (OR-al) Pertaining to the mouth.

orbit (OR-bit) The bony socket that holds the eyeball.

orchiectomy (or-kee-ECK-toh-mee) Removal of one or both testes.

orchiopexy (OR-kee-oh-PEK-see) Surgical fixation of a testis in the scrotum.

orchitis (or-KIE-tis) Inflammation of the testis. Also called *epididymoorchitis.*

organ (OR-gan) Structure with specific functions in a body system.

organelle (OR-gah-nell) Part of a cell having a specialized function(s).

organophosphate (OR-ga-no-FOS-fate) Organic phosphorus compound used as an insecticide.

origin (OR-ih-gin) Fixed source of a muscle at its attachment to bone.

oropharynx (OR-oh-FAIR-inks) Region at the back of the mouth between the soft palate and the tip of the epiglottis.

orthopedic (or-thoh-PEE-dik) Pertaining to the correction and cure of deformities and diseases of the musculoskeletal system; originally, most of the deformities treated were in children. Also spelled *orthopaedic.*

orthopedist (or-thoh-PEE-dist) Specialist in orthopedics.

orthopnea (or-THOP-nee-ah) Difficulty in breathing when lying flat.

orthotic (or-THOT-ik) Orthopedic appliance used to correct an abnormality.

orthotist (or-THOT-ist) Maker and fitter of orthopedic appliances.

os (OS) Opening into a canal; for example, the cervix.

osmosis (oz-MOH-sis) The passage of water across a cell membrane.

ossicle (OS-ih-kel) A small bone, particularly relating to the three bones in the middle ear.

osteoarthritis (OS-tee-oh-ar-THRIE-tis) Chronic inflammatory disease of the joints with pain and loss of function.

osteoblast (OS-tee-oh-blast) Bone-forming cell.

osteoclast (OS-tee-oh-klast) Bone-removing cell.

osteocyte (OS-tee-oh-site) Bone-maintaining cell.

osteogenesis (OS-tee-oh-JEN-eh-sis) Creation of new bone.

osteogenesis imperfecta (OS-tee-oh-JEN-eh-sis im-per-FEK-tah) Inherited condition in which bone formation is incomplete, leading to fragile, easily broken bones.

osteogenic sarcoma (OS-tee-oh-JEN-ik sar-KOH-mah) Malignant tumor originating in bone-producing cells.

osteomalacia (OS-tee-oh-mah-LAY-shee-ah) Soft, flexible bones lacking in calcium (rickets).

osteomyelitis (OS-tee-oh-my-eh-LIE-tis) Inflammation of bone tissue.

osteopathy (OS-tee-OP-ah-thee) Medical practice based on maintaining the structural integrity of the musculoskeletal system.

osteopenia (OS-tee-oh-PEE-nee-ah) Decreased calcification of bone.

GLOSSARY

osteoporosis (OS-tee-oh-poh-ROH-sis) Condition in which the bones become more porous, brittle, and fragile and are more likely to fracture.

osteosarcoma (OS-tee-oh-sar-KOH-mah) Cancer arising in bone-forming cells.

ostomy (OS-toh-mee) Surgery to create an artificial opening into a tubular structure.

otitis media (oh-TIE-tis MEE-dee-ah) Inflammation of the middle ear.

otolith (OH-toh-lith) A calcium particle in the vestibule of the inner ear.

otologist (oh-TOL-oh-jist) Medical specialist in diseases of the ear.

otomycosis (OH-toh-my-KOH-sis) Fungal infection of the external ear.

otorhinolaryngologist (OH-toh-RIE-noh-LAH-rin-GOL-oh-jist) Ear, nose, and throat medical specialist.

otosclerosis (oh-toh-skler-OH-sis) Hardening at the junction of the stapes and oval window that causes loss of hearing.

otoscope (OH-toh-skope) Instrument for examining the ear.

otoscopic (oh-toh-SKOP-ik) Pertaining to examination with an otoscope.

otoscopy (oh-TOS-koh-pee) Examination of the ear.

ovarian (oh-VAIR-ee-an) Pertaining to the ovary.

ovary (OH-va-ree) One of the paired female egg-producing glands.

ovulation (OV-you-LAY-shun) Release of an oocyte from a follicle.

oxyhemoglobin (OK-see-HEE-moh-GLOH-bin) Hemoglobin in combination with oxygen.

oxytocin (OK-see-TOH-sin) Pituitary hormone that stimulates the uterus to contract.

P

pacemaker (PACE-may-ker) Device that regulates cardiac electrical activity.

palate (PAL-uht) Roof of the mouth.

palatine (PAL-ah-tine) Bone that forms the hard palate and parts of the nose and orbits.

palliative care (PAL-ee-ah-tiv KAIR) Care that relieves symptoms and pain without curing.

pallor (PAL-or) Paleness of the skin.

palm (PAHLM) The flat anterior surface of the hand.

palpate (PAL-pate) To examine with the fingers and hands.

palpation (pal-PAY-shun) An examination with the fingers and hands.

palpitation (pal-pih-TAY-shun) Forcible, rapid beat of the heart felt by the patient.

palsy (PAWL-zee) Paralysis or paresis from brain damage.

pancreas (PAN-kree-as) Lobulated gland, the head of which is tucked into the curve of the duodenum.

pancreatic (pan-kree-AT-ik) Pertaining to the pancreas.

pancreatitis (PAN-kree-ah-TIE-tis) Inflammation of the pancreas.

pancytopenia (PAN-sigh-toh-PEE-nee-ah) Deficiency of all types of blood cells.

panendoscopy (pan-en-DOS-koh-pee) Examination of the inside of the esophagus, stomach, and upper duodenum using a flexible fiber-optic endoscope.

panhypopituitarism (pan-HIGH-poh-pih-TYU-ih-tah-rizm) Deficiency of all the pituitary hormones.

Pap test (PAP TEST) Examination of cells taken from the cervix.

papilla (pah-PILL-ah) Any small projection. Plural *papillae*.

papilledema (pah-pill-eh-DEE-mah) Swelling of the optic disc in the retina.

papilloma (pap-ih-LOH-mah) Benign projection of epithelial cells.

papule (PAP-yul) Small, circumscribed elevation on the skin.

para (PAH-rah) Abbreviation for number of deliveries.

paralysis (pah-RAL-ih-sis) Loss of voluntary movement.

paralyze (PAR-ah-lize) To make incapable of movement.

paranasal (PAR-ah-NAY-zal) Adjacent to the nose.

paranoid (PAIR-ah-noyd) Having delusions of persecution.

paraphimosis (PAR-ah-fi-MOH-sis) Condition in which a retracted prepuce cannot be pulled forward to cover the glans.

paraplegia (par-ah-PLEE-jee-ah) Paralysis of both lower extremities.

parasite (PAR-ah-site) An organism that attaches itself to, lives on or in, and derives its nutrition from another species.

parasympathetic (par-ah-sim-pah-THET-ik) Pertaining to division of the autonomic nervous system; has opposite effects of the sympathetic division.

parathyroid (pair-ah-THIGH-royd) Endocrine glands embedded in the back of the thyroid gland.

paraurethral (PAR-ah-you-REE-thral) Situated around the urethra.

parenchyma (pah-RENG-kih-mah) Characteristic functional cells of a gland or organ that are supported by the connective tissue framework.

parenteral (pah-REN-ter-al) Giving medication by any means other than the gastrointestinal tract.

paresis (par-EE-sis) Partial paralysis.

paresthesia (par-es-THEE-zee-ah) An abnormal sensation; for example, tingling, burning, pricking. Plural *paresthesias*.

parietal (pah-RYE-eh-tal) Pertaining to the wall of an organ or a body cavity.

parietal bones (pah-RYE-eh-tal BOHNZ) Bones that form the bulging sides and roof of the cranium.

parietal lobe (pah-RYE-eh-tal LOBE) Area of the brain under the parietal bone.

parity (PAIR-ih-tee) Number of deliveries.

Parkinson disease (PAR-kin-son diz-EEZ) Disease of muscular rigidity, tremors, and a masklike facial expression.

paronychia (par-oh-NICK-ee-ah) Infection alongside the nail.

parotid (pah-ROT-id) Parotid gland is the salivary gland beside the ear.

paroxysmal (par-ok-SIZ-mal) Occurring in sharp, spasmodic episodes.

particle (PAR-tih-kul) A small piece of matter.

particulate (par-TIK-you-let) Relating to a fine particle.

patella (pah-TELL-ah) Thin, circular bone in front of the knee joint and embedded in the patellar tendon. Also called the *kneecap*.

patent (PAY-tent) Open.

patent ductus arteriosus (PAY-tent DUK-tus ar-TEER-ee-oh-sus) An open, direct channel between the aorta and the pulmonary artery.

pathogen (PATH-oh-jen) A disease-causing microorganism.

pathologic fracture (path-oh-LOJ-ik FRAK-chur) Fracture occurring at a site already weakened by a disease process, such as cancer.

pathologist (pah-THOL-oh-jist) A specialist in pathology (study of disease or characteristics of a particular disease).

pathology (pah-THOL-oh-jee) Medical specialty dealing with the structural and functional changes of a disease process; *or* the cause, development, and structural changes in disease.

pectoral (PEK-tor-al) Pertaining to the chest.

pectoral girdle (PEK-tor-al GIR-del) Incomplete bony ring that attaches the upper limb to the axial skeleton.

pedal (PEED-al) Pertaining to the foot.

pediatrician (PEE-dee-ah-TRISH-an) Medical specialist in pediatrics.

pediculosis (peh-dick-you-LOH-sis) An infestation with lice.

pelvic (PEL-vic) Pertaining to the pubic bone.

pelvis (PEL-vis) A cup-shaped cavity, as in the pelvis of the kidney; *or* a cup-shaped ring of bone.

penis (PEE-nis) Conveys urine and semen to the outside.

pepsin (PEP-sin) Enzyme produced by the stomach that breaks down protein.

pepsinogen (pep-SIN-oh-jen) Converted by HCl in stomach to pepsin.

peptic (PEP-tik) Relating to the stomach and duodenum.

perforated (PER-foh-ray-ted) Punctured with one or more holes.

perforation (per-foh-RAY-shun) Erosion that progresses to become a hole through the wall of a structure.

perfuse (per-FYUSE) To force blood to flow through a lumen or a vascular bed.

pericarditis (PER-ih-kar-DIE-tis) Inflammation of the pericardium, the covering of the heart.

pericardium (per-ih-KAR-dee-um) Structure around the heart.

perimeter (peh-RIM-eh-ter) An edge or border.

perimetrium (per-ih-MEE-tree-um) The covering of the uterus; part of the peritoneum.

perinatal (per-ih-NAY-tal) Around the time of birth.

perineum (PER-ih-NEE-um) Area between the thighs, extending from the coccyx to the pubis.

periodontal (PER-ee-oh-DON-tal) Around a tooth.

periodontitis (PER-ee-oh-don-TIE-tis) Inflammation of tissues around a tooth.

periorbital (per-ee-OR-bit-al) Pertaining to tissues around the orbit.

periosteum (PER-ee-OSS-tee-um) Fibrous membrane covering a bone.

peripheral (peh-RIF-er-al) Pertaining to the periphery or external boundary.

peripheral vision (peh-RIF-er-al VIZH-un) Ability to see objects as they come into the outer edges of the visual field.

periphery (peh-RIF-eh-ree) Outer part of a structure away from the center.

peristalsis (per-ih-STAL-sis) Waves of alternate contraction and relaxation of the intestinal wall to move food along the digestive tract.

peritoneum (per-ih-toh-NEE-um) Membrane that lines the abdominal cavity.

peritonitis (PER-ih-toh-NIE-tis) Inflammation of the peritoneum.

peritubular (PER-ih-TOO-byu-lar) Surrounding the small renal tubules.

permeable (PER-mee-ah-bull) Allows passage of substances through a membrane.

pernicious anemia (per-NISH-us ah-NEE-mee-ah) Chronic anemia due to lack of vitamin B_{12}.

peroneal (pair-uh-NEE-al) Pertaining to the lateral part (fibula) of the lower leg, or the nerve named after it.

pertussis (per-TUSS-is) Infectious disease with a spasmodic, intense cough ending on a whoop (stridor). Also known as *whooping cough*.

pes planus (PES PLAY-nuss) A flat foot with no plantar arch.

pessary (PES-ah-ree) Appliance inserted into the vagina to support the uterus.

pesticide (PES-tih-side) Agent for destroying flies, mosquitoes, and other pests.

petechia (peh-TEE-kee-ah) Pinpoint capillary hemorrhagic spot in the skin. Plural *petechiae*.

petit mal (peh-TEE MAL) Old name for an absence seizure.

Peyronie disease (pay-ROH-nee diz-EEZ) Penile bending and pain on erection.

phacoemulsification (FAK-oh-ee-mul-sih-fih-KAY-shun) Technique used to fragment the center of the lens into very tiny pieces and suck them out of the eye.

phagocytize (FAG-oh-site-ize) Ingest foreign particles and cells.

phagocytosis (FAG-oh-sigh-TOH-sis) Process of ingestion and destruction.

phalanx (FAY-lanks) A bone of a finger or toe. Plural *phalanges*.

pharmacist (FAR-mah-sist) Person licensed by the state to prepare and dispense drugs.

pharmacology (far-mah-KOL-oh-jee) Science of the preparation, uses, and effects of drugs.

pharmacy (FAR-mah-see) Facility licensed to prepare and dispense drugs.

pharyngitis (fair-in-JIE-tis) Inflammation of the pharynx.

pharynx (FAIR-inks) Air tube from the back of the nose to the larynx.

phenotype (FEE-noh-type) A visible trait.

pheochromocytoma (fee-oh-KROH-moh-sigh-TOH-mah) Adenoma of the adrenal medulla secreting excessive catecholamines.

pheomelanin (FEE-oh-mel-ah-nin) The lighter form of melanin.

pheromone (FER-oh-moan) Substance that carries and generates a physical attraction for other people.

phimosis (fi-MOH-sis) Condition in which the prepuce cannot be retracted.

phlebitis (fleh-BIE-tis) Inflammation of a vein.

phlegm (FLEM) Abnormal amounts of mucus expectorated from the respiratory tract.

phobia (FOH-bee-ah) Pathologic fear or dread.

phosphatase (FOS-fah-tase) Enzyme that liberates phosphorus.

photocoagulation (foh-toh-koh-ag-you-LAY-shun) The use of light (laser beam) to form a clot.

photophobia (foh-toh-FOH-bee-ah) Fear of the light because it hurts the eyes.

photoreceptor (foh-toh-ree-SEP-tor) A photoreceptor cell receives light and converts it into electrical impulses.

photosensitivity (foh-toh-sen-sih-TIV-ih-tee) Condition in which light produces pain in the eye.

physiatrist (fih-ZIE-ah-trist) Specialist in physical medicine.

physiatry (fih-ZIE-ah-tree) Physical medicine.

physical medicine (FIZ-ih-cal MED-ih-sin) Diagnosis and treatment by means of remedial agents, such as exercises, manipulation, and heat.

physical therapy (FIZ-ih-cal THAIR-ah-pee) Use of remedial processes to overcome a physical defect. Also known as *physiotherapy.*

pia mater (PEE-ah MAY-ter) Delicate inner layer of the meninges.

pineal (PIN-ee-al) Pertaining to the pineal gland.

pink eye (PINK EYE) Conjunctivitis.

pinna (PIN-ah) Another name for *auricle.* Plural *pinnae.*

pituitary (pih-TOO-ih-tair-ee) Pertaining to the pituitary gland.

placenta (plah-SEN-tah) Organ that allows metabolic interchange between the mother and the fetus.

plaque (PLAK) Patch of abnormal tissue.

plasma (PLAZ-mah) Fluid, noncellular component of blood.

plasma cell (PLAZ-mah SELL) Cell derived from B lymphocytes and active in formation of antibodies.

platelet (PLAYT-let) Cell fragment involved in the clotting process. Also called *thrombocyte.*

pleura (PLUR-ah) Membrane covering the lungs and lining the ribs in the thoracic cavity. Plural *pleurae.*

pleurisy (PLUR-ih-see) Inflammation of the pleura.

plexus (PLEK-sus) A weblike network of joined nerves. Plural *plexuses.*

plica (PLEE-cah) Fold in a mucous membrane. Plural *plicae.*

pneumatic (new-MAT-ik) Pertaining to a structure filled with air.

pneumoconiosis (new-moh-koh-nee-OH-sis) Fibrotic lung disease caused by the inhalation of different dusts.

pneumonectomy (NEW-moh-NEK-toh-mee) Surgical removal of a whole lung.

pneumonia (new-MOH-nee-ah) Inflammation of the lung parenchyma.

pneumothorax (new-moh-THOR-aks) Air in the pleural cavity.

podiatrist (poh-DIE-ah-trist) Practitioner of podiatry.

podiatry (poh-DIE-ah-tree) Specialty concerned with the diagnosis and treatment of disorders and injuries of the foot.

poikilocytic (POY-kee-loh-SIT-ik) Pertaining to an irregular-shaped RBC.

poliomyelitis (POH-lee-oh-MY-eh-LIE-tis) Inflammation of the gray matter of the spinal cord, leading to paralysis of the limbs and muscles of respiration.

pollutant (poh-LOO-tant) Substance that makes an environment unclean or impure.

pollution (poh-LOO-shun) Condition that is unclean, impure, and a danger to health.

polycystic (pol-ee-SIS-tik) Composed of many cysts.

polycythemia vera (POL-ee-sigh-THEE-me-ah VEH-rah) Chronic disease with bone marrow hyperplasia and an increase in the number of RBCs and blood volume.

polydipsia (pol-ee-DIP-see-ah) Excessive thirst.

polyhydramnios (POL-ee-high-DRAM-nee-os) Too much amniotic fluid.

polymenorrhea (POL-ee-men-oh-REE-ah) More than normal frequency of menses.

polymorphonuclear (POL-ee-more-foh-NEW-klee-ar) White blood cell with a multilobed nucleus.

polyneuropathy (POL-ee-nyu-ROP-ah-thee) Disorder affecting many nerves.

polyp (POL-ip) Mass of tissue that projects into the lumen of the bowel.

polyphagia (pol-ee-FAY-jee-ah) Excessive eating.

polysaccharide (pol-ee-SACK-ah-ride) A combination of many saccharides; for example, starch.

polysomnography (pol-ee-som-NOG-rah-fee) Test to monitor brain waves, muscle tension, eye movement, and oxygen levels in the blood as the patient sleeps.

polyuria (pol-ee-YOU-ree-ah) Excessive production of urine.

pons (PONZ) Part of the brainstem.

popliteal (pop-LIT-ee-al) Pertaining to the back of the knee.

popliteal fossa (pop-LIT-ee-al FOSS-ah) The hollow at the back of the knee.

portal; portal vein (POR-tal VANE) The vein that carries blood from the intestines to the liver.

postcoital (post-KOH-ih-tal) After sexual intercourse.

posterior (pos-TEER-ee-or) Pertaining to the back surface of the body; situated behind.

postictal (post-IK-tal) Occurring after a seizure.

postmature (post-mah-TYUR) Infant born after 42 weeks of gestation.

postmaturity (post-mah-TYUR-ih-tee) Condition of being postmature.

postpartum (post-PAR-tum) After childbirth.

postpolio syndrome (PPS) (post-POH-lee-oh SIN-drome) Progressive muscle weakness in a person previously affected by polio.

postprandial (post-PRAN-dee-al) Following a meal.

postpubescent (post-pyu-BESS-ent) After the period of puberty.

posttraumatic (post-traw-MAT-ik) Occurring after and caused by trauma.

posture (POSS-chur) The carriage of the body as a whole and the position of the limbs.

Pott fracture (POT FRAK-chur) Fracture of the lower end of the fibula, often with fracture of the tibial malleolus.

precancerous (pree-KAN-sir-us) Lesion from which a cancer can develop.

precursor (pree-KUR-sir) Cell or substance formed earlier in the development of the cell or substance.

preeclampsia (pree-eh-KLAMP-see-uh) Hypertension, edema, and proteinuria during pregnancy.

pregnancy (PREG-nan-see) State of being pregnant.

prehypertension (pree-HIGH-per-TEN-shun) Precursor to hypertension.

premature (pree-mah-TYUR) Occurring before the expected time; for example, an infant born before 37 weeks of gestation.

prematurity (pree-mah-TYUR-ih-tee) Condition of being premature.

prenatal (pree-NAY-tal) Before birth.

prepatellar (pree-pah-TELL-ar) In front of the patella.

prepuce (PREE-puce) Fold of skin that covers the glans penis.

presbyopia (prez-bee-OH-pee-ah) Difficulty in nearsighted vision occurring in middle and old age.

preterm (PREE-term) Baby delivered before 37 weeks of gestation. Also called *premature.*

prevention (pree-VEN-shun) Process undertaken to prevent occurrence of a disease or health problem.

previa (PREE-vee-ah) Anything blocking the fetus during its birth; for example, an abnormally situated placenta, *placenta previa.*

priapism (PRY-ah-pizm) Persistent erection of the penis.

primary care (PRY-mah-ree KAIR) Comprehensive and preventive health care services that are the first point of care for a patient.

primigravida (pree-mih-GRAV-ih-dah) First pregnancy.

primipara (pree-MIP-ah-ruh) Woman who has given birth for the first time.

prion (PREE-on) Small infectious protein particle.

proctitis (prok-TIE-tis) Inflammation of the lining of the rectum.

proctoscopy (prok-TOSS-koh-pee) Examination of the inside of the anus by endoscopy.

progesterone (proh-JESS-ter-ohn) Hormone that prepares the uterus for pregnancy.

progestin (pro-JESS-tin) A synthetic form of progesterone.

prognathism (PROG-nah-thizm) Condition of a forward-projecting jaw.

prognosis (prog-NO-sis) Forecasting of the probable course of a disease.

prolactin (proh-LAK-tin) Pituitary hormone that stimulates the production of milk.

prolactinoma (proh-lak-tih-NOH-mah) Prolactin-producing tumor.

prolapse (proh-LAPS) The falling or slipping of a body part from its normal position.

proliferate (proh-LIF-eh-rate) To increase in number through reproduction.

pronate (PROH-nate) Rotate the forearm so that the surface of the palm faces posteriorly in the anatomical position.

pronation (proh-NAY-shun) Process of lying facedown or of turning a hand or foot with the volar (palm or sole) surface down.

prone (PRONE) Lying facedown, flat on your belly.

prophylaxis (pro-fih-LAX-is) Prevention of disease.

prostaglandin (PROS-tah-GLAN-din) Hormone present in many tissues, but first isolated from the prostate gland.

prostate (PROS-tate) Organ surrounding the beginning of the urethra.

prostatectomy (pross-tah-TEK-toh-mee) Surgical removal of the prostate.

prostatitis (pross-tah-TIE-tis) Inflammation of the prostate.

prosthesis (pros-THEE-sis) A manufactured substitute for a missing or diseased part of the body.

protease (PROH-tee-aze) Group of enzymes that break down protein.

protection (proh-TEK-shun) Defense against attack or invasion.

protein (PRO-teen) Class of food substances based on amino acids.

proteinuria (pro-tee-NYU-ree-ah) Presence of protein in urine.

prothrombin (proh-THROM-bin) Protein formed by the liver and converted to thrombin in the blood-clotting mechanism.

proton pump inhibitor (PPI) (PROH-ton PUMP in-HIB-ih-tor) Agent that blocks production of gastric acid.

protooncogene (pro-toh-ONG-koh-jeen) A normal gene involved in normal cell growth.

provisional diagnosis (proh-VISH-un-al die-ag-NOH-sis) A temporary diagnosis pending further examination or testing. Also called *preliminary diagnosis.*

proximal (PROK-sih-mal) Situated nearest to the center of the body.

pruritus (proo-RYE-tus) Itching.

psoriasis (so-RYE-ah-sis) Rash characterized by reddish, silver-scaled patches.

psychedelic (sigh-keh-DEL-ik) Agent that intensifies sensory perception.

psychiatric (sigh-kee-AH-trik) Pertaining to psychiatry.

psychiatrist (sigh-KIE-ah-trist) Licensed medical specialist in psychiatry.

psychiatry (sigh-KIE-ah-tree) Diagnosis and treatment of mental disorders.

psychoactive (sigh-koh-AK-tiv) Able to alter mood, behavior, and/or cognition.

psychoanalysis (sigh-koh-ah-NAL-ih-sis) Method of psychotherapy.

psychoanalyst (sigh-koh-AN-ah-list) Practitioner of psychoanalysis.

psychological (sigh-koh-LOJ-ik-al) Pertaining to psychology.

psychologist (sigh-KOL-oh-jist) Licensed specialist in psychology.

psychology (sigh-KOL-oh-jee) Scientific study of the human mind and behavior.

psychopath (SIGH-koh-path) Person with antisocial personality disorder.

psychosis (sigh-KOH-sis) Disorder causing mental disruption and loss of contact with reality.

psychosomatic (sigh-koh-soh-MAT-ik) Pertaining to disorders of the body usually resulting from disturbances of the mind.

psychotherapist (sigh-koh-THAIR-ah-pist) Practitioner of psychotherapy.

GLOSSARY

psychotherapy (sigh-koh-THAIR-ah-pee) Treatment of mental disorders through communication.

ptosis (TOH-sis) Sinking down of an eyelid or an organ.

puberty (PYU-ber-tee) Process of maturing from child to young adult capable of reproducing.

pubic (PYU-bik) Pertaining to the pubis.

pubis (PYU-bis) Bony front arch of the pelvis of the hip. Also called *pubic bone.*

puerperium (pyu-er-PEE-ree-um) Six-week period after birth in which the uterus involutes.

pulmonary (PULL-moh-NAIR-ee) Pertaining to the lungs and their blood supply.

pulmonologist (PULL-moh-NOL-oh-jist) Medical specialist in puimonary disorders.

pulp (PULP) Dental pulp is the connective tissue in the cavity in the center of the tooth.

pupil (PYU-pill) The opening in the center of the iris that allows light to reach the lens. Plural *pupillae.*

Purkinje fibers (per-KIN-jee FIE-bers) Network of nerve fibers in the myocardium.

purpura (PUR-pyu-rah) Skin hemorrhages that are red initially and then turn purple.

purulent (PURE-you-lent) Showing or containing a lot of pus.

pustule (PUS-tyul) Small protuberance on the skin that contains pus.

pyelitis (pie-eh-LIE-tis) Inflammation of the renal pelvis.

pyelogram (PIE-el-oh-gram) X-ray image of renal pelvis and ureters.

pyelonephritis (PIE-eh-loh-neh-FRIE-tis) Inflammation of the kidney and renal pelvis.

pyloric (pie-LOR-ik) Pertaining to the pylorus.

pylorus (pie-LOR-us) Exit area of the stomach.

pyorrhea (pie-oh-REE-ah) Purulent discharge.

pyrexia (pie-REK-see-ah) An abnormally high body temperature or fever.

pyromania (pie-roh-MAY-nee-ah) Morbid impulse to set fires.

Q

quadrant (KWAD-rant) One-quarter of a circle.

quadrantectomy (kwad-ran-TEK-toh-mee) Surgical excision of a quadrant of the breast.

quadriceps femoris (KWAD-rih-seps FEM-or-is) An anterior thigh muscle with four heads.

quadriplegia (kwad-rih-PLEE-jee-ah) Paralysis of all four limbs.

R

radial (RAY-dee-al) Pertaining to the forearm.

radiation (ray-dee-AY-shun) A spreading out, as of anatomical parts.

radical (RAD-ih-kal) Extensive, as in complete removal of a diseased part.

radioactive (RAY-dee-oh-AK-tiv) Spontaneously emitting alpha, beta, or gamma rays.

radioactive iodine (RAY-dee-oh-AK-tiv EYE-oh-dine) Any of the various tracers that emit alpha, beta, or gamma rays.

radiologist (ray-dee-OL-oh-jist) Medical specialist in the use of x-rays and other imaging techniques.

radiology (ray-dee-OL-oh-jee) The study of medical imaging.

radionuclide (RAY-dee-oh-NYU-klide) Radioactive agent used in diagnostic imaging.

radiotherapy (RAY-dee-oh-THAIR-ah-pee) Treatment using radiation.

radius (RAY-dee-us) The forearm bone on the thumb side.

rale (RAHL) Crackle heard through a stethoscope when air bubbles through liquid in the lungs. Plural *rales.*

raphe (RAY-fee) Line separating two symmetrical structures.

reabsorption (ree-ab-SORP-shun) The taking back into the blood of substances that had previously been filtered out from it.

recombinant DNA (ree-KOM-bin-ant DEE-en-a) DNA (deoxyribonucleic acid) altered by inserting a new sequence of DNA into the chain.

rectocele (REK-toh-seal) Hernia of the rectum into the vagina.

rectum (RECK-tum) Terminal part of the colon from the sigmoid to the anal canal.

recurrent (ree-KUR-ent) Symptoms or lesions returning after an intermission.

reflex (REE-fleks) An involuntary response to a stimulus.

reflux (REE-fluks) Backward flow.

regenerate (ree-JEN-eh-rate) Reconstitution of a lost part.

regimen (REJ-ih-men) Program of treatment.

regulate (REG-you-late) To control the way in which a process progresses.

regurgitate (ree-GUR-jih-tate) To flow backward; for example, through a heart valve.

regurgitation (ree-gur-jih-TAY-shun) The flow of material in backwards direction. In the digestive system, it means to expel contents of the stomach into the mouth, short of vomiting.

rehabilitation (REE-hah-bil-ih-TAY-shun) Therapeutic restoration of an ability to function as before.

remission (ree-MISH-un) Period in which there is a lessening or absence of the symptoms of a disease.

renal (REE-nal) Pertaining to the kidney.

renin (REE-nin) Enzyme secreted by the kidney that causes vasoconstriction.

replicate (REP-lih-kate) To produce an exact copy.

replication (rep-lih-KAY-shun) Reproduction to produce an exact copy.

reproductive (ree-pro-DUC-tiv) Relating to the process by which organisms produce offspring.

resection (ree-SEK-shun) Removal of a specific part of an organ or structure.

residual (ree-ZID-you-al) Pertaining to anything left over.

resistance (ree-ZIS-tants) Ability of an organism to withstand the effects of an antagonistic agent.

resorption (ree-SORP-shun) Loss of substance, such as bone.

respiration (RES-pih-RAY-shun) Fundamental process of life used to exchange oxygen and carbon dioxide.

respiratory (RES-pir-ah-TOR-ee) Relating to the process of exchanging oxygen and carbon dioxide.

restorative rehabilitation (ree-STOR-ah-tiv REE-hah-bil-ih-TAY-shun) Promote renewal of health and strength.

rete testis (REE-teh TES-tis) Network of tubules between the seminiferous tubules and the epididymis.

retention (ree-TEN-shun) Holding back in the body what should normally be discharged (e.g., urine).

reticulum (reh-TIK-you-lum) Fine network of cells in the medulla oblongata.

retina (RET-ih-nah) Light-sensitive innermost layer of the eyeball.

retinaculum (ret-ih-NAK-you-lum) Fibrous ligament that keeps the tendons in place on the wrist so that they do not "bowstring" when the forearm muscles contract.

retinoblastoma (RET-in-oh-blas-TOH-mah) Malignant neoplasm of primitive retinal cells.

retinoid (RET-ih-noyd) A class of keratolytic agents.

retinopathy (ret-ih-NOP-ah-thee) Degenerative disease of the retina.

retraction (ree-TRAK-shun) A pulling back, as a pulling back of the intercostal spaces and the neck above the clavicle.

retrograde (RET-roh-grade) Reversal of a normal flow; for example, back from the bladder into the ureters.

retroverted (REH-troh-vert-ed) Tilted backward.

retrovirus (REH-troh-VIE-rus) Virus that replicates in a host cell by converting its RNA core into DNA.

Reye syndrome (RAY SIN-drome) Encephalopathy and liver damage in children following an acute viral illness; linked to aspirin use.

rhabdomyolysis (RAB-doh-my-oh-LIE-sis) Destruction of muscle to produce myoglobin.

rhabdomyosarcoma (RAB-doh-MY-oh-sar-KOH-mah) Cancer derived from skeletal muscle.

rheumatoid arthritis (RA) (RHU-mah-toyd ar-THRIE-tis) Disease of connective tissue, with arthritis as a major manifestation.

rhinitis (rye-NIE-tis) Inflammation of the nasal mucosa. Also called *coryza.*

rhinoplasty (RYE-noh-plas-tee) Surgical procedure to change the size or shape of the nose.

rhonchus (RONG-kuss) Wheezing sound heard on auscultation of the lungs; made by air passing through a constricted lumen. Plural *rhonchi.*

ribosome (RYE-bo-sohm) Structure in the cell that assembles amino acids into protein.

rickets (RIK-ets) Disease due to vitamin D deficiency, producing soft, flexible bones.

Rinne test (RIN-eh TEST) Test for conductive hearing loss.

root (ROOT) Fundamental or beginning part of a structure.

rosacea (roh-ZAY-she-ah) Persistent erythematous rash of the central face.

rotator cuff (roh-TAY-tor CUFF) Part of the capsule of the shoulder joint.

Roux-en-Y (ROO-on-Y) Surgical procedure to reduce the size of the stomach.

ruga (ROO-gah) A fold, ridge, or crease. Plural *rugae.*

rupture (RUP-tyur) Break or tear of any organ or body part.

S

sacral (SAY-kral) In the neighborhood of the sacrum.

sacroiliac joint (SAY-kroh-ILL-ih-ak JOYNT) The joint between the sacrum and the ilium.

sacrum (SAY-krum) Segment of the vertebral column that forms part of the pelvis.

sagittal (SAJ-ih-tal) Pertaining to the vertical plane through the body, dividing it into right and left portions.

saliva (sa-LIE-vah) Secretion in the mouth from salivary glands.

salpingectomy (sal-pin-JEK-toh-mee) Surgical removal of fallopian tube(s).

salpingitis (sal-pin-JIE-tis) Inflammation of the uterine tube.

saphenous (SAF-ih-nus) Relating to the saphenous vein in the thigh.

sarcoidosis (sar-koy-DOH-sis) Granulomatous lesions of the lungs and other organs; cause is unknown.

sarcoma (sar-KOH-mah) A malignant tumor originating in connective tissue.

sarcopenia (sar-koh-PEE-nee-ah) Progressive loss of muscle mass and strength in aging.

scab (SKAB) Crust that forms over a wound or sore during healing.

scabies (SKAY-bees) Skin disease produced by mites.

scapula (SKAP-you-lah) Shoulder blade. Plural *scapulae.*

scar (SKAR) Fibrotic seam that forms when a wound heals.

schizoid (SKITZ-oyd) Withdrawn, socially isolated.

schizophrenia (skitz-oh-FREE-nee-ah) Disorder of perception, thought, emotion, and behavior.

Schwann cell (SHWANN SELL) Connective tissue cell of the peripheral nervous system that forms a myelin sheath.

sciatic (sigh-AT-ik) Pertaining to the sciatic nerve or sciatica.

sciatica (sigh-AT-ih-kah) Pain from compression of L5 or S1 nerve roots.

scintigraphy (sin-TIG-rah-fee) Recording of radioactivity with a special camera.

sclera (SKLAIR-ah) Fibrous outer covering of the eyeball and the white of the eye.

scleritis (sklair-RIE-tis) Inflammation of the sclera.

scleroderma (sklair-oh-DERM-ah) Thickening and hardening of the skin due to new collagen formation.

sclerose (skleh-ROZE) To harden or thicken.

sclerotherapy (SKLAIR-oh-THAIR-ah-pee) To collapse a vein by injecting a solution into it to harden it.

scoliosis (skoh-lee-OH-sis) An abnormal lateral curvature of the vertebral column.

scrotum (SKROH-tum) Sac containing the testes.

seasonal affective disorder (SEE-zon-al af-FEK-tiv dis-OR-der) Depression that occurs at the same time every year, often in winter.

sebaceous glands (se-BAY-shus GLANDZ) Glands in the dermis that open into hair follicles and secrete an oily fluid called sebum.

seborrhea (seb-oh-REE-ah) Excessive amount of sebum.

sebum (SEE-bum) Waxy secretion of the sebaceous glands.

secrete (seh-KREET) To release or give off, as substances produced by cells.

secretin (se-KREE-tin) Hormone produced by the duodenum to stimulate pancreatic juice.

sedative (SED-ah-tiv) Agent that calms nervous excitement.

sedentary (sed-en-TAIR-ee) Accustomed to little exercise or movement.

segment (SEG-ment) A section of an organ or structure.

segmentectomy (seg-men-TEK-toh-mee) Surgical excision of a segment of a tissue or organ.

seizure (SEE-zhur) Event due to excessive electrical activity in the brain.

self-examination (SELF-ek-zam-ih-NAY-shun) The examination of part of one's own body.

self-mutilation (self-myu-tih-LAY-shun) Injury or disfigurement made to one's own body.

semen (SEE-men) Penile ejaculate containing sperm and seminal fluid.

semilunar (sem-ee-LOO-nar) Appears like a half moon.

seminal vesicle (SEM-in-al VES-ih-kull) Sac of the ductus deferens that produces seminal fluid.

seminiferous tubule (sem-ih-NIF-er-us TU-byul) Coiled tubes in the testes that produce sperm.

seminoma (sem-ih-NOH-mah) Neoplasm of germ cells of a testis.

senescence (seh-NES-ens) The state of being old.

senile (SEE-nile) Characteristic of old age.

senility (seh-NIL-ih-tee) Old age.

sensorineural hearing loss (SEN-sor-ih-NYUR-al HEER-ing LOSS) Hearing loss caused by lesions of the inner ear or the auditory nerve.

sensory (SEN-soh-ree) Having the function of sensation; relating to structures of the nervous system that carry impulses to the brain.

septum (SEP-tum) A wall dividing two cavities. Plural *septa*.

serosa (seh-ROH-sa) Outermost covering of the alimentary tract.

serotonin (ser-oh-TOH-nin) A neurotransmitter in the central and peripheral nervous systems.

serous (SEER-us) Thicker and less transparent than water.

serum (SEER-um) Fluid remaining after removal of cells and fibrin clot.

shock (SHOCK) Sudden physical or mental collapse or circulatory collapse.

shunt (SHUNT) A bypass or diversion of fluid, such as blood.

sibling (SIB-ling) Brother or sister.

sigmoid (SIG-moyd) Sigmoid colon is shaped like an "S."

sigmoidoscopy (sig-moi-DOS-koh-pee) Endoscopic examination of the sigmoid colon.

sign (SINE) Physical evidence of a disease process.

silicosis (sil-ih-KOH-sis) Fibrotic lung disease from inhaling silica particles.

sinoatrial (SA) node (sigh-noh-AY-tree-al NODE) The center of modified cardiac muscle fibers in the wall of the right atrium that acts as the pacemaker for the heart rhythm.

sinus (SIGH-nus) Cavity or hollow space in a bone or other tissue.

sinus rhythm (SIGH-nus RITH-um) The normal (optimal) heart rhythm arising from the sinoatrial node.

sinusitis (sigh-nuh-SIGH-tis) Inflammation of the lining of a sinus.

skeletal (SKEL-eh-tal) Pertaining to the bones.

smegma (SMEG-mah) Oily material produced by the glans and prepuce.

Snellen letter chart (SNEL-en LET-er CHART) Test for acuity of distance vision.

snore (SNOR) Noise produced by vibrations in the structures of the nasopharynx.

sociopath (SOH-see-oh-path) Person with antisocial personality disorder.

soleus (SOH-lee-us) Large muscle of the calf.

somatic (soh-MAT-ik) Relating to the body in general; *or* pertaining to a division of the peripheral nervous system serving the skeletal muscles.

somatoform (soh-MAT-oh-form) Physical symptoms occurring without identifiable physical cause.

somatostatin (SOH-mah-toh-STAT-in) Hormone that inhibits release of growth hormone and insulin.

somatotropin (SOH-mah-toh-TROH-pin) Hormone of the anterior pituitary that stimulates growth of body tissues. Also called *growth hormone.*

sonographer (so-NOG-rah-fer) The technician who performs a sonogram.

spasmodic (spaz-MOD-ik) Having intermittent spasms or contractions.

spastic (SPAS-tik) Increased muscle tone on movement.

specificity (spes-ih-FIS-ih-tee) State of having a fixed relation to a particular entity.

sperm (SPERM) Mature male sex cell. Also called *spermatozoon.*

spermatic (SPER-mat-ik) Pertaining to sperm.

spermatid (SPER-mah-tid) A cell late in the development process of sperm.

spermatocele (SPER-mat-oh-seal) Cyst of the epididymis that contains sperm.

spermatogenesis (SPER-mat-oh-JEN-eh-sis) The process by which male germ cells differentiate into sperm.

spermatozoa (SPER-mat-oh-ZOH-ah) Sperm (plural of *spermatozoon*).

spermicidal (SPER-mih-SIDE-al) Pertaining to sperm.

spermicide (SPER-mih-side) Agent that destroys sperm.

sphenoid bone (SFEE-noyd BONE) Wedge-shaped bone that forms part of the base of the cranium and the orbits.

spherocyte (SFEER-oh-site) A spherical cell.

spherocytosis (SFEER-oh-sigh-TOH-sis) Presence of spherocytes in the blood.

sphincter (SFINK-ter) Band of muscle that encircles an opening; when it contracts, the opening squeezes closed.

sphygmomanometer (SFIG-moh-mah-NOM-ih-ter) Instrument for measuring arterial blood pressure.

spina bifida (SPY-nah BIH-fih-dah) Failure of one or more vertebral arches to close during fetal development.

spina bifida cystica (SPY-nah BIH-fih-dah SIS-tik-ah) Meninges and spinal cord protrude through the absent vertebral arch and have the appearance of a cyst.

spina bifida occulta (SPY-nah BIH-fi-dah oh-KUL-tah) The deformity of the vertebral arch is not apparent from the skin surface.

spiral fracture (SPY-ral FRAK-chur) A fracture in the shape of a coil.

spirochete (SPY-roh-keet) Spiral-shaped bacterium causing a sexually transmitted disease (syphilis).

spirometer (spy-ROM-eh-ter) An instrument used to measure respiratory volumes.

spirometry (spy-ROM-eh-tree) Use of a spirometer.

spleen (SPLEEN) Vascular, lymphatic organ in the left upper quadrant of the abdomen.

splenectomy (spleh-NEK-toh-mee) Surgical removal of the spleen.

splenomegaly (spleh-noh-MEG-ah-lee) Enlarged spleen.

spondylosis (spon-dih-LOH-sis) Degenerative osteoarthritis of the spine.

spongiosum (spun-jee-OH-sum) Spongelike tissue.

sputum (SPYU-tum) Matter coughed up and spat out by individuals with respiratory disorders.

squamous cell (SKWAY-mus SELL) Flat, scalelike epithelial cell.

stage (STAYJ) Definition of the extent and dissemination of a malignant neoplasm.

staging (STAY-jing) Process of determining the extent of the distribution of a neoplasm.

stapes (STAY-pees) Inner (medial) one of the three ossicles of the middle ear; shaped like a stirrup.

status epilepticus (STAT-us ep-ih-LEP-tik-us) A recurrent state of seizure activity lasting longer than a specific time frame (usually 30 minutes).

stem cell (STEM SELL) Undifferentiated cell found in a differentiated tissue that can divide to yield the specialized cells in that tissue.

stenosis (steh-NOH-sis) Narrowing of a canal or passage, as in the narrowing of a heart valve.

stent (STENT) Wire mesh tube used to keep arteries open.

stereopsis (ster-ee-OP-sis) Three-dimensional vision.

stereotactic (STER-ee-oh-TAK-tik) Pertaining to a precise three-dimensional method to locate a lesion.

sterile (STER-ill) Free from all living organisms and their spores; *or* unable to fertilize or reproduce.

sternum (STIR-num) Long, flat bone forming the center of the anterior wall of the chest.

steroid (STER-oyd) Large family of chemical substances found in many drugs, hormones, and body components.

stethoscope (STETH-oh-skope) Instrument for listening to cardiac and respiratory sounds.

stimulant (STIM-you-lant) Agent that excites or strengthens functional activity.

stimulation (stim-you-LAY-shun) Arousal to increased functional activity.

stoma (STOH-mah) Artificial opening.

strabismus (strah-BIZ-mus) A turning of an eye away from its normal position.

strain (STRAIN) Overstretch or tear in a muscle or tendon.

stratum basale (STRAH-tum ba-SAL-eh) Deepest layer of the epidermis, from which the other cells originate and migrate.

streptokinase (strep-toh-KIE-nase) An enzyme that dissolves clots.

striated muscle (STRIE-ay-ted MUSS-el) Another term for *skeletal muscle.*

striation (strie-AY-shun) Stripes.

stricture (STRICK-shur) Narrowing of a tube.

stridor (STRIE-door) High-pitched noise made when there is a respiratory obstruction in the larynx or trachea.

stroke (STROHK) Acute clinical event caused by an impaired cerebral circulation.

stroma (STROH-mah) Connective tissue framework that supports the parenchyma of an organ or gland.

subarachnoid space (sub-ah-RAK-noyd SPASE) Space between the pia mater and the arachnoid membrane.

subclavian (sub-CLAY-vee-an) Underneath the clavicle.

subcutaneous (sub-kew-TAY-nee-us) Below the skin. Also known as *hypodermic.*

subdural (sub-DUR-al) Located in the space between the dura mater and the arachnoid membrane.

sublingual (sub-LING-wal) Underneath the tongue.

subluxation (sub-luk-SAY-shun) An incomplete dislocation in which some contact between the joint surfaces remains.

submandibular (sub-man-DIB-you-lar) Underneath the mandible.

submucosa (sub-mew-KOH-sa) Tissue layer underneath the mucosa.

suicidal (SOO-ih-SIGH-dal) Wanting to kill oneself.

sulcus (SUL-cuss) Groove on the surface of the cerebral hemispheres that separates gyri. Plural *sulci.*

superior (soo-PEE-ree-or) Situated above.

supinate (SOO-pih-nate) Rotate the forearm so that the surface of the palm faces anteriorly in the anatomical position.

supination (soo-pih-NAY-shun) Process of lying face upward or turning an arm or foot so that the palm or sole is facing up.

supine (soo-PINE) Lying face up, flat on your spine.

suprapubic (SOO-prah-PYU-bik) Above the symphysis pubis.

surfactant (ser-FAK-tant) A protein and fat compound that creates surface tension to hold lung alveolar walls apart.

susceptible (suh-SEP-tih-bull) Capable of being affected by.

suture (SOO-chur) Place where two bones are joined together by a fibrous band continuous with their periosteum, as in the skull; *or* a stitch to hold the edges of a wound together. Plural *sutures.*

sympathetic (sim-pah-THET-ik) Pertaining to the part of the autonomic nervous system operating at the unconscious level.

sympathy (SIM-pa-thee) Appreciation and concern for another person's mental and emotional state.

symphysis (SIM-feh-sis) Two bones joined by fibrocartilage. Plural *symphyses.*

symptom (SIMP-tum) Departure from normal health experienced by the patient.

symptomatic (simp-toh-MAT-ik) Pertaining to the symptoms of a disease.

synapse (SIN-aps) Junction between two nerve cells, or a nerve fiber and its target cell, where electrical impulses are transmitted between the cells.

synchondrosis (sin-kon-DROH-sis) A rigid articulation (joint) formed by cartilage. Plural *synchondroses.*

syncope (SIN-koh-peh) Temporary loss of consciousness and postural tone due to diminished cerebral blood flow.

syndesmosis (sin-dez-MOH-sis) A rigid articulation (joint) formed by ligaments. Plural *syndesmoses*.

syndrome (SIN-drohm) Combination of signs and symptoms associated with a particular disease process.

synovial (sih-NOH-vee-al) Pertaining to synovial fluid and synovial membrane.

synthesis (SIN-the-sis) The process of building a compound from different elements.

synthetic (sin-THET-ik) Built up or put together from simpler compounds.

syphilis (SIF-ih-lis) Sexually transmitted disease caused by a spirochete.

syringomyelia (sih-RING-oh-my-EE-lee-ah) Abnormal longitudinal cavities in the spinal cord that cause paresthesias and muscle weakness.

systemic (sis-TEM-ik) Relating to the entire organism.

systemic lupus erythematosus (sis-TEM-ik LOO-pus er-ih-THEE-mah-toh-sus) Inflammatory connective tissue disease affecting the whole body.

systole (SIS-toh-lee) Contraction of the heart muscle.

T

tachycardia (tak-ih-KAR-dee-ah) Rapid heart rate (above 100 beats per minute).

tachypnea (tak-ip-NEE-ah) Rapid breathing.

tactile (TAK-tile) Relating to touch.

talipes (TAL-ip-eez) Deformity of the foot involving the talus.

talus (TAY-luss) The tarsal bone that articulates with the tibia to form the ankle joint.

tampon (TAM-pon) Plug or pack in a cavity to absorb or stop bleeding.

tamponade (tam-poh-NAID) Pathologic compression of an organ such as the heart.

tangent (TAN-jent) Sudden change of course.

tangentiality (tan-jen-shee-AL-ih-tee) Disturbance in thought processes, which move rapidly from one topic to another.

tarsus (TAR-sus) The collection of seven bones in the foot that form the ankle and instep; *or* the flat fibrous plate that gives shape to the outer edges of the eyelids.

tartar (TAR-tar) Calcified deposit at the gingival margin of the teeth. Also called *dental calculus*.

taste (TAYST) Sensation from chemicals on the taste buds.

Tay-Sachs disease (TAY-SAKS diz-EEZ) Congenital fatal disorder of fat metabolism.

temporal bones (TEM-por-al BONES) Bones that form the sides and part of the base of the cranium.

temporal lobe (TEM-por-al LOBE) Posterior two-thirds of the cerebral hemispheres.

temporomandibular joint (TMJ) (TEM-por-oh-man-DIB-you-lar JOYNT) The joint between the temporal bone and the mandible.

tendinitis (ten-dih-NIE-tis) Inflammation of a tendon. Also spelled *tendonitis*.

tendon (TEN-dun) Fibrous band that connects muscle to bone.

tenosynovitis (TEN-oh-sine-oh-VIE-tis) Inflammation of a tendon and its surrounding synovial sheath.

teratogen (TER-ah-toh-jen) Agent that produces fetal deformities.

teratogenesis (TER-ah-toh-JEN-eh-sis) Process involved in producing fetal deformities.

teratoma (ter-ah-TOH-mah) Neoplasm of a testis or ovary containing multiple tissues from other sites in the body.

testicle (TES-tih-kul) One of the male reproductive glands. Also called *testis*.

testis (TES-tis) A synonym for testicle. Plural *testes*.

testosterone (tes-TOSS-ter-ohn) Powerful androgen produced by the testes.

tetanus (TET-ah-nuss) A disease with painful, tonic, muscular contractions caused by the toxin produced by *Clostridium tetani*.

tetany (TET-ah-nee) Severe muscle twitches, cramps, and spasms.

tetralogy of Fallot (TOF) (teh-TRAL-oh-jee OV fah-LOH) Set of four congenital heart defects occurring together.

thalamus (THAL-ah-mus) Mass of gray matter underneath the ventricle in each cerebral hemisphere.

thalassemia (thal-ah-SEE-mee-ah) Group of inherited blood disorders that produce a hemolytic anemia.

thenar (THAY-nar) The fleshy mass at the base of the thumb.

therapeutic (THAIR-ah-PYU-tik) Relating to the treatment of a disease or disorder.

therapist (THAIR-ah-pist) Professional trained in the practice of a particular therapy.

therapy (THAIR-ah-pee) Systematic treatment of a disease, dysfunction, or disorder.

thoracentesis (THOR-ah-sen-TEE-sis) Insertion of a needle into the pleural cavity to withdraw fluid or air. Also called *pleural tap*.

thoracic (thor-ASS-ik) Pertaining to the chest (thorax).

thoracoscopy (thor-ah-KOS-koh-pee) Examination of the pleural cavity with an endoscope.

thoracotomy (thor-ah-KOT-oh-mee) Incision through the chest wall.

thrombin (THROM-bin) Enzyme that forms fibrin.

thrombocyte (THROM-boh-site) Another name for *platelet*.

thrombocytopenia (THROM-boh-sigh-toh-PEE-nee-ah) Deficiency of platelets in circulating blood.

thromboembolism (THROM-boh-EM-boh-lizm) A piece of detached blood clot (embolus) blocking a distant blood vessel.

thrombolysis (throm-BOL-ih-sis) Dissolving a thrombus (clot).

thrombophlebitis (THROM-boh-fleh-BIE-tis) Inflammation of a vein with clot formation.

thrombosis (throm-BOH-sis) Formation of a thrombus.

thrombus (THROM-bus) A clot attached to a diseased blood vessel or heart lining.

thrush (THRUSH) Infection with *Candida albicans*.

thymectomy (thigh-MEK-toh-mee) Surgical removal of the thymus gland.

thymoma (thigh-MOH-mah) Benign tumor of the thymus gland.

thymus (THIGH-mus) Endocrine gland located in the mediastinum.

thyroid (THIGH-royd) Endocrine gland in the neck; *or* a cartilage of the larynx.

thyroid hormone (THIGH-royd HOR-mohn) Collective term for the two thyroid hormones, T_3 and T_4.

thyroid storm (THIGH-royd STORM) Medical crisis and emergency due to excess thyroid hormones.

thyroidectomy (thigh-roy-DEK-toh-mee) Surgical removal of the thyroid gland.

thyroiditis (thigh-roy-DIE-tis) Inflammation of the thyroid gland.

thyrotoxicosis (THIGH-roh-tok-sih-KOH-sis) Disorder caused by excessive thyroid hormone production.

thyrotropin (thigh-roh-TROH-pin) Hormone from the anterior pituitary gland that stimulates function of the thyroid gland.

thyroxine (thigh-ROK-seen) Thyroid hormone T_4, tetraiodothyronine.

tibia (TIB-ee-ah) The larger bone of the lower leg.

tic (TIK) Sudden, involuntary, repeated contraction of muscles.

tic douloureux (TIK duh-luh-RUE) Painful, sudden, spasmodic involuntary contractions of the facial muscles supplied by the trigeminal nerve. Also called *trigeminal neuralgia.*

tinea (TIN-ee-ah) General term for a group of related skin infections caused by different species of fungi.

tinnitus (TIN-ih-tus) Persistent ringing, whistling, clicking, or booming noise in the ears.

tissue (TISH-you) Collection of similar cells.

tolerance (TOL-er-ants) The capacity to become accustomed to a stimulus or drug.

tomography (toh-MOG-rah-fee) Radiographic image of a selected slice of tissue.

tone (TONE) Tension present in resting muscles.

tongue (TUNG) Mobile muscle mass in the mouth; bears the taste buds.

tonic-clonic seizure (TON-ik-KLON-ik SEE-zhur) Generalized seizure due to epileptic activity in all or most of the brain.

tonometer (toh-NOM-eh-ter) Instrument for determining intraocular pressure.

tonometry (toh-NOM-eh-tree) The measurement of intraocular pressure.

tonsil (TON-sill) Mass of lymphoid tissue on either side of the throat at the back of the tongue.

tonsillectomy (ton-sih-LEK-toh-mee) Surgical removal of the tonsils.

tonsillitis (ton-sih-LIE-tis) Inflammation of the tonsils.

topical (TOP-ih-kal) Medication applied to the skin to obtain a local effect.

torsion (TOR-shun) The act or result of twisting.

Tourette syndrome (tur-ET SIN-drome) Disorder of multiple motor and vocal tics.

toxic (TOK-sick) Pertaining to a toxin.

toxicity (tok-SIS-ih-tee) The state of being poisonous.

toxin (TOK-sin) Poisonous substance formed by a cell or organism.

trachea (TRAY-kee-ah) Air tube from the larynx to the bronchi.

trachealis (tray-kee-AY-lis) Pertaining to the trachea.

tracheostomy (tray-kee-OST-oh-mee) Surgical opening into the windpipe, usually so that a tube can be inserted to assist breathing.

tracheotomy (tray-kee-OT-oh-mee) Incision made into the trachea to create a tracheostomy.

tract (TRAKT) Bundle of nerve fibers with a common origin and destination.

tranquilizer (TRANG-kwih-lie-zer) Agent that calms without sedating or depressing.

transcriptionist (tran-SCRIP-shun-ist) One who makes the copy of dictated material.

transdermal (trans-DER-mal) Going across or through the skin.

transducer (trans-DYU-sir) Device that converts energy from one form to another.

transfusion (trans-FYU-zhun) Transfer of blood or a blood component from donor to recipient.

transplant (TRANZ-plant) The tissue or organ used; *or* the act of transferring tissue from one person to another.

transplantation (TRANZ-plan-TAY-shun) The moving of tissue or an organ from one person or place to another.

transverse (trans-VERS) Pertaining to the horizontal plane dividing the body into upper and lower portions.

transverse fracture (trans-VERS FRAK-chur) A fracture perpendicular to the long axis of the bone.

tremor (TREM-or) Small, shaking, involuntary, repetitive movements of hands, extremities, neck, or jaw.

triceps brachii (TRY-sepz BRAY-kee-eye) Muscle of the arm that has three heads or points of origin.

Trichomonas **(trik-oh-MOH-nas)** A parasite causing a sexually transmitted disease.

trichomoniasis (TRIK-oh-moh-NIE-ah-sis) Infection with *Trichomonas vaginalis.*

tricuspid (try-KUSS-pid) Having three points; a tricuspid heart valve has three flaps.

trigeminal (try-GEM-in-al) Fifth (V) cranial nerve, with its three different branches supplying the face.

triglyceride (trie-GLISS-eh-ride) Any of a group of fats containing three fatty acids.

triiodothyronine (trie-EYE-oh-doh-THIE-roh-neen) Thyroid hormone T_3.

trimester (TRY-mes-ter) One-third of the length of a full-term pregnancy.

triplegia (try-PLEE-jee-ah) Paralysis of three limbs.

trochlear (TROHK-lee-ar) Fourth (IV) cranial nerve; supplies one muscle of the eye.

tropic (TROH-pik) Tropic hormones stimulate other endocrine glands to produce hormones.

trypsin (TRIP-sin) Enzyme that breaks down protein.

tuberculosis (too-BER-kyu-LOH-sis) Infectious disease that can infect any organ or tissue.

tumor (TOO-mer) Any abnormal swelling.

tunica (TYU-nih-kah) A layer in the wall of a blood vessel or other tubular structure.

tunica vaginalis (TYU-nih-kah vaj-ih-NAHL-iss) Covering, particularly of a tubular structure. The tunica vaginalis is the sheath of the testis and epididymis.

turbinate (TUR-bin-ate) Another name for the nasal conchae on the lateral walls of the nasal cavity.

tympanic (tim-PAN-ik) Pertaining to the tympanic membrane or tympanic cavity.

tympanostomy (tim-pan-OS-toh-mee) Surgically created new opening in the tympanic membrane to allow fluid to drain from the middle ear.

U

ulcer (ULL-cer) Erosion of an area of skin or mucosa.

ulcerative (UL-sir-ah-tiv) Marked by an ulcer or ulcers.

ulna (UL-nah) The medial and larger bone of the forearm.

ulnar (UL-nar) Pertaining to the ulna or any of the structures (artery, vein, nerve) named after it.

ultrasonography (UL-trah-soh-NOG-rah-fee) Delineation of deep structures using sound waves.

ultrasound (UL-trah-sownd) Use of very-high-frequency sound waves.

umbilical (um-BIL-ih-kal) Pertaining to the umbilicus or the center of the abdomen.

umbilicus (um-BIL-ih-kus) Pit in the abdomen where the umbilical cord entered the fetus.

unipolar disorder (you-nih-POLE-ar dis-OR-der) Depression.

uranium (you-RAY-nee-um) Radioactive metallic element.

urea (you-REE-ah) End product of nitrogen metabolism.

uremia (you-REE-mee-ah) The complex of symptoms arising from renal failure.

ureter (you-REET-er) Tube that connects the kidney to the urinary bladder.

ureteroscope (you-REE-ter-oh-skope) Endoscope to view the inside of the ureter.

ureteroscopy (you-REE-ter-OS-koh-pee) Examination of the ureter.

urethra (you-REE-thra) Canal leading from the bladder to outside.

urethritis (you-ree-THRIE-tis) Inflammation of the urethra.

urethrotomy (you-ree-THROT-oh-mee) Incision of a stricture of the urethra.

urinalysis (you-rih-NAL-ih-sis) Examination of urine to separate it into its elements and define their kind and/or quantity.

urinary (YUR-in-air-ee) Pertaining to urine.

urination (yur-ih-NAY-shun) The act of passing urine.

urine (YUR-in) Fluid and dissolved substances excreted by the kidney.

urologist (you-ROL-oh-jist) Medical specialist in disorders of the urinary system.

urology (you-ROL-oh-jee) Medical specialty of disorders of the urinary system.

urticaria (ur-tih-KARE-ee-ah) Rash of itchy wheals (hives).

uterus (YOU-ter-us) Organ in which an egg develops into a fetus.

uvea (YOU-vee-ah) Middle coat of the eyeball—includes the iris, ciliary body, and choroid.

uveitis (you-vee-IE-tis) Inflammation of the uvea.

uvula (YOU-vyu-lah) Fleshy projection of the soft palate.

V

vaccination (vak-sih-NAY-shun) Administration of a vaccine.

vaccine (vak-SEEN) Preparation to generate active immunity.

vagina (vah-JIE-nah) Female genital canal extending from the uterus to the vulva.

vaginal (VAJ-in-al) Pertaining to the vagina.

vaginitis (vah-jih-NIE-tis) Inflammation of the vagina.

vaginosis (vah-jih-NOH-sis) Any disease of the vagina.

vagus (VAY-gus) Tenth (X) cranial nerve; supplies many different organs throughout the body.

varicocele (VAIR-ih-koh-seal) Varicose veins of the spermatic cord.

varicose (VAIR-ih-kos) Characterized by or affected with varices.

varix (VAIR-iks) Dilated, tortuous vein. Plural *varices*.

vasectomy (vah-SEK-toh-mee) Excision of a segment of the ductus deferens.

vasoconstriction (VAY-soh-con-STRIK-shun) Reduction in diameter of a blood vessel.

vasodilation (VAY-soh-die-LAY-shun) Increase in diameter of a blood vessel.

vasopressin (vay-soh-PRESS-in) Pituitary hormone that constricts blood vessels and decreases urine output. Also called *antidiuretic hormone (ADH)*.

vasovasostomy (VAY-soh-vay-SOS-toh-mee) Reanastomosis of the ductus deferens to restore the flow of sperm. Also called *vasectomy reversal*.

vegetative (VEJ-eh-tay-tiv) Functioning unconsciously as plant life is assumed to do.

vein (VANE) Blood vessel carrying blood toward the heart.

vena cava (VEE-nah KAY-vah) One of the two largest veins in the body. Plural *venae cavae*.

venogram (VEE-noh-gram) Radiograph of veins after injection of radiopaque contrast material.

venous (VEE-nus) Pertaining to venous blood or the venous circulation.

ventilation (ven-tih-LAY-shun) Movement of gases into and out of the lungs.

ventral (VEN-tral) Pertaining to the belly or situated nearer to the surface of the belly.

ventricle (VEN-trih-kel) A cavity of the heart or brain.

venule (VEN-yule) Small vein leading from the capillary network.

vermiform (VER-mih-form) Worm shaped; used as a descriptor for the appendix.

vernix caseosa (VER-niks kay-see-OH-sah) Cheesy substance covering the skin of the fetus.

verruca (ver-ROO-cah) Wart caused by a virus.

vertex (VER-teks) Topmost point of the vault of the skull.

vertigo (VER-tih-goh) Sensation of spinning or whirling.

vesicle (VES-ih-kull) Small sac containing liquid; for example, a blister or semen.

vestibule (VES-tih-byul) Space at the entrance to a canal.

vestibulectomy (ves-tib-you-LEK-toh-mee) Surgical excision of the vulva.

vestibulocochlear (ves-TIB-you-loh-KOK-lee-ar) Eighth (VIII) cranial nerve; carrying information for the senses of hearing and balance.

villus (VILL-us) Thin, hairlike projection, particularly of a mucous membrane lining a cavity. Plural *villi.*

virilism (VIR-ih-lizm) Development of masculine characteristics by a woman or girl.

virulent (VIR-you-lent) Extremely toxic or pathogenic.

virus (VIE-rus) Group of infectious agents that require living cells for growth and reproduction.

visceral (VISS-er-al) Pertaining to the internal organs.

viscosity (vis-KOS-ih-tee) The resistance of a fluid to flowing.

viscous (VISS-kus) Sticky; resistant to flow.

visual acuity (VIH-zhoo-wal ah-KYU-ih-tee) Sharpness and clearness of vision.

vital signs (VIE-tal SIGNS) A procedure during a physical examination in which temperature (T), pulse (P), respirations (R), and blood pressure (BP) are measured to assess general health and cardiorespiratory function.

vitamin (VIE-tah-min) Essential organic substance necessary in small amounts for normal cell function.

vitiligo (vit-ill-EYE-go) Nonpigmented white patches on otherwise normal skin.

vitreous humor (VIT-ree-us HEW-mor) A gelatinous liquid in the posterior cavity of the eyeball with the appearance of glass.

vocal (VOH-kal) Pertaining to the voice.

void (VOYD) To evacuate urine or feces.

voluntary muscle (VOL-un-tare-ee MUSS-el) Muscle that is under the control of the will.

vomer (VOH-mer) Lower nasal septum.

vulva (VUL-vah) Female external genitalia.

vulvodynia (vul-voh-DIN-ee-uh) Chronic vulvar pain.

vulvovaginitis (VUL-voh-vaj-ih-NIE-tis) Inflammation of the vagina and vulva.

W

Weber test (VAY-ber TEST) Test for sensorineural hearing loss.

whiplash (WHIP-lash) Symptoms caused by sudden, uncontrolled extension and flexion of the neck, often in an automobile accident.

white matter (WITE MATT-er) Regions of the brain and spinal cord occupied by bundles of axons.

whooping cough (WHO-ping KAWF) Infectious disease with spasmodic, intense cough ending on a whoop (stridor). Also called *pertussis.*

Wilms tumor (WILMZ TOO-mor) Cancerous kidney tumor of childhood. Also known as *nephroblastoma.*

wound (WOOND) Any injury that interrupts the continuity of skin or a mucous membrane.

X

xenograft (ZEN-oh-graft) A graft from another species. Also known as *heterograft.*

Y

yolk sac (YOKE SACK) Source of blood cells and future sex cells for the fetus.

Z

zygote (ZIE-goht) Cell resulting from the union of the sperm and egg.

Ischemia, 334–336
Ischemic, 335
Ischemic strokes, 286
Ischia, 491
Ischial, 491
Ischium, 490, 491
Ishihara color system, 556, 558, 559
Islet cells, 130, 131
Islets of Langerhans, 616, 617
Isotope, 604, 605
Isotopic, 605
Isotopic thyroid scans, 604
Isthmus, 220, 221
ITP, 382, 390
IUD, 232
IV, 248, 290, 728
IVC, 342
IVF, 33, 34, 238, 239
IVP, 156, 164, 170

J

Jaeger reading cards, 556, 557
Jaundice, 124–126, 128, 129
  breast feeding failure, 126
  breast milk, 126
  physiologic, 126
Jejunal, 121
Jejunum, 102, 120, 121
Joint capsule, 42
Joints, 12, 470–503
  ankle and foot, 498–499
  classes of, 470–471
  diseases of, 474–475
  elbow, 482–483
  hand, 520–521
  hip and thigh, 492–493
  knee, 42, 66–43, 494–497
  movement of, 472–473
  sacroiliac, 490, 491
  shoulder, 518–519
  surgical procedures for, 500
  temporomandibular, 478, 479
  wrist, 520–521
JRA, 488
Jugular, 343
Juvenile, 489
Juvenile rheumatoid arthritis (JRA), 488

K

Kaposi sarcoma, 414, 415
Karyotype, 46, 47
Kegel exercises, 172, 173
Keloid, 88, 89
Kennedy, John F., 608, 610

Keratectomy, 558, 559
Keratin, 66, 67
Keratinocytes, 66, 67
Keratolytic, 92, 93
Keratomileusis, 559
Keratoses, 90, 91
Keratosis, 91
Keratotomy, 559
Kernicterus, 250, 251
Ketoacidosis, 171, 621
Ketone formation, 620
Ketones, 170, 171, 621
Ketosis, 171, 621
Keynotes, W-21
Kidneys, 156, 157
  anatomy and physiology of, 158–159
  disorders of, 160–163
  functions of, 158
Kidney transplant, 172
Killer T cells, 402
Kleptomania, 642, 643
Knee, 12
Knee joint, 40, 494–495
  connective tissues in, 42–43
  surgical procedures, 500
KUB, 164, 170
Kyphosis, 476, 477
Kyphotic, 477

L

L, 366
Labia, 213
Labia majora, 212
Labia minora, 212
Labium, 213
Labor, 244, 246, 247
Laboratory technician, 398
Labrum, 492, 493
Lab tests, 644
Labyrinth, 570, 571
Labyrinthitis, 571
Laceration, 88, 89
Lacrimal, 478, 479, 541
Lacrimal apparatus, 540
Lacrimal ducts, 540
Lacrimal gland, 540
Lacrimal sac, 540
Lactase, 106, 107, 134, 135
Lactate, 255
Lactation, 254, 255
Lacteals, 132, 133
Lactiferous, 255
Lactiferous ducts, 254
Lactiferous sinus, 254
Lactose, 106, 107, 135

Lactose intolerance, 106, 134
Lacuna, 465
Lacunae, 464, 465
Lanugo, 244, 245
Laparoscope, 103, 234, 235
Laparoscopic, 102, 103, 612
Laparoscopic radical nephrectomy, 155
Laparoscopy, 103, 202, 234, 235
Large cell carcinoma, 682
Large intestine, 102
  disorders of, 138–139
  structure and functions of, 136–137
Laryngeal, 429
Laryngitis, 434, 435
Laryngopharynx, 432, 433
Laryngoscope, 434, 435
Laryngotracheobronchitis, 434, 435
Larynx, 115, 429
  anatomy of, 428
  deglutition and, 114
  functions and disorders of, 434–435
Laser, 88, 89
Laser ablation, 604
Laser-assisted in situ keratomileusis
    (LASIK), 558
Laser corneal surgery, 558
Laser surgery, 238, 554
Laser therapy, 90
Last menstrual period (LMP), 236
Lateral, 495
Lateral collateral ligament (LCL), 494
Lateral flexion, 472
Lateral menisci, 494
Lateral rotation, 472
Lateral view, 708
Latex, 72, 73
Latin words, 12
Latissimus dorsi, 520, 521
Lavage, 140, 141, 689
Laxative, 144, 145
LCC-ST, 192
LCL, 494
LDL, 348
Lead, 686
Lead poisoning, 162
Learners
  active, W-6, W-7, W-9
  types of, W-13
Learning
  commitment to, W-13
  contextual approach to, W-4
  medical language, W-11
Learning outcomes, W-2, W-17, W-18
LEEP, 232, 238
Left common carotid artery, 340
Left lower quadrant (LLQ), 52